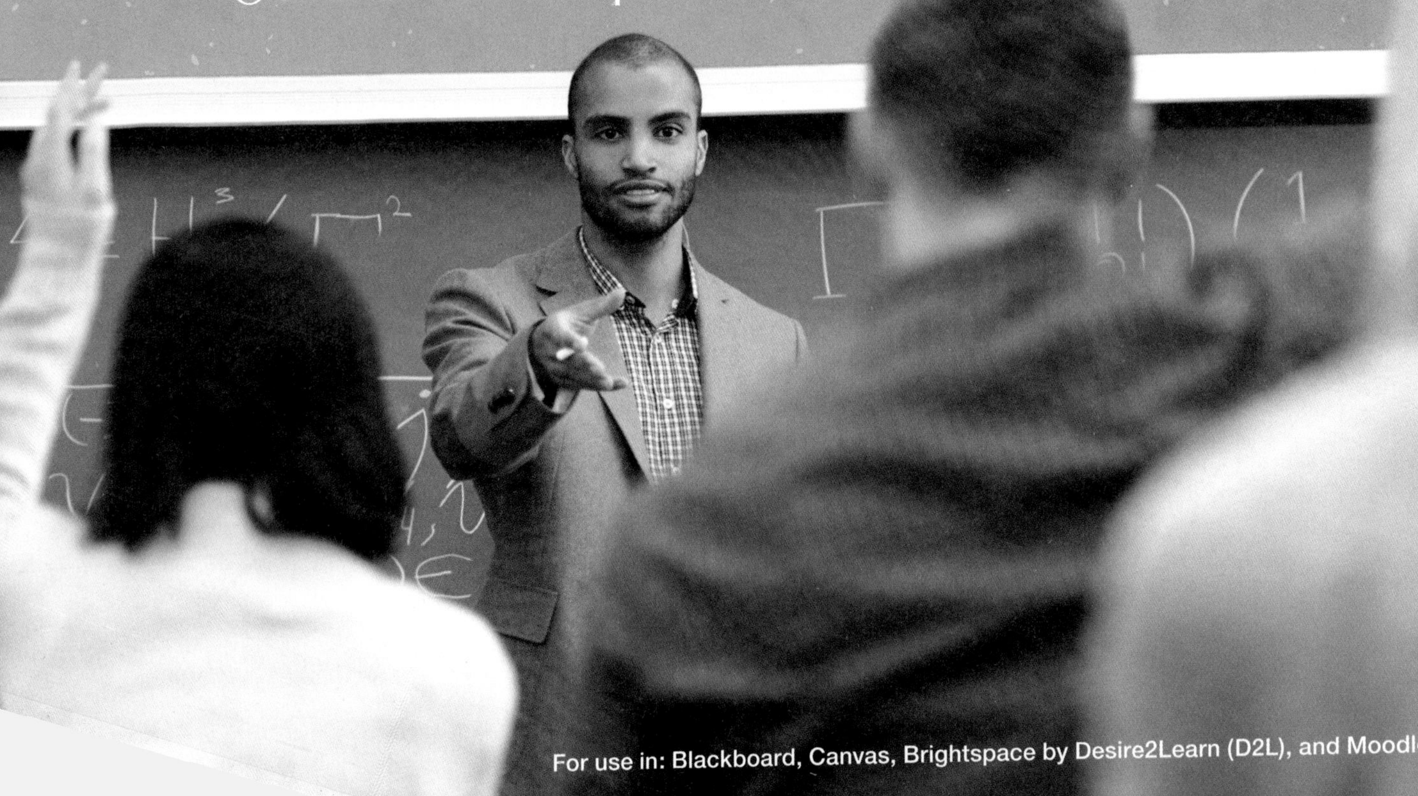

The Hallmark Features

A COMPLETE LEARNING PACKAGE

SAGE Premium Video in the Interactive eBook boosts student comprehension and bolsters analysis.

- **FIGURES BROUGHT TO LIFE ANIMATIONS** demonstrate concept processes with animated versions of select illustrations and are accompanied by easy-to-follow narrations.

- **IT'S A MYTH! BOXES** dispel the many misperceptions that often circulate concerning brain and behavior.

- **APPLICATIONS BOXES** explore key concepts in more depth and provide students with examples of how some of the findings and information presented in the chapters can be used in real-life settings.

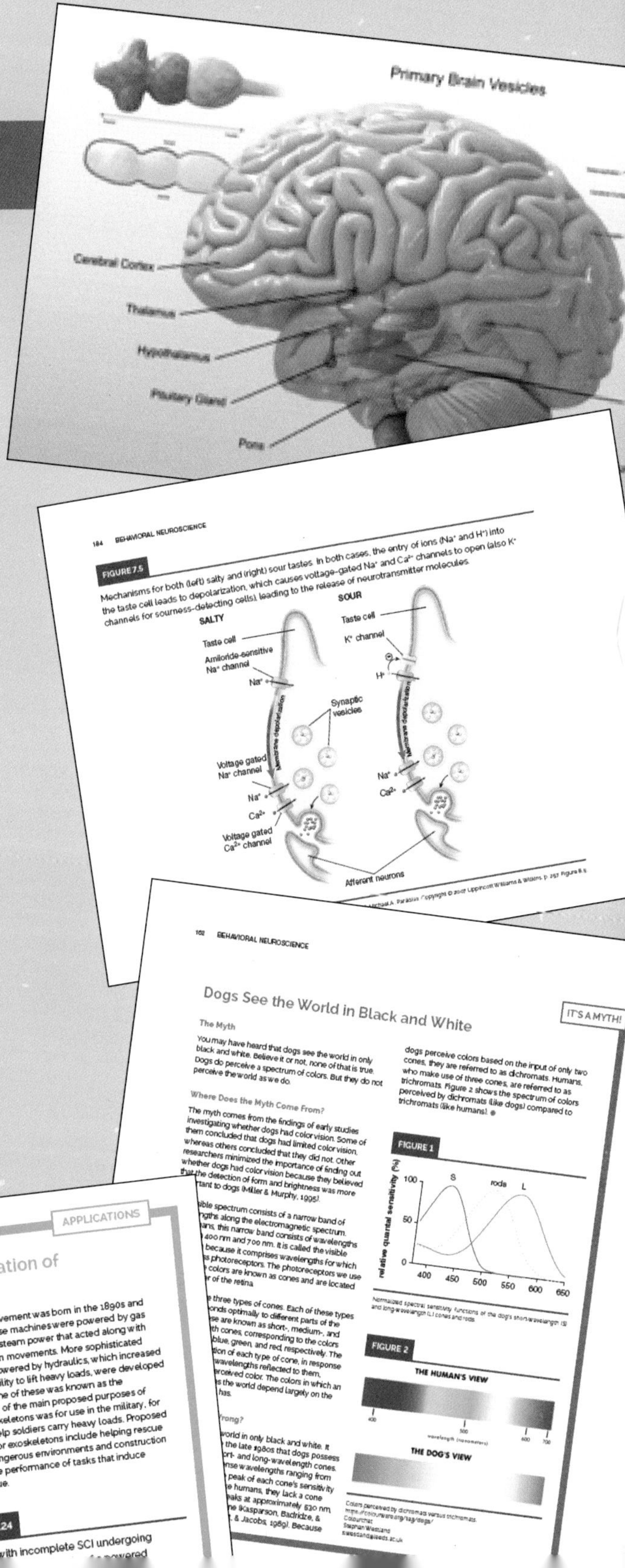

Sara Miller McCune founded SAGE Publishing in 1965 to support the dissemination of usable knowledge and educate a global community. SAGE publishes more than 1000 journals and over 600 new books each year, spanning a wide range of subject areas. Our growing selection of library products includes archives, data, case studies and video. SAGE remains majority owned by our founder and after her lifetime will become owned by a charitable trust that secures the company's continued independence.

Los Angeles | London | New Delhi | Singapore | Washington DC | Melbourne

BEHAVIORAL NEUROSCIENCE

To Marilyn, my life-long love and partner and the wonderful step children she gave me, April and Sam, who through their love, acceptance, and often tolerance supported me throughout the writing of this textbook.

BEHAVIORAL NEUROSCIENCE

Essentials and Beyond

Stéphane Gaskin

Dawson College

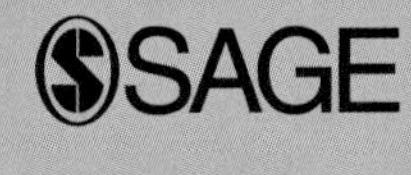

Los Angeles | London | New Delhi
Singapore | Washington DC | Melbourne

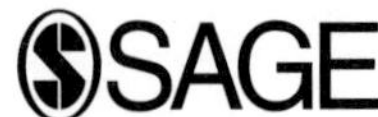

FOR INFORMATION:

SAGE Publications, Inc.
2455 Teller Road
Thousand Oaks, California 91320
E-mail: order@sagepub.com

SAGE Publications Ltd.
1 Oliver's Yard
55 City Road
London EC1Y 1SP
United Kingdom

SAGE Publications India Pvt. Ltd.
B 1/I 1 Mohan Cooperative Industrial Area
Mathura Road, New Delhi 110 044
India

SAGE Publications Asia-Pacific Pte. Ltd.
18 Cross Street #10-10/11/12
China Square Central
Singapore 048423

Medical illustrations created by Body Scientific International.

Printed in Canada

Library of Congress Cataloging-in-Publication Data

Names: Gaskin, Stephane, author.

Title: Behavioral neuroscience : essentials and beyond / Stephane Gaskn, Dawson College.

Description: Thousand Oaks, California : SAGE Publishing, [2021] | Includes bibliographical references and index.

Identifiers: LCCN 2019032654 | ISBN 9781544393803 (paperback) | ISBN 9781071802069 (Looseleaf) | ISBN 9781506391465 (epub) | ISBN 9781506391472 (epub) | ISBN 9781506391496 (pdf)

Subjects: LCSH: Psychobiology.

Classification: LCC QP360 .G378 2020 | DDC 612.8—dc23
LC record available at https://lccn.loc.gov/2019032654

Acquisitions Editor: Abbie Rickard
Content Development Editor: Emma Newsom
Editorial Assistant: Elizabeth Cruz
Production Editor: Tracy Buyan
Copy Editor: Amy Marks
Typesetter: C&M Digitals (P) Ltd.
Proofreader: Christine Dahlin
Indexer: Judy Hunt
Cover Designer: Gail Buschman
Marketing Manager: Katherine Hepburn

This book is printed on acid-free paper.

20 21 22 23 24 10 9 8 7 6 5 4 3 2 1

BRIEF CONTENTS

DETAILED CONTENTS

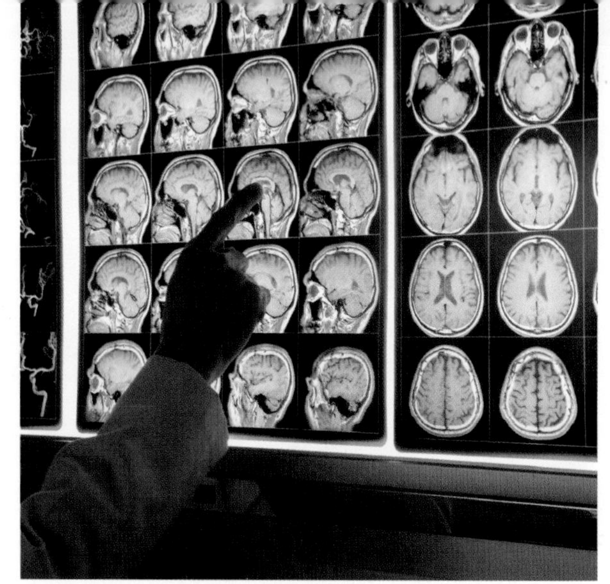
iStock.com/whitehoune

iStock.com/solvod

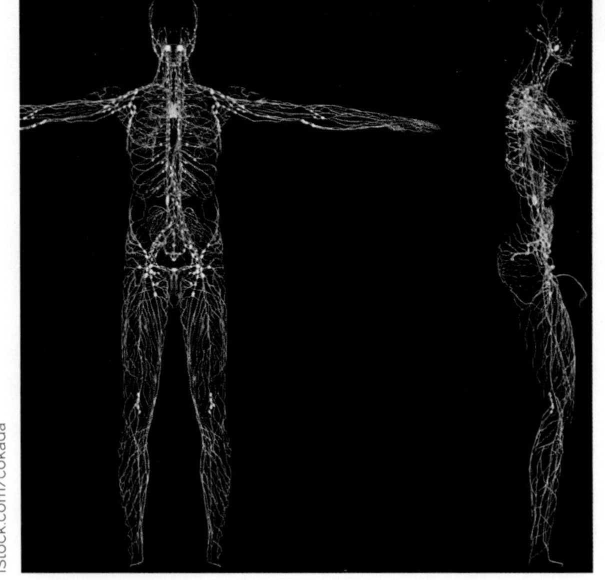
iStock.com/cokada

iStock.com/BraunS

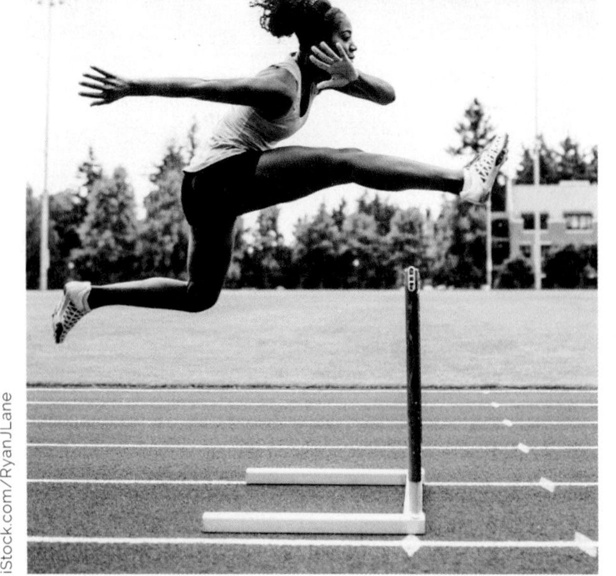
iStock.com/RyanJLane

PeopleImages/istockphoto

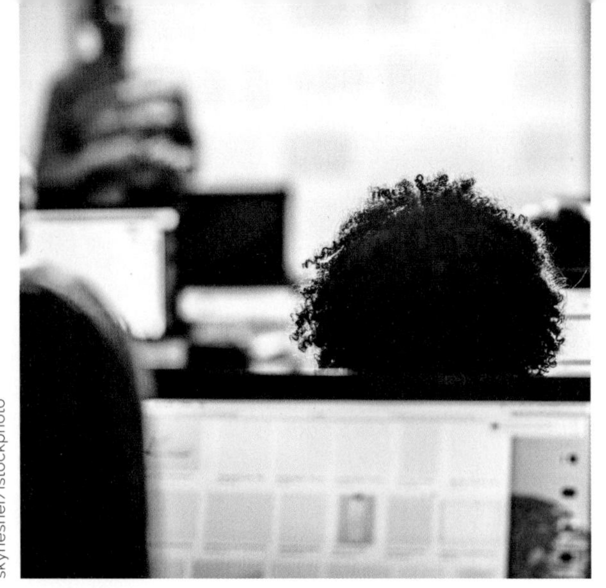
skynesher/istockphoto

Gugurat/istockphoto

PREFACE

At the time of writing this textbook, I had been teaching psychology and behavioral neuroscience at both Dawson College and Concordia University. Until about 2013, I had taught only neuroscience courses. This included the fundamentals of behavioral neuroscience, the neurobiology of learning and memory, the fundamentals of neuropsychology, as well as the neurobiology of sensation and perception. In 2013, the psychology department at Dawson College decided to add a brain and behavior course to its curriculum. I was given the honor of putting together and teaching the very first offering of the course. The course was a welcome addition and is well appreciated by psychology students, who before then were taught psychology strictly as a social science. From my experience in teaching the fundamentals of behavioral neuroscience to first-year psychology students, I had noticed the gap in knowledge that existed between the strictly psychological aspects of behavior and its neurobiological basis. I have always found this to be quite appalling considering the current state of science, in which behavior could more than ever be explained partly through the study of the complex webs of interactions that exist between biological and environmental influences. Therefore, studying psychology strictly as a social science can only lead to an incomplete understanding of the forces that shape behavior as well as the cognitive and emotional processes that accompany it.

The idea for writing a brain and behavior textbook came to me several years ago. However, the topic about which to write it, and the opportunity to do so, only came to me with the introduction of the brain and behavior course I was given the opportunity to teach at Dawson. I thought that most textbooks I used at university would be too advanced for the college student, who for the most part were taking their first steps in studying psychology and who did not necessarily make the link between neuroscience and psychology. I then decided that I would teach from my own notes, which I had prepared during the summer preceding the term in which I was to teach the course. One day, at the beginning of that term, and as I was preparing one of my first classes, a sales representative from one of the major textbook companies peeked over my shoulder and asked me what I was doing. I replied that I was writing out notes for use in the newly created brain and behavior class. The sales representative asked if I was planning to write a textbook. This was all I needed. I took the idea and ran with it. It was then that I decided to embark on a textbook-writing adventure that spanned the next five years.

OVERVIEW

Chapters, Modules, and Units

This textbook contains 15 chapters. The chapters are divided into modules, which are further subdivided into units. I chose this format because I have found that it makes it easy for instructors to assign students specific topics by referring to any given module or unit of the textbook. I find this formula to be useful when, as in most cases, instructors are limited in the number of chapters or topics they can cover during a single term.

Research Blends With Foundational Studies

I wanted the textbook to contain a mix of classic studies from years past and some of the most recent evidence up to the time of writing. This is made evident in the text by the frequent descriptions and explanations of specific studies and their results. I found it important to formally cite each study rather than leave both the student and the instructor to wonder where the explanations came from, which is a problem I have encountered from time to time in several textbooks. This is made obvious by the frequent in-text citations and the extensive list of references at the end of the book.

Chapter Features

Module Summaries and Review Questions

Each of the modules is followed by a summary of the material presented in the module. Students can use these summaries in two ways. They can use the summaries to review the key points presented in the chapter. They can also read the summaries before reading the chapters to form an overall mental schema of the chapters to which the more specific content can be added. Each module is also followed by questions designed to test the students' retention and understanding of the module's material.

Boxed Material

The chapters in the printed version of the book do not contain much boxed material or other special features. This is simply because research has shown that, although these features add flashiness and color to the text, they do not enhance learning compared to the material covered by the regular text. Therefore, only two types of boxed material are included in each chapter: "It's a Myth!" and "Applications."

It's a Myth! Another goal that I had for this textbook was to debunk some of the common myths surrounding brain-behavior relationships. To do so, I include in each chapter an "It's a Myth!" box, in which I present and explain a myth relevant to the chapter material.

Applications. I have also thought it useful to provide students with an "Applications" box at the end of each chapter. This box explores some of the chapter's material in more depth and provides students with examples of how the findings and information presented in the chapter can be used in real-life settings. These boxes promote a deeper understanding of the topics and can spark student interest, with the hope that they may encourage students to pursue further studies in behavioral neuroscience.

Coverage of Language

The text does not contain a chapter or module dedicated to language. The omission of this aspect of human behavior is in no way due to any prejudice against the field on my part or due to any perception that it isn't an important topic. I instead chose to expand the coverage on sensory processing, compared to other behavioral neuroscience textbooks, to include two chapters. I find this to be important because not all programs of study in which this book will be used offer a course on sensation and perception. This also left room for an entire chapter on social neuroscience.

CHAPTER BY CHAPTER

Chapter 1—Behavioral Neuroscience: Understanding Brain-Behavior Relationships

Chapter 1 comprises four modules:

- **1.1 What Is Behavioral Neuroscience?** This module introduces students to behavioral neuroscience. In Unit 1, behavioral neuroscience is defined as the study of brain-behavior relationships. In Unit 2, students will be given a quick tour of the brain so as to immediately provide context for the remaining topics. This brief overview of the brain is followed, in Unit 3, by a succinct exploration of the various levels of analysis or perspectives from which behavioral neuroscientists can view behavior. This exploration provides students with concrete examples of scientific studies performed at each level. Unit 4 focuses on the genetics and environmental factors that govern behavior.
- **1.2 The Evolution of Brain-Behavior Relationships** This module briefly reviews evolutionary theory and natural selection (Unit 1) and then applies these concepts to the evolution of brain-behavior relationships (Unit 2).
- **1.3 The Origins of Behavioral Neuroscience** This module adds an historical perspective to the study of brain-behavior relationships. This ranges from the views held in antiquity, in Unit 1, to questions relating to the so-called mind-body problem in Unit 2. Finally, Unit 3 traces the history of how neuroscientists came to accept the idea of localization of function, a key idea in the study of brain-behavior relationships.
- **1.4 Studying Brain-Behavior Relationships Today** This module explores how brain-behavior relationships are viewed and studied today. This ranges from the study of brain-damaged patients, in Unit 1, to the use of techniques that manipulate and measure brain activity in Unit 2. Finally, Unit 3 introduces students to the various fields of study related to behavioral neuroscience as well as examples of studies performed in each one of these fields.

Chapter 2—Neurons and Glia

Chapter 2 comprises four modules:

- **2.1 Putting Neurons Into Context** Through this module, students will understand the place of neurons in the historical context of their discovery and of the different types of cells within the body. Unit 1 introduces students to the different types of tissues and cells in the body. Unit 2 briefly traces the history of how neurons came to be seen as the basic functioning units of the nervous system. Unit 3 describes some of the methods used to study neurons. Unit 4 brings students up to date on the latest findings concerning the estimated number of neurons in the brain compared to the number of nonneuronal cells, as well as the method used to arrive at these estimates.
- **2.2 The Structure of Neurons** This module is dedicated to understanding the structure of neurons as well as their diversity. Unit 1 introduces students to the prototypical neuron, its basic parts, and their functions. Unit 2 addresses the wide variety of neurons that exist across species.

- **2.3 The Action Potential** This module explores the action potential, which consists of the electrical impulses by which neurons communicate. Unit 1 is dedicated to understanding basic chemistry, which is necessary for an understanding of the action potential. The ways in which action potentials are generated and propagated through neurons are explored in Units 2 and 3, respectively.
- **2.4 Glia** This module examines glia, the nonneuronal cells of the nervous system. In Unit 1, students learn that glia, once believed to act only as the glue or matrix that held neurons together, play an important role in neuronal function. Unit 2 explores the wide variety of glia as well as the many functions they are believed to play in the functioning of the nervous system.

Chapter 3—The Synapse, Neurotransmitters, Drugs, and Addiction

Chapter 3 comprises three modules:

- **3.1 The Synapse** This module is dedicated to understanding what occurs at the synapse, which is the point of communication between neurons. Unit 1 defines and describes the synapse. In Unit 2, students are introduced to the details of the processes and events that occur at synapses. Unit 3 is dedicated to providing students with a basic understanding of how neurons integrate messages from thousands of other neurons to produce a response. Unit 4 explores the variety in the types of synapses that exist in the nervous system.
- **3.2 Neurotransmitters** This module explores neurotransmitters, the chemicals used by neurons to communicate with each other as well as with other types of cells. In Unit 1, students will learn about what neurotransmitters are and how they are subdivided into several classes. Unit 2 explores some of the roles played by neurotransmitters and how they function within systems.
- **3.3 Drugs and Drug Addiction** The aim of this module is for students to understand how drugs affect the nervous system and how drugs can lead to addiction. Unit 1 familiarizes students with how drugs of abuse are defined and how they are subdivided into classes. Unit 2 introduces students to the concepts that define drug addiction, such as tolerance and withdrawal. The neurobiological basis by which people become addicted to drugs is discussed in Unit 3. Finally, Unit 4 examines some of the neurobiological mechanisms by which commonly abused drugs exert their effects.

Chapter 4—The Nervous System

Chapter 4 comprises three modules:

- **4.1 Central Nervous System Development** This module focuses on the development of the central nervous system. Unit 1 describes the events that occur in the days following fertilization, which leads to the formation of the germ layers that give rise to all of the tissues of the body. In Unit 2, the focus turns to the development of the germ layer that gives rise to nervous tissue. This is followed, in Unit 3, by an exploration of the development of the brain itself from primary vesicles.
- **4.2 The Fully Developed Brain** This module examines the structures and functions of the fully developed nervous system. Various brain structures and their functions are discussed in Units 1 to 3. Unit 4 explores the structure and function of the spinal cord, whereas Unit 5 focuses on the brain's defense mechanisms, including how it is protected from the entry of potentially dangerous molecules, physical injury, and infections. Finally, Unit 6 briefly explores how the brain's hemispheres are differentially involved in behavior. Concepts such as cerebral dominance and handedness are also discussed.
- **4.3 The Peripheral Nervous System** This module is dedicated to the understanding of the peripheral nervous system. The divisions of the peripheral nervous system, which consists of the somatic and autonomic nervous systems, are discussed in Units 1 and 2, respectively.

Chapter 5—Neurodevelopment, Neuroplasticity, and Aging

Chapter 5 comprises three modules:

- **5.1 Neurodevelopment** This module provides students with a basic understanding of neurodevelopment. In Unit 1, students will learn about the events that occur from the generation of new neurons to their migration to specific brain areas where they will become the brain's cortical layers. Unit 2 discusses the mechanisms through which neurogenesis occurs in the adult brain.
- **5.2 Neuroplasticity** This module is dedicated to neuroplasticity, which is the ability of the brain to change itself with experience. Unit 1 introduces students to the concept of neuroplasticity. They will learn about the different types of neuroplastic changes within

the brain. Neuroplastic changes are expressed as the remodeling of neurons, changes in the efficacy of synapses, and changes in cortical organization. These forms of neuroplasticity are discussed in Units 2, 3, and 4, respectively. Unit 5 explores what occurs when neuroplastic changes in the brain are exaggerated.

- **5.3 The Aging Brain: Adolescence and Old Age** This module explores the changes in the brain that occur naturally during the aging process and those that occur in the diseased brain. Normal changes that occur in the brains of adolescents as well as associated behavioral changes are discussed in Unit 1. Unit 2 covers the brain changes that occur normally as one approaches old age. Unit 3 is dedicated to abnormal aging of the brain due to disease processes, describing the most common form of dementia, Alzheimer's disease.

Chapter 6—Sensation and Perception 1: Vision and Hearing

Chapter 6 comprises two modules:

- **6.1 Vision** This module is dedicated to the neurobiological processes that give rise to the visual experience. In Unit 1 of this module, the physical properties of light are briefly discussed followed by an exploration of the early visual system, which makes possible the transmission of information conveyed by wavelengths of light to the brain. Unit 2 deals with how information, in the form of wavelengths along the electromagnetic spectrum, is converted (or transduced) into patterns of nerve impulses. Unit 3 briefly discusses the patterns of neuronal connections that result in the acuity and sensitivity of the visual system. In Unit 4, students will learn how specific patterns of stimulation of neurons in the visual system represent the beginnings of how the brain will eventually make sense of visual stimulation. This is followed, in Unit 5, by how color perception is thought to occur. In Unit 6, students will learn how processing of visual information in various brain areas is performed.
- **6.2 Hearing** This module introduces students to some of the neurobiological processes involved in auditory perception. The physical and perceptual dimensions of sound are discussed in Unit 1, followed by a description of the auditory system in Unit 2. How the brain processes auditory stimulation to give rise to the experience and interpretation of sounds is discussed in Unit 3.

Chapter 7—Sensation and Perception 2: Taste, Smell, and Touch

Chapter 7 comprises three modules:

- **7.1 Taste** This module provides students with an understanding of the basic constituents of taste perception. In Unit 1, students will learn that taste is experienced after chemical molecules bind to specialized receptors in the mouth, triggering patterns of nerve impulses analyzed within the brain. Unit 2 provides students with a description of taste receptors. Unit 3 covers the mechanisms by which taste receptors function as well as how the different subtypes of taste receptors are activated by the different chemicals found in food. Unit 4 explores how the activation of taste receptors leads to the perception of the myriad tastes we can experience.
- **7.2 Smell** This module is dedicated to the understanding of smell. In Unit 1, students will come to a basic understanding of what constitutes the perception of smell. This includes learning that the experience of smell begins when airborne molecules bind to specialized receptors deep within the nasal cavity and trigger patterns of nerve impulses that are ultimately analyzed by the brain. The nature and function of these receptors are explored in Unit 2. In Unit 3, students will learn how these patterns of nerve impulses are analyzed within the brain to produce the perception of the variety of smells that we can experience. Unit 4 explores how animals release chemicals known as pheromones, which create specific behavioral reactions in the individuals that detect them.
- **7.3 Touch** In this module students will explore the sense of touch. In Unit 1, students will learn that the sense of touch is an umbrella term that constitutes several bodily senses. Unit 2 surveys the variety of touch receptors that exist as well as how each one functions. Unit 3 covers the way in which touch receptors transmit information to the brain. Unit 4 explores the pathways by which tactile information travels to the brain and where in the brain this information is analyzed to produce touch perception. Finally, the goal of Unit 5 is to provide students with an understanding of how touch information can also convey the perception of pain.

Chapter 8—Sensorimotor Systems

Chapter 8 comprises three modules:

- **8.1 This Is What Makes You Move** This module is dedicated to the basic understanding of the mechanics of movement. Unit 1 provides a survey of the types of muscles in the body. This is followed, in Unit 2, by a look at the way in which muscles are innervated by motor neurons. Unit 3 covers the way in which this innervation leads to muscle contraction.

- **8.2 Spinal Control of Movement** This module explores the role played by the spinal cord in the production of movement. In Unit 1, students will learn how reflexive movements are produced by interactions between neurons within the spinal cord. This is followed, in Unit 2, by an exploration of how movements that are rhythmic and highly automated, such as walking, are generated.
- **8.3 Cortical Control of Movement and Sensorimotor Integration** This module is dedicated to learning how the cortex controls movement by integrating sensory information from the body. Unit 1 briefly explores how movement is constantly adjusted in response to information from bodily sensations. Unit 2 explains how information makes it to the muscles through different pathways to produce movement, and Unit 3 explores the ways in which various cortical areas are involved in processing information that produces voluntary movements. Finally, in Unit 4, all of what was learned in this chapter is summarized to provide students with a global understanding of how movement is produced.

Chapter 9—Motivation: Theories, Temperature Regulation, Energy Balance, and Sleep

Chapter 9 comprises three modules:

- **9.1 Theories of Motivation** This module introduces students to well-known theories of motivation. Unit 1 defines motivation and gives examples of motivated behaviors. Unit 2 briefly explains a theory of motivation based on the reduction of needs, known as need reduction theory. Unit 3 introduces a theory of motivation that links levels of physiological arousal to performance and personality. Unit 4 explores prominent theories about the neurological basis of the link between motivation and pleasure seeking and reward.
- **9.2 Physiological Mechanisms** This module is dedicated to the physiological mechanisms that underlie temperature regulation (Unit 1) and energy balance (Unit 2). This includes a description of the neurobiological mechanisms, including the involvement of hormones, neurotransmitters, and specific brain areas that keep body temperature and the amount of energy available to organisms in check, in an effort to ensure their survival.
- **9.3 Regulation of Sleep and Wakefulness** This module explores the world of sleep. Unit 1 describes sleep as well as how it is studied in the laboratory. Unit 2 explores how waking and sleeping are regulated by circadian and homeostatic mechanisms. Finally, Unit 3 explores the brain areas and neurotransmitter systems involved in regulating waking and sleeping.

Chapter 10—Hormones: Social and Reproductive Behavior

Chapter 10 comprises three modules:

- **10.1 What Are Hormones?** This module defines hormones and differentiates them from neurotransmitters, which form the basis of another type of chemical communication. This is achieved in Unit 1. Unit 1 also traces the history of the study of hormones and their effect on behavior. Unit 2 surveys the different types of hormones. Unit 3 distinguishes between steroid and nonsteroid hormones, with an explanation and examples of how steroid hormones are used to enhance athletic performance and how they can potentially have significant effects on behavior. Unit 4 examines the actions of specific types of hormones.
- **10.2 Hormones and Behavior** This module focuses on the role played by hormones in social behavior. Unit 1 focuses on three aspects of social behavior: social recognition, pair bonding, and parenting. Unit 2 focuses on the role played by hormones on sexual and reproductive behavior.
- **10.3 Organizing Effects of Hormones and Sexual Orientation** This module explains the role played by hormones in determining gender and gender-specific sexual behavior early in development (Unit 1) and also examines sexual orientation (Unit 2).

Chapter 11—Emotions

Chapter 11 comprises four modules:

- **11.1 What Are Emotions?** This module aims at defining emotions. Unit 1 defines emotions and distinguishes between emotional experience and emotional expression. Unit 2 introduces students to prominent theories of emotions.

- **11.2 Emotions: Where in the Brain?** This module is dedicated to the neurobiological basis of emotions. Unit 1 explores the brain networks thought to be involved in emotional processing. Unit 2 focuses on the role played by the amygdala in animal models of emotional processing, and Unit 3 explores the role of the amygdala in emotional processing in humans.
- **11.3 Emotions and Decision Making: Beyond the Amygdala** This module explores the role played by emotions in decision making. Unit 1 focuses on the role of the prefrontal cortex in emotional processing and on case studies in which emotional processing and decision making were impaired following brain damage. Unit 2 presents and explains a theory that suggests emotions play a central role in the decision-making process.
- **11.4 Aggression** This module focuses on the neurobiological basis of aggression. Unit 1 defines aggression, and Unit 2 presents a brief historical overview of the brain regions thought to be involved in aggressive behavior. Unit 3 describes a theory that implicates the role of hormones in aggressive behavior.

Chapter 12—Memory and Memory Systems

Chapter 12 comprises five modules:

- **12.1 Memory and Memory Systems** This module is dedicated to defining memory and how memory is subdivided into multiple subsystems. Unit 1 provides a definition of memory. Unit 2 introduces students to the concept that memories are formed in stages. Unit 3 explains that different storage mechanisms, or registers, are involved in the formation of memories, including the concept that information can be stored from a brief period lasting only seconds to a period lasting a lifetime. Unit 4 is dedicated to understanding working memory.
- **12.2 Long-Term Memory** The focus of this module is on long-term memory. Unit 1 provides a definition of long-term memory and describes the various types of long-term memories that exist. Unit 2 explores the neurobiological basis of long-term memories and introduces historic case studies that contributed to the discovery of the brain areas involved in the formation of long-term memories.
- **12.3 Memory Consolidation** This module introduces students to the concept of memory consolidation. This is achieved in Unit 1. This is followed, in Unit 2, by a description and explanation of different theories proposed to account for how memories stabilize over time.
- **12.4 Navigating Through Space: Spatial Memory** This module is dedicated to the study of spatial memory. Unit 1 focuses on the role of the hippocampus in spatial memory. The various tasks used to test the role played by the hippocampus in spatial memory are presented and explained. In Unit 2, students learn about the discovery of specialized neurons that are differentially involved in mapping space. This is followed, in Unit 3, by a comparison of the role played by the hippocampus in spatial and object-recognition memory.
- **12.5 Learning: The Acquisition of Memories** This module describes and explains the molecular events thought to be involved in simple forms of learning. Unit 1 provides a definition of learning. This is followed by descriptions and explanations of the neurobiological processes involved in nonassociative learning (Unit 2) and associative learning (Unit 3) through the use of a simple animal model. Unit 4 introduces students to the neuroplastic processes that occur at synapses that result in learning.

Chapter 13—Attention and Consciousness

Chapter 13 comprises two modules:

- **13.1 Attention** This module introduces students to basic concepts in attention and its neurobiological basis. Unit 1 defines attention and different types of attentional processes. Unit 2 explores some of the basic concepts and models of attention. This unit also introduces students to some of the classic studies of attention. Unit 3 is dedicated to the study of some of the neurobiological processes that underlie attentional processes through learning about key studies aimed at discovering them. Unit 4 familiarizes students with the disorders of attention.
- **13.2 Consciousness** This module introduces students to the study of consciousness and its neural correlates. Unit 1 defines consciousness. Unit 2 explores the problems that make up the study of consciousness, including whether the mind is similar to a computer. Unit 3 reviews some of the classic studies that sought to uncover the neural correlates and the contents of consciousness. Unit 4 describes and explains a theory that aims to explain consciousness. Unit 5 discusses disorders of consciousness, including coma and unresponsive wakefulness.

Unit 6 explores the possibility that individuals who seemingly lack consciousness may be somewhat conscious and able to respond to the external world if proper methods are used to assess their consciousness. Finally, Unit 7 tackles the question of whether we have free will by examining two key studies providing evidence that brain activity that is predictive of an action may occur before an individual becomes conscious of the decision to perform the action.

Chapter 14—Psychological Disorders

Chapter 14 comprises five modules:

- **14.1 What Is a Psychological Disorder?** This module introduces students to the nature of psychological disorders. Unit 1 describes what consists of a psychological disorder. Unit 2 explains how psychological disorders cannot be attributed to a single cause but instead result from multiple interacting forces that include both genetic and environmental factors. Some of the types of studies performed to uncover these interactions are also described.
- **14.2 Anxiety Disorders and Posttraumatic Stress Disorder** This module introduces students to the general characteristics of anxiety disorders and posttraumatic stress disorder. A general definition of anxiety disorders is provided in Unit 1 and the often-confused states of fear and anxiety are differentiated. Unit 2 explores the neurobiological basis of anxiety disorders. Unit 3 defines posttraumatic stress disorder and describes some of its symptoms, and Unit 4 describes the neurobiological basis of the disorder.
- **14.3 Obsessive-Compulsive Disorder** This module is dedicated to obsessive-compulsive disorder. The symptoms of obsessive-compulsive disorder are described in Unit 1, whereas some of its neurobiological basis is presented in Unit 2.
- **14.4 Major Depressive Disorder** This module familiarizes students with major depressive disorders. Unit 1 briefly describes the symptoms of major depressive disorder. Unit 2 focuses on the neurobiological factors believed to play a role in the development of major depressive disorder. This unit also provides a brief historical outlook of the development of the drugs used to treat major depressive disorder.
- **14.5 Schizophrenia** The focus of this module is on schizophrenia. The different types of symptoms that characterize schizophrenia, such as hallucinations and delusions, are described in Unit 1. Unit 2 discusses the brain abnormalities thought to be present in the brains of people suffering from schizophrenia.

Chapter 15—Social Neuroscience

Chapter 15 comprises six modules:

- **15.1 What Is Social Neuroscience?** This module describes the field of social neuroscience. Unit 1 provides students with a definition of social neuroscience, including how its study is an outgrowth of the combination of social psychology and cognitive neuroscience. Unit 2 describes and explains the perspectives from which social neuroscientists study behavior.
- **15.2 Self-Awareness** This module is dedicated to self-awareness. Self-awareness is defined in Unit 1. Unit 2 explores different components of self-awareness and the different brain areas associated with each component.
- **15.3 Theory of Mind and Empathy** This module introduces students to the concept of theory of mind. Theory of mind is defined in Unit 1. Unit 2 presents different theories concerning how a theory of mind is generated in the brain. Unit 3 explores how having a theory of mind is related to the ability to show empathy.
- **15.4 Social Pain** This module explores the concept of social pain, which is defined in Unit 1. Unit 2 explores how a relationship between social pain and physical pain may exist in that they share a common neurobiological basis.
- **15.5 Altruism** This module is dedicated to altruism. Unit 1 defines altruism and presents models that seek to explain it. Unit 2 focuses on the neurobiological basis thought to underlie altruistic behaviors.
- **15.6 Cooperation and Trust** This module explores cooperation and trust. Unit 1 explains how cooperation and trust can be studied by having people participate in tasks based on game theory. Unit 2 describes the brain regions activated while people are engaged in such tasks.

ANCILLARIES

SAGE Edge

SAGE Edge offers a robust online environment featuring an impressive array of tools and resources for review, study, and further exploration, keeping both instructors and students on the cutting edge of teaching and learning. Go to **edge.sagepub.com/gaskin** to access the companion site.

SAGE Edge for Instructors

SAGE Edge for Instructors supports teaching by making it easy to integrate quality content and create a rich learning environment for students. This password-protected site gives instructors access to a full complement of resources to support and enhance their behavioral neuroscience course. The following chapter-specific assets are available on the teaching site:

- A **test bank** provides a diverse range of questions as well as the opportunity to edit any question and/or insert personalized questions to effectively assess students' progress and understanding.
- Sample **course syllabi** for semester and quarter courses provide suggested models for structuring a course.
- Editable, chapter-specific **PowerPoint slides** offer complete flexibility for creating a multimedia presentation for the course.
- An **instructor's manual** includes lecture notes that summarize key concepts by chapter, in addition to discussion questions and classroom activity suggestions.
- **SAGE Coursepacks** make it easy to import our quality instructor and student content into your school's learning management system (LMS). Intuitive and simple to use, SAGE Coursepacks allow you to customize course content to meet your students' needs. Learn more at sagepub.com/coursepacks.

SAGE Edge for Students

SAGE Edge for Students provides a personalized approach to help students reach their coursework goals in an easy-to-use learning environment. To maximize students' understanding of behavioral neuroscience and to promote critical thinking, we have provided the following chapter-specific student resources on the open-access portion of **edge.sagepub.com/gaskin**.

- Mobile-friendly **flashcards** strengthen understanding of key terms and concepts.
- Mobile-friendly **practice quizzes** allow for independent assessment by students of their mastery of course material.
- **Learning objectives** reinforce the most important material.
- **Multimedia content** includes online resources that appeal to students with different learning styles.

Original Artwork and Animations

Carefully curated original artwork includes figures and illustrations designed to enhance and explore core concepts and current research. Select figures are further explored in animations. These animations illustrate concepts by showing the identified process visually, along with a step-by-step narration. These are available in the Interactive eBook.

Interactive eBook

An easy-to-follow Interactive eBook provides access to the same content and page layout of the traditional printed book but in a flexible digital format. Animations exploring select figures and concepts from the text are located within the Interactive eBook.

ACKNOWLEDGMENTS

The writing of a textbook was for me a monumental task. For me, undertaking, persisting at, and completing this task would not have been possible without the passion I have for the field of behavioral neuroscience. This passion found its beginnings during my undergraduate years at Concordia University in Montréal, where I worked in the laboratory of Zalman Amit at the Center for Studies in Behavioral Neurobiology (CSBN). I therefore thank Zalman for giving me my first opportunity. While in this lab, I worked on many studies, most of which were published in scientific journals. My passion for the field was fueled further by my master's supervisor, Dave Mumby, also at the CSBN, and by Ph.D. supervisor Norman White at McGill University. I would also like to thank Larry Squire and Robert Clark at the University of California, San Diego, who gave me the opportunity to work with them as a postdoctoral researcher.

I also thank my colleagues in the psychology department at Dawson College, with whom I have shared my ideas about the format and contents of the textbook. I especially thank my colleague Rajesh Malik with whom I always had stimulating and motivating scientific conversations over the years, which helped me get through the task of writing when it seemed to be overwhelming. Of course, the writing of a behavioral neuroscience textbook would never have come to life without having the opportunity to teach. I also owe a special thanks to Valerie Turner, who was chair of the psychology department when I began writing the book, for giving me the opportunity to teach the very first brain and behavior course officially offered at Dawson College.

I also extend my deepest gratitude to Marilyn Tardif not only for significantly contributing to my postdoctoral work but also for her sound advice concerning some of the content and readability of the text.

Finally, I would like to thank all of the folks at SAGE, including Reid Hester, Abbie Rickard, Mitch Yapko, Emma Newsom, and Elizabeth Cruz, who have made the production of this textbook possible. I also thank all of those, listed below, who participated in making this textbook a reality by reviewing its chapters and providing extremely useful and constructive comments:

Jeffrey S. Bedwell, University of Central Florida

Tom Byrne, Massachusetts College of Liberal Arts

Amy Camodeca, The Pennsylvania State University, Beaver Campus

Suzanne Clerkin, Purchase College, State University of New York

Ann D. Cohen, University of Pittsburgh School of Medicine

Heidi E. Day, University of Colorado Boulder

Steven I. Dworkin, Western Illinois University

Amanda El Bassiouny, Spring Hill College

Tifani Fletcher, West Liberty University

Kara I. Gabriel, Central Washington University

Lily Halsted, Queens University of Charlotte

Christopher Hayashi, Southwestern College

Justin C. Hulbert, Bard College

Spencer L. MacAdams, University of South Carolina

Maura Mitrushina, California State University, Northridge

Daniel Montoya, Fayetteville State University

Joseph H. Porter, Virginia Commonwealth University

Erin Rhinehart, Susquehanna University

Amy L. Salmeto-Johnson, Graceland University

Dennis J. Trickett, University of the Cumberlands

Lucy J. Troup, University of the West of Scotland

Stephen Weinert, Cuyamaca College

Xiaojuan Xu, Grand Valley State University

ABOUT THE AUTHOR

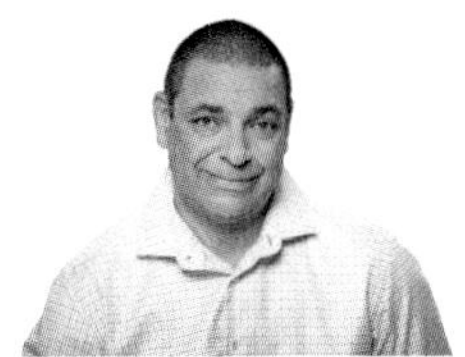

Stéphane Gaskin is a psychology professor at Dawson College in Montréal. He is also a lecturer at Concordia and McGill universities. Over the past 15 years, Stéphane has taught a variety of psychology courses at both college and university, including courses on general psychology, sensation and perception, the neurobiology of learning and memory, abnormal psychology, learning, human neuropsychology, and behavioral neuroscience. He has taught the very first brain and behavior course officially offered at Dawson College. Stéphane obtained both his bachelor's and master of psychology degrees at Concordia University. For his master's degree, Stéphane's research focused on the role of the hippocampus in spatial and object-recognition memory. He then pursued and obtained a Ph.D. degree at McGill University, where he studied the interaction between various brain areas such as the hippocampus, amygdala, and striatum in learning to approach cues associated with appetitive stimuli. Stéphane then pursued his studies as a postdoctoral researcher at both the University of California in San Diego and Concordia University in Montréal. Much of Stéphane's research has been published in international scientific journals and presented at the Society for Neuroscience's annual conferences.

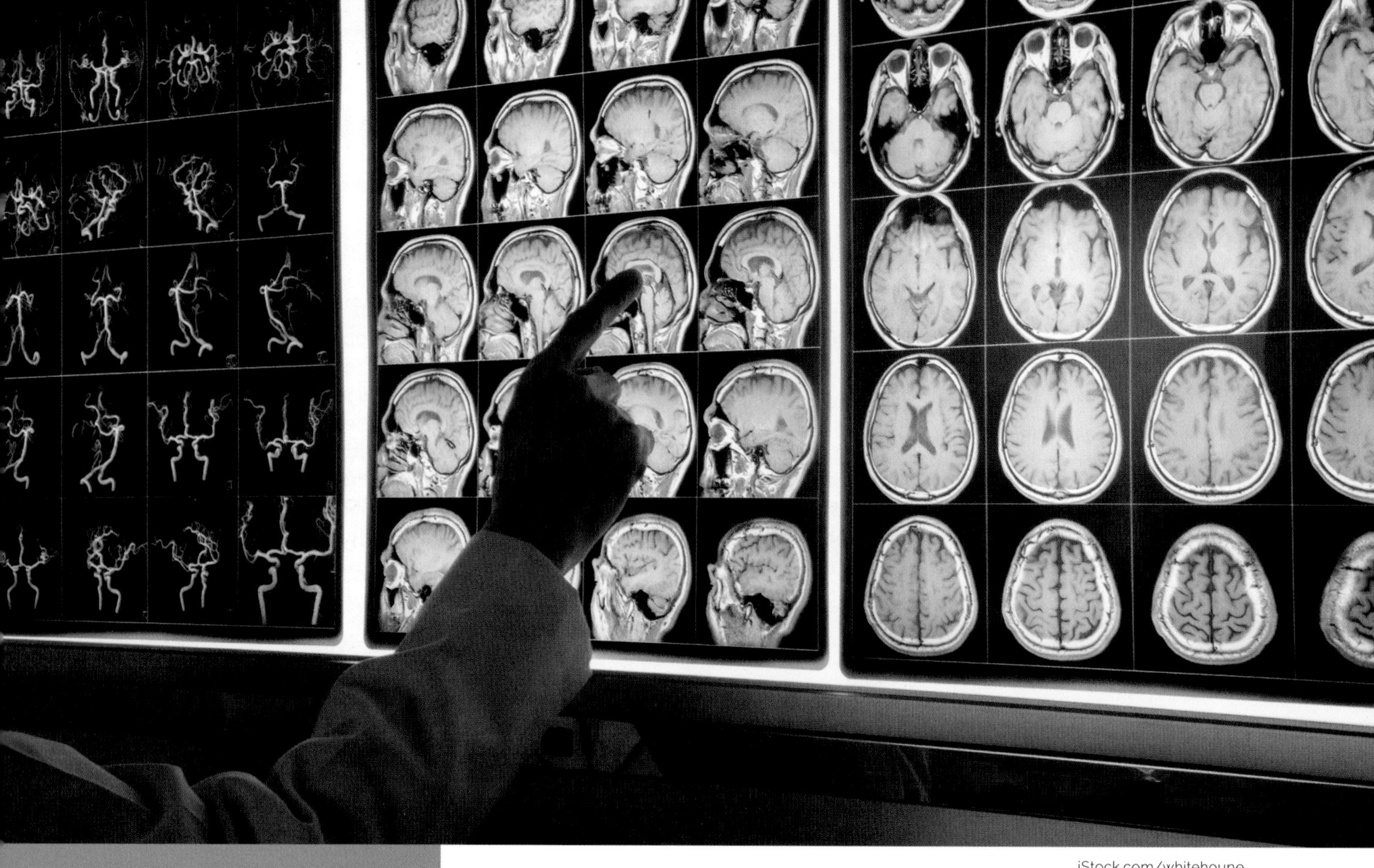

iStock.com/whitehoune

1 Behavioral Neuroscience

Understanding Brain-Behavior Relationships

Chapter Contents

Learning Objectives

1.1.1 Know and understand what constitutes the study of brain-behavior relationships.

1.1.2 Have a broad understanding of the global structural aspects of the brain and some of its basic functions.

1.1.3 Explain the different levels of analysis that constitute the study of brain-behavior relationships.

1.1.4 Understand the basics of how genes influence behavior and how the environment influences genes.

1.2.1 Explain the concept of natural selection.

1.2.2 Understand the adaptive variations that gave rise to brain-behavior relationships.

1.3.1 Describe some of the views associated with brain function throughout antiquity.

1.3.2 Explain the philosophical roots that underlie the relationship between brain and body.

1.3.3 Understand how the idea that brain functions are localized to specific areas developed.

1.4.1 Explain how the study of brain-damaged patients can inform neuroscientists about brain-behavior relationships.

1.4.2 Describe how brain-behavior relationships can be inferred by lesioning, stimulating, and measuring the brain's activity.

1.4.3 Define the different fields of study related to behavioral neuroscience.

Brain-Behavior Relationships: From Holes in the Head to Brain Imaging

In the 1860s, American diplomat, archeologist, collector, and popular writer Ephraim George Squier (1821–1888) was shown an ancient skull. The skull was discovered at an ancient Inca burial site in Peru. One notable peculiarity of the skull was a large rectangular-shaped hole located near its front and on its top. Squier took the skull as evidence that the ancient Peruvians performed some type of brain surgery. Over the years, many more such skulls, dating back to the time of the Inca empire (1400–1532), and much earlier (800–100 B.C.E.), have been discovered on the coast of Peru. A slew of similar skulls have also been found at sites around the world. What is intriguing about those skulls is that the holes in them show signs of healing. This means that the holes were not inflicted during battle and were not meant to kill. Rather, the holes seemed to have been made purposely by the scraping, drilling, or boring of the skull bone, a procedure known as trepanation. Some of the skulls even showed evidence of postoperative treatments, such as the holes being covered with plaques made of metal or bone. Why did ancient civilizations practice trepanation? Several theories have been proposed in an attempt to answer this question. On the one hand, the holes may have been bored for spiritual reasons. For example, discs made of cranial bones may have been believed to ward off demons. The holes may also have been bored into the skulls to permit the release of spirits thought to cause mental illness. On the other hand, trepanation may have served some therapeutic purpose. For example, it may have been used in the treatment of seizures, headaches, diseases, and skull fractures. Trepanation was also used in ancient Greece and Rome. For example, Greek physician Hippocrates (460–370 B.C.E.) used trepanation to release intracranial pressure due to the swelling of the brain following injury. Galen (130–210 C.E.), physician to the gladiators, refined the technique.

Today, trepanation or, as it is commonly called, craniotomy is used to gain access to the brain in the treatment of various conditions such as epilepsy, aneurysms, or the removal of tumors. Modern craniotomy procedures bear little resemblance to their ancient counterparts. They can be performed under the guidance of computers and imaging methods so that the hole is drilled at a precise location over the brain area in need of treatment. A brain area can even be examined by drilling a small hole into the skull through which a lighted scope with a camera is inserted. In addition, brain-behavior relationships can be inferred by brain imaging methods that permit neuroscientists to observe the brain's activity while an individual is performing a task, and behaviors can be elicited by electrically stimulating the brain.

INTRODUCTION

In this chapter, you will be introduced to the study of brain-behavior relationships, also known as behavioral neuroscience. After having defined and explored some of the branches of behavioral neuroscience, you will get a quick tour of the brain, including its main structures and the specialized cells of which it is composed. Brain-behavior relationships can be better understood if they are studied from multiple perspectives. Therefore, neuroscientists study brain-behavior relationships from the perspectives of interacting molecules within brain cells, the functioning of brain cells themselves, and the interaction between systems in the brain, cognition, and social behavior. Brain-behavior relationships can also be understood as the outcome of an evolutionary process that resulted in adaptations that permit animals to survive in their environments. Finally, understanding the progress made in the quest to learn about brain-behavior relationships requires you to look at some of the major figures and discoveries throughout the history of neuroscience. We will survey these main historical figures and discoveries, followed by the methods used to study brain-behavior relationships today. You will also learn about the different fields of study that are related to behavioral neuroscience, as well as some of the fields that benefit from behavioral neuroscience research findings.

1.1 What Is Behavioral Neuroscience?

Module Contents

Learning Objectives

1.1.1 Know and understand what constitutes the study of brain-behavior relationships.

1.1.2 Have a broad understanding of the global structural aspects of the brain and some of its basic functions.

1.1.3 Explain the different levels of analysis that constitute the study of brain-behavior relationships.

1.1.4 Understand the basics of how genes influence behavior and how the environment influences genes.

1.1.1 THE STUDY OF BRAIN-BEHAVIOR RELATIONSHIPS

>> LO 1.1.1 Know and understand what constitutes the study of brain-behavior relationships.

Key Terms

- **Behavioral neuroscience:** The scientific study of how brain activity influences behavior.
- **Overt behavior:** Behavior that is readily observable such as reaching out for a cup of coffee.
- **Covert behavior:** Behavior that cannot readily be observed, such as thinking, remembering, paying attention, experiencing emotions, and a range of others.
- **Cognitive neuroscience:** A branch of behavioral neuroscience that focuses on the processes within the brain that are associated with cognitive functions such as reasoning, problem solving, memory, and attention.
- **Affective neuroscience:** A branch of behavioral neuroscience in which researchers focus on the neurobiological processes that underlie emotions.
- **Social neuroscience:** A branch of behavioral neuroscience that focuses on the neurobiological processes of social behaviors such as those involved in empathy, affiliation, and morality.
- **Decision neuroscience:** A branch of behavioral neuroscience that focuses on the neurobiological basis of choice behavior; sometimes known as neuroeconomics.
- **Teratogens:** Factors that can cause malformations of the embryo.
- **Fetal alcohol spectrum disorders (FASDs):** A group of disorders associated with a mother drinking alcohol during pregnancy, which affects the development of the baby; characterized by abnormal facial features, short height, low body weight, low intelligence, and behavioral problems.

Behavioral neuroscience is the scientific study of how brain activity influences behavior. The study of behavioral neuroscience includes the study of how the brain is involved in both overt and covert behavior. **Overt behavior** refers to readily observable behavior such

FIGURE 1.1

The woman on the left is engaged in covert behavior. That is, she may be remembering, deciding, or planning. However, it is difficult to infer what is going on inside her mind by examining her overt behavior (sitting at home seemingly looking outside a window). By contrast, the woman on the right is engaged in overt behavior for which what she is covertly experiencing can more easily be inferred.

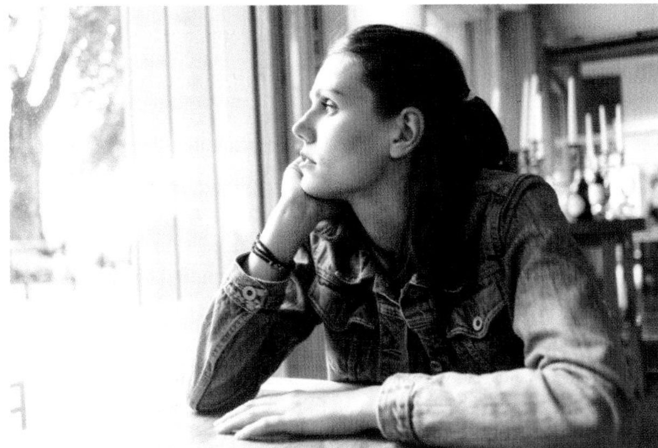

iStock.com/Vladimir Vladimirov

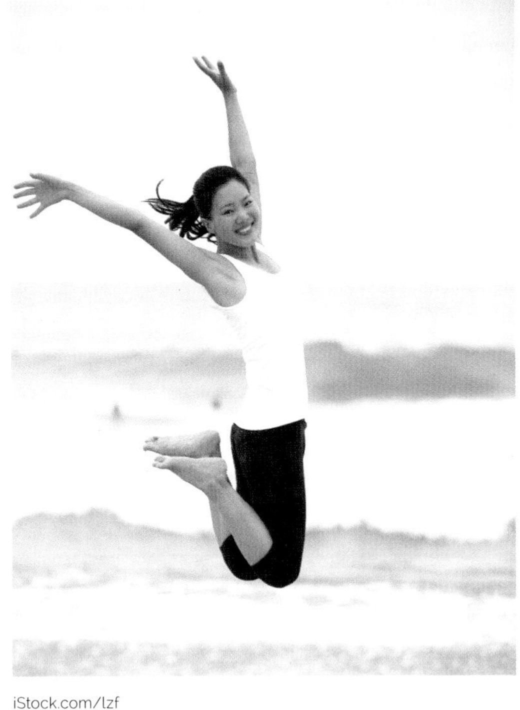

iStock.com/lzf

as reaching out to grab a cup of freshly brewed coffee, behaving aggressively, or bursting out in laughter. **Covert behavior** refers to behavior that cannot readily be observed, such as remembering, experiencing emotions, dreaming, lying, reading silently, and a range of others (Figure 1.1). Of course, overt behaviors often inform us about covert behavior, such as when we infer that someone is thinking about a sad event (covert) when crying (overt) or that someone is remembering what was studied (covert) while taking an exam (overt).

Behavioral neuroscientists—the scientists who study brain-behavior relationships—may sometimes be more specific about what they study. For example, in **cognitive neuroscience**, the focus of study is on the processes within the brain that are associated with cognitive functions such as reasoning, problem solving, memory, and attention (Baars & Gage, 2010). In **affective neuroscience**, researchers focus on brain processes associated with the experience and expression of emotions (Dalgleish, 2004). In **social neuroscience**, researchers are interested in the brain processes involved in socially based functions such as empathy, affiliation, and morality (Decety & Keenan, 2006). Behavioral neuroscientists may also be interested in the brain processes involved in choice behavior, in what is known as **decision neuroscience**, sometimes called neuroeconomics (Doya, 2008).

The Importance of Environment and Experience

Behavioral neuroscientists are aware that behavior is influenced by environmental factors and life experiences. For example, expressing and experiencing fear requires both changes occurring in the brain and a situation perceived as a threat. Environmental factors also influence normal brain development. For example, stimulation of the senses is required for the normal development of brain areas that process sensory information.

A slew of environmental factors can adversely affect brain development. Some of these factors may take the form of substances (various chemicals or drugs) known as **teratogens** that can potentially cause birth defects. For example, a woman who consumes alcohol while pregnant puts her developing baby at risk for **fetal alcohol spectrum disorders (FASDs)**. Babies born with FASDs have varying degrees of abnormal facial features, short height, low body weight, low intelligence, and behavioral problems (Figure 1.2) (Wilhoit, Scott, & Simecka, 2017). Sadly, an estimated 1 in 100 babies in the United States is born with features of FASDs, the most preventable cause of developmental disabilities and birth defects (Lyons, 2016). See the "It's a Myth!" feature in Chapter 5 for more on this topic.

FIGURE 1.2

A child with FASD, which is characterized by abnormal facial features as well as short height and low body weight. FASD is also associated with low intelligence and behavioral problems.

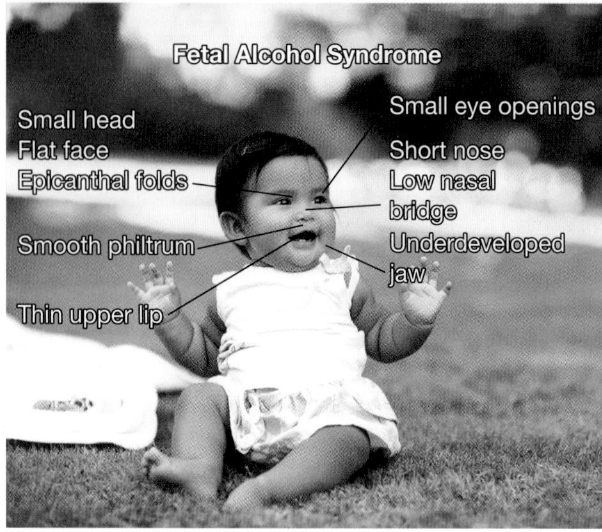
Fetal Alcohol Syndrome
Small head
Flat face
Epicanthal folds
Smooth philtrum
Thin upper lip
Small eye openings
Short nose
Low nasal bridge
Underdeveloped jaw

iStock.com/mmg1design

1.1.2 A QUICK LOOK AT THE BRAIN

>> **LO 1.1.2 Have a broad understanding of the global structural aspects of the brain and some of its basic functions.**

Key Terms

- **Lateral view:** The surface of the brain as viewed from one of its sides.
- **Cortex:** The outermost layer of the brain.
- **Lobes:** Anatomical subdivisions of the brain.
- **Gyri:** Ridges (or bumps) on the surface of the cortex.
- **Sulci:** Grooves that separate the gyri.
- **Fissures:** Large grooves that can be used to delineate cortical areas.
- **Sylvian fissure:** The fissure that separates the frontal lobe from the temporal lobe.
- **Superior view:** The brain as viewed from the top.
- **Hemispheres:** The two halves of the brain.
- **Sagittal view:** A lateral view of the brain with one of the hemispheres missing.
- **Corpus callosum:** The thick bundle of fibers that connect the two hemispheres, permitting them to communicate with each other.
- **Inferior view:** The brain as viewed from the bottom.
- **Neurons:** Cells that perform the major computational functions of the nervous system.
- **Glia:** Cells that support neuronal function and clear debris, toxins, and bacteria from the brain.

General Structure and Views of the Brain

The average human brain weighs about 1.36 kilograms (3 lb.) and has a volume of 1,273.6 cm^3 for men and 1,131.1 cm^3 for women (Allen, Damasio, & Grabowski, 2002). Different views of the human brain are shown in Figure 1.3. The top left of the figure shows a **lateral view** of the brain, which means that only one of its sides is visible. From this view, the main superficial parts of the brain can be seen. The outermost layer of the brain is called the **cortex**, which is Latin for "bark" or "shell." What can also be seen is how the brain is divided into different parts called **lobes**. These are the frontal, temporal, parietal, and occipital lobes. As you will learn in Chapter 4, each one of these lobes is associated with a particular set of functions. The first thing that may strike you about the cortex is its pattern of bumps and grooves. The bumps are known as **gyri** (singular: *gyrus*) and the grooves are known as **sulci** (singular: *sulcus*), about which we will have more to say in Chapter 4. Some of the sulci in the cortex are larger than others. These are known as **fissures**. For example, the **Sylvian fissure** separates the frontal lobe from the temporal lobe.

Two structures at the back of the brain are prominent. One is the *cerebellum*, which is Latin for "small brain," and the other is the brainstem. The cerebellum is involved in the coordination of movements. Areas in the brainstem are involved in sleep, wakefulness, and vital functions such as respiration and heartbeat. The bottom left shows a **superior view** (or dorsal view) of the brain, which simply means that it is seen from the top. Most prominent from this view is the fact that the brain has two halves, called **hemispheres** (left and right), separated by the interhemispheric (or longitudinal) fissure. Also visible is the central sulcus, which separates the frontal lobe from the parietal lobe.

The top right of the figure shows a **sagittal view** of the brain. This view shows the brain as if one of the hemispheres was removed and then shown as a lateral view. This view shows the center of the brain. That is, other regions not visible from the surface can now be seen. This includes a structure of the brainstem called the *pons*, which is Latin for "bridge." The pons relays signals from the cerebellum to the cortex. Also visible are the midbrain and the thalamus. The midbrain contains areas important for perception and motivation, whereas the thalamus relays information from the senses to the appropriate area in the cortex. The optic chiasm is where the nerves bringing visual information to the brain from each eye meet, some crossing over to the opposite side of the brain while others remain on the same side. Also visible is the **corpus callosum**, which is a thick bundle of fibers

FIGURE 1.3

Different views of the brain.

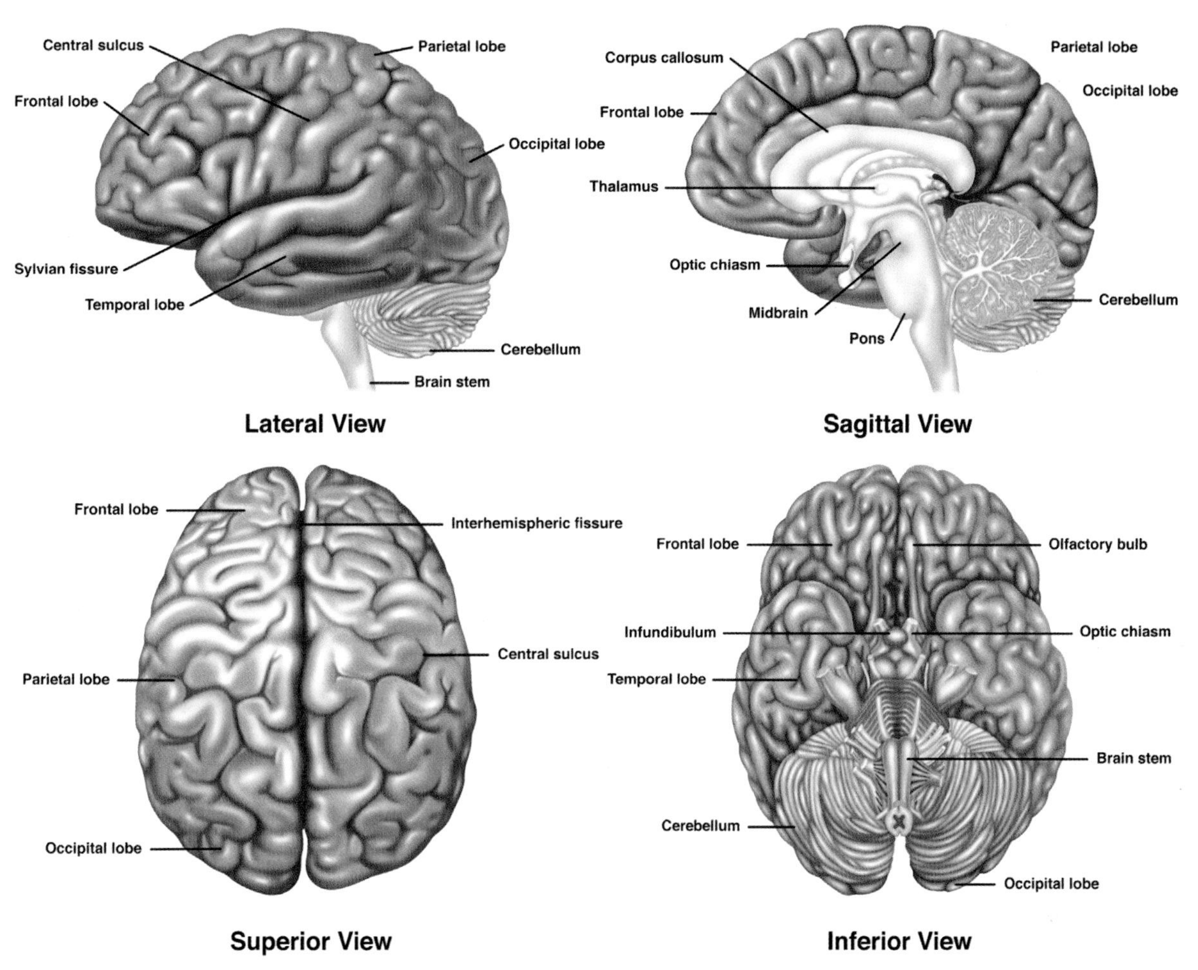

Gwen Shockey/SCIENCE SOURCE

that connect the two hemispheres, permitting them to communicate with each other.

The bottom right of the figure shows an **inferior view** (or ventral view) of the brain, which simply means that it is viewed from the bottom. This view shows the olfactory bulb, which is where information from the sense of smell is first analyzed. Also visible from this view is the infundibulum, which connects the hypothalamus and pituitary gland (not shown), which we will have much to say about in Chapter 10.

Brain Cells

Like all tissues in the body, the brain is made up of its own kinds of cells. There are two major types of cells in the brain, neurons and glia. **Neurons** are the basic functional units of the brain. They communicate with other cells through electrical messages known as action potentials. Other cells with which neurons communicate include muscle and gland cells. It is this interaction between neurons and other cells that makes moving, thinking, emotions, and learning possible.

Glia come in many forms, each playing specific roles, from providing immune defense to the brain (Plog & Nedergaard, 2018) to ensuring that neurons communicate in an efficient manner (Verkhratsky & Nedergaard, 2018).

Neurons and glia are illustrated in Figure 1.4. You can see that neurons have two main parts, a cell body and a tail-like extension called an axon. The neurons' electrical messages are conveyed through their axons. The glia that you see in the figure are specialized in coating the axons with a fatty substance called myelin, which increases their electrical conductivity. Much more is said about neurons and glia in Chapter 2. The details by which neurons communicate are explored in Chapter 3.

FIGURE 1.4

Neurons and glia (insert to the top right of the brain). Neurons (dark blue) are the basic functional units of the brain. Two major parts of a neuron are the cell body, which has extensions called dendrites that receive messages from other neurons, and a tail-like extension called an axon, through which electrical messages called action potentials travel. Also shown are two types of glia. Astrocytes (light blue), which serve diverse functions, and oligodendrocytes (green), which insulate axons by coating them with myelin (pink).

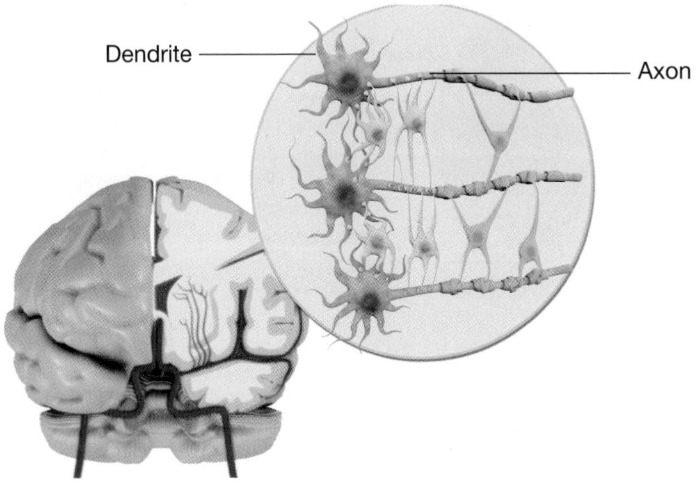

GUNILLA ELAM/SCIENCE SOURCE

IT'S A MYTH!

Left Brained/Right Brained

Are you left brained or right brained? Have you ever heard this question being asked? Chances are that you have. The idea that the left and right hemispheres of the brain are specialized for different types of thinking is pervasive in movies and magazines and on websites and social media.

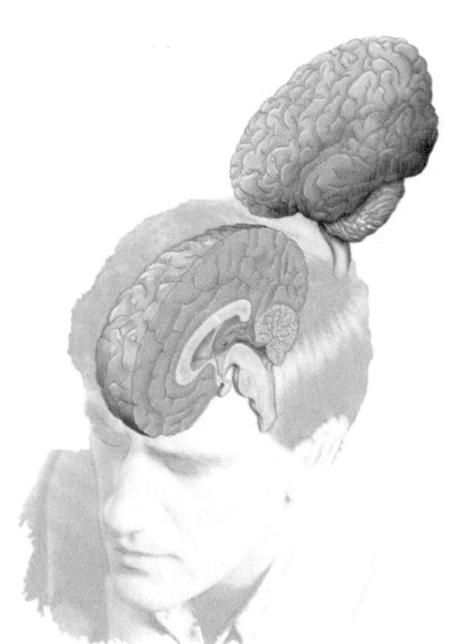

Sun Sentinel/Tribune News Service/Getty Images

It is true that the left and right hemispheres of the brain were found to be involved in different functions. For example, in most people, the left hemisphere is associated with speech and the logical thinking skills required for processing verbal and numerical information. It is also the hemisphere that leads to analytical thinking, such as extracting details or the single parts that make up the structure of a whole. The left hemisphere's propensity to think logically and to be analytical means that it takes things quite literally. This means that the left hemisphere is incapable of getting the punchline of jokes or understanding the true meaning of common everyday sayings. For example, when you hear the expression "He kicked the bucket," you know that this means that a person has died. However, if you had only the left hemisphere of your brain, you would wonder why someone had literally kicked a bucket.

By contrast, the right hemisphere is associated with nonverbal and visuospatial skills. It processes information holistically instead of extracting meaning from the analysis of individual parts. For example, it is the right hemisphere that understands that someone has died when you hear the phrase "He kicked the bucket." The right hemisphere is also the one to which creativity is attributed.

The Myth

The myth states that some people are predominantly "left brained" and others "right brained" and that your left or right "brainedness" dictates your thinking style and personality. You are more likely left brained if you are the type to become an engineer, whereas you are more likely right brained if you are the artistic type.

Where Does the Myth Come From?

The source of the myth can be attributed at least partly to Arthur Ladbroke Wigan (1785–1847), who described the two hemispheres of the brain as independent entities thinking in different ways, in his book *A New View of Insanity: Duality of the Mind*. He wrote that the two halves of the brain usually cooperate but that they may work against each other in mental illness. This idea gained momentum after Paul Broca, in the 1860s, and Carl Wernicke, in the 1870s, found that different functions may be controlled by either the left or right hemisphere. They found that speech and the understanding of language were controlled by the left hemisphere, which became known as the dominant hemisphere.

However, the greatest boost to the myth came in the 1960s and 1970s, when neuropsychologist Roger Sperry studied the behavior of patients in whom the corpus callosum had been intentionally severed to limit the spread of epileptic seizures from one hemisphere to the other. These patients, who became known as split-brain patients, were assessed for their ability to process information presented to either one of the hemispheres at a time. For example, when Sperry asked split-brain patients to identify a hidden object held in their right hand, they could easily do so. However, if the object was held in the left hand, they were unable to name it. This was because limbs are controlled by the hemisphere opposite to the body part. Therefore, to name an object in the left hand, the information processed by the right hemisphere has to be transferred to the left hemisphere, which controls language, through the corpus callosum, which was cut in the split-brain patients. In contrast, the information from an object held in the right hand is directly represented in the left hemisphere, through which the object can be named. Further experiments with split-brain patients showed that the right hemisphere was superior at processing visuospatial and emotional information.

Why Is the Myth Wrong?

Although the left and right hemispheres appear to be specialized for processing different types of information when isolated in experimental studies, this does not mean that they function independently of each other with their very own thinking styles. There is no scientific evidence that the way people think—or their personalities—is determined by one hemisphere dominating over the other. In fact, when researchers examined the brain scans of 1,011 individuals, they found that the study participants could not be classified on the basis of whether they used one hemisphere more than the other (Nielsen, Zielinski, Ferguson, Lainhart, & Anderson, 2013). ●

1.1.3 LEVELS OF ANALYSIS: PUTTING BRAIN-BEHAVIOR RELATIONSHIPS IN PERSPECTIVE

>> LO 1.1.3 Explain the different levels of analysis that constitute the study of brain-behavior relationships.

Key Terms

- **Level of analysis:** Refers to the location, scale, or size of what is being studied.
- **Molecular level of analysis:** The study of the workings of the nervous system using methods that permit the study of the genes and the chemistry of proteins within neurons.
- **Cellular level of analysis:** The study of the morphology and physiological properties of cells within the nervous system.
- **Systems level of analysis:** The study of how the activity in patterns of neuronal connections gives rise to overt and covert behaviors and how information is encoded and stored in the patterns of connections between neurons that are part of functional systems.
- **Cognitive level of analysis:** The study of the neurobiological basis of higher mental processes.
- **Social level of analysis:** The study of how neurobiological processes are involved in social behavior.

To have a broad understanding of brain-behavior relationships, one must know how they can be studied from different **levels of analysis**, as illustrated in Figure 1.5. A level of analysis refers to the location, scale, or size of what is being studied. For example, behavioral neuroscientists can study brain-behavior relationships at the

FIGURE 1.5

Behavioral neuroscientists are interested in studying behavior at the molecular, cellular, systems, cognitive, and social levels of analysis.

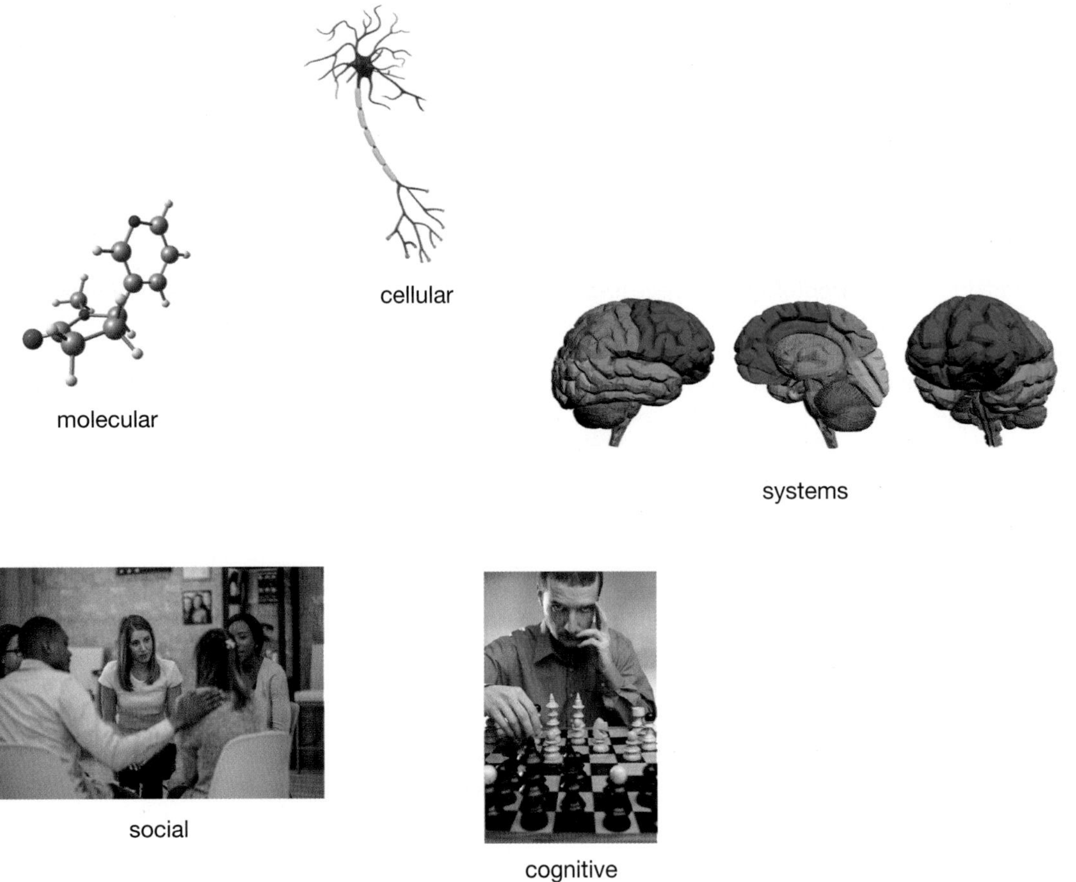

(Clockwise from top left) iStock.com/ollaweila; iStock.com/3drenderings; iStock.com/Slim3D; iStock.com/dulezidar; iStock.com/FatCamera

molecular, cellular, systems, cognitive, and social levels of analysis. Let's take a look at what it means to study brain-behavior relationships at each of these levels.

At the **molecular level of analysis**, neuroscientists are interested in studying the brain using methods that permit them to study the genes and the chemistry of proteins within neurons. This may include the study of how genes and the chemistry of proteins can be altered by environmental influences (see the next unit for a description of genes).

For example, researchers found that different genes respond to specific types of environmental stressors in rats, whereas other genes respond to stress regardless of its source (Jacobson, Kim, Patro, Rosati, & McKinnon, 2018). The researchers reported that they could tell which rats were exposed to stress by studying the expression of a subset of their genes. In addition, by looking at the expression of other genes, they could tell the type of stressors to which the rats were exposed.

At the **cellular level of analysis**, neuroscientists are interested in studying the morphology and physiological properties of cells within the brain. This includes studying how the integrity of certain types of cells is crucial for proper functioning of the brain. For example, scientists studying the brain at the cellular level found that the degeneration of what are known as gatekeeper cells, which control the flow of blood inside the brain, is partly responsible for Alzheimer's disease, in which people suffer a slow decline in memory and other thinking skills (Kisler et al., 2017).

At the **systems level of analysis**, neuroscientists are interested in how activity in patterns of neuronal connections gives rise to overt and covert behaviors. They are also interested in how information is encoded and stored in the patterns of connections between neurons that are part of functional systems (e.g., the visual system, motor systems, memory systems) and the possible interactions that exist between them. For example, researchers found that networks of neurons in a part of the brain called the entorhinal cortex are involved in representing time in rats as they encode new experiences. They proposed that this information is combined with the memory for places and objects, which is encoded by networks of neurons in other brain areas (Tsao et al., 2018).

At the **cognitive level of analysis**, neuroscientists are interested in the neurobiological basis of higher mental processes. This includes the processes involved in language, attention, self-awareness, consciousness, and mental imagery. For example, researchers found that interpreters, who perform the simultaneous translation of one language into another, have hyperconnectivity between the frontal parts of the two hemispheres of their brains compared to non-language experts who speak more than one language (C. Klein, Metz, Elmer, & Jancke, 2018).

At the **social level of analysis**, neuroscientists are interested in how neurobiological processes are involved in social behavior. For example, researchers have found that prosocial behavior in adolescents was associated with levels of activity in a part of the brain called the anterior cingulate cortex (Okada et al., 2019).

1.1.4 A CLOSER LOOK AT THE MOLECULAR LEVEL: GENETICS

>> LO 1.1.4 **Understand the basics of how genes influence behavior and how the environment influences genes.**

Key Terms

- **Genetics:** The study of inherited traits and their variation.
- **Genes:** Once referred to as the basic functional units of heredity, genes are sequences of deoxyribonucleic acid (DNA), some of which code for proteins.
- **Deoxyribonucleic acid (DNA):** A molecule composed of sequences of smaller molecules called nucleotides, bound together by molecules of sugar and phosphate.
- **Phenotype:** The characteristic traits observed in individuals resulting from the interactions between their genotype and the environment.
- **Genotype:** Every individual's unique genetic constitution.
- **Behavioral genetics:** The field of study that seeks to understand how the variation of a trait in a population is related to the variation of genes within that population.
- **Heritability estimates:** The proportion of variation in a trait that can be accounted for by genetic variation in a population.
- **Epigenetics:** The study of changes in gene expression with no changes in DNA sequences, which can occur naturally or through the influence of environmental factors.

Genetics is the study of inherited traits and their variation. **Genes** are often defined as being the basic functional units of heredity. However, this definition of genes is not accurate. We now know that such basic units of heredity do not exist (Portin & Wilkins, 2017). Rather, genes are sequences of what is known as **deoxyribonucleic acid (DNA)**, which resides in the nucleus of every cell in the body. Some genes contain the instructions for building proteins. Other genes are noncoding and are involved in regulating protein synthesis along with a host of other functions (Pennisi, 2012). Estimates of the number of human genes have changed over the years (Salzberg, 2018). One of the latest counts sets the number of human genes at 43,162, of which 20,352 code for protein (Pertea et al., 2018).

DNA is a molecule composed of sequences of smaller molecules called nucleotides, which are bound together by molecules of sugar and phosphate. DNA takes the form of two strands bound together in a double helix. Nucleotides differ from each other only by the nature of what is known as a nitrogenous base. There are four nitrogenous bases. These are adenine, thymine, guanine, and cytosine. The nitrogenous bases bind the two single strands of DNA by forming base pairs. Base pairs are not formed randomly. That is, adenine is always paired with thymine and guanine is always paired with cytosine. DNA is present in almost all living organisms. The only exceptions to this are found in certain viruses (Hiyoshi, Miyahara, Kato, & Ohshima, 2011).

As shown in Figure 1.6, the sequences of DNA that compose genes are contained in what are known as chromosomes. In humans, each cell has 23 pairs of chromosomes. Twenty-two of those pairs are called autosomes, whereas one pair consists of the sex chromosomes (male XY and female XX), which determine gender. Figure 1.7 shows a picture of an individual's set of chromosomes in what is called a karyotype. The information contained in DNA dictates the synthesis of proteins. The variations in the proteins synthesized give rise to the differences in **phenotype**, which are the characteristic traits observed in individuals resulting from their **genotype**.

The influence that genes have in the synthesis of proteins depends on how they interact with the environment. Traits, whether physical or psychological, are considered to be the product of these interactions (Moore & Shenk, 2017). This means that there are no single genes or combinations of genes that, by themselves, directly result in the development of any given trait.

How Genes Are Transmitted From Parent to Offspring

Cells replicate through division. There are two types of cell divisions: mitosis and meiosis. Mitosis refers to the division of somatic cells (the ones that compose the various tissues of the body). Genes are passed on to the next generation through the division of sex cells (the ones present in the ovaries of females and testes of males) in a process called meiosis. Meiosis leads to the

FIGURE 1.6

Organisms are made up of cells, each of which contains an identical set of genes.

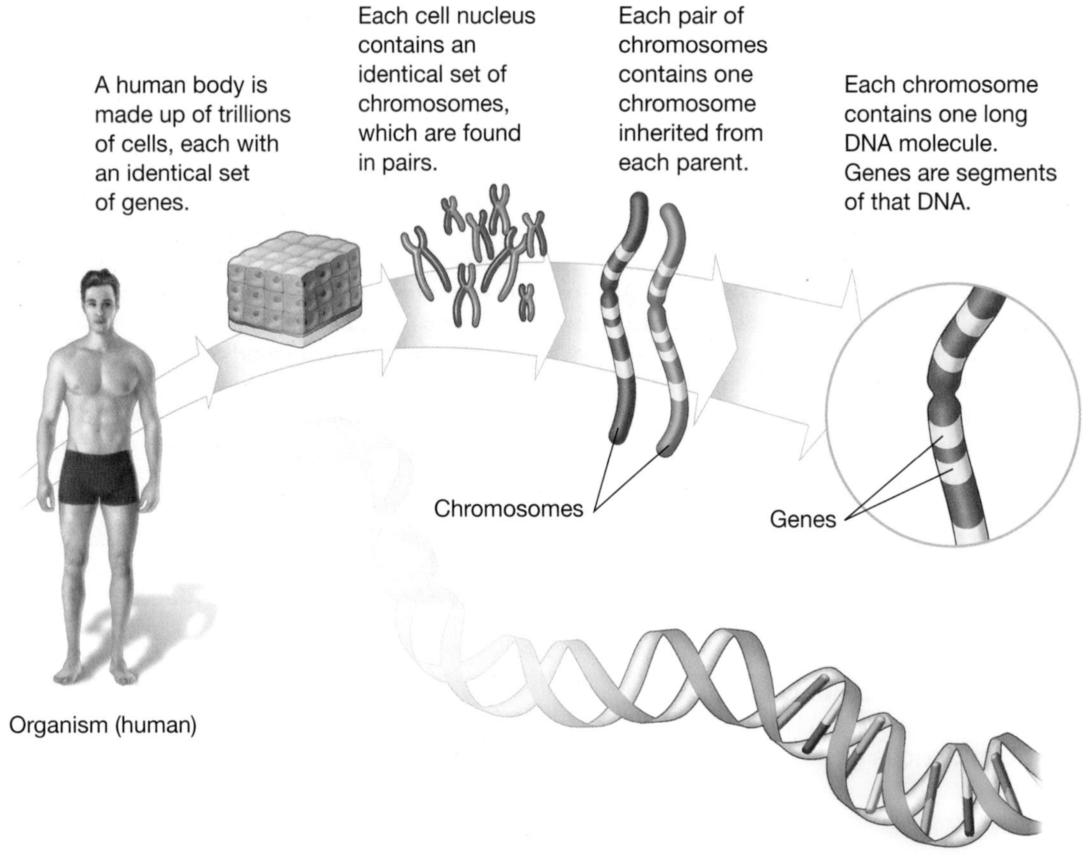

A human body is made up of trillions of cells, each with an identical set of genes.
Each cell nucleus contains an identical set of chromosomes, which are found in pairs.
Each pair of chromosomes contains one chromosome inherited from each parent.
Each chromosome contains one long DNA molecule. Genes are segments of that DNA.
Chromosomes
Genes
Organism (human)

Carolina Hrejsa/Body Scientific Intl.

FIGURE 1.7

Human karyotype. Humans have 23 pairs of chromosomes, which include 22 pairs of autosomes and one pair of sex chromosomes (X,Y).

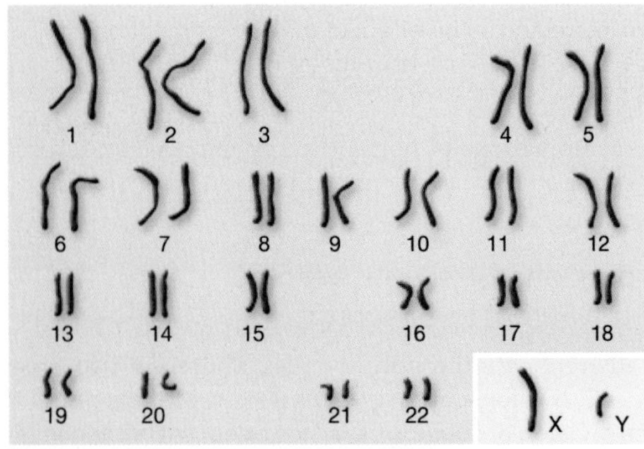

U.S. National Library of Medicine

creation of cells having only half of the total number of chromosomes. For example, in humans, out of a total of 46 chromosomes in somatic cells, each sex cell ends up with 23 chromosomes. Therefore, half of the genes you have inherited came from the set of 23 chromosomes provided by your mother and the other half came from the set provided by your father.

Behavioral Genetics

Behavioral genetics is the field of study that seeks to understand how the variation of a trait in a population is related to the variation of genes within that population. As a student of behavioral neuroscience, why should you be interested? Because behavioral geneticists consider how variations in brain function are related to variations of genes within a population.

Behavioral geneticists are interested not only in how genes contribute to behavior but also in how genes interact with environmental factors to produce behavior. Environmental factors include social and cultural factors, child-rearing practices, level of acceptance, social and cultural factors, as well as educational level (Kawamoto & Endo, 2015; Menardo, Balboni, & Cubelli, 2017). For behavioral geneticists, environmental factors also include biological factors such as nutrients, hormones, viruses, and bacteria.

To get a clue about how much of the variation of a trait can be accounted for by genetic variation in a population, behavioral geneticists compute what are known as **heritability estimates**. For example, the heritability estimate for personality was found to be 40%. This means that variation in gene composition accounts for 40% of the variation in personality in the population and that environmental factors account for 60% of the differences (Vukasovic & Bratko, 2015).

Behavioral geneticists are also interested in the heritability estimates of psychological disorders. For example, the heritability of alcohol use disorder was found to be approximately 50% (Verhulst, Neale, & Kendler, 2015). In another study, researchers found that the heritability estimates for minor and major depression are 37% and 46%, respectively (Corfield, Yang, Martin, & Nyholt, 2017).

Epigenetics

Epigenetics is the study of changes in gene expression with no changes in DNA sequences. Epigenetic changes occur naturally. However, they are also triggered by environmental factors and give rise to certain behavioral characteristics (Goldberg, Allis, & Bernstein, 2007). For example, social environment in early life can alter the expression of genes. In a study published in 2004, rat pups who experienced high levels of licking, grooming, and nursing by their mothers had a more moderate response to stress than rat pups that did not experience such high levels of maternal care. The researchers found that higher levels of maternal care created this difference by changing the expression of a gene involved in regulating how the brain is affected by glucocorticoids, which are chemicals released by the adrenal glands in times of stress (Weaver et al., 2004).

You might now wonder whether these epigenetic changes in the expression of genes are passed on to the next generations. The answer to this question is yes. For example, trauma-related epigenetic changes in Holocaust survivors who were imprisoned and tortured in concentration camps during World War II were passed on to their children (Yehuda et al., 2016). Even acquired fears may be inherited. Another study found that male mice trained to fear the smell of cherry blossoms through pairing it with an electric shock had offspring that feared the same smell (Dias & Ressler, 2014).

MODULE SUMMARY

Behavioral neuroscience is the study of brain-behavior relationships. Behavior can be overt, as when actions can be observed directly; or covert, as when behavior cannot be observed directly, such as remembering, reading silently, and dreaming. Behavioral neuroscience includes cognitive neuroscience, affective neuroscience, social neuroscience, and decision neuroscience. Brain-behavior relationships can be studied from different perspectives and at different scales called levels of analysis. These are the molecular, cellular, systems, cognitive, and social levels of analysis.

Genetics is the study of inherited traits and their variations. These inherited traits and characteristics are carried within genes. Genes are located on chromosomes. Humans have 23 pairs of chromosomes: 22 pairs of autosomes and one pair of sex chromosomes. Chromosomes are made of strands of DNA. The set of genes carried by an individual is called the genotype. The inherited traits as a result of the expression of those genes are called the phenotype. However, phenotypes are not determined by genes alone but by the interaction between genes and environmental influences.

Behavioral geneticists are interested in how variations of a trait in a population can be explained by the variation of genes within the same population. They are also known to compute heritability estimates, which estimate the proportion of the variance of a trait that is due to the variation of genes. In epigenetics, researchers are interested in the effect of the environment on the expression of genes. Studies have found that experiences in the early social environment can induce changes in gene expression. In addition, these changes can be passed on to the next generation.

TEST YOURSELF

1.1.1 Explain what the study of brain-behavior relationships consists of.

1.1.2 Describe the main structural aspects of the brain and some of the functions associated with each of the areas you read about.

1.1.3 Name and describe the levels of analysis that constitute the study of brain-behavior relationships.

1.1.4 Briefly explain how phenotypes result from the interactions between genes and environment.

1.2 The Evolution of Brain-Behavior Relationships

Module Contents

1.2.1 Natural Selection

1.2.2 Neuroecology: How Natural Selection Accounts for Brain-Behavior Relationships

Learning Objectives

1.2.1 Explain the concept of natural selection.

1.2.2 Understand the adaptive variations that gave rise to brain-behavior relationships.

1.2.1 NATURAL SELECTION

>> LO 1.2.1 Explain the concept of natural selection.

Key Terms

- **Descent with modification:** The idea that current forms of life evolved from preexisting forms.
- **Natural selection:** The process by which evolution can be explained.

Many of life's characteristics are truly striking. Have you ever marveled over the fact that animals are remarkably well adapted to their environments? For example, kangaroo rats can survive in the desert without ever drinking water by extracting moisture from the seeds that they eat (Tracy & Walsberg, 2000); notothenioid fish, which live in the freezing conditions of the Antarctic, produce a protein that acts as an "antifreeze," binding to water crystals in their blood (Cheng & Detrich, 2007); and the amazing cuttlefish changes its color to blend with its surroundings, allowing it to escape predators (Chiao, Chubb, & Hanlon, 2015).

English naturalist Charles Darwin (1809–1882) sought to find a scientific explanation for these adaptations. He proposed that current forms of life evolved from preexisting forms in what is known as **descent with modification**. Much of his amazement was cultivated on his voyage to the Galápagos Islands on the ship *H.M.S. Beagle*. Among many observations, he noted that finches varied considerably in the form of their beaks, and the way in which they used them, from island to island. He found that the form of their beaks seemed to have adapted to the types of food they ate on their respective islands: seeds, flowers, buds, or insects (Figure 1.8).

FIGURE 1.8

Darwin found that different varieties of finches lived on the different islands of the Galápagos. The finches were distinguished by the shapes of their beaks, which were adapted to the types of foods they ate on their respective islands.

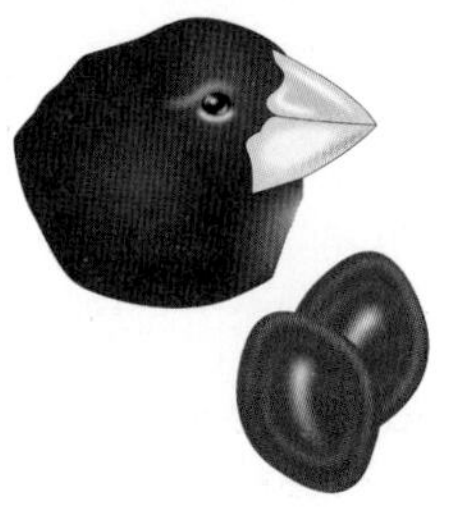

Large ground finch (seeds)

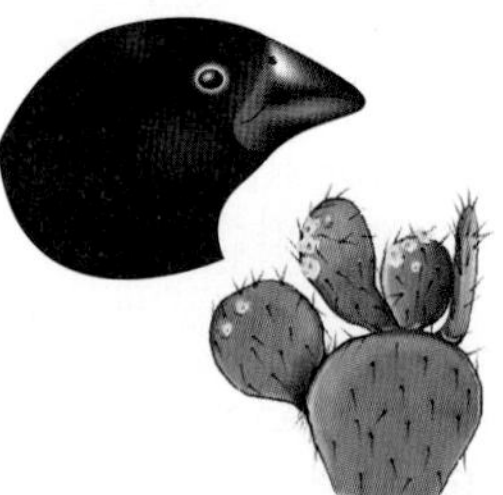

Cactus finch (cactus fruit and flowers)

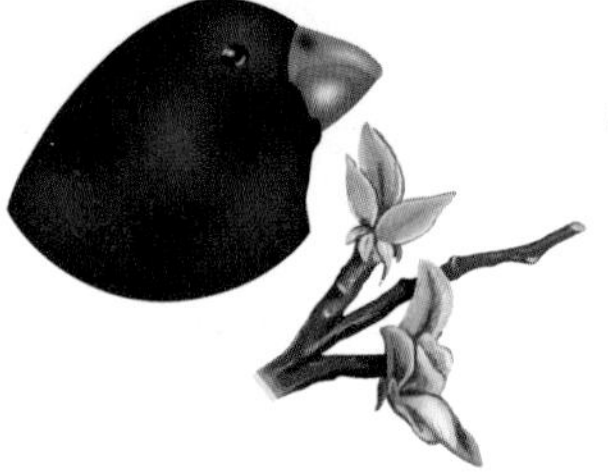

Vegetarian finch (buds)

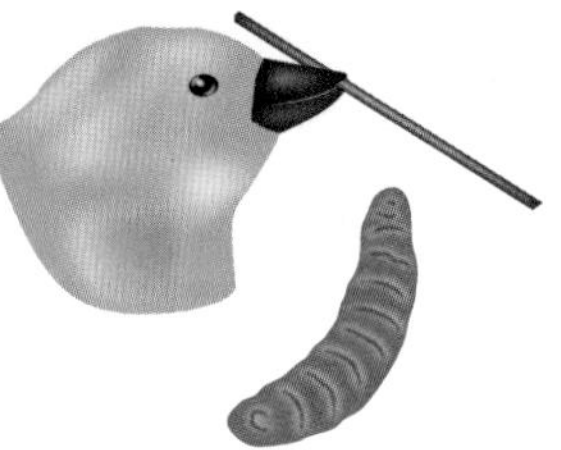

Woodpecker finch (insects)

Amanda Tomasikiewicz/Body Scientific Intl.

How can species be so well adapted to their environments? Darwin proposed that some of an animal's offspring possess characteristics that will make them more suited to their environment than others, giving them a survival advantage and, therefore, making them more likely to pass on those characteristics to subsequent generations. This process is known as **natural selection** (Darwin, 1859).

Natural selection can be summarized by two observations and inferences made by Darwin:

Observations

1. Members of a population often vary in inherited traits.
2. All species can produce more offspring than the environment can support.

Inferences

1. Some individuals will have inherited traits that will give them a survival advantage and higher

probability of reproducing than individuals that do not have those traits.

2. This survival advantage and higher reproductive probability will lead to the accumulation of those traits in subsequent generations.

1.2.2 NEUROECOLOGY: HOW NATURAL SELECTION ACCOUNTS FOR BRAIN-BEHAVIOR RELATIONSHIPS

>> LO 1.2.2 Understand the adaptive variations that gave rise to brain-behavior relationships.

Key Terms

- **Neuroecology:** The field that studies relationships between the brain and ecologically relevant behaviors and how they may have evolved through natural selection.
- **High vocal center (HVC):** The brain area at the center of a song-learning system in song birds.
- **Exaptation:** The adaptation of a trait that differs from the one it was selected for.

After reading about the adaptations of animals to their environments, you may be left wondering how natural selection can account for brain-behavior relationships. **Neuroecology** is the field of study in which researchers are interested in these types of relationships. For example, neuroecologists study the adaptive variations in the relationships that exist between cognition, sensory, and motor processes, and the brain, with respect to how organisms interact with their environment (Riffell & Rowe, 2016; Sherry, 2006). Neuroecologists have focused on several examples demonstrating that natural selection contributed to brain-behavior relationships in animals.

One of the most often cited examples is that of the relationship between the development of a brain area known as the **high vocal center (HVC)** and song learning in male song birds such as zebra finches and canaries. The HVC is part of a larger system known as the "song system" (Nottebohm, 2005; Nottebohm, Stokes, & Leonard, 1976; Wild, 1997). This system is involved in both song learning and the vocalization of songs. Researchers found that the song system is larger in males than in females and that the size of the HVC and other regions of the song system are enlarged during the spring breeding season. The enlargement of the HVC region in the spring coincides with the production of birdsongs, which are used to attract mates and to ward off rivals. How is this related to natural selection? Females were found to prefer to mate with males that sing at a high rate and that have a large repertoire of songs relative to those that do not. It is not difficult to apply the observations and inferences made by Darwin to this situation (see the previous unit). That is, males with a better developed song system would have been selected for and have greater reproductive success. Consequently, the genes associated with the development of effective song systems were passed on to later generations.

Another often-cited adaptation related to a brain-behavior relationship is that of a number of bird species that store food in hundreds or even thousands of caches (hiding places) over the course of a year. The birds are then able to retrieve the food from the caches, which are widely dispersed in their environment, anywhere from several days to several months after hiding it. This obviously requires an uncanny ability to remember spatial locations. Memory for spatial locations, otherwise known as spatial memory, is dependent on a brain area called the hippocampus (discussed at length in Chapter 12). The hippocampus of food-storing birds was found to be larger (relative to their brain and body size) than the hippocampus of birds that do not store their food. Further, the hippocampus of food-storing birds increases in size during the autumn and winter. This coincides with when food-storing birds cache the most food, due to the rarity of insects and plant seeds during those months (Sherry & Hoshooley, 2010).

However, not every behavior can be said to have arisen through natural selection. For example, the human brain is good at remembering email addresses or learning to use computers even if it obviously did not evolve to do so. For this reason, some researchers think that the brains of our early ancestors evolved general rules to deal with certain tasks that we can now apply to modern-day problems. This is known as **exaptation**, which is the adaptation of a trait that differs from the one it was selected for (Gould & Vrba, 1982; S. B. Klein, Cosmides, Tooby, & Chance, 2002; Sherry & Schacter, 1987). It is also worth noting that, as discussed earlier, changes in an organism's gene expression can be passed on to subsequent generations through epigenetic changes.

MODULE SUMMARY

Animals are remarkably well adapted to their environments. In addition, different species of animals share many life-supporting characteristics. At the same time, an enormous diversity of organisms exists. Charles Darwin sought to find a scientific explanation for those facts. He proposed that current forms of life evolved from preexisting forms in what is known as descent with modification. The mechanism by which he thought this occurred is known as natural selection.

Neuroecology is the field that studies relationships between the brain and ecologically relevant behaviors and how they may have evolved through natural selection. Several examples of such relationships and how they may have been selected for exist, namely, the high vocal center and song learning in song birds and the size of the hippocampus in food-storing birds.

Not all behaviors can be said to have evolved through natural selection. Some behaviors may have evolved to solve ancient problems but are well adapted to solve modern-day problems. The adaptation of a trait for uses that differ from what it was selected for is known as exaptation.

TEST YOURSELF

1.2.1 Explain the concept of natural selection.

1.2.2 Discuss how variations in brain structures evolved to give rise to brain-behavior relationships. Give two examples.

1.3 The Origins of Behavioral Neuroscience

Module Contents

1.3.1 Antiquity

1.3.2 The Mind-Body Problem

1.3.3 Localization of Function

Learning Objectives

1.3.1 Describe some of the views associated with brain function throughout antiquity.

1.3.2 Explain the philosophical roots that underlie the relationship between brain and body.

1.3.3 Understand how the idea that brain functions are localized to specific areas developed.

1.3.1 ANTIQUITY

>> LO 1.3.1 Describe some of the views associated with brain function throughout antiquity.

Key Term

- **Edwin Smith Papyrus:** A medical papyrus that seems to have been written around 1600 B.C.E., during the third dynasty of pharaohs.

The Egyptians

Today we know that the brain is the source of all of our faculties. However, this has not always been the case. In 1862, an archeologist named Edwin Smith (1822–1906) bought an ancient Egyptian papyrus, which became known as the **Edwin Smith Papyrus** (Figure 1.9). The papyrus seems to have been written around 1600 B.C.E., during the third dynasty of pharaohs. Smith kept the papyrus until his death without ever having it translated. The papyrus was eventually translated by another archeologist, James Henry Breasted (1865–1935). Once translated the papyrus revealed itself to be an ancient medical text. In it are descriptions of injuries sustained during building projects and battles.

Some of the injuries described in the papyrus involve head injuries. From the description of the injuries, it is evident that Egyptians knew that brain damage could affect bodily functions ranging from hand-eye coordination problems to paralyzed limbs. However, they thought the heart was the seat of the soul and all of the functions we attribute to the brain today. In fact, so little was thought of the brain that, after death, it was removed through the nostrils with an iron hook and thrown away.

The Greeks

In early Greece there was no room for people's ability to control their own fates. Humans were believed to be created and controlled by gods, much the same way that puppeteers control their puppets. Eventually, the Greeks became more aware of their place in nature and gradually began to think of themselves as free individuals devoid of the tight grip that the gods held on them. People also started to think differently about disease, seeking more naturalistic causes and treatments for them rather than explanations and treatments based on religion.

Central to this change was Hippocrates (460–370 B.C.E.), who treated people according to the laws of nature. Contrary to the Egyptians, Hippocrates firmly believed that the brain, and not the heart, was the seat of all mental

FIGURE 1.9

The Edwin Smith Papyrus (left) and archeologist James Henry Breasted (right), who translated it.

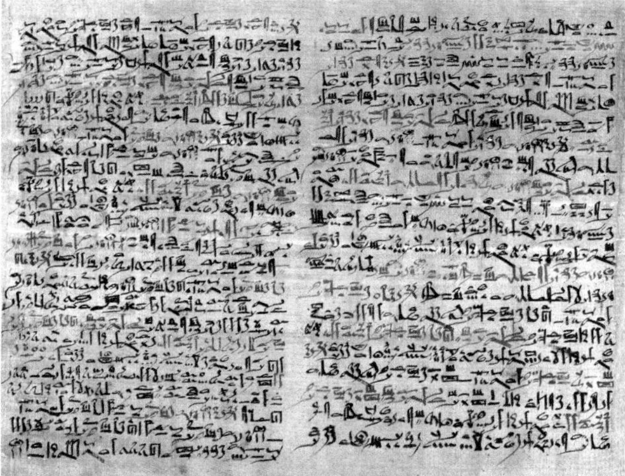

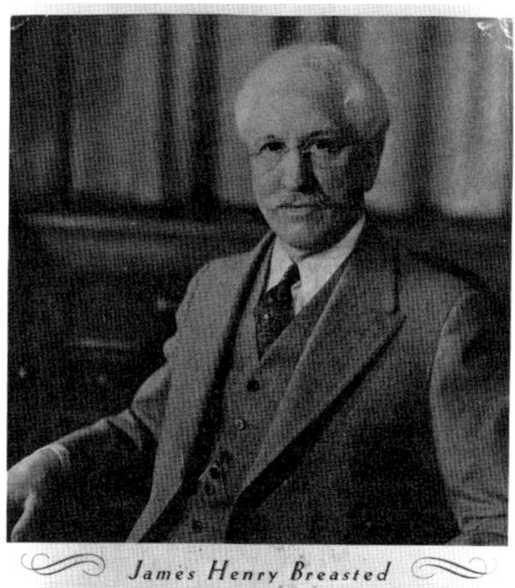

(left) Pictures From History/Newscom; (right) Library of Congress/Corbis Historical/Getty Images

faculties. This was contrary to the belief of the great philosopher Aristotle (384–322 B.C.E.), who thought that the heart was at the center of all faculties. Aristotle believed that the brain served only as a radiator to cool the blood heated by the seething heart (E. Clarke & Stannard, 1963).

Hippocrates believed that the brain interpreted stimuli from the outside world, giving rise to perception. He identified the brain as the center for consciousness, intelligence, and willpower; and he found the cause of epilepsy to be brain malfunction, rather than divine intervention.

For religious reasons, autopsies were forbidden in Greece in Hippocrates's day. Therefore, it is thought that he learned much about brain-behavior relationships by examining soldiers who sustained head wounds. For example, he noticed that wounds to the head often resulted in convulsions, paralysis, and loss of speech.

Dissections of human cadavers weren't permitted until after Hippocrates's death, with the softening of religious taboos. This allowed Alexandrian anatomists Herophilus of Chalcedon (335–280 B.C.E.) and Erasistratus (304–250 B.C.E.) to perform hundreds of

FIGURE 1.10

Galen (left), who dissected sheep's brains (right), thought that the cerebrum was ideal to pick up sensations, whereas the cerebellum controlled the muscles.

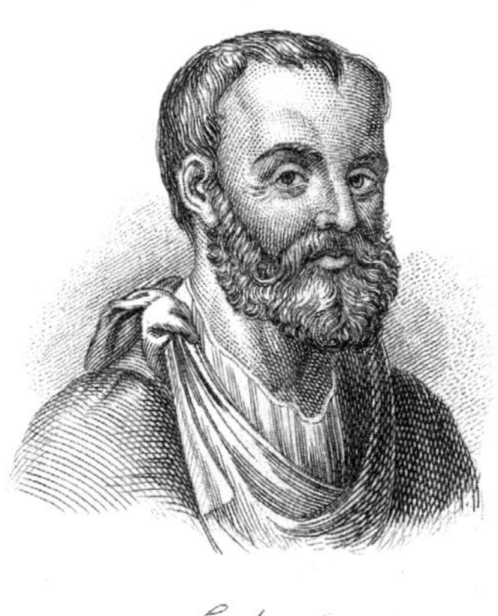

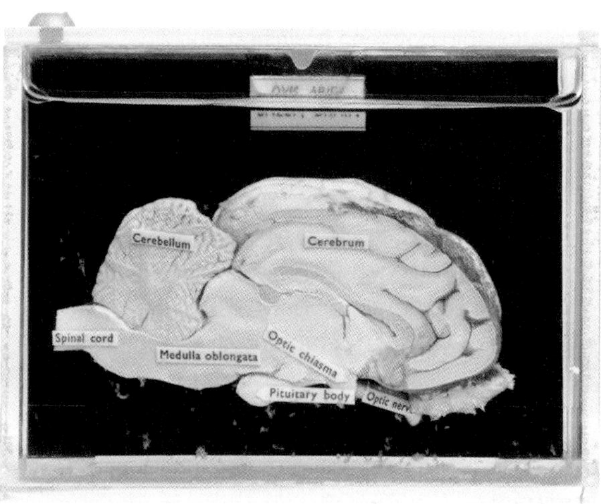

(left) Wellcome Library, London. Wellcome Images via Wikimedia Commons; (right) Gregory Davies/SCIENCE SOURCE

such dissections. Herophilus thought that the soul was housed in the fourth ventricle because of the number of motor nerves that leave that area. For his part, Erasistratus attributed the superior intellect of humans to the higher number of circumvolutions (folds) on the cortex compared to other animals. The Greek physician Galen (130–210 C.E.) pointed out that this attribution was wrong, remarking that donkeys possess highly circumvoluted brains but are among the stupidest animals (C. U. Smith, 2010).

Galen practiced in Rome and had a predicament similar to that of Hippocrates. Human autopsies were not permitted in the Rome of his day. Galen then studied the bodies of dead soldiers and of those he encountered by chance. Because the bodies he found were often in a state of decomposition, it was impossible to study soft organs such as the brain. For this reason, Galen turned to dissecting animals. Galen's dissections provided much knowledge about the nervous system. For example, he described the cranial nerves, which go from the brain to the face and upper body. He also differentiated between motor and sensory nerves.

Some of Galen's many findings made him believe that the brain was the seat of the mind. One of his observations made this obvious to him. He noticed that the nerves associated with the sense organs could all be traced to the brain, not the heart. Galen also related the brain to function after dissecting sheep brains (Figure 1.10). He observed that the front part of the brain, the cerebrum, was fleshy and soft, which would make it ideal to soak up sensations, whereas the back of the brain, the cerebellum, was hard and therefore controlled the muscles (Rocca, 2003). Although his explanations for how perception and movement relate to the brain were wrong, his conclusions were correct. That is, the cerebrum is involved in perceptions and the cerebellum plays an important role in movement.

1.3.2 THE MIND-BODY PROBLEM

>> LO 1.3.2 Explain the philosophical roots that underlie the relationship between brain and body.

Key Terms

- **Mind-body problem:** The age-old philosophical question concerning how the mind, which is immaterial, interacts with the material body.
- **Dualism:** The philosophical position that mind and body are distinct and that they could exist independently of each other.
- **Fluid-mechanical theory:** The idea that movement can be explained by the movement of fluids, called animal spirits, through hollow tubes in the body.

The **mind-body problem** reflects an age-old philosophical question: How does the mind, which is immaterial, interact with the material body? Many positions regarding the relationship between mind and body have been proposed. Here we focus on the position held by philosopher and mathematician René Descartes (1596–1650).

Descartes believed that the mind and the body were distinct and that they could exist independently of each other, a position called **dualism**. Descartes thought that properties of the mind cannot be ascribed to material objects. He included in this category not only stones and plants but also nonhuman animals.

According to what is known as the **fluid-mechanical theory**, Descartes believed that nonhuman animals were mere automata, whose actions can be likened to robots and driven by simple reflexes (Descartes & Schuyl, 1662). These reflexes he explained by the movement of fluids, called animal spirits, through hollow tubes in the body (Figure 1.11).

FIGURE 1.11

Descartes's model of simple reflexes. Putting a foot near a flame causes particles emanating from the flame (A) to pull on the skin on your foot (B). This pulling on the skin stretches a little thread (C). The thread being pulled opens the entrance (*e*) to a pore (*d*). The open pore permits animal fluids to flow into it from a cavity within the brain (F). From the cavity, these animal spirits flow down the tube to the muscles, pulling the foot away from the flame.

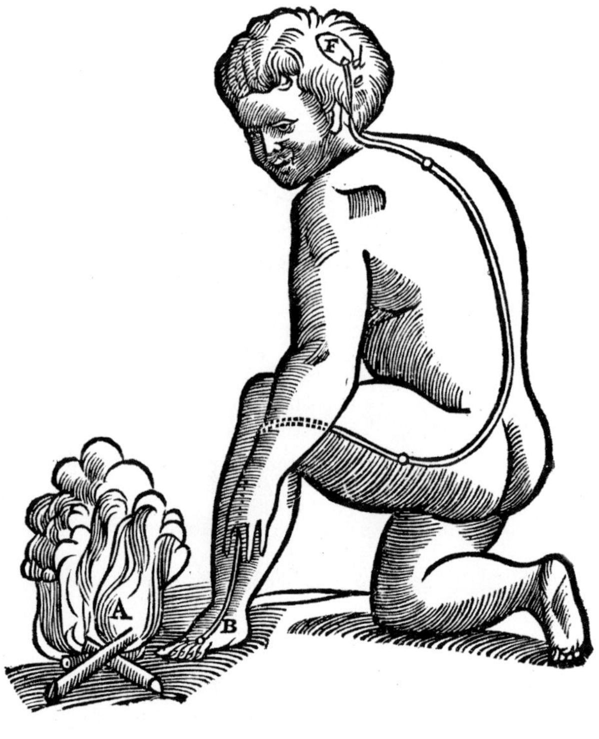

Print Collector/Hulton Archive/Getty Images

Descartes believed that humans partly functioned this way as well. Contrary to humans, however, he thought that animals, devoid of a mind, could not reason, lacked self-consciousness, and were incapable of language. For Descartes, all of the qualities that we think of as being distinctively human required a God-given soul (or mind), which animals lacked. He thought that the immaterial soul interacted with the pineal gland, which conferred on humans the unique abilities to have free will and to perform voluntary actions.

He thought the pineal gland to be ideal for interacting with the soul because it is a singular structure sitting at the midline of the brain. He also thought that its being suspended, small, and light made it easy to be moved by the immaterial soul. He believed that, in response to sensory experiences and innate ideas, the soul caused the pineal gland to tip, releasing and directing animal spirits through the nerves to control the body (Figure 1.12).

Of course, today's scientists have long since dispensed with the idea of animal spirits and the hollow tubes through which they travel. The pineal gland that Descartes thought was the seat of the soul is now known to produce a chemical called melatonin, which is involved in regulating physiological processes on a 24-hour cycle (known as a circadian rhythm and discussed in more detail in Chapter 9). Descartes's hollow tubes are now known as nerves, and what flows through them are not animal spirits but, rather, electrical impulses called nerve impulses or action potentials, discussed in Chapter 2.

FIGURE 1.12

Descartes's example of how the soul interacted with the body via the pineal gland. When light enters the retina, it triggers the opening of valves behind the eyes, which permits animal spirits to enter tubules connected to the pineal gland. In turn, the pineal gland releases and directs animal spirits to focus the eyes.

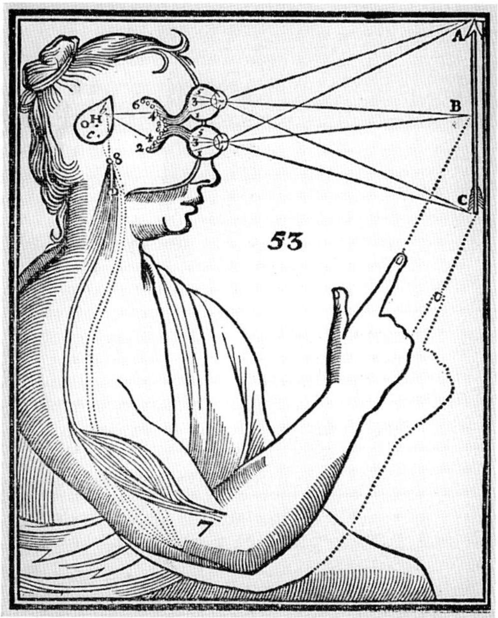

Hulton Archive/Getty Images

1.3.3 LOCALIZATION OF FUNCTION

>> LO 1.3.3 Understand how the idea that brain functions are localized to specific areas developed.

Key Terms

- **Localization of function:** The theory that individual brain areas are dedicated to distinct functions.
- **Phrenology:** The idea that bumps on the skull reflect the size of the underlying brain region, which is associated with a particular faculty.
- **Aphasia:** The loss of an individual's ability to speak.
- **Cerebral dominance:** The idea that the left hemisphere is dominant in the control of speech function.
- **Broca's area:** The area of the third convolution of the left frontal lobe, associated with speech production.
- **Topographical map:** A map, within the brain, that represents different areas of the body in an orderly way.

Modern ideas of brain-behavior relationships began with observations that individual brain areas seemed to be dedicated to distinct functions. This idea became known as the theory of **localization of function**, first proposed in the 1740s by scientist and philosopher Emanuel Swedenborg (1688–1772). However, the best-known early proponent of localization of function was German anatomist Franz Joseph Gall (1758–1828) (Simpson, 2005).

When he was nine years old, Gall noticed that classmates who excelled at memorizing verbal material had large protruding eyes, compared to those who were not as good at doing so. Gall believed that the brain area responsible for verbal memory was enlarged in these students and was located right behind the eyes. Gall then went on to localize myriad other mental functions to particular brain areas, 27 in all. Gall also believed that the bumps on the skull reflected the size of the underlying brain

FIGURE 1.13

A phrenological map showing the areas associated with various faculties.

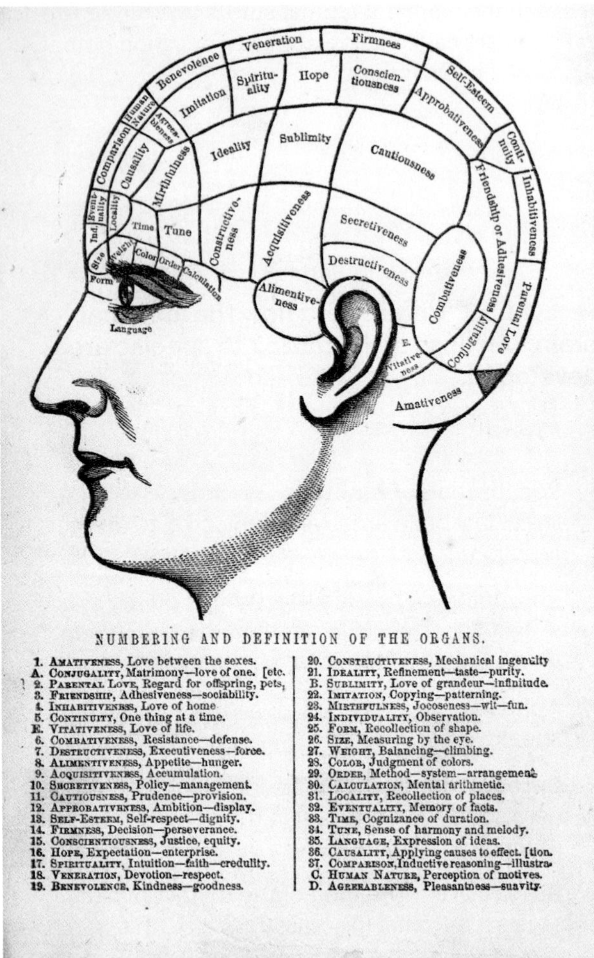

istock.com/cjp

region, which was associated with a particular faculty (Figure 1.13). Therefore, he believed that the larger the bump on the skull, the more the faculty represented by the underlying brain area was developed in that individual. Gall studied the patterns of bumps on the skulls of the extremes in society, from people of great talent and intelligence to people considered intellectually challenged and criminals.

Veneration
Firmness
Benevolence
Spirituality
Hope
Conscientiousness
Self-Esteem
Approbativeness
Imitation
Ideality
Sublimity
Cautiousness
Comparison
Causality
Mirthfulness
Continuity
Inhabitiveness
Friendship or Adhesiveness
Secretiveness
Destructiveness
Combativeness
Acquisitiveness
Constructiveness
Time
Tune
Alimentiveness
Parental Love
Amativeness
Language
NUMBERING AND DEFINITION OF THE ORGANS.
1. Amativeness, Love between the sexes.
A. Conjugality, Matrimony—love of one. [etc.
2. Parental Love, Regard for offspring, pets,
3. Friendship, Adhesiveness—sociability.
4. Inhabitiveness, Love of home
5. Continuity, One thing at a time.
E. Vitativeness, Love of life.
6. Combativeness, Resistance—defense.
7. Destructiveness, Executiveness—force.
8. Alimentiveness, Appetite—hunger.
9. Acquisitiveness, Accumulation.
10. Secretiveness, Policy—management.
11. Cautiousness, Prudence—provision.
12. Approbativeness, Ambition—display.
13. Self-Esteem, Self-respect—dignity.
14. Firmness, Decision—perseverance.
15. Conscientiousness, Justice, equity.
16. Hope, Expectation—enterprise.
17. Spirituality, Intuition—faith—credulity.
18. Veneration, Devotion—respect.
19. Benevolence, Kindness—goodness.
20. Constructiveness, Mechanical ingenuity
21. Ideality, Refinement—taste—purity.
B. Sublimity, Love of grandeur—infinitude.
22. Imitation, Copying—patterning.
23. Mirthfulness, Jocoseness—wit—fun.
24. Individuality, Observation.
25. Form, Recollection of shape.
26. Size, Measuring by the eye.
27. Weight, Balancing—climbing.
28. Color, Judgment of colors.
29. Order, Method—system—arrangement.
30. Calculation, Mental arithmetic.
31. Locality, Recollection of places.
32. Eventuality, Memory of facts.
33. Time, Cognizance of duration.
34. Tune, Sense of harmony and melody.
35. Language, Expression of ideas.
36. Causality, Applying causes to effect. [tion.
37. Comparison, Inductive reasoning—illustra-
C. Human Nature, Perception of motives.
D. Agreeableness, Pleasantness—suavity.

Over the years, Gall assessed the skulls of hundreds of people and kept a record of the mental and personality characteristics he concluded they possessed from his assessments. Later, one of Gall's students, Johann Spurzheim (1776–1832), expanded the list of faculties proposed by Gall to 33 and coined the term ***phrenology***, which is Greek for "mental science" or "science of the mind."

Gall's ideas were soon refuted by French physiologist Marie-Jean-Pierre Flourens (1794–1867), who found, by lesioning the cortex of several species of animals, that specific functions were not associated with the brain areas that Gall had assigned to them. He instead found that what affected function in animals was the size of the lesion but not the specific area damaged (J. M. Pearce, 2009).

Localization of Language

Although Gall's theory of relating bumps on the skull to parts of overdeveloped cortex, which represented specific functions, was refuted, the idea of localization of function lived on. It gained momentum when French physician Jean-Baptiste Bouillaud (1796–1881) pointed to the fact that many patients with diseases of the brain displayed motor disturbances, such as paralysis of an arm or a leg. He also noted that loss of speech often accompanied damage to the left frontal lobes (Finger, 2000).

In 1861, Ernest Auburtin (1825–unknown year of death), Bouillaud's son-in-law, reported on several cases in which damage to the frontal lobes resulted in speech impairments. In one of the cases, a patient who attempted suicide by shooting himself in the head found himself with the bone covering the frontal lobes completely blown off, leaving them exposed. His intelligence as well as his speech remained intact. However, as he spoke, pressure applied to his exposed frontal lobes with the back of a large spatula caused his speech to be interrupted mid-word. His speech returned to normal once the pressure applied by the spatula was removed.

Soon after, Auburtin issued the challenge that he would renounce localization of function theory if a case of loss of speech without frontal lobe damage were found. The challenge was taken up by French physician, anatomist, and anthropologist Paul Broca (1824–1880) (Figure 1.14, left). Broca had a patient named Mr. Leborgne, nicknamed "Tan," because this is the sound he made when attempting to give his name. Leborgne had suffered from epilepsy since he was young and lost his ability to speak (a condition called *aphémie* by Broca but later renamed **aphasia**). Broca invited Auburtin to come and examine the patient. Upon his examination, he concluded that Leborgne must have sustained damage to the frontal lobes.

After Leborgne's death, Broca performed an autopsy on him and found that he had progressive damage to his left frontal lobe (in the third convolution). This finding convinced many to accept the up-to-then widely contested localization of function theory. Following Leborgne's autopsy, Broca found several more cases of aphasia, all associated with damage to the left frontal lobe. When damage to only the right frontal lobe was found, the ability to speak was not affected. Broca suggested that the left hemisphere dominated

FIGURE 1.14

Photograph of Paul Broca (left) and the location of Broca's area in the left frontal lobe (right).

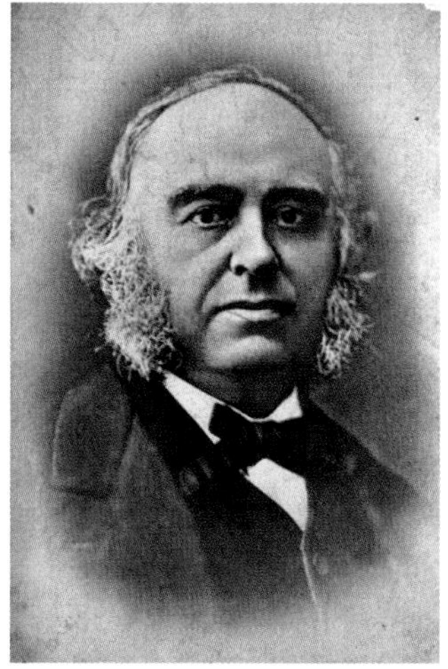

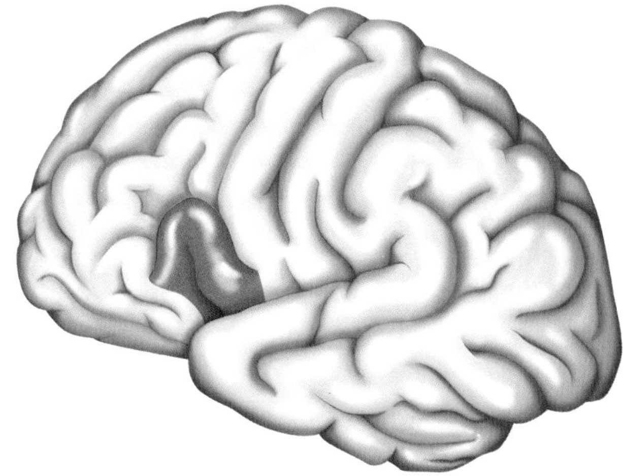

(left) U.S. National Library of Medicine; (right) BSIP/Science Source

over the right hemisphere in controlling speech function. This led to the concept known today as **cerebral dominance**. The area in the left frontal lobe that was associated with speech production became known as **Broca's area** (Figure 1.14, right).

Motor Representations in the Cortex

The idea that functions were localized to specific areas of the cortex went well beyond Broca's reported cases of aphasia in patients with damage to the left frontal lobe. For example, British neurologist John Hughlings Jackson (1815–1911) hypothesized that the brain had sensory and motor functions. He based this idea on his observations that, during epileptic seizures, convulsions spread from one part of the body to another in sequential order. From this, he concluded that a representation of the body must exist in the brain (Jackson, 1958).

Jackson's conclusions were confirmed by German anatomist Gustav Fritsch (1838–1927) and psychiatrist Eduard Hitzig (1838–1907). Both independently observed that electrical stimulation of the brain led to the movement of various body parts. As a psychiatrist, Hitzing noticed that electrically stimulating the head in some of his patients produced eye movements. As a battlefield surgeon, Fritsch noticed that while he was dressing an open wound on one side of a soldier's head, the limbs on the opposite side of the body moved (Carlson & Devinsky, 2009).

In 1870, Fritsch and Hitzig conducted an experiment to test whether motor functions were localized to particular areas of the cortex. They electrically stimulated the exposed cortex of dogs to see if this would result in movements of the body. The electrical stimulation produced twitching of the muscles on the side opposite from the hemisphere that was stimulated, and stimulation of different parts of the cortex caused different muscles to twitch. They also found that the stimulated cortex formed a **topographical map** of the body, in that different body parts projected to the cortex in an orderly way.

Later, Scottish neurologist David Ferrier (1843–1928) extended Fritsch and Hitzig's finding and the number of areas that can be excited by electrical current. He found that electrically stimulating the cortex of several animals caused them to engage in natural movements such as walking, grabbing, and scratching. He also found that stimulating specific areas of the cortex caused the body to move in ways that imitated that of epileptic patients as described by Jackson (Finger, 2000).

Relatively closer to our times, American Canadian neurosurgeon Wilder Penfield (1891–1976) electrically stimulated the brains of patients undergoing surgery to treat epilepsy. As he was doing so, he asked patients to report what they were experiencing. This was possible because the patients remained awake during surgery. Depending on where he applied the electrical current, Penfield caused specific areas of the body to twitch. However, sometimes the stimulation caused paralysis of parts of the body (Feindel, 1982). Through these experiments, Penfield found that a motor map, similar to the one discovered by Fritsch and Hitzig in dogs, also existed in humans, which became known as the motor homunculus (discussed at greater length in Chapter 8). Figures 1.15a–c show the topographic maps drawn by Fritsch and Hitzing and by Penfield.

FIGURE 1.15

Topographical maps of the brain of dogs by (a) David Ferrier and (b) Fritsch and Hitzig; and (c) topographical map of the human brain discovered by Wilder Penfield.

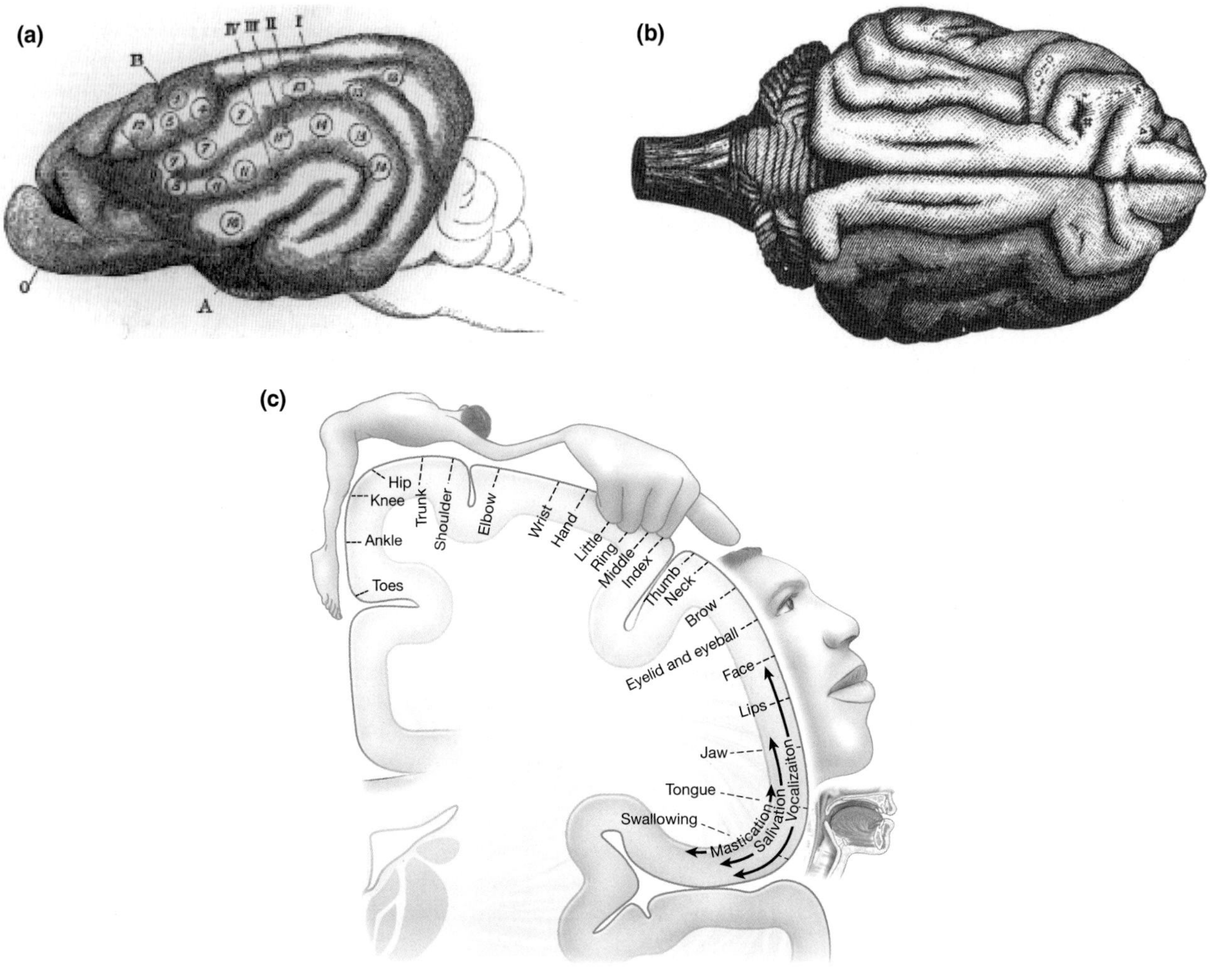

(a) David Ferrier via Wikimedia Commons; (b) Eduard Hitzig und Gustav Fritsch via Wikimedia Commons; (c) Adapted from *The Cerebral Cortex of Man*, Penfield and Rasmussen. © 1950 Gale, a part of Cengage Learning, Inc.

MODULE SUMMARY

Ideas about the relationships between the brain and behavior have been around since antiquity. Head injuries were described in an ancient Egyptian medical papyrus known as the Edwin Smith Papyrus, written in about 1600 B.C.E. From reading the papyrus it is obvious that the Egyptians of the day knew that brain injury can affect bodily function. However, they thought that the heart and not the brain was the seat of the soul and all of the functions we today attribute to the brain. In contrast, the ancient Greek physician Hippocrates believed that the brain and not the heart was responsible for all mental faculties. Aristotle clung to the view that the heart was at the center of mental faculties and that the brain only served to cool the blood. Galen, a Greek physician who practiced in Rome, noticed that the nerves from the sense organs all led to the brain and not the heart, making it obvious to him that the brain was the seat of the mind. Galen also concluded that the cerebrum processes information from the senses and that the cerebellum controls the muscles.

The mind-body problem is an age-old question as to how the mind, which is immaterial, can interact with the material brain. Philosopher and mathematician René Descartes believed that the mind and body were distinct and that they existed independently of each other, a position known as dualism. Descartes believed that simple reflexes could be explained by the movements of fluids through hollow tubes in the body, in what became known as the fluid-mechanical theory. Descartes believed that animals had no soul. Therefore, he believed that all of their behaviors were reflexive. However, he thought that humans were special in that they have a soul. Descartes thought that the soul interacted with the brain in the pineal gland.

Localization of function is the idea that different functions are controlled by specific brain areas. One of the first proponents of this idea was Franz Joseph Gall. Gall believed that the bumps on the skull reflected the abilities for which the underlying cortex was responsible. He thought that the size of a bump related to the extent to which the underlying ability was developed within a person. This practice became known as phrenology. French physician Paul Broca found that many of his patients who suffered from aphasia also had damage to the left frontal lobe. This gave the idea of localization of function a great boost. The idea was bolstered further when Gustav Fritsch and Eduard Hitzig found that electrical stimulation of the cortex of dogs produced twitching in the side of the body opposite to which the stimulation was applied and that the stimulated cortex formed a topographical map of the body. These results were extended by David Ferrier, who found that electrically stimulating the cortex of animals can also cause more complex movements. Wilder Penfield electrically stimulated the brains of patients undergoing surgery to treat epilepsy and found that a motor map, similar to the one discovered by Fritsch and Hitzig in dogs, also existed in humans.

TEST YOURSELF

1.3.1 Discuss the views associated with brain function that prevailed throughout antiquity.

1.3.2 What are some of the philosophical roots that underlie the thinking about the relationship between brain and body?

1.3.3 Trace the history of the idea that brain functions are localized to specific areas.

1.4 Studying Brain-Behavior Relationships Today

Module Contents

Learning Objectives

1.4.1 Explain how the study of brain-damaged patients can inform neuroscientists about brain-behavior relationships.

1.4.2 Describe how brain-behavior relationships can be inferred by lesioning, stimulating, and measuring the brain's activity.

1.4.3 Define the different fields of study related to behavioral neuroscience.

1.4.1 BRAIN-DAMAGED PATIENTS AND STRUCTURAL BRAIN IMAGING

>> LO 1.4.1 Explain how the study of brain-damaged patients can inform neuroscientists about brain-behavior relationships.

Key Terms

- **Traumatic brain injury:** An injury that results from a blow to the head or from an object penetrating the skull.

- **Structural brain imaging:** Imaging techniques that permit the detection of brain injury.
- **Magnetic resonance imaging (MRI):** A method by which an image of any part of the body can be created with the use of a powerful magnetic field and the emission of a resonant frequency.
- **Computed tomography (CT scan):** A method in which X-ray images are taken from many angles and processed by a computer to produce virtual cross-sections, permitting the examination of structures deep within the brain.

The least invasive way to learn about brain-behavior relationships is to study people who have sustained **traumatic brain injury**. A traumatic brain injury can result from a blow to the head or from an object penetrating the skull (Lunetta, Ohberg, & Sajantila, 2002). Another way in which a person's brain can be damaged is through the progression of neurodegenerative disease such as Alzheimer's disease (Vemuri & Jack, 2010) or Parkinson's disease (Lehericy, Sharman, Dos Santos, Paquin, & Gallea, 2012). The brain can also be damaged by a stroke, in which the flow of blood either to the entire brain or to a specific part of the brain has been cut off.

In any case, the changes in behavior or deficits observed in people who have experienced any of these conditions can inform neuroscientists as to which brain areas are likely to be damaged. Also, once the type of brain damage is known, researchers can use this knowledge to predict what types of tasks a person may have difficulties with and design studies to test their predictions. However, the study of brain-damaged patients may not be informative enough to determine the precise location of the brain damage responsible for a given change in behavior or deficit. This is because the brain damage observed in those conditions is often not restricted to any single brain area.

The brain damage caused by these conditions can be observed through **structural brain imaging**. The brain imaging methods most commonly used in these conditions are **magnetic resonance imaging (MRI)** and **computed tomography (CT scan)**. Magnetic resonance imaging is a method by which an image of any part of the body can be created. The area of interest for our purposes is, of course, the brain. An MRI scanner creates an image of the brain by subjecting it to a very powerful magnetic field (the "M" in MRI). This powerful magnetic field induces the nuclei of certain atoms to align. Then, a pulse of radio frequency (the "R" in MRI), which is just right for the nuclei of hydrogen atoms (resonance), is briefly emitted. This pulse alters the alignment of the atoms that resulted from exposure to the magnetic field. The energy from the pulse is absorbed by the nuclei of the atoms. Then the pulse is turned off and the nuclei release that energy and realign with the magnetic field. The release of this energy is detected by the scanner and forms the basis of the image (the "I" in MRI). Remember that MRI does not include the use of X-ray radiation. Figure 1.16a compares MRI scans of a normal brain with that of someone suffering from Alzheimer' disease.

In contrast to MRI, a CT scan makes use of X-ray technology. However, it differs from a regular X-ray examination in that X-ray measurements are taken from many angles. The images are processed by a computer and virtual cross-sections are produced, which permits the examination of structures deep within the brain. A CT scan can also permit the detection of brain damage such as a cerebral infarction, which is an area of dead tissue due to the blockage or narrowing of an artery (Figure 1.16b).

FIGURE 1.16

(a) MRI scans comparing a brain of a normal elderly person (left) with that of a patient suffering from Alzheimer's disease (right). (b) A CT scan of a cerebral infarction due to the blockage or narrowing of an artery.

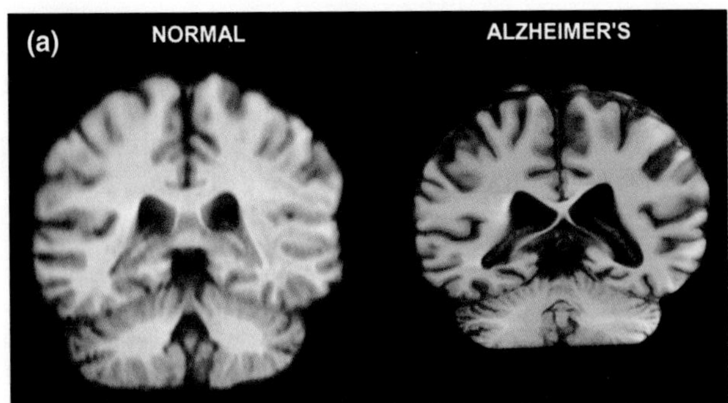

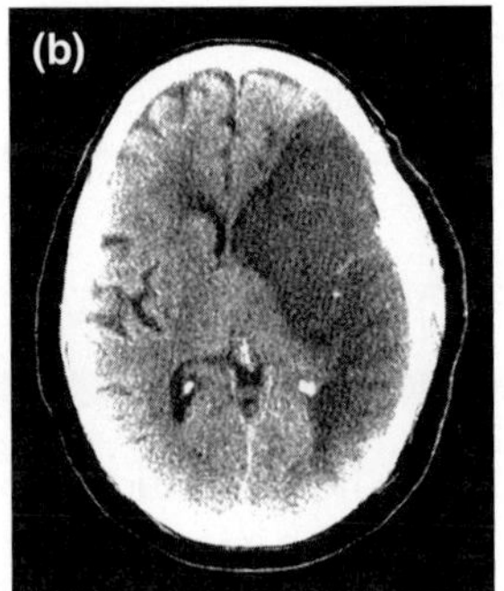

(a) TheVisualMD/Science Source; (b) Living Art Enterprises, LLC/Science Source

1.4.2 LESIONING, STIMULATING, AND MEASURING THE BRAIN'S ACTIVITY

>> LO 1.4.2 Describe how brain-behavior relationships can be inferred by lesioning, stimulating, and measuring the brain's activity.

Key Terms

- **Manipulation technique:** A technique in which the structure or function of the brain is altered and the resulting effects on behavior are observed.
- **Measurement technique:** A technique in which the brain activity of subjects is measured while they are engaged in some behavioral task with the aim of identifying brain areas that might be involved in its performance.
- **Functional brain imaging:** An imaging technique that permits the measurement of subjects' brain activity while performing a task.
- **Lesioning:** Creating brain damage in experimental animals to determine the functions of particular areas.
- **Deep brain stimulation (DBS):** Inferring the functions of a particular brain area through the administration of a low-voltage electrical current to that area.
- **Transcranial magnetic stimulation (TMS):** Inferring the functions of a particular brain area through the application of a magnetic field over a brain area of interest from the top of the skull.
- **Optogenetics:** The field in which genetics and optics are combined to use light-sensitive molecules to control cellular activity.
- **Functional magnetic resonance imaging (fMRI):** Inferring brain function using MRI technology to image the brain in a way that detects the amount of oxygen used by neurons.
- **Positron emission tomography (PET):** An imaging method in which brain function is inferred by detecting the consumption of glucose by neurons.
- **Electroencephalography (EEG):** A method in which brain function is inferred by detecting differences in the electrical energy emitted from different brain areas.
- **Event-related potentials (ERP):** Small voltage changes, called waveforms, in brain areas responsive to specific events or stimuli.
- **Magnetoencephalography (MEG):** A method in which brain function is inferred by detecting differences in the electromagnetic fields emitted from different brain areas.
- **Intracellular recording:** A method by which tiny electrodes are inserted directly inside neurons to record their electrical activity.
- **Microelectrode:** A tiny electrode used to measure the electrical activity of neurons.
- **Single-unit recording:** A method by which the electrical activity of a single neuron can be recorded.
- **Extracellular recording:** A method by which a microelectrode is inserted into the fluid surrounding neurons to record electrical currents generated by the neurons in the electrode's vicinity.

In addition to studying the behavioral and cognitive deficits suffered by brain-damaged patients with the help of structural brain imaging, there are two main classes of techniques used by behavioral neuroscientists to study brain-behavior relationships. These consist of manipulation and measurement techniques (Huettel, Song, & McCarthy, 2014). With **manipulation techniques**, the structure or function of the brain is altered and the resulting effects on behavior are observed. With **measurement techniques**, the brain activity of subjects is measured while they are engaged in some behavioral task, with the aim of identifying brain areas that might be involved in its performance (Figure 1.17). For this reason, measurement techniques are also known as **functional brain imaging**. In this unit, we will review the most commonly used manipulation and measurement techniques.

Manipulation Techniques

Lesions

You have just read that studying brain-damaged patients may not inform researchers about specific brain areas responsible for changes in behaviors or deficits. Behavioral neuroscientists can circumvent this problem by **lesioning** specific brain areas in experimental animals and then testing them on various behavioral tasks. Brain lesions can also be induced by administering drugs directly into a brain area of interest or by passing an electrical current through it.

Brain Stimulation

In a procedure called **deep brain stimulation (DBS)**, the functions of a specific brain area can be assessed or enhanced through electrical stimulation. This is done by administering a low-voltage electrical current through electrodes implanted in a brain area or areas of interest. This neurosurgical treatment involves the implantation

FIGURE 1.17

Brain-behavior relationships can be studied using manipulation and measurement techniques.

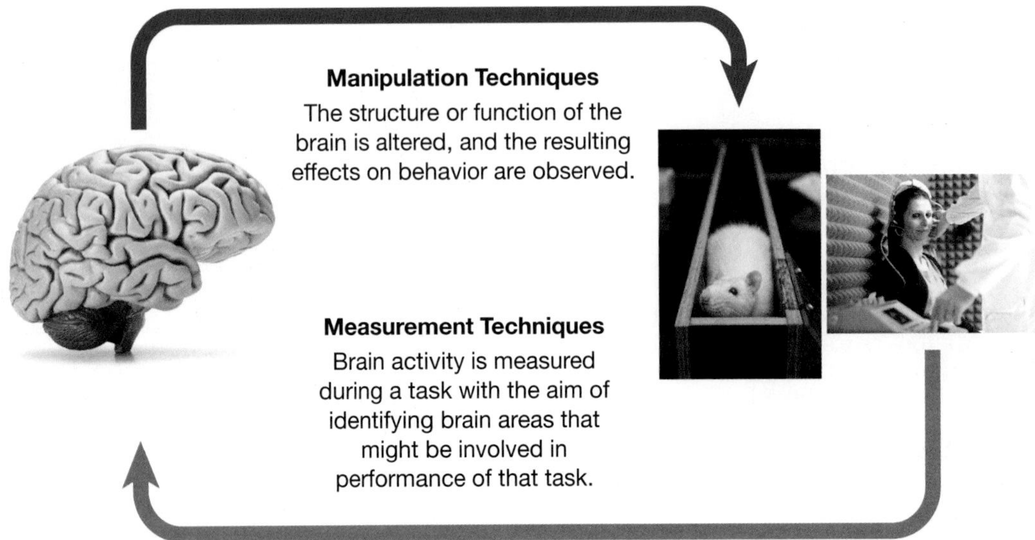
Manipulation Techniques
The structure or function of the brain is altered, and the resulting effects on behavior are observed.
Measurement Techniques
Brain activity is measured during a task with the aim of identifying brain areas that might be involved in performance of that task.

(Left to right) iStock.com/DNY59; iStock.com/ibreakstock; iStock.com/kaisersosa67

of electrodes in the brain, through the scalp (illustrated in Figure 1.18). The electrodes are connected to a pulse generator implanted below the skin. Clinicians then use a computer that communicates with the device to set the strength and frequency of the stimulation. For example, researchers found that electrically stimulating the temporal cortex, an area important for memory (see Chapter 12), enhanced subjects' ability to recall lists of words, compared to subjects who did not receive the stimulation (Ezzyat et al., 2018; Kucewicz et al., 2018).

DBS can also be administered through electrodes implanted in the subthalamic nucleus (or other brain areas) in the treatment of people with Parkinson's disease, a disorder characterized by shaking, slowness of movement, and rigidity (Mohammed, Bayford, & Demosthenous, 2018; Okun, 2012). DBS is also used to administer electrical stimulation to the ventral striatum in patients who have treatment-resistant obsessive-compulsive disorder (Greenberg et al., 2010). DBS is also being tested for use in the treatment of major depression (Drobisz & Damborska, 2019). Obsessive-compulsive disorder and major depression are discussed further in Chapter 14.

Another way to manipulate brain functioning is through the application of a magnetic field over a brain area of interest from the top of the skull. This method is known as **transcranial magnetic stimulation (TMS)** (illustrated in Figure 1.19). In TMS, electrical current is run through a coil of wires shaped like a figure-eight, which results in the production of a magnetic field. The coil of wires is then placed next to the skull over the brain region scientists are interested in studying. In this way, the magnetic field, produced by the electrified coil, can stimulate or inhibit the neurons in the brain region of interest. Whether neurons are stimulated or inhibited depends on the frequency of the magnetic field. The researchers using TMS can then deduce the importance of a certain brain region to specific tasks by examining the effects that TMS has on the performance of those tasks.

Temporary Inactivation

Sometimes neuroscientists want to compare the functions of a brain area when it is functioning normally to when it is not functioning normally. For this purpose, they can inject a drug that temporarily inactivates a specific brain area. Animals can then be tested on behavioral tasks while the brain area is inactivated and tested again once the drug has worn off.

Another way in which the functions of a specific brain area can be tested in animals is by turning neurons on or off using light in a method known as **optogenetics** (see "Applications" at the end of Chapter 2). Optogenetics is the field in which genetics and optics are combined to use light-sensitive molecules to control cellular activity. This may involve making neurons responsive to light by altering their genetic makeup. The use of optogenetics is a relatively new way of manipulating the brain. Similar to temporary inactivation, optogenetics can be used to temporarily activate or deactivate neurons in particular brain areas and then observe the resulting effects on task performance.

Certain organisms, such as bacteria, have cells that contain light-sensitive proteins. Some frequencies of light—for example, blue light—activate their cells. Other frequencies—for example, yellow light—deactivate them.

FIGURE 1.18

(a) Patient set up with a deep brain stimulation (DBS) device. (b) X-ray of the head and neck of a patient fitted with a DBS device.

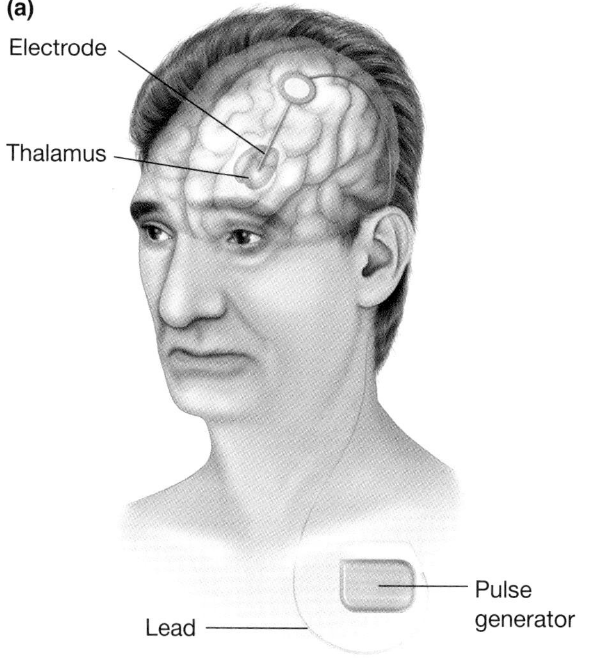

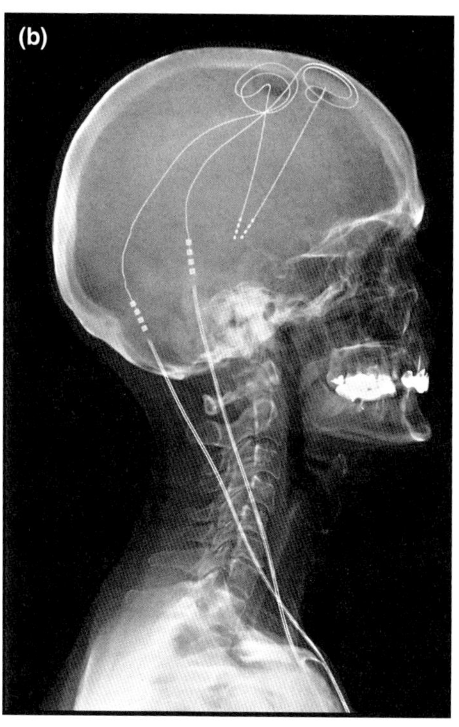

(a) Amanda Tomasikiewicz/Body Scientific Intl.; (b) Living Art Enterprises/Science Source

FIGURE 1.19

Person receiving transcranial magnetic stimulation (TMS).

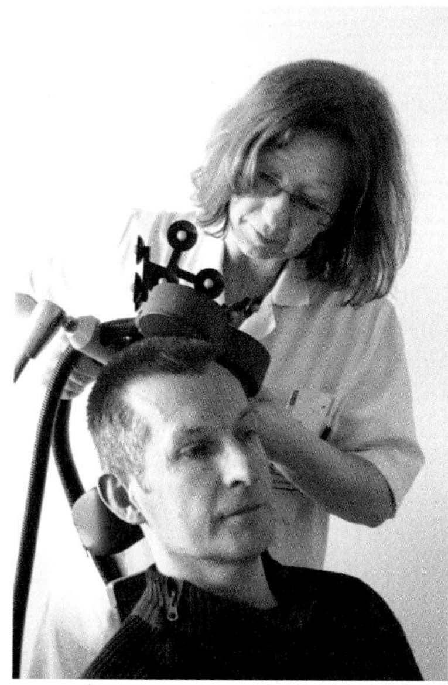

Amélie Benoist/SCIENCE SOURCE

To activate or deactivate neurons in experimental animals with lights of different colors, scientists attach the genes for the light-sensitive proteins of these bacteria to harmless viruses. These viruses are then injected into the brain of animals where it is incorporated into the animals' neurons. To activate or deactivate the neurons with light, scientists drill small holes in the skulls of animals, through which they can lower light-emitting diodes (LEDs) of different frequencies into the brain area(s) of interest.

Measurement Techniques

Functional Magnetic Resonance Imaging (fMRI)

As you just read, some of the methods used by neuroscientists involve manipulating the brain in some way and then observing the effects resulting from the manipulation. However, brain-behavior relationships can also be inferred by observing the brain in action. One of the most popular methods to do this is called **functional magnetic resonance imaging (fMRI)**. An fMRI scanner can image the brain with the use of a strong magnetic field and can also detect the amount of oxygen used by neurons. A person's brain can therefore be scanned while the individual performs a behavioral task. The neurons in the brain areas associated with the performance of the given task will consume more oxygen than areas that are least involved in the task. This difference in oxygen consumption by neurons is fed into a computer program and can be visualized by the experimenter (Figure 1.20a).

Positron Emission Tomography

Another popular method of imaging the brain is known as **positron emission tomography (PET)**. A PET scan detects the consumption of glucose by neurons. Participants in a PET study are injected with glucose molecules attached to a radioactive element called an isotope, which decays over time. They are then given a behavioral task while their brain is being scanned. Neurons use glucose for energy. Therefore, the neurons within the brain areas that are activated by the performance of the task consume more glucose, which as we just mentioned is attached to a radioactive isotope. The radioactively tagged glucose goes all over the brain. As the isotope decays, it emits what is known as a positron. When a positron meets an electron, they annihilate each other, which results in the release of energy. More of this energy will be detected in the brain areas associated with the performance of the task, relative to areas that are not. As with fMRI, this information is fed into a computer program and visualized by the experimenter (Figure 1.20b).

Electroencephalography

Electroencephalography (EEG), shown in Figure 1.21a, is a method by which the flow of electrical currents produced by the communication between neurons in the brain is detected by electrodes placed on the scalp. The electrodes are placed above all regions of the skull in order to record from various regions of the brain.

When neurons communicate with each other, waves of electrical currents, commonly called brainwaves, are produced. These are picked up by the electrodes. Researchers can then examine the pattern of brain activity while the subject performs a particular task.

Through this method scientists have also discovered that the brain produces wavelengths of different frequencies and amplitudes, depending on a person's state of consciousness. For example, I presume you are presently alert and awake while reading this text or when you attend classes. Alertness and waking states are associated with high-frequency wavelengths of low amplitude. When you are sleeping, presumably not in class, your brain emits wavelengths of low frequency with high amplitude. However, when you are dreaming, your brain emits wavelengths that look more like the ones emitted while awake, which are of high frequency and low amplitude. Figure 1.21b shows how different types of wavelengths are associated with different stages of sleep (for details about the brainwaves generated in different states of consciousness, see Chapter 9).

EEG is also used to measure what are known as **event-related potentials (ERPs)**. ERPs are small voltage changes, called waveforms. ERPs are detected when many neurons fire in synchrony in response to events in an individual's environment. These events can be part of an individual's external or internal environment. Events can be sensory, cognitive, or motor. Therefore, ERPs can be used to investigate the role of the brain in processing sensory, motor, and cognitive information.

Different types of events trigger different types of waveforms. Studying ERPs permits neuroscientists

FIGURE 1.20

Images of the brain obtained through (a) fMRI and (b) PET scan. The relative activity of brain areas is represented by different colors. Areas of higher activity are represented by warm colors such as red, orange, and yellow, whereas areas of lower activity are represented by blueish and violet colors.

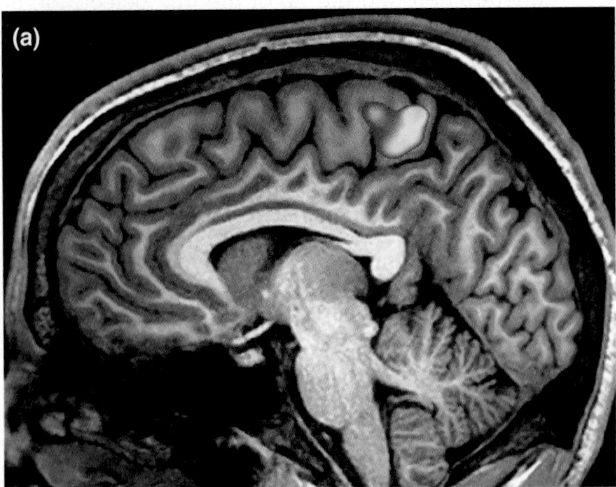

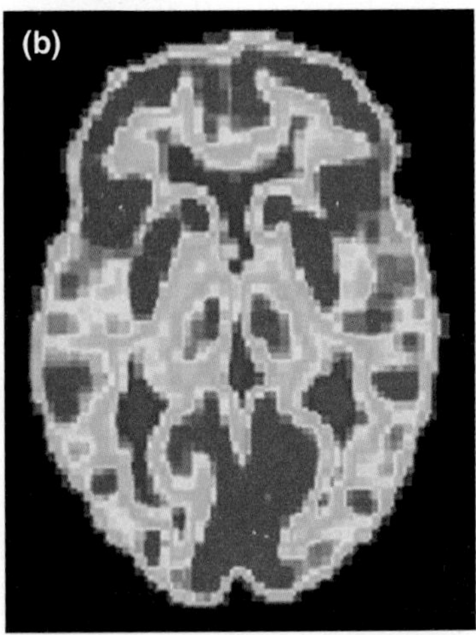

(a) Living Art Enterprises/SCIENCE SOURCE; (b) National Institute of Aging/NIH/SCIENCE SOURCE

FIGURE 1.21

(a) Woman undergoing an EEG. (b) Brain waves measured by EEG are associated with different stages of sleep.

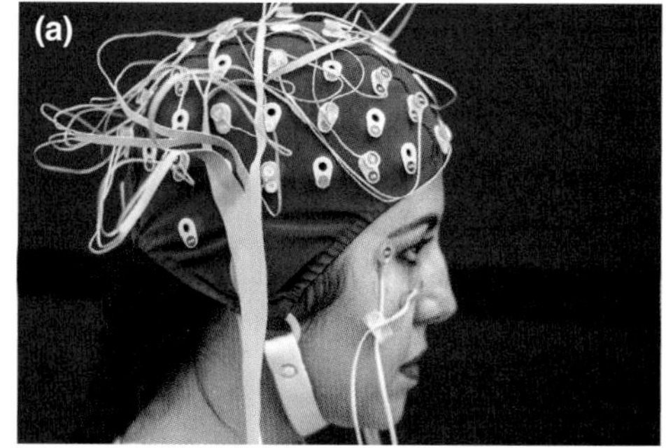

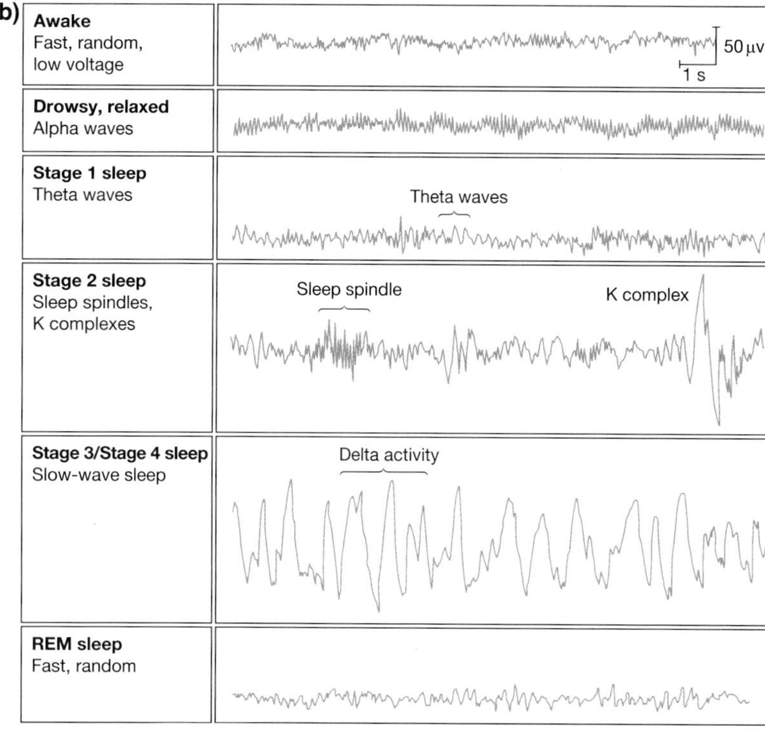

(a) iStock.com/Latsalomao; (b) From *Current Concepts: The Sleep Disorders*, P. Hauri, Kalamazoo, MI: Upjohn, 1982.

to learn about how different brain areas are involved in language, memory, and attentional processes. Neuroscientists may also use ERPs to study abnormal functioning that occurs in various psychiatric disorders such as in schizophrenia, substance abuse, and anxiety disorders (Sur & Sinha, 2009).

ERPs are usually measured from the scalp (scalp ERP). However, on rare occasions an electrode can be inserted directly within a brain structure (intracranial ERP). This type of ERP is rare and is usually done to assess the electrical activity in a particular brain area before brain surgery.

A similar method known as **magnetoencephalography (MEG)** measures the magnetic fields produced by communicating neurons, instead of the electrical fields measured by EEG. The advantage of MEG over EEG is that intervening tissue has very little effect on the clarity of the magnetic signal compared to the electrical signal. Wherever electrical current is present, there is also a magnetic field. Therefore, the source of the signal detected by MEG is the same as in EEG.

However, the signals generated by magnetic fields are very weak. For this reason, they are easily interfered with by magnetic fields generated by computers, elevators, and other electrical machines or instruments present in the environment. Therefore, MEG recordings have to be done in a special room that blocks out environmental magnetic fields.

Electrophysiological Measurements

Neuroscientists are sometimes interested in measuring the electrical activity of individual neurons. This is done through **intracellular recording**, which involves inserting a tiny metal wire called a **microelectrode** directly inside a neuron to measure the current that flows through it. This method is often referred to as **single-unit recording**. Electrodes may also be placed in the fluid outside of neurons and the electrical activity generated around the tip of the microelectrode is measured. This method is known as **extracellular recording**.

1.4.3 FIELDS OF STUDY RELATED TO BEHAVIORAL NEUROSCIENCE

>> LO 1.4.3 **Define the different fields of study related to behavioral neuroscience.**

Key Terms

- **Neuroanatomy:** The scientific study of the structures and organization of the nervous system.

- **Neurochemistry:** The scientific study of how chemicals in the brain are synthesized and involved in brain function.
- **Neuroendocrinology:** The scientific study of how hormones, which are chemicals that control important bodily functions, interact with the nervous system.
- **Neuropathology:** The scientific study of the changes in the brain that occur when it becomes diseased.
- **Neuropharmacology:** The scientific study of how drugs and other agents already inside the brain affect the function of cells.
- **Neuropsychopharmacology:** The scientific study of how drugs produce psychotropic effects.
- **Neurophysiology:** The scientific study of brain function by using various methods to stimulate, measure, or record the activity of individual brain cells or entire brain areas.
- **Neuropsychology:** The scientific study of how psychological functions are localized in certain brain areas.

The study of behavioral neuroscience draws from and influences the study of many related areas. One of these areas is **neuroanatomy**. Neuroanatomy is the study of the structure and organization of the nervous system. The study of neuroanatomy results in a greater understanding of how the brain functions, how it is shaped by environmental influences, and how it changes throughout development (Lerch et al., 2017).

Whereas neuroanatomists are interested in charting the nervous system's structure and organization, neuroscientists who study **neurochemistry** are interested in how chemicals in the brain are synthesized and involved in brain function. Findings from the study of neurochemistry can inform neuroscientists on many brain processes, such as those involved in learning (Hakim & Keay, 2018) and in the development of disorders (Rajagopal, Huang, Michael, Kwon, & Meltzer, 2018).

In the field known as **neuroendocrinology**, neuroscientists are interested in how hormones, which are chemicals that control important bodily functions, interact with the nervous system. The study of neuroendocrinology can inform neuroscientists on the basis of many types of behaviors, including those involved in feeding (Edwards & Abizaid, 2017) and reproduction (Mani & Oyola, 2012).

Neuroscientists who study **neuropathology** are mostly interested in the changes in the brain that occur when it becomes diseased. For example, the study of neuropathology provides valuable insight into the processes involved in Alzheimer's disease (Mostafavi et al., 2018) and Parkinson's disease (Dickson, 2018).

Neuropharmacology is the field in which neuroscientists study how drugs and other agents affect the functioning of neurons. One of the aims of neuropharmacology is to discover drugs that may one day be used in the treatment of neurological and psychological disorders (Yeung, Tzvetkov, & Atanasov, 2018). Neuropharmacologists may also be interested in how drugs can act as environmental risk factors in the development of psychological disorders. For example, it was found that exposure to cannabis and stress during adolescence may increase the probability that someone will suffer from excessive anxiety, characterized by exaggerated fears (Saravia et al., 2019).

In **neuropsychopharmacology**, neuroscientists study how drugs produce psychotropic effects, that is, how they affect a person's mind, emotions, and behavior through their actions in the brain. For example, it was found that the drug lysergic-acid diethylamide (LSD) and other drugs produce visual hallucinations (seeing things that are not really there) by increasing the activity of the brain chemical called serotonin (Kraehenmann et al., 2017), which you will learn about in Chapter 3, and by increasing the excitation of a variety of brain areas related to vision (Kometer & Vollenweider, 2018).

In the study of **neurophysiology**, neuroscientists may also be interested in learning about brain function by using various methods to stimulate, measure, or record the activity of individual brain cells or entire brain areas. For example, several studies have shown that exercise has positive effects on mood and cognition. Neurophysiological studies have provided evidence for the neurobiological basis of these effects by showing that exercise increases activity in relevant brain areas (Basso & Suzuki, 2017).

Finally, some neuroscientists are interested in studying how psychological functions are localized in certain brain areas. Such is the field of **neuropsychology**. Neuropsychologists can learn about the localization of functions by creating damage to specific brain areas in experimental animals and testing them on a task relevant to the function of interest. Neuropsychologists also acquire knowledge about brain function by studying people who have suffered brain damage. Neuropsychologists can also relate activity in certain brain areas, measured by various imaging methods, to specific functions. For example, it was found that people with damage to a part of the brain called the prefrontal cortex are impaired in understanding the emotions of others (A. Perry et al., 2017).

Who Is Interested in Findings From Behavioral Neuroscience?

The fields of study just described are considered to be subfields of neuroscience. However, people in other fields of study and professions that do not necessarily engage in neuroscience research may be interested in the findings that emanate from behavioral neuroscience. This includes neurologists, who are trained to diagnose and treat disorders of the nervous system; psychiatrists, who are trained to diagnose and treat mental disorders; and neurosurgeons, who are trained to perform surgery on the nervous system. The list also includes psychologists, professors, various health practitioners, and many more.

Graduates from university programs in behavioral neuroscience or neuroscience in general can find employment in a variety of more or less related fields. Lists of these fields can be found on the websites of various universities. For example, the following link is to the Careers in Neuroscience website of Princeton University: https://pni.princeton.edu/undergraduate-concentration/careers-neuroscience.

MODULE SUMMARY

Today, brain-behavior relationships are studied in many different ways. For example, patients who have suffered brain damage through various ways can be studied and the kind and extent of their brain damage can be related to impairments in behavioral tasks. The extent of the brain damage can be assessed by imaging methods such as magnetic resonance imaging and computed tomography. Scientists can find out whether a given brain area is related to some behavioral function by lesioning specific brain areas of experimental animals and then testing them on behavioral tasks to see if the lesion caused any kind of impairment in function. The same areas can also be stimulated to see whether any change in behavior can be observed. The brain can be stimulated in several ways. These include electrical brain stimulation and transcranial magnetic stimulation. Neurons in specific brain areas can also be turned off temporarily by the administration of drugs that can inactivate them. Furthermore, neurons can be turned either on or off by genetically altering them to make them responsive to light in what is known as optogenetics.

Brain activity can be related to behavior through methods that permit neuroscientists to observe the extent to which brain areas are used in the performance of behavioral tasks. These include functional magnetic resonance imaging, electroencephalography, and magnetoencephalography. Finally, neuroscientists can also record the electrical activity of individual neurons by inserting a tiny electrode either inside individual neurons to measure their electrical activity or in the fluid in which neurons bathe to measure the electrical current flowing near the electrode. This activity is related to the behavior being performed by the animal at the time of recording.

Fields of study related to behavioral neuroscience include neuroanatomy, neurochemistry, neuroendocrinology, neuropathology, neuropharmacology, neuropsychopharmacology, neurophysiology, and neuropsychology. Finally, many practitioners, who do not necessarily engage in research, may also be interested in findings from the study of behavioral neuroscience. These include neurologists, psychiatrists, neurosurgeons, professors, and various health practitioners.

TEST YOURSELF

1.4.1 Explain how the study of brain-damaged patients informs neuroscientists about brain-behavior relationships.

1.4.2 How are brain-behavior relationships inferred by lesioning, stimulating, and measuring the brain's activity?

1.4.3 Name and differentiate between the areas related to behavioral neuroscience.

APPLICATIONS

Brain Imaging as a Lie Detector: Not So Fast!

You have probably seen it in many movies and television series. A crime suspect is hooked up to devices measuring blood pressure, pulse, and skin conductivity. The purpose is to determine whether the individual is lying. This procedure is known as the polygraph test. The polygraph test does not directly measure whether someone is lying but, rather, measures the physiological reactions triggered when someone fails to tell the truth. Although the polygraph is great for enhancing movie drama, its results are inadmissible in the courtroom as evidence of someone's guilt. This is because of problems

(Continued)

(Continued)

associated with interpreting the results of a polygraph test. That is, no pattern of physiological reactions is known to be associated exclusively with lying. For example, heightened physiological reactions may not necessarily be indicative of a lie but may instead indicate that the person is simply nervous about the test. In contrast, a lack of reaction may be due to a subject's being exceptionally calm while lying. Within this context, the question arose as to whether more valid physical correlates of lying could be developed.

Enter functional magnetic resonance imaging (fMRI). Functional magnetic resonance imaging is used in both research and medicine to observe how brain activity is related to cognitive and behavioral function. It does so by measuring the amount of oxygen taken up by neurons while an individual performs a task. Neurons in brain areas most solicited by the task consume more oxygen than other areas, which is detected by the scanner and taken as evidence that the area is involved in the performance of the task.

Among many other questions related to brain-behavior relationships, some neuroscientists are trying to determine whether fMRI can be used to detect whether someone is lying and whether fMRI can become a superior method to the polygraph. If so, will the results obtained through fMRI ever become admissible evidence in a court of law? Before this happens, much more evidence will be needed regarding the validity and reliability of findings relating fMRI results to lying. That is, do the results truly reflect lying and not some other cognitive functions, and can the results be reliably replicated? So far neuroscientists have no evidence that either of these conditions has been met.

The quest to find out whether fMRI can be used as a lie detector began in the early 2000s when psychiatrist Daniel D. Langleben and colleagues (2002) administered the guilty knowledge test (GKT) to subjects while their brains were being imaged by fMRI. The GKT involves asking participants to answer no in response to questions to which both the participant and the experimenter know the answer to be yes. Langleben's hypothesis was that because lying requires an individual to inhibit giving a truthful response, areas of the brain associated with response inhibition, namely, the prefrontal and cingulate cortex, should be activated when an individual is lying. The study confirmed Langleben's hypothesis in that there was a significant difference in the pattern of brain areas activated in participants when telling the truth and when being deceitful. Since that time, several studies using fMRI have identified brain areas that are consistently activated when someone is lying. As shown in Figure 1.22, these include the lateral areas such as the medial frontal gyrus (MFG), inferior parietal lobule (IPL), and the insula in the inferior frontal gyrus

FIGURE 1.22

Is this the brain of a liar? Results of a study in which fMRI was used to detect deception. Areas in orange are consistently activated across studies when lying.

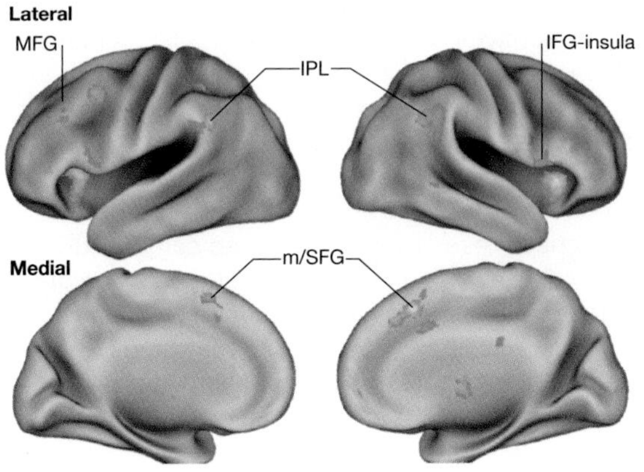

Farah, M.J., et al. (2014). Functional MRI-based lie detection: scientific and societal challenges. *Nature Reviews Neuroscience* 15: 123–131. With permission from Springer Nature.

(IFG-insula). They also include medial areas of the brain such as the medial and superior frontal gyrus (m/SFG) (Farah, Hutchinson, Phelps, & Wagner, 2014).

However, the results of those studies must be interpreted with caution because many other factors could have contributed to the brain activation observed in individuals while they were lying. These include memory and attentional processes related to the experimental setup and procedures used in the studies. For example, in one study, simply getting the instructions to lie increased brain activity. In another study, subjects were asked to pretend to steal objects, hide them, and lie about having taken them, leading to the possibility that brain activity may reflect memory for objects in addition to activation related to deception (Gamer, Klimecki, Bauermann, Stoeter, & Vossel, 2012).

In addition to these possible confounds, neuroscientists have come up with several hurdles that would need to be dealt with. For example, questions still remain as to whether laboratory conditions under which these fMRI studies are conducted reflect real-life situations, in which individuals are asked questions about real-life moral violations, the answers to which could result in them going to jail. Another question has to do with whether patterns of results while being deceptive generalize to different populations, such as those defined by age group, profession, or the presence of mental illness.

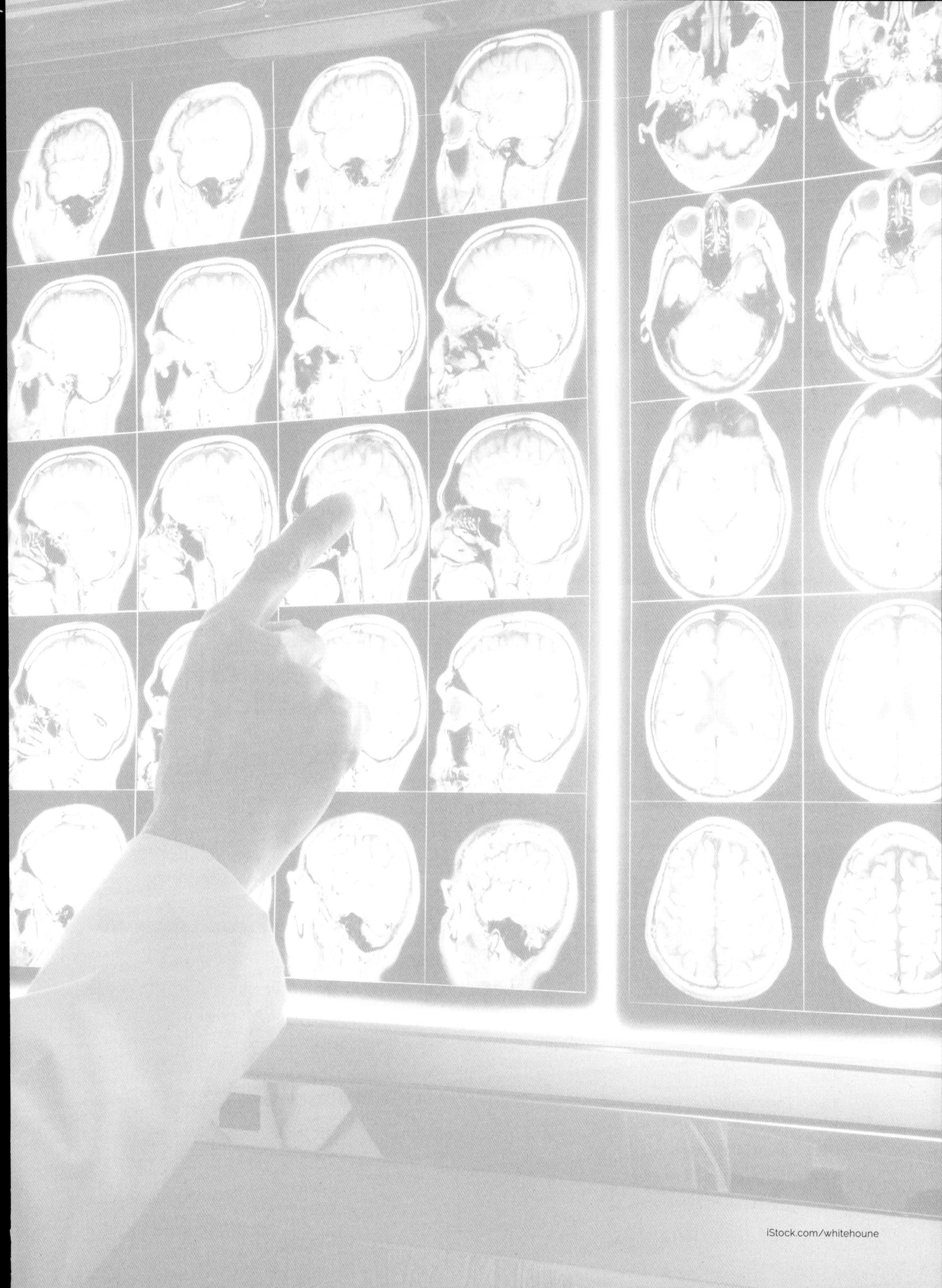
iStock.com/whitehoune

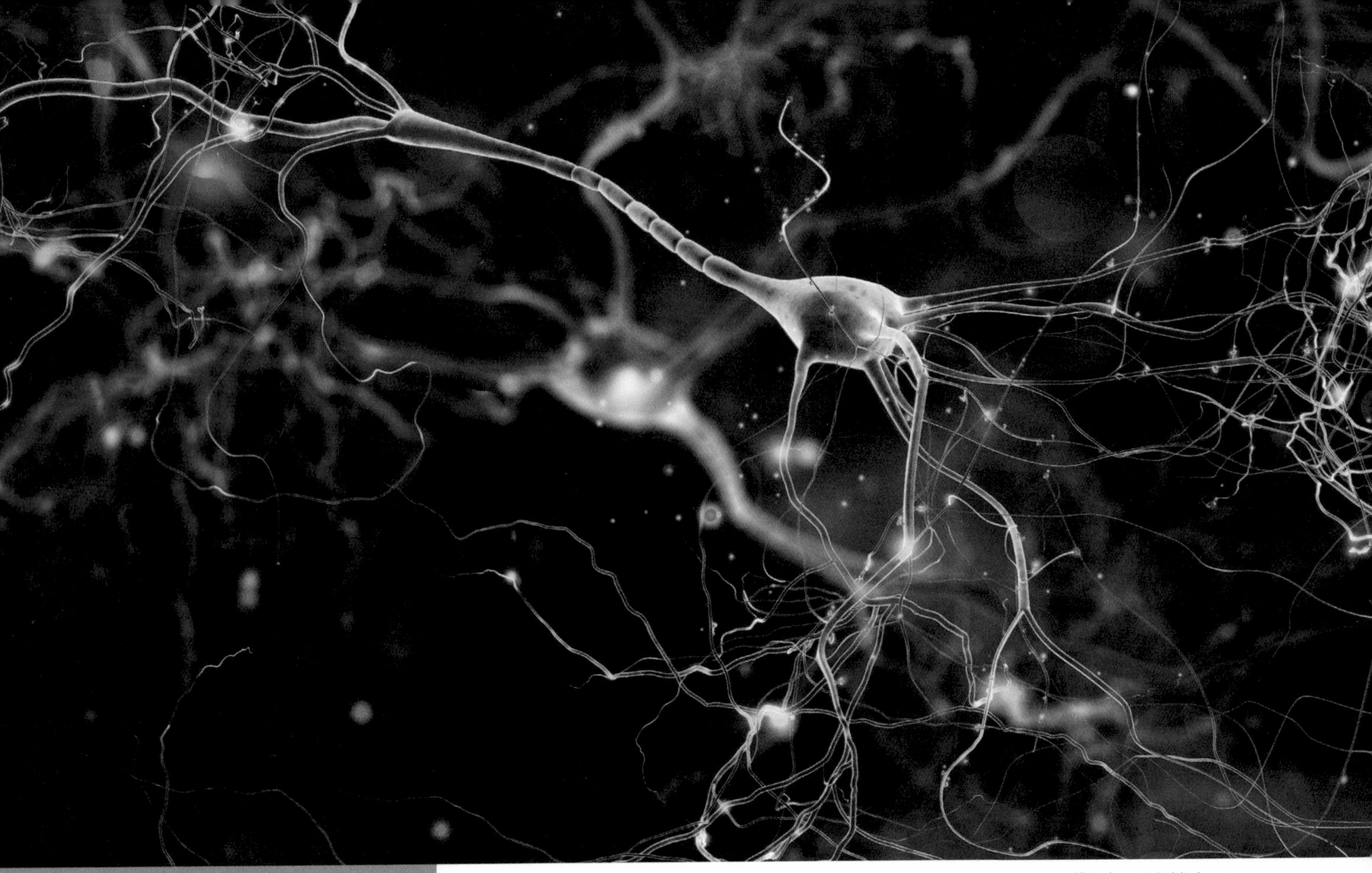

iStock.com/whitehoune

2 Neurons and Glia

Chapter Contents

Learning Objectives

2.1.1 Explain where neurons fit in with the other types of cells in the body.

2.1.2 Explain the cell theory and the neuron doctrine.

2.1.3 Describe the methods used to study neurons.

2.1.4 Explain what scientists have learned from having accurate estimates of the numbers of neurons in the brains of humans and other animals.

2.2.1 Describe the prototypical neuron and explain the roles of its parts.

2.2.2 Describe the ways by which neurons can be differentiated.

2.3.1 Explain the forces of diffusion and electrostatic pressure and how they are involved in the movement of ions across the cell membrane.

2.3.2 Explain how action potentials are initiated.

2.3.3 Explain how action potentials are propagated down the axons of neurons.

2.4.1 Describe the initial discovery of glia and the role initially assigned to them.

2.4.2 Explain the functions of the different types of glia.

The Black Mamba: A Potentially Deadly Encounter

The intact functioning of the nervous system depends on proper functioning of neurons. Neurons are specialized cells that communicate by generating electrical currents called action potentials. The generation of these action potentials depends on the flow of electrically charged molecules, called ions, back and forth from the outside to the inside of neurons. The two ions most implicated in the generation of action potentials are sodium and potassium. Interference with the flow of these ions can have drastic consequences for the functioning of the nervous system.

Poisons that attack the nervous system are known as neurotoxins. The ingestion of neurotoxins can seriously disrupt functioning of the nervous system and can ultimately lead to death. Neurotoxins can be synthetic chemicals, but they are also part of the self-defense mechanisms of many plants and animals. Fortunately, we tend to stay away from those. However, deadly encounters with such organisms do occur. For example, in the spring of 2008, a young man named Nathan Layton was on a safari-training course in South Africa. Some of the professors of the college he was attending captured a black mamba snake to use in a demonstration. Layton stood nearby as the snake was being transferred from container to container. The snake suddenly sprang upward and bit one of Layton's fingers. About 20 minutes later, Layton complained of blurred vision, slipped into a coma, and died.

The venom in the black mamba is composed of dendrotoxins. Dendrotoxins are a class of neurotoxins. These toxins block the flow of potassium out of neurons, resulting in muscle paralysis, disruption of heart muscle contraction, and respiratory failure.

INTRODUCTION

In this chapter, you will learn about the cells of the nervous system: neurons and glia. The brain contains billions of neurons and just about the same number of glia. Each one of these neurons can communicate with thousands of others, resulting in an extensive network of connectivity. Through communicating with each other, neurons permit us to sense our environment and appreciate music, good food, and works of art. This extensive network of connectivity is also responsible for the wide range of emotions that we experience and for encoding the information that results in our memories. You will also learn about glia, the other billions of cells that are crucial for the day-to-day maintenance and functioning of the nervous system, brain development, and communication between neurons.

2.1 Putting Neurons Into Context

Module Contents

2.1.1 The Place of Neurons Within the Body

2.1.2 Cell Theory and the Neuron Doctrine

Learning Objectives

2.1.1 Explain where neurons fit in with the other types of cells in the body.

2.1.2 Explain the cell theory and the neuron doctrine.

2.1.3 Describe the methods used to study neurons.

2.1.4 Explain what scientists have learned from having accurate estimates of the numbers of neurons in the brains of humans and other animals.

2.1.1 THE PLACE OF NEURONS WITHIN THE BODY

>> LO 2.1.1 Explain where neurons fit in with the other types of cells in the body.

Key Terms

- **Nervous tissue:** Tissue that makes up the nervous system. It is composed of neurons and glia.
- **Central nervous system:** The division of the nervous system that includes the brain and the spinal cord.
- **Peripheral nervous system:** The nervous tissue that connects to the muscles and organs of the body.

The body is made up of four types of tissues: connective, epithelial, muscle, and nervous tissue. Connective tissue binds, separates, and connects other types of tissues. Connective tissue makes up the bones, blood, ligaments, and tendons of the body. Epithelial tissue forms the outer layer of the skin and lines the cavities of the body, such as the digestive and respiratory systems. Muscle tissue forms the muscles that move the body, make the heart beat, and move food through the digestive tract. Finally, **nervous tissue** makes up the nervous system, which includes the **central nervous system**, consisting of the brain and spinal cord, and the **peripheral nervous system**, consisting of the nervous tissue that connects to the muscles and organs of the body. (The divisions of the nervous system are discussed at length in Chapter 4.)

All tissues are composed of specific types of cells. For example, connective tissue includes bone cells called osteocytes and blood cells called hematocytes. Epithelial tissue includes skin cells called squamous cells, and the liver has cells called hepatocytes. Muscle tissue is composed of muscle cells called myocytes. Nervous tissue is composed of neurons and glia, which are the focus of prime interest to neuroscientists. Neurons communicate with other neurons, muscle, and organs and perform the major computational functions of the nervous system, whereas glia support neuronal function and clear debris, toxins, and bacteria from the brain. The types of tissue and the cells associated with them are listed in Table 2.1.

TABLE 2.1

The Tissues of the Body and an Example of the Cells of Which They Are Composed

TISSUE	FUNCTION	CELL
Connective tissue	Makes up the bones, blood, ligaments, and tendons of the body	Bone (osteocytes)
Epithelial tissue	Makes up the outer layer of the skin and lines the cavities of the body, such as the digestive and respiratory systems	Skin (squamous cells)
Muscle tissue	Makes up the muscles that move the body, make the heart beat, and move food through the digestive tract	Muscle (myocytes)
Nervous tissue	Makes up the nervous system, which includes the brain, spinal cord, and nerves that connect to the muscles and organs of the body	Nervous system (neurons)

Images (top to bottom): iStock.com/Dr_Microbe; iStock.com/tonaquatic; iStock.com/JOSE LUIS CALVO MARTIN & JOSE ENRIQUE GARCIA-MAURINO MUZQUIZ; iStock.com/bestdesigns

2.1.2 CELL THEORY AND THE NEURON DOCTRINE

>> LO 2.1.2 Explain the cell theory and the neuron doctrine.

Key Terms

- **Cell theory:** The idea that the cell is the basic functional unit of all living things.
- **Reticular theory:** The idea that the neurites (axons and dendrites) of neurons fuse with the neurites of other neurons in a neural net.
- **Neuron doctrine:** The idea that the cell theory is applicable to neurons.

The **cell theory**, proposed in 1838 by German physiologist Theodor Schwann (1810–1882), states that the cell is the basic functional unit of all living things. At the time, however, the cell theory did not seem to apply to neurons. With the use of increasingly more powerful microscopes, it was observed that neurons have several parts, but it was not known how these parts were linked to each other.

In the late 1800s, Camillo Golgi (1843–1946) invented a staining method that permitted researchers to clearly observe all the parts of neurons (cell body, axon, and dendrites) and how they relate to each other. This became known as the Golgi stain and involved immersing nervous tissue into a silver nitrate solution. Figure 2.1 shows a Golgi-stained neuron.

Despite researchers being able to study the structure of neurons, it still was not clear whether the cell theory applied to neurons. The neurites (axons and dendrites) of neurons seemed to fuse with the neurites of other neurons in a neural net. This idea, known as the **reticular theory**, was championed by Golgi and many others.

In 1888, Santiago Ramón y Cajal (1852–1934), highly skilled in drawing neurons (Figure 2.2), studied the neurons in the cerebellum of a chick using an improved version of the Golgi stain. He observed that the axons of neurons always led up to the dendrites of other neurons but that they were not continuous with them in that they did not touch. Ramón y Cajal concluded that, like other cells of the body, neurons are basic and independent functional units. This meant that the cell theory was also applicable to neurons. The idea that the cell theory applies to neurons is known as the **neuron doctrine**. Together, Golgi's and Ramón y Cajal's contributions earned them a shared Nobel prize in 1906. In the following decades, observations made through increasingly powerful microscopes supported the neuron doctrine.

FIGURE 2.1

A Golgi-stained neuron.

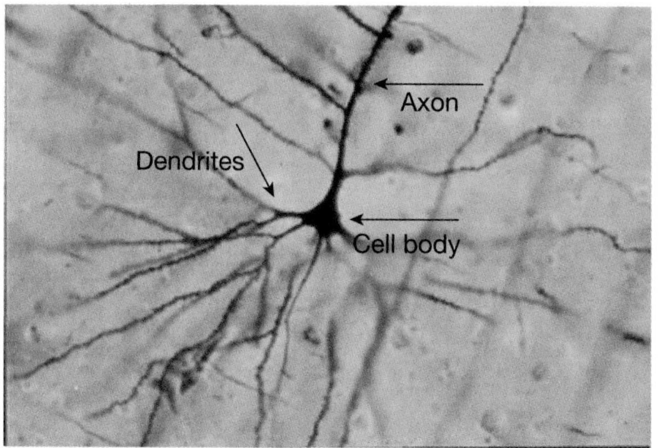

Bob Jacobs, Laboratory of Quantitative Neuromorphology, Department of Psychology, Colorado College.

FIGURE 2.2

Santiago Ramón y Cajal's drawing of neurons in a rabbit's hippocampus (as you will learn later, the hippocampus is an area of the brain important for memory).

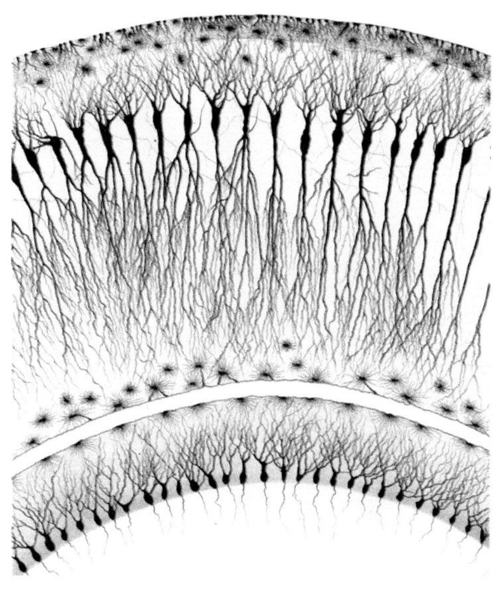

SCIENCE SOURCE

2.1.3 STUDYING NEURONS

>> LO 2.1.3 Describe the methods used to study neurons.

Key Terms

- **Histology:** The scientific study of cells and tissues.

- **Microscopy:** The field that uses microscopes to see objects that are not visible to the naked eye.
- **Microtome:** A laboratory instrument used to cut extremely thin sections of tissue.

Neuroscientists use several methods to study neurons. These include histology and microscopy. **Histology** is the scientific study of cells and tissues using special staining techniques combined with microscopy. **Microscopy** is the field that uses microscopes to see objects that are not visible to the naked eye.

To be able to clearly see neurons through a microscope, thin sections of brain tissue are cut, mounted on glass slides, and stained. However, the brain has the consistency of Jell-O. Therefore, sectioning it in its natural state is extremely difficult. To solve this problem, a method of fixing (hardening) the brain by soaking it in paraformaldehyde was devised. Extremely thin sections of the brain, micrometers thin (1 micrometer [μm] = 1 millionth of a meter), are made with the use of a **microtome**. Before being sectioned, the brain is frozen and sometimes embedded in a waxy substance. Figure 2.3a shows a technician using a microtome.

The sections of the brain are then mounted on microscope slides and treated with various types of stains. The Golgi stain, invented by Camillo Golgi, shown in Figure 2.1, is but one of these stains. You have already seen that the Golgi stain clearly shows the cell body, axon, and dendrites of neurons. The type of stain used depends on the types of cells and cell components a researcher is interested in studying. For example, a stain called cresyl violet is used to highlight the cell body (Figure 2.3b) but does not clearly identify axons and dendrites.

2.1.4 THE NUMBER OF NEURONS AND GLIA IN THE BRAIN

>> LO 2.1.4 **Explain what scientists have learned from having accurate estimates of the numbers of neurons in the brains of humans and other animals.**

Key Term

- **Isotropic fractionation:** A method by which the number of cells in a brain area of interest can be estimated.

Various sources of information (including textbooks) state that the brain contains 100 billion neurons and 10 times as many glial cells (F. Doetsch, 2003; Kandel, Schwartz, & Jessell, 2000). However, recent research does not support these numbers. For example, using a method known as **isotropic fractionation**, neuroscientist Suzana Herculano-Houzel and colleagues found that the human brain contains, on average, 86.06 billion neurons and 84.61 billion glia (Azevedo et al., 2009; Herculano-Houzel, 2014). Isometric fractionation involves reducing brain areas of interest to a solution. The number of neurons and glia in an area of interest can then be estimated by the application of special stains that differentiate between them. Figure 2.4 shows a cross-section of a human brain with its distribution of neurons and glia, referred to as non-neuronal cells.

FIGURE 2.3

(a) A microtome being used to cut sections of a rodent brain. (b) A brain section stained with cresyl violet. Note the visibility of the cell nuclei compared with their axons and dendrites.

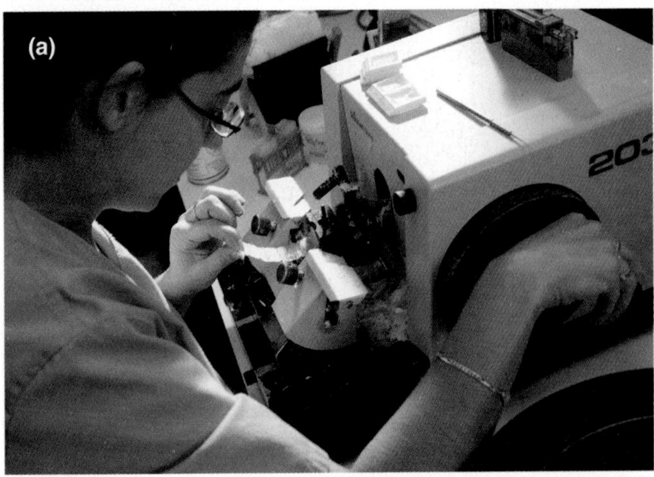

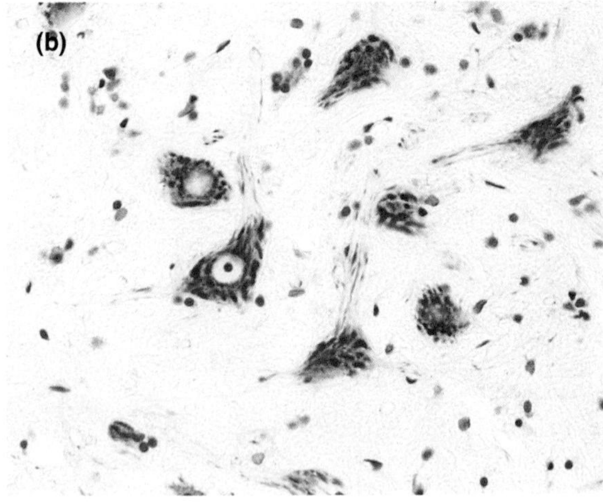

(a) age fotostock / Alamy Stock Photo; (b) Jose Luis Calvo/Science Source

FIGURE 2.4

Number of neurons and non-neuronal cells in the whole human brain and by brain area. B = billion; non-neur = non-neuronal cells, or glia.

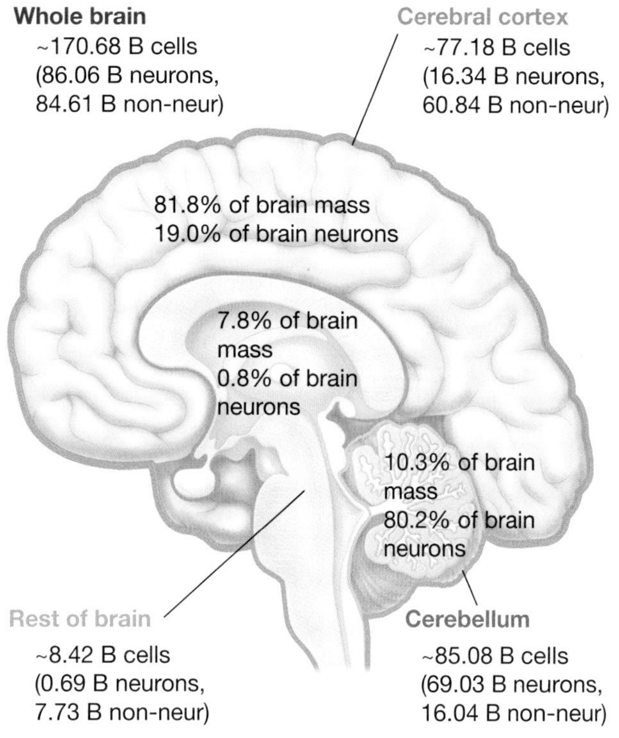

Amanda Tomasikiewicz/Body Scientific Intl.

It is also widely believed that the differences in cognitive abilities across species of animals are related to brain size or to the number of neurons. However, recent studies show that these beliefs make no sense if humans are to be considered as the smartest animals. Compared to the brains of other species, the human brain neither is the largest nor does it contain the highest number of neurons. For example, elephants have a bigger and heavier brain (about 4.6 kilograms compared to about 1.5 kilograms for the human brain) with more neurons (about 258 billion) than humans have (about 86 billion). Rather, differences in intelligence between species may be related to the number of neurons located in the cerebral cortex. Elephants have significantly more neurons than humans but only about 5.93 billion are in the cerebral cortex. In contrast, the human cerebral cortex contains about 16 billion neurons (see Olkowicz et al., 2016, for a comparison in brain size, total number of neurons, and number of neurons concentrated in the cerebral cortex across birds and mammals).

IT'S A MYTH!

No New Neurons

The Myth

The adult brain is incapable of generating new neurons.

Where Does the Myth Come From?

The origin of this myth can be traced back to Santiago Ramón y Cajal, the father of the neuron doctrine. In

(Continued)

(Continued)

his 1913 book *Degeneration and Regeneration of the Nervous System*, Ramón y Cajal stated that new neurons could not be generated after birth (Ramón y Cajal, DeFelipe, & Jones, 1991). He could not conceive how new neurons could be integrated into already well-established networks. Regarding the nervous system, he claimed that "everything may die and nothing may be regenerated." This dogma persisted in the minds of neuroscientists for many years, often in the face of contrary evidence. Even today, the "no new neurons" myth is still very much present in the general population.

Why Is the Myth Wrong?

It is true that neurons do not replicate through cell division. This is because they lack the molecular machinery needed to do so. However, in the 1960s, Joseph Altman discovered that neurogenesis (the generation of new neurons) occurs in postnatal guinea pigs, even though they are born with nearly adult-sized brains. He found that this occurred in the hippocampus, a brain structure known to be important for memory (Altman, 1962). Altman's findings were largely ignored, as often occurs when a new finding contradicts the prevailing view. Altman's report was followed by a series of findings that made neurogenesis more difficult to ignore. In the 1980s, Fernando Nottebohm and colleagues discovered neurogenesis in the brains of song birds (Alvarez-Buylla, Ling, & Nottebohm, 1992; Nottebohm, 1989). By the late 1990s, it was known that adult neurogenesis occurred in at least two brain areas: the hippocampus and the olfactory bulb. Several studies show that neurogenesis in the hippocampus is related to the formation of new memories (Hung, Hsiao, & Gean, 2014; Ko et al., 2009).

Today, the search for the functions of neurogenesis continues. For example, it was found that chronic stress, which can lead to major depression, inhibits neurogenesis in the hippocampus. In contrast, antidepressant drugs were found to increase neurogenesis (Anacker, 2014; Mahar, Bambico, Mechawar, & Nobrega, 2014; Ruiz et al., 2018). ●

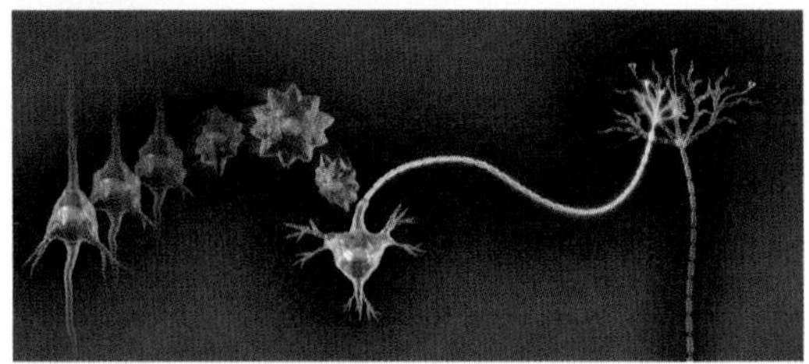

Henning Dalhoff/Bonnier Publications/SCIENCE SOURCE

MODULE SUMMARY

The body is made up of many different types of tissues, each composed of specialized types of cells. The tissue of most interest to neuroscientists is nervous tissue. Nervous tissue is composed of two types of cells: neurons and glia. Neurons are responsible for the computational functions of the nervous system, which permit us to sense our environment, move around, experience emotions, and form memories. Glia support neuronal function and clear debris, toxins, and bacteria from the brain.

The cell theory states that the cell is the basic functional unit of all living things. It was once believed that neurons did not conform to the cell theory in that axons and dendrites of different neurons were thought to be continuous with each other in a neural net. This is known as the reticular theory. It was later discovered that the cell theory did apply to neurons. This is known as the neuron doctrine.

Neuroscientists study neurons using histological methods, in which they use special staining techniques, and microscopy. The human brain was once thought to contain 100 billion neurons and 10 times as many glia. However, recent studies show that the human brain contains about 86 billion neurons and approximately the same number of glia.

TEST YOURSELF

2.1.1 Describe how neurons and glia are but other types of cells in the body and explain what they are responsible for.

2.1.2 Explain the cell theory and the neuron doctrine.

2.1.3 Describe the methods used to study neurons.

2.1.4 How many neurons and glia are presently thought to be in the human brain? How does that differ from previous thinking? In what way is the number of neurons thought to account for the complexity of human behavior as compared to other species?

2.2 The Structure of Neurons

Module Contents

Learning Objectives

2.2.1 Describe the prototypical neuron and explain the roles of its parts.

2.2.2 Describe the ways by which neurons can be differentiated.

2.2.1 THE PROTOTYPICAL NEURON

>> LO 2.2.1 Describe the prototypical neuron and explain the roles of its parts.

Key Terms

- **Action potential:** Also known as a nerve impulse; the conduction of an electrical charge within a neuron.
- **Neurotransmitter:** A chemical messenger released from neurons; used to communicate with other neurons and other types of cells in the body.
- **Soma:** Also called the cell body or perikaryon; contains the nucleus and organelles found in other cell types.
- **Nucleus:** The part of the cell that contains deoxyribonucleic acid (DNA), which codes for proteins.
- **Dendrite:** An outgrowth of the neuron at which connections between neurons are typically made.
- **Axon:** An outgrowth of neurons through which action potentials are conducted.
- **Axon hillock:** The point of contact between the soma and the beginning of the axon.
- **Axon terminal:** The part of the axon farthest from the cell body; stores and releases neurotransmitters.
- **Synaptic cleft:** The tiny gap that exists between neurons.
- **Ligand:** Neurotransmitters or other chemicals, such as drugs, that bind to neurotransmitter receptors.
- **Ligand-gated ion channels:** Channels that open in response to the binding of ligands to their receptors.
- **Synapse:** The site of communication between neurons or between neurons and other types of cells.
- **Presynaptic neuron:** The neuron that releases neurotransmitter molecules into the synaptic cleft.
- **Postsynaptic neuron:** The neuron located across the synaptic cleft.
- **Myelin sheath:** Fatty tissue that insulates axons.
- **Oligodendrocytes**: Myelin-producing glia in the central nervous system.
- **Schwann cells:** Myelin-producing glia in the peripheral nervous system.
- **Neuronal membrane:** The cellular membrane of neurons.
- **Cytoskeleton:** The collection of filaments and tubules that gives the cell its shape, rigidity, and ability to move.
- **Microtubules:** The largest of the cytoskeletal elements.
- **Actin filaments:** Also called microfilaments; the smallest of the cytoskeletal elements.
- **Intermediate filaments:** Also called neurofilaments; of intermediate size between microtubules and actin filaments.
- **Axoplasmic transport:** The transport of materials from one part of the cell to another via microtubules.

Figure 2.5a shows a prototypical neuron. As we explore their basic structures, keep in mind that neurons communicate through electrical impulses called **action potentials**, also known as nerve impulses, which are examined in depth later in the chapter. Action potentials result in the release of **neurotransmitters** onto specialized receptors situated on target cells. Target cells can be other neurons, muscle cells, or the cells of internal organs.

Neurotransmitters are chemical messengers that are released by neurons as well as being synthesized and stored within them. Many neurotransmitters are known to exist. Each neurotransmitter is associated with certain functions in both the central and

FIGURE 2.5

(a) A prototypical neuron. (b) Comparison between a photomicrograph of dendrites and a digital image of tree branches. (c) Images of a dendrite along with three-dimensional reconstruction of its spines (in red, center). The white dots represent the locations at which the spines insert into the dendrite (left and right).

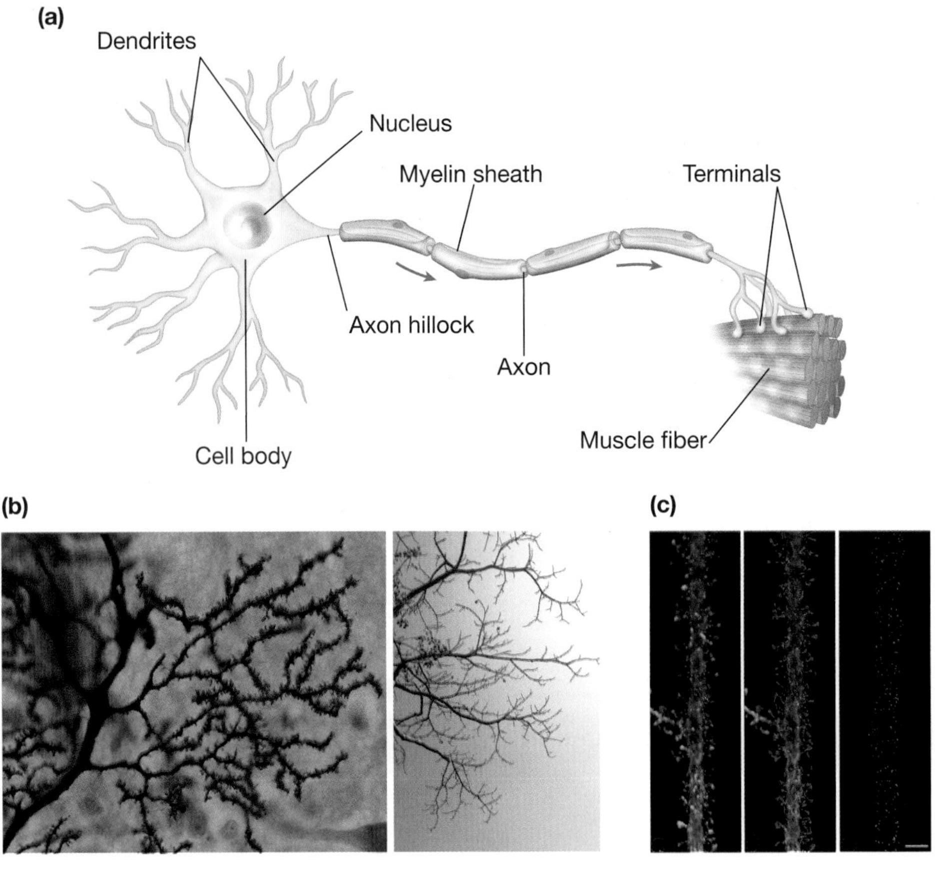

(b) *left:* Jose Luis Calvo/Science Source; *right:* iStock.com/Siewwy84; (c) Morales, J., et al. (2014). Random Positions of Dendritic Spines in Human Cerebral Cortex. *Journal of Neuroscience 34*(30), 10078–10084. With permission from The Society for Neuroscience.

peripheral nervous systems. Neurotransmitters are discussed at length in Chapter 3.

The Structure of Neurons

The Soma (or Cell Body)

The **soma** is the part of the neuron that contains the **nucleus** of the neuron as well as many organelles, which are structures that carry out the cell's functions. The soma can measure anywhere from 5 μm to 100 μm in diameter, depending on the type of neuron. The nucleus contains deoxyribonucleic acid (DNA), which codes for proteins (see Chapter 1).

Dendrites

Dendrite is the Greek word for "tree." Dendrites are outgrowths of neurons at which connections between neurons are typically made. They have receptors to which neurotransmitters bind. Each type of neurotransmitter binds to its own type of receptor. As an analogy, think of receptors as keyholes and neurotransmitters as the keys that fit them. Through binding to these receptors, some neurotransmitters can trigger neurons to generate action potentials, whereas other neurotransmitters can prevent neurons from firing action potentials.

Dendrites have small outgrowths called dendritic spines. Figure 2.5c shows a three-dimensional reconstruction of a dendrite with its spines (Morales et al., 2014). Dendritic spines have neurotransmitter receptors. This increases the number of connections dendrites can make with other neurons. They undergo plastic changes in response to experience, which underscores their importance in learning and memory (see Chapter 5 for a discussion of neuroplasticity). Abnormalities in dendritic spines may be related to developmental problems, such as the learning difficulties and cognitive deficits found in individuals with fragile X syndrome, a genetic disorder caused by an abnormality on the X chromosome (Comery et al., 1997; K. Han et al., 2015). Figure 2.5b compares a digital image of dendrites, taken through a microscope (photomicrograph), with an image of tree branches. Can you tell which is which?

The Axon

The **axon** joins the soma to the axon terminals, the parts of the axon farthest away from the soma. Action potentials are initiated at the **axon hillock**, which is the point of contact between the soma and the beginning of the axon. A bundle of axons in the central nervous system (situated in the brain and spinal cord) is called a tract. A bundle of axons in the peripheral nervous system (that connects to the muscles and internal organs) is referred to as a nerve.

Axons can be very long, up to 1.5 meters in length or more. The longest nerve in the human body is the sciatic nerve, which runs from the lower back to the foot. Have you ever heard of sciatica? It is a painful condition in which the sciatic nerve is pinched by a displaced disc in the lower vertebral column. People with sciatica can experience pain down the leg and sometimes all the way down to their toes.

Axon Terminals

Axon terminals (Figure 2.6) are situated at the end of the axon. They contain packets of neurotransmitters called synaptic vesicles. In response to action potentials reaching the axon terminals, calcium enters the terminal and synaptic vesicles bind to the neuronal membrane and release their contents of neurotransmitters into the tiny gap that exists between neurons, known as the **synaptic cleft**. The neurotransmitters then bind to receptors of the neuron across the synaptic cleft. These receptors are on channels that open in response to the binding of neurotransmitters. Neurotransmitters and other chemicals that bind to receptors are known as **ligands**. Because of this, these channels are known as **ligand-gated ion channels**.

The site of communication between neurons or between neurons and other types of cells is known as the **synapse**. Thus, the neuron releasing the neurotransmitters is referred to as the **presynaptic neuron**, whereas the neuron that receives the neurotransmitters, on the other side of the synaptic cleft, is referred to as the **postsynaptic neuron**. You will learn much more about this process in Chapter 3.

FIGURE 2.6

A synapse.

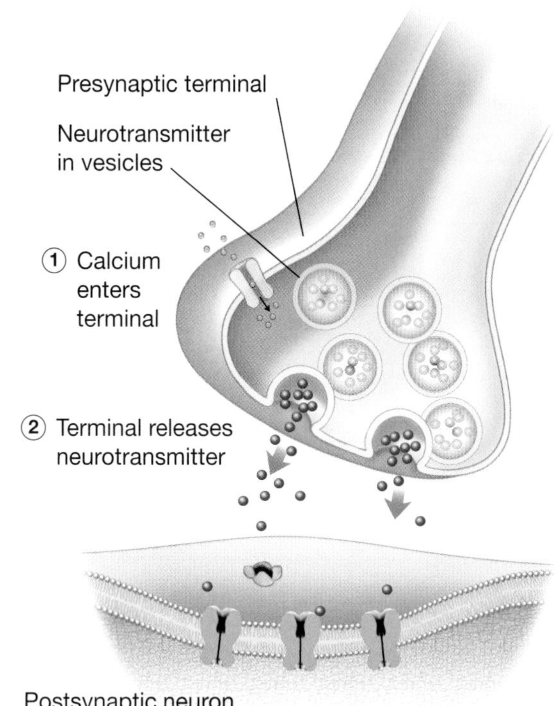

The Myelin Sheath

The **myelin sheath** is a fatty tissue that insulates axons. It contributes to how well neurons conduct action potentials. This is similar to the insulation of a power cord, without which current would not make it very far. The myelin sheath is not continuous through the entire length of the axon. There are frequent breaks in the sheath known as nodes of Ranvier, named after the French anatomist Louis-Antoine Ranvier (1835–1922). These breaks are about 1 μm in length and occur at intervals of about 1–2 μm. They are the sites at which action potentials are regenerated.

The myelin sheath is produced by glia. The myelin-producing glia in the central nervous system, which includes the brain and spinal cord, are called **oligodendrocytes**. In the peripheral nervous system, which controls your muscles and organs, the myelin-producing glia are called **Schwann cells**, named after Theodor Schwann, who, as you read earlier, proposed the cell theory. The process by which glial cells insulate axons is illustrated later in the chapter, in Figure 2.24.

The Neuronal Membrane

The **neuronal membrane** (Figure 2.7) consists of a phospholipid bilayer, as the molecules that compose it form two layers. The term *phospholipid* is derived from two words: *phosphate* and *lipid* (*lipos* is Greek

FIGURE 2.7

The neuronal membrane with its phospholipid bilayer. Also shown, spanning the membrane, is an ion channel and a water-filled pore through which ions enter or exit the neuron.

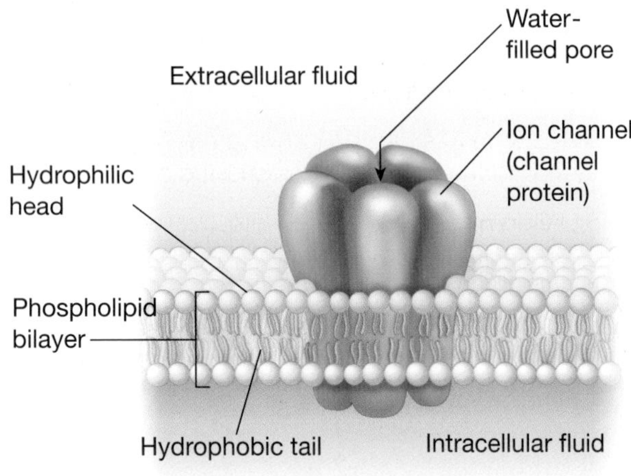

Carolina Hrejsa/Body Scientific Intl.

for “fat”). The phospholipid molecules each have a head and a tail. The head of each molecule is hydrophilic, meaning water loving and that it readily interacts with water, whereas the tail of each molecule is hydrophobic, meaning water fearing and that it does not interact with water. Remember that oil and water do not mix.

The molecules are oriented so that the hydrophobic tail of each molecule faces the tail of another molecule. The hydrophilic heads of the molecules bathe in the extracellular and intracellular fluids. This arrangement keeps water and various particles either on the outside or on the inside of the neuron. Embedded within this membrane are proteins that form channels across the membrane, also seen in Figure 2.7. These channels are semipermeable and permit the movement of molecules in and out of the neuron. Channels come in many types, each type letting in or out of the cell certain molecules called ions, such as sodium or potassium, through a water-filled pore.

The Cytoskeleton

The word **cytoskeleton** literally means “skeleton of the cell.” This is because it gives the cell its shape, rigidity, and ability to move. There are three types of cytoskeletal elements: microtubules, actin filaments, and intermediate filaments (Figure 2.8). **Microtubules** are the largest of the cytoskeletal elements. Microtubules are held together by tubulin-associated protein (TAU). **Actin filaments** (also called microfilaments) are the smallest of the cytoskeletal elements. They also run through axons and dendrites, but, in addition, they are fastened to the inside of the cell’s membrane.

Intermediate filaments (also called neurofilaments) are of intermediate size between microtubules and actin filaments. They are present in dendrites but more numerous in axons. They are essential in preserving the axon’s diameter and play an important role in maintaining the velocity of action potentials.

Axoplasmic Transport

The microtubules act as railroad tracks for the transport of materials from one part of the cell to another. This type of transport is called **axoplasmic transport**. Materials such as organelles, lipids, or proteins are transported in vesicles along microtubules by what look like little “legs.” These “legs” are made of the proteins kinesin and dynein. In anterograde transport, kinesin carries materials from the soma toward the axon terminals. In retrograde transport, dynein carries materials from axon terminals to the soma (Figure 2.9).

Pathology of the cytoskeleton can lead to neuropsychiatric disorders. The most widely known of these disorders is Alzheimer’s disease, in which people suffer progressively more severe memory loss and other cognitive problems. In Alzheimer’s disease, the TAU

FIGURE 2.8

The cytoskeleton. Three different elements make up the cytoskeleton: actin filaments, intermediate filaments, and microtubules.

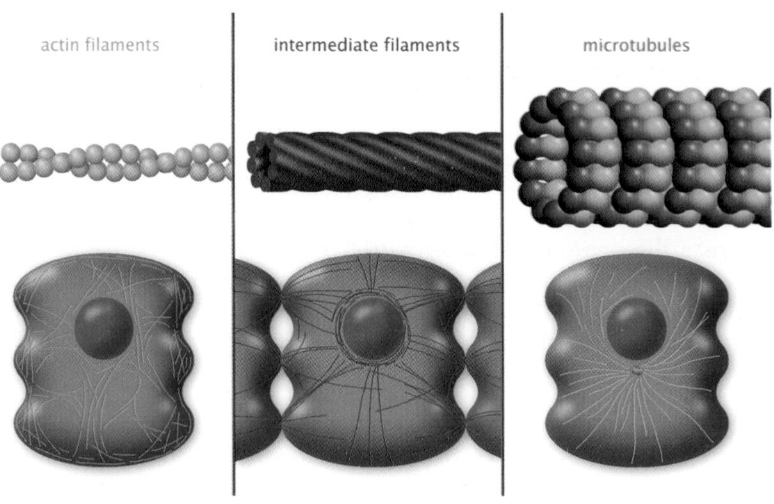

Art for Science/Science Source

FIGURE 2.9

Axoplasmic transport.

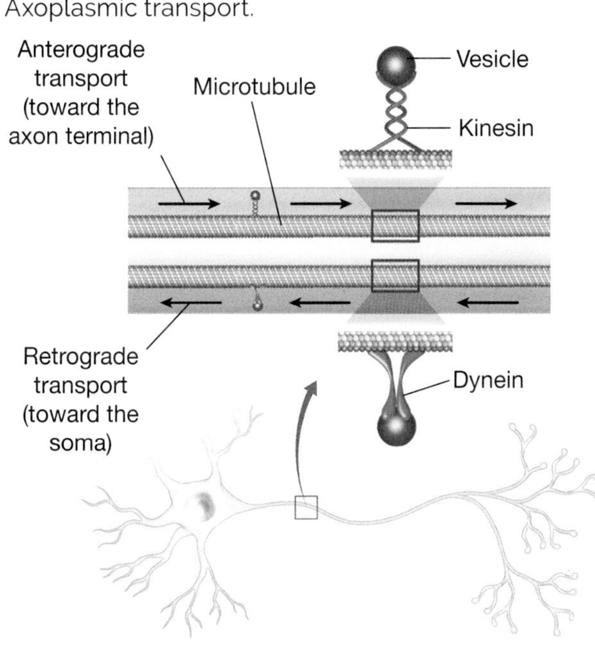

Amanda Tomasikiewicz/Body Scientific Intl.

protein is hyperphosphorylated, meaning that it takes on additional phosphate groups. This change in structure of the TAU protein prevents it from binding with microtubules. This causes the microtubules to collapse into tangles known as neurofibrillary tangles and loose aggregates of TAU known as paired-helical filaments. Alzheimer's disease is discussed in Chapter 5.

2.2.2 THE DIVERSITY OF NEURONS

>> LO 2.2.2 Describe the ways by which neurons can be differentiated.

Key Terms

- **Sensory neuron:** A neuron that carries sensory information from the peripheral nervous system to the central nervous system.
- **Motor neuron:** A neuron that carries movement information from the central nervous system to the peripheral nervous system.
- **Interneuron:** A neuron that connects sensory neurons to motor neurons.
- **Bipolar neuron:** A neuron that has a single dendrite and axon, each exiting opposite sides of the soma.
- **Unipolar neuron:** A neuron with only one process that flows uninterrupted by the soma.
- **Multipolar neuron:** A neuron that has many dendrites sticking out of one side of the soma and an axon sticking out of the other side.
- **Pyramidal neuron:** A type of neuron that has the appearance of a pyramid.
- **Stellate cell:** A neuron in which the disposition of the dendrites gives it a star-shaped appearance.
- **Rosehip neuron:** A recently discovered type of neuron with unknown function that is found in humans but not in rodents.

Diverse types of neurons exist. Neurons can be differentiated by their function; their morphology; the architecture of their dendrites; and the type of neurotransmitters they synthesize, store, and release. Neurons also show considerable diversity across species.

Differences in Function

Functional differences between neurons are illustrated in the reflex arc (Figure 2.10). Movement is often produced involuntarily. For example, when the body makes contact with a painful stimulus, muscles contract automatically to move the affected part of the body away from the stimulus. This is known as a withdrawal reflex.

FIGURE 2.10

The reflex arc.

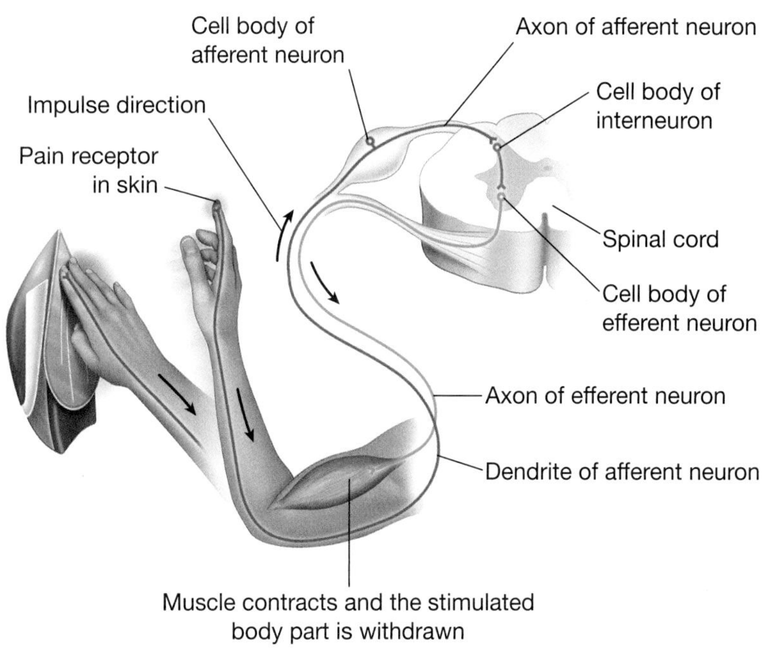

Amanda Tomasikiewicz/Body Scientific Intl.

FIGURE 2.11

(a) Morphological variation in neurons, as described in the text. (b) Photomicrograph of a pyramidal cell (left) and a stellate cell (right). (c) Computer reconstructions of diverse neurons across species: (A) rat neocortex Martinotti cell, (B) rat neocortex bipolar cell, (C) rat neocortex pyramidal cell, (D) mouse neocortex pyramidal cell, (E) mouse hippocampus Schaffer collateral-associated neuron, (F) mouse cerebellum Golgi cell, (G) cat brainstem vertical cell, (H) rat olfactory bulb deep short-axon cell, (I) mouse neocortex Cajal-Retzius cell, (J) mouse retina ganglion cell, (K) spiny lobster stomatogastric ganglion motor neuron, (L) rat hippocampus granule cell, (M) mouse cerebellum Purkinje cell, and (N) rat neocortex interneuron. (d) Anatomical reconstruction of a rosehip neuron.

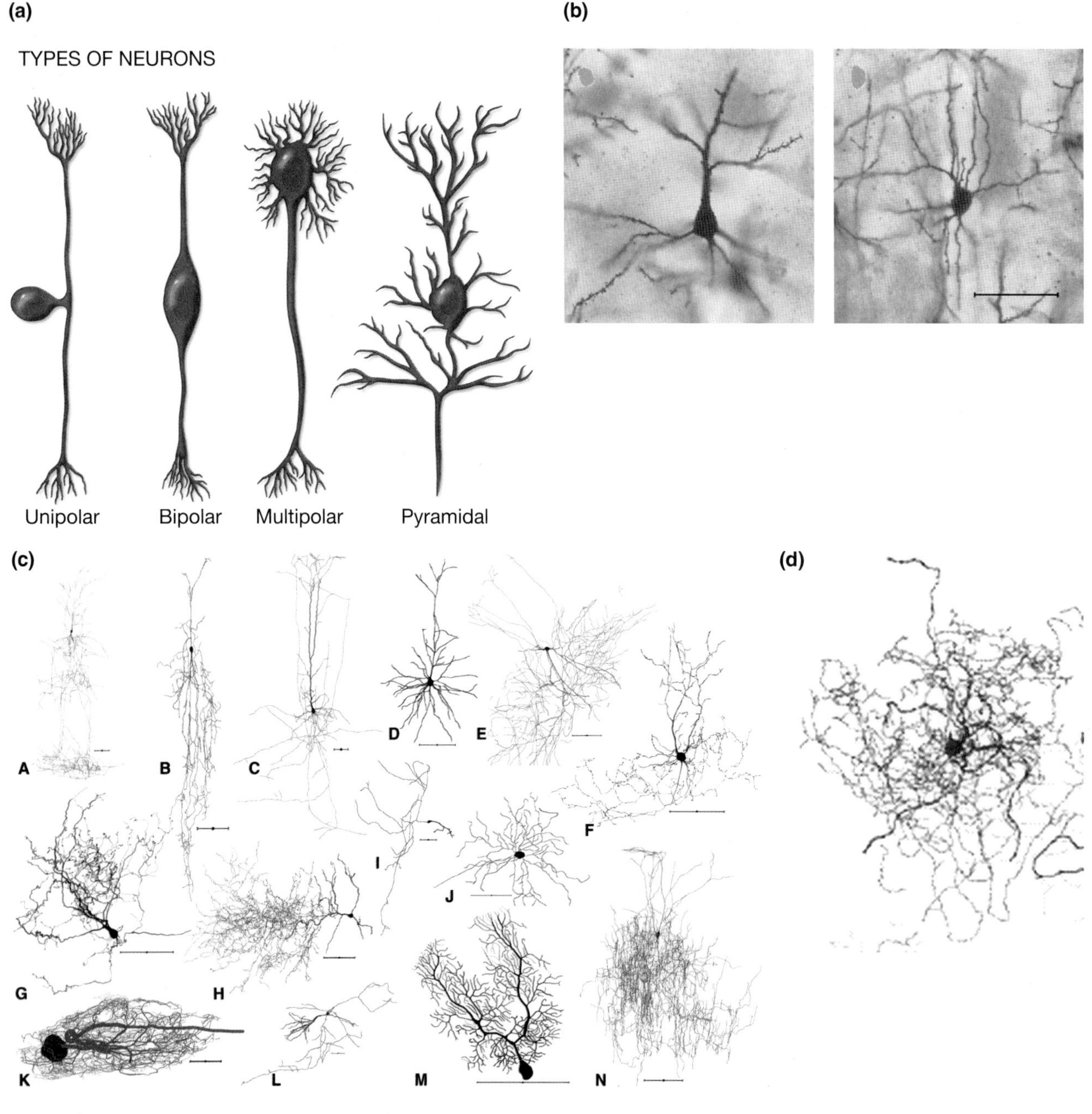

(a) Monica Schroeder/Science Source; (b) Parekh, R., & Ascoli, G. A. (2013). Neuronal morphology goes digital: a research hub for cellular and system neuroscience. *Neuron, 77*(6), 1017–38; (c) Parekh, R., & G.A. Ascoli. (2013). Neuronal morphology goes digital: a research hub for cellular and system neuroscience. *Neuron 77*(6), 1017–1038. With permission from Elsevier; (d) Boldog, E. et al. (2018). Transcriptomic and morphophysiological evidence for a specialized human cortical GABAergic cell type. *Nature Neuroscience 21*(9): 1185–1195. With permission from Springer Nature.

Unlike voluntary movement, reflexes do not require the brain for their execution. In a reflex arc (such as the one seen in Figure 2.10), three types of neurons, differentiated by their functions, are involved. These are sensory neurons, motor neurons, and interneurons. **Sensory neurons**, also known as afferent neurons (*afferent* means to carry information toward), bring information from sensory receptors, which are part of the peripheral nervous system, toward the brain and spinal cord, which constitute the central nervous system. **Motor neurons**, also known as efferent neurons (*efferent* means carrying information away from), carry information away from the brain and spinal cord to cause muscles to contract. To summarize, sensory neurons carry sensory information from the peripheral nervous system to the central nervous system, and motor neurons carry information from the central nervous system to the peripheral nervous system. **Interneurons** mediate the connections between sensory and motor neurons.

Morphological Variations

Variations in the morphology of neurons are illustrated in Figure 2.11a. **Bipolar neurons** have a single dendritic tree and axon each exiting from opposite sides of the soma. Think of the North and South Poles of Earth with a dendrite coming out of the north and an axon coming out of the south. Bipolar neurons are quite rare. They are found only in the auditory and visual systems. **Unipolar neurons** have a single process that flows uninterrupted by the soma. That is, the dendrite and the axon are continuous. Unipolar neurons have an axon that splits into two branches. One branch, the central branch, exits the cell body and enters the dorsal root of the spinal cord. The other branch, the peripheral branch, collects sensory information from the receptors in muscles, skin, and joints. These are typical of sensory neurons.

Multipolar neurons have many dendrites sticking out of one side of the soma and an axon sticking out of the other side. These are typical of motor neurons and interneurons. The prototypical neuron illustrated at the beginning of this chapter is a multipolar neuron.

Variations in Dendrite Architecture

Pyramidal neurons have a pyramid-shaped soma with a single dendrite arising from the top of the pyramid and several branching dendrites emanating from its base (right image in Figure 2.11a and left image in Figure 2.11b). **Stellate cells** are typically interneurons. They are called stellate cells because the disposition of their dendrites gives them a star-shaped appearance (right image in Figure 2.11b).

Variations in Neurotransmitter Type

Neurons can also be differentiated by the neurotransmitters they synthesize, store, and release. That is, different neurons synthesize, store, and release particular neurotransmitters. We discuss neurotransmitters and the mechanisms by which neurons use them to communicate in Chapter 3.

Diversity in Neurons Across Species

Figure 2.11c shows computer reconstructions of the diversity in neurons that exist across species (Parekh & Ascoli, 2013). The majority of neurons shown in Figure 2.11c are from rodents (rats and mice). New types of neurons continue to be discovered. For example, an entire new class of neurons was discovered in the neocortex, hippocampus, and olfactory bulb (Tripathy, Burton, Geramita, Gerkin, & Urban, 2015). More recently, a type of neuron called a **rosehip neuron** (so called because it looks like the fruit of a rose bush) was discovered in the neocortex of humans (Boldog et al., 2018) (Figure 2.11d). What is fascinating about these neurons is that they do not appear to exist in rodents. However, the exact functions of rosehip neurons are still a mystery to neuroscientists. This is important to know since rodents are the animals used most frequently for modeling behavior and cognition. As a result, a greater understanding of the neurobiological basis of human cognition, behavior, and psychological disorders might come from discovering neurons that are unique to humans.

MODULE SUMMARY

The soma (or cell body) is the part of the neuron that mostly resembles other cells. It contains the nucleus and various organelles. The nucleus codes for proteins. Neurons have an axon and many dendrites. Axons attach to the soma at the axon hillock and carry information in the form of action potentials. Action potentials travel down the axon until they reach the axon terminals, where they trigger the release of neurotransmitters into the synaptic cleft. The neurotransmitters released by neurons bind to receptors located on the dendrites of other neurons. Dendrites have small outgrowths known as dendritic spines, on which additional receptors are located. Dendritic spines greatly increase the connections a neuron can make with other neurons. Axons are insulated by a fatty tissue called the myelin sheath, which increases the conductivity. The myelin sheath is interrupted periodically at what are known as nodes of Ranvier.

The neuronal membrane keeps water and other soluble molecules from traveling in and out of the neuron. To enter or exit the neuron, ions pass through channels, selective to each ion. The shape, rigidity, and mobility of neurons are provided by the cytoskeleton, which is made up of three elements: microtubules, intermediate filaments, and actin filaments. Microtubules are also used in axoplasmic transport. Anterograde transport is the transport of molecules from the soma toward the axon terminals, and retrograde transport is the transport of molecules from the axon terminals toward the soma. Alzheimer's disease may be due to pathology of the cytoskeleton.

Neurons can be differentiated by their function, as can be demonstrated in a reflex arc. For example, sensory neurons carry information from the body to the spinal cord, where they communicate with motor neurons through interneurons, which send electrical signals to the muscles. Neurons also come in a variety of shapes: unipolar, bipolar, and multipolar neurons; pyramidal cells; and stellate cells. Neurons also show diversity across species. Finally, neurons can be differentiated by the neurotransmitters they synthesize, store, and release.

TEST YOURSELF

2.2.1 On a sheet of paper, draw a prototypical neuron and label its parts. Describe the function of each part.

2.2.2 Describe the ways in which neurons can be differentiated.

2.3 The Action Potential

Module Contents

Learning Objectives

2.3.1 Explain the forces of diffusion and electrostatic pressure and how they are involved in the movement of ions across the cell membrane.

2.3.2 Explain how action potentials are initiated.

2.3.3 Explain how action potentials are propagated down the axons of neurons.

2.3.1 A LITTLE BIT OF CHEMISTRY

>> LO 2.3.1 Explain the forces of diffusion and electrostatic pressure and how they are involved in the movement of ions across the cell membrane.

Key Terms

- **Ion:** An electrically charged particle.
- **Diffusion:** The process by which molecules tend to move from an area of high concentration to an area of low concentration.
- **Electrostatic pressure:** The phenomenon by which ions that are of the same charge repel each other and ions that are of opposite charge attract each other.
- **Resting membrane potential:** The difference in charge between the inside and the outside of the neuron when not conducting action potentials.
- **Equilibrium potential:** The voltage across the membrane (V_m) at which the forces of electrostatic pressure and diffusion counteract each other.

As with any other cell, neurons bathe in fluid and are fluid filled. The fluid outside the neuron is called extracellular fluid; the fluid inside the neuron is referred to as intracellular fluid. **Ions**, which are electrically charged particles, float around inside these fluids. Some ions have a net positive electrical charge, whereas other ions have a net negative electrical charge. The charge of the ion is indicated by the appropriate superscript (+ or –). Ions with a net positive electrical charge are known as cations, whereas ions with a net negative electrical charge are known as anions. You need to know something about ions to understand how action potentials are initiated and propagated down the axon of a neuron.

Ions result from dissolving molecules, such as sodium chloride (NaCl) (otherwise known as table salt) into water. As shown in Figure 2.12, when NaCl is dissolved in water, Na^+ and Cl^- are pulled apart, resulting in free Na^+ ions and Cl^- ions surrounded by water molecules. There are other types of ions within the extracellular and intracellular fluids, for example, potassium (K^+), calcium (Ca^{2+}), and hydrogen (H^+). For now, we will mostly focus our attention on only two of them, Na^+ and K^+.

Diffusion and Electrostatic Pressure: Two Forces of Nature in Action

When a neuron is not conducting an action potential, Na^+ is 10 times more concentrated in the extracellular fluid than it is in the intracellular fluid. In contrast, K^+ is 20 times more concentrated in the intracellular fluid than it is in the extracellular fluid. This difference in the concentration of ions between the outside and the

FIGURE 2.12

Table salt (NaCl) molecules dissolving in water, resulting in Na^+ and Cl^- ions surrounded by spheres of hydration.

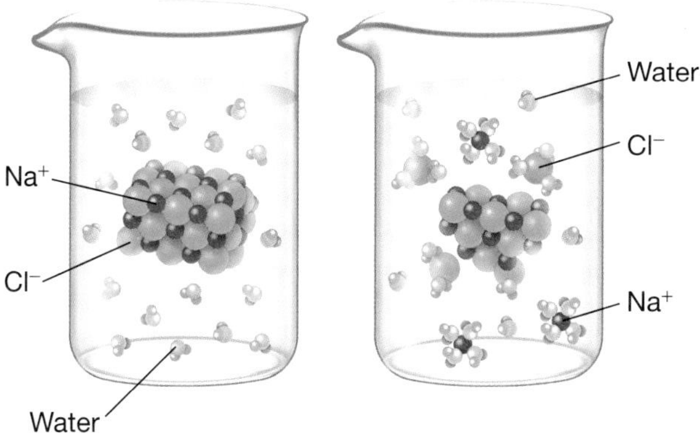

Amanda Tomasikiewicz/Body Scientific Intl.

inside of the neuron (concentration gradient) sets up the condition for diffusion to occur. **Diffusion**, illustrated in Figure 2.13a, is the process by which solutes (substances dissolved in water) move from an area of high concentration to an area of low concentration. For example, when milk is poured into a cup of coffee, it is initially concentrated in one area. It then moves throughout the whole cup. The milk is said to move down its concentration gradient. That is, it moves from an area in which it is more concentrated to an area in which it is less concentrated.

The inside of the neuron is electrically negative relative to the outside. This difference in electrical charge between the inside and the outside of the neuron sets up the condition for a second force—called **electrostatic pressure**, also known as the electrical force—to come into play. Electrostatic pressure creates the phenomenon by which ions that are of the same charge (+ + or – –) repel each other and ions that are of opposite charge (+ –) attract each other.

Cations and anions are also attracted to other sources of opposite electrical charge. For example, imagine that electrodes from the positive and negative poles of a battery are lowered into a beaker of water (Figure 2.13b). An electrode from the positive pole (anode) of the battery is lowered into the beaker on one side, and an electrode from the negative pole (cathode) of the battery is lowered into the beaker on the other side.

Imagine, also, that a permeable membrane was lowered into the beaker in between the two electrodes (the anode and the cathode). Now, imagine that channels permeable to Na^+ are inserted into the membrane. In which direction will the Na^+ ions flow? The answer is that they will flow from the side with the positive electrode to the side of the membrane with the negative electrode. There are two reasons for this. First, the Na^+ ions will flow down their concentration gradient, that is, from the area in which they are more concentrated to the area in which they are least concentrated, a case of diffusion. Second, because the Na^+ ions have a net positive electrical charge (anion), they will be drawn to the side of the membrane that was rendered electronegative

FIGURE 2.13

The forces of diffusion and electrostatic pressure. (a) In diffusion, solutes move from an area of high concentration to an area of lower concentration until the concentrations are balanced. (b) Electrostatic pressure causes ions with a net negative charge (anions) to be attracted to a positive electrical charge (anode) while ions with a net positive charge (cations) are attracted to a negative charge (cathode).

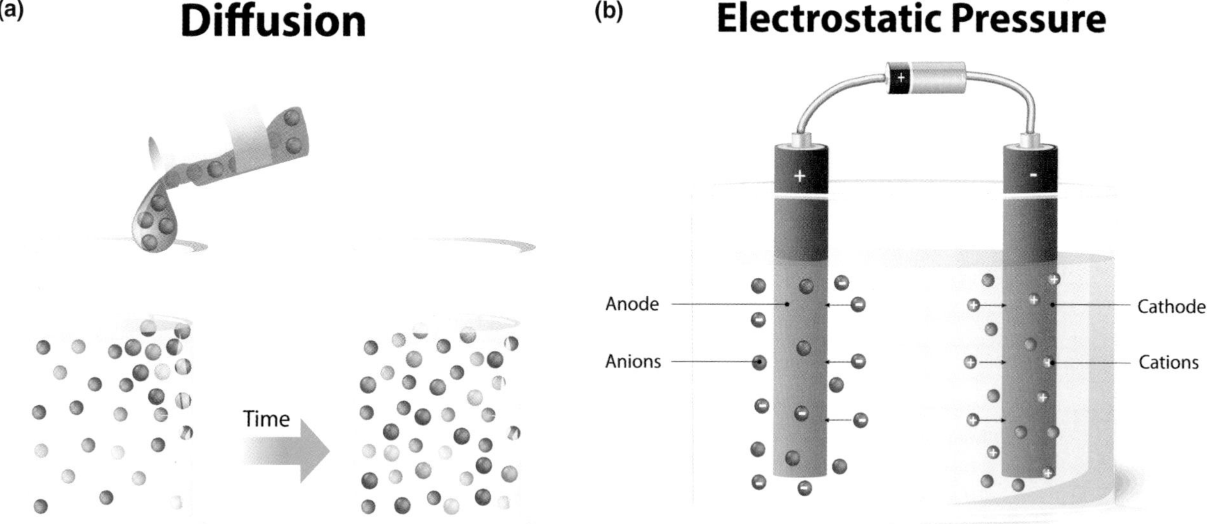

(a) iStock.com/ttsz; (b) iStock.com/ttsz

by the presence of the negative electrode. This is due to electrostatic pressure. This, of course, would also happen if channels permeable to K^+ were put in place. Ions with a net negative charge (cations), such as chloride (Cl^-), would move in the opposite direction.

The Resting Membrane Potential, Voltage, and Conductivity

The **resting membrane potential** refers to the difference in charge between the inside and the outside of the neuron when it is at rest, that is, when it is not generating action potentials. My favorite analogy for this is a car battery like the one illustrated in Figure 2.14a. A car battery, like any other battery, stores energy. You wouldn't know it just by looking at one. But you could hook up wires to the battery's positive and negative poles, marked, respectively, by a "+" and a "–," and then hook up both of these wires to a motor or anything else you want the battery to power.

The fact that one pole of the battery is marked with a "+" and the other is marked with a "–" means that there is a difference in electrical charge between the two poles. This difference in charge is measured in volts. For a standard car battery, the difference in charge between the negative and positive poles is about 12 volts (Figure 2.14a). If we used shoelaces to hook the poles of the battery to an engine, nothing would happen. This is because shoelaces have no conductivity. Conductivity is the ability of a material to conduct electricity.

The same goes for neurons. However, instead of a difference in charge between two poles, the difference in charge is across the membrane between the inside and the outside of the neuron (voltage across the membrane = V_m). The resting membrane potential, that is, the difference in charge between the inside and the outside of the neuron when it is not conducting action potentials is approximately –70 millivolts (mV) (Figure 2.14b).

What about conductivity? For the car battery, conductivity depends on how well current flows from its positive pole, through the engine, to the negative pole. We mentioned that shoelaces have no conductivity. Therefore, if you use shoelaces to hook up your car battery, you will not get anywhere. This is because the conductivity of shoelaces is "0." However, if you use electrical wires, the engine will start (provided the battery is not dead). This is because the conductivity of the cables is more than "0."

In neurons, conductivity depends on the number of ion channels that are open. Remember that channels are made of proteins that span the membrane. When many Na^+ channels are open, conductivity for Na^+ is high; when many channels are closed, conductivity for Na^+ is low. When conductivity for Na^+ is high, Na^+ ions flow freely into the neuron through diffusion.

The Equilibrium Potential

As mentioned earlier, K^+ is 20 times more concentrated inside the neuron than it is outside the neuron. This

FIGURE 2.14

The voltage of a car battery versus that of a neuron at rest. (a) A voltmeter can be used to measure the voltage of a car battery. (b) To measure the voltage across the membrane of a neuron, two thin electrodes are used. One electrode records the electrical charge outside the neuron and the other records the charge inside the neuron. For a neuron at rest, this difference is –70 millivolts (mV).

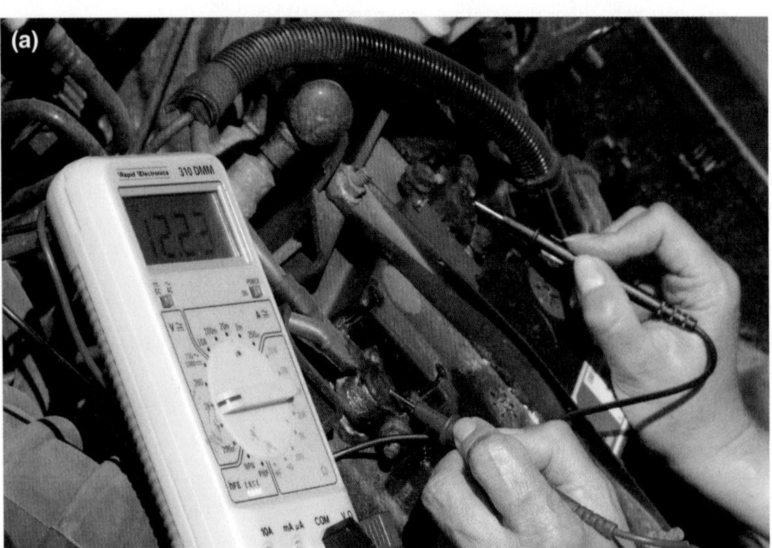

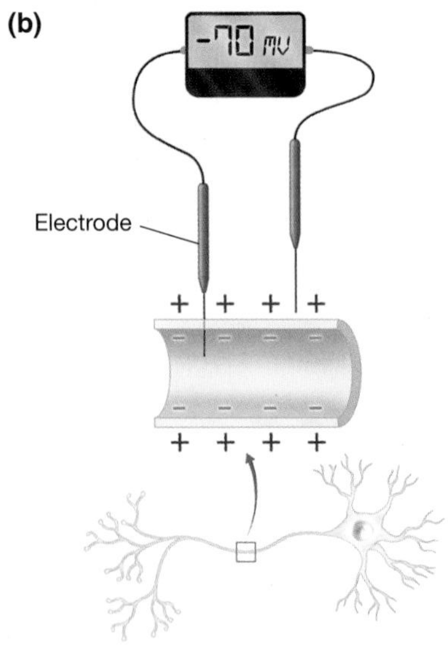

(a) David Forster / Alamy Stock Photo; (b) Amanda Tomasikiewicz/Body Scientific Intl.

FIGURE 2.15

(a) The chemical driving force of diffusion and the electrical driving force of electrostatic pressure. (b) The equilibrium potential for several ions. The concentration of the ions inside and outside neurons is shown in micromoles per liter of water (a mole is a measure of the weight of molecules in chemistry; it is the molecular weight in grams).

(a)

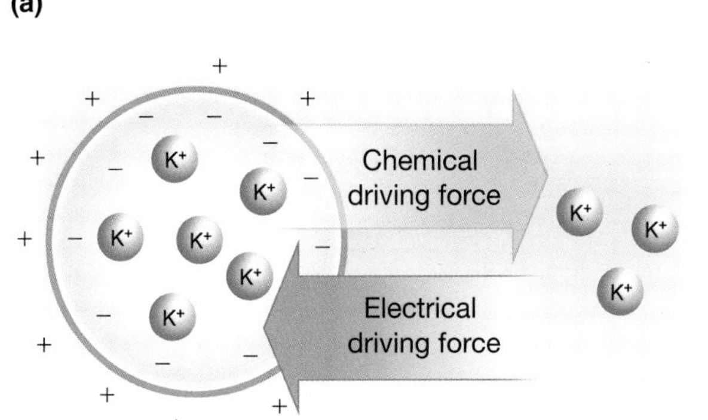

(b)

ION	CONCENTRATION (mmol/L OF H_2O) INSIDE CELL	OUTSIDE CELL	EQUILIBRIUM POTENTIAL (mV)
Na+	15.0	150.0	+60
K+	150.0	7.5	–90
Cl–	9.0	125.0	–70

Resting membrane potential = –70 mV

(a) Carolina Hrejsa/Body Scientific Intl.

means that, when K^+ channels are open, K^+ will diffuse down its concentration gradient from the inside to the outside of the neuron (Figure 2.15a). However, as K^+ leaves the neuron, the inside of the neuron will become more electronegative relative to the outside of the neuron. This will eventually cause K^+ ions to be drawn back into the neuron due to electrostatic pressure. Remember! Opposites attract.

The V_m at which electrostatic pressure counteracts diffusion is known as the **equilibrium potential** (E_{ion}). For K^+ ions, the V_m at which this occurs is –90 mV or E_{K+} = –90 mV; for Na^+ ions, it is +60 mV (E_{Na+} = +60 mV). Every ion has its own equilibrium potential, as shown in Figure 2.15b. The maintenance of the resting membrane potential is highly dependent on E_{K+} as many K^+ channels are open when the neuron is at rest.

Key Terms

- **Depolarization:** To reduce polarity (i.e., to make less negative); the inside of the neuron becomes less electrically negative relative to the outside.
- **Activation threshold**: The minimal amount of depolarization that must occur for an

FIGURE 2.16

The phases of the action potential.

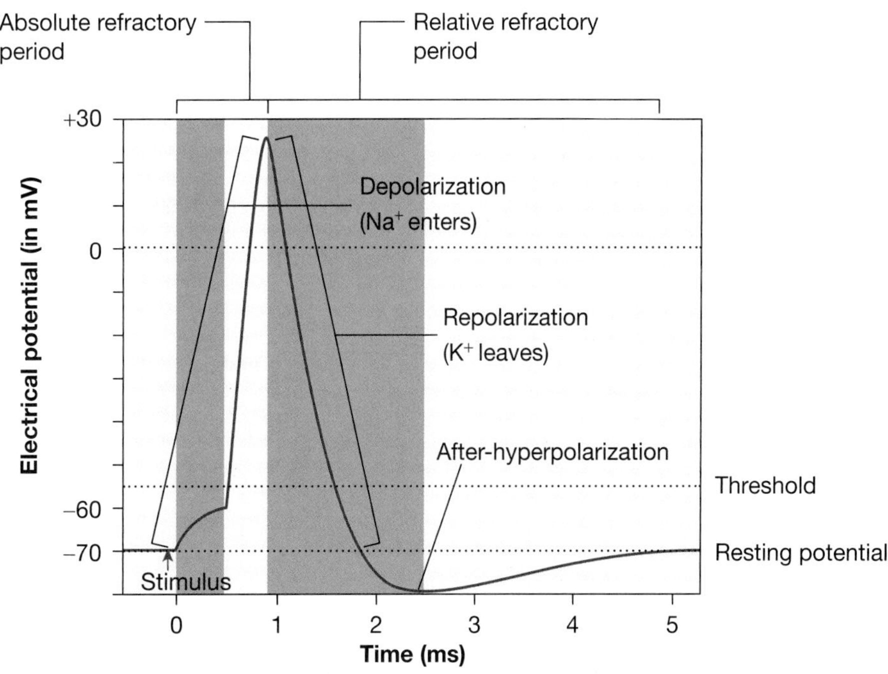

2.3.2 INITIATION OF ACTION POTENTIALS

>> LO 2.3.2 **Explain how action potentials are initiated.**

FIGURE 2.17

The sodium-potassium pump. (1) ATP powers the pump by giving up one of its phosphate molecules, becoming ADP. (2) Three Na^+ ions are sequestered by the pump. (3) The Na^+ ions are transferred out of the neuron and two K^+ ions are sequestered by the pump. (4) The K^+ ions are transferred to the inside of the neuron.

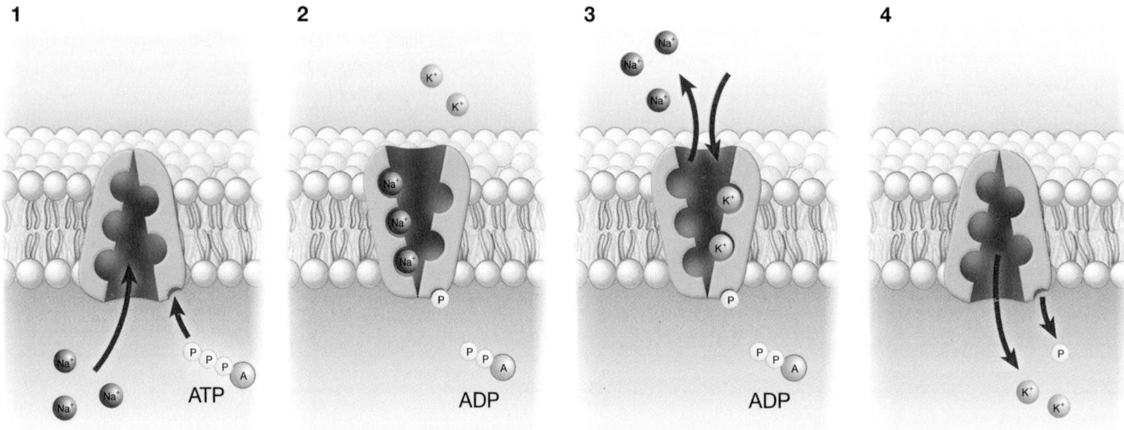

Carolina Hrejsa/Body Scientific Intl.

FIGURE 2.18

Current intensity and the frequency of action potentials. As stated in the all-or-none law, current intensity does not result in an action potential that reaches a higher voltage (+30 mV) once it has crossed the threshold. Instead, stimulus intensity is related to the frequency of action potentials.

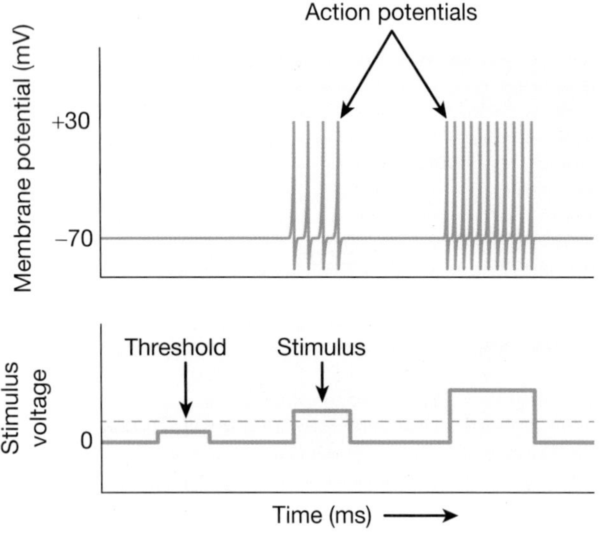

Carolina Hrejsa/Body Scientific Intl.

action potential to be initiated, which is about −55 mV.

- **Absolute refractory period:** The voltage at which further depolarization of the neuron is impossible and another action potential cannot be initiated in that neuron.
- **Relative refractory period:** The period when initiation of another action potential is possible but is difficult to induce.
- **All-or-none law:** The fact that more stimulation than is necessary for the neuron to be depolarized to threshold will not result in a stronger action potential.

We are finally ready to put together all that you have learned so that you can understand how an action potential is generated. A stimulus such as pressure on the skin is felt because it causes Na^+ channels to open, resulting in action potentials moving up your arm, through your spinal cord, and to your brain. Action potentials are initiated because the opening of these channels increases conductivity for Na^+. Since Na^+ is more concentrated on the outside of the neuron, this causes Na^+ to flow down its concentration gradient and to enter the neuron by the force of diffusion. The entry of Na^+ into the neuron causes the membrane to undergo **depolarization**, which means that the inside of the neuron becomes less electrically negative relative to the outside. Depolarization of the membrane causes other Na^+ channels to open. This is associated with the rising phase of the action potential (Figure 2.16). However, an action potential will be generated only if this depolarization crosses what is known as the **activation threshold**. The activation threshold, which refers to the minimal amount of depolarization that must occur for an action potential to be initiated, is about −55 mV.

Once the depolarization of the membrane crosses the activation threshold, it continues well past the point where V_m = 0 mV. This is referred to as the overshoot. When V_m reaches approximately +30 mV, K^+

FIGURE 2.19

Stretch-activated channels can be opened (a) by the stretch of the cell membrane itself, (b) by the displacement of cytoskeletal elements, or (c–d) by interacting with proteins inside and outside the neuron, which can sense deformation (modified from Del Valle et al., 2012). (e) A deactivated voltage-gated Na^+ channel. Ion channels have a selectivity filter, which makes them permeable only to certain ions (in this case, Na^+ ions). Voltage-gated channels also have voltage sensors (white rectangles with plus signs).
(f) Depolarization of the membrane (for example, from resting membrane potential to the threshold) is detected by the voltage sensors, causing the channel to open, and Na^+ enters the neuron. (g) An inactivation gate then closes the channels until the channel is once again deactivated.

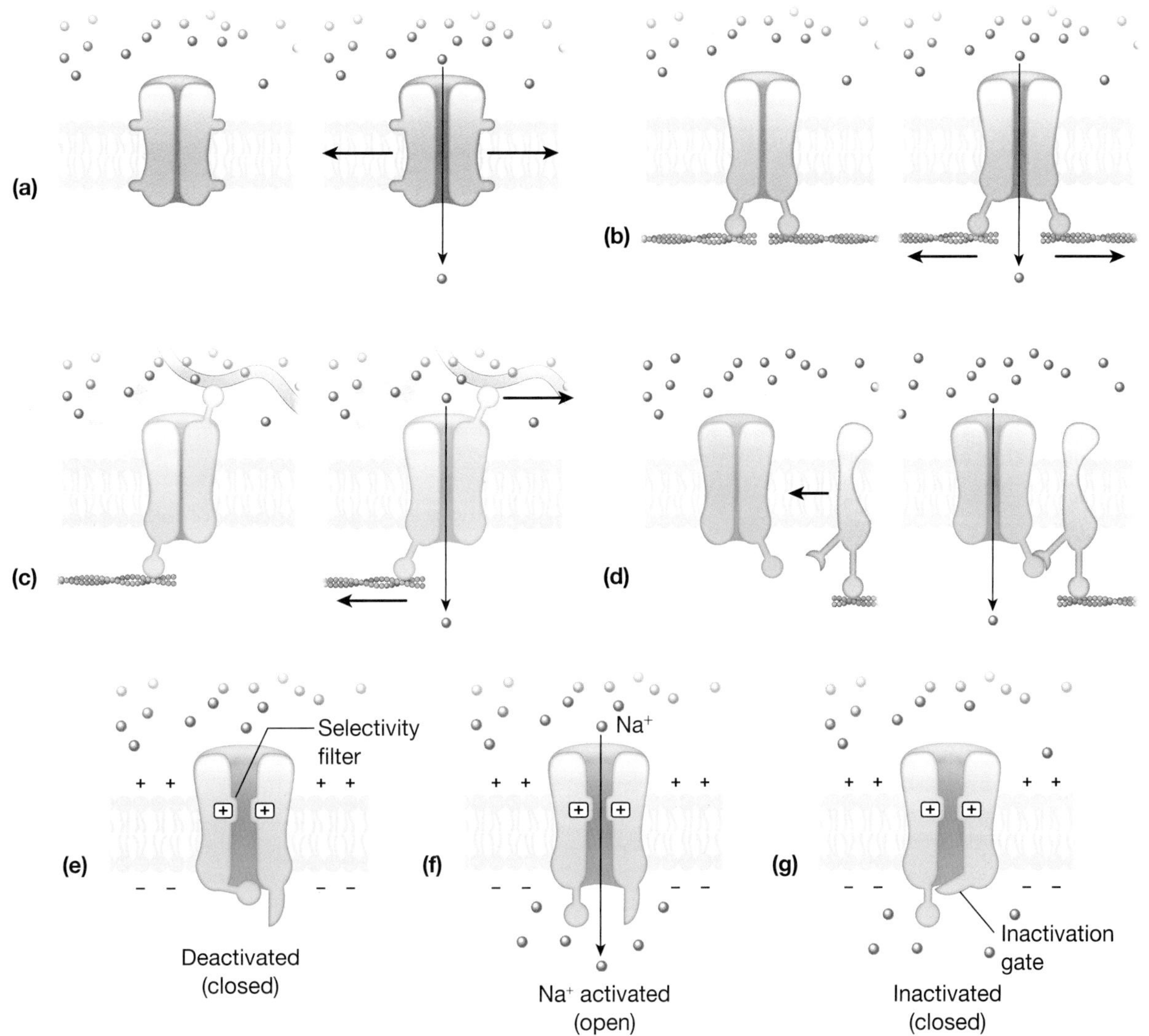

Carolina Hrejsa/Body Scientific Intl.

channels open and K^+ ions flow down their concentration gradient to the outside of the neuron. At about the same time, Na^+ channels close and Na^+ can no longer enter the neuron. The outward movement of K^+ causes the voltage of the neuron to repolarize (to become more negative).

Because Na^+ channels are quickly inactivated after the initiation of an action potential, another action potential cannot be generated in the same neuron for a period of about 1 millisecond (ms). This is called the **absolute refractory period**. With the exit of K^+, voltage across the membrane of the neuron drops drastically, toward the resting membrane potential and beyond. This is the falling phase of the action potential, which is associated with repolarization.

The point at which voltage across the membrane is more negative than the resting membrane potential (−70 mV) is called undershoot, also known as after-hyperpolarization. During the period that covers repolarization and after-hyperpolarization, initiation of another action potential is possible, but it is difficult to induce. This is called the **relative refractory period**.

We are now confronted with a problem. There is a reversal of the concentration gradients for Na^+ and K^+. That is, there is now a greater concentration of K^+ ions on the outside of the neuron than there is on the inside of the neuron and a greater concentration of Na^+ ions on the inside than there is on the outside. The original concentration gradients must quickly be restored because the initiation of an action potential depends on the original ratios of Na^+ and K^+ ions with respect to the inside and the outside of the neuron. Restoration of the original concentration gradients is achieved by sodium-potassium pumps (Figure 2.17). Contrary to the forces of diffusion and electrostatic pressure, this is an active process that requires energy in the form of adenosine triphosphate (ATP), the energy currency of cells. For each molecule of ATP that is broken down into adenosine diphosphate (ADP), the sodium-potassium pump transfers three Na^+ ions out of the neuron and two K^+ ions back into the neuron.

Once the depolarization of the membrane crosses the activation threshold, all action potentials are of the same amplitude. That is, there is no such thing as a stronger or weaker action potential. Either a neuron fires an action potential or it does not. This is referred to as the **all-or-none law**. However, an intense stimulus, such as a punch on the arm versus a gentle stroke, will result in a higher frequency of action potentials. Therefore, the intensity of a stimulus is signaled not by the amplitude of action potentials but by their frequency (Figure 2.18).

You have learned how the entry of Na^+ through specialized channels triggers the initiation of action potentials. However, not much was said about the nature of these channels. As mentioned earlier, some channels open in response to mechanical deformations of the skin. These are known as stretch-gated or mechanosensitive channels, which mediate the sense of touch, discussed in Chapter 7. Others open or close in response to a change in voltage across the neuronal membrane. These are referred to as voltage-gated ion channels. These channels open or close in response to changes in voltage across the neuronal membrane. For example, you learned that Na^+ and K^+ channels open or close during the different phases of an action potential. These are referred to as voltage-gated Na^+ and voltage-gated K^+ channels. Other channels open through interacting with specific neurotransmitters. These are known as neurotransmitter-gated channels and are discussed in Chapter 3. Figure 2.19 illustrates how different types of stretch-activated and voltage-gated channels function.

2.3.3 PROPAGATION OF ACTION POTENTIALS

>> LO 2.3.3 **Explain how action potentials are propagated down the axons of neurons.**

Key Terms

- **Orthodromic conduction:** Movement of an action potential from the soma to the axon terminal.
- **Antidromic conduction:** Movement of an action potential toward the cell body.
- **Saltatory conduction:** Propagation of an action potential down an axon by jumping from one node of Ranvier to another.
- **Multiple sclerosis:** An autoimmune disease in which the myelin sheath is destroyed.

Figure 2.20 shows how an action potential is propagated down the axon of a neuron from the point of its initiation. As you already know, the entry of Na^+ ions through its channels causes the depolarization of the neuronal membrane. In addition, the Na^+ ions that have just entered the neuron diffuse down the axon away from the channel through which they entered. This causes the depolarization of the patch of membrane ahead of the channel, which triggers the opening of voltage-gated Na^+ channels. In this way, the action potential is continuously regenerated down the axon until it gets to the axon terminals. Depolarization of the axon terminal triggers the opening of voltage-gated Ca^{2+} channels. The entry of Ca^{2+} into the axon terminal triggers the release of a neurotransmitter into the synaptic cleft, which stimulates or inhibits

FIGURE 2.20

Propagation of an action potential. Following their entry into the neuron, Na^+ ions diffuse in both directions within the axon. This is followed by the exit of K^+ ions and the diffusion of Na^+ down the axon, depolarizing the patch of membrane ahead of where it initially entered, which in turn causes voltage-gated Na^+ channels to open. Another action potential is thus initiated.

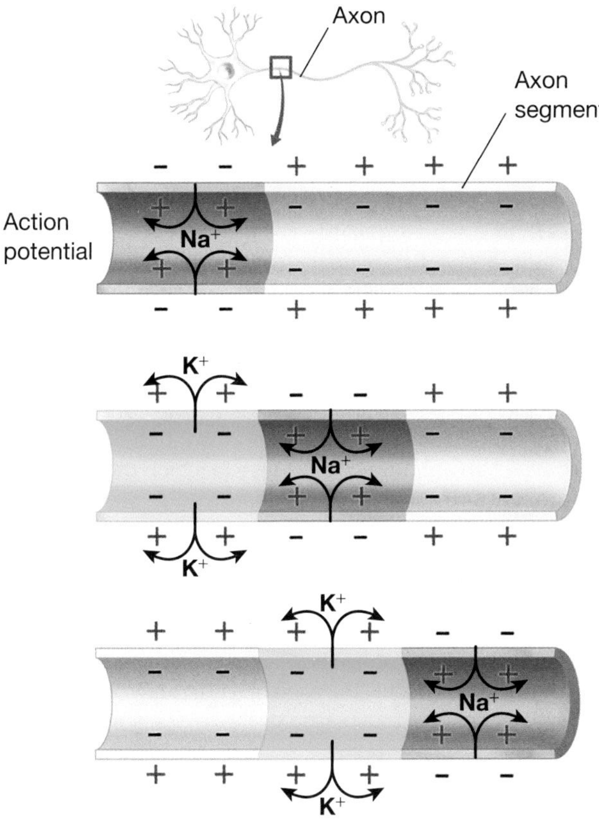

Amanda Tomasikiewicz/Body Scientific Intl.

FIGURE 2.21

Saltatory conduction. The myelin sheath is not continuous throughout the axon. It is interrupted by the nodes of Ranvier. Many voltage-gated Na^+ channels are present at the nodes of Ranvier, which permits the regeneration of action potentials. The depolarization of the membrane by the entry of Na^+ ions quickly spreads through the insulated part of the axon to again be regenerated at the following node.

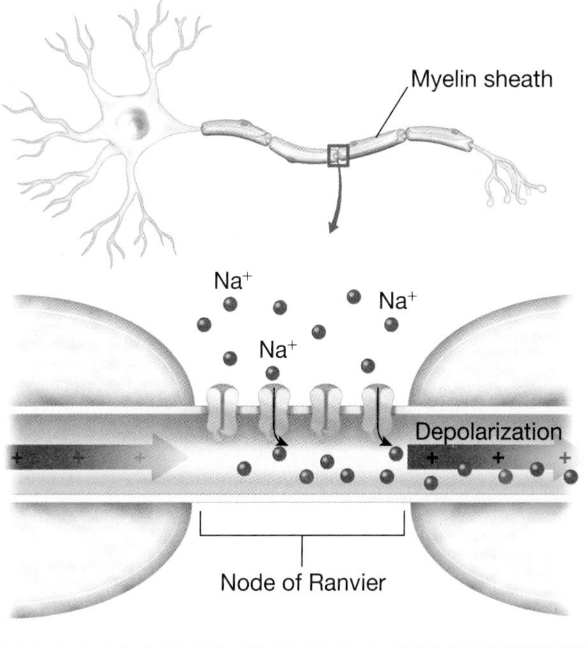

Amanda Tomasikiewicz/Body Scientific Intl.

the neuron or any other target cell the neuron is communicating with, a process discussed in Chapter 3.

Action potentials move through the axon in only one direction, from soma to the axon terminals. This is known as **orthodromic conduction**. Although Na^+ ions diffuse in both directions after entering the neuron, the patch of membrane before the point of entry is still in the absolute refractory period, during which no new action potential can be generated. **Antidromic conduction** refers to an action potential moving in the opposite direction, toward the cell body. However, this does not normally occur in neurons and can be achieved only in the laboratory.

The propagation of an action potential is facilitated by the myelin sheath, which insulates axons. One often-cited analogy for the insulation of axons provided by myelin is that of tape around a leaky garden hose. Without myelin, much of the current, flowing down the axon, escapes through the membrane, like water escapes through holes in a leaky garden hose. A break in the myelin sheath occurs at regular intervals called nodes of Ranvier, as mentioned earlier. At these intervals, a concentration of Na^+ channels can be found, where the action potential is regenerated. Depolarization of the membrane speeds down the covered part of the axon until the next node, to again be regenerated, a process called **saltatory conduction**, illustrated in Figure 2.21. In a devastating disease called **multiple sclerosis**, the myelin sheath is recognized as being foreign by the immune system and is progressively destroyed.

MODULE SUMMARY

The neuronal membrane is a phospholipid bilayer that keeps water and other molecules either on the outside or the inside of the neuron. The neuronal membrane has proteins that form channels that let specific ions in and out of the neuron. Two forces are at play in the exchange of ions across the neuronal membrane: diffusion and electrostatic pressure. The neuron at rest maintains a certain voltage (–70 mV). This voltage is called the resting membrane potential. Voltage is the difference in charge between the inside and the outside of the neuron.

Neurons communicate through generating electrical current in what are known as action potentials. Action potentials result from the movement of Na^+ and K^+ in and out of neurons. When channels selective for Na^+ open, Na^+ diffuses into the neuron due to its higher concentration on the outside relative to the inside of the neuron. This causes the membrane of the neuron to depolarize. This change in voltage causes Na^+ channels to close and K^+ channels to open. This causes K^+ to diffuse out of the neuron due to its higher concentration on the inside of the neuron relative to the outside, resulting in the repolarization of the neuron. This is followed by a period of hyperpolarization when the membrane voltage is below that of the resting membrane potential. The restoration of the initial relative concentrations of Na^+ and K^+ on the outside and inside of the neuron is performed by sodium-potassium pumps. Once a neuron reaches the threshold of voltage change during the depolarization of its membrane, it will generate an action potential. Every action potential is of equal intensity. This is known as the all-or-none law. The absolute refractory period refers to a period of 1 ms during which a new action potential cannot be generated. During the relative refractory period, which covers the periods of repolarization and after-hyperpolarization, a new action potential can be generated but is more difficult to induce.

Channels can be opened in a variety of ways. They can be stretch activated, voltage gated, or neurotransmitter gated. Depolarization of the axon terminals triggers the opening of voltage-gated Ca^{2+} channels. The entry of Ca^{2+} into the axon terminals triggers the release of neurotransmitters. These neurotransmitters then bind to specialized receptors on the postsynaptic neuron. Action potentials can travel only in the direction of the soma to the axon terminals. This is known as orthodromic conduction. Conduction in the opposite direction, from axon terminals to the soma, is known as antidromic conduction and can be achieved only in the laboratory. Myelin—the fatty tissue produced by oligodendrocytes in the central nervous system and Schwann cells in the peripheral nervous system—speeds up the conduction of nerve impulses through saltatory conduction. Multiple sclerosis is an autoimmune disease in which the myelin sheath that surrounds axons is destroyed.

TEST YOURSELF

2.3.1 What are the forces of diffusion and hydrostatic pressure?

2.3.2 Explain how an action potential is generated, and then name and describe each phase of an action potential.

2.3.3 Describe and explain how action potentials are propagated down the axon of a neuron. Make sure to include the role played by the myelin sheath.

2.4 Glia

Module Contents

2.4.1 Putting Glia Into Context

2.4.2 The Functions of Glia

Learning Objectives

2.4.1 Describe the initial discovery of glia and the role initially assigned to them.

2.4.2 Explain the functions of the different types of glia.

2.4.1 PUTTING GLIA INTO CONTEXT

>> LO 2.4.1 Describe the initial discovery of glia and the role initially assigned to them.

Key Terms

- ***Nervenkitt*:** German word for "nerve cement"; used by Rudolf Virchow to describe the role of glia.
- **Migration:** The process during which young neurons make their way to the superficial layers of the cortex.

So far you have learned about neurons and how they transmit information in the form of action potentials. However, as mentioned at the beginning of the chapter, neurons are not the only cells in the nervous system. The brain, with its approximately 86 billion neurons, contains just about as many glia (Azevedo et al., 2009).

The term *glia* was coined in 1858 by biologist Rudolf Virchow (1821–1902). *Glia* is Greek for "glue." Virchow chose this term for the non-neuronal cells of the nervous system because of his belief that they acted as "nerve cement" (German, ***nervenkitt***), lying between neurons and holding them together.

Today, we know that glia play many roles in the functioning of the nervous system. For example, depending on their type, they can clean up damaged tissue, cover axons with myelin, participate in neurotransmission, associate themselves with blood vessels to isolate the brain from potential toxins, and guide the **migration** of neurons to their proper brain area during development. The diversity of glia was first recognized in the 1920s.

2.4.2 THE FUNCTIONS OF GLIA

>> LO 2.4.2 **Explain the functions of the different types of glia.**

Key Terms

- **Phagocytosis:** The engulfing of particles by the membrane of a cell.
- **Apoptosis:** Organized cell death that results from cellular injury.
- **Phosphatidylserine:** A chemical marker that appears on dying cells, marking them for engulfment by microglia.
- **Lysosome:** An organelle that contains digestive enzymes.
- **Neuroplasticity:** The brain's ability to change with experience.

Microglia

Microglia are small in size, as their name suggests. They are activated when damage to nervous tissue occurs. For example, they play an important role in cleaning up damaged tissue and cell debris following a stroke, through the process of **phagocytosis** (*phago-* comes from the Greek word *phagein*, meaning "to devour") (Figure 2.22). A stroke occurs when an artery that brings blood up into the brain is clogged or ruptured. This causes some neurons to die by **apoptosis**, which is a form of organized cell death, because of a lack of oxygen and nutrients carried by the blood.

As a cell dies, it sends a chemical signal, which permits microglia to find it. This has been referred to as the "find me" phase. Another marker, consisting of a phospholipid (**phosphatidylserine**) that appears on the apoptotic cell surface, triggers the microglia to engulf the apoptotic cell. This has been referred to as the "eat me" phase. **Lysosomes**, which contain digestive enzymes, are drawn toward the apoptotic cell now sequestered in a vacuole (compartment) called a phagosome. The apoptotic cell is then digested within a phagolysosome, which is a phagosome that contains a lysosome. This has been referred to as the "digest me" phase (Brown & Neher, 2014; Ravichandran, 2010; Sierra, Abiega, Shahraz, & Neumann, 2013).

Macroglia

Macroglia are subdivided into many types. These are typically larger cells. Some of them are found

FIGURE 2.22

The three phases of phagocytosis: find me, eat me, and digest me.

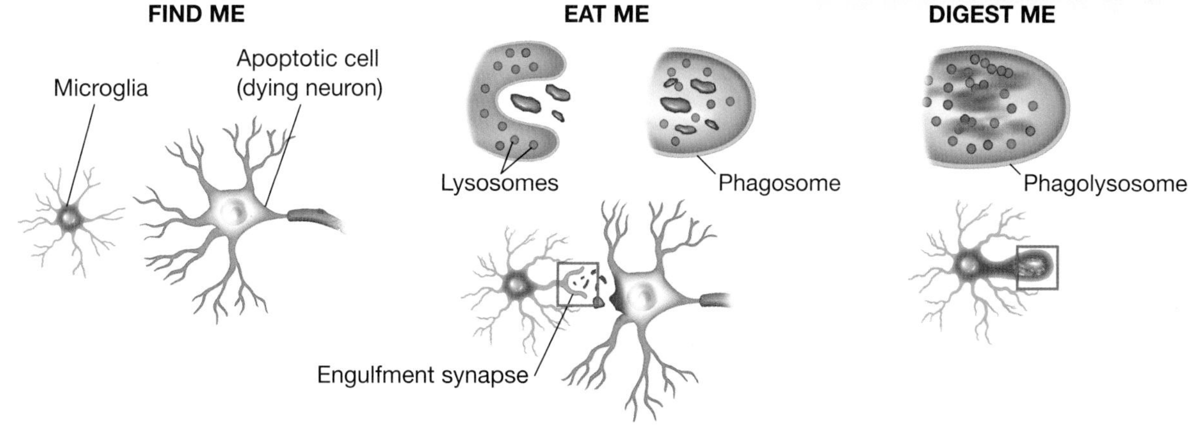

Amanda Tomasikiewicz/Body Scientific Intl.

exclusively in the central nervous system and others in the peripheral nervous system. These include astrocytes, radial glia, oligodendrocytes, and Schwann cells.

Astrocytes. Astrocytes clear increasing levels of K^+ from the extracellular fluid due to nearby neurotransmission (remember that K^+ leaves the neuron during action potentials). This action is made possible due to the high permeability of astrocytes to K^+ ions. The K^+ that flowed inside the astrocyte is then spread out to more distant areas. This process is referred to as K^+ spatial buffering (Kofuji & Newman, 2004). Astrocytes were also found to play an important role in cleansing the brain of bacteria, cellular debris, and toxins (Iliff et al., 2012). In addition, astrocytes are an important part of the blood-brain barrier (discussed in Chapter 4), which keeps potentially dangerous molecules from entering the brain.

We also know that astrocytes play an active role in neurotransmission and neuroplasticity. **Neuroplasticity** refers to the brain's ability to change with experience, such as during learning (a topic covered in detail in Chapter 12). An example of neuroplasticity is the strengthening of highly active synapses between neurons. Astrocytes can sense the release of neurotransmitters at active synapses, leading them to increase their intracellular levels of Ca^{2+}. This increase in Ca^{2+} levels causes astrocytes to release a neurotransmitter (also known as gliotransmitter) into the synapse, which in turn increases the amount of neurotransmitter released by the presynaptic neuron (N. J. Allen, 2014; Santello, Cali, & Bezzi, 2012).

Radial Glia. Radial glia play a crucial role during development of the central nervous system, more precisely during neuron migration, the process during which young neurons make their way to the superficial layers of the cortex (Rakic, 1972; Zheng & Yuan, 2008). Radial glia act as scaffolds for newly created neurons to follow. Figure 2.23 shows a young neuron climbing up the appendage of a radial glia The role played by radial glia in neurodevelopment is discussed further in Chapter 5.

FIGURE 2.23

Radial glia serve as scaffolds for migrating newly created neurons to the superficial layers of the cortex.

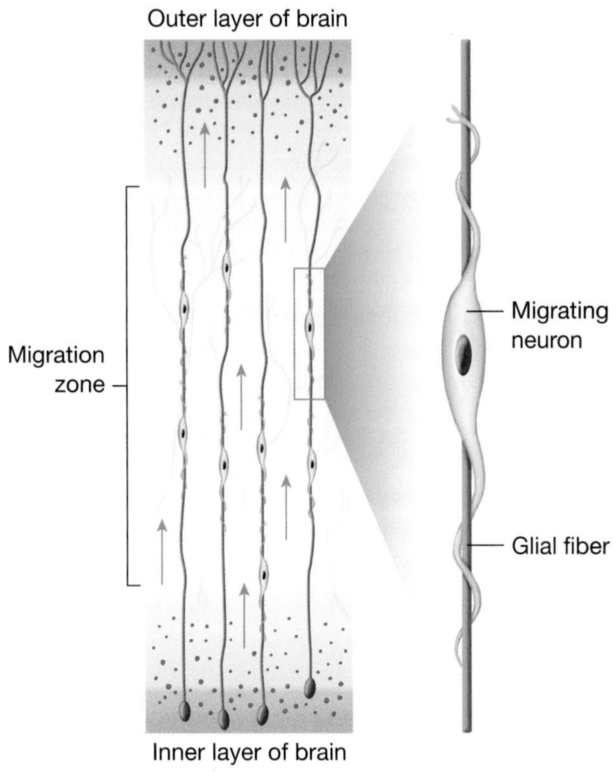

Adapted from illustration by Lydia Kibiuk, © 1995.

Oligodendrocytes and Schwann Cells. Oligodendrocytes produce and wrap the axons of neurons with myelin, which insulates axons in the central nervous system. The myelination process begins when an oligodendrocyte extends an appendage to an axon. Cytoplasm flows from the oligodendrocyte toward the axon to produce the myelin lamellae (Figure 2.24). Schwann cells are the glia that produce myelin for neurons of the peripheral nervous system. The process by which Schwann cells myelinate neurons in the peripheral nervous system differs from that of oligodendrocytes in the central nervous system. For example, a Schwann cell can myelinate only a single axon, whereas a single oligodendrocyte can myelinate up to 60 different axons.

MODULE SUMMARY

Glia is the Greek word for "glue." The term was coined by Rudolf Virchow to reflect his belief that glia acted as nerve cement that kept neurons together. In the 1920s, it was discovered that neurons come in many different types: microglia, astrocytes, and oligodendrocytes and Schwann cells. We now know that the role of glia is much more extensive than previously thought. Microglia clean up dead tissue and cellular debris through the process of phagocytosis. Astrocytes regulate the chemical environment of neurons and participate in the strengthening of synapses between neurons. Radial glia guide the migration of neurons to the superficial layers of the cortex during development. Oligodendrocytes and Schwann cells produce the myelin that insulates the axons of neurons in the central nervous system and peripheral nervous system, respectively.

FIGURE 2.24

Oligodendrocytes and the myelin sheath. (a) An oligodendrocyte projects its appendages onto the axon of a neuron. Cytoplasm is excreted by the oligodendrocyte, producing the myelin lamellae. (b) Cross-section of an axon showing its myelin sheath.

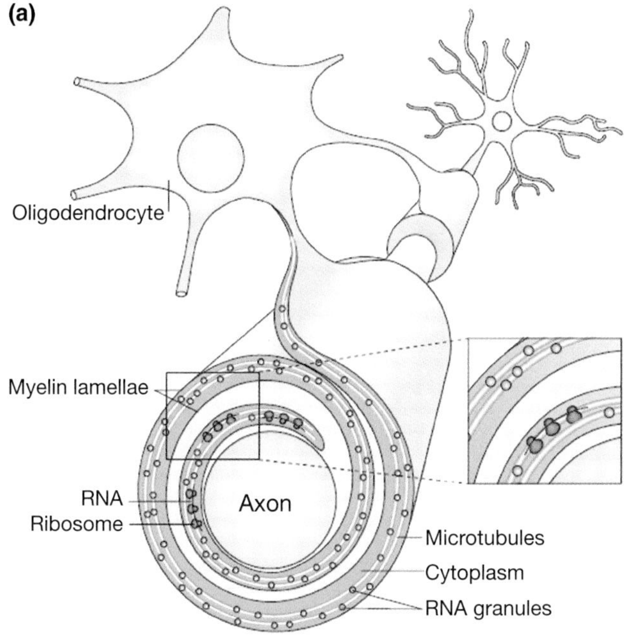

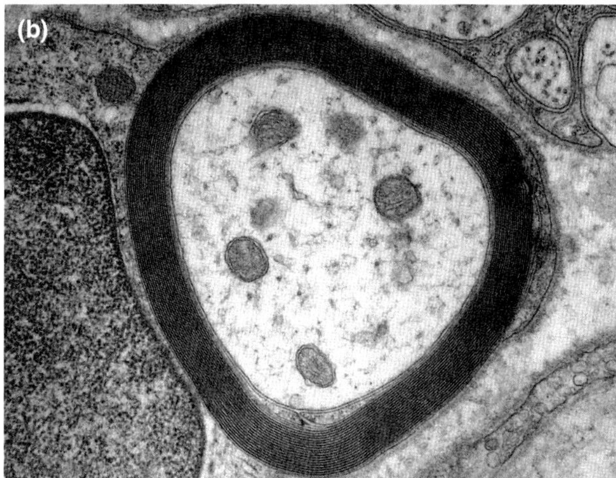

(a) Sherman, D. and P. Brophy. (2005). Mechanisms of axon ensheathment and myelin growth. *Nature Reviews Neuroscience* 6(9): 683–690. With permission from Springer Nature; (b) Scott Camazine / Alamy Stock Photo

TEST YOURSELF

2.4.1 Describe the roles initially assigned to glia.

2.4.2 Explain the functions of the different types of glia.

APPLICATIONS

Optogenetics

Neuroscientists have been manipulating the flow of action potentials in neurons for decades. This has traditionally been done through the electrical stimulation of neurons or the use of drugs that can increase or decrease the flow of ions in and out of neurons.

Although these methods have proved to be extremely useful, neither can be used to target restricted sets of neurons. This kind of specificity has been achieved through optogenetics. Optogenetics is a method in which pulses of light are used to control the flow of action potentials within specific populations of neurons.

It has been known since the 1960s that certain microorganisms such as some algae and bacteria produce light-responsive proteins, called opsins, that regulate the electric charge across the membranes

(Continued)

(Continued)

of their cells. In the early 2000s, researchers found that the algae *Chlamydomonas* and *Volvox carteri* have light-activated sodium channels, now known as channelrhodopsin-2 (ChR2) and channelrhodopsin-1 (VChR1), respectively. It was also found that the bacterium *Natronomonas pharaonis* has light-activated chloride pumps (similar to sodium-potassium pumps). These chloride pumps are activated through the opsin called halorhodopsin (NpHR).

Action potentials are generated through the depolarization created by the flow of sodium ions into a neuron. In contrast, the flow of chloride ions into a neuron causes it to hyperpolarize, making it less likely

FIGURE 2.25

Top: Some of the microorganisms from which opsins are obtained. Middle: Different opsins are sensitive to different wavelengths of light, resulting in the opening of sodium (Na^+) channels or the activation of chloride (Cl^-) pumps. Bottom: The relative response of each of the opsins to different wavelengths of light.

Microbe

Wavelength (nanometers)

470 nm

535 nm

589 nm

589 nm

Channel

Na^+

Cl^-

ChR2 channelrhodopsin allows positive sodium ions to pass in response to blue light.

VChR1 channelrhodopsin responds to some wavelengths of green and yellow light.

NpHR halorhodopsin regulates the flow of negative chloride ions in response to yellow light.

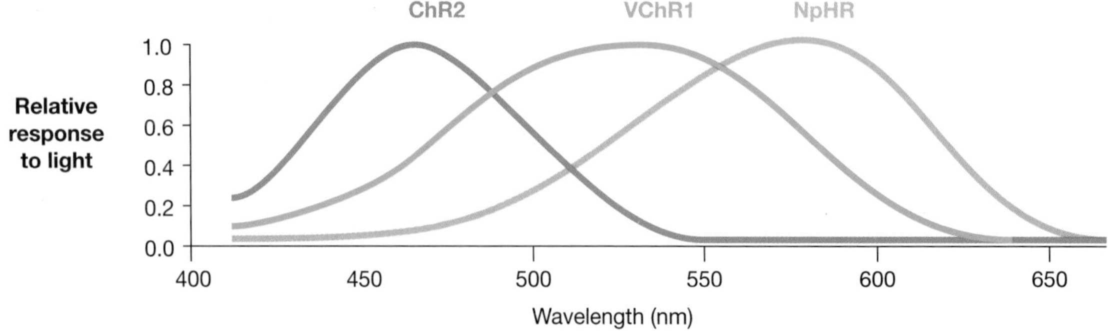

Carolina Hrejsa/Body Scientific Intl.

to generate action potentials. The stage was set to figure out a way to use this knowledge to turn neurons on and off at will.

How Did They Do It?

Researchers identified the sequence of genes that produces light-activated channels. The next step was to figure out a way to incorporate these channels into the neurons of living animals. Neuroscientist Karl Deisseroth at Stanford University achieved this with the use of transfection. Transfection is a method by which genetic material from one organism can be incorporated into the cells of another organism. To do this, the gene responsible for light-activated channels is spliced into the genes of a harmless virus, known as a viral vector. The virus is then injected into the neurons of an animal, which will now produce its own light-activated channels.

As illustrated in Figure 2.25, each channel is mostly activated with lights of a different wavelength. When activated, ChR2 and VChR1 channels increase the flow of sodium ions into neurons, leading to their depolarization. NpHR-activated pumps increase the flow of chloride ions into the neuron, leading to their hyperpolarization. Once the genes coding for the light-activated channels and pumps are expressed, light of different wavelengths can be delivered to the brain with a fiber-optic cable. ●

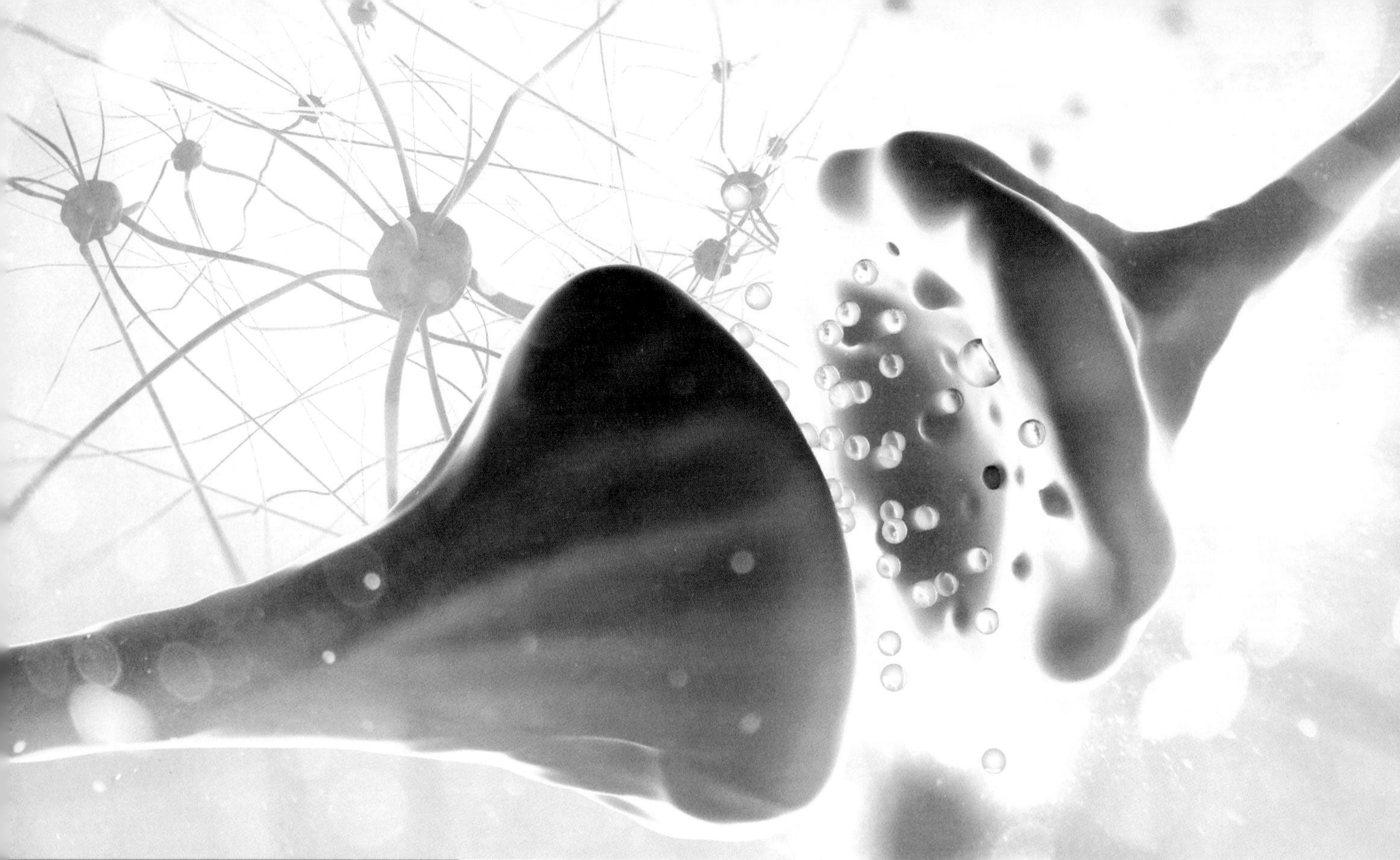

iStock.com/solvod

3 The Synapse, Neurotransmitters, Drugs, and Addiction

Chapter Contents

Learning Objectives

3.1.1 Describe and explain what constitutes a synapse.

3.1.2 Describe what occurs at a synapse.

3.1.3 Explain what constitutes synaptic integration.

3.1.4 Describe the varieties of synapses.

3.2.1 Explain what a neurotransmitter is and identify the criteria that qualify a chemical as being a neurotransmitter.

3.2.2 Identify the different classes of neurotransmitters as well as their pathways, functions, and receptors.

3.3.1 Define what constitutes a psychoactive drug.

3.3.2 Define and explain drug addiction.

3.3.3 Identify and explain the neurobiological models of addiction.

3.3.4 Describe the neurobiological mechanisms of some commonly abused drugs.

A Chemical Attack

In April 2017, a chemical attack was unleashed on the citizens of northern Syria. Photographs of dead bodies and of people suffering terrible seizures made the headlines in media outlets all over the world. The chemical apparently used in the attack was the nerve agent sarin. Several nerve agents were originally developed as insecticides but were soon after developed for military use. The targets of many nerve agents are neurotransmitters, the chemicals used by neurons to communicate with each other as well as with other cells of the body. The target of sarin is the neurotransmitter acetylcholine. Acetylcholine is the neurotransmitter released from motor neurons onto muscle cells, causing them to contract. Acetylcholine is also the neurotransmitter that counteracts the increased physiological activity, such as increased heart rate, triggered by potential threats in the environment. Concentrations of acetylcholine are normally kept in check through its degradation by an enzyme known as acetylcholinesterase. This prevents muscles from contracting excessively and also prevents acetylcholine from overcompensating for the increased physiological response to potential threats. Sarin and other nerve agents bind to part of the acetylcholinesterase molecule and make it inactive. As a result, the effects of acetylcholine on muscle cells go unchecked, leading to uncontrollable twitching, paralysis, and possible respiratory failure. In addition, rising levels of acetylcholine result in drooling, sweating, nausea, vomiting, and abdominal pain.

INTRODUCTION

So far, you have learned how neurons conduct action potentials down the lengths of their axons and that the arrival of action potentials at axon terminals results in the release of a neurotransmitter, which is used to communicate with other neurons as well as with other types of cells. In this chapter, you will learn what occurs once neurotransmitter molecules are released onto neurons being communicated with. You will begin by discovering what constitutes the sites of connection between communicating neurons and what happens once a neuron has communicated with another cell through the release of a neurotransmitter. You will then learn about neurotransmitters, the classes into which they are subdivided, and how they carry out various functions in the nervous system. Finally, we will explore how people become addicted to drugs and how commonly abused drugs produce their effects on the nervous system.

3.1 The Synapse

Module Contents

Learning Objectives

3.1.1 Describe and explain what constitutes a synapse.

3.1.2 Describe what occurs at a synapse.

3.1.3 Explain what constitutes synaptic integration.

3.1.4 Describe the varieties of synapses.

3.1.1 WHAT IS A SYNAPSE?

>> LO 3.1.1 **Describe and explain what constitutes a synapse.**

Key Terms

- **Presynaptic element:** The axon terminals of the presynaptic neuron.
- **Postsynaptic element:** The areas that contains neurotransmitter receptors on the post-synaptic neuron.
- **Active zones:** The areas of the presynaptic axon terminal where synaptic vesicles bind to the axon terminal's membrane.
- **Postsynaptic densities:** Areas of the dendrite on which receptors are located.
- **Membrane differentiations:** The combination of the active zones of the presynaptic axon terminals and postsynaptic densities of the postsynaptic dendrites.
- **Axodendritic synapse:** A synapse between an axon and a dendrite.
- **Axoaxonic synapse:** A synapse between two axons.
- **Axosomatic synapse:** A synapse between an axon and a cell body.
- **Dendrodendritic synapse:** A synapse between two dendrites.

The arrival of action potentials at axon terminals of neurons triggers the release of chemical messengers known as neurotransmitters. Several types of neurotransmitters exist. Neurotransmitters can be differentiated by their molecular structures and their actions on the nervous system. Following their release, neurotransmitters cross a tiny gap, approximately 20–40 nanometers wide (a nanometer [nm] is one billionth of a meter) called the synaptic cleft (Ahmari & Smith, 2002). Neurotransmitters then bind to receptors located on other neurons or other types of cells—such as those of muscles, glands, and organs—to control their functions. The site at which neurons communicate with other cells is known as the synapse.

The neuron releasing a neurotransmitter into the synaptic cleft is referred to as the presynaptic neuron. The neuron across the synaptic cleft, which contains the receptors onto which the neurotransmitter binds, is referred to as the postsynaptic neuron. The synapse includes the **presynaptic element**, which consists of the axon terminals of the presynaptic neuron, the synaptic cleft, and the **postsynaptic element**, which are the areas that contain neurotransmitter receptors on the postsynaptic neuron.

The areas of a presynaptic neuron's axon terminals, from which neurotransmitters are released, are called **active zones**. The areas of a postsynaptic neuron's dendrites on which receptors are located are called **postsynaptic densities**. Together, the active zones of the presynaptic neuron and postsynaptic densities of the postsynaptic neuron are referred to as **membrane differentiations**.

Neurons can form several different kinds of synapses. A synapse can exist between the axon of a presynaptic neuron and a dendrite, an axon, or the cell body of a postsynaptic neuron. Synapses can also occur between a dendrite on the presynaptic neuron and a dendrite on the postsynaptic neuron. These different kinds of synapses are known, respectively, as **axodendritic**, **axoaxonic**, **axosomatic**, and **dendrodendritic** synapses (Figure 3.1a). Figure 3.1b shows a prototypical axodendritic synapse.

3.1.2 WHAT OCCURS AT A SYNAPSE?

>> LO 3.1.2 **Describe what occurs at a synapse.**

Key Terms

- **Synaptic vesicles:** Membrane-bound vesicles that contain small-molecule neurotransmitters.
- **Neurosecretory granules:** Membrane-bound vesicles that contain large-molecule neurotransmitters.
- **Transporters:** Proteins that transport neurotransmitters and other molecules across cellular membranes.
- **Docking:** The process by which synaptic vesicles align to the area from which they will release the neurotransmitters they contain.
- **Exocytosis:** The process by which molecules are exported out of a cell.
- **Endocytosis:** The process by which molecules are taken up into a cell.
- **Ionotropic receptors:** Receptors located on ion channels that directly affect the cell's function.
- **Neurotransmitter-gated ion channels:** Channels that open in response to the binding of a neurotransmitter to receptors located on the channel.
- **Metabotropic receptors:** Receptors located on proteins embedded in the neuronal membrane

FIGURE 3.1

(a) Types of synapses (not shown is a dendrodendritic synapse). (b) Close-up of an axodendritic synapse.

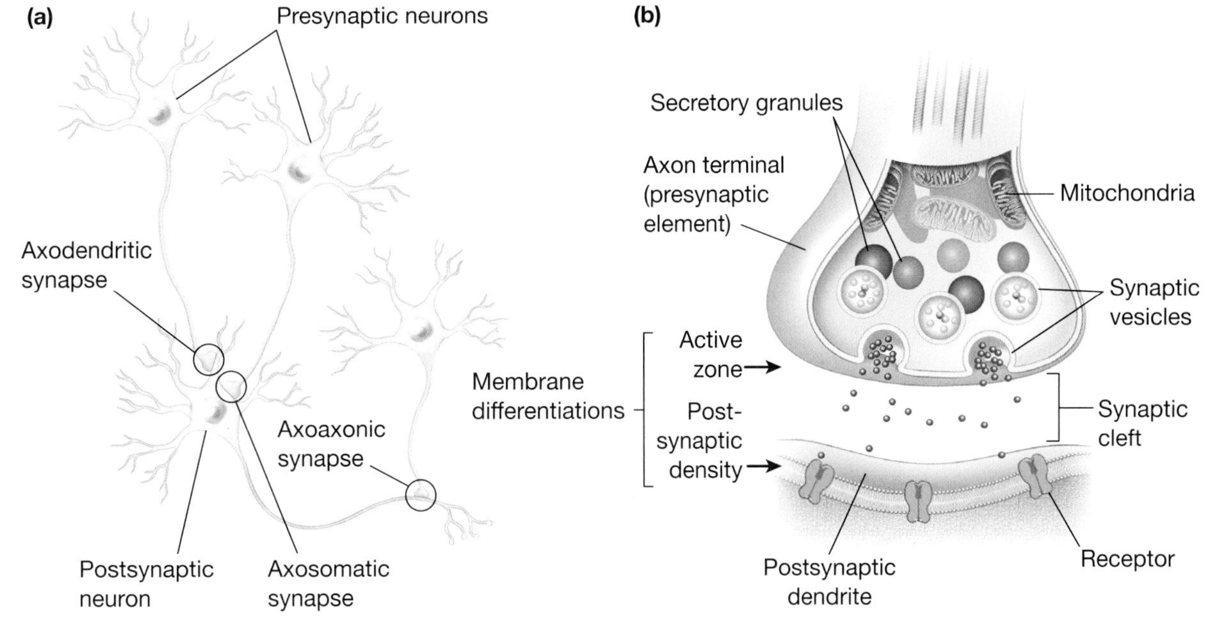

Amanda Tomasikiewicz/Body Scientific Intl.

that do not form channels but indirectly affect the cell's function.

- **G-protein**: A protein that, when activated, travels on the inside of the neuron, where it can influence its function.
- **G-protein-coupled receptor:** A type of receptor to which a G-protein is attached.
- **Shortcut pathway:** A pathway by which activated G-proteins can bind to ion channels from inside the cell.
- **Second messenger cascade:** The process by which a G-protein activates an effector enzyme, which in turn can synthesize molecules known as second messengers.

Remember from the preceding unit that a synapse is the point of communication between neurons or other types of cells. What occurs at a synapse can be subdivided into two sets of events. There are presynaptic events, which occur within presynaptic neurons, and postsynaptic events, which occur within postsynaptic neurons.

Presynaptic Events

Neurotransmitter molecules are stored in one of two types of vesicles located within axon terminals. What are known as small-molecule neurotransmitters are stored in membrane-enclosed sacs approximately 39.5 nm in diameter called **synaptic vesicles** (Qu, Akbergenova, Hu, & Schikorski, 2009). What are known as large-molecule neurotransmitters are stored in larger vesicles called **neurosecretory granules**. Other differences between these two types of neurotransmitters are discussed shortly.

Synaptic vesicles are produced in the soma of neurons. They are transported down to the axon terminals by the protein kinesin, which, as mentioned in Chapter 2, is responsible for anterograde transport (moving materials along microtubules from the soma to axon terminals). Proteins called **transporters**, which carry molecules across cellular membranes, then load the synaptic vesicles with small-molecule neurotransmitters, which are themselves synthesized from precursor molecules with the help of synthetic enzymes. Next, the synaptic vesicles make their way to the active zones. As you learned in the preceding unit, these are sites from which they will eventually be released.

When action potentials reach the axon terminals, depolarization of the neuronal membrane causes Ca^{2+} channels to open. The entry of Ca^{2+} causes synaptic vesicles to align to the area from which they will release the neurotransmitters they contain, in a process known as **docking**. Further entry of Ca^{2+} into the axon terminals causes the synaptic vesicles to fuse to the membrane and to release their contents of neurotransmitters into the synaptic cleft through **exocytosis**, the process by which molecules are exported out of a cell. The vesicles are then recovered through the reverse process of **endocytosis** and reloaded with a neurotransmitter.

The process by which large-molecule neurotransmitters are released is similar except that they are synthesized and processed by the endoplasmic reticulum and loaded into neurosecretory granules by the Golgi apparatus, within the soma of neurons. They are then transported to the axon terminals by axoplasmic transport.

Postsynaptic Events

The chemical structure of particular neurotransmitter molecules permits them to bind only to certain receptors, similar to how only exact copies of a single key can open a lock. Some of these receptors form ion channels, which, as you learned in Chapter 2, directly control the flow of ions across the neuronal membrane. These are known as **ionotropic receptors**. When bound to by neurotransmitters, ion channels open or close. Ion channels that respond to the binding of a neurotransmitter are known as **neurotransmitter-gated ion channels**. Other receptors are located on proteins that do not form channels but are embedded in the postsynaptic membrane. These indirectly affect the cell's function by triggering a cascade of events inside the cell. These are known as **metabotropic receptors** (Coutinho & Knopfel, 2002).

Many plants contain chemicals whose molecules are similar enough to a neurotransmitter to be a ligand of its receptor. In fact, all psychoactive drugs are ligands. The effects of these drugs are due to the actions of naturally occurring ligands in a large variety of plants. Examples include marijuana, cocaine, and morphine. A range of other drugs are ligands created in the laboratory. You will learn much more about the actions of drugs on the nervous system later in this chapter. For now, we will focus our attention on the two types of receptors mentioned earlier: ionotropic and metabotropic receptors.

Ionotropic Receptors

When a neurotransmitter binds to a transmitter-gated ionotropic receptor (Figure 3.2), it induces that receptor's channel to open or close by changing its shape. These receptors control various ion channels, such as Na^+ or Cl^-. The effect that the binding of a neurotransmitter to its receptor has on the cell depends on the channel's ion selectivity. For example, binding to a Na^+ channel results in the flow of Na^+ ions into the neuron, causing it to depolarize. In contrast, the binding of a neurotransmitter to receptors located on a Cl^- channel results in a flow of Cl^- ions into the neuron, causing it to hyperpolarize.

Metabotropic Receptors

In contrast to ionotropic receptors, metabotropic receptors are not located on ion channels. Instead,

FIGURE 3.2

An ionotropic receptor. Ionotropic receptors are located on ion channels known as neurotransmitter-gated channels. These channels open by changing their shapes in response to the binding of a neurotransmitter to its receptor.

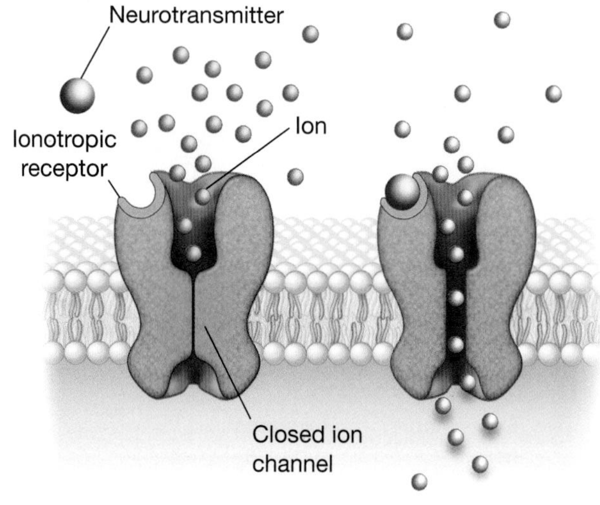

Carolina Hrejsa/Body Scientific Intl.

when a neurotransmitter binds to a metabotropic receptor, a protein attached to the inside of the cell membrane is activated. This protein is called guanine nucleotide-binding protein, or simply **G-protein**. Receptors to which G-proteins are attached are called **G-protein-coupled receptors**. When activated, G-proteins travel on the inside of the neuron and influence its function. For example, in what is known as the **shortcut pathway** (Figure 3.3a), activated G-proteins bind to ion channels from inside the cell and cause it to open. Such a channel is said to be G-protein gated.

Another way in which metabotropic receptors influence cell function is through a **second messenger cascade** (Figure 3.3b), in which a G-protein activates an effector enzyme, which in turn can synthesize molecules known as second messengers. These second messengers can then interact with proteins to influence intracellular events.

An example of a second messenger cascade is the cyclic adenosine monophosphate (cAMP)-dependent pathway. In a cAMP-dependent pathway, a G-protein activates an effector enzyme called adenylyl cyclase. Once activated, adenylyl cyclase catalyzes the synthesis of cAMP, which is a second messenger. The presence of cAMP then activates protein kinase (PKA), which activates other proteins that can influence gene transcription in the nucleus of the cell. As you will learn in Chapter 12, this process is important to the formation of new memories.

FIGURE 3.3

Metabotropic receptors. (a) The shortcut pathway. (b) The second messenger cascade.

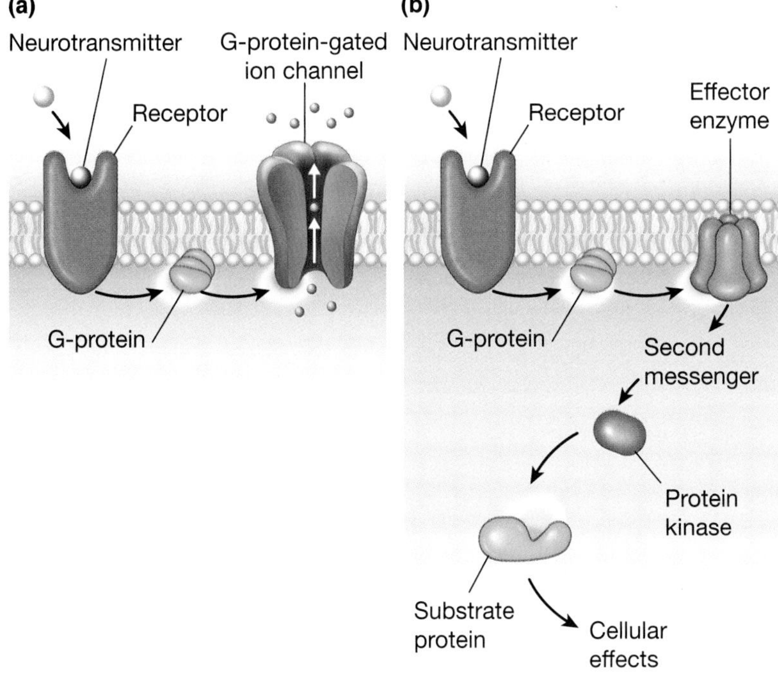

Amanda Tomasikiewicz/Body Scientific Intl.

For a long time, it was believed that axon terminals were only the sites of release for neurotransmitters and that receptors were located only on postsynaptic neurons. However, it is now known that receptors are also located on presynaptic axon terminals (Schlicker & Feuerstein, 2017). The role of some of these receptors is to regulate the release of neurotransmitters by the presynaptic neuron through a negative feedback loop. Think of a thermostat that regulates the temperature in your home. When the temperature rises, it turns down the heating to attain a comfortable level. Conversely, when the temperature drops, it turns up the heating. Autoreceptors act in a similar way. When neurotransmitter levels in the synaptic cleft are too high, they bind to the autoreceptors, which signal the presynaptic neuron to stop releasing neurotransmitters.

Neurotransmitter Removal

The neurotransmitters released into the synaptic cleft are permitted to remain there for only a short period. This is because neurotransmitter receptors become unresponsive when overly stimulated. This would spell disaster for the communication between neurons as signals from the presynaptic neurons would no longer have an effect on the postsynaptic cell. Also, prolonged activation of receptors may be excitotoxic, which means that it can lead to the death of neurons as a result of overstimulation. Three mechanisms exist to prevent this from happening: diffusion, degradation, and reuptake.

Diffusion. Neurotransmitters are removed from the synaptic cleft by diffusing away into extracellular fluid, where they are absorbed by glial cells (Bergles, Diamond, & Jahr, 1999).

Degradation. Once dissociated from their receptors, neurotransmitters are degraded by enzymes. For example, the enzyme monoamine oxidase (MAO) degrades, as its name suggests, the neurotransmitters of a class known as the monoamines, which you will learn about in more detail later in the chapter. Another neurotransmitter, known as acetylcholine, is degraded within the synaptic cleft into choline and acetic acid by the enzyme acetylcholinesterase (Figure 3.4). Acetylcholinesterase is the enzyme rendered inactive by nerve agents, the focus of the chapter's opening vignette. For this reason, neuroscientists are hard at work in an attempt to find an antidote to these agents (Kuca, Bajgar, & Kassa, 2019; Quinn, 2018). Drugs that block the actions of acetylcholinesterase, resulting in more acetylcholine being available to bind to receptors, are used in the treatment of Alzheimer's disease (discussed in Chapter 5). These drugs are known as acetylcholinesterase inhibitors, sometimes referred to as cholinesterase inhibitors (Shah, Dar, Dar, Ganie, & Kamal, 2017).

Reuptake. Neurotransmitters may also be reuptaken by the neuron that released them. The mechanism by which this occurs involves what are known as transporters (Olivares-Banuelos, Chi-Castaneda, & Ortega, 2019). Transporters are proteins that form channels across cell membranes. Many drugs, including those used in the treatment of psychological disorders, act through blocking the reuptake of neurotransmitters. The administration of these drugs results in more of the neurotransmitter being available in the synapse to bind to receptors. For example, some drugs block the reuptake of the neurotransmitter serotonin and/or norepinephrine in the treatment of major depression (a topic we will come back to in Chapter 14). These are commonly known as selective serotonin reuptake inhibitors (SSRIs) and serotonin/norepinephrine reuptake inhibitors (SNRIs) (Weilburg, 2004).

FIGURE 3.4

The degradation of acetylcholine. The enzyme acetylcholinesterase (AChE) degrades acetylcholine into choline and acetic acid.

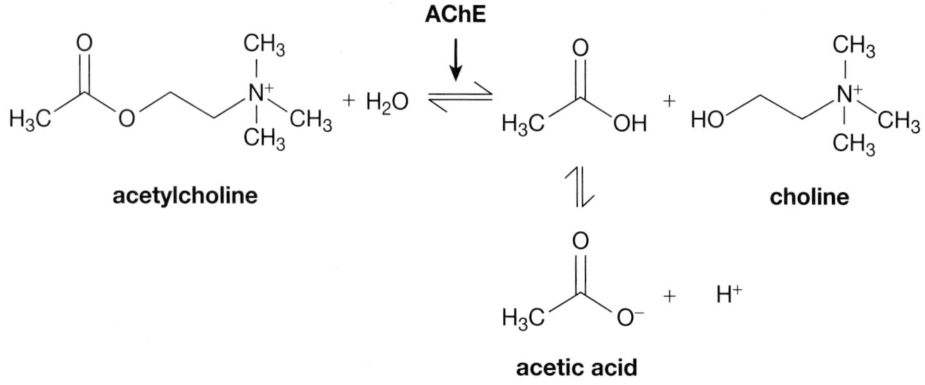

3.1.3 SYNAPTIC INTEGRATION

>> LO 3.1.3 **Explain what constitutes synaptic integration.**

Key Terms

- **Excitatory neurotransmitter:** A neurotransmitter that binds to receptors that trigger the opening of Na^+ channels, which results in the depolarization of the neuronal membrane.
- **Inhibitory neurotransmitter:** A neurotransmitter that binds to receptors that trigger the opening of Cl^- channels, which results in the hyperpolarization of the neuronal membrane.
- **Synaptic integration:** The computational process that a neuron performs to determine whether it will be more or less likely to fire an action potential.
- **Postsynaptic potential:** The change in voltage of the neuronal membrane due to the entry of Na^+ or Cl^- into a neuron.
- **Excitatory postsynaptic potential (EPSP):** A postsynaptic potential that causes the voltage of the membrane to move toward the activation threshold.
- **Inhibitory postsynaptic potential (IPSP):** A postsynaptic potential that causes the voltage of the neuronal membrane to move away from and below the activation threshold and even below the resting membrane potential.
- **Summation:** The processes of summing the input of neurons in the form of EPSPs or IPSPs, which may or may not result in the firing of action potentials.
- **Temporal summation:** When several postsynaptic potentials that follow each other with little delay are added together at the same synapse.
- **Spatial summation:** When several postsynaptic potentials that occur at the same time but at different synapses are added together.

You learned in Chapter 2 that an action potential is triggered when the entry of Na^+ into a neuron causes the neuronal membrane to depolarize beyond the activation threshold. You also learned that the activation threshold is approximately −55 mV. In the preceding unit, you learned that the entry of ions into a neuron can be triggered by the binding of a neurotransmitter to receptors. You also learned that a neurotransmitter can do this directly by binding to an ionotropic receptor or indirectly by binding to a metabotropic receptor.

A neurotransmitter that binds to receptors that trigger the opening of Na^+ channels, which results in the depolarization of the neuronal membrane, is referred to as an **excitatory neurotransmitter**. A neurotransmitter that binds to receptors that trigger the opening of Cl^- channels, which results in the hyperpolarization of the neuronal membrane, is referred to as an **inhibitory neurotransmitter**.

A single neuron can receive thousands of inputs from other neurons. On average, the number of synapses per neuron was estimated to range from 1,000 to 30,000 (Cherniak, 1990; Rockland, 2002). Some of these inputs are mediated by excitatory neurotransmitters, which form excitatory synapses. However, the same neuron also receives inputs mediated by inhibitory neurotransmitters, which form inhibitory synapses. These synapses hyperpolarize the neuronal membrane, making it less likely to fire action potentials. So, what is the neuron to do? To fire or not to fire? The answer is that the neuron adds up the excitatory and inhibitory messages it receives from other neurons. If the amount of excitation outweighs the amount of inhibition, the neuron will be more likely to fire an action potential. The computational process that a neuron performs to determine whether it will be more or less likely to fire an action potential is known as **synaptic integration**.

Postsynaptic Potentials

The change in voltage of the neuronal membrane due to the entry of Na^+ or Cl^- into a neuron is referred to as a **postsynaptic potential**. A postsynaptic potential that causes the voltage of the membrane to move toward the activation threshold is called an **excitatory postsynaptic potential (EPSP)**. A postsynaptic potential that causes the voltage of the neuronal membrane to move away from and below the activation threshold, and even below the resting membrane potential, is called an **inhibitory postsynaptic potential (IPSP)**. The difference between an EPSP and an IPSP is illustrated in Figure 3.5.

Students often confuse postsynaptic potentials and action potentials, but there are two main differences between the two. First, a postsynaptic potential could be either a depolarization or a hyperpolarization of the neuronal membrane. An action potential results in depolarization that crosses the neuron's activation threshold. Second, the depolarization associated with a single postsynaptic potential (you now know that this is an EPSP) is too small to cross the activation threshold and is short lived compared to an action potential.

Summation

A single postsynaptic potential changes the membrane voltage by approximately 1 mV (Yasunami, Kuno, & Matsuura, 1988). Therefore, EPSPs must add up to muster enough voltage to depolarize the neuronal membrane beyond the activation threshold (about -55 mV) at which an action potential can occur (Platkiewicz & Brette, 2010). This is known as **summation**. Two types of summation exist: temporal and spatial.

In 1906, British neurophysiologist Charles Scott Sherrington (1857–1952) observed that pinching one of a dog's legs resulted in a withdrawal reflex (D. Levine, 2007; Sherrington, 1906b). He also noticed that, on some occasions, the pinch was not intense enough to produce the reflex. However, if he repeatedly pinched the dog's leg in close succession, at the same place and with the same intensity, the reflex was observed. This is known as **temporal summation**, which occurs when several postsynaptic potentials that follow each other with little delay are added together at the same synapse. Sherrington also observed that several pinches, which by themselves did not give rise to the reflex, given at different places on the dog's leg at the same time resulted in the reflex. This is known as **spatial summation**, which occurs when several postsynaptic potentials that occur at the same time but at different synapses are added together. Similarly, IPSPs must also add up to cause enough hyperpolarization to prevent action potentials from occurring. Temporal and spatial summation are illustrated in Figure 3.6.

3.1.4 THE VARIETIES OF SYNAPSES

>> LO 3.1.4 **Describe the varieties of synapses.**

Key Terms

- **Afferent pathway:** A pathway through which trains of action potentials course through sensory neurons in the direction of the spinal cord.
- **Efferent pathway:** A pathway through which trains of action potentials course through motor neurons in the direction of the periphery.
- **Polysynaptic pathway:** A pathway to a response that requires more than one synapse.
- **Monosynaptic pathway:** A pathway to a response that requires only one synapse.

FIGURE 3.5

EPSP (left) and IPSP (right).

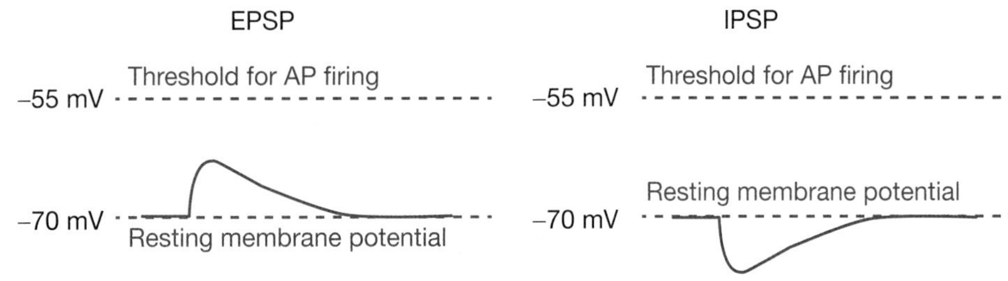

FIGURE 3.6

Temporal summation: (1) A single EPSP results in a small depolarization of the membrane but is not strong enough to produce an action potential. (2) and (3) Several EPSPs can combine to reach the activation threshold. Spatial summation: (4) Depolarization can also reach the activation threshold when several EPSPs occurring at different synapses are added together. Temporal summation of IPSPs: (5) and (6) The summation of IPSPs results in hyperpolarizations that take the neuronal membrane potential away from the activation threshold.

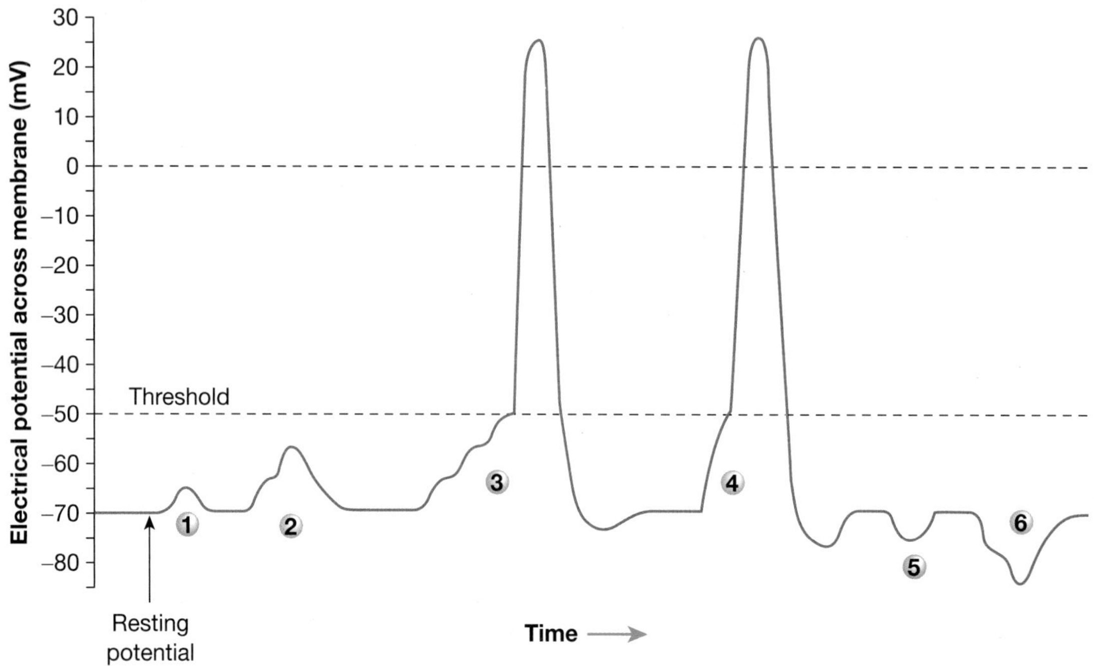

- **Neuromuscular junction:** The synapse between a motor neuron and a muscle cell.
- **Junctional folds:** Deep indentations in the membranes of muscle cells that are rich in neurotransmitter receptors.
- **Gap junctions:** The points of connection between presynaptic and postsynaptic neurons at electrical synapses.
- **Connexins:** Proteins that allow the passage of ions from one neuron to the other at electrical synapses.

Are Synapses Chemical or Electrical?

For some time, controversy existed as to whether communication between neurons occurred through chemical messengers (i.e., neurotransmitters) or through the direct transfer of electrical current from one neuron to another. The proponents of chemical transmission were said to be of the "soup" school, whereas the proponents of electrical transmission were said to be of the "spark" school.

The seeds that led to settling this controversy were planted in the early 1900s when British biologist Henry Dale (1875–1968) observed that a drug can interrupt the normal beating of the heart. This led Dale to hypothesize that neural transmission was chemical. Dale's hypothesis was tested in the 1920s by German pharmacologist Otto Loewi (1873–1961). He did so by conducting a clever experiment (Figure 3.7), which is famously said to have come to him in a dream. Loewi electrically stimulated the vagus nerve entering a frog's heart, which was bathed in fluid. As he expected, the heartbeat slowed (it was known that stimulation of the vagus nerve slows the heart). He then pumped some of the fluid, in which the heart was bathed, into fluid in which a second frog's heart was bathed. Guess what happened? The beat of the second heart also slowed.

This convinced Loewi that, upon stimulation, the vagus nerve released a chemical into the fluid in which the first heart was bathed. Pumping some of that fluid into the fluid in which the second heart was bathed transferred the same chemical into it, having the same effect it did on the first heart. Because the chemical was released by the vagus nerve, Loewi named it *vagusstoff* (German for "substance of the vagus nerve").

Loewi then stimulated the accelerator nerve of the first heart. He then accelerated the beating of the second heart by applying to it some of the fluid from the first heart. He called the chemical that accelerated the heart *acceleranstoff* ("substance that accelerates"). Dale

FIGURE 3.7

Otto Loewi's frog-heart experiment.

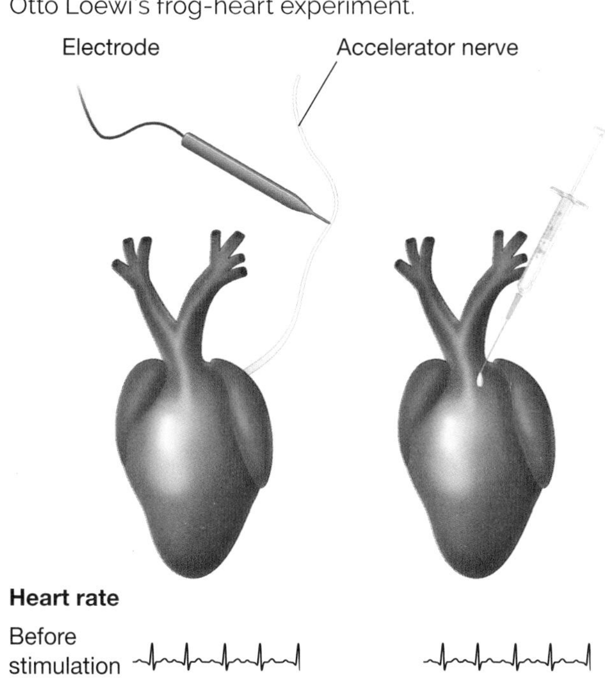

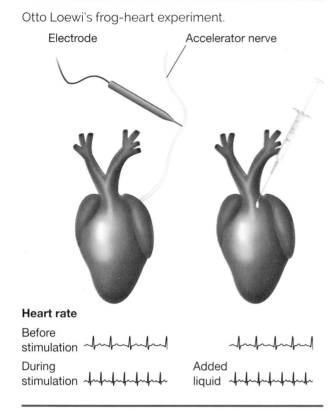

identified *vagusstoff* as what we now know as the neurotransmitter acetylcholine. *Acceleranstoff* was later identified by Swedish physiologist Ulf von Euler (1905–1933) as the neurotransmitter we now know as norepinephrine.

Synapses Within the Reflex Arc

Sherrington inferred the presence of synapses by studying the reflex arc in dogs. In a reflex arc, a stimulus such as touching a hot iron causes heat-sensitive Na^+ channels on sensory receptor cells to open. This causes a train of action potentials to course through what is known as the **afferent pathway** to the spinal cord.

Within the spinal cord, the axons of sensory neurons form synapses with interneurons, which in turn form synapses with motor neurons. The action potentials initiated in motor neurons course through what is known as the **efferent pathway** to the periphery. This causes muscles to contract, permitting the hand to be withdrawn from the painful stimulus.

Sherrington discovered that for muscle flexion to go unopposed, extensor muscles need to be inhibited. How is this achieved? The answer is that sensory neurons also form inhibitory synapses with motor neurons that connect to the extensor muscles (i.e., the triceps). Sherrington inferred the presence of synapses when he measured the distance a nerve impulse must travel from the point of stimulation on a dog's skin through the spinal cord and to the muscles. He measured the speed of conduction through the reflex arc to be 15 m/s (meters per second). This was in sharp contrast to the speed of conduction known at the time, 40 m/s. How did Sherrington account for this discrepancy? He hypothesized that the process must be slowed down where neurons communicate with each other, that is, at synapses.

The reflex arc contains two synapses: one from the sensory neuron to an interneuron, and another from the interneuron to the motor neuron. When a neuronal pathway, such as the one that composes the reflex arc, includes more than one synapse, it is said to be **polysynaptic**. Not that all reflexes are polysynaptic. For example, the patellar reflex (also known as the knee-jerk reflex), induced by your doctor when tapping the areas just below your knee, includes only one synapse: between a sensory neuron and a motor neuron. When a neuronal pathway includes only one synapse, it is said to be **monosynaptic**.

The Neuromuscular Junction

The synapse between a motor neuron and a muscle cell is known as the **neuromuscular junction**. Figure 3.8 illustrates a neuromuscular junction. One muscle cell is stimulated by only one motor neuron. The precise area at which the motor neurons synapse on the muscle cell is called the motor endplate. The neuromuscular

FIGURE 3.8

The neuromuscular junction. Top: A motor neuron forming synapses with muscle cells (fibers). Middle: Close-up of the motor endplate. Bottom: Close-up of the synapse at the neuromuscular junction.

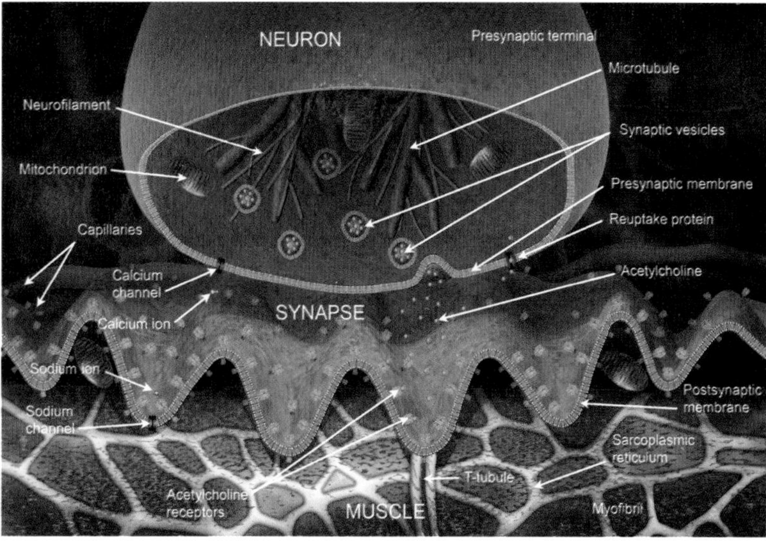

Carol and Mike Werner/Science Source

junction synapse differs significantly from the synapses that occur between neurons in the central nervous system (the innervation of muscles is in the peripheral nervous system). The membranes of muscle cells have deep indentations known as **junctional folds**. The active zones from the axon terminals of motor neurons line up above the folds. Each one of these junctional folds contains many receptors and Na^+ channels.

The neurotransmitter released from motor neurons' axon terminals is acetylcholine, the one that Loewi found to slow frog hearts. However, at the neuromuscular junction, acetylcholine is excitatory. Another difference between neuromuscular junction synapses and those in the central nervous system is that when acetylcholine binds to the receptors within the junctional folds, it gives rise to strong EPSPs (or endplate potentials) compared to those in the central nervous system. You learned earlier that a postsynaptic potential in the central nervous system, in the form of either an EPSP or an IPSP, causes a change in the membrane voltage of only about 1 mV. To result in an action potential in the central nervous system, EPSPs must add up through temporal and spatial summation. In contrast, a single EPSP at the neuromuscular junction causes a depolarization of about 70 mV. This is enough to depolarize the membrane beyond the activation threshold, which, as you learned, is about −55 mV. In addition, the neurotransmitter molecules that fall in the folds are guaranteed to interact with receptors, causing the opening of Na^+ channels. Together, these two factors make the synapse at the neuromuscular junction fail-safe.

The Electrical Synapse

Through his ingenious frog-heart experiment, Loewi discovered that the transmission of information between neurons was chemical. However, it was later discovered that some synapses are electrical. They occur at sites called **gap junctions** (Rozental, Giaume, & Spray, 2000). At gap junctions, synapses are lined with proteins called **connexins**, which allow the passage of ions from one neuron to the other. Transmission through these gap junctions is extremely fast because current passes directly from one neuron to the other. Like chemical synapses, they can either be excitatory or inhibitory. The differences between chemical and electrical synapses are illustrated in Figure 3.9. Although the bulk of synapses in the central nervous system are chemical, ongoing research is showing that gap junctions may play a larger role than was previously thought (Dong, Liu, & Li, 2018).

FIGURE 3.9

Comparison between an electrical synapse (left) and a chemical synapse (right).

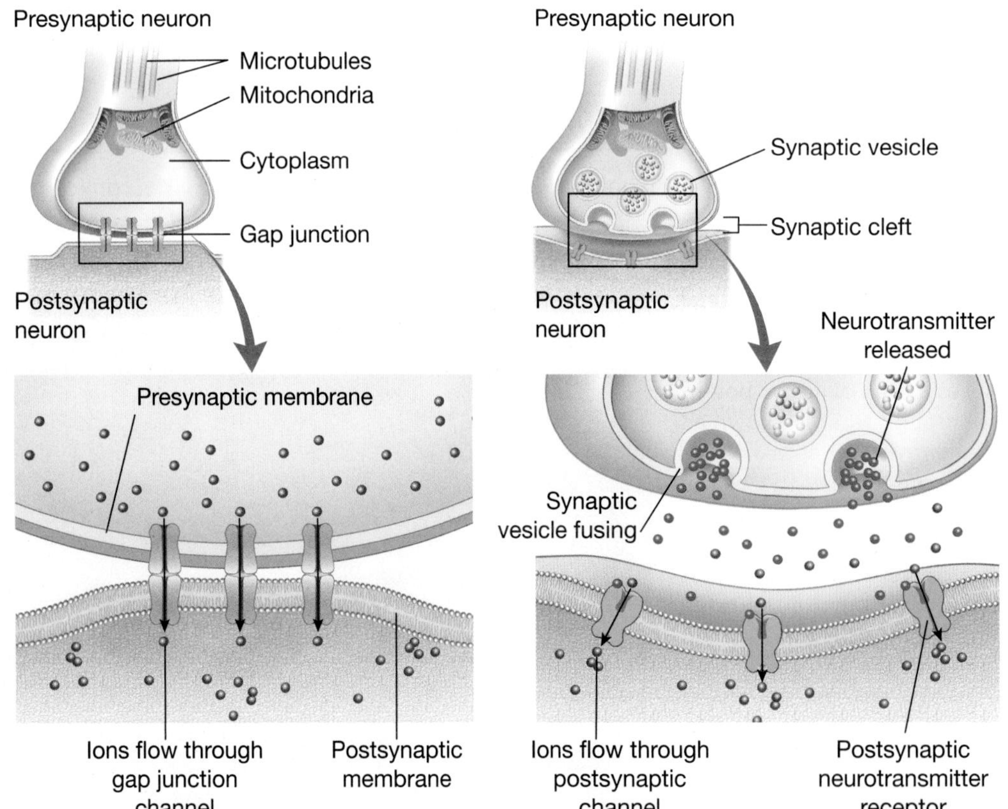

Amanda Tomasikiewicz/Body Scientific Intl.

MODULE SUMMARY

The synapse is the point at which neurons communicate with each other and with other types of cells. Neurons do not communicate with other cells through direct contact. They are separated by a tiny gap known as the synaptic cleft. They communicate with other cells through the release of neurotransmitters into the synaptic cleft onto receptors located on the cells they communicate with. The neuron that releases a neurotransmitter into the synaptic cleft is referred to as the presynaptic neuron. The cell that receives the neurotransmitter onto its receptors is referred to as the postsynaptic neuron.

Neurotransmitters can consist of small or large molecules. Both types are loaded into vesicles: synaptic vesicles for small-molecule neurotransmitters and neurosecretory granules for large-molecule neurotransmitters. These vesicles bind to the membrane of the presynaptic axon terminals and are released into the synaptic cleft through the process of exocytosis upon the arrival of action potentials into the axon terminals. The neurotransmitters cross the synaptic cleft and bind to receptors located on postsynaptic cells. There are two broad types of receptors: ionotropic and metabotropic receptors. Ionotropic receptors are located on ion channels and directly cause the opening of these channels. Metabotropic receptors indirectly affect a cell's function when they are bound with neurotransmitters, by the activation of G-proteins, which in turn activate second messengers. Neurotransmitters are cleared from the synaptic cleft in three ways: by diffusion, degradation, and reuptake. Specialized receptors, called autoreceptors, are located on the presynaptic neuron. Their function is to regulate the amount of neurotransmitter released by the presynaptic neuron. This may occur through a negative feedback loop.

The opening of channels permits charged ions to enter the postsynaptic cells. When charged ions enter postsynaptic cells, they create what are known as postsynaptic potentials, which are subthreshold depolarizations or hyperpolarizations of the postsynaptic cell. These differ from action potentials in which depolarization has crossed the activation threshold. Positively charged ions such as Na^+ depolarize the neuron in what are called excitatory postsynaptic potentials (EPSP). Negatively charged ions such as Cl^- hyperpolarize the postsynaptic cell in what are called inhibitory postsynaptic potentials (IPSP), making it less likely that the cell will fire an action potential. Although a single postsynaptic potential cannot give rise to an action potential, EPSPs can add up to result in a change in voltage that crosses the activation threshold. Adding together EPSPs or IPSPs is called summation. Summation can be temporal, in which several small depolarizations are induced in succession at the same synapse, or spatial, in which small depolarizations are induced at different synapses at the same time.

Significant controversy once existed surrounding the question of whether synapses were chemical or electrical. Otto Loewi was the first scientist to provide evidence that synapses were chemical. Sherrington inferred the presence of synapses when he found that the velocity of nerve conduction in the reflex arc was 15 m/s, which was significantly slower than the speed of 40 m/s known at the time. Neuronal pathways can include more than one synapse; these are known as polysynaptic pathways. Other neuronal pathways include only one synapse; these are known as monosynaptic pathways. Some motor neurons form synapses with muscle cells at neuromuscular junctions. Transmission of acetylcholine at the neuromuscular junction gives rise to EPSPs that are stronger than in the rest of the nervous system; this transmission is referred to as being fail-safe. We now know that electrical synapses exist, occurring at gap junctions where ions pass from one neuron to another.

TEST YOURSELF

3.1.1 What constitutes a synapse?

3.1.2 Describe what occurs at the synapse. Be sure to describe both presynaptic and postsynaptic events.

3.1.3 What constitutes synaptic integration?

3.1.4 Name and describe the varieties of synapses. How do they differ from each other?

3.2 Neurotransmitters

Module Contents

Learning Objectives

3.2.1 Explain what a neurotransmitter is and identify the criteria that qualify a chemical as being a neurotransmitter.

3.2.2 Identify the different classes of neurotransmitters as well as their pathways, functions, and receptors.

3.2.1 WHAT ARE NEUROTRANSMITTERS?

>> LO 3.2.1 Explain what a neurotransmitter is and identify the criteria that qualify a chemical as being a neurotransmitter.

So far you have learned about synapses, the point at which neurons communicate with each other as well as with other types of cells. You have also learned that most synapses are chemical. However, not much attention has yet been paid to the chemical messengers that make this communication possible. These chemical messengers are known as neurotransmitters. Neurotransmitters are chemicals that are released from neurons to affect a specific target. As you learned earlier, these targets are receptors located on other neurons or on other types of cells, such as the ones located on muscles, glands, and organs.

Because different substances in the nervous system can have similar actions, a substance must meet four criteria to qualify as being a neurotransmitter:

1. The substance must be synthesized in the presynaptic neuron.
2. The substance must be present in presynaptic terminals and have an effect on its postsynaptic target.
3. When experimentally applied, the substance must mimic the effects of the substance that is naturally released by the neuron.
4. A mechanism must exist for the substance to be cleared from the synaptic cleft.

Let's summarize seven key points that you should already know about neurotransmitters:

1. Neurotransmitters are chemical messengers that are synthesized, stored, and released by neurons.
2. There are two broad types of neurotransmitters: small-molecule neurotransmitters and large-molecule neurotransmitters.
3. Small-molecule neurotransmitters are synthesized in axon terminals and stored in synaptic vesicles, whereas large-molecule neurotransmitters are synthesized in the cell body and stored in neurosecretory granules.
4. Neurotransmitters are released into the synaptic cleft by presynaptic neurons through the process of exocytosis.
5. Neurotransmitters travel across the synaptic cleft and bind to receptors, mostly located on the dendrites of postsynaptic neurons.
6. Neurotransmitters could be excitatory or inhibitory. They are excitatory when they trigger EPSPs and inhibitory when they trigger IPSPs.
7. Neurotransmitters are also released onto types of cells other than neurons, for example, muscle cells, cells of internal organs, and glands.

3.2.2 NEUROTRANSMITTER SYSTEMS: PATHWAYS, FUNCTIONS, AND RECEPTORS

>> LO 3.2.2 Identify the different classes of neurotransmitters as well as their pathways, functions, and receptors.

Key Terms

- **Myasthenia gravis:** An autoimmune disease in which the body's immune system destroys the receptors for acetylcholine at the neuromuscular junction.
- **Clostridium botulinum:** A bacterium found in improperly conserved foods. It is better known as botulinum toxin.
- **Nigrostriatal pathway:** The pathway through which dopaminergic neurons project from the substantia nigra to the striatum.
- **Mesocorticolimbic pathway:** The pathway through which dopaminergic neurons project from the ventral-tegmental area. It is subdivided into the mesocortical and mesolimbic pathways.
- **Tuberoinfundibular pathway:** The pathway through which dopaminergic neurons project from the arcuate nucleus of the hypothalamus.
- **Parkinson's disease:** A neurodegenerative brain disease in which dopamine neurons in the substantia nigra die, giving rise to the inability of affected individuals to smoothly control their movements.
- **Mesocortical pathway:** The part of the mesocorticolimbic pathway that runs from the ventral-tegmental area to the prefrontal cortex.

- **Mesolimbic pathway:** The part of the mesocorticolimbic pathway that runs from the ventral-tegmental area to the nucleus accumbens, amygdala, and hippocampus.
- **Molecular coincidence detector:** A receptor that regulates the activity of a channel by detecting two events that are occurring in temporal proximity.
- **Allosteric modulation**: When different chemicals can regulate the activity of a channel by each having their own receptor site on that same channel.
- **Ligand-binding assay:** Adding a radioactive label to a molecule to trace its location in the tissue.
- **Retrograde signaling:** The process by which the activity of a neuron is regulated by a chemical messenger released by its postsynaptic target neuron.

Neurotransmitters can be subdivided into (a) small-molecule neurotransmitters, (b) large-molecule neurotransmitters, and (c) lipid neurotransmitters. Other types of neurotransmitters also exist, including gases such as nitric oxide, carbon monoxide, and sodium hydroxide, which serve diverse functions such as in the dilation of blood vessels and possibly the control of anxiety, sexual behavior, and aggression. Another type of neurotransmitter, the purine neurotransmitters, includes the inhibitory neurotransmitter adenosine. However, due to space considerations, these are not covered in the text.

Small-Molecule Neurotransmitters

Amines. The amines are small-molecule neurotransmitters that include acetylcholine, dopamine, norepinephrine, epinephrine, and serotonin. All of the amines, except for acetylcholine, are derived from a precursor amino acid (amino acids are molecules that serve as building blocks for proteins). Acetylcholine is derived from acetyl-coenzyme A and choline, a component of our diets. With the exception of acetylcholine, the amine neurotransmitters are subdivided further into the biogenic amines, which include the catecholamines and serotonin. The catecholamines are dopamine, norepinephrine (also known as noradrenaline), and epinephrine (also known as adrenaline). The catecholamines have as their precursor the amino acid tyrosine, whereas serotonin has for its precursor the amino acid tryptophan. Neurotransmitters are synthesized in steps. Each step is catalyzed by enzymes and gives rise to a variety of neurotransmitters.

Acetylcholine: Pathways and Functions

The cholinergic pathway (the pathway for acetylcholine) originates in two groups of cells (Figure 3.10). One of these groups forms what is known as the medial-septal system, which includes the medial septal nuclei and the nucleus basalis of Meynert of the basal forebrain. From there, cholinergic neurons project widely through the cortex and to the hippocampus. The other group is located in the pontomesencephalic tegmentum. These cholinergic neurons project to the thalamus, where they regulate sensory information on its way to the cortex.

FIGURE 3.10

The cholinergic pathway. Cholinergic neurons are organized into two systems: the medial-septal system, which also includes the nucleus of Meynert, and the pontomesencephalo-tegmental complex system.

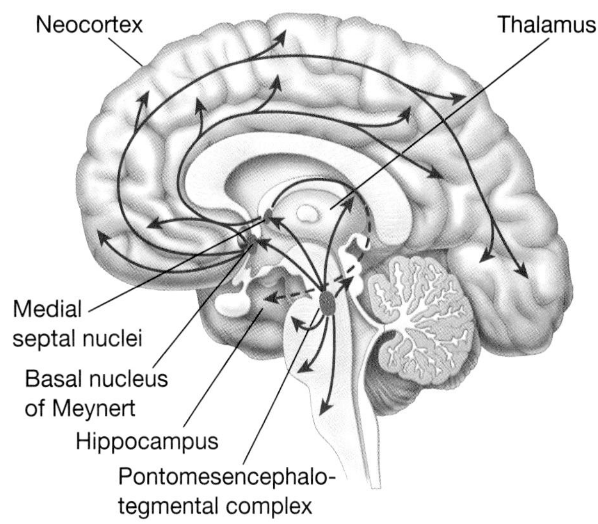

Acetylcholine in the medial-septal system plays an important role in cognitive processes, such as those involved in memory and attention (Hasselmo, 2006; Klinkenberg, Sambeth, & Blokland, 2011). This is believed to be so because cholinergic neurons, in the basal forebrain, have a large number of connections to the hippocampus, which, as you will learn in detail in Chapter 12, is known to be important for memory. In addition, disrupting the cholinergic input to the hippocampus results in impaired memory (Haam & Yakel, 2017). As you will read about in Chapter 5, the number of cholinergic neurons in the basal forebrain is significantly reduced in Alzheimer's disease, a neurodegenerative condition in which people suffer irreversible loss in memory and other cognitive functions (Grothe et al., 2014).

Acetylcholine is also the neurotransmitter used by motor neurons at the neuromuscular junction. In the autoimmune disease **myasthenia gravis**, the body's immune system destroys the receptors for acetylcholine at the neuromuscular junction. This disease is characterized by weakness of the muscles. Some of the symptoms include drooping eyelids or corners of the mouth, smoothed forehead, slurred speech, and weakness in the arms and legs (Figure 3.11a).

FIGURE 3.11

(a) The hallmark signs of myasthenia gravis include drooping eyelids, smoothing of the forehead, and drooping of the corners of the mouth. (b) A woman receives an injection of Botox, which when injected locally smooths out wrinkles.

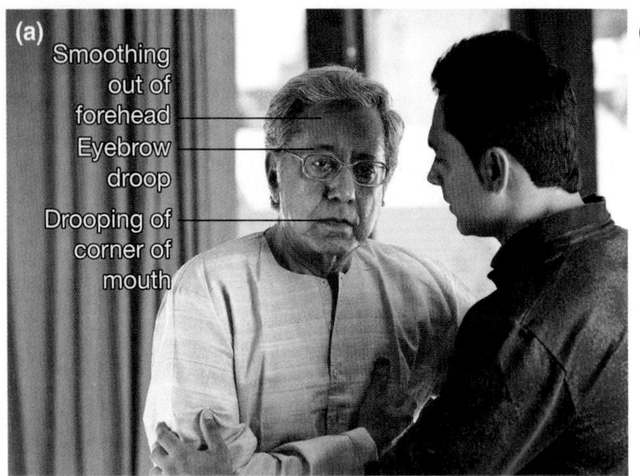

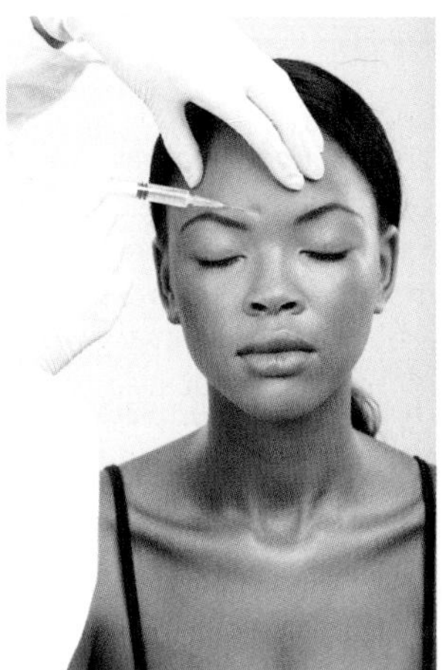

(a) iStock.com/triloks; (b) iStock.com/michaeljung

Have you ever heard of **Clostridium botulinum**? It is a bacterium found in improperly conserved foods. It is better known as botulinum toxin. When ingested, it blocks the release of acetylcholine from neurons at the neuromuscular junction. This results in muscle paralysis. It is the most powerful toxin known. If you have not heard about it, it also goes by the name of Botox. When injected locally, Botox paralyzes facial muscles for a certain length of time, smooths out wrinkles, and makes people look younger (Figure 3.11b).

Acetylcholine Receptors

Acetylcholine binds to nicotinic receptors at the neuromuscular junction, which causes your muscles to contract. Acetylcholine also binds to muscarinic receptors at the heart, causing it to slow down. These receptors got their names because nicotine, the drug present in the tobacco plant, and muscarine, a toxic substance that comes from a certain variety of mushrooms, are agonists of both types of receptors, respectively (Figure 3.12). The drug curare is a nicotinic receptor antagonist, whereas the drug atropine is a muscarinic receptor antagonist.

Dopamine: Pathways and Functions

As shown in Figure 3.13, dopaminergic neurons originate in three pathways: the **nigrostriatal pathway**, the **mesocorticolimbic pathway**, and the **tuberoinfundibular pathway**. Of the three pathways, we will focus only on the nigrostriatal pathway and the mesocorticolimbic pathway. Regarding the tuberoinfundibular pathway, it originates in neurons of the arcuate nucleus of the hypothalamus and it regulates milk production, through the release of the hormone prolactin from the pituitary gland (see Chapter 10).

The nigrostriatal pathway contains dopaminergic neurons that project from the substantia nigra to the striatum. These projections are important for regulating voluntary movement and the learning of motor skills. In the neurodegenerative disorder **Parkinson's disease**, dopamine neurons in the substantia nigra die, giving rise to the inability of affected individuals to smoothly control their movements.

The mesocorticolimbic pathway is subdivided further into the **mesocortical pathway** and the **mesolimbic pathway**. Dopaminergic neurons in the mesocortical pathway project from the ventral-tegmental area (VTA) to the prefrontal cortex. The prefrontal cortex is known to be important for executive functions. Executive

FIGURE 3.12

Nicotinic and muscarinic acetylcholine receptors. Nicotine can bind to and activate acetylcholine receptors at the neuromuscular junction, whereas muscarine can bind to and activate acetylcholine receptors in the heart. In contrast, curare and atropine block the actions of acetylcholine at nicotinic and muscarinic receptors, respectively.

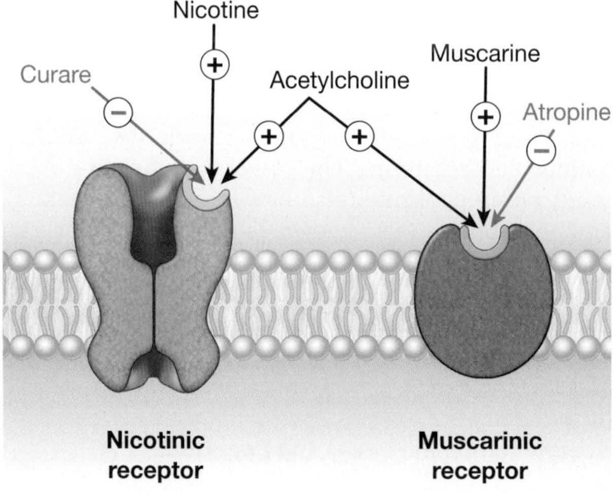

Carolina Hrejsa/Body Scientific Intl.

functions include goal-directed behavior, working memory, and attention. The prefrontal cortex is also involved in the selection of behaviors that are appropriate to the context. For example, it may be appropriate to put your feet up on your desk when you are at home, but you surely refrain from doing so when at your friend's house (Ott & Nieder, 2019).

The selection of contextually appropriate behaviors (i.e., not putting your feet up on your friend's desk), which requires behavioral flexibility, depends on the gating of sensory information by the prefrontal cortex. That is, sensory information in the form of the sight of a desk is held in working memory (a limited amount of information held for a short time [see Chapter 12]) and matched with the context in which it is located, your friend's house. This information is then relayed to other brain areas responsible for generating motor commands. The functions of the prefrontal cortex involved in this process depend on the input of dopamine neurons of the mesocortical pathway (Vijayraghavan, Major, & Everling, 2017).

Dopaminergic neurons in the mesolimbic pathway project from the VTA to the nucleus accumbens, amygdala, and hippocampus. The mesolimbic pathway plays a role in the control of emotional states and motivation. It is often referred to as the brain reward pathway (Wise, 2002) but has more recently been called the dopamine motive system. This is because its role may have more to do with the anticipation of a reward and how strongly the reward is associated with the cues that predict it (Berridge & Robinson, 2016; Volkow, Wise, & Baler, 2017). The brain reward pathway is discussed in the context of drug addiction later in this chapter and as it relates to motivated behaviors in general in Chapter 9.

The excess of dopamine neurotransmission in the mesolimbic pathway is thought to contribute to some of the symptoms of schizophrenia (a psychological disorder discussed in Chapter 14), such as hallucinations and delusions. Other symptoms of schizophrenia such as cognitive deficits and blunted emotional reactions are thought to be due to a decrease in dopamine in the mesocortical pathway (da Silva Alves, Figee, van Amelsvoort, Veltman, & de Haan, 2008; Pogarell et al., 2012).

Dopamine Receptors

There are five known dopamine receptors subtypes: D_1, D_2, D_3, D_4, and D_5. These subtypes are subdivided further into two subclasses, the D1-like subclass and the D2-like subclass. The D1-like subclass includes D_1 and D_5 receptors, whereas the D2-like subclass includes the D_2, D_3, and D_4 receptors. All dopamine receptors are G-protein-coupled receptors (see Figure 3.4 and accompanying text).

The subclasses can be differentiated by their structure and by the agonist and antagonist drugs that bind to them. Remember from Unit 3.1.2 that when bound to by a neurotransmitter, G-protein-coupled receptors (such as dopamine receptors) interact with second messengers, which can trigger a cascade of events inside the neuron. One such second messenger is cAMP (see Figure 3.3). D1-like and D2-like receptors can also be differentiated by their effects on cAMP. D1-like receptors stimulate the production of cAMP, whereas D2-like receptors inhibit its production. The behavioral functions of dopamine depend on the subtype of receptor to which it binds.

FIGURE 3.13

The dopaminergic pathways. Dopamine spreads through the brain via two pathways: the nigrostriatal pathway, projecting from the substantia nigra to the striatum, and the mesocorticolimbic pathway, projecting from the ventral-tegmental area to the frontal lobes (mesocortical) and limbic structures such as the amygdala, nucleus accumbens, and hippocampus (mesolimbic pathway). Only the nigrostriatal and mesocortical pathways are shown here.

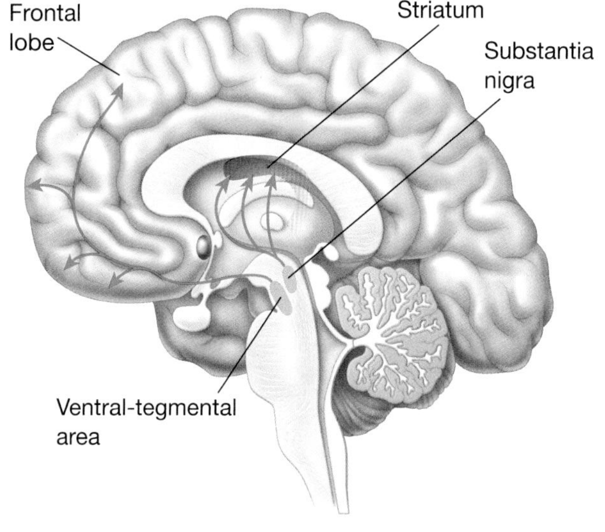

Norepinephrine: Pathways and Functions

Norepinephrine is produced by neurons in the locus coeruleus (an area located in the brainstem) that project to the cortex, spinal cord, cerebellum, temporal lobe, hypothalamus, and thalamus (Figure 3.14). Norepinephrine is important for regulating wakefulness (R. Brown, Basheer, McKenna, Strecker, & McCarley, 2012), as discussed in Chapter 9. It is also the neurotransmitter used to activate the sympathetic nervous system, which drives bodily changes such as accelerated heart rate, constriction of the blood vessels, and increased rate of respiration. These responses are associated with what is known as the "fight or flight" response, which is covered in more detail in Chapter 4.

Norepinephrine also plays an important role in cognitive functions through projections to the prefrontal cortex (Borodovitsyna, Flamini, & Chandler, 2017). Dysfunctions in the noradrenergic system are associated with a range of disorders, including depression, schizophrenia, anxiety disorders, Alzheimer's disease,

FIGURE 3.14

The noradrenergic pathway. Norepinephrine is produced by neurons in the locus coeruleus that project to the cortex, spinal cord, cerebellum, temporal lobe, hypothalamus, and thalamus.

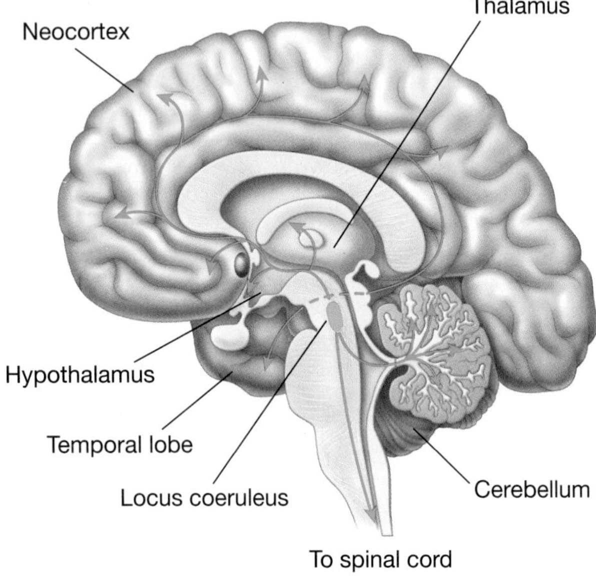

and Parkinson's disease (Borodovitsyna et al., 2017; Moret & Briley, 2011).

Norepinephrine Receptors (Adrenergic Receptors)

Norepinephrine receptors are known as adrenergic (or noradrenergic) receptors. Like the receptors for dopamine, adrenergic receptors are G-protein-coupled receptors. There are nine known subtypes of adrenergic receptors. These are subdivided into three categories: alpha-1 (α1), alpha-2 (α1), and beta (β) receptors. Alpha-1 and -2 receptors are the most abundant adrenergic receptors in the brain. Their activation is thought to play a role in attention and in the formation of memories (Sirvio & MacDonald, 1999). These receptors are also located in smooth muscles such as in the stomach, intestines, and bladder, and in the muscles that line the blood vessels. When activated, these receptors cause muscles to contract and blood vessels to become constricted (vasoconstriction), which is the constriction or narrowing of blood vessels. Beta receptors are primarily active in the periphery and contribute to the fight or flight response generated by the sympathetic nervous system (see Chapter 4).

Serotonin: Pathways and Functions

The cell bodies of serotonergic neurons are located in the raphe nuclei, within the brainstem. The

IT'S A MYTH!

Dopamine Is the "Pleasure Neurotransmitter"

The Myth

Dopamine is often referred to as the "pleasure neurotransmitter" in the media. A slew of media articles report the cause of addiction—including to drugs, shopping, food, guns, and sex—to be the intense pleasure induced by these activities, through the excessive release of dopamine.

Contrary to popular belief, however, dopamine is not the "pleasure neurotransmitter." In fact, scientists have found that dopamine release is associated with the *expectancy* of receiving a reward more than receipt of a reward itself. In addition, dopamine is involved in other functions. Finally, other brain chemicals have been found to be released in response to the receipt of a reward. Hence, dopamine scarcely deserves the title of "pleasure neurotransmitter."

Where Does the Myth Come From?

In the 1960s, neuroscientists James Olds and Peter Milner found that rats would repeatedly press a lever to receive electrical brain stimulation. In fact, rats quickly appeared to become addicted to pressing the bar to receive the stimulation. The area stimulated was found to be associated with the release of dopamine in the nucleus accumbens, which became part of what is known as the brain's reward system.

Why Is the Myth Wrong?

Dopamine neurons project to the brain through three pathways: the nigrostriatal pathway, the mesocorticolimbic pathway, and the tuberoinfundibular pathway. When discussing dopamine as the "pleasure neurotransmitter," what is being referred to is the so-called brain reward pathway. In this pathway, known as the mesocorticolimbic pathway, dopamine neurons originate in the ventral-tegmental area (VTA).

However, the role of dopamine in the other two pathways is comparatively rarely mentioned in the media. For example, the nigrostriatal pathway is involved in the production of movement, whereas the tuberoinfundibular pathway is involved in lactation by signaling the release of the hormone prolactin from the pituitary gland. The myth is also wrong because scientists now know that dopamine is involved in the anticipation of pleasure and for creating feelings of "wanting" rather than feelings of "liking" (Berridge & Robinson, 2016; Robinson & Berridge, 1993, 2008). In addition, feelings of pleasure are associated with a variety of other brain chemicals. Chemicals such as endorphins (which bind to opiate receptors) and anandamide (which binds to cannabinoid receptors) are the ones associated with the delivery of a reward itself.

Researchers even found that dopamine is released during aversive events (events that are not pleasurable). For example, in one study (L. Clark, Lawrence, Astley-Jones, & Gray, 2009), participants were given a gambling task in which they played a virtual slot machine, while their brains were imaged by functional magnetic resonance imaging (fMRI). The slot machine was rigged so that the experimenters controlled the number of times the symbols almost aligned (near misses) versus the number of times they did not (full misses). Experimenters also controlled the extent to which the participants felt they exerted control over the outcome of the game. They did this by either having the participants physically press a button setting the wheels into motion (perceived control) or having a computer set the wheels in motion (no control).

The researchers found that near misses were rated as more aversive than full misses. However, activity in the areas of the mesocorticolimbic pathway was significantly higher when the participants experienced near misses than when they experienced full misses, even if near misses were rated as being more aversive. They also found that this effect occurred only in the condition in which participants perceived having control over the outcome. ●

serotonergic pathway is illustrated in Figure 3.15. Neurons of the raphe nuclei are subdivided into two main groups known as the rostral group and the caudal group. The neurons in the rostral group reside in the rostral pons and project to the cortex, hypothalamus, thalamus, basal ganglia, and temporal lobes. The neurons in the caudal group reside in the caudal pons and project to the spinal cord, brainstem, and cerebellum.

Serotonin (also known as 5-hydroxytriptamine [5-HT]) is involved in the regulation of mood, sleep, and appetite. There is also evidence that serotonin plays a role in the brain's reward system by increasing the firing of dopamine neurons in the VTA (Wang et al., 2019). Dysfunctions in the serotonergic system are thought to be involved in various psychiatric disorders such as depression, schizophrenia, and those linked to anxiety such as obsessive-compulsive disorder, all of which we discuss in Chapter 14 (Zmudzka, Salaciak, Sapa, & Pytka, 2018). Serotonergic dysfunctions have also been linked to a variety of cognitive deficits, including memory loss, poor concentration, and impaired learning and executive functions (Svob Strac, Pivac, & Muck-Seler, 2016). Overactivation of serotonin receptors is associated with the psychedelic effects of hallucinogenic drugs such as lysergic-acid diethylamide (LSD) and psilocybin, the active compound found in magic mushrooms (Madsen et al., 2019).

Serotonin Receptors

Serotonin receptors form seven different families. The serotonin receptor families as well as their types (G-protein-coupled or ionotropic [ligand-gated]) are shown in Table 3.1. As you can see in the table, all but one of the families (5-HT_3) are G-protein-coupled receptors. Also shown in the table are their respective mechanisms in terms of decreasing or increasing levels of second messengers such as cAMP, inositol triphosphate (IP_3), and diacylglycerol (DAG). The behavioral, emotional, cognitive, and physiological roles of serotonin depend on the activity of these receptors.

FIGURE 3.15

The serotonergic pathway. Serotonergic neurons send projections to widespread areas in the nervous system, including the cortex, spinal cord, hypothalamus, thalamus, basal ganglia, temporal lobes, and cerebellum.

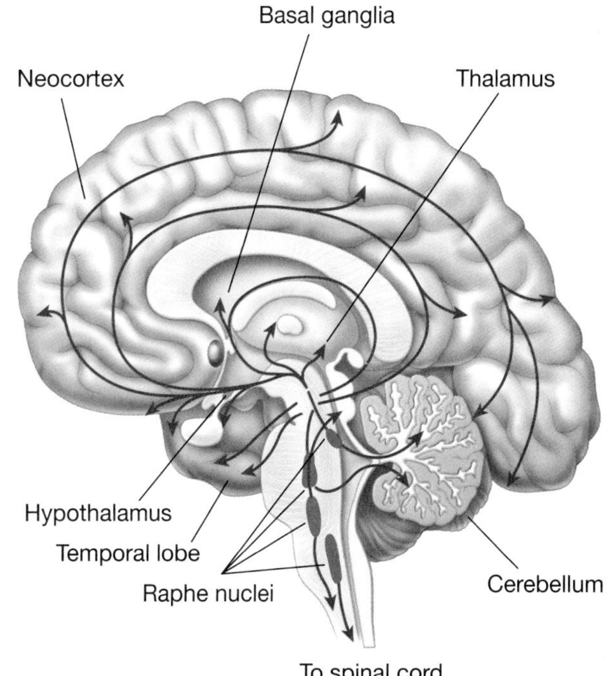

TABLE 3.1

Serotonergic Receptor Families, Types, and Mechanisms

SEROTONIN RECEPTORS			
FAMILY	TYPE	MECHANISM	POTENTIAL
5-HT_1	G-protein coupled	Decreasing cellular levels of cAMP	Inhibitory
5-HT_2	G-protein coupled	Increasing cellular levels of IP_3 and DAG	Excitatory
5-HT_3	Ligand-gated Na^+ and K^+ cation channel	Depolarizing plasma membrane	Excitatory
5-HT_4	G-protein coupled	Increasing cellular levels of cAMP	Excitatory
5-HT_5	G-protein coupled	Decreasing cellular levels of cAMP	Inhibitory
5-HT_6	G-protein coupled	Increasing cellular levels of cAMP	Excitatory
5-HT_7	G-protein coupled	Increasing cellular levels of cAMP	Excitatory

Amino Acid Neurotransmitters. Amino acid neurotransmitters are nonessential amino acids. Contrary to essential amino acids like tyrosine and tryptophan (the precursors of catecholamines and serotonin, respectively), they are not taken into the body through the diet. They are synthesized within the body. The main amino acid neurotransmitters are glutamate, glycine, and gamma-aminobutyric acid (GABA). Glutamate is synthesized from the amino acid glutamine. Glycine is itself an amino acid. GABA is not an amino acid itself but is synthesized from glutamate. The chemical reactions, mediated by enzymes, that give rise to glutamate from glutamine and the reactions that mediate the synthesis of GABA from glutamate are illustrated in Figure 3.16.

Glutamate

Glutamate is the most abundant excitatory neurotransmitter in the brain. Glutamate neurotransmission is concentrated mostly in the anterior cingulate cortex, the middle of the frontal lobes, and the hippocampus. Some evidence shows that it has a mesocorticolimbic pathway that parallels that of dopamine (Yamaguchi, Wang, Li, Ng, & Morales, 2011). Glutamate transmission is important for the formation of long-term memories (Sachser, Haubrich, Lunardi, & de Oliveira Alvares, 2017) (a topic discussed in Chapter 12). However, abnormally high levels of glutamate can damage neurons and even lead to their death. The toxicity of abnormally high levels of glutamate is linked to neurodegenerative disorders such as Parkinson's disease and Alzheimer's disease, as well as amyotrophic

FIGURE 3.16

The steps by which glutamate is synthesized from the amino acid glutamine and by which GABA is synthesized from glutamate.

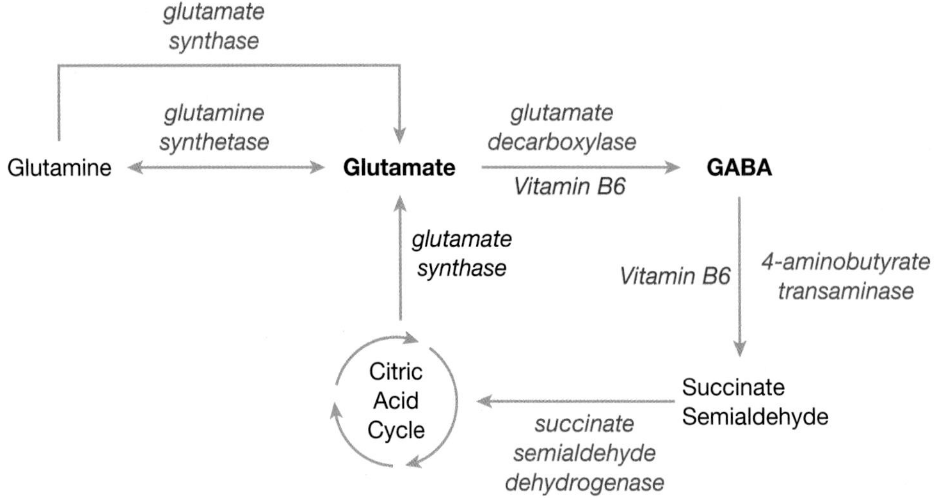

lateral sclerosis (ALS, also known as Lou Gehrig's disease) (Lau & Tymianski, 2010).

By contrast, lower than normal glutamate neurotransmission is thought to be a factor in the development of schizophrenia. Evidence for this comes from the observation that drugs that block glutamate neurotransmission, such as phencyclidine (PCP) and ketamine, give rise to schizophrenia-like symptoms (Frohlich & Van Horn, 2014).

The Glutamate Receptors

Figure 3.17 shows how the neurotransmitter glutamate can bind to at least three receptors: AMPA (α-amino-3-hydroxy-5-methyl-4-isoxazole propionate), NMDA (N-methyl-D-aspartate), and kainite receptors. Most of the excitatory neurotransmission in the nervous system occurs through AMPA and NMDA receptors. AMPA-gated receptors are permeable to Na+, and a large depolarization of the neuronal membrane occurs when they are open. Where you find AMPA receptors, NMDA receptors are nearby.

NMDA receptors differ from AMPA receptors in that their channels are permeable to Ca^{2+} in addition to Na^+. Another difference is that they are voltage gated. At resting membrane potential, the NMDA-receptor channel is blocked by magnesium (Mg^{2+}). This Mg^{2+} block prevents Na^+ and Ca^{2+} from entering the cell even if the binding of glutamate to the receptor opens the channel. So how does the NMDA receptor get rid of the Mg^{2+} block? The depolarization caused by the binding of glutamate to the AMPA channel causes the Mg^{2+} to pop out of the channel. This is shown in Figure 3.18.

For this reason, the NMDA receptor is known as a **molecular coincidence detector**. This is because for it to admit Na^+ and Ca^{2+} into the cell, two events need to occur in close temporal proximity: (a) the binding of glutamate to NMDA receptors and (b) depolarization of the membrane due to binding of glutamate to AMPA receptors.

Gamma-Aminobutyric Acid (GABA)

Gamma-aminobutyric acid (GABA) is the most abundant inhibitory neurotransmitter in the central nervous system. The main role of GABA is to silence the activity of neurons. GABA is also thought to play a role in the regulation of fear and anxiety (Crestani et al., 1999). There is also evidence for a mesocorticolimbic pathway for GABA (Crestani et al., 1999). As you will read later in this chapter, drugs that relieve anxiety and that can put you to sleep increase levels of GABA.

FIGURE 3.17

The three types of glutamate receptors: AMPA, NMDA, and kainate.

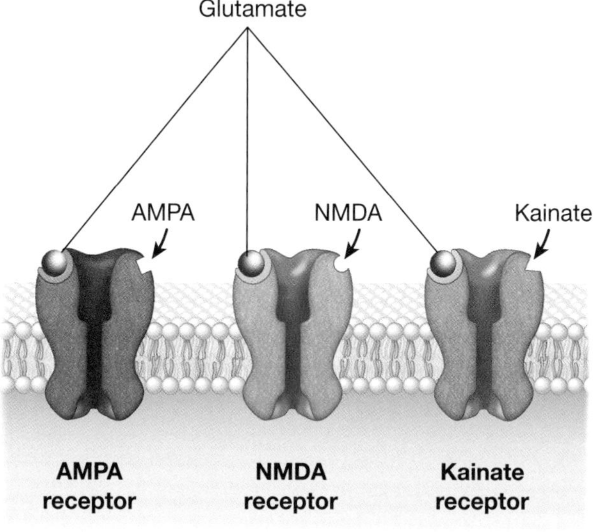

Carolina Hrejsa/Body Scientific Intl.

FIGURE 3.18

Mechanism for NMDA receptor opening. (a) At resting membrane potential, an Mg^{2+} block prevents Na^+ and Ca^{2+} from entering the neuron. (b) Upon depolarization of the membrane, due to the entry of Na^+ and Ca^{2+} through AMPA receptors, the Mg^{2+} block is removed and Na^+ and Ca^{2+} can enter the neuron. Also shown is the resulting efflux of K^+.

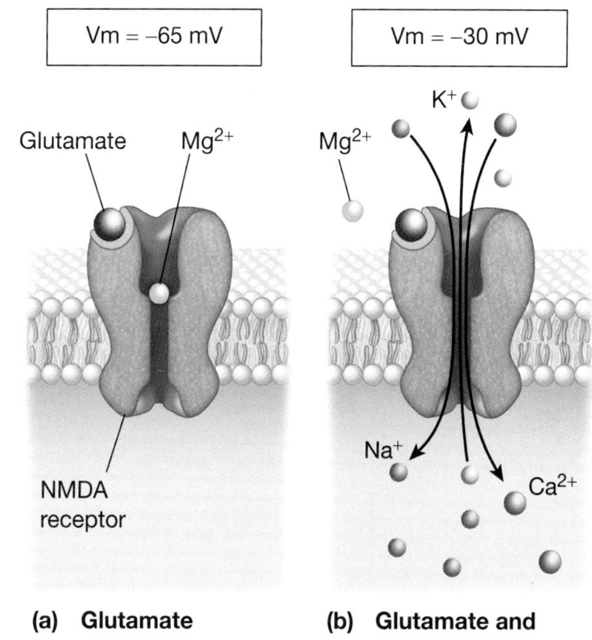

Carolina Hrejsa/Body Scientific Intl.

The GABA Receptors

GABA is an inhibitory neurotransmitter. GABA receptors are associated with Cl^- channels. The entry of Cl^- (an ion with a negative charge) leads to the hyperpolarization of neurons, making them less likely to fire. Some Cl^- channels are special in that they have different receptor sites for different chemicals. For example, in addition to GABA receptors, Cl^- channels have binding sites for drugs such as alcohol and other depressant drugs including barbiturates (sleeping pills), benzodiazepines (antianxiety medications), and general anesthetics. Such a channel is said to be regulated by **allosteric modulation** (Figure 3.19).

Glycine

Glycine is another inhibitory neurotransmitter. It is the major inhibitory neurotransmitter in the brainstem and spinal cord. During the rapid eye movement (REM) stage of sleep, your body is relatively paralyzed through a loss of muscle tone. You do most of your dreaming in REM sleep. One of the reasons for this is probably to prevent you from acting out your dreams. Researchers found that a deficiency in glycine might be responsible for REM sleep behavior disorder (see Chapter 9). People with this disorder are not paralyzed during REM sleep and, therefore, act out their dreams, which means they may talk, yell, punch, or kick in their dreams (Fraigne, Torontali, Snow, & Peever, 2015).

Large-Molecule Neurotransmitters

Neuroactive Peptides. Neuroactive peptides are large-molecule neurotransmitters. As mentioned earlier, neuroactive peptides are produced in the cell body, where they are stored in what are called neurosecretory granules. Only then are they transported to the axon terminals. This differs from small-molecule neurotransmitters that are both synthesized and uploaded in synaptic vesicles within axon terminals. Neuroactive peptides are released from neurons only after multiple action potentials. Neuroactive peptides can bind to receptors on neurons located in widespread areas away from the neurons that release them. The duration of their effects is also longer than that of small-molecule neurotransmitters.

There are at least 150 neuroactive peptides. Their role centers around the regulation of hunger, thirst, and pain. The most common neuroactive peptides are the opioid peptides. There are at least three opioid peptides: β-endorphin, enkephalin, and dynorphin. The opioid peptides have wide-ranging effects, including pain analgesia, reward mediation such as in drug addiction, and modulation of emotions and responses to stress. Just like the other neurotransmitters you learned about earlier, neuroactive peptides arise from precursor molecules.

The precursor molecule for β-endorphin is known as proopiomelanocortin (POMC), pro-enkephalin A for enkephalin, and prodynorphin for dynorphin (Chavkin, Shoemaker, McGinty, Bayon, & Bloom, 1985).

FIGURE 3.19

An allosterically modulated Cl^- channel.

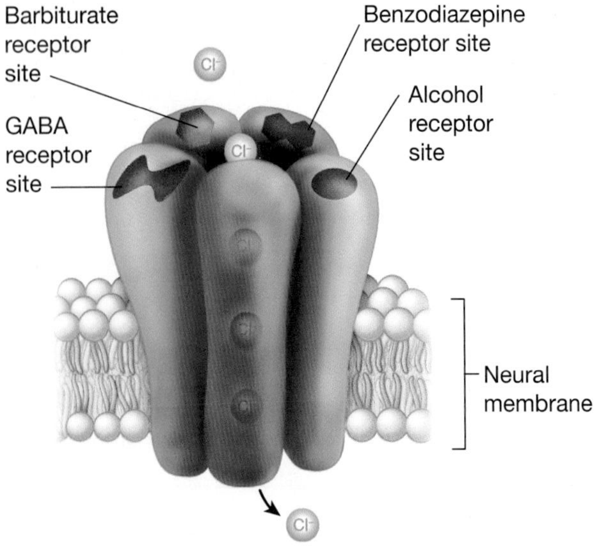

The Opioid Receptors. In the 1970s, neuroscientists Solomon Snyder and Candace Pert set out to discover how morphine produces its painkilling effects (Snyder & Pasternak, 2003). They did so with a method called a **ligand-binding assay**. This involved adding a radioactive label to morphine and applying it to brain sections of guinea pigs. They then looked through a microscope to determine where the radiolabeled morphine ended up and found that the morphine bound to specific receptors in the brain. These are now known as opioid receptors. They then realized that a brain chemical bound to the same receptors as the morphine. Morphine binds to the same receptor as endorphins because both molecules have a portion that fits into the same receptor.

We now know that there are at least three different types of opioid receptors. These are the mu (μ), delta (δ), and kappa (κ) receptors. Opioid receptors are G-protein-coupled receptors. Each receptor is associated with certain effects and is known to be bound to by specific opioid peptides (Pathan & Williams, 2012). The μ receptor is the primary mediator of the rewarding effects of drugs and is mostly bound to by β-endorphin. They are widely expressed in the brain's reward pathway, which includes the VTA and the nucleus accumbens. The δ receptor, mostly bound to by enkephalin, also plays a role in reward but significantly less so than the μ receptor. Both receptors are also involved in analgesia. The κ receptor is mostly bound to by dynorphin and is involved in regulating mood and stress. It is also thought to play a role in consciousness (Stiefel, Merrifield, & Holcombe, 2014).

Lipid Neurotransmitters Endocannabinoids. Like other neurotransmitters, endocannabinoids play an important role in the brain and are involved in various

FIGURE 3.20

The steps by which the lipid neurotransmitters anandamide (AEA) and 2-srachidonoglycerol (2-AG) are synthesized. (a) N-acetyltransferase and N-acyl phosphatidylethanolamine phospholipase D (NAPE-PLD) are enzymes that catalyze the reactions in the synthesis of AEA. The initial step in the synthesis of AEA produces another endocannabinoid known as N-arachidonoyl. (b) Phospholipase Cβ and DAG lipase catalyze the reactions in the synthesis of 2-AG. The initial step in the synthesis of 2-AG produces the second messenger DAG.

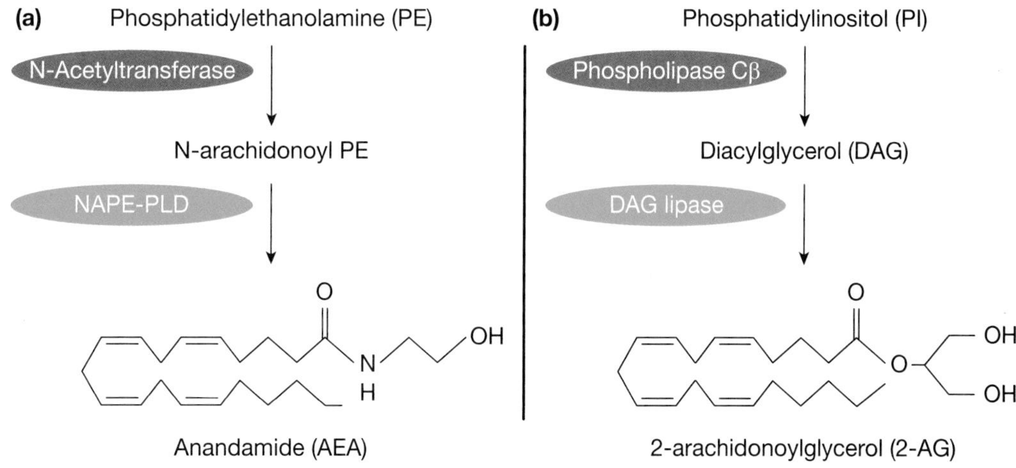

neurobiological processes, including the ones necessary for learning and memory (Marsicano & Lafenetre, 2009), appetite (Kirkham, 2005), sleep (Prospero-Garcia, Amancio-Belmont, Becerril Melendez, Ruiz-Contreras, & Mendez-Diaz, 2016), and the regulation of emotional states. It is also thought that the endocannabinoid system modulates the contents of dreams (Murillo-Rodriguez, Pastrana-Trejo, Salas-Crisostomo, & de-la-Cruz, 2017). Dysfunctions within the endocannabinoid system have been associated with disorders such as anxiety, depression, and schizophrenia (Pacher, Batkai, & Kunos, 2006). There are at least two endocannabinoids: anandamide and 2-arachidonoylglycerol (2-AG). The precursor molecule to anandamide is known as phosphatidylethanolamine (PE), and the precursor molecule to 2-AG is phosphatidylinositol (PI). Both are phospholipids, which are made up of fatty acids, glycerol, and phosphate. As with the other neurotransmitters, the synthesis of lipid neurotransmitters requires steps marked by reactions catalyzed by enzymes. The steps and the enzymes involved are illustrated in Figure 3.20. As you can see in Figure 3.20, the initial step in the synthesis of anandamide produces another endocannabinoid known as N-arachidonoyl, whereas the initial step in the synthesis of 2-AG produces the second messenger DAG.

Cannabinoid Receptors. There are two main types of cannabinoid receptors: CB_1 and CB_2 receptors. Most CB_1 receptors are found in the brain and other parts of the nervous system. CB_2 receptors are also found in diverse organs such as the spleen, liver, heart, and kidneys, where endocannabinoids help regulate biological functions. The activation of CB_1 receptors by

FIGURE 3.21

Retrograde signaling by endocannabinoids.

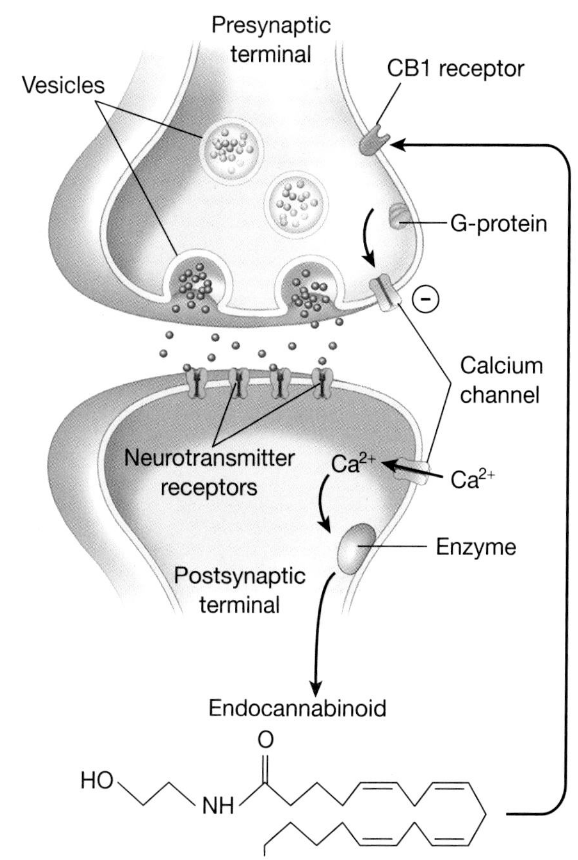

Carolina Hrejsa/Body Scientific Intl.

anandamide is thought to be involved in the sensation of pleasure or "liking" discussed in the next module (Mahler, Smith, & Berridge, 2007; M. R. Mitchell, Berridge, & Mahler, 2018).

These receptors are bound to by the neurotransmitter anandamide. Activation of CB_1 receptors inhibits the firing of neurons on which these receptors are present through **retrograde signaling** (Figure 3.21). Retrograde signaling is a process by which the activity of a neuron is regulated by a chemical messenger released by its postsynaptic target neuron (Lu & Mackie, 2016). In the endocannabinoid system, this occurs when the entry of Ca^{2+} in the postsynaptic neuron, in response to being stimulated by the presynaptic neuron, activates an enzyme that stimulates the production of endocannabinoids. These endocannabinoids then travel up to the presynaptic neuron where they bind to CB_1 receptors. The binding of endocannabinoids to CB_1 receptors, which are G-protein-coupled receptors, causes the closing of Ca^{2+} channels. This results in the inhibition of neurotransmitter release by the presynaptic neuron. For example, if an excitatory connection exists between two neurons, retrograde signaling will reduce the amount by which the postsynaptic neuron is stimulated.

MODULE SUMMARY

Neurotransmitters are chemical messengers by which neurons communicate. There are four specific criteria for a substance to be called a neurotransmitter: It must be synthesized and released by the presynaptic neuron; it must be present in axon terminals and affect a postsynaptic target; it must mimic the naturally occurring substance when experimentally applied; and there must be mechanisms to remove it from the synaptic cleft. There are three classes of neurotransmitters: large molecule, small molecule, and lipid. The neurons that produce and release specific neurotransmitters are organized into systems that bear the name of the neurotransmitter. Some neurotransmitters are known to be involved in disorders or diseases of the nervous system, for example, acetylcholine in Alzheimer's disease, dopamine in schizophrenia and Parkinson's disease, and serotonin in depression and other psychiatric disorders.

Neurotransmitter receptors were first discovered using the ligand-binding assay method, by which a molecule is radiolabeled and its location in brain tissue is traced. Each neurotransmitter is associated with its own receptors, but there are different types of receptors for the same neurotransmitter. For example, nicotine binds to receptors at the muscles where it is excitatory, whereas muscarine binds to receptors at the heart where it is inhibitory. Glutamate binds to three types of receptors: AMPA, NMDA, and kainite. NMDA receptors are molecular coincidence detectors. That is, they activate the channel they are associated with only when both the binding of glutamate to NMDA receptors and depolarization induced by the binding of glutamate to AMPA receptors occur in temporal proximity. Cl^- channels are regulated by allosteric modulation, meaning they can be regulated by several different substances. For example, the entry of Cl^- into a channel can be induced by the binding of GABA, alcohol, benzodiazepines, or barbiturates, each to their own receptors.

TEST YOURSELF

3.2.1 Give a definition of a neurotransmitter as well as the criteria for a substance to be considered a neurotransmitter.

3.2.2 (a) Name the different classes of neurotransmitters and the neurotransmitters in each class. (b) Describe the pathways for different neurotransmitters. (c) Describe the functions in which each of the neurotransmitters you learned about are implicated. (d) Describe the receptors for each of the neurotransmitters. What type of receptors are they? Are there any subtypes?

3.3 Drugs and Drug Addiction

Module Contents

3.3.1 What Is a Drug?

3.3.2 Drug Addiction

3.3.3 Neurobiological Models of Drug Addiction

3.3.4 Mechanisms of Action of Commonly Abused Drugs

Learning Objectives

3.3.1 Define what constitutes a psychoactive drug.

3.3.2 Define and explain drug addiction.

3.3.3 Identify and explain the neurobiological models of addiction.

3.3.4 Describe the neurobiological mechanisms of some commonly abused drugs.

3.3.1 WHAT IS A DRUG?

>> LO 3.3.1 Define what constitutes a psychoactive drug.

Key Terms

- **Drug:** A chemical or mixture of chemicals that alters physiological function.
- **Euphoria:** An enhanced sense of pleasure, excitement, and well-being.
- **Psychoactive drugs:** Drugs that can give rise to feelings of euphoria and altered perceptions.
- **Stimulants:** Drugs that speed activity in the central and peripheral nervous systems.
- **Depressants:** Drugs that slow activity in the central and peripheral nervous systems.
- **Hallucinogens:** Drugs that alter perceptions to the point of creating hallucinations.
- **Opiates:** Powerful painkillers that also provide feelings of intense feelings of pleasure, well-being, and calm.
- **Antagonists:** Drugs that block the actions of a neurotransmitter by binding to its receptors.
- **Agonists:** Drugs that bind to receptors to mimic the effects of the neurotransmitter that normally binds to it.
- **Inverse agonists:** Drugs that bind to a neurotransmitter receptor but exert opposite effects.
- **Reuptake inhibitors:** Drugs that inhibit the reuptake of a neurotransmitter by the neuron that released it.

A **drug** is a chemical or mixture of chemicals that can alter physiological function and structure. Some drugs affect mood, thinking, and behavior. They provide the user with what is commonly referred to as a "high." This includes an enhanced sense of pleasure, excitement, and well-being known as **euphoria**. They may also alter perceptions and give rise to hallucinations and/or bodily illusions. Such drugs are known as **psychoactive drugs**. Psychoactive drugs, such as cocaine, marijuana (in most states), and ecstasy, can only be obtained illegally. Others, such as alcohol, nicotine, and caffeine, are commonly used and are legal. Still other drugs, such as painkillers and antianxiety drugs, typically can only be obtained with a physician's prescription. However, these drugs also find their way to the streets and are purchased through the illicit drug market.

Psychoactive drugs can be divided into four broad categories: stimulants, depressants, hallucinogens, and opiates. **Stimulants** speed things up in the nervous system. They include drugs such as caffeine, cocaine, amphetamine, and nicotine. **Depressants** slow things down in the nervous system. They include drugs such as alcohol, antianxiety drugs, and sleeping pills. **Hallucinogens** alter perceptions by giving rise to hallucinations. Some hallucinogens also have stimulant properties. They include drugs such as LSD, mescaline, and psilocybin. Some hallucinogens also produce a sensation of the mind being dissociated from the body. These are known as dissociative drugs. They include ketamine and PCP. **Opiates** are powerful painkillers that also provide intense feelings of pleasure, well-being, and calm. These drugs include heroin, morphine, and codeine.

All psychoactive drugs exert their effects by altering the functions of neurotransmitter systems. They do so by their ability to bind to the same receptors as naturally occurring brain chemicals. Some drugs are ligands that block the actions of a neurotransmitter by binding to its receptors. These drugs are known as **antagonists**. Other drugs bind to receptors to mimic the effects of the neurotransmitter that normally binds to it. These drugs are known as **agonists**. Still other drugs bind to a neurotransmitter receptor but exert opposite effects. Such drugs are known as **inverse agonists**.

Some drugs can also exert their effects by inhibiting the reuptake of a neurotransmitter by the neuron that released it. These drugs are known as **reuptake inhibitors**. Some drugs can also inhibit the enzyme that destroys the neurotransmitters, making more of that neurotransmitter available at the synapse. Another way in which drugs can act is by inhibiting or facilitating the release of a neurotransmitter. Finally, drugs can affect the processes of synthesis, transport, or storage of neurotransmitters within neurons.

3.3.2 DRUG ADDICTION

>> LO 3.3.2 Define and explain drug addiction.

Key Terms

- **Drug abuse**: Using drugs in a way that causes physical and/or psychological harm to self or to others.
- **Addiction:** Drug abuse that is characterized by the presence of tolerance and withdrawal symptoms.
- **Tolerance**: The phenomenon by which a person needs to take increasingly large amounts of a drug to experience the same effects.
- **Dispositional tolerance:** When the body becomes progressively better at breaking down and eliminating the drug.

- **Behavioral tolerance:** When a person has learned to compensate for the drug's effects.
- **Functional tolerance:** When neurons progressively become adjusted to the effects of a drug.
- **Cell-adaptation theory:** The idea that functional tolerance occurs when neurons become progressively adjusted to the effects of a drug.
- **Withdrawal:** Occurs with the cessation of the use of a drug once the nervous system has adjusted to the drug's presence. Depending on the drug, withdrawal symptoms may include nausea, headaches, weakness, and body aches.
- **Anhedonia:** The inability to feel pleasure.

Almost everyone either uses drugs or has used drugs in the past. If you enjoy a cup of coffee in the morning, you are using a drug. However, you are not alone. It is estimated that 85% of Americans use a caffeinated beverage at least once a day (D. C. Mitchell, Knight, Hockenberry, Teplansky, & Hartman, 2014). People may use drugs socially, to manage pain, or for recreational purposes. Often, using drugs in such ways does not lead to undesirable consequences. However, people can also use drugs in ways that cause physical and/or psychological harm to themselves or to others who are affected by their behavior. Such a pattern of drug use is known as **drug abuse**.

Tolerance and Withdrawal

The most widely accepted signs of drug **addiction** are the presence of tolerance and/or withdrawal symptoms. **Tolerance** is the phenomenon by which a person needs to take increasingly large amounts of a drug to have the same effect. There are three types of tolerance: dispositional, behavioral, and functional tolerance.

Dispositional tolerance occurs when the body becomes progressively better at breaking down and eliminating a drug. **Behavioral tolerance** occurs when a person has learned to compensate for a drug's effects. For example, a person may still be able to walk a straight line even after drinking a substantial amount of alcohol. **Functional tolerance** occurs when neurons become progressively adjusted to the effects of a drug. This is known as the **cell-adaptation theory**.

To help you understand functional tolerance, imagine that someone repeatedly takes a stimulant. Stimulants accelerate activity in the nervous system. This is akin to stepping on a car's accelerator, or gas pedal. Now, to adjust for the acceleration, the nervous system responds by slowing things down. This is akin to stepping on the brakes. With repeated exposures to the stimulant, the nervous system becomes better at slowing things down, or stepping on the brakes. Therefore, progressively more drug is needed to produce the same effects. Can you think of a similar analogy to explain functional tolerance to a depressant drug?

Withdrawal symptoms occur with the cessation of the use of a drug once the nervous system has adjusted to it. Depending on the drug, withdrawal symptoms may include nausea, headaches, weakness, and body aches. It also often includes psychological symptoms, such as anxiety, depression, and irritability. The withdrawal symptoms of a drug are often the opposite of the drug's effect. For example, the withdrawal symptoms associated with a stimulant include depressed nervous system activity. For example, people withdrawing from cocaine report what is known as the "cocaine blues," which is characterized by feeling depressed and **anhedonia**, which refers to the inability to feel pleasure. This happens because of functional tolerance. As you will read later in this chapter, cocaine is a dopamine reuptake inhibitor. Therefore, taking cocaine results in the greater availability of dopamine to bind to receptors at synapses. To compensate for this effect, progressively less dopamine is released from neurons. Therefore, with cocaine cessation, the person is left with neurons that produce very little dopamine.

People withdrawing from alcohol, a depressant drug, may experience what is known as delirium tremens, which is partly characterized by hyperactivity of the nervous system. Why does this happen? As you will read later in this chapter, the main mechanism of action of alcohol is to bind to GABA receptors. Remember that GABA is an inhibitory neurotransmitter. Therefore, it slows down activity in the nervous system. The nervous system adjusts to this effect by the additional release of glutamate, an excitatory neurotransmitter. With alcohol cessation, inhibition is removed from the nervous system but the extra excitation that was compensating for the inhibition is still there. In fact, the nervous system excitation during delirium tremens is so intense that it may be dangerous to withdraw from alcohol and other depressant drugs without medical supervision.

The accelerator and brake-pedal analogy used to explain functional tolerance is also helpful in understanding why withdrawal symptoms are often experienced as the opposite effects of a drug. For example, after an individual has used a stimulant for a while (stepping on the accelerator), the nervous system has learned to slow things down (by stepping on the brake pedal). However, after the cessation of stimulant use (taking the foot off the accelerator), it takes a while for the nervous system to speed things up again (taking the foot off the brake).

3.3.3 NEUROBIOLOGICAL MODELS OF DRUG ADDICTION

>> LO 3.3.3 Identify and explain the neurobiological models of addiction.

Key Terms

- **Positive reinforcement:** When a behavior produces a pleasurable or desirable outcome, increasing the probability that the behavior that produced the outcome will be repeated.

- **Natural reinforcers:** Activities or events that naturally provide pleasure, such as food, sex, or having a good time with friends.
- **Intracranial self-stimulation:** A procedure in which animals are trained to press a lever to receive electrical stimulation through electrodes implanted in these areas.
- **Brain reward areas:** Brain areas that provide a sense of pleasure when stimulated.
- **Negative reinforcement:** When a behavior removes an aversive or unwanted outcome, increasing the probability that it will be repeated.
- **Cycle of addiction:** A theory that views addiction as progressing through three stages.
- **Circuit of addiction:** A circuit of brain areas associated with the stages of the cycle of addiction.
- **Incentive-salience theory**: The theory in which two components of motivated behaviors, "wanting" and "liking," are involved in the development of drug addiction and the stimulation of dopamine pathways is not responsible for the pleasurable effects of drugs.
- **Wanting:** Strong cravings and drug-seeking behavior observed in the addicted person when exposed to environmental cues associated with taking the drug.
- **Liking:** Linked to the pleasurable sensations experienced by users when they have taken a drug.

Positive Reinforcement

Researchers interested in why people become addicted to drugs have proposed several theories. Some researchers emphasize the role of **positive reinforcement** in the initiation and continuation of drug-taking behavior (Wise & Koob, 2014). Positive reinforcement occurs when a behavior produces a pleasurable or desirable outcome, increasing the probability that the behavior that produced the outcome will be repeated. Drugs are viewed as powerful reinforcers. To these researchers, drugs stimulate the brain's dopamine pathways (associated with reward and pleasure) more strongly than do **natural reinforcers**, such as good food, sex, or having a good time with friends. In addition, the pleasurable sensations produced by drugs strengthen the memory of the drug-taking experience. This strong memory for the experience is what contributes to the creation of the strong cravings and drug-seeking behaviors observed in addicted individuals.

The reinforcing effects of psychoactive drugs are partly due to their actions on the mesocorticolimbic dopamine pathway, which links the VTA to the nucleus accumbens. The mesocorticolimbic pathway is part of a larger pathway called the medial forebrain bundle (MFB), which courses through several brain areas, including the hypothalamus, septum, and striatum. In the early 1950s, James Olds and Peter Milner at McGill University discovered that, using a procedure called **intracranial self-stimulation**, rats could be trained to press a lever to receive electrical stimulation through electrodes implanted in these areas (discussed in the context of general motivation in Chapter 9).

The stimulation seemed incredibly rewarding to the rats, so much so that they would press the bar to exhaustion. This led neuroscientists to propose the existence of **brain reward areas**. In the ensuing years, researchers discovered that electrical stimulation of these areas produced the release of dopamine in the nucleus accumbens. Since then, dopamine has often been considered to be the neurotransmitter that controls the pleasure system (but see this chapter's "It's a Myth!" box). The rewarding effects of drugs are also mediated by other neurotransmitters such as serotonin, cannabinoids, and opioids.

Negative Reinforcement

Another theory states that positive reinforcement plays an important role in the first stage of addiction but that what keeps the person addicted is the avoidance of the withdrawal symptoms that occur when the person has not taken the drug for some time. This emphasizes the role of **negative reinforcement** in drug addiction (Wise & Koob, 2014). Negative reinforcement occurs when a behavior removes an aversive or unwanted outcome, increasing the probability that it will be repeated. According to this theory, addiction consists of a three-stage cycle, referred to as the **cycle of addiction** (Herman & Roberto, 2015), illustrated in Figure 3.22. Each of the stages is associated with activity in certain brain areas, which together are known as the **circuit of addiction**:

Stage 1 (binge/intoxication): During this stage, positive reinforcement predominates. The person takes the drug for its reinforcing effects, that is, because of the way it makes him or her feel. It can also make the user more productive, provide pain relief, or reduce anxiety. At this stage, drug intake may be impulsive. That is, it may be risky and inappropriate for the situation. The brain regions implicated during this stage include the VTA, striatum, and cerebellum.

Stage 2 (withdrawal/negative affect): This is the stage at which negative reinforcement predominates. At this stage, the person experiences withdrawal symptoms and now takes the drug to avoid those symptoms. The person may find it difficult to experience the pleasurable effects of the drug. Drug-taking behavior has also shifted from being impulsive to being compulsive; that is, it may now be out of control without regard to any of the negative consequences that result from the use of the drug. The amygdala is one of the brain areas responsible for how a person feels during that stage.

Stage 3 (preoccupation/anticipation): This is the stage in which the person experiences intense cravings for the drug, accompanied by constant drug-seeking behaviors. The brain areas implicated during this stage include the prefrontal cortex and hippocampus.

FIGURE 3.22

The three-stage cycle of addiction.

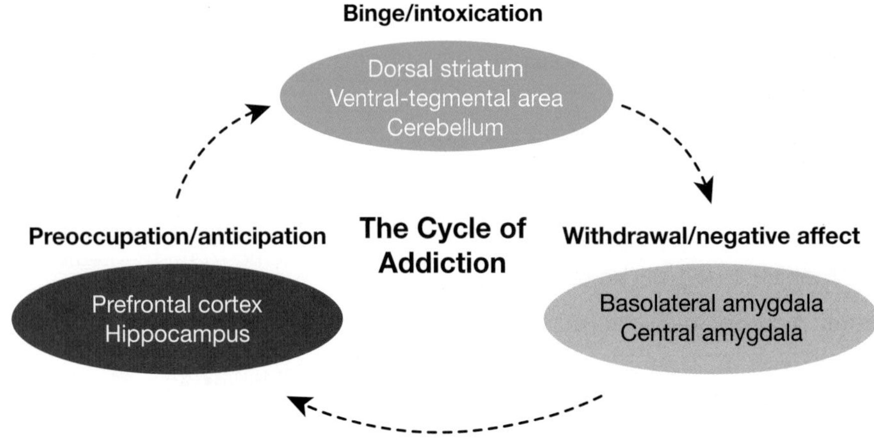

Herman, M. A., & M. Roberto. (2015). The addicted brain: understanding the neurophysiological mechanisms of addictive disorders. *Frontiers in Integrative Neuroscience 9*, 18.

Incentive-Salience Theory

In what is known as the **incentive-salience theory** (or incentive-sensitization theory, discussed in Chapter 9 in the greater context of motivation), researchers have proposed that the stimulation of dopamine pathways is not responsible for the pleasurable effects of drugs (Berridge & Robinson, 2016; Robinson & Berridge, 1993, 2008). Instead, they believe that two components of motivated behaviors—"wanting" and "liking"—are involved in the development of drug addiction. They define **wanting** as the strong cravings and drug-seeking behavior observed in the addicted person when exposed to environmental cues (object, places, or people) associated with taking the drug. These researchers believe that, through association of these cues with the drug's effect, the cues have become extremely salient (noticeable) and difficult to ignore. It is this wanting component that they found to be associated with the mesocorticolimbic system, which includes the ventral tegmental area, prefrontal cortex, amygdala, large areas of the nucleus accumbens, and the striatum.

They define **liking** as the pleasurable sensations (in other words, the "high" and euphoria) that the user experiences when taking the drug. They believe that liking is not related to the dopamine pathways but, instead, is restricted to small areas of the nucleus accumbens, prefrontal cortex, ventral pallidum, brainstem, and insula referred to as "hedonic hotspots." As opposed to wanting, these hotspots are stimulated not by dopamine but by opioids and endocannabinoids. The brain areas involved in wanting and liking are illustrated in Figure 3.23.

FIGURE 3.23

Brain areas involved in wanting and liking. In incentive-sensitization theory, wanting is associated with the mesocorticolimbic dopamine system (orange arrows). Liking is associated with "hedonic hotspots" (areas connected by the green line).

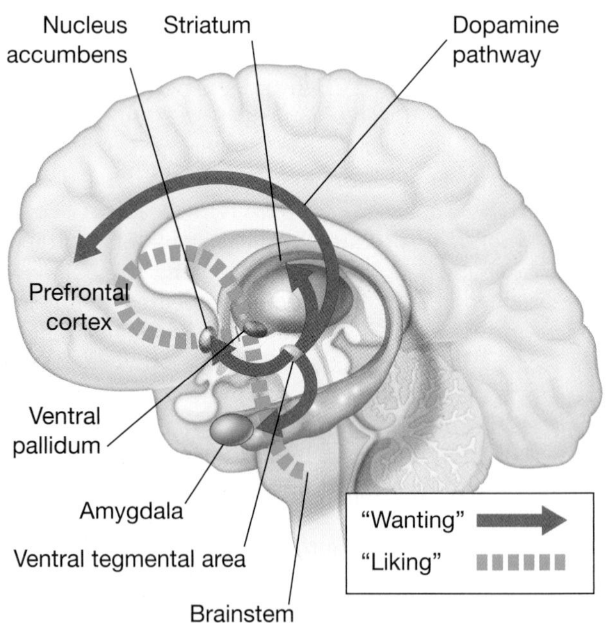

Carolina Hrejsa/Body Scientific Intl.

Interestingly, as wanting grows, liking diminishes over time. This can be observed by the difference in the way a drug affects a nonaddicted person versus a person who is addicted to the drug. A nonaddicted person may like the effects of a drug but does not lose appreciation for natural reinforcers, retains self-control, and has no cravings for the drug. In contrast, the addicted person likes the drug progressively less, loses appreciation for natural reinforcers, and loses control over the use of the drug. The addicted person also experiences intense cravings for the drug.

FIGURE 3.24

(a) Conditioned place-preference paradigm. (b) Self-administration paradigm.

(a)

a) Conditioning with neutral substance (saline) in one compartment

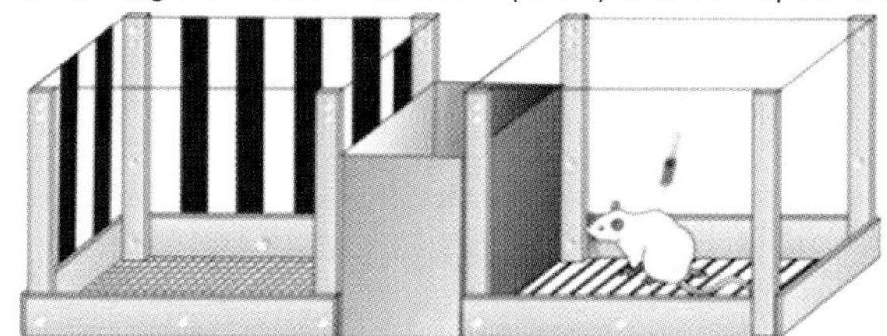

b) Conditioning with drug in opposite compartment

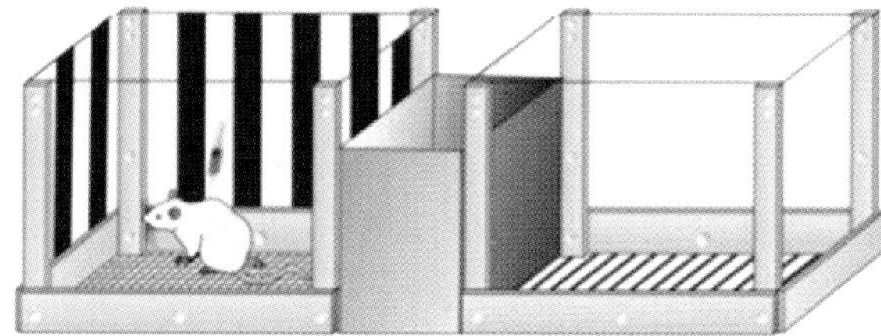

c) Place preference testing

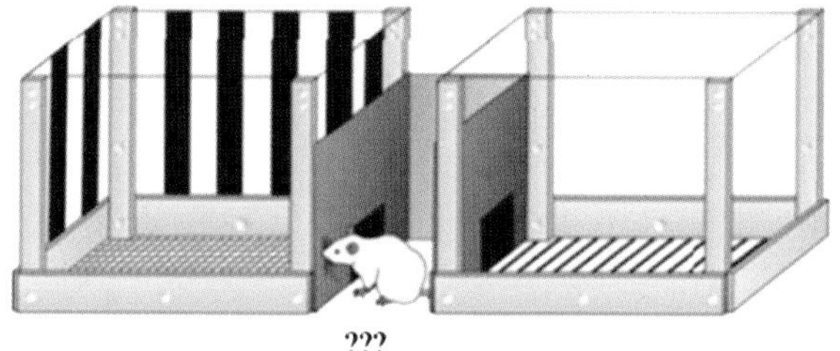

(b)

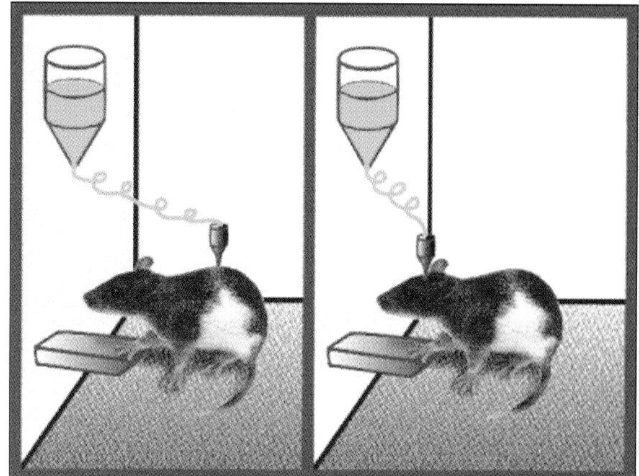

(a) From "Conditioning of Addiction," M. Foster Olive and Peter Kalivas. In *Addiction Medicine: Science and Practice*, A. Johnson Bankole, ed., 2011. Reprinted by permission of Springer; (b) National Institute of Drug Abuse.

Animal Models of Addiction

Today researchers use several methods to study drug addiction. This includes animal models (Carr, Phillips, & Fibiger, 1988; Garcia Pardo, Roger Sanchez, De la Rubia Orti, & Aguilar Calpe, 2017). Two widely used models are the conditioned place-preference (CPP) paradigm and the drug self-administration paradigm. In the CPP paradigm, illustrated in Figure 3.24a, an animal is confined to one of two distinct compartments and injected with a saline solution (salt water). The animal is then moved to the other compartment, where it is injected with an addictive drug (e.g., cocaine). Next, the animal is given a choice between spending time in the compartment in which it was given saline or the compartment in which it was given the drug. Typically, animals will spend more time in the compartment in which they received the drug. This shows that the animal has learned that the specific context in which the drug was given became associated with the drug's effects. This is similar to how humans can be drawn to places where they previously experienced the effects of a drug.

In the self-administration paradigm, illustrated in Figure 3.24b, an animal is trained to perform an action in order to receive a drug. Many variants of this paradigm exist. Typically, animals are taught to press a lever to receive a drug. The drug can be administered orally, directly into the bloodstream, or into a specific brain area. The purpose of this type of paradigm is to study how drugs reinforce the behaviors that lead to their delivery.

3.3.4 MECHANISMS OF ACTION OF COMMONLY ABUSED DRUGS

>> LO 3.3.4 **Describe the neurobiological mechanisms of some commonly abused drugs.**

Key Terms

- **Sedative hypnotics:** Drugs that can relieve anxiety as well as having the potential to induce sleep.
- **Opioid:** Any drug that interacts with opiate receptors.
- **Endogenous opioids:** Opioids that are naturally present in the nervous system.

Nicotine

Nicotine, classified as a stimulant, acts by binding to the subset of acetylcholine receptors known as nicotinic receptors (discussed in Unit 3.2.2, on neurotransmitters). Nicotinic receptors are located on dopamine neurons in both the VTA and the nucleus accumbens, which as you just learned are part of the brain's reward circuit. The addictive effects of nicotine are therefore thought to involve the activation of these areas. However, nicotinic receptors are found all over the brain. In one study, psychiatrist Arthur Brody and colleagues used a positron emission tomography (PET) scanning technique to visualize the extent to which the binding of nicotine to nicotinic receptors in various brain areas was related to the number of cigarettes smoked and cravings for nicotine. The brain areas studied were the thalamus, brainstem, and cerebellum (Brody et al., 2006).

Brody and colleagues injected participants with a radioactively labeled ligand for nicotinic receptors after which their brains were imaged by a PET scan. While in the scanner, participants either did not smoke or smoked 0.1 (1 puff), 0.3 (3 puffs), 1.0, or 3.0 cigarettes. Before the participants smoked, the radioactively labeled ligand bound to a high percentage of receptors in all three regions of interest. However, 3.1 hours after smoking, nicotine had displaced a percentage of the ligand bound to receptors in proportion to the amount of smoking. That is, the more smoking the participants did, the more binding to the nicotinic receptors by nicotine occurred in all areas studied. Smoking one or two puffs resulted in nicotine occupying 50% of the receptors, whereas smoking one whole cigarette or more resulted in the occupation of more than 88% of the receptors.

A reduction in nicotine cravings occurred only when participants smoked one or more cigarettes or when at least 88% of the receptors were bound to by nicotine. The results suggest that to avoid withdrawal symptoms, smokers must maintain a minimum of 88% occupancy of nicotinic receptors.

Alcohol and Other Depressants

Alcohol

Alcohol is a depressant drug, also called a **sedative hypnotic**. At low doses, alcohol reduces anxiety, which reflects its sedative effects. However, at higher doses, alcohol can put you to sleep, its hypnotic effect. These effects of alcohol are due to its ability to bind to its own receptor on Cl^- channels, which potentiates the inhibitory effects of GABA (Matsuzawa & Suzuki, 2002).

FIGURE 3.25

The pharmacological effects of alcohol (1–6) and the naltrexone (7). NAc = nucleus accumbens.

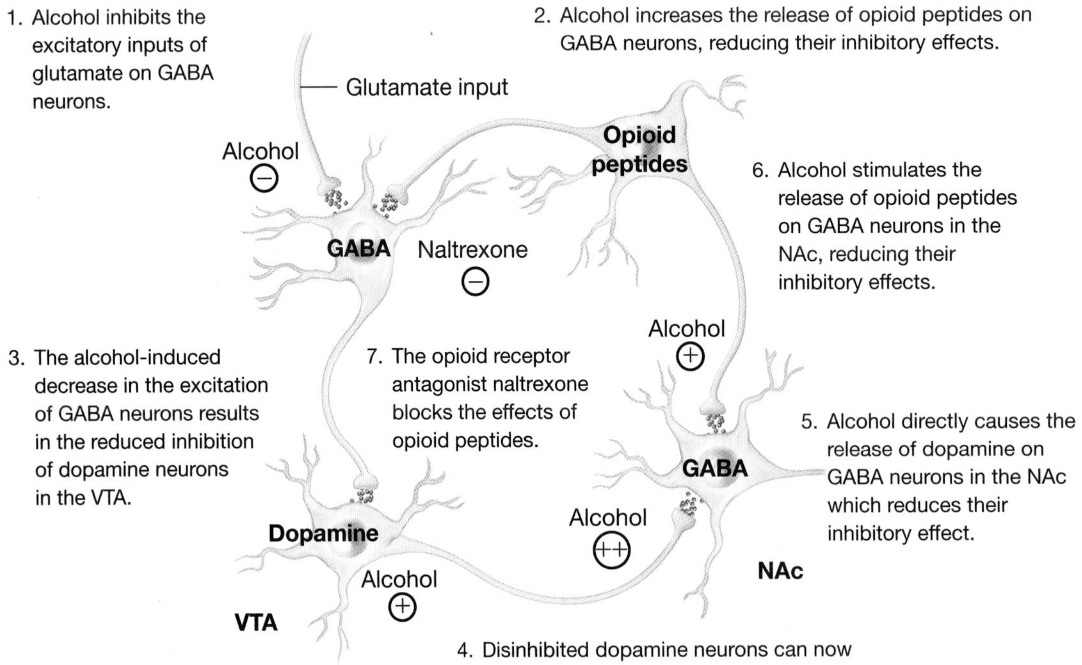

1. Alcohol inhibits the excitatory inputs of glutamate on GABA neurons.
2. Alcohol increases the release of opioid peptides on GABA neurons, reducing their inhibitory effects.
Glutamate input
Alcohol
Opioid peptides
6. Alcohol stimulates the release of opioid peptides on GABA neurons in the NAc, reducing their inhibitory effects.
GABA
Naltrexone
Alcohol
3. The alcohol-induced decrease in the excitation of GABA neurons results in the reduced inhibition of dopamine neurons in the VTA.
7. The opioid receptor antagonist naltrexone blocks the effects of opioid peptides.
5. Alcohol directly causes the release of dopamine on GABA neurons in the NAc which reduces their inhibitory effect.
GABA
Dopamine
Alcohol
NAc
Alcohol
VTA
4. Disinhibited dopamine neurons can now better inhibit GABA neurons in the NAc.

Amanda Tomasikiewicz/Body Scientific Intl.

The rewarding effects of alcohol include a general feeling of well-being and euphoria. As shown in Figure 3.25 (numbers 1–6), alcohol affects the brain's reward system in a variety of ways. Alcohol inhibits the release of glutamate on GABA neurons. This results in a reduction of the release of GABA, which as you know is inhibitory, on dopamine neurons in the VTA. This, in turn, results in an increase in dopamine release in the nucleus accumbens (Nicola & Malenka, 1997).

In addition, alcohol increases the release of opioid peptides (such as endorphins), which directly inhibit the firing of GABA neurons. This is another way in which the inhibition of dopamine neurons in the VTA is removed. This effect is blocked by the administration of naltrexone, which is an opioid receptor antagonist (see this chapter's "Applications" box to read about how naltrexone is used as a pharmacological therapy for alcohol addiction).

Opioid peptides are also released onto GABA neurons within the nucleus accumbens, directly reducing their inhibitory influence in this area (Chieng & Williams, 1998). Alcohol also directly increases the release of dopamine into the nucleus accumbens by dopamine neurons in the VTA.

Other Sedative-Hypnotics (Benzodiazepines, Non-Benzodiazepine Sleep Medications, and Barbiturates)

Other sedative-hypnotics are used as prescription medications. These include benzodiazepines, non-benzodiazepine sleep medications, and barbiturates. These drugs have effects that are similar to those of alcohol. In fact, they also exert their effects by each binding to their own receptors located on Cl^- channels. Benzodiazepines are mostly used to treat anxiety. They include drugs such as

FIGURE 3.26

Retrograde signaling and THC. Dopamine neurons in the nucleus accumbens release endocannabinoids (AEA, 2-AG). These endocannabinoids travel back to presynaptic neurons and inhibit their ability to release neurotransmitters (e.g., GABA and glutamate) by binding to CB_1 receptors. THC (gray rectangles) mimics the effects of endocannabinoids by binding to the same receptors. This results in the removal of GABA's inhibitory effects on dopamine neurons, explaining the rewarding properties of marijuana.

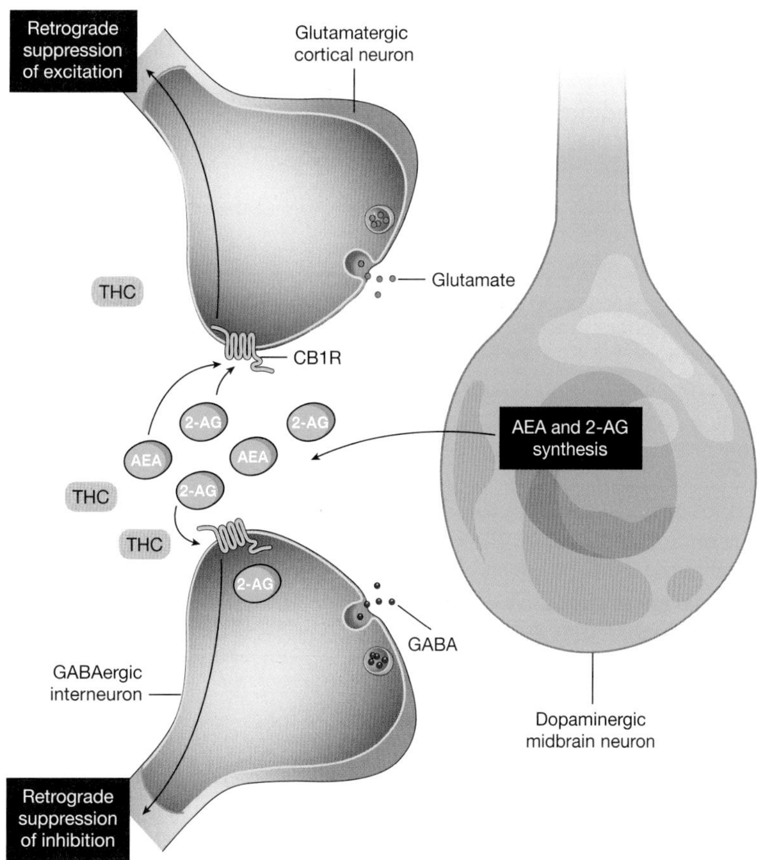

Bloomfield, M.A., et al. (2016). The effects of Delta9-tetrahydrocannabinol on the dopamine system. *Nature 539*(7629): 369–377. With permission from Springer Nature.

alprazolam (Xanax), diazepam (Valium), and lorazepam (Ativan). The binding of benzodiazepines to their receptors increases the frequency at which the associated Cl^- channels open. Non-benzodiazepine sleep medications also bind to benzodiazepine receptors but are used to treat insomnia. These include zolpidem (Ambien), eszopiclone (Lunesta), and zaleplon (Sonata). Barbiturates include drugs such as phenobarbital and pentobarbital. Their effects are longer lasting than those of benzodiazepines. Barbiturates are used mainly to treat insomnia. However, they are used less frequently due to their higher potential for addiction. The binding of barbiturates to their receptors increases the length of time for which Cl^- channels are open.

Marijuana

Marijuana does not fit neatly into any drug class. This is because it has both depressant and excitatory effects on the nervous system. In addition, at high doses, marijuana can have hallucinogenic effects. Marijuana refers to the dried flowers, leaves, and stems of the cannabis plant. The cannabis plant contains more than 100 chemicals known as phytocannabinoids (Aizpurua-Olaizola et al., 2016; ElSohly, Radwan, Gul, Chandra, & Galal, 2017). Marijuana is usually smoked in the form of rolled cigarettes called "joints" or "blunts." However, marijuana can also be consumed with the use of vaporizers or by eating foods (including candies, cookies, and brownies) that contain delta-9 tetrahydrocannabinol (THC), the primary psychoactive cannabinoid. The effects of marijuana vary from user to user but generally include altered visual and auditory experiences and an altered sense of time. When taken in high doses, marijuana can cause hallucinations, delusions, and paranoia. Marijuana users also experience changes in mood, difficulties in thinking and problem solving, and impaired short-term memory. The sensory distortions experienced by users may be due to suppressed neurotransmission in the brain's sensory areas, whereas short-term memory deficits may be due to reduced neurotransmission in the hippocampus and prefrontal cortex (Lorenzetti, Solowij, & Yucel, 2016). Contrary to popular belief, marijuana is not a harmless drug (see the "It's a Myth!" box in Chapter 12).

THC produces its psychotropic effects by binding to CB_1 cannabinoid receptors located all over the brain (Hu & Mackie, 2015). As illustrated in Figure 3.26, the rewarding effects of marijuana are thought to be caused initially by the binding of THC molecules to CB_1 receptors located on GABAergic neurons, resulting in their inhibition, through retrograde signaling. This in turn removes their inhibitory effects on dopamine neurons within the nucleus accumbens (Bloomfield, Ashok, Volkow, & Howes, 2016).

Opioids

The term **opioid** refers to any drug that interacts with opiate receptors. The term *opiate* is reserved for opioids that are synthesized from the opium poppy. These are opium, morphine, codeine, and heroin. Although heroin is not synthesized directly from the poppy, it is synthesized from morphine and is therefore also considered an opiate.

Synthetic or semisynthetic drugs, such as oxycodone, hydromorphone, and fentanyl, that are designed to work in the same way as opiates are simply designated as opioids. Opioids mimic the effects of **endogenous opioids**, such as endorphins, enkephalins, and dynorphins and have an extreme potential for addiction.

As with alcohol, the rewarding effects of opioids occur through the inhibition of GABAergic neurons in the VTA. This, in turn, removes GABA's inhibition on dopaminergic neurons in the VTA, resulting in increased dopamine release in the nucleus accumbens (Margolis, Hjelmstad, Fujita, & Fields, 2014) (Figure 3.27).

FIGURE 3.27

(1) Opioids such as morphine bind to opioid receptors located on GABAergic neurons.
(2) GABAergic neurons are therefore inhibited and their inhibitory effect on dopaminergic neurons in the nucleus accumbens is removed. (3) This results in an increase of dopamine release in the nucleus accumbens.

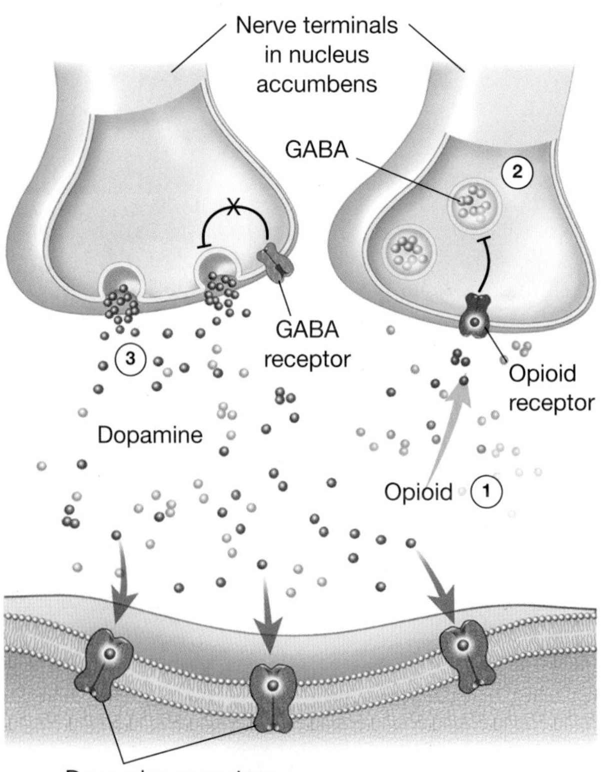

Amanda Tomasikiewicz/Body Scientific Intl.

Other Stimulants (Cocaine, Amphetamine, and Methamphetamine)

Cocaine users typically experience euphoria, increased energy, heightened attention, and intensified emotions. Cocaine is a dopamine reuptake inhibitor. That is, it prevents transporters from taking dopamine back into the neuron that released it. This results in more dopamine being available to bind to receptors on postsynaptic neurons (Fowler, Volkow, Kassed, & Chang, 2007).

The rewarding effects of cocaine are attributed to the higher concentrations of dopamine released in the nucleus accumbens. The increase in the amounts of norepinephrine and serotonin contributes to the rewarding effects of cocaine by facilitating the firing of dopamine neurons. The increases in locomotor activity (speedy effects) observed in cocaine users is due to increased levels of norepinephrine (Cooper, Robison, & Mazei-Robison, 2017). The effects of amphetamine and methamphetamine are like those of cocaine but are significantly longer lasting. However, unlike cocaine, they do not block the reuptake of dopamine, norepinephrine, and serotonin but, instead, increase the release of those neurotransmitters from presynaptic neurons.

MODULE SUMMARY

A drug is defined as a substance that can alter physiological function. Psychoactive drugs give rise to a sense of euphoria and may produce altered sensory perceptions. Drugs are subdivided into several classes: stimulants, depressants, and hallucinogens. All drugs of abuse produce their effects by acting on neurotransmitter systems. Drugs can affect the synthesis, transport, storage, release, degradation, or reuptake of neurotransmitters. A drug can be an agonist to the extent that it mimics the actions of a neurotransmitter. A drug can also be an antagonist to the extent that it blocks the actions of a neurotransmitter.

Drug addiction is a pattern of drug abuse in which people lose control of the use of a drug. Addiction is also characterized by the presence of tolerance and withdrawal symptoms. Tolerance is the phenomenon in which people need to take progressively more of a drug to feel the same effects. There are three types of tolerance: dispositional tolerance, in which the body becomes progressively better at eliminating the drug; behavioral tolerance, in which a person becomes better at compensating for the drug's effects, such as walking in a straight line while drunk; and functional tolerance, in which neurons become less responsive to the drug. Withdrawal symptoms are feelings of illness that occur with the cessation of drug intake once the body has adjusted to its presence.

There are several neurobiological models of addiction. One model is based on positive reinforcement, which states that people keep taking drugs because of the pleasurable sensations they produce by stimulating the brain's reward areas. Another model, the cycle of addiction, is based on negative reinforcement. It states that people take the drug for positive reinforcement at the beginning of the cycle of drug addiction but eventually take the drug only to avoid experiencing withdrawal symptoms. Yet another theory, called the incentive-salience theory, states that drug addiction includes feelings of "wanting" and "liking," each linked to different brain chemicals and areas. This theory states that cues associated with the use of the drug induce feelings of wanting, which are linked to traditional reward areas of the brain and the neurotransmitter dopamine. The feelings of liking are associated with other brain chemicals associated with pleasure, such as endorphins and anandamide. To better understand addiction, researchers have developed animal models. These include the conditioned place-preference paradigm and a variety of self-administration models.

People use many drugs. Some drugs, such as nicotine and alcohol, are more commonly used and abused than others and can be obtained legally. Other drugs can be obtained legally with a physician's prescription. These include painkillers, sleeping pills, and some stimulants used to treat various conditions. Some of the drugs used to treat certain conditions and usually prescribed by a physician are also obtained illegally and have a high potential for addiction. Finally, all addictive drugs act on the brain areas responsible for feeling pleasure, such as the nucleus accumbens and the ventral-tegmental area.

TEST YOURSELF

3.3.1 Define a psychoactive drug.

3.2.2 Define drug addiction. What are the signs that someone is addicted to a drug?

3.3.3 Name and explain the different neurobiological models of drug addiction.

3.3.4 Discuss the effects and mechanisms of action of some commonly abused drugs.

APPLICATIONS

Pharmacological Treatments for Drug Addiction

Many factors could explain why someone starts and continues to use drugs. Not everyone who uses drugs becomes addicted to them. However, people who do become addicted often cause significant harm to themselves and others who must live with the consequences of their behavior. Fortunately, it is possible for an addicted person to stop using a drug. Addiction is complex; therefore, the reasons why someone becomes addicted and whether that individual is successful at recovering from drug addiction depends on many interacting factors, including genetic, social, emotional, behavioral, and neurobiological factors.

Other factors such as the drug(s) to which the person is addicted, the context in which the person lives, age, culture, work, family conditions, and the individual's psychological state must also be considered. There is no "one-size-fits-all" approach to treating drug addiction. Even so, many treatment programs share the following goals:

- Stop taking the drug
- Remain drug free
- Resume normal occupational and family functioning

A successful drug treatment program consists of the following steps:

- Detoxification
- Behavioral counseling
- Pharmacological treatment (medication)
- Treatment of cooccurring mental health issues
- Long-term follow-up to prevent relapse

Each of these steps is equally important for the treatment of drug addiction. However, here we focus strictly on pharmacological treatments.

During the detoxification phase, the period in which the addicted person first abstains from the drug, an individual may suffer from withdrawal symptoms and experience intense cravings for the drug.

The withdrawal symptoms the person experiences are due to the brain's ability to adjust to the drug while the person is taking it. The intense cravings stem from changes in the brain's reward system, which makes the person extremely sensitive to the cues associated with taking the drug.

The role of pharmacological treatments is to reduce the extent to which the person experiences withdrawal symptoms as well as reducing cravings for the drug. Pharmacological treatments are typically considered for opioid, nicotine, and alcohol addiction.

Opioid Addiction

Opioids produce their pleasurable effects by binding to opioid receptors in the brain, mimicking the effects of naturally occurring opioids such as endorphins and enkephalins. The binding of opioids to these receptors removes the inhibition on dopamine neurons, which results in a greater amount of dopamine being released in the nucleus accumbens, which is part of the brain's reward system. The opioids to which people become addicted include the street drug heroin and medications usually obtained only through a physician's prescription or while hospitalized (e.g., oxycodone, codeine, and fentanyl).

Opioid Receptor Agonists

The drugs used to treat opioid addiction also act on opioid receptors. Some of these drugs are opioids themselves and are therefore opioid-receptor agonists. Although they bind to opioid receptors, they do not provide the "high" associated with the drug to which the person is addicted. This helps the individual to abstain from the drug by reducing withdrawal symptoms and cravings. Examples of these drugs are methadone and buprenorphine.

Opioid Receptor Antagonists

Other drugs, such as naltrexone, are opioid-receptor antagonists. That is, they bind to opioid receptors but block opioids from binding to them. This means that an addicted person would not feel the effects of the drug should it be consumed again. It is used for people who have already been detoxified. Its purpose is to reduce cravings and drug-seeking behaviors.

Nicotine Addiction

Nicotine binds to and stimulates nicotinic acetylcholine receptors in the brain. In turn, cholinergic neurons directly activate dopamine release in the nucleus accumbens.

Nicotine Replacement Therapy

The first type of pharmacological treatment for nicotine addiction was nicotine replacement therapy (NRT). The idea behind NRT is to provide the user with nicotine in decreasing doses to ease withdrawal symptoms and cravings while abstaining from the drug. Nicotine can be delivered via a chewing gum, lozenge, nasal spray, or transdermal patch.

Nicotinic Receptor Agonists

The drug varenicline (Chantix) was introduced recently. Varenicline is a nicotinic receptor partial agonist. This means that it binds to nicotinic receptors but to a lesser degree. This permits the drug to lessen withdrawal symptoms without nicotine's stimulating effects.

Nicotine Vaccine

Nicotine vaccines are currently being investigated. A nicotine vaccine would trigger an immune response from the body. This means that any nicotine present in the bloodstream would be sequestered by antibodies and prevented from entering the brain, which means that rewarding effects of smoking would be eliminated.

Alcohol Addiction

Alcohol produces its antianxiety and sedative effects by enhancing the neurotransmission of the inhibitory neurotransmitter GABA.

Opioid Receptor Antagonists

Alcohol's rewarding effects are due to its indirect action on dopamine release in the nucleus accumbens. By binding to opioid receptors, alcohol removes the inhibitory effects of GABA on dopamine neurons.

Accordingly, one pharmacological treatment strategy for dealing with alcohol addiction is with the opioid receptor antagonist naltrexone, as can be used for opioid addiction. This strategy reduces cravings for alcohol and was shown to be effective in reducing relapse.

Another drug, acamprosate, can be used to reduce the occurrence of insomnia, anxiety, and restlessness associated with alcohol withdrawal.

Aversion Therapy

Finally, alcohol addiction can be treated with aversion therapy using a drug called disulfiram (Antabuse). Alcohol is normally metabolized in the body into acetaldehyde. Acetaldehyde is further metabolized by an enzyme and eliminated. Acetaldehyde, if permitted to build up in the body, produces unpleasant symptoms such as headaches, nausea, and vomiting.

Disulfiram prevents the breakdown of acetaldehyde, resulting in its build-up in the body. Therefore, a person who drinks alcohol while taking disulfiram is exposed to these symptoms. The main challenge in using disulfiram as a pharmacological treatment is getting the person to comply. ●

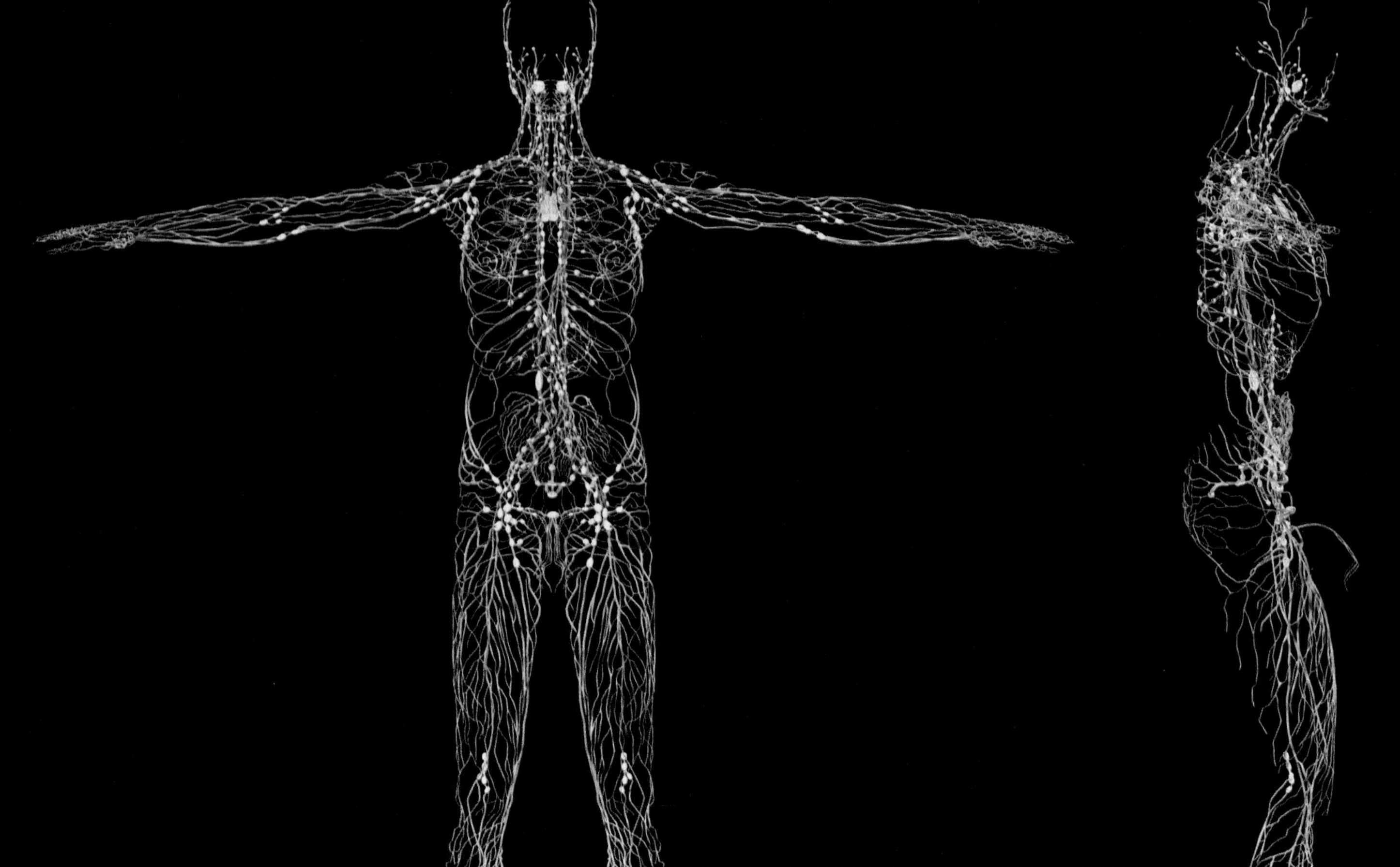

iStock.com/cokada

4 The Nervous System

Chapter Contents

Learning Objectives

4.1.1 Describe the process of gastrulation.

4.1.2 Describe the process of neurulation.

4.1.3 Explain how the neural tube differentiates into the brain's primary vesicles.

4.2.1 Identify the major structures of the telencephalon and some of their functions.

4.2.2 Identify the major structures of the diencephalon and some of their functions.

4.2.3 Identify the major structures of the midbrain and the hindbrain and some of their functions.

4.2.4 Describe the structure of the spinal cord and how it transmits information to and from the brain.

4.2.5 Describe the different protective layers of the brain and how they work.

4.2.6 Explain how each hemisphere of the brain is associated with different functions.

4.3.1 Explain the functions of the somatic nervous system.

4.3.2 Explain the functions of the autonomic nervous system.

Carolyn Pioro: From Trapeze Artist to Quadriplegic

September 20, 2005, marked the day of a dramatic change in trapeze artist Carolyn Pioro's life. Her "big act" consisted of swinging through the air while hanging onto a bar, letting go and flipping for a revolution, and then being caught by the wrists by a catcher, hanging upside down from his own bar. On that day, however, instead of Pioro being caught, her body collided with the catcher's. This sent her spinning as she fell head first into a safety net below, breaking her neck and severing her spinal cord, the bundle of nerve fibers that run up and down the middle of the back. The fall left her paralyzed from the shoulders down.

Sensations coming from your body and motor commands from your brain to your body make their way through your spinal cord. It follows that damage to the spinal cord impairs sensory and motor function in the body below the point at which the spinal cord has been damaged. The extent of the paralysis depends on the amount of damage done to the nerves of the spinal cord. For Pioro, damage to her spinal cord was almost total. But because of an early intervention, she retained the ability to breathe on her own, speak, and shrug her shoulders. The condition in which Pioro found herself is known as quadriplegia, also known as tetraplegia. When damage occurs lower in the spinal cord, only the lower body may be affected, a condition known as paraplegia. Pioro is now a journalist who writes about body image and the media.

INTRODUCTION

Figure 4.1 shows the divisions of the nervous system. The nervous system is subdivided into the central nervous system (CNS) and the peripheral nervous system (PNS). The CNS consists of the brain and spinal cord. The PNS is subdivided into the somatic nervous system (SNS) and the autonomic nervous system (ANS). The SNS consists of the nerve fibers that connect to your skin, muscles, and joints. The ANS regulates the functions of your organs and glands. These are the functions that you never have to think about, like breathing, your heartbeat, or the dilation of your pupils. The ANS is subdivided further into the sympathetic and parasympathetic nervous systems. The sympathetic nervous system activates your body by interacting with your various organs and glands, whereas the parasympathetic nervous system calms your body back down. In this chapter, we will take a closer look at each one of these systems. We begin, however, with an overview of how the CNS develops after conception.

4.1 Central Nervous System Development

Module Contents

FIGURE 4.1

Divisions of the nervous system.

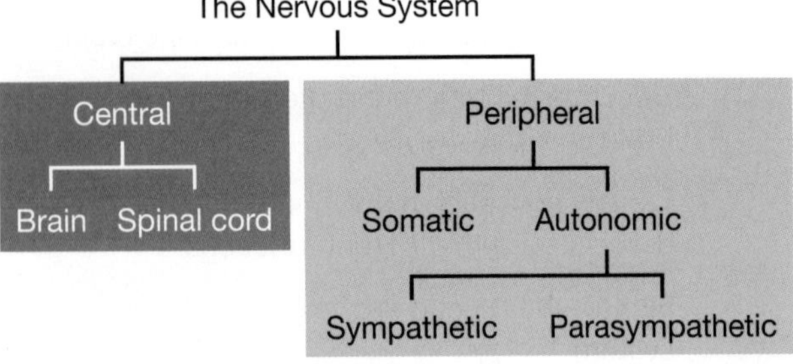

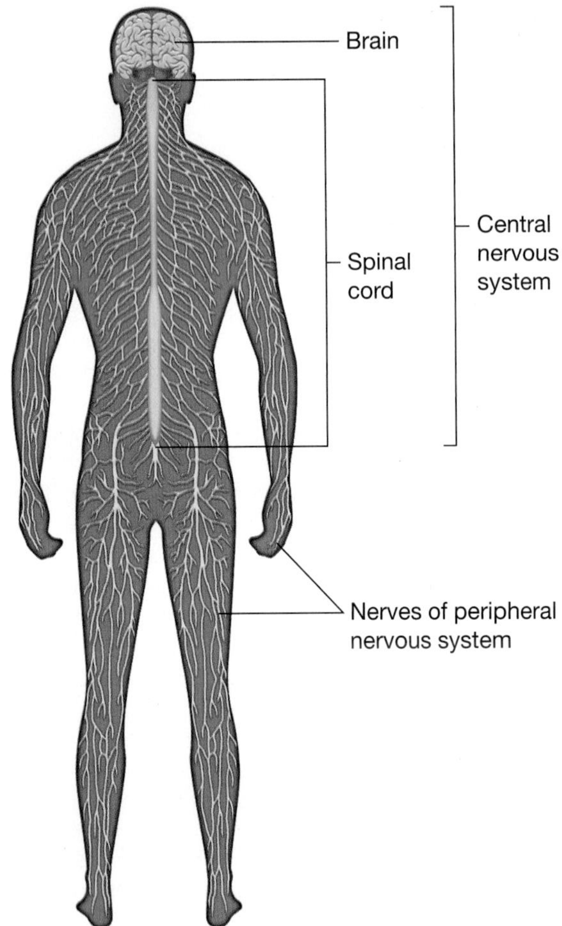

Adapted from *Biological Foundations of Human Behavior*, by J. Wilson, 2003, Belmont, CA: Wadsworth.

Learning Objectives

4.1.1 Describe the process of gastrulation.

4.1.2 Describe the process of neurulation.

4.1.3 Explain how the neural tube differentiates into the brain's primary vesicles.

4.1.1 GASTRULATION

>> LO 4.1.1 **Describe the process of gastrulation.**

Key Terms

- **Blastocyst:** A fluid-filled ball that contains a mass of cells.
- **Embryonic disk:** The mass of cells that develop within the blastocyst.
- **Gastrula:** The structure that develops from the blastocyst and forms the germ layers.
- **Gastrulation:** The process by which the blastocyst develops into the gastrula.
- **Germ layers:** Three layers of cells that develop into the different tissues of the body.
- **Ectoderm:** The germ layer that develops into the nervous system and the skin.
- **Mesoderm:** The germ layer that gives rise to the muscles, skeleton, some of the internal organs, and the circulatory system.
- **Endoderm:** The germ layer that gives rise to the digestive system, lungs, and glands.

Shortly after fertilization, about five days in humans, a fluid-filled ball known as the **blastocyst** begins to form (Figures 4.2a and 4.2b). Inside this ball, a mass of cells known as the **embryonic disk** becomes a new organism. Next, the blastocyst develops into what is known as the **gastrula**, through the process of **gastrulation**. The gastrula forms three layers of cells, known as **germ layers** (Figure 4.2c). The germ layers are known as the ectoderm, mesoderm, and endoderm. Each of these layers develops into a different type of tissue, giving rise to the different parts of the body.

As shown in Figure 4.2d, the **ectoderm** gives rise to the nervous system and the skin; the **mesoderm** gives rise to the muscles, skeleton, some of the internal organs, and the circulatory system; and the **endoderm** gives rise to the digestive system, lungs, and glands (Moore, Persaud, & Torchia, 2016). For obvious reasons (because this book is mainly about the brain), we will focus mostly on the ectoderm, which is responsible for the development of the nervous system.

FIGURE 4.2

Gastrulation: The process by which a hollow ball of cells called the blastocyst is transformed into the gastrula, which contains the germ layers that are to become the different tissues of the body. (a) Artist conception of the blastocyst (the mass of cells at the bottom is the embryonic disk). (b) Light micrograph of a human blastocyst. (c) Gastrula with its germ layers, consisting of the endoderm, mesoderm, and ectoderm (also shown is the blastopore, which is the opening by which the cavity of the gastrula communicates with the exterior). (d) The three germ layers with the corresponding types of tissue to which they each give rise.

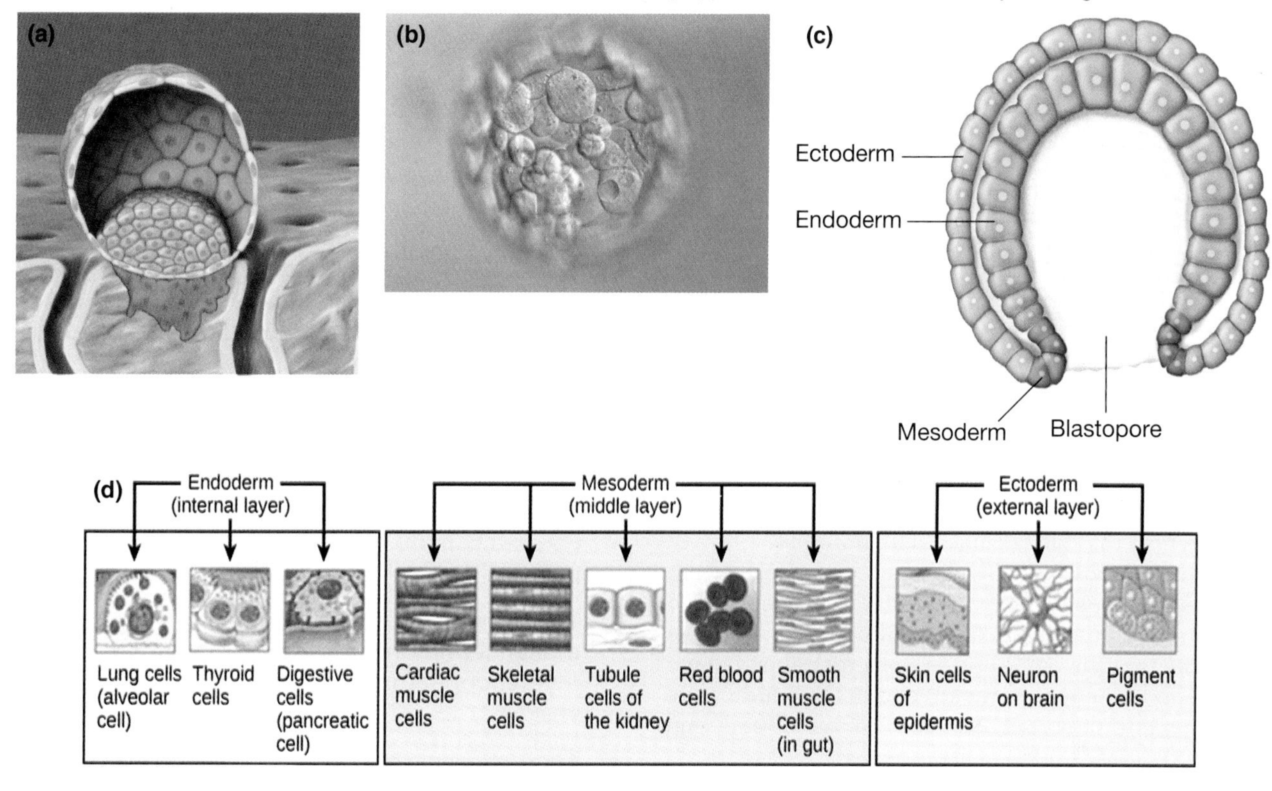

(a) QA International/Science Source; (b) Pascal Goetgheluck/Science Source; (c) Liana Bauman/Body Scientific Intl.; (d) OpenStax College, Fertilization and Early Embryonic Development. October 17, 2013. .

4.1.2 NEURULATION

>> LO 4.1.2 **Describe the process of neurulation.**

Key Terms

- **Neurulation:** The process by which the neural tube is formed, which gives rise to the central nervous system.
- **Neural folds:** Risen edges of the ectoderm, which fuse together to form the neural tube.
- **Neural groove:** The depression in the central region of the ectoderm caused by the neural folds.
- **Neural plate:** The region that spans the neural folds along with the neural groove.
- **Notochord:** A flexible, rodlike structure made out of cells from the mesoderm, which serves as the skeleton of the embryo until the formation of the vertebrae.
- **Neural crest:** Made from migrating cells of the ectoderm; gives rise to the peripheral nervous system.
- **Somites:** Protrusions on either side of the neural tube formed by the mesoderm, which give rise to the vertebrae and associated skeletal muscles.

The central nervous system arises from the neural tube. The developmental process by which the neural tube is formed is known as **neurulation** (Darnell & Gilbert, 2017). Shortly after the formation of the gastrula (described in the preceding unit), the edges of the ectoderm rise and become what are known as the **neural folds**. This results in a depression in the central

FIGURE 4.3

The process of neurulation.

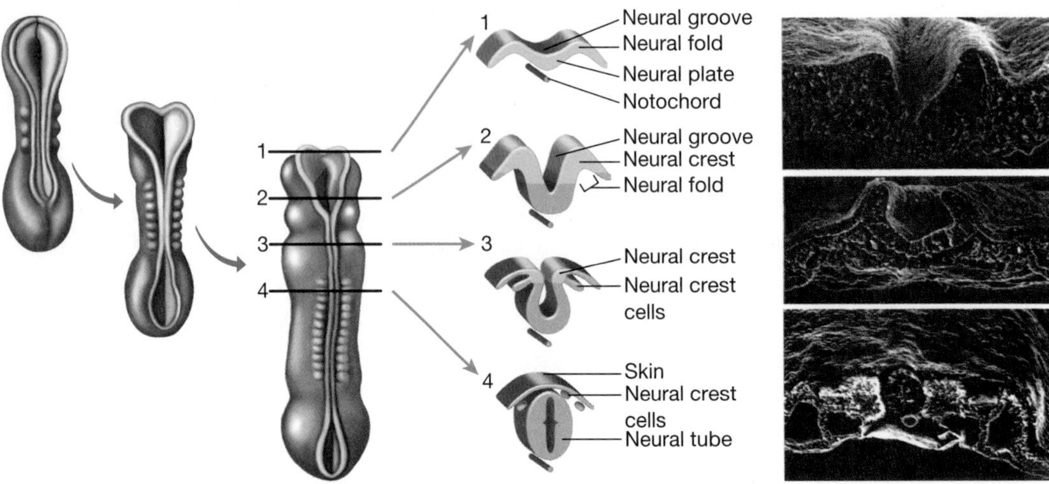

Kathryn Tosney

region, known as the **neural groove**. The region that spans the neural folds along with the neural groove is known as the **neural plate**. The **notochord**, which is a flexible, rodlike structure made out of cells from the mesoderm, serves as the skeleton of the embryo until the vertebrae form. This is illustrated in Figure 4.3. Note that the neural plate has a rostral end and a caudal end. The rostral (head) end of the neural plate develops into the brain, whereas the caudal (tail) end develops into the spinal cord.

The neural folds, which are at the edges of the neural plate move toward each other and fuse. The fusion of the neural folds occurs first in the middle of the neural plate. The fusion then progresses from the middle toward the rostral and caudal ends. The completion of this process gives rise to the neural tube. As the neural folds fuse, some of the cells from the ectoderm migrate to both sides of the neural tube and form the **neural crest**. The cells from the neural crest give rise to the peripheral nervous system.

In addition, the mesoderm forms protrusions, called **somites**, on either side of the neural tube. The 33 vertebrae of the spinal column, as well their associated skeletal muscles, develop from the somites.

4.1.3 DIFFERENTIATION OF THE NEURAL TUBE INTO THE PRIMARY BRAIN VESICLES

>> LO 4.1.3 **Explain how the neural tube differentiates into the brain's primary vesicles.**

Key Terms

- **Forebrain, midbrain, hindbrain:** The three primary brain vesicles.
- **Telencephalon, diencephalon, mesencephalon, metencephalon, myelencephalon:** The five secondary brain vesicles.
- **Tectum:** A subdivision of the mesencephalon involved in producing reflexive eye movements, pitch perception, and the spatial localization of sounds.
- **Tegmentum:** A subdivision of the midbrain involved in motor coordination and the regulation of pain. It also contains the ventral-tegmental area, which is part of the brain's reward system.

Approximately 25 days after conception, the neural tube begins to expand. Its rostral end expands at a quicker rate than the caudal end and differentiates into the three primary vesicles of the brain. The three primary vesicles are the **forebrain**, **midbrain**, and **hindbrain** (Figure 4.4a). After about 40 days, the primary vesicles subdivide into five secondary vesicles. These are the telencephalon, diencephalon, mesencephalon, metencephalon, and the myelencephalon (Figure 4.4b).

The **telencephalon** gives rise to the brain's hemispheres, which consist of the cerebral cortex. The telencephalon also gives rise to the basal ganglia, the olfactory bulb, the hippocampus, and the amygdala. The **diencephalon** consists of the thalamus

FIGURE 4.4

(a) The primary vesicles of the brain. (b) The subdivisions of the primary vesicles into secondary vesicles, including the spinal cord. (c) The fully developed human brain.

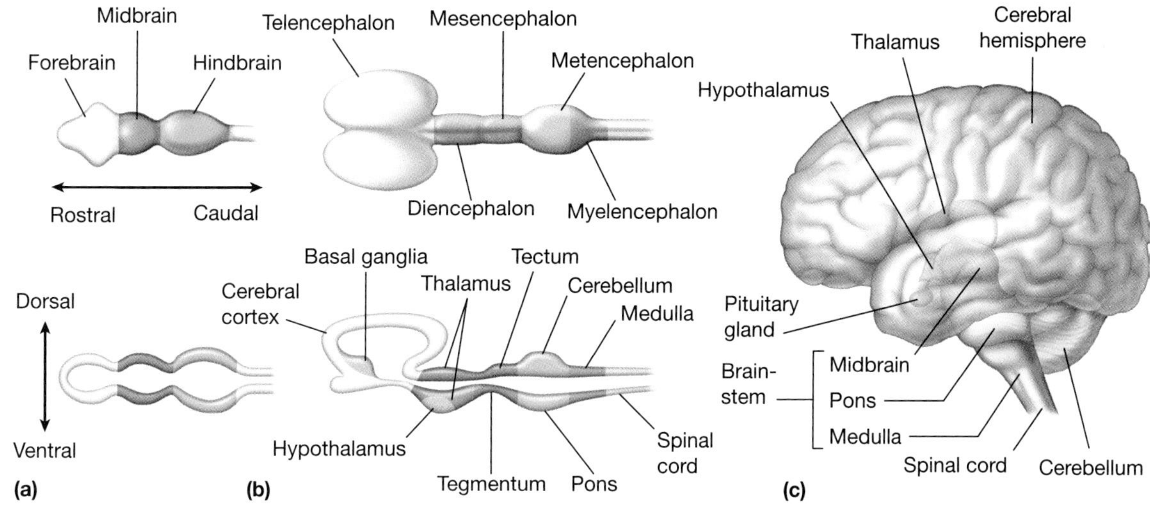

Carolina Hrejsa/Body Scientific Intl.

and the hypothalamus. The **mesencephalon** (sometimes referred to as the midbrain) subdivides into the tectum and tegmentum. The **tectum** consists of the superior colliculus and inferior colliculus. The **tegmentum** contains the periaqueductal gray matter, the substantia nigra, and the red nucleus. To remember these regions, simply remember the colors gray, black (nigra), and red. The hindbrain is subdivided into the metencephalon and the myelencephalon. The **metencephalon** consists of the cerebellum and the pons, whereas the **myelencephalon** consists of the medulla (sometimes called the medulla oblongata). Figure 4.4c shows the fully developed human brain.

IT'S A MYTH!

Vaccines Cause Autism

The Myth

A prominent myth that has persisted for more than 20 years is that the measles, mumps, and rubella (MMR) vaccine causes autism (now known as autism spectrum disorder, or ASD). This myth has contributed a great deal to the fear that some parents have about immunizing their children against dangerous diseases, putting their own children and the population at risk. At the same time, scientific studies have *never* found a link between vaccines and ASD. This is a stark reminder of the importance of basing health-related decisions on scientific evidence rather than on reported stories propagated through the Internet, social media, magazines, and other unreliable sources of information.

What Is Autism Spectrum Disorder?

Autism spectrum disorder is a neurodevelopmental disorder characterized by impairments in social interaction as well as in language and communication skills. It also includes the performance of rigid and repetitive behaviors. Its prevalence in the United States in 1 in 68 births, and the signs typically appear during early childhood. There are many probable causes of ASD, including genetic variations, overconnectivity between neurons, underconnectivity between brain regions, environmental factors, and impairments in white fiber connectivity. There is presently no cure for ASD. Therapeutic interventions are aimed at enhancing cognitive skills, learning rate, attention control, communication skills, and speech development.

(Continued)

(Continued)

What Is a Vaccine?

A vaccine is a compound, also known as a biological preparation, made from biological organisms that help the immune system combat germs (viruses and bacteria) that can potentially cause serious diseases. It does so because the preparation contains the germ that causes the disease it is designed to combat. This primes the immune system to react more effectively the next time in encounters the germ. The germ present in the vaccine can be in different forms, depending on the type of vaccine. Some vaccines contain the live but weakened version of the germ. These are known as live-attenuated vaccines. These include vaccines for yellow fever, smallpox, chicken pox, and MMR (the one implicated in the myth). Other vaccines contain a dead version of the germ. These are known as inactivated vaccines and are used for the prevention of hepatitis A, the flu, polio, and rabies. Other vaccines use key pieces of the germ. These are used to prevent hepatitis B, whooping cough, shingles, and several other diseases. Finally, some vaccines contain a toxin that is produced by the germ. These vaccines prevent diphtheria and tetanus. Other types of vaccines, including DNA vaccines, are being developed.

In addition to germs, vaccines contain several other agents. These may include thimerosal (which contains ethyl mercury—more on that shortly), formaldehyde, aluminum, antibiotics, gelatin, and monosodium glutamate (MSG). Thimerosal, gelatin, and MSG are used as preservatives, which prolong a vaccine's shelf-life considerably and keep them effective through varying temperatures. They also prevent bacterial and fungal infections of the vaccines. Formaldehyde and antibiotics are used to inactivate viruses and to detoxify any toxins that may make their way into the vaccine. Aluminum makes the vaccine more effective in triggering an immune response. By themselves, these agents have been linked to health problems, but the small amounts the vaccines contain do not present any significant risks.

Where Does the Myth Come From?

The myth that vaccines cause neurological disorders is nothing new. Throughout history, vaccines have been claimed to cause epilepsy, multiple sclerosis, schizophrenia, and several other neurological disorders (Gasparini, Panatto, Lai, & Amicizia, 2015). However, no scientific evidence has ever existed to support those claims.

In 1998, the medical journal *The Lancet* published a study by British gastroenterologist Andrew Wakefield and colleagues that suggested the MMR vaccine caused what they called "regressive autism" (i.e., appearing after previously typical development). *The Lancet* retracted the study in 2010 on the grounds of conflict of interest. Wakefield had attempted to produce his own vaccine and was engaged in a lawsuit against companies that produced the MMR vaccine. Wakefield's medical license was later revoked by the United Kingdom's General Medical Council.

In an article published in 2011, the *British Medical Journal* found Wakefield's reported findings on the links between vaccines and autism to be deliberate fraud (Godlee, Smith, & Marcovitch, 2011). It became evident that, in Wakefield's study, only one out of the nine children whose cases he reported really developed "regressive autism." Wakefield was also found to have lied about the health status of the children before the study. He had claimed that none of the children previously had developmental difficulties, but it turned out that five of them did.

The main culprit contained within vaccines was purported to be thimerosal, the mercury-based preservative and antibacterial agent mentioned earlier. However, there has never been evidence that mercury causes any harm in the doses contained in vaccines. Despite this, thimerosal was removed from nearly all vaccines in 1999 (including the MMR vaccine). The only exception is for the vaccine for influenza, in which the risk of infection is higher because it is administered from multidose vials. This precautionary measure was misinterpreted by the public as an admission that thimerosal caused autism.

In 2005, *Rolling Stone* and *Salon* magazines published an article suggesting that the government orchestrated a cover-up of the link between thimerosal and autism. After multiple corrections, *Salon* removed the article from its website in 2011, though *Rolling Stone* did not. The MMR myth got a boost in 2016, with the release of the documentary *Vaxxed*, directed by Wakefield himself. The documentary also alleged that the Centers for Disease Control and Prevention (CDC) covered up a study that showed a link between the MMR vaccine and autism. This was nothing but another falsehood. The study in question had stated that the rates of vaccination in a group of older kids were higher in those with ASD. However, the kids in that group were in a preschool education program attended by children who already had ASD, and in which there were immunization requirements.

Why Is the Myth Wrong?

In 2014, a meta-analysis (a study that combines the results of many studies) was published that summarized the results of 10 studies examining the link between the MMR vaccine and ASD. Altogether, the meta-analysis included results from nearly 1.3 million children, and it found no evidence of any relationship between the MMR vaccine and ASD, between thimerosal and ASD, or between ASD and mercury (Taylor, Swerdfeger, & Eslick, 2014). ●

MODULE SUMMARY

The blastocyst, which is formed about five days after fertilization in humans, is a fluid-filled ball that contains a mass of cells called the embryonic disk, which will become the organism. The embryonic disk contains three germ layers: (1) the ectoderm, which gives rise to the nervous system and the skin; (2) the mesoderm, which gives rise to the muscles, skeleton, some of the internal organs, and the circulatory system; and (3) the endoderm, which gives rise to the digestive system, lungs, and glands. It does so through the process of gastrulation.

The neural tube, which is formed by the process of neurulation, gives rise to the nervous system. The edges of the ectoderm become what are known as the neural folds, neural groove, and neural plate. The neural folds fuse to form the neural crest. The mesoderm forms protrusions, called somites, on either side of the neural tube, which give rise to the vertebrae of the spinal cord and their associated skeletal muscles. The neural tube expands and develops into the three primary vesicles of the brain. During differentiation, these become the forebrain, midbrain, and hindbrain.

The primary vesicles subdivide into five secondary vesicles. The forebrain subdivides into the telencephalon and diencephalon. The telencephalon gives rise to the brain's hemispheres, basal ganglia, olfactory bulb, hippocampus, and amygdala. The diencephalon develops into the thalamus and hypothalamus. The mesencephalon (or midbrain) develops into the tectum and tegmentum. The tectum is subdivided further into the superior colliculus and inferior colliculus. The tegmentum contains the periaqueductal gray matter, the substantia nigra, the red nucleus, and the ventral-tegmental area. The hindbrain consists of the metencephalon, which contains the cerebellum and the pons, whereas the myelencephalon contains the medulla (sometimes called the medulla oblongata).

TEST YOURSELF

4.1.1 Describe the process of gastrulation.

4.1.2 What is the neural tube? What is the gastrula, and how does it develop into the neural tube?

4.1.3 Name and describe the three primary and five secondary vesicles of the brain.

4.2 The Fully Developed Brain

Module Contents

Learning Objectives

4.2.1 Identify the major structures of the telencephalon and some of their functions.

4.2.2 Identify the major structures of the diencephalon and some of their functions.

4.2.3 Identify the major structures of the midbrain and the hindbrain and some of their functions.

4.2.4 Describe the structure of the spinal cord and how it transmits information to and from the brain.

4.2.5 Describe the different protective layers of the brain and how they work.

4.2.6 Explain how each hemisphere of the brain is associated with different functions.

4.2.1 THE STRUCTURES AND FUNCTIONS OF THE FOREBRAIN: THE TELENCEPHALON

>> LO 4.2.1 **Identify the major structures of the telencephalon and some of their functions.**

Key Terms

- **Executive functions:** Brain functions, attributed to the frontal lobes, that include planning, judgment, attention, problem solving, working memory, and decision making.

- **Mirror neurons:** Neurons in the premotor cortex that are activated when performing an action or when watching another individual perform the same action.
- **Proprioception:** The ability to know the relative position of one's own body parts.

Figure 4.5 shows a comparison of the brains of different species. Despite the similarities that exist between these brains, there are also obvious differences. The most obvious difference is in their relative sizes. Another is the extent to which the cortices of different species are circumvoluted by the patterns of ridges and grooves on their surfaces, which are known as gyri (singular, *gyrus*) and sulci (singular, *sulcus*), respectively. You may wonder about the functions of such circumvolutions. Their purpose may be to augment the surface area of the cortex. That is, more neurons can be packed into a highly circumvoluted brain, such as that of humans, monkeys, and chimpanzees, than in the brains of armadillos, cats, rats, and rabbits. As an analogy, think about how much could be written on the surface of a marble versus a long shoelace and then think about trying to fit each of those in a box of the same size. Much more information can be written on the long shoelace, which can then be folded over many times (representing the brain's convolutions) to fit in the box.

FIGURE 4.5

Brains of different species.

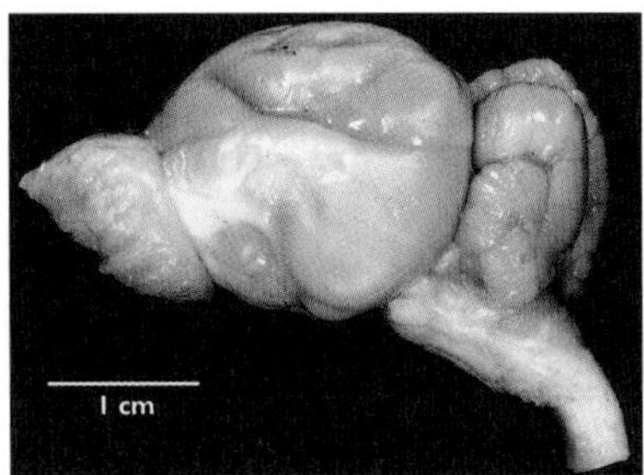

Armadillo brain.

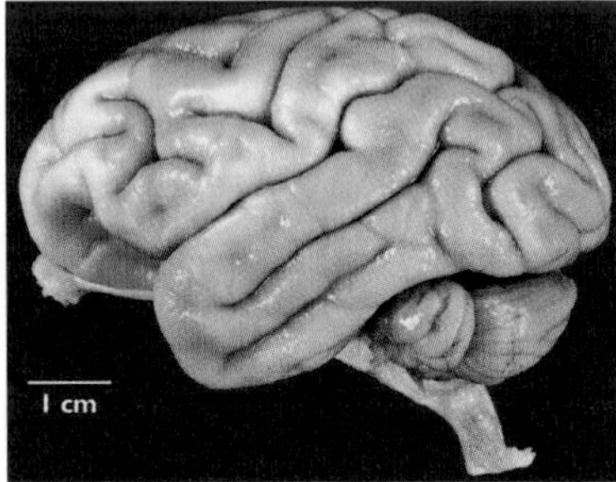

Monkey brain.

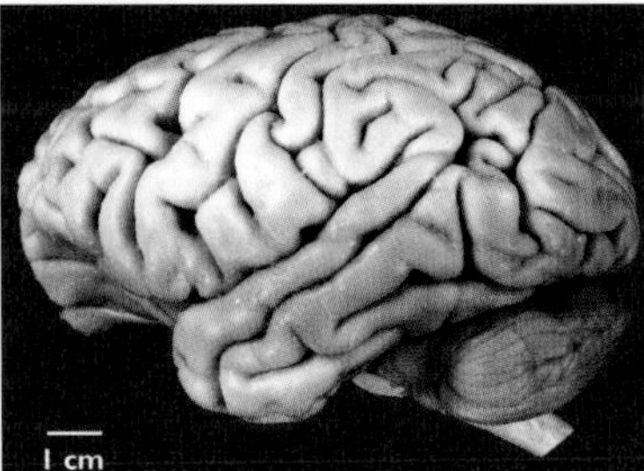

Chimpanzee brain.

National Museum of Health and Medicine

It is still not well understood how sulci and gyri develop. One hypothesis is that gyri are regions that grow at a high rate and rise above the sulci (Lefevre & Mangin, 2010). Another hypothesis is that axons of neurons pull interconnected cortical areas closer together, giving rise to the gyri (Herculano-Houzel, Mota, Wong, & Kaas, 2010). Finally, there is now evidence that gyri form because gray matter (areas consisting of cell bodies) grows faster than white matter (nerve fibers). This results in gray matter being compressed, making it accumulate in the mounds we recognize as gyri (Tallinen, Chung, Biggins, & Mahadevan, 2014; G. Xu et al., 2010).

Sulci and gyri also play different roles in the connectivity between neurons. Neurons located within gyri communicate with neurons within other distant gyri and neurons in nearby sulci. At the same time, neurons within sulci communicate directly with nearby gyri and indirectly, through gyri, with more distant brain areas (F. Deng et al., 2014). As you will read later, gyri and sulci also serve as anatomical landmarks and their names are sometimes used to designate specific areas. For example, the primary motor cortex, covered in the next section, is also known as the precentral gyrus.

As mentioned earlier, the brain develops into the three major parts: the forebrain, the midbrain, and the hindbrain. You also learned that the forebrain consists of the telencephalon and the diencephalon. The telencephalon consists of the cortex, basal ganglia, amygdala, and hippocampus. As you can see in Figure 4.6, the cortex is subdivided into four lobes: frontal lobes, parietal lobes, temporal lobes, and occipital lobes. The basal ganglia, hippocampus, and amygdala are not visible by looking at the surface of the brain. This is because they lie below the cortex. For this reason, they are sometimes referred to as subcortical structures. Each lobe and subcortical structure has been associated with certain functions. We turn our attention first to the functions of the areas contained within the telencephalon, followed by those contained in the diencephalon, which consists of the thalamus and the hypothalamus.

The Forebrain (Telencephalon)

The Frontal Lobes

The frontal lobes are responsible for what are called **executive functions**. These functions make us

FIGURE 4.6

The lobes of the brain (also shown are the cerebellum and the brainstem).

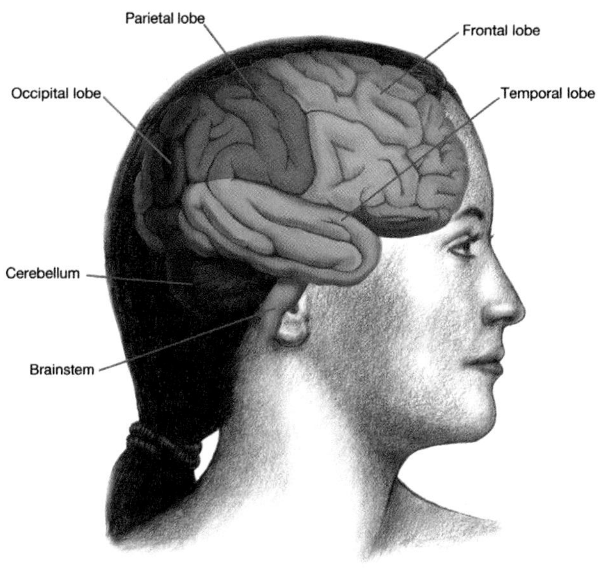

Spencer Sutton/Science Source

distinctively human. Executive functions include planning, judgment, attention, problem solving, working memory, and decision making. The frontal lobes are also involved in behavioral inhibition, ensuring you behave properly in social situations. For example, when you are having dinner at a relative's house, you presumably do not start swearing uncontrollably while starting a food fight with your aunt. This is taken for granted, but people with damage to the frontal lobes may act this way. The frontal lobes are also involved in processing emotions (Bechara, Damasio, & Damasio, 2000). We have learned a lot about the functions of the frontal lobes by studying brain-damaged patients. The most famous of these patients was Phineas Gage, a railroad worker who was the victim of a terrible accident (discussed in Chapter 11).

The left frontal lobe contains the area responsible for speech production, known as Broca's area (after neurologist Paul Broca [see Chapter 1]). Damage to this area causes considerable deficits in the production of speech (Stinnett & Zabel, 2018). However, we now know that speech production requires interactions among several brain areas (Flinker et al., 2015). Figure 4.7 shows the location of Broca's area in the left frontal lobe.

The frontal lobes also house the precentral gyrus, also called the primary motor cortex, or M1. This area is situated at the back of your frontal lobes and is responsible for moving your body (Figure 4.8). The primary

FIGURE 4.7

Broca's area.

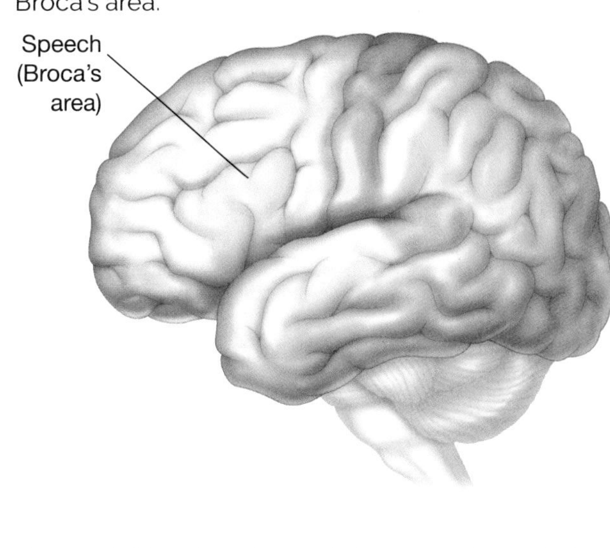

motor cortex is organized into a topographic map of the body, which is commonly represented as a homunculus (little man) (see Figure 1.15c in Chapter 1 and Figure 8.14a in Chapter 8).

As you learned in Chapter 1, this map of your body was discovered by Wilder Penfield, a famous Canadian neurosurgeon, in the 1950s. He observed that, while patients were undergoing surgery, he could electrically

FIGURE 4.8

The primary motor cortex (precentral gyrus or M1).

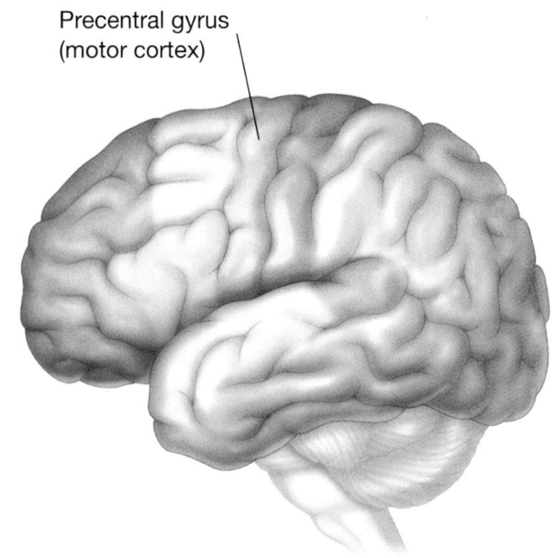

stimulate parts of a patient's motor cortex and observe parts of the patient's body move. The same body parts always moved in response to stimulation of the same areas (Schott, 1993).

In front of the primary motor cortex is another area that controls movement called the premotor cortex. However, this area does so in a different way than does the primary motor cortex. This area plans movements ahead of time. It is also responsible for the completion of sequences of movements. The premotor cortex is also the home of some fascinating neurons. These neurons, called **mirror neurons**, were discovered in the premotor cortex in monkeys (Rizzolatti & Craighero, 2004). Mirror neurons are activated when a monkey watches another monkey perform an action or when the monkey performs the same action itself. Mirror neurons are discussed at some length in Chapter 8.

The Parietal Lobes

The parietal lobes take over from where the primary motor cortex of the posterior frontal lobes leaves off. Just posterior to the central sulcus we find the postcentral gyrus, also called the primary somatosensory cortex, or S1 (Figure 4.9). The primary somatosensory cortex contains another homunculus. It is responsible for your sensations of touch, pressure, pain, and temperature.

The posterior part of the parietal cortex is involved in **proprioception**, which is the ability to sense the position of and movement of your body. The posterior parietal cortex acts in conjunction with other cortical areas to combine proprioceptive and visual information to accurately represent the position of your limbs. The posterior parietal cortex contains maps of space from a person-centered point of view. This means that it maps the location of objects relative to different body parts,

FIGURE 4.9

Location of the primary somatosensory cortex within the parietal lobe and the somatosensory homunculus.

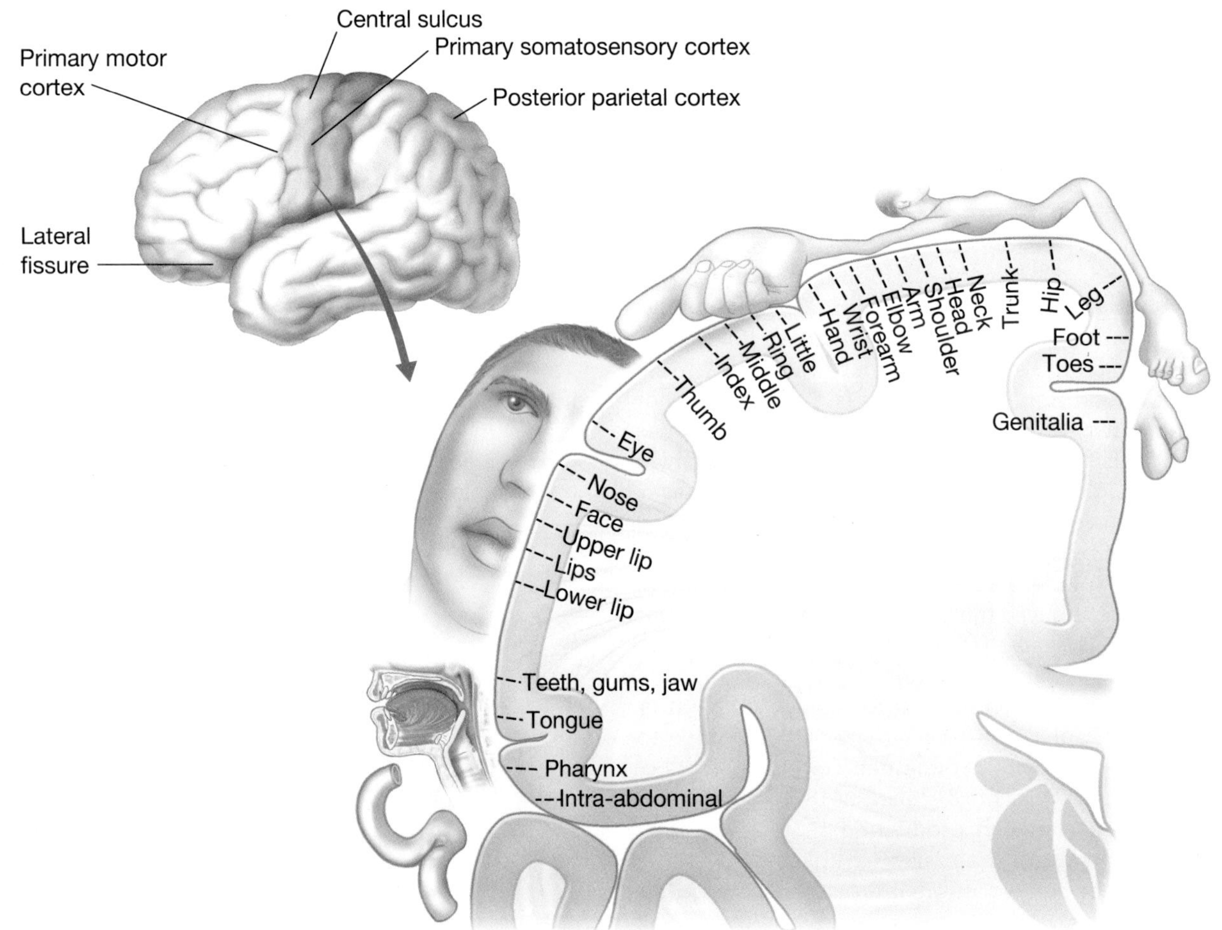

which permits you to orient your limbs in the proper position and orientation to complete various tasks (Limanowski & Blankenburg, 2016). This includes accurately reaching for objects and producing the appropriate types of grips that are best for grasping different objects. It is also thought to be involved in the planning of hand-specific actions (Valyear & Frey, 2015). The posterior parietal cortex is also involved in sensorimotor integration, which is the process of producing a motor output in response to sensory input (Andersen & Buneo, 2003).

The posterior parietal cortex was also found to integrate allocentric spatial information, which refers to the location of objects in the environment relative to each other, with egocentric spatial information, which refers to the location of cues relative to the self, for spatial navigation (Whitlock, Sutherland, Witter, Moser, & Moser, 2008). Another part of the parietal cortex, the medial parietal region is thought to be involved in "route knowledge," which is expressed by the ability to make the correct turns along a route to get to your destination, without being consciously aware of it (Sato, Sakata, Tanaka, & Taira, 2006). The parietal cortex and its functions are discussed in more detail in Chapter 8.

FIGURE 4.10

Ocular dominance columns: Some of the cells in V1 are organized into columns specialized in analyzing features of the environment. For example, cells in particular columns respond best to particular line orientations. Other cells, responsible for color vision, are organized into columns called blobs.

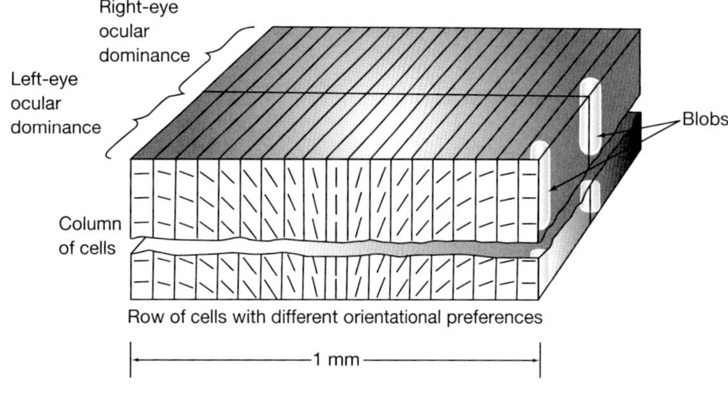

The Temporal Lobes

The temporal lobes are located right below the frontal and parietal lobes, across the lateral fissure (shown in Figure 4.9). If you were to poke sticks into your ears (don't try this at home!) and continue all the way through, you would soon get to your temporal lobes. The temporal lobes are the home of the primary auditory cortex, where sounds are analyzed. It is in the primary auditory cortex that physical features of the environment such as frequencies and amplitudes of sound waves are interpreted as pitch and loudness (auditory perception is covered in Chapter 6).

The front-most part of the temporal lobes contains Wernicke's area, which is important for understanding language. Information about language acquired by Wernicke's area is relayed to Broca's area for the proper production of speech. Speech sounds can be produced without this input from Wernicke's area, but these sounds would not qualify as language. People with damage to Wernicke's area suffer from Wernicke's aphasia, in which they can only produce unintelligible speech (Bogen & Bogen, 1976). However, as we mentioned for speech production, we now know that speech comprehension relies on a broader network of brain areas (Binder, 2017). The temporal lobes are also important for memory and the recognition of objects, as you will learn in Chapter 12.

The Occipital Lobes

The occipital lobes house the primary visual cortex, or V1. The primary visual cortex is where visual information is first analyzed. Here physical information from the environment, in the form of light waves, is first interpreted into visual experience. Some of the cells in the primary visual cortex are organized into columns, known as ocular dominance columns (Figure 4.10). They exist for both the right eye and the left eye.

Ocular dominance columns are specialized in analyzing particular features of the environment such as the orientation of lines or the direction of movement. Area V1 sends information to other brain areas, including the parietal and temporal lobes, where other features of the environment are analyzed. Some neurons are organized in cylindrical shapes called blobs. These neurons are responsible for color perception.

In 1959, Canadian researcher David Hubel and Swedish neurophysiologist Torsten Wiesel recorded the electrical activity in some of the cells in the primary visual cortex of cats. They found that some cells were activated when lines of a particular orientation were presented to the cats on a screen, and other cells were activated when lines of a particular orientation and moving in a particular direction were presented (Hubel & Wiesel, 1959, 2009). This discovery earned the pair the Nobel Prize in 1981. You will learn much more about the functions of V1 in Chapter 6.

Subcortical Structures

Subcortical structures are parts of the brain that lie below the cortex. These include the basal ganglia,

FIGURE 4.11

The location of the basal ganglia, hippocampus, and amygdala.

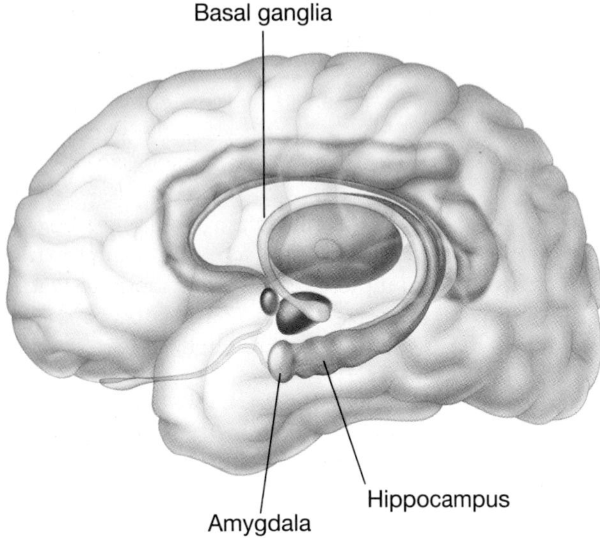

Carolina Hrejsa/Body Scientific Intl.

the hippocampus, and the amygdala (Figure 4.11). Some of their functions are discussed in the sections that follow.

The Basal Ganglia

The basal ganglia consist of several nuclei, which are collections of cell bodies in the central nervous system. The nuclei that compose the basal ganglia consist of the dorsal striatum (which includes the caudate nucleus and putamen), the ventral striatum (which includes the nucleus accumbens), and the substantia nigra. The basal ganglia are involved in the smooth execution of movement and in the selection of appropriate actions. They are also involved in habit learning, such as when you learned to turn right or left automatically after exiting the classroom; and procedural learning, such as when an athlete has learned to go through a complex sequence of movements automatically, without giving it any thought.

Dysfunctions of the basal ganglia give rise to devastating neurological disorders (Yanagisawa, 2018). For example, in Parkinson's disease, neurons in the substantia nigra die, depriving the dorsal striatum of its dopaminergic inputs. The symptoms of Parkinson's disease include shaking and rigidity of movements. The death of neurons in the dorsal striatum is responsible for Huntington's disease, which results in uncontrollable movements. Dysfunctions of the basal ganglia are also thought to be involved in Tourette's syndrome, which is characterized by chronic multiple tics; in the development of drug addiction (Chapter 3); and in obsessive-compulsive disorder (Chapter 14).

The Hippocampus

The hippocampus lies against the medial line of the temporal lobe. It gets its name because of its resemblance to a seahorse, which belongs to the genus hippocampus—*hippos*, from the Greek "horse," and *kampos*, meaning "sea monster." The hippocampus is known to play a special role in memory. People and animals with damage to the hippocampus have trouble acquiring, storing, and retrieving certain types of memories (Squire, Genzel, Wixted, & Morris, 2015), such as those of past episodes of their lives (Wixted et al., 2018).

The hippocampus is also important for successfully navigating in and learning about one's spatial environment. Canadian researchers John O'Keefe and Lynn Nadel discovered that the hippocampus has cells that are activated when a rat finds itself in a familiar environment. These are known as place cells (O'Keefe & Nadel, 1978). The role played by the hippocampus in memory is discussed at greater length in Chapter 12.

The Amygdala

The amygdala is an almond-shaped structure (*amygdala* is Greek for "almond") that is deeply interconnected with the hippocampus. The amygdala is mostly known for its involvement in processing emotions. People and animals with damage to the amygdala do not process emotions normally. For example, if rats are placed in a box in which they receive a foot shock after hearing a tone, they will freeze upon hearing that tone again even without getting a shock. This reaction is taken as an indication of fear (M. Davis, 1992).

However, rats that have sustained damage to the amygdala will not react to the tone—as though they could not make a connection between the tone and the shock. In humans, amygdala damage may render it difficult to experience emotions or to be able to recognize emotions on people's faces (Tranel, Gullickson, Koch, & Adolphs, 2006). We will discuss the amygdala's role in emotions at greater lengths in Chapter 11.

4.2.2 THE STRUCTURES AND FUNCTIONS OF THE FOREBRAIN: THE DIENCEPHALON

>> LO 4.2.2 **Identify the major structures of the diencephalon and some of their functions.**

Key Term

- **Homeostasis:** The tendency of biological systems to maintain a stable internal environment in response to stimuli that challenge stability.

The diencephalon consists of the thalamus and the hypothalamus. The location of these two structures is shown in Figure 4.12.

The Thalamus

The thalamus is situated midway between the front and back of the brain, just below the cortex. The thalamus acts as a relay station between your sensory receptors and the brain areas responsible for interpreting those sensations. That is, information from your senses of hearing, vision, taste, and touch are routed through the thalamus to the auditory, visual, gustatory, and somatosensory cortices, respectively. There is one exception, however. Information about smell first goes directly to the olfactory bulb. Although the thalamus is often described as being a relay station, it is important for a range of other functions, such as movement, the regulation of sleep-wake cycles (Chapter 9), emotional states (Chapter 11), and consciousness (Chapter 13) (Kumar, van Oort, Scheffler, Beckmann, & Grodd, 2017). As shown in Figure 4.13, the thalamus is subdivided into several nuclei, each involved in certain functions.

The Hypothalamus

As its name implies (*hypo* meaning "below"), the hypothalamus is situated right below the thalamus. The hypothalamus is a complex structure that is considered the master gland of the body. It plays many roles—too many to enumerate here. Briefly, it regulates many of your body's functions. It is the major player in **homeostasis**, which is the tendency of biological systems to maintain a stable internal environment in response to stimuli that challenge stability. For example, when you have not had enough water to drink, your blood volume is lowered. This is sensed by the thirst center in your hypothalamus, which causes you to feel thirsty. The hypothalamus will also increase your production of a hormone called vasopressin, which is then released by your pituitary gland, causing your kidneys to retain more water from your blood. The hypothalamus also regulates body temperature. It creates bodily responses according to whether you are getting too hot or too cold. For example, it causes your body to warm up by making you shiver when you are too cold and makes you sweat when you are too hot.

The hypothalamus also has an area called the suprachiasmatic nucleus, which regulates circadian rhythms (Hastings, Brancaccio, & Maywood, 2014). This means that it regulates functions that are repeated in cycles that last about a day. The hypothalamus controls the release of many hormones. The role of the hypothalamus in homeostasis is discussed in Chapter 9. The hypothalamus also plays an important role in sexual and reproductive behaviors, which are discussed in Chapter 10.

FIGURE 4.12

Location of the thalamus and hypothalamus.

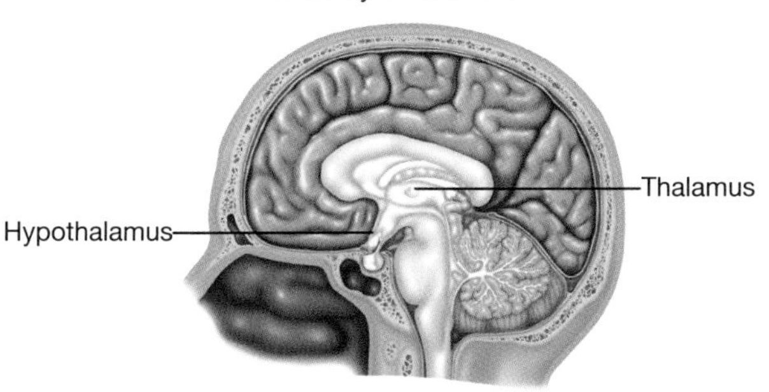

Gwen Shockey/Science Source

FIGURE 4.13

The thalamus is subdivided into several nuclei, each involved in particular functions.

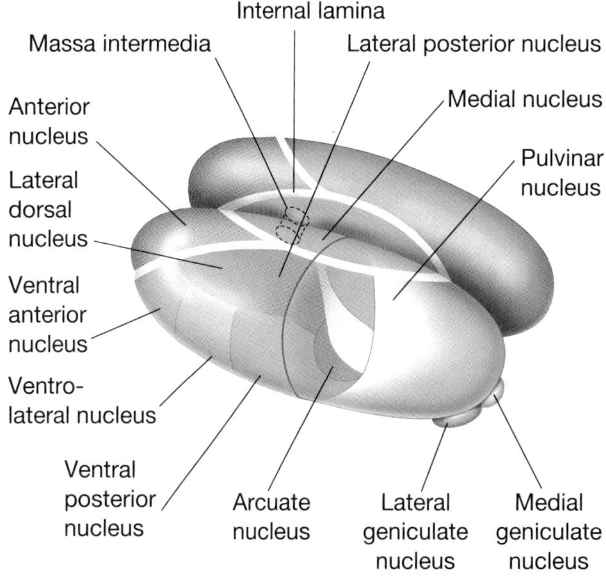

Amanda Tomasikiewicz/Body Scientific Intl.

4.2.3 THE MIDBRAIN AND THE HINDBRAIN

>> LO 4.2.3 Identify the major structures of the midbrain and the hindbrain and some of their functions.

Key Terms

- **Superior colliculus:** Also referred to as the optic tectum because it plays an important role in controlling eye movements.
- **Inferior colliculus:** A part of the tectum that plays a role in processing auditory information.

The midbrain consists of the tectum and the tegmentum. The hindbrain consists of the cerebellum, pons, and medulla. Figure 4.14 shows the location of each of these structures.

Tectum

Tectum means "roof." In the brain, the tectum is the roof of the mesencephalon. The tectum can be subdivided in two areas: the superior colliculus and the inferior colliculus. The **superior colliculus** is often referred to as the optic tectum because it plays an important role in controlling eye movements. The **inferior colliculus** processes auditory information.

Tegmentum

The tegmentum plays an important role in movement and reward. It houses the substantia nigra (also considered part of the basal ganglia), which produces dopamine, a neurotransmitter important for movement. As mentioned earlier, in Parkinson's disease, neurons in the substantia nigra that produce dopamine are dying off (Damier, Hirsch, Agid, & Graybiel, 1999). The tegmentum also houses the ventral-tegmental area, which is involved in reward processes, such as those involved in the motivation for food and drug intake (see Chapters 3 and 9).

FIGURE 4.14

The midbrain and the hindbrain (cerebellum, pons, and medulla).

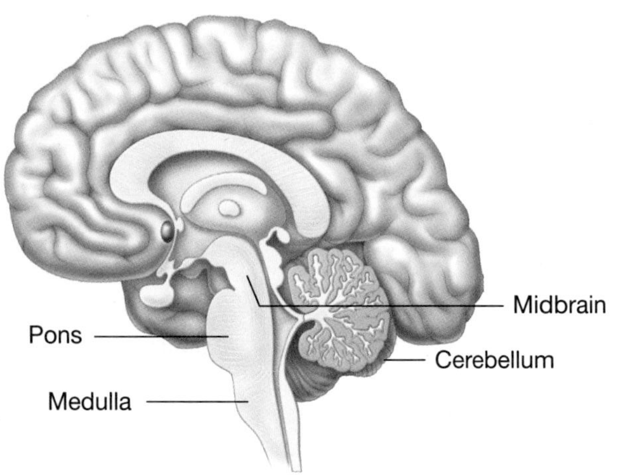

The Hindbrain

The Cerebellum. *Cerebellum* literally means "small brain." The cerebellum is important for motor coordination (discussed in Chapter 8) (Schmahmann & Pandya, 1997). People with damage to the cerebellum cannot properly adjust their ongoing movements or coordinate their limbs very well. The cerebellum is also involved in learning automatic motor responses. For example, after your friend has sprayed you with a garden hose, you will automatically raise your hands in a defensive posture when a hose is pointed at you. This is an example of classical conditioning, which is discussed in Chapter 12.

The cerebellum is also thought to play an important role in cognitive functions. It is believed to have an important role in organizing and coordinating thoughts (Ito, 2008) and is thought to regulate the speed, capacity, and consistency of cognitive functions (Buckner, 2013; Schmahmann, 1991).

The Pons. The pons (Latin for "bridge") relays signals between the cortex and the cerebellum. It is important for maintaining vital functions such as respiration. It is also involved in consciousness, sleep, and arousal.

The Medulla. The medulla regulates vital functions such as breathing and heartbeat.

4.2.4 THE SPINAL CORD

>> LO 4.2.4 Describe the structure of the spinal cord and how it transmits information to and from the brain.

Key Terms

- **Foramen magnum:** The hole at the base of the skull through which the spinal cord passes.
- **Spinal nerves**: Pairs of nerves that carry information to and from parts of the body.
- **Ascending fibers:** Nerves through which sensory information travels to the brain.
- **Descending fibers:** Nerves that carry information from the brain.

- **Upper motor neurons:** Motor neurons that carry information from the brain.
- **Lower motor neurons:** Motor neurons that innervate the muscles.
- **Paraplegia:** Loss of the use of and sensation in the lower limbs that results from damage to the lower parts of the spinal cord.
- **Quadriplegia (also known as tetraplegia):** Loss of the use of and sensation in both upper and lower limbs that results from damage to the upper spinal cord.

The spinal cord is the other part of the central nervous system that, like the brain, is encased in bone. It runs up and down your back, protected by your vertebrae. It enters the skull through a large hole at its base, called the **foramen magnum**, where it connects to the medulla. The spinal cord receives sensory messages from your body and transmits this information to your brain. The spinal cord also carries messages from your brain to your body. It can also function independently of your brain; for example, in the execution of reflexes. The spinal cord is subdivided into 33 segments: 8 cervical, 12 thoracic, 5 lumbar, 5 sacral, and 3 coccygeal. Each segment, except for two of the coccygeal segments, contains a pair of nerves known as the **spinal nerves**. The coccygeal segments have only one pair of nerve for all three segments (Figure 4.15). An area of the skin that is connected to a spinal nerve is referred to as a dermatome (discussed in detail in Chapter 7).

The cervical segments innervate your neck, shoulders, and arm muscles. The thoracic segments innervate the muscles of your chest, back, and midsection, as well as your breathing muscles. The thoracic segments also innervate, among other organs, your heart, lungs, gallbladder, pancreas, spleen, and kidneys. The lumbar segments innervate the muscles of your lower back, thighs, legs, calves, and feet. They also innervate your large intestines, appendix, reproductive organs, bladder, and prostate. The sacral segments innervate the hips, buttocks, thighs, and leg muscles. The coccygeal segment innervates the perineum, which includes the anogenital area.

Sensory nerve fibers enter the spinal cord, carrying information to the brain, through what are known as the dorsal nerve roots. Motor nerve fibers, carrying information from the brain to the body, exit the spinal cord through what are known as the ventral nerve roots (Figure 4.16). The dorsal and ventral roots are composed of gray matter, the cell bodies of neurons. The axons of these neurons, which carry information to and from the brain, compose the white matter.

Nerves through which sensory information travel to the brain are called **ascending fibers**. Nerves that carry information from the brain to the body are referred to as **descending fibers**. Motor neurons that carry information from the brain are called **upper motor neurons**. These upper motor neurons connect to **lower motor neurons**, the neurons that innervate your muscles. Upper motor neurons never leave the CNS. Injury to the spinal cord can lead to a significant loss in sensory and motor function.

Loss in sensory and motor function occurs in parts of the body that are below the site of the injury. For example, damage to the lowest part of the spinal cord (coccygeal) may only result in paralysis of

FIGURE 4.15

The spinal cord is subdivided into 33 segments: 8 cervical, 12 thoracic, 5 lumbar, 5 sacral, and 3 coccygeal. The nerves from the bottom segments of the spinal cord extend in such a way that they resemble a horse's tail, hence, the term *cauda equina*, which is Latin for "horse tail." Also note the filum terminale, which is a strand of fibrous tissue that extends from the coccygeal segments.

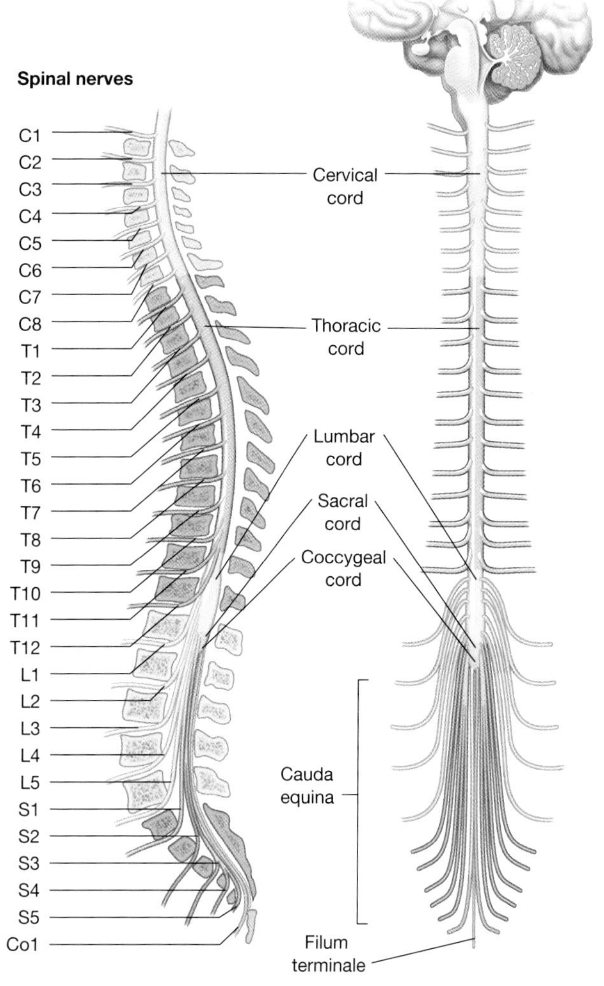

Carolina Hrejsa/Body Scientific Intl.

FIGURE 4.16

Cross-section of the spinal cord.

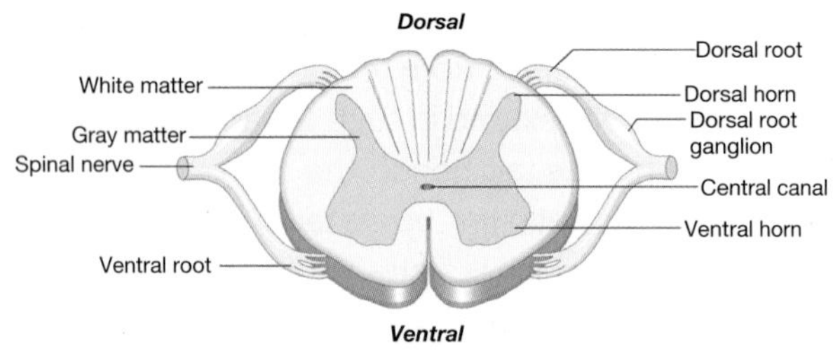

Krystal Thompson/Science Source

the legs. Damage higher up in the spinal cord (lumbar or thoracic) may also result in a loss of control of the muscles of the bladder. This condition is called **paraplegia** (Figure 4.17a). With damage even higher up in the spinal cord (cervical), the loss of function can also include both arms. This condition is called **quadriplegia** (Figure 4.17b), as this chapter's opening vignette described.

FIGURE 4.17

Depictions of quadriplegia (top) and paraplegia (bottom).

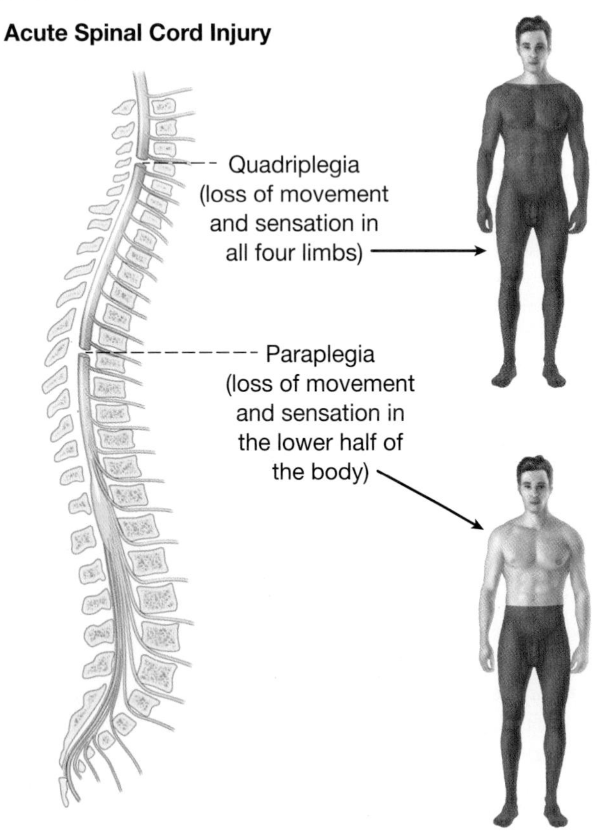

Carolina Hrejsa/Body Scientific Intl.

4.2.5 THE PROTECTED BRAIN

>> **LO 4.2.5 Describe the different protective layers of the brain and how they work.**

Key Terms

- **Meninges:** Three membranes that envelop the brain (and spinal cord): the pia mater, the arachnoid mater, and the dura mater.
- **Cerebrospinal fluid (CSF):** Fluid that cushions the brain and spinal cord.
- **Blood-brain barrier:** The protective barrier formed by the cells of the brain's blood vessels, which block or slow the passage of harmful molecules to the brain.
- **Central canal:** The hollow center of the spinal cord.
- **Ventricles:** Hollow areas of the brain in which cerebrospinal fluid is produced.

Your central nervous system is protected at three different levels: the **meninges**, the **cerebrospinal fluid (CSF)**, and the **blood-brain barrier**. Each of these protective barriers is described in the sections that follow.

The Meninges

Figure 4.18a shows how your brain and spinal cord are enveloped by what are known as the meninges, which consist of three membranes: the pia mater, the arachnoid mater, and the dura mater, which are Greek terms for "soft mother," "spidery mother," and "tough mother," respectively. The pia mater is the one that adheres the most closely to the surface of the CNS. It is also the most delicate but impermeable to CSF, which we discuss in the next section. The arachnoid mater looks like a spider web. Below the arachnoid mater is the subarachnoid space, which contains blood vessels and CSF. The dura mater is the hardest and most closely adheres to the skull. It is thick and nonelastic. Also visible in Figure 4.18a is a layer of sheetlike tissue called aponeurosis, which attaches the muscles of the skull, and the periosteum, which covers the surface of all bones.

The Cerebrospinal Fluid

The CSF fills the subarachnoid space and the hollow center of the spinal cord called the **central canal**. The CSF is produced in hollow spaces in the brain called **ventricles**. There are four ventricles (Figure 4.18b): two

FIGURE 4.18

The protected brain. The brain has three protective layers: (a) the meninges; (b) the CSF, which fills the subarachnoid space and is stored in the brain's ventricles; and (c) the blood-brain barrier.

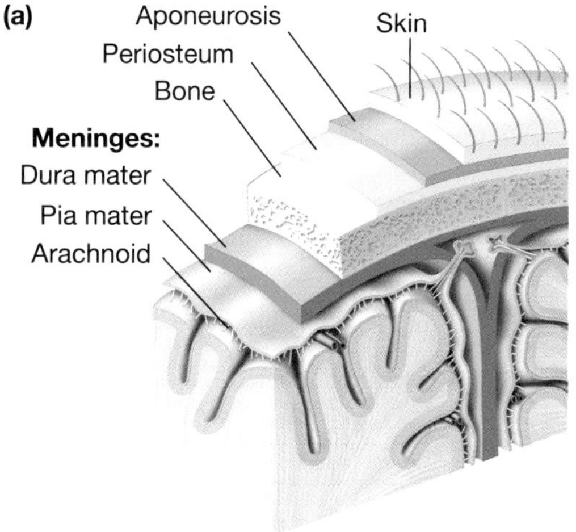

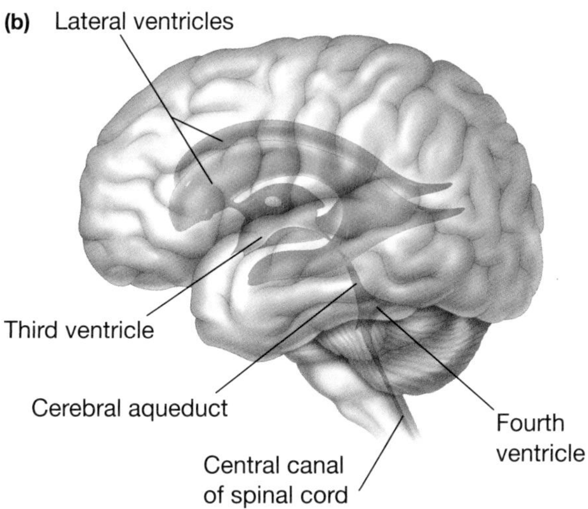

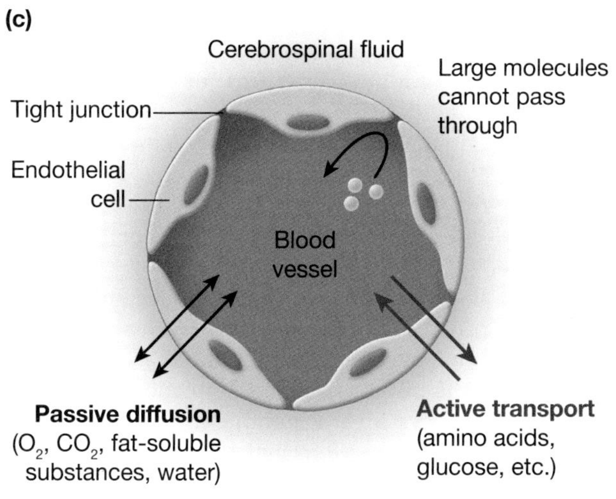

lateral ventricles, the third ventricle, and the fourth ventricle. The third and fourth ventricles are connected by the cerebral aqueduct. Cerebrospinal fluid is produced in the choroid plexus (Greek for "braided membrane"). The role of the CSF is to cushion and support the brain and spinal cord.

The Blood-Brain Barrier

The cells (endothelial cells) of the brain's blood vessels are packed more tightly than the cells in the blood vessels elsewhere in your body. They are sealed in a narrow band called tight junctions. This arrangement, called the blood-brain barrier, blocks or slows the passage of large and potentially harmful molecules into the brain (Figure 4.18c). Only small and fat-soluble molecules, such as oxygen and carbon dioxide, and certain drugs can make it through by simple diffusion. In contrast, water-soluble molecules, such as amino acids and glucose, must be actively transported across the wall of the blood vessels.

Some drugs can cross the blood-brain barrier but do so slowly. One such drug is morphine, a powerful painkiller. Heroin, a derivative of morphine, was designed to cross the blood-brain barrier more readily; however, it is not used in medicine due to its high potential for addiction.

Another example involves dopamine. As you learned earlier, in Parkinson's disease, dopamine neurons in the substantia nigra die. The drug prescribed to treat Parkinson's is a precursor of dopamine called levodopa (L-dopa). Neurons inside the brain then use L-dopa to produce more dopamine. Why not just administer dopamine to Parkinson's patients? The answer is that it does not cross the blood-brain barrier.

4.2.6 HEMISPHERIC SPECIALIZATION

>> LO 4.2.6 **Explain how each hemisphere of the brain is associated with different functions.**

Key Terms

- **Hemispheric asymmetry:** When functions are associated with either the right or left hemisphere.
- **Handedness:** The preferred usage of one hand over the other.
- **Split-brain patients:** Patients who have been subjected to the removal of the corpus callosum.

The forebrain, as mentioned earlier, is composed of two hemispheres, the right and left hemispheres. The hemispheres are connected to each other by a thick bundle of nerve fibers called the corpus callosum. The corpus callosum is used to send information from one side of the brain to the other.

Each of the two hemispheres has been found to perform different functions (Corballis, 2009). This is known as **hemispheric asymmetry**. Table 4.1 shows the functions associated with either the right or left hemisphere. The right hemisphere is responsible for your creative side and makes you understand things holistically. It is your right hemisphere that enables you to understand figures of speech, such as knowing that the expression "He kicked the bucket" means that someone has died (see "It's a Myth!" in Chapter 1).

The right hemisphere processes spatial information. It is mostly involved when navigating through the environment, assembling pictures, and rotating objects mentally. The left hemisphere is more analytical. It is mostly involved in tasks requiring perceptual speed, manual precision, mathematical calculation, and linguistic abilities. It takes things literally. For example, to your left hemisphere, the expression "He kicked the bucket" literally means that someone has kicked a bucket.

TABLE 4.1

Hemispheric Asymmetry

DOMINANT HEMISPHERE (LEFT HEMISPHERE)	NONDOMINANT HEMISPHERE (RIGHT HEMISPHERE)
Verbal (speech)	Nonverbal
Linguistic description	Spatial concepts (comprehension)
Reading, writing, drawing, and associated functions of language; grammatical language using script	Musical (some elements of music)
Mathematical	Geometrical
Sequential	Recognition of faces
Analytical	Pictorial language
Direct link to the consciousness	Temporal synthesis Expressing emotions, reading emotions Global holistic processing Understanding of metaphors Discrimination of shapes (e.g., picking out a camouflaged object)
Positive emotions (joy, gratitude, hope)	Negative emotions (ashamed, lied, abused)
FUNCTIONS SHARED BY BOTH HEMISPHERES	
Sensations on both sides of the face Sounds heard by both ears Pain Hunger	

Source: Agrawai, D., et al. (2014). Split brain syndrome: One brain but two conscious minds? *Journal of Health Research and Reviews in Developing Countries 1*(2): 27–33. With permission from Wolters Kluwer Medknow Publications.

Cerebral Dominance

Broca, who discovered that control of speech was situated in the left hemisphere, observed that there was a relationship between **handedness** (the preferred usage of one hand over the other) and the speech area in the brain. That is, in right-handers, the speech area was most often located in the left hemisphere. Broca took this as an indication that right-handers had an inborn dominance by the left hemisphere. What about left-handers? Well, he also discovered that in some left-handers the speech area was located in the left hemisphere and in others it was in the right hemisphere. The hemisphere that contained the language area became known as the dominant hemisphere.

Split-Brain Patients

Much of what we know about the functions of each hemisphere comes to us from the study of **split-brain patients**. Split-brain patients are people whose corpus callosum has been severed (cut) in order to relieve them of recurring epileptic seizures, which are bouts of uncontrollable brain activity that can give rise to uncontrollable movements or changes in consciousness. Why does severing the corpus callosum alleviate the seizures? Seizures sometimes begin in one hemisphere and travel to the other hemisphere via the corpus callosum. Severing the corpus callosum prevents the spreading of seizures from one hemisphere to another.

Roger Sperry (1961) made some intriguing discoveries while studying split-brain patients. In one experiment, split-brain patients were made to stare at a point in the middle of a screen. Objects were then presented either on the right side of the screen (in the patient's right visual field) or on the left side of the screen (in the patient's left visual field). Because of the way the neurons that carry information from the retina to the brain are wired, images in the patient's right visual field were projected to the left hemisphere and images in the patient's left visual field were projected to the right hemisphere (Figure 4.19). (The patterns of connections between the retina and the visual cortex are discussed at greater length in Chapter 6.)

When the image of an object was presented in the subject's right visual field, meaning it was processed by the left hemisphere, split-brain patients could easily name it. This is because the left hemisphere also contained their speech area. When the image of an object was presented in the left visual field, meaning it was processed by the right hemisphere, subjects could not name the object. To be able to name an object processed in the right hemisphere, information about it would

FIGURE 4.19

Neuronal connections from the retina to the visual cortex. Images presented to the right visual field are processed in the left hemisphere, and images presented to the left visual field are processed in the right hemisphere.

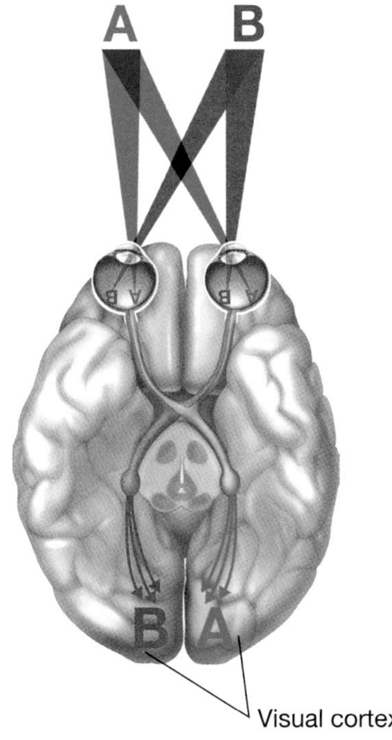

FIGURE 4.20

Sperry's split-brain experiment.

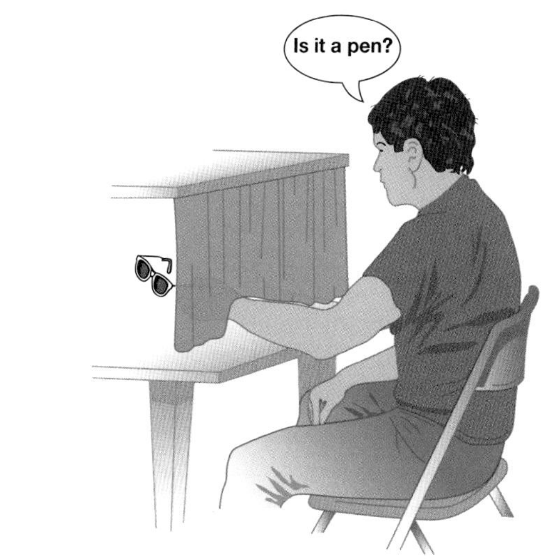

have had to cross over to the speech area located in the subject's left hemisphere via the corpus callosum.

In addition, split-brain patients could not name objects held in the left hand when hidden from view (Figure 4.20). Similar to what happens with stimuli presented to the left visual field, information about an object held in the left hand is processed in the right hemisphere. For the object to be named, information about the object has to cross over, via the corpus callosum, to the left hemisphere, where the speech area is located.

Handedness

Many theories have been put forward in an attempt to explain handedness, but none is completely satisfactory. Many of them have to do with the question of why a majority of people are right-handed. These theories are based on several lines of research, including evolutionary, environmental, and genetic research.

In the late 1970s, experimental support was provided to Broca's observation of the relationship between handedness and the location of the speech area in the brain. This support was provided by experiments that made use of what became known as the Wada test. The Wada test was developed by Juhn Atsushi Wada to guide neurosurgeons in not damaging the language area of patients undergoing brain surgery (Wada & Rasmussen, 2007). In short, a subject is asked to count repeatedly from 1 to 20 while holding up both arms. At the same time, sodium amytal, a barbiturate used as an anesthetic, is injected into one of the patient's two carotid arteries, which pass through the neck and carry blood to the brain. This anesthetizes only one of the hemispheres because each carotid artery supplies blood to only one hemisphere. If the drug is injected into the left hemisphere and the patient can no longer count and drops the right arm, the person's speech area is located in the left hemisphere and the individual is right-handed, which accounts for the majority of the findings.

Using the Wada test, researchers found that the speech area was located in the left hemisphere in 95% of right-handers; in the other 5%, the speech area was located in the right hemisphere. The control of speech was located in the left hemisphere for 70% of left-handers. In only 15% of left-handers was the speech area located in the right hemisphere. Another 15% of left-handers showed mixed dominance (Rasmussen & Milner, 1977).

MODULE SUMMARY

The brain developed into three major sections: the forebrain, the midbrain, and the hindbrain. The forebrain gave rise to the telencephalon and the diencephalon.

The telencephalon consists of four lobes: the frontal, temporal, parietal, and occipital lobes, as well as the entire neocortex, basal ganglia, hippocampus, and amygdala. The diencephalon gave rise to the thalamus and hypothalamus. The midbrain consists of the tectum and tegmentum. The hindbrain contains the cerebellum, pons, and medulla. The spinal cord carries information from the body to the brain and from the brain to the body. The central nervous system is protected at three different levels, the meninges, the cerebrospinal fluid, and the blood-brain barrier. The right and left hemispheres of the brain are connected to each other by a thick bundle of fibers called the corpus callosum. Each of the two hemispheres performs different functions. The right hemisphere is responsible for creativity and processing spatial information, whereas the left hemisphere is more analytical. Split-brain patients are people whose corpus callosum has been cut in order to relieve them from recurring epileptic seizures. Broca discovered that handedness had something to do with cerebral dominance.

TEST YOURSELF

4.2.1 Name the structures of the telencephalon and explain their functions.

4.2.2 Name the structures of the diencephalon and explain their functions.

4.2.3 Name the structures of the mesencephalon, metencephalon, and myelencephalon and explain their functions.

4.2.4 Explain the structure of the spinal cord, how it is involved in the transmission of information, and the effects of spinal cord damage.

4.2.5 Name and explain the three different levels at which the brain is protected.

4.2.6 What are some of the differences in the way the left and right hemispheres process information?

4.3 The Peripheral Nervous System

Module Contents

Learning Objectives

4.3.1 Explain the functions of the somatic nervous system.

4.3.2 Explain the functions of the autonomic nervous system.

The PNS consists of the parts of the nervous system that are outside of the central nervous system. This includes the somatic and autonomic nervous systems. The PNS also includes the cranial nerves, which are involved in transmitting information from the senses of vision, taste, and hearing. They are also involved in the control of facial muscles and regulate several physiological processes. Although the CNS and the PNS are treated as separate systems, they are functionally and physiologically interrelated. For example, the PNS has axons for which the cell bodies are contained within the spinal cord, which, as you know, is part of the CNS.

4.3.1 THE SOMATIC NERVOUS SYSTEM

>> LO 4.3.1 Explain the functions of the somatic nervous system.

Key Terms

- **Dorsal roots:** Areas through which sensory neurons enter the spinal cord.
- **Ventral roots:** Areas through which motor neurons exit the spinal cord.
- **Reflex arc:** A loop of information that begins with the activation of sensory neurons and ends with muscle contraction, through the activation of motor neurons.

The somatic nervous system (SNS) refers to the part of the PNS that is responsible for the voluntary control of movement. It consists of a collection of nerve fibers that enter and exit the spinal cord. Sensory neurons convey sensory information from your skin, muscles, joints, tendons, blood vessels, and organs. Near the spinal cord, each of the spinal nerves splits in two. Sensory neurons, also known as afferent neurons, enter the back of the spinal cord through the **dorsal roots**. Motor neurons, also known as efferent neurons, move your muscles and exit the front of the spinal cord through the **ventral roots** (see Figure 4.16).

An interaction between your CNS and PNS occurs when the doctor tests your patellar reflex by hitting your patellar tendon (just below your kneecap) with a rubber hammer. This results in a message being sent through sensory neurons up your thigh (PNS), which then connect with ascending fibers in the spinal cord that carry the information to your brain (CNS). An interaction between your PNS and CNS also occurs when you voluntarily move your arm—a message is sent from your motor cortex down your spinal cord (CNS) and connects with a motor neuron that, in turn, connects with your arm muscles (PNS).

The Reflex Arc

Continuing with the preceding example, in which the doctor tests your patellar reflex, you surely noticed that your leg automatically lifts from its resting position. It does so a split second before you feel the hit of the hammer below your knee, which relies on a signal going to your brain. The reason your leg lifts from its resting position is that the sensory neuron activated by the stroke of the hammer forms a synapse with an interneuron within your spinal cord, which in turn forms a synapse with a motor neuron. This motor neuron forms a synapse with one of the muscle cells responsible for contracting the thigh muscle. This is known as the **reflex arc** (Figure 4.21).

FIGURE 4.21

The reflex arc. The hammer stretches the tendon, causing a reflexive contraction of the extensor muscle and a kicking motion.

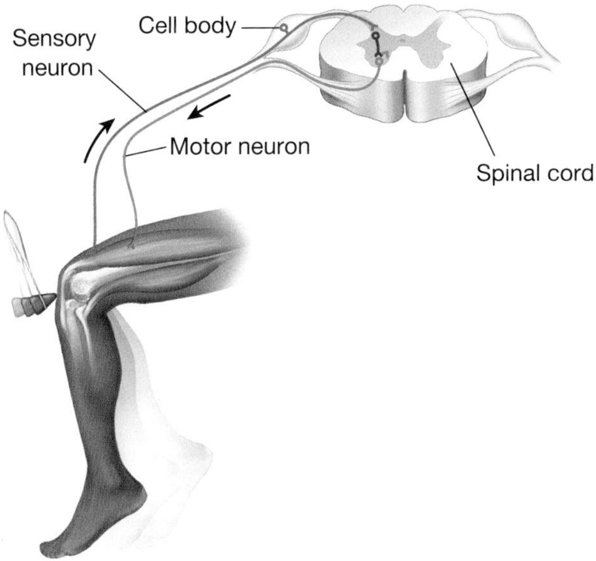

4.3.2 THE AUTONOMIC NERVOUS SYSTEM

>> LO 4.3.2 **Explain the functions of the autonomic nervous system.**

Key Terms

- **Involuntary muscles:** Muscles that are not under conscious control.
- **Sympathetic nervous system:** Gets your body ready for action; often referred to as the "fight-or-flight" system.
- **Parasympathetic nervous system:** Counters the activity of the sympathetic nervous system by slowing things down; often referred to as the "rest-and-digest" system.
- **Ganglia:** A collection of cell bodies.
- **Preganglionic fibers:** Fibers that exit the spinal cord and enter ganglia.
- **Postganglionic fibers:** Fibers that exit ganglia and enter the spinal cord.

As its name suggests, the autonomic nervous system (ANS) is autonomous. It performs the bodily functions that you do not have to think about. The ANS controls your smooth muscles, which are muscles that are not under conscious control. These are known as **involuntary muscles**. You have these types of muscles in your intestines, blood vessels, bladder, and urinary tract. The ANS also controls your heart, lungs, and liver. Your glands are also under the control of your ANS. The ANS is highly involved in homeostasis, which means that it balances and coordinates activity in your body. For example, it regulates blood chemistry, respiration, circulation, and digestion.

The ANS is subdivided into the sympathetic nervous system and the parasympathetic nervous system, which act in opposition to each other. The **sympathetic nervous system** gets your body ready for action. For this, it is often referred to as the "fight-or-flight" system. For example, if someone were to walk into your classroom and yell "fire," several physiological responses would occur in your body. Think of what some of these responses might be. Chances are that you thought about some obvious things like your heartbeat and your respiration accelerating. Depending on how convincing the person was, you might also start to sweat. However, some more subtle things would also happen. For example, glucose would be released from your liver to be used as energy for your muscles, the smooth muscles in your intestines would slow down and digestion would come to a crawl, and your pupils would dilate.

FIGURE 4.22

The autonomic nervous system.

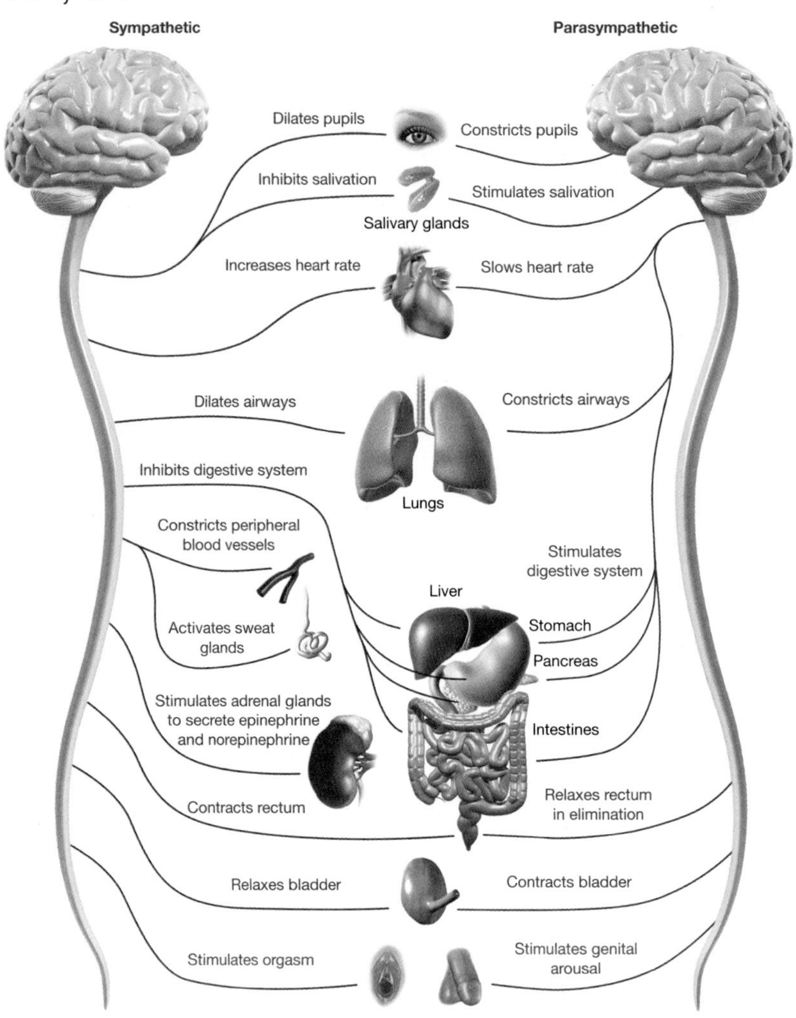

The PNS counters the activity of the sympathetic nervous system by bringing autonomic activity back to normal. Contrary to the sympathetic nervous system, the **parasympathetic nervous system** is often referred to as the "rest-and-digest" system. This is because its actions are contrary to those of the sympathetic nervous system.

Figure 4.22 illustrates the effects that the sympathetic and parasympathetic nervous systems have on the organs of the body. Sympathetic fibers exit the spinal cord from its thoracic and lumbar segments, whereas parasympathetic fibers exit the spinal cord from its cranial and sacral segments.

Both the sympathetic and parasympathetic fibers connect with collections of cell bodies called **ganglia**, which lie outside the spinal cord. These are known as **preganglionic fibers**. From these ganglia, other fibers connect with the organs involved in the activating effects. These are known as **postganglionic fibers**.

The sympathetic and parasympathetic nervous systems also differ in the neurotransmitters that they use. Both the preganglionic and postganglionic fibers of the parasympathetic nervous system use acetylcholine. However, in the sympathetic nervous system, the preganglionic fibers use acetylcholine but the postganglionic fibers use norepinephrine. One exception to this is the adrenal medulla, which is innervated by preganglionic fibers of the sympathetic nervous system and uses acetylcholine as a neurotransmitter.

The Cranial Nerves

So far, we have seen that nerve fibers that are part of the peripheral nervous system originate either from the brainstem or from different sections of the spinal cord. There is, however, an exception to this arrangement. The peripheral nervous system also includes the innervation of the cranial nerves (Figure 4.23). Contrary to the spinal nerves, which originate in the spinal cord, cranial nerves originate in the brain. There are 12 pairs of cranial nerves.

FIGURE 4.23

The cranial nerves.

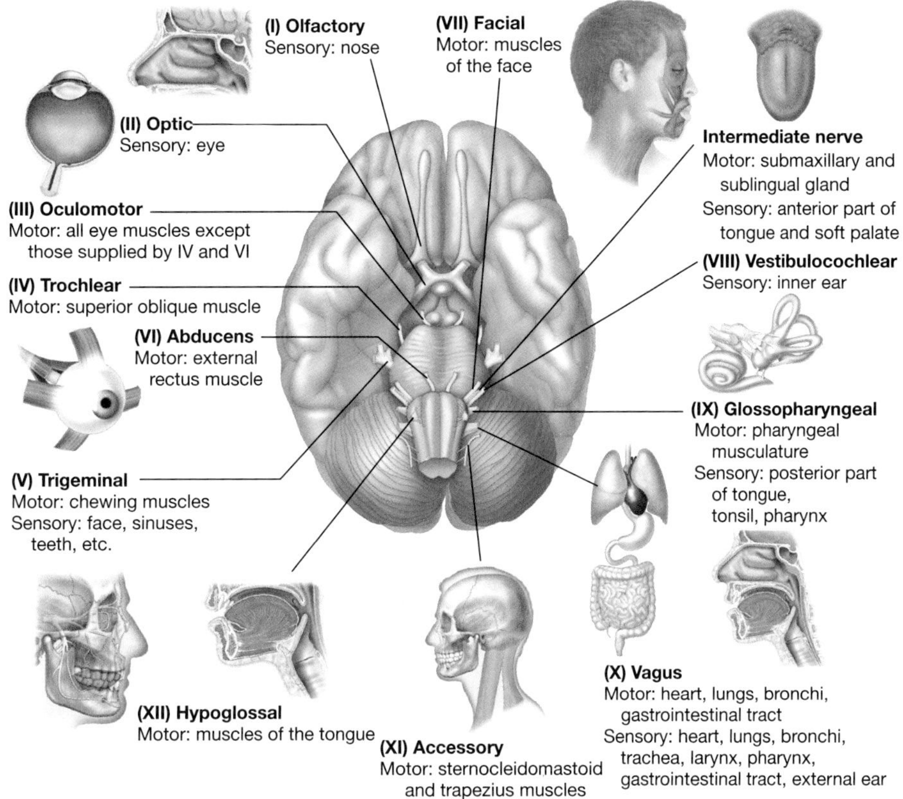

Encyclopaedia Britannica/Contributor/Universal Images Group/Getty

Each was given both a name and a number. Some of these nerves transmit information from the senses of smell, vision, hearing, balance, and taste. Cranial nerve I is the olfactory nerve, and cranial nerve II is the optic nerve. The nerve for hearing and balance is cranial nerve VIII, also called the vestibuloacoustic nerve. Information about taste is transmitted through several of the cranial nerves: the trigeminal (cranial nerve V), facial (cranial nerve VII), glossopharyngeal (cranial nerve IX), and vagus nerves (cranial nerve X).

Other cranial nerves are involved in movement. Eye movements are produced by the oculomotor (cranial nerve III), trochlear (cranial nerve IV), and abducens nerves (cranial nerve VI). The facial nerve also transmits motor information to the muscles of the face. The swallowing reflex is transmitted by the glossopharyngeal nerve. The spinal accessory nerve (cranial nerve XI) stabilizes the head and the neck. The muscles of the tongue are innervated by the hypoglossal (cranial nerve XII).

The cranial nerve with the most complex set of connections is the vagus nerve. The vagus nerve plays an important role in the PNS. It slows the heart and regulates the activity of internal organs. It also controls your laryngeal muscles, which produce speech.

MODULE SUMMARY

The somatic nervous system (SNS) refers to the part of the peripheral nervous system that is responsible for the voluntary control of movement. It consists of the autonomic nervous system (ANS), which controls involuntary muscles and automatic processes such as regulating blood chemistry, respiration, circulation, and digestion. The ANS is subdivided into the sympathetic and parasympathetic nervous systems. The sympathetic nervous system is also known as the fight-or-flight system and gets the body ready for action. The parasympathetic nervous system is also known as the rest-and-digest system and returns the body to a relaxed state. There are 12 pairs of cranial nerves, all originating from the brain. Some cranial nerves relay information from the senses of smell, vision, hearing, balance, and taste. Other cranial nerves are involved in movement of the eyes and face as well as the swallowing reflex. The vagus nerve (cranial nerve X) has the most complex set of connections. It plays an important role, slowing the heart and regulating the activity of internal organs.

TEST YOURSELF

4.3.1 Describe the somatic nervous system. What does it consist of, and what are its functions?

4.3.2 What are the divisions of the autonomic nervous system? What are its functions?

APPLICATIONS

Powered Exoskeletons in the Rehabilitation of Patients With Spinal Cord Injury

There are 17,700 new cases of spinal cord injury (SCI) every year in the United States (National Spinal Cord Injury Statistical Center, 2018) and 500,000 cases a year worldwide (World Health Organization, 2013). The severity of SCI varies between individuals. Tetraplegia (also known as quadriplegia) refers to spinal cord damage above the first thoracic vertebra, which means that, depending on the extent of injury (complete or incomplete), the patient loses sensation and the ability to move the body below the neck. Paraplegia (which can also be complete or incomplete) refers to injury to the lower thoracic, lumber, or sacral segments of the spinal cord, which results in the lack of sensation and the ability to move the lower extremities. The leading causes of SCI (in order of frequency) are car crashes, falls, acts of violence (such as gunshot wounds), sports, and recreational injuries.

Individuals with SCI show varying degrees of paralysis of the trunk muscles, resulting in their lack of ability to maintain enough postural stability to sit or stand, and many lose the ability to walk independently. Fewer than 1% of SCI patients experience complete recovery (National Spinal Cord Injury Statistical Center, 2018).

Treatment and rehabilitation for SCI patients includes locomotor training, respiratory muscle training, bodyweight-supported gait training, and neuromuscular electrical stimulation. In any case, the treatment and rehabilitation of SCI is long, arduous, and expensive (Nas, Yazmalar, Sah, Aydin, & Ones, 2015).

What Is a Powered Exoskeleton?

The word *exoskeleton* literally means "external skeleton." Unlike humans and other animals, insects such as grasshoppers and cockroaches as well as crustaceans such as crabs and lobsters have their skeletons on the outside of their bodies. The idea that exoskeletons could be built to fit humans in order to assist with movement was born in the 1890s and early 1900s. These machines were powered by gas compression or steam power that acted along with the person's own movements. More sophisticated exoskeletons powered by hydraulics, which increased the wearer's ability to lift heavy loads, were developed in the 1960s. One of these was known as the Hardiman. One of the main proposed purposes of powered exoskeletons was for use in the military, for example, to help soldiers carry heavy loads. Proposed civilian uses for exoskeletons include helping rescue workers in dangerous environments and construction workers in the performance of tasks that induce muscle fatigue.

FIGURE 4.24

A patient with incomplete SCI undergoing rehabilitation with the help of a powered exoskeleton.

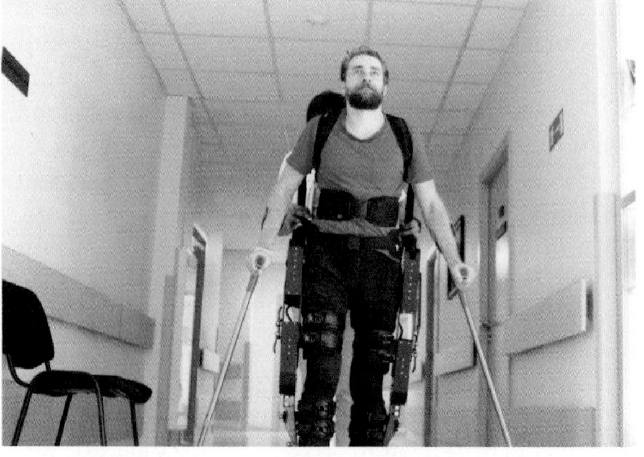

iStock.com/chudakov2

In recent years, the use of powered exoskeletons has become a promising option in the treatment and rehabilitation of people with incomplete SCI. Several companies have developed powered exoskeletons to help people with SCI improve balance, walking distance, and speed.

In a recent study, patients with incomplete SCI underwent powered exoskeleton training three or four days per week for a total of 100 hours. At first, the device was set to provide a maximal level of assistance, which was progressively reduced based on the patient's individual performance. The patient's performance was video-recorded while walking along a 10-meter walkway. The results showed that 100 hours of training with the powered exoskeleton resulted in improvements in the patient's walking speed, the time needed to take a step, and the length of the patient's steps (Ramanujam et al., 2018).

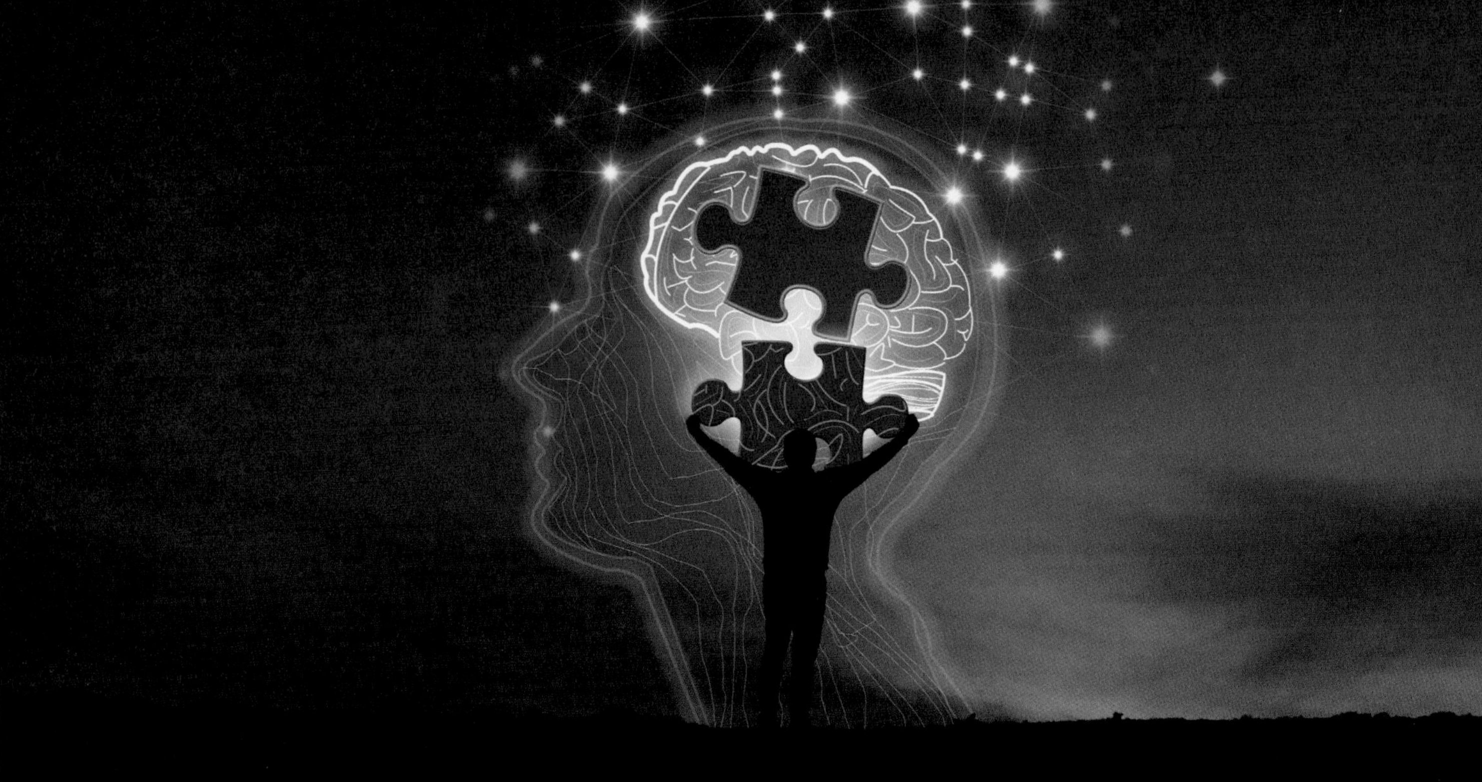

iStock.com/Urupong

5 Neurodevelopment, Neuroplasticity, and Aging

Chapter Contents

Learning Objectives

5.1.1 Explain neurogenesis and the concepts of proliferation, differentiation, migration, and synaptogenesis.

5.1.2 Discuss what is meant by adult neurogenesis, where it is known to occur in the brain, and why it is important.

5.2.1 Define neuroplasticity.

5.2.2 Explain structural remodeling and identify the types of stimulation by which it can be induced.

5.2.3 Define synaptic plasticity and explain the different ways in which it occurs.

5.2.4 Define and differentiate functional and structural plasticity.

5.2.5 Explain how cortical plasticity may not always be adaptive by being exaggerated.

5.3.1 Describe the neurobiological basis for the association between adolescence and risk-taking and impulsive behavior.

5.3.2 Explain the cognitive declines that occur during normal aging of the brain.

5.3.3 Describe the cognitive declines due to a disease process (Alzheimer's) in the aged brain.

Massive Cortical Reorganization: The Case of Zion Harvey

When he was only two years old, Zion Harvey suffered sepsis due to a staphylococcal infection. Sepsis occurs when the immune system goes into overdrive to deal with infection. When this happens, the flow of blood can be severely restricted by exaggerated clotting. This means that tissues of the body are not getting proper nourishment and are at risk of dying. Dead tissue must be removed. Sometimes, sepsis is so severe as to be life threatening and entire limbs must be amputated. Zion had both hands and feet amputated, in addition to being the recipient of a kidney transplant. Remarkably, Zion learned to eat, write, and play video games without hands. He was also able to walk, run, and even jump with the help of prosthetic feet.

In 2015, when he was eight years old, Zion was the first child to successfully undergo a double hand transplant. The operation was performed at the Children's Hospital in Philadelphia and lasted more than 10 hours. After the operation, Zion took some time to adjust to his new hands. However, eight months after the surgery, he could use scissors and was able to write with crayons. One year later, he could use a baseball bat.

Throughout Zion's recovery, his brain was monitored periodically by MRI. After all, the hand area of Zion's somatosensory cortex had been deprived of sensory information from the hands since he was two years old. An intriguing question concerned how Zion's brain reorganized to adapt to this new reality and whether further reorganization occurred after new hands were connected.

The findings were astounding. Soon after the surgery, researchers found that Zion's somatosensory cortex had reorganized in a way that reflected the fact that the hand area was no longer receiving stimulation. In fact, the hand area now responded to stimulation of the lips. It looked as though, because it lacked stimulation, the hand area was invaded by the face area. The hand area began to be active again after the nerves to his new hands were connected. About seven months later, the face and hand areas resegregated, in that the hand area responded to stimulation of the hands and not to stimulation of the lips.

INTRODUCTION

The case of Zion Harvey is testimony to the remarkable ability of the brain to reorganize itself in response to experience. Such an example of massive cortical reorganization, known as functional neuroplasticity, is the focus of this chapter's second module. The chapter also explores how changes occur at synapses and in the cortex and how these changes are due to experience with one's environment. In the final units of the chapter, you will learn how the brain changes during normal aging as well as the changes in behavior and cognitive functions associated with the aging brain. We will also take a look at how the brain can change due to disease processes such as those observed in Alzheimer's disease. But, first, we will briefly explore the beginnings of the nervous system itself, exemplified by the generation of new neurons and their journey to where they will take up permanent residence in the brain.

5.1 Neurodevelopment

Module Contents

Learning Objectives

5.1.1 Explain neurogenesis and the concepts of proliferation, differentiation, migration, and synaptogenesis.

5.1.2 Discuss what is meant by adult neurogenesis, where it is known to occur in the brain, and why it is important.

5.1.1 NEUROGENESIS, CELL PROLIFERATION, MIGRATION, DIFFERENTIATION, AND SYNAPTOGENESIS

>> LO 5.1.1 Explain neurogenesis and the concepts of proliferation, differentiation, migration, and synaptogenesis.

Key Terms

- **Neurogenesis:** The creation of new neurons, which first occurs during embryological development and then continues throughout life.
- **Neural stem cells:** Cells that emerge from the ectoderm and produce progenitor cells.
- **Proliferation:** The stage during which neural stem cells multiply.
- **Common progenitor cells:** Cells that give rise to neuronal and glial progenitor cells, which differentiate into neurons and glia.
- **Differentiation:** The process by which progenitor cells give rise to neurons and glia.
- **Neuroblasts:** Immature neurons that differentiate from neuronal progenitor cells.
- **Glioblasts:** Immature glial cells that differentiate from neuronal progenitor cells.
- **Radial migration:** The process by which cells reach their destination by sliding along processes extended by radial glia.
- **Tangential migration:** The process by which cells reach their destination by sliding across one glial cell to another.
- **Corticogenesis:** The process by which the cortex develops from the generation of neuronal and glial progenitor cells.
- **Chemoaffinity hypothesis:** The idea that axons find their way to their targets by following a chemical signal.
- **Growth cone:** Processes at the tip of growing axons that possess a structure capable of changing its structure in response to chemical signals.
- **Filopodia:** Thin membranes that protrude from the axon's cytoplasm and are part of its growth cone.
- **Lamellipodia:** A thin sheetlike membrane that is part of an axon's growth cone.
- **Chemotaxis:** The guidance of growth cones by chemical cues.
- **Chemoattraction:** The attraction of growth cones toward chemical cues.
- **Chemorepulsion:** The repulsion of growth cones away from a chemical source.
- **Contact guidance:** The guidance of growth cones induced by direct contact with chemicals.
- **Contact attraction:** The attraction of growth cones through direct contact with chemicals.
- **Contact repulsion:** The repulsion of growth cones through direct contact with chemicals.
- **Synaptogenesis**: The formation of new synapses in developing and adult brains.
- **Cell-adhesion molecules (CAMs):** Molecules that play a crucial role in synapse formation.

Neurogenesis refers to the creation of new neurons. Neurogenesis first occurs during embryological development and then continues throughout life. In Chapter 4, you learned about the process of gastrulation. Gastrulation marks the stage at which the blastocyst, a cell mass that will become the embryo, reorganizes into the germ cell layers that give rise to the different tissues of the body. These are the ectoderm, the mesoderm, and the endoderm.

FIGURE 5.1

Neurogenesis.

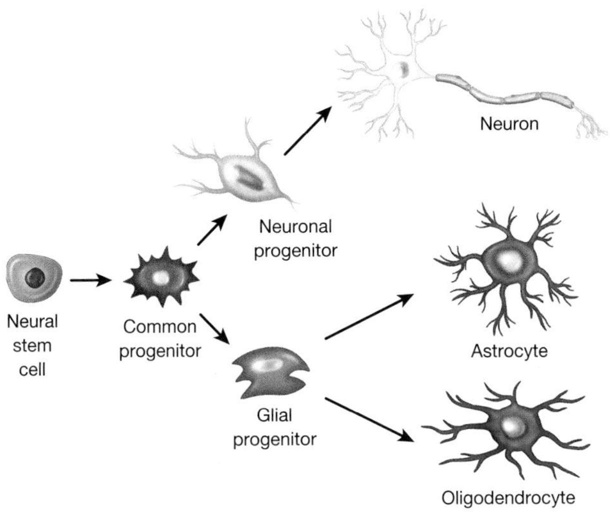

Amanda Tomasikiewicz/Body Scientific Intl.

FIGURE 5.2

Radial migration.

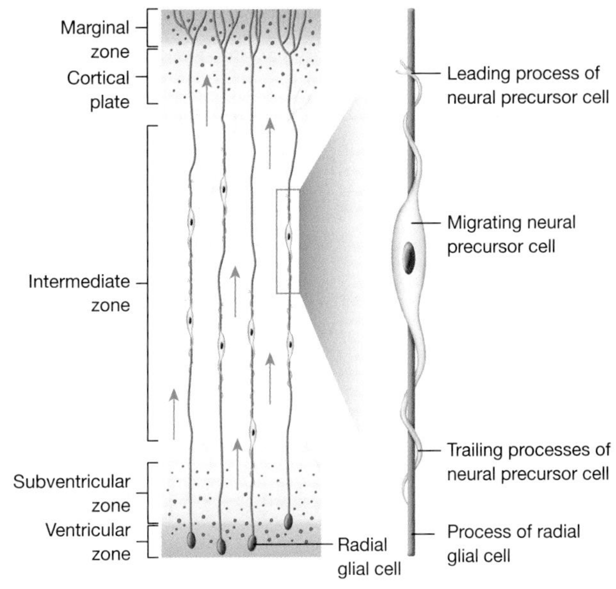

Adapted from illustration by Lydia Kibiuk. © 1995.

The cell lines that initially give rise to all the cells of the central nervous system emerge from the ectoderm. These are known as **neural stem cells**. These cells multiply during a stage known as **proliferation**. They have the ability for self-renewal, meaning that they give rise to other neural stem cells. However, when neural stem cells divide, they also produce what are known as **common progenitor cells**. In turn, these give rise to neuronal and glial progenitor cells. In the further process of **differentiation**, progenitor cells give rise to the variety of neurons and glia (e.g., astrocytes and oligodendrocytes) of the central nervous system (Bystron, Blakemore, & Rakic, 2008). This is illustrated in Figure 5.1.

Most neural stem cells, as well as neuronal and glial progenitor cells, reside in embryonic tissues called the ventricular zone, so named because of its proximity to what is to become the brain's ventricles. From there, immature neurons (**neuroblasts**) and glia (**glioblasts**) travel to the area of the brain where they will reside for life, in a process referred to as migration.

Migration is the mechanism by which the cortex and other brain structures are formed (Figure 5.2). There are two main types of migration: radial migration and tangential migration. In **radial migration**, cells get to their destination by sliding along processes extended by radial glia, which themselves are neural progenitors

FIGURE 5.3

Corticogenesis.

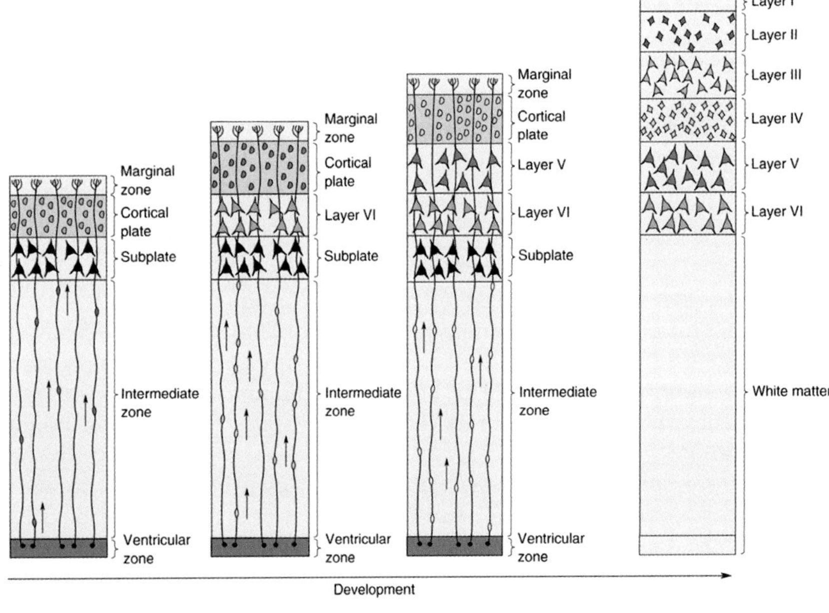

From *Neuroscience: Exploring the Brain* 4th Edition, Bear, Connors, and Paradiso, 2016. Reprinted with permission from Wolters Kluwer.

(Noctor, Martinez-Cerdeno, Ivic, & Kriegstein, 2004) (also discussed in Chapter 2). The processes extended by radial glia originate in the ventricular zone and span across other embryonic zones (i.e., subventricular zone, intermediate zone, cortical plate) all the way to the topmost layer known as the marginal zone. In humans, 90% of immature cells migrate through radial migration (Letinic, Zoncu, & Rakic, 2002). In **tangential migration**, cells reach their destination by sliding across one glial cell to another, following a parallel path along the ventricular zone (Nakajima, 2007; O'Rourke, Sullivan, Kaznowski, Jacobs, & McConnell, 1995).

Radial and tangential migration were once each associated with the production of different types of neurons. It was thought that glutaminergic pyramidal neurons migrated radially and that GABAergic inhibitory neurons migrated tangentially. However, we now know that glutaminergic pyramidal neurons can also migrate tangentially (Barber & Pierani, 2016).

The cortex is composed of six layers. Each layer consists largely of pyramidal cells (see Chapter 2 for types of neurons). The cells within the six layers form functional circuits with neurons from the various layers of a given area and with neurons located in other parts of the brain.

The process by which the cortex develops from the generation of neuronal and glial progenitor cells is known as **corticogenesis**. We now take a look at how radial migration is involved in this process (Figure 5.3). The first cells to migrate away from the ventricular zone form what is known as the subplate. Next, neurons that will form the cortical layers migrate past the subplate and form what is called the cortical plate. Which of the six layers they form depends on their time of arrival at the cortical plate. The layers of the cortex are added from the inside out. That is, cells that arrived first form layer VI. The cells arriving second, third, fourth, fifth, and sixth form layers V, IV, III, II, and I, respectively. Once the process is completed, neurons from the subplate disappear.

Differentiation

As mentioned earlier, neuroblasts have already started to differentiate into recognizable neurons during migration. This occurs through neurite outgrowth. The neurites of a neuron comprise the axon and dendrites. Figure 5.4 shows the outgrowth of neurites of hippocampal neurons of 18-day fetal rats (Dotti, Sullivan, & Banker, 1988).

The development of neurites was observed over a seven-day period. Early on, neurites extend from the cell body. As you can see in Figure 5.4a, one of the neurites appears to be more elongated than the others. This one becomes the axon, and shorter neurites become the dendrites. The axon also gives rise to branches called axon collaterals (Figure 5.4e).

FIGURE 5.4

Differentiation of a pyramidal neuron grown in culture. (a) By the end of day 1, neurites extending from the cell body could be observed. One of these neurites appeared more elongated than the others (A) and becomes the axon. The other shorter neurites (D1-D3) are destined to become dendrites. (b) By the end of day 2, the axon underwent further elongation and gave rise to axon collaterals (A1-A2), giving the cell the characteristic shape of a pyramidal neuron. (c) By the end of the third day, the dendrites had remained the same length but axon collateral A2 gained in length. (d) At the end of day 5, the cell continued to grow into its characteristic shape and a new axon (A3) had extended. (e) Finally, on day 7, a new axon (A4) as well as a new collateral had branched out of collateral A3 (A3-1).

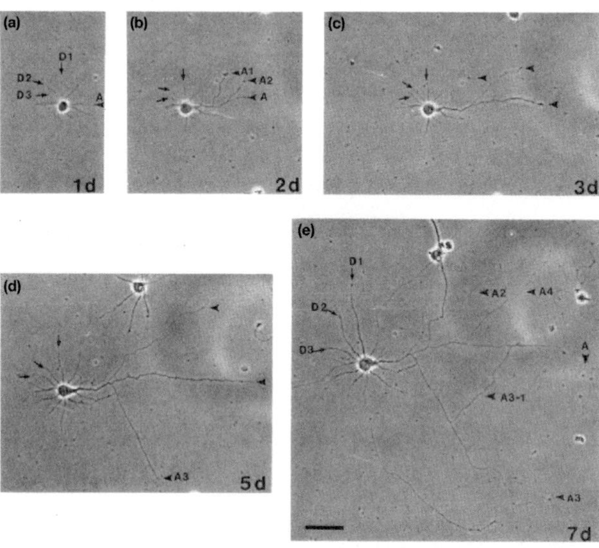

Axon Guidance

Once cells have differentiated into neurons, their axons begin their journey toward their targets, which are the neurons with which they will form synapses. For example, retinal neurons must make their way from the back of the eye to the thalamus. How do axons achieve the feat of accurately reaching their targets amid the thousands of possible connections they could make? This is an important question to answer if we are to understand how different patterns of connectivity between neurons give rise to organized behavior.

Remarkably, until the 1940s, many neuroscientists did not believe that organized behavior depended on any particular patterns of connections between neurons. However, neuroscientist Roger Sperry (1913–1994) set out to show that the specificity of connections was important and that learning alone cannot account for behavior. He did so in a set of remarkable experiments (Sperry, 1956). In one of these experiments, Sperry rotated the eyes of newts (a type of salamander) by 180 degrees (Sperry, 1944b). This completely reversed their vision. Newts subjected to the eye rotations dug into the sand at the bottom of the aquarium when bait was hung above them, turned their heads toward the rear when the bait was hung in front of them and lunged forward when the bait was presented to their backs. The newts never learned to adjust to their new reality for as long as two

FIGURE 5.5

Evidence for chemoaffinity. (a) Optics (top): The normal field of view of a frog. The image is inverted on the retina but right side up in the tectum. Connectivity (middle): The nerves exiting the anterior retina connect to the posterior tectum (green line). The nerves exiting the posterior retina connect to the anterior tectum (orange line). The nerves exiting the dorsal retina connect to the ventral part of the tectum (blue line). The nerves exiting the ventral retina connect to the dorsal tectum (yellow line). Action (bottom): The frog accurately tracks a fly. (b) Optics (top): Field of view of a frog with rotated eyes. The image is inverted in both the retina and the tectum. Connectivity (middle): The cut retinal nerves grew back to their original site in the tectum even though the eyes were rotated. Action (bottom): The frog could still not accurately track the fly in its field of view.

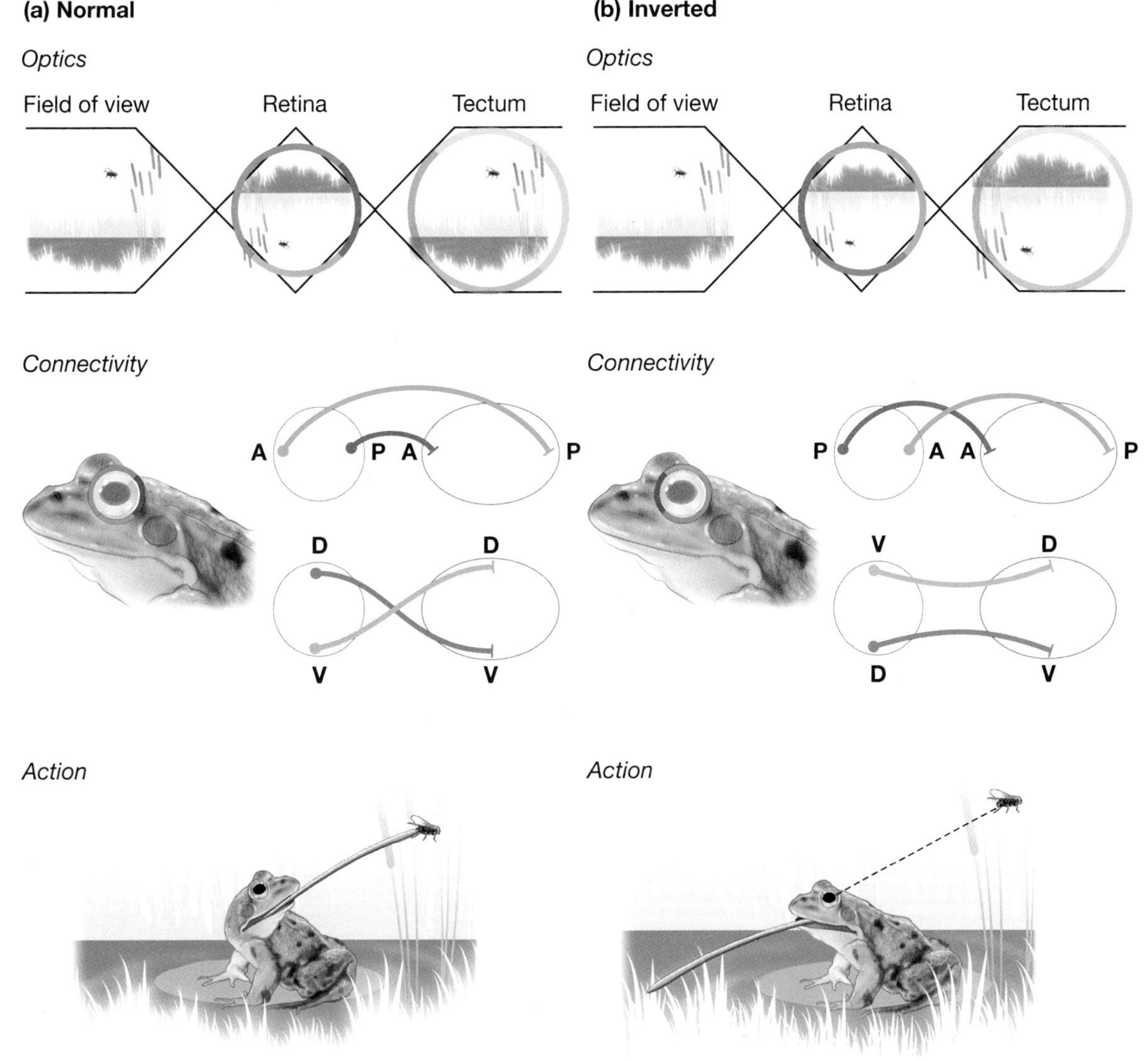

Carolina Hrejsa/Body Scientific Intl.

years. However, their vision normalized as soon as their eyes were rotated back to their original positions.

Sperry's demonstrations that specific connections were required for normal behavior were convincing. However, the question remained as to how the specific connections were formed. In 1892, Santiago Ramón y Cajal hypothesized that axons found their way to their targets by following a chemical trail. Roger Sperry was a proponent of Ramón y Cajal's idea and found evidence for it in the 1960s.

He did so by conducting the experiment illustrated in Figure 5.5. Figure 5.5a (top) shows the field of view (including a fly) of a normal frog. The image is inverted in the retina and right side up in the tectum. Figure 5.5a (middle) shows the connection between the nerves of a frog's retina and the optic tectum. You can see that the nerves exiting the anterior retina normally connect to the posterior tectum and that nerves exiting the posterior retina normally connect to the anterior tectum. You can also see that the nerves exiting the dorsal retina connect to the ventral part of the tectum and that nerves exiting the ventral retina connect to the dorsal tectum. Figure 5.5a (bottom) shows that this pattern of connection permits the frog to accurately track the fly in its field of view.

To test whether axons followed a chemical trail to their destinations, Sperry rotated the frog's eyes and cut the nerves exiting the retina. He then observed whether they grew back to the same areas of the tectum (Sperry, 1944a). The point of rotating the eyes was so that the axons would have to find another route to their destination. Figure 5.5b (top) shows the field of view of a frog with rotated eyes. The image is inverted in both the retina and the tectum. Figure 5.5b (middle) shows that the nerves from the anterior retina, which had been cut, grew back to the posterior tectum and nerves from the posterior retina grew back to the anterior tectum even if they had to follow a different path to get there. The same was observed of nerves from the dorsal and ventral retina that grew back to the ventral and dorsal tectum, respectively. Figure 5.5b (bottom) shows that, because of its rotated eyes, the frog could not accurately track the fly.

How did the fibers from the retina, which had been cut, find their way back to the same area of the tectum to which they connected? Sperry concluded from those findings that neurons in the tectum must emit chemical signals that label their types and positions. According to Sperry, the retinal fibers followed these chemical signals to navigate their way to their target neurons within the tectum. The idea that axons find their way to their targets by following a chemical signal became known as the **chemoaffinity hypothesis**.

The Growth Cone

The next challenge was to discover the mechanism by which neuronal fibers followed a chemical trail to their targets. The tip of growing axons possesses a structure capable of changing its structure in response to chemical signals. This permits axons to grow in the direction of target cells while the cell body remains in place. This structure, illustrated in Figure 5.6, is known as the **growth cone**.

The growth cone's ability to move forward and navigate through the cell's environment is dependent on a set of structures within it. It contains thin membranes that protrude from the axon's cytoplasm called **filopodia** (singular, *filopodium*), which extend from a thin sheetlike membrane called **lamellipodia**.

As you can also see in Figure 5.6, the growth cone can be subdivided into three domains: a peripheral domain, a central domain, and a transition zone. The peripheral domain (P-domain) contains bundles of long F-actin filaments (actin is a protein that forms filaments ["F" stands for filament]). These bundles of F-actin form the filopodia. In addition, a network of branched F-actin forms the lamellipodia.

The central domain (C-domain) contains microtubules that are continuous from the axon shaft and associate themselves with the filopodia. The transition zone (T-domain) forms a boundary between the P- and C-domains. It is composed of contractile structures called F-actin arcs, which form a semicircular ring within the T-domain.

Filopodia have receptors that sense the neuron's environment for chemical cues, which guide the axon's movements toward its targets at a distance. The guidance of growth cones by chemical cues is known as **chemotaxis**. Some of these chemical cues attract growth cones to move toward them in a process known as **chemoattraction**. Other chemicals cause growth cones to move away from them; this is known as **chemorepulsion**.

FIGURE 5.6

The growth cone can be subdivided into three domains: a peripheral domain (P-domain), a central domain (C-domain), and a transition zone (T-zone). The growth cone's ability to move forward and navigate through the cell's environment is dependent on a set of structures in each one of these domains. These include filopodia, lamellipodia, and microtubules (MT) from the axon's shaft.

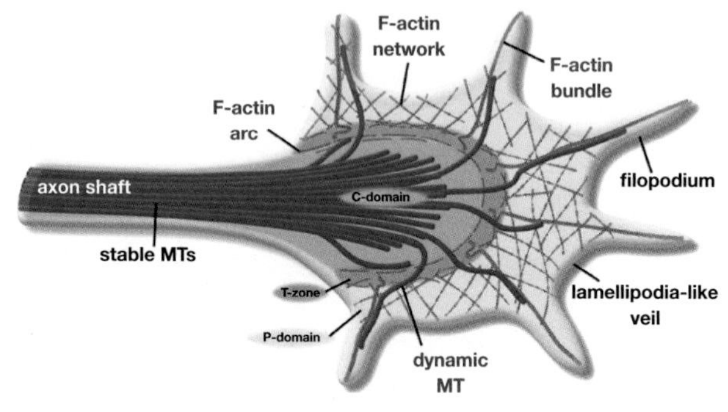

Lowery, L.A. & V. Van Vactor. (2009). The trip of the tip: understanding the growth cone machinery. *Nature Reviews Molecular Cell Biology 10*(5): 332–343. With permission from Springer Nature.

We will not get into the cast of chemicals that are involved with chemoattraction and chemorepulsion. Other works cover these topics in detail (Price, 2011).

In addition to being guided by distant chemical cues, growth cones are also guided by local chemical cues—found on the surface of other cells or in the extracellular matrix—with which they must come into direct contact. Guidance by chemicals with which growth cones must come into direct contact is known as **contact guidance**. When growth cones encounter these chemicals, they are either attracted or repelled. This is known as **contact attraction** and **contact repulsion**, respectively. The four types of guidance cues are illustrated in Figure 5.7.

FIGURE 5.7

Growth cones are guided by multiple types of chemical cues.

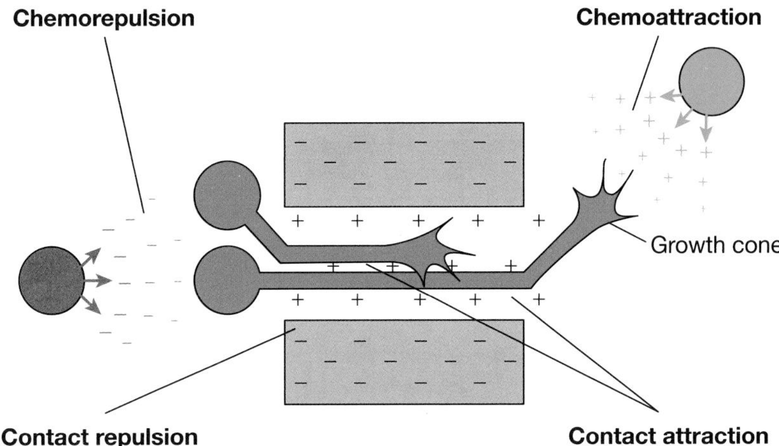

Growth Cone Motility

You may be wondering about the mechanisms by which growth cones turn toward or away from chemical cues, that is, how chemoattraction and chemorepulsion work. Figure 5.8 illustrates a growth cone turning toward an attractive chemical cue (green). As you saw in Figure 5.7, F-actin is the main component of filopodia and lamellipodia. The microtubules, which enter the growth cone from the axon shaft, known as dynamic microtubules (dynamic MT), spread out randomly in the P-domain of the growth cone.

When the growth cone encounters an attractant, F-actin molecules polymerize, meaning they come together to form a large chain. This increases the number (filopodial dilation) and length of the filopodia on the side where a chemoattractant is detected. In contrast, filopodia withdraw from the side where no chemoattractant is detected. At the same time, microtubules, which at first spread randomly within the growth cone, also polymerize and associate with the F-actin in the filopodia on the side of the chemoattractant, which stabilizes the filopodia, making it turn in one direction (Dent & Gertler, 2003; Mortimer, Fothergill, Pujic, Richards, & Goodhill, 2008).

FIGURE 5.8

How filopodia move.

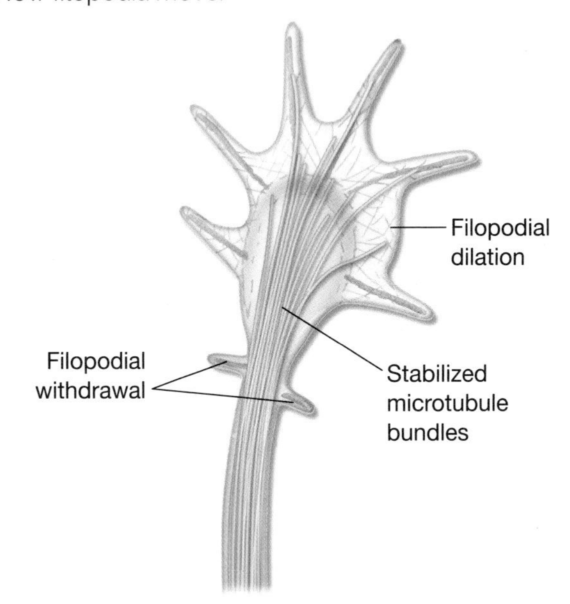

Liana Bauman/Body Scientific Intl.

Synaptogenesis

So far, you have learned about some of the key processes involved in brain development, from the formation of the neural tube to the proliferation, migration, and differentiation of neurons. You have also just learned about how axons of neurons find their way to their target cells with the help of growth cones. However, another step is necessary to lead to the brain's functionality that gives rise to your sensation and perception of environmental information, the range of emotions that you experience, the perception of who you are, your ability to learn, and the myriad experiences that you remember. This step marks the formation of connections between neurons at synapses.

As described in detail in Chapter 3, synapses are the sites where neurons communicate with target cells. Such communication is typically defined as occurring through the junction between the axon terminals of a presynaptic neuron and the dendrites of a postsynaptic neuron. The formation of new synapses in developing and adult brains is known as **synaptogenesis**. Synapses are created in four stages. These are filopodial outgrowth, specification and induction, synapse formation, and synapse stabilization, which includes synapse selection and synapse withdrawal (Figure 5.9 a–d2).

FIGURE 5.9

The stages of synaptogenesis.

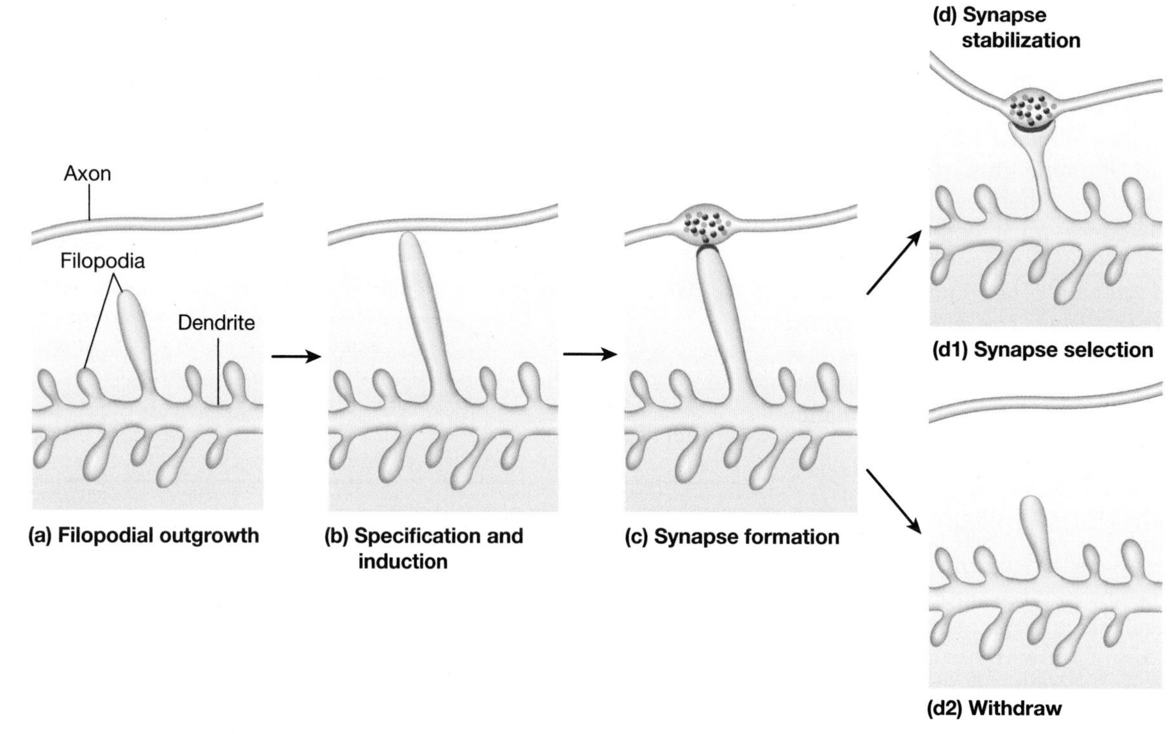

Amanda Tomasikiewicz/Body Scientific Intl.

During specification and induction, filopodia grow out of postsynaptic dendrites to extend toward passing axons. The growth cones of these axons and the filopodia of dendrites express several molecules that play a crucial role in synapse formation. These are known as **cell-adhesion molecules** (CAMs). Growth cones express a CAM known as neurexin, whereas the filopodia express neuroligin.

Synapse formation occurs when a growth cone is close enough to a filopodium. The neurexin in growth cones binds to the neuroligin expressed by the dendritic filopodia. Binding of neurexin to neuroligin causes calcium channels to open, leading to an influx of Ca^{2+}. This influx of Ca^{2+} induces the formation of dendritic spines, which will eventually express neurotransmitter receptors and form the site of excitatory synapses.

Synapses are stabilized with the addition of neurexin in the presynaptic cell when stimulated consistently. Synapses that are not stimulated are disassembled and the dendritic filopodia withdraw. As shown in Figure 5.10, neural networks become increasingly complex over the first two years of life (Conel, 1939). By adulthood, each of the brain's more than 80 billion neurons will form an astonishing average of 7,000 synapses (Drachman, 2005).

FIGURE 5.10

The development of neural networks over the first two years of life.

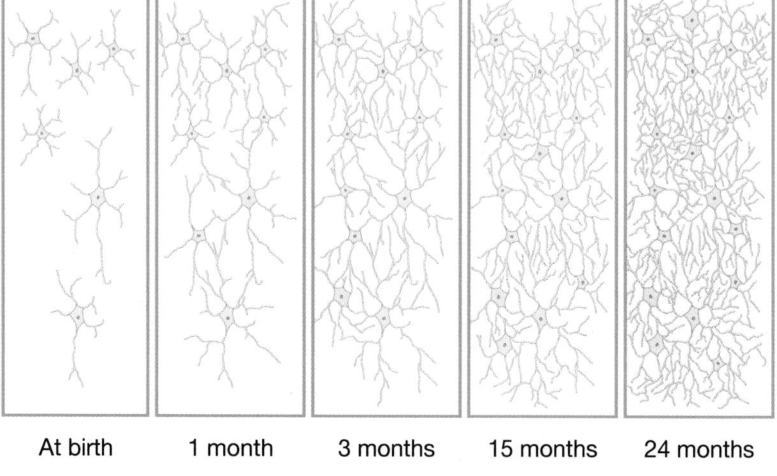

Liana Bauman/Body Scientific Intl.

IT'S A MYTH!

It's Okay to Have a Drink While Pregnant

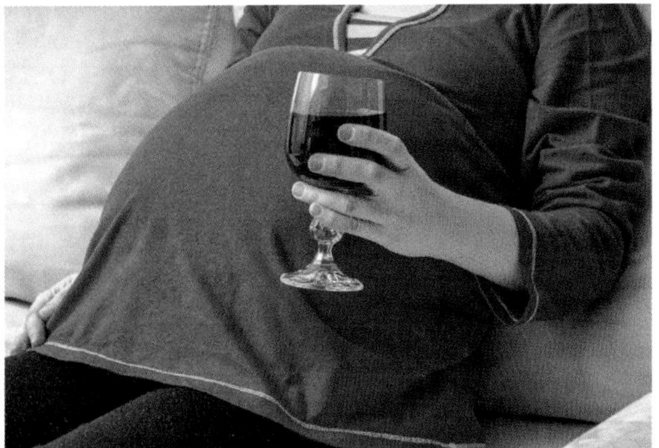

iStock.com/vchal

The Myth

You may have heard that consuming a small amount of alcohol while pregnant can do no harm to the baby, but you should know that there is no safe amount of alcohol that one can consume during pregnancy. Alcohol is a known teratogen. A teratogen is defined as an agent that can cause damage to the developing embryo and fetus. Like anything else that the mother ingests, alcohol reaches the baby through the placenta.

Where Does the Myth Come From?

Opinions differ on the topic, even among physicians, with some obstetricians believing that small amounts of alcohol are harmless. Some studies have shown no harm with small amounts of alcohol consumed, but even the authors of those studies warn that the findings may not be generalized to the whole population but may be relevant only to the characteristics of the participants involved in their studies.

Why Is the Myth Wrong?

This myth is wrong because no amount of alcohol has been determined to be safe for pregnant women to consume (National Center on Birth Defects and Developmental Disabilities, 2004). Drinking while pregnant unnecessarily exposes the developing fetus to fetal alcohol spectrum disorders (FASDs), a set of related conditions observed in the offspring of mothers who consumed alcohol during pregnancy. The most severe of these disorders is fetal alcohol syndrome (FAS). It is characterized by a pattern of impaired growth and alterations in the development of the nervous system. FAS also includes significant impairments in cognitive functioning related to memory, language, communication, attention, planning, and reasoning. Children with FAS also show patterns of hyperactivity and problems with motor coordination. The other FASDs, known as partial fetal alcohol syndrome and alcohol-related neurodevelopmental disorder, are less severe forms of FAS. Whether a child is born with FAS or one of the other forms is related to the amount of alcohol the mother consumes (Berk, 2018, pp. 84–85).

What Happens in the Brain?

Brain abnormalities in FAS are plentiful. Babies born with FAS have a small head, a condition known as microcephaly, which is associated with an underdeveloped brain. Typical of FAS are smaller than normal frontal lobes and structural abnormalities in the cerebellum, caudate, hippocampus, and other areas of the temporal lobes, which includes abnormally low numbers of neurons and glia (E. Moore, Migliorini, Infante, & Riley, 2014; Norman, Crocker, Mattson, & Riley, 2009).

How Does Alcohol Cause Fetal Alcohol Syndrome?

Consuming alcohol during pregnancy can decrease the survival rate and proliferation of progenitor neurons, which is what may account for the observed microcephaly. In addition, alcohol impairs neuron migration and synaptogenesis. Impaired migration may account for the structural abnormalities and low numbers of neurons and glia in the neocortex and hippocampus (Guerri, Bazinet, & Riley, 2009).

So, if you think having a drink while pregnant is okay . . . think again. ●

Myelination

Another important step in the development of the nervous system is that of myelination. Myelination is achieved by glial cells. Myelin increases the rate at which neurons conduct action potentials. Myelination begins shortly after birth within the spinal cord and spreads quickly to other parts of the brain. The process by which glial cells myelinate neurons is explained in Chapter 2.

5.1.2 ADULT NEUROGENESIS

>> LO 5.1.2 Discuss what is meant by adult neurogenesis, where it is known to occur in the brain, and why it is important.

Key Terms

- **Adult neural stem/progenitor cells (NSPCs):** Cells that give rise to adult neurogenesis. They have been found mainly in the dentate gyrus of the hippocampus and the subventricular zone.
- **Subventricular zone (SVZ):** The area that lines the walls of the lateral ventricles and contains NSPCs that generate neurons that migrate to the olfactory bulb.
- **Subgranular zone (SGZ):** The area located near the dentate gyrus (DG) of the hippocampus, which contains NSPCs that generate neurons that migrate to the DG and differentiate into what are known as granule cells.

Neurogenesis occurs not only during the prenatal period but also throughout life. This was not thought to be possible until it was discovered by Joseph Altman in postnatal guinea pigs with nearly adult-sized brains (Altman & Das, 1967). Then, in the 1980s, Fernando Nottebohm and colleagues discovered neurogenesis in the brains of songbirds (Goldman & Nottebohm, 1983).

In adults, new neurons are generated by what are known as **adult neural stem/progenitor cells (NSPCs)**. NSPCs were found to exist in two brain areas. These are the **subventricular zone (SVZ)**, situated in the walls of the lateral ventricles, and the **subgranular zone (SGZ)**, located near the dentate gyrus (DG) of the hippocampus.

The neurons generated in the SVZ migrate to the olfactory bulb. The neurons generated in the SGZ migrate to the DG and differentiate into what are known as granule cells. However, it is still debated whether neurogenesis occurs in the human olfactory bulb (Huart, Rombaux, & Hummel, 2019). More recent studies have shown that adult neurogenesis may also occur in the hypothalamus (D. A. Lee et al., 2012; Recabal, Caprile, & Garcia-Robles, 2017).

Neurons migrating from the SVZ are thought to be involved in the discrimination of new odors and in replacing olfactory neurons. Neurogenesis in the DG is thought to be involved in the formation of new memories. As will be discussed in detail in Chapter 12, the hippocampus is highly involved in the formation of new memories. The addition of new neurons in the DG of the hippocampus may permit new memories to be stored without interfering with the maintenance of older memories. Without neurogenesis, the same set of neurons would have to maintain old memories as well as participate in the formation of new ones (W. Deng, Aimone, & Gage, 2010).

MODULE SUMMARY

Neurogenesis refers to the birth of new neurons, which occurs during embryological development but also continues throughout life. Cell lines that give rise to all cells of the nervous system are known as neural stem cells, some of which keep multiplying by a process known as proliferation. Some give rise to common progenitor cells. These in turn give rise to neurons and glia. The variety in the types of cells in the nervous system arises through the process of differentiation. Neuronal and glial progenitors reside within the ventricular zone, from which they travel to the brain areas in which they will reside through the process of migration. These cells make it all the way up to the top cortical layer called the marginal zone. The first cells that migrate away from the ventricular zone form the subplate, followed by cells that form the cortical plate. During migration, immature neurons known as neuroblasts differentiate into recognizable neurons through the outgrowth of neurites. Once they have differentiated, axons grow toward the target neurons onto which they will form synapses.

The idea that axons make it to their targets by following chemical messages is known as the chemoaffinity hypothesis. Evidence for the chemoaffinity hypothesis was provided by Roger Sperry in the 1960s by performing experiments with newts and frogs. Axons follow chemical trails by extending a growth cone. Guidance cues for growth cones include chemoattraction, chemorepulsion, and contact guidance. The formation of synapses between neurons occurs through the process of synaptogenesis, which consists of four stages: filopodial outgrowth, specification and induction, synapse formation, and synapse stabilization.

Neurogenesis is not confined to prenatal development but occurs throughout life. Adult neurogenesis has been shown to occur in the dentate gyrus of the hippocampus and in the subventricular zone. Neurons generated in the dentate gyrus are important for the formation of new memories, whereas neurons generated in the subventricular zone migrate to the olfactory bulb, where they are involved in olfactory discrimination and in the formation of new olfactory neurons. Neurogenesis has also been observed in the hypothalamus and possibly also occurs in the neocortex.

TEST YOURSELF

5.1.1 Explain what is meant by the following terms: (a) neurogenesis, (b) proliferation, (c) migration, (d) differentiation, and (e) synaptogenesis.

5.1.2 Explain the concept of neurogenesis and how it is not confined to the prenatal period. In what parts of the brain has it been found to occur?

5.2 Neuroplasticity

Module Contents

Learning Objectives

5.2.1 Define neuroplasticity.

5.2.2 Explain structural remodeling and identify the types of stimulation by which it can be induced.

5.2.3 Define synaptic plasticity and explain the different ways in which it occurs.

5.2.4 Define and differentiate functional and structural plasticity.

5.2.5 Explain how cortical plasticity may not always be adaptive by being exaggerated.

5.2.1 WHAT IS NEUROPLASTICITY?

>> LO 5.2.1 **Define neuroplasticity.**

Neuroplasticity refers to the brain's ability to change its structure and function (Zilles, 1992). The term *neuroplasticity* was first used by Santiago Ramón y Cajal to describe changes in the structure of the adult brain that were not due to any kind of disease process (Ramón y Cajal et al., 1991). In the 1960s, the term *neuroplasticity* was used to refer to morphological changes (changes in shape) observed in neurons of the hippocampus in response to psychological stress induced by forced restraint (Y. Watanabe, Gould, & McEwen, 1992).

5.2.2 STRUCTURAL REMODELING

>> LO 5.2.2 **Explain structural remodeling and identify the types of stimulation by which it can be induced.**

Key Terms

- **Structural remodeling:** Changes in the structure of neurons in response to the activity of other neurons or stimulation from the external environment.
- **Forced restraint:** A condition in which animals are forcibly restrained to measure the effects of chronic stress.
- **Attentional set shifting task:** A task that measures attention and cognitive flexibility.

Neuroplasticity occurs when neurons are stimulated by the activity of other neurons. This activity may be spontaneous but is often triggered by events in the environment. In response, neurons may undergo **structural remodeling** such as a change in their numbers of dendritic spines or in the length of their dendrites. (Remember that dendritic spines are protrusions from dendrites onto which synapses with other neurons are formed.)

We will now look at how environmental factors play a role in the structural remodeling of neurons. Three of these factors are environmental enrichment, learning, and environmental stress.

Environmental Enrichment

In the late 1940s, eminent psychologist Donald Hebb (1904–1985) found that rats reared as pets performed better at solving mazes than rats raised in standard laboratory conditions. Hebb attributed the superior problem-solving ability of these rats to enriched experience, which facilitated their learning (Hebb, 1949).

In the 1970s, psychologist William Greenough (1944–2013) conducted a study in which recently weaned rats were housed in three different conditions: an enriched condition (EC), in which rats interacted with various objects; in pairs (social condition [SC]); or individually (IC) for a period of 30 days. Greenough wanted to find out whether experience would result in the formation of new neuronal connections in the visual cortex. What he found was astounding. Rats housed in the EC developed larger dendritic fields in neurons of the visual cortex (Volkmar & Greenough, 1972). He later found that rats housed in the EC had more synapses per neuron (Turner & Greenough, 1985) than SC or IC rats.

Myriad studies have found that environmental enrichments of all sorts induce plastic changes in neurons (Nithianantharajah & Hannan, 2006). For example, environmental sensory enrichment, visual or somatosensory, induces neuroplasticity in the visual cortex and somatosensory cortex, respectively. Cognitive stimulation—such as the creation of spatial maps, recognizing objects, and attentional processes—induces neuroplastic changes in the hippocampus and neocortex. Motor activity, such as running in a wheel, promotes neuroplastic changes in the motor cortex and cerebellum (Figure 5.11).

FIGURE 5.11

Environmental sensory enrichment. Visual stimuli induce neuroplasticity in the visual cortex (orange), somatosensory stimuli induce neuroplasticity in the somatosensory cortex (red), cognitive stimulation induces neuroplastic changes in the hippocampus and neocortex (blue), and motor activity promotes neuroplastic changes in the motor cortex and cerebellum (green).

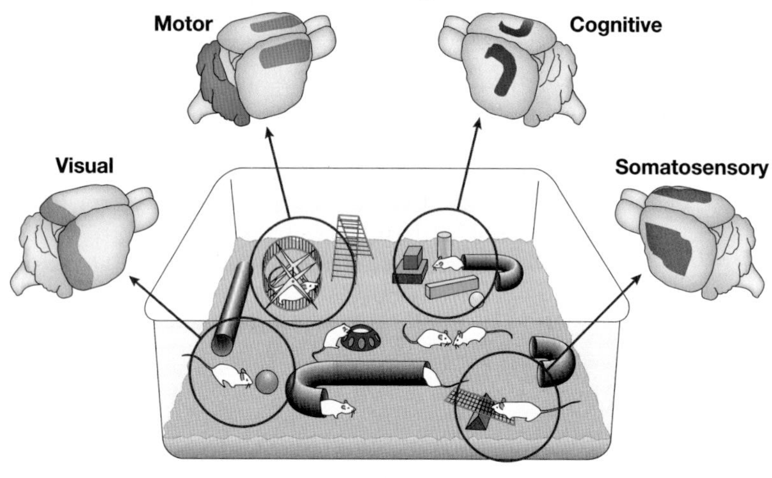

Nithianantharajah, J. & A. Hannan. (2006). Enriched environments, experience-dependent plasticity and disorders of the nervous system. *Nature Reviews Neuroscience* 7(9): 697–709. With permission from Springer Nature.

FIGURE 5.12

(a) Motor task in which mice had to learn to reach through a plastic opening to get a food reward. (b) Dendrites in the motor cortex of the mice learning the task underwent significant remodeling.

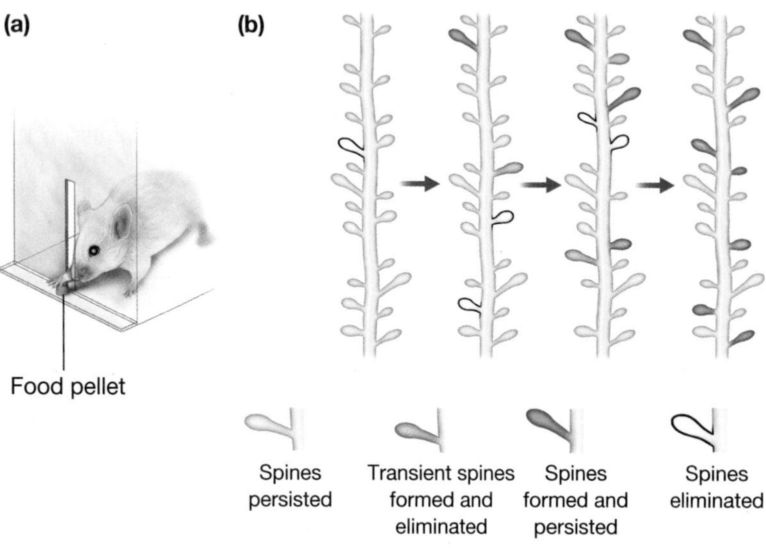

Amanda Tomasikiewicz/Body Scientific Intl.

Learning

Researchers have also found that structural remodeling is necessary for learning. For example, neuroscientist Tonghui Xu and colleagues found that learning a motor task involved the structural remodeling of dendrites in mice (Xu et al., 2009). In this task, the mice had to reach through an opening in a plastic enclosure to retrieve a food pellet (Figure 5.12a).

As shown in Figure 5.12b, dendrites in the motor cortex of the mice learning the task underwent significant remodeling. The observed changes occurred within the hour following initiation of training. Some of the spines already present persisted (yellow), but others were eliminated (orange). New spines were formed that persisted after training (purple), whereas others formed but were eliminated (black outline).

You may wonder why this pattern of remodeling occurs. For example, why do some of the spines persist when others are eliminated? Why are some spines formed and persist whereas other newly formed spines are eliminated? This is how the brain creates and stabilizes new memories. At the beginning, many more spines are created than is necessary. Over time, some of the connections formed by the new spines may become redundant, and keeping unnecessary connections may interfere with the connectivity associated with memories that are already stored.

Environmental Stress

Structural remodeling of neurons may also underlie cognitive impairments due to chronic stress. For example, in one study, researchers subjected rats to **forced restraint** 6 hours/day for 21 days (Liston et al., 2006). They subjected rats to an **attentional set shifting task**, which is a task that measures attention and cognitive flexibility. In this study, rats were required to shift their attention from one stimulus to another to obtain a food reward. Rats subjected to forced restraint were impaired in doing so. As shown in Figures 5.13b and 5.13c, the same rats had significant reductions in the length of apical dendrites in the anterior cingulate cortex (Figure 5.13a). In contrast, the apical dendrites of the orbitofrontal cortex of the same rats showed an increase in length compared to control rats. This led the authors to conclude that

FIGURE 5.13

(a) Location of the anterior cingulate cortex (ACg) and orbitofrontal cortex (OFC) in the brain of rats. (b) Apical dendrites of neurons in the ACg of control rats (blue) and stressed rats (red). (c) Apical dendrites of the OFC of control (blue) and stressed rats (red). (d) Typical pyramidal neuron from the OFC. The apical dendrite is indicated by the arrow, and the axon is indicated by the arrowheads.

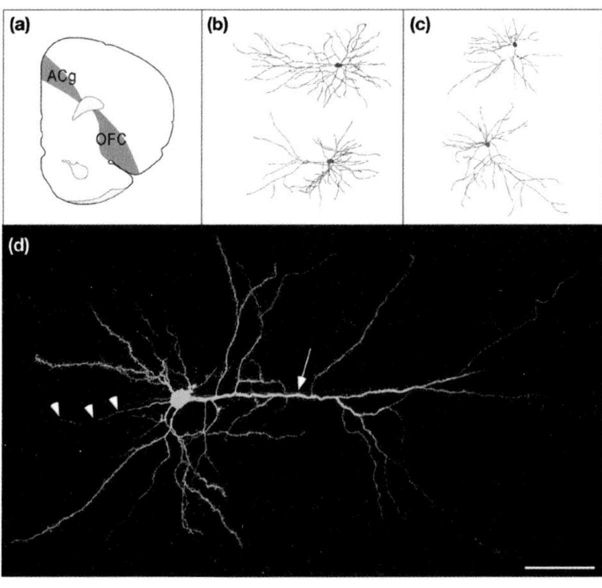

Liston, C., et al. (2006). Stress-induced alterations in prefrontal cortical dendritic morphology predict selective impairments in perceptual attentional set-shifting. *Journal of Neuroscience 26*(30): 7870–7874. With permission from The Society for Neuroscience.

stress-induced changes in the shape of dendrites might contribute to the impairments in attention found in depression and anxiety disorders.

5.2.3 SYNAPTIC PLASTICITY

>> LO 5.2.3 Define synaptic plasticity and explain the different ways in which it occurs.

Key Terms

- **Synaptic plasticity:** Changes in the efficacy of synapses.
- **Short-term plasticity:** Changes in synaptic strength that occur within a matter of milliseconds to a few minutes and are thought to be the basis for short-term memory and decision making.
- **Long-term plasticity:** Changes in synaptic efficacy that last more than a few minutes and are thought to be the basis for the formation of long-term memories.

You read in the preceding unit that learning and the stabilization of memories involves structural remodeling. Another form of plasticity, necessary for learning and storing information, is known as **synaptic plasticity**. Synaptic plasticity refers to a change in the efficacy of synapses. This change may take the form of either an increase or a decrease in the strength of connections between neurons.

Synaptic plasticity occurs in several ways (Ho, Lee, & Martin, 2011). Repeated stimulation of a synapse can induce (a) an increase in the amount of neurotransmitter release by the presynaptic neuron (Regehr, 2012); (b) a change in the size of the postsynaptic membrane and in the number and sensitivity of receptors on the postsynaptic neuron (Mayford, Siegelbaum, & Kandel, 2012); (c) a general increase in the size of the synapse on both the presynaptic and postsynaptic sides; or (d) the enlargement or branching of dendritic spines of the postsynaptic neuron, which increases the area onto which the synapse can form (Schulz, 1997; Toni, Buchs, Nikonenko, Bron, & Muller, 1999). These changes result in stronger postsynaptic potentials. (Recall from Chapter 3 that postsynaptic potentials are small depolarizations of postsynaptic neurons that do not cause the firing of action potentials. Also remember that postsynaptic potentials from different synapses can add up to result in the generation of action potentials in the postsynaptic neuron.) In the hippocampus, repeated stimulation leads to hippocampal neurogenesis (Epp, Chow, & Galea, 2013).

Neuroscientists distinguish between two forms of synaptic plasticity. These are known as short-term plasticity and long-term plasticity. **Short-term plasticity** refers to changes in synaptic strength that occur within a matter of milliseconds to a few minutes. The changes induced by short-term synaptic plasticity are only temporary; the state of the synapse returns to normal quickly if the presynaptic neuron is no longer stimulated. Short-term synaptic plasticity is thought to be involved in decision making (Deco, Rolls, & Romo, 2010) and short-term memory (Barak, Tsodyks, & Romo, 2010). In contrast, **long-term plasticity** refers to changes in synaptic efficacy that last more than a few minutes. Long-term synaptic plasticity is thought to be the basis for the formation of long-term memory (Lamsa & Lau, 2018). In Chapter 12, you will learn that long-term plasticity is the result of what is known as long-term potentiation, in which synapses are strengthened, and long-term depression, in which synapses are weakened (Connor & Wang, 2016; Mayford et al., 2012).

5.2.4 CORTICAL PLASTICITY

>> LO 5.2.4 Define and differentiate functional and structural plasticity.

Key Terms

- **Functional plasticity:** Functional changes in a brain area to compensate for damage to another area or changes in the body.
- **Structural plasticity:** Changes in brain structure that occur in response to the extensive practice of motor or cognitive skills.
- **Phantom limb:** The phenomenon in which amputees report retaining sensation of a missing limb.
- **Phantom pain:** The phenomenon in which a patient experiences pain in a phantom limb.

You just learned that environmental enrichment, learning, and chronic stress can induce neuroplastic changes in neurons and in the strength of synapses. In this unit we look at how neuroplastic changes can also occur in the cortex. Some of the changes in the cortex include changes in the function(s) of any given cortical area. This is one of two types of cortical plasticity known as **functional plasticity**. Functional plasticity is observed in patients who have had a limb amputated or when damage to sensory nerves prevents information from a part of the body to make it to the brain.

Other changes include changes in the structure of cortical areas or in the organization of nerve fibers that run through them. This type of cortical plasticity is known as **structural plasticity**. Structural plasticity involves changes in cortical thickness or gray matter volume in any given brain area. Structural plasticity is observed in response to the extensive practice of motor or cognitive skills. In the sections that follow, we review cases in which both functional and structural plasticity were observed.

FIGURE 5.14

(a) Representation of the digits of the hand on the left cheek of patient DS. (b) Rearranged representation of the digits six months after amputation. (c) The somatosensory homunculus showing that the representation of the digits is adjacent to the face representation. (d) Brain imaging results using magnetoencephalography, showing normal representations of the arm (blue), face (red), and hand (green) in the right hemisphere with the areas representing the arm and hand invaded by the representation (covered up with red) in the left hemisphere.

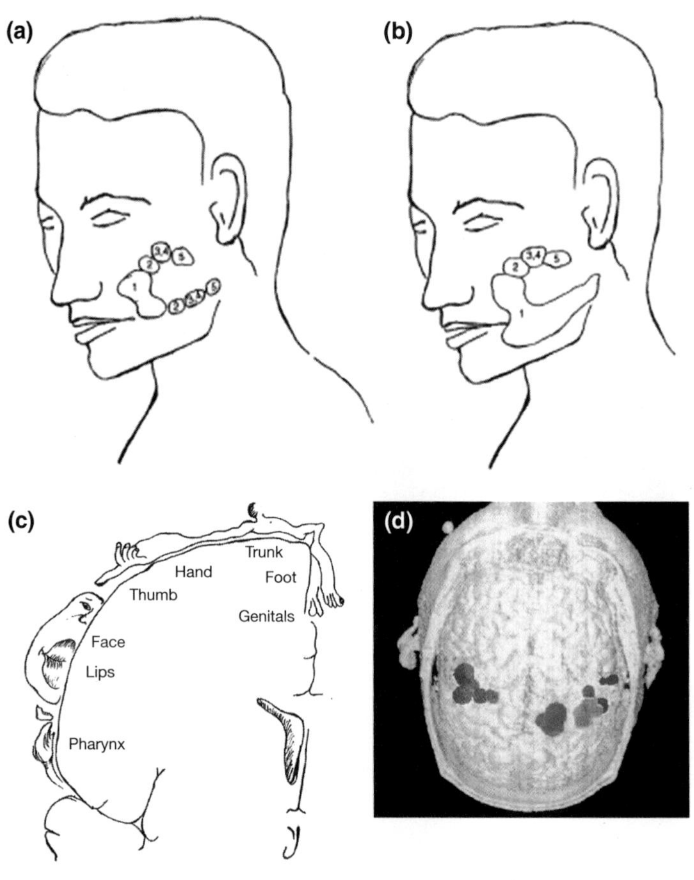

Ramachandran, V.S. & W. and Hirstein. (1998). The perception of phantom limbs. *Brain 121*(Pt 9): 1603–1630. With permission from Oxford University Press.

Functional Plasticity

Remarkable examples of cortical functional plasticity have been observed in people who have had a limb amputated (Ramachandran & Hirstein, 1998). One of the most famous cases is that of a man, known as DS, whose right arm was amputated following a motorcycle accident. DS experienced what is known as **phantom limb**, a condition in which a patient still feels the presence of an amputated limb. These patients may also experience **phantom pain**, which is the perception of pain in the missing limb.

When DS was asked to point to the source of his phantom, he pointed to the empty space where his hand would have been if it had not been amputated. As intriguing as this already is, DS also reported feeling the fingers of the missing hand when stroked across his left cheek (the limbs of one side of the body are represented in the opposite side of the brain [see Chapter 8]). The representation of the fingers on his cheek is illustrated in Figure 5.14a. Figure 5.14b shows how the map rearranged itself six months later.

How did this happen? As can be seen by looking at the homunculus in Figure 5.14c, the area of the somatosensory cortex that represents the fingers is immediately adjacent to the face area. It was therefore hypothesized that DS felt his missing fingers while being stroked across the cheek because the adjacent face area expanded to include the area that used to respond to stimulation of the fingers. The face area had thus acquired a new functional property.

Evidence for this came from a study in which the somatosensory cortex of a patient with a similar amputation to that of DS was imaged by magnetoencephalography (MEG) (Ramachandran, 1993). Figure 5.14d shows the representation of the patient's right and left arms in the somatosensory cortex (remember, left arm to the right and right arm to the left). Therefore, the normal representation is on the right (arm, blue; face, red; and hand, green). However, on the left side, you can see that the areas that usually represent the arm and hand are almost completely covered with red.

In this chapter's opening vignette, you read about the case of Zion Harvey who underwent a double hand transplant at age eight after having his hands amputated due to a staphylococcal infection when he was two years old. Because Zion didn't have hands, the hand area of his somatosensory cortex had presumably stopped being stimulated. Researchers wanted to understand how Zion's somatosensory cortex responded to the amputation of his hands and then to the transplanted hands (Gaetz et al., 2018). To do so, they stimulated Zion's lips and right index finger while his brain was being imaged by MRI and observed the responses in the corresponding areas of the somatosensory cortex (lip cortex and the right index finger area [RD2], respectively) compared to an age-matched control subject (Figure 5.15a).

FIGURE 5.15

The case of Zion Harvey. (a) Typical response of the somatosensory cortex to stimulation of the lips. RD2 (area outlined in black) represents the right index finger. The area outlined in blue represents the lip area. Stimulation of the lip results in activity in the lip area (as indicated by the patch of red color) but not in RD2. (b) Zion's area RD2 responded to stimulation of the lips one month and eight days after receiving his new hands (left). Seven months and 18 days later, stimulation of the lip now activated only the lip area, and stimulation of the right index finger stimulated RD2 normally (right).

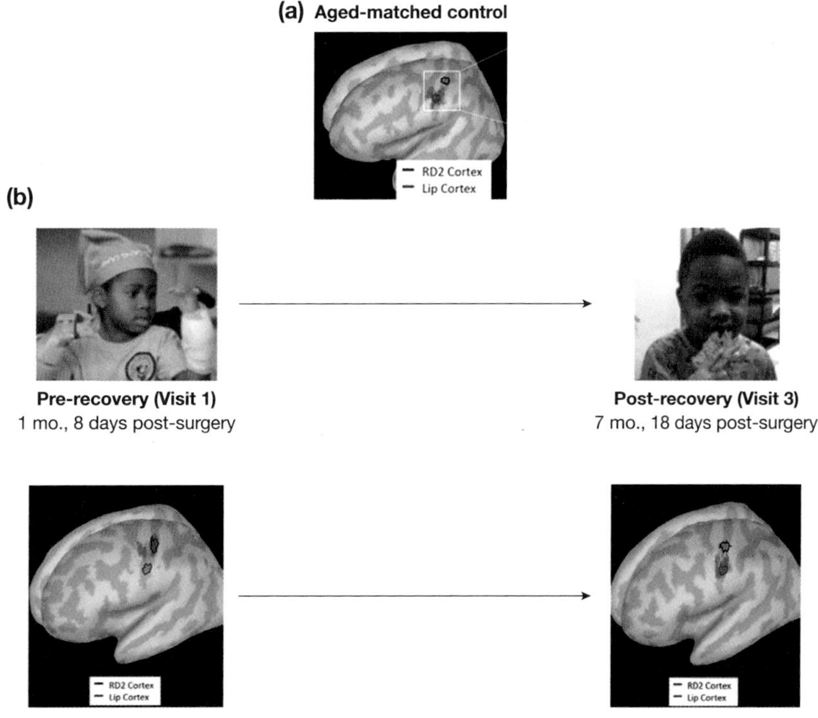

Gaetz, W., et al. (2017). Massive cortical reorganization is reversible following bilateral transplants of the hands: evidence from the first successful bilateral pediatric hand transplant patient. *Annals of Clinical and Translational Neurology* 5(1): 92–97. With permission from John Wiley & Sons.

One month and eight days after receiving his new hands, Zion's RD2 area responded to stimulation of the lips. This indicated that because of lack of stimulation of the right index finger (due to the amputation), the lip area reorganized in such a way that it responded to stimulation of that finger (Figure 5.15b [left]). However, seven months and 18 days later, Zion's somatosensory cortex underwent "massive reorganization" in that stimulation of the lip now activated only the lip area and stimulation of the right index finger stimulated RD2 normally (Figure 5.15b [right]).

Structural Plasticity

Structural plasticity has been observed in many studies. For example, it was found that regions of cortex associated with the playing of a musical instrument expand and/or become more responsive (Amunts et al., 1997; Y. Han et al., 2009). Structural plasticity has also been found in regions associated with the practice of sports (Jacini et al., 2009; A. Pearce, Thickbroom, Byrnes, & Mastaglia, 2000).

In fact, structural plasticity is likely to occur in brain areas associated with the extended practice of any skill. For example, neuroscientist Bogdan Draganski and colleagues explored whether structural plasticity, represented by an increase in the volume of gray matter (which consists of cell bodies), would occur in the cortex of participants who learned to juggle versus subjects who did not learn to juggle (Draganski et al., 2004). Participants in the juggling group were given three months to learn the "three-ball cascade" (Figure 5.16). The brains of the participants who both learned and did not learn to juggle were scanned by MRI at the beginning of the study. A second scan was performed once they became successful three-ball jugglers, and a third scan was performed three months later.

The first scan revealed no differences in gray matter between the brains of the participants in the juggling group versus the participants who did not learn to juggle. However, the second scan, performed after the subjects learned to juggle, revealed a significant increase in gray matter in the juggling group. Such an increase in gray matter volume was not found in the non-juggling group. As shown in Figure 5.16, increases in gray matter were found bilaterally in the left posterior intraparietal sulcus and in the medial temporal area. Why those areas? Would we not expect changes in motor areas? First, let's look at the functions of the areas that did show changes. The medial temporal area is highly involved in the processing of visual motion information used to construct motor commands (Dursteler & Wurtz, 1988). The intraparietal sulcus is involved in the intention and planning of specific movements (Andersen & Buneo, 2002). Both of these functions are highly relevant to juggling skills. The researchers suggested that there were no changes in motor areas because the subjects in both groups already had good motor skills before the study started.

Compensatory Enhancement of Senses

You may have heard that the loss of one sense is compensated by other senses becoming more acute.

FIGURE 5.16

MRI images in sagittal, coronal, and horizontal views (a–c) of the areas that showed changes in gray matter for the jugglers and non-jugglers. (d) Increases in gray matter in participants, as shown by three separate brain scans, when first learning to juggle, once they became successful, and three months later.

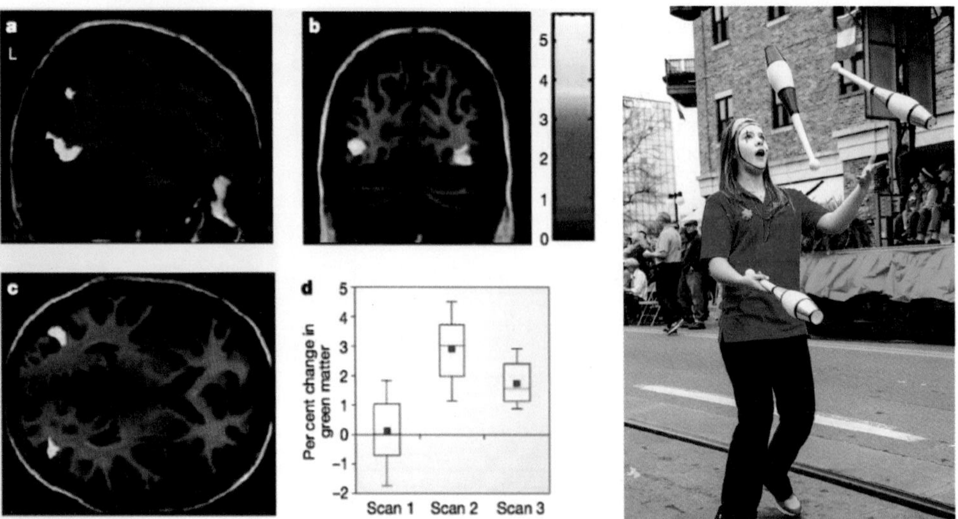

(a–c) Draganski, B., Gaser, C., Busch, V., Schuierer, G.R., Bogdahn, U., & May, A. (2004). Changes in grey matter induced by training. *Nature*, 427, 311–312; (d) iStock.com/erniedecker.

There is much evidence that this is true and that these changes are reflected in functional changes in the relevant cortical areas. For example, it was shown that blind individuals are better at discriminating textures by touch compared to sighted individuals (Gurtubay-Antolin & Rodriguez-Fornells, 2017). Blind individuals have also demonstrated superior performance in auditory pitch and speech discrimination compared to the sighted (Arnaud, Gracco, & Menard, 2018; Gougoux et al., 2004). Deaf individuals have also been shown to be better than the hearing at detecting motion (Shiell, Champoux, & Zatorre, 2014).

This compensatory effect by the other senses may reflect functional plasticity induced by increased use of another sense. For example, using electrophysiological recordings, neuroscientist Alvaro Pascual-Leone found that the sensorimotor cortex on the side representing the finger area used to read Braille was larger in blind participants one year after Braille training. The area was also significantly larger than in control subjects who did not learn to read Braille (Pascual-Leone & Torres, 1993).

5.2.5 WHEN CORTICAL PLASTICITY GOES OVERBOARD

>> LO 5.2.5 Explain how cortical plasticity may not always be adaptive by being exaggerated.

Key Terms

- **Focal task-specific dystonia:** A movement disorder that interferes with movements involved in highly practiced tasks.
- **Synergy:** The co-contraction of body parts as a unit due to a lack of inhibition of adjacent cortical representations.
- **Sensorimotor retuning:** A neuromuscular treatment used to reduce abnormal movements during instrument play in musicians with focal hand dystonia.

You have learned that neuroplastic changes in the cortex can be amazingly adaptive. However, sometimes neuroplasticity causes problems. One of these problems is known as **focal task-specific dystonia (FTSD)**. FTSD is a movement disorder that interferes with movements involved in highly practiced tasks. Such tasks include the extensive practice of musical instruments, the use of tools, the practice of a sport, and writing.

The typical symptoms of FTSD are involuntary movements and muscle cramping. Much of the research on FTSD has been done on musicians. Involuntary movements may be due to hypofunctioning inhibitory processes in the motor system. This might explain why a pianist affected by FTSD may not be able to inhibit the movements of a finger adjacent to the one hitting a specific note, leading to impaired performance. In this case, the lack of inhibition leads to the co-contraction of both correct and incorrect fingers when intending to strike a specific piano key. The same kind of impairment can occur in musicians playing stringed instruments, where a fine discrimination must be achieved between the fingers intended to play specific notes on the neck of a violin.

What specifically is happening in the brains of people with FTSD? You may have guessed that people with FTSD have developed maladaptive body representations. Indeed, people with FTSD have altered representations of the body parts that have been trained extensively. Figure 5.17 shows how the normal representations of digits are separated by sharp boundaries (left). In contrast, these boundaries are blurred (middle) in a stringed instrument player with FTSD. There is also reduced inhibition of the representations of the muscles surrounding the ones that control the trained body part. This results in them being contracted together as though they were one. This is known as **synergy**.

How can FTSD be treated? People with FTSD can potentially be helped through a treatment called **sensorimotor retuning** (SMR) (Enke & Poskey, 2018). The method has been described for use with wind-instrument players, pianists, and guitarists. For pianists and guitarists, the treatment consists of immobilizing any finger other than the dystonic one with the

FIGURE 5.17

Focal task-specific dystonia. Normal representations of digits are separated by sharp boundaries (left). In a stringed instrument player with FTSD, the boundaries are blurred (middle). After sensorimotor retuning, the boundaries are restored right).

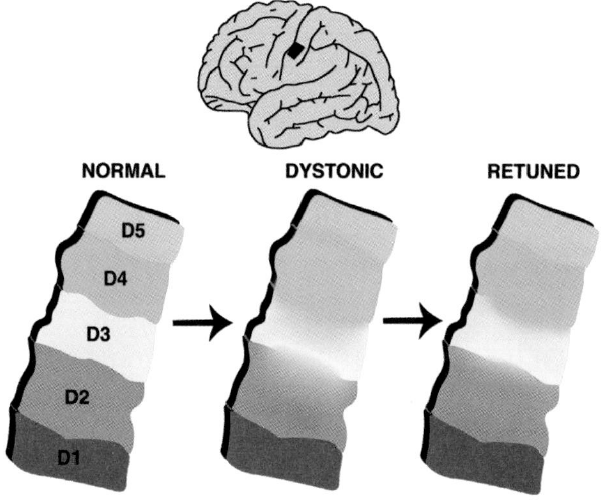

Nudo, R.J. (2002). Retuning the misfiring brain. *Proceedings of the National Academy of Sciences USA 100*(13): 7425–7427. Copyright 2003 National Academy of Sciences, U.S.A. Reprinted with permission.

use of a splint. The patient must then practice moving the dystonic finger repetitively in combination with one of the other free fingers in sequence. The patient is instructed to practice the procedure for up to two and a half hours per day for an entire year (Candia et al., 2002). After SMR, the boundaries between the digit representations in the somatosensory cortex are normalized (Figure 5.17, right).

MODULE SUMMARY

Neuroplasticity refers to the brain's ability to change its structure and function in response to experience or damage to itself or to the body. Structural remodeling refers to changes in the structure of neurons in response to the activity of other neurons or stimulation from the external environment. In the 1940s, Donald Hebb found that rats reared as pets were better than lab rats at solving mazes. He attributed their superior ability to having enriched experiences. In the 1970s, William Greenough found that rats raised in enriched conditions had larger dendritic fields in the visual cortex as well as more synapses per neuron than rats raised in standard conditions. These findings have been replicated and showed structural remodeling in brain areas relevant to the types of enrichment to which animals were subjected (visual, somatosensory, spatial, object exploration, and motor activity). Structural remodeling also occurs during the learning of various tasks and includes changes in the length of dendrites in the anterior cingulate cortex and orbitofrontal cortex.

Changes in the strength of synapses require changes in the efficiency of synapses. This is known as synaptic plasticity. Synaptic plasticity includes changes in the amount of neurotransmitter released at synapses, changes in the number and sensitivity of receptors on the postsynaptic neuron, and changes in the size of synapses. Neuroscientists differentiate between short-term synaptic plasticity, which is associated with short-term memory and decision making, and long-term synaptic plasticity, which is associated with the formation of long-term memories. Changes in the cortex include functional and structural plasticity. Functional plasticity refers to changes in the function of cortical areas, whereas structural plasticity refers to changes in the structure of cortical areas.

A remarkable example of functional plasticity is phantom limb, a phenomenon in which amputees report retaining sensation of the missing limb. A classic case of structural plasticity was reported in the 1990s where the representation of the right versus the left hand differed in the somatosensory cortex of violin players. There is evidence that people who lose one of their senses become better at using other senses. For example, neuroplastic changes have been observed in the finger area of the somatosensory cortex of Braille-reading individuals compared to those who do not read Braille. It was also shown that deaf individuals had enhanced attention to visual stimuli compared to those with normal hearing. Cortical plasticity can also go overboard in a condition known as focal task-specific dystonia.

TEST YOURSELF

5.2.1 Define neuroplasticity and discuss its different types.

5.2.2 What is structural remodeling? Discuss how it can be induced.

5.2.3 What is synaptic plasticity? Explain the ways in which it occurs as well as the difference between short-term and long-term synaptic plasticity.

5.2.4 Explain functional and structural plasticity by distinguishing between the two types and by giving an example for each one.

5.2.5 What is focal task-specific dystonia? What are its symptoms, and how can it be induced?

5.3 The Aging Brain: Adolescence and Old Age

Module Contents

Learning Objectives

5.3.1 Describe the neurobiological basis for the association between adolescence and risk-taking and impulsive behavior.

5.3.2 Explain the cognitive declines that occur during normal aging of the brain.

5.3.3 Describe the cognitive declines due to a disease process (Alzheimer's) in the aged brain.

5.3.1 THE ADOLESCENT BRAIN AND BEHAVIOR

>> LO 5.3.1 Describe the neurobiological basis for the association between adolescence and risk-taking and impulsive behavior.

Key Terms

- **Risk-taking behaviors:** Behaviors that carry potential for harm such as unprotected sexual activity, sexting, smoking, alcohol and illegal substance use, dangerous driving, and various illegal activities.
- **Impulse control:** The ability to inhibit thoughts and actions that lead to immediate gratification in favor of those that are oriented toward the fulfillment of goals.
- **Frontostriatal circuit:** A network of brain areas highly involved in impulse control, which includes the inferior frontal gyrus and the ventrolateral prefrontal cortex and the striatum.

You have undoubtedly heard that adolescents are typically rebellious, irresponsible, and lacking impulse control and that they engage in risky behaviors. You may also have heard that adolescents are more at risk, than other age groups, for depression, eating disorders, and suicide (Berk, 2018). You also need to know, however, that although many adolescents face important challenges, the great majority of people get through adolescence without experiencing major psychological disturbances.

The extent to which these disturbances are experienced depends on environmental, biological, social, and psychological factors. In this module, we focus on the adolescent brain with regard to risk-taking behaviors and deficits in impulse control (Casey, Jones, & Hare, 2008).

Risk-taking behaviors in adolescents include unprotected sexual activity, sexting, smoking, drug use, dangerous driving, and various illegal activities. By contrast, **impulse control** refers to the ability to inhibit inappropriate thoughts, emotions, and actions, such as those that lead to immediate gratification in favor of those that are oriented toward the fulfillment of long-term goals. This is especially difficult when actions geared toward fulfilling a long-term goal compete with activities that are immediately rewarding. For example, as you sit there writing a paper due the following week, it may be difficult for you to resist the temptation to play your favorite video game or to check the number of "likes" for your latest posts on social media.

Risky behaviors, which can result from low impulse control, have been suggested to be due to early-maturing and overactive dopamine-rich areas of the brain, such as the ventral striatum. The ventral striatum signals the value of rewards (see Chapter 9), which means that new and exciting stimuli exert a stronger pull on adolescents than on children and adults, making adolescents more likely to act impulsively. In contrast, the network of brain areas that keeps the influence of the ventral striatum in check, through cognitive control, is thought to be relatively immature and less functional in adolescents (Galvan et al., 2006). This network, known as the **frontostriatal circuit**, is important for impulse control (Dalley, Mar, Economidou, & Robbins, 2008). The areas that make up this circuit include the inferior frontal gyrus, ventrolateral prefrontal cortex, and striatum.

The relatively immature frontostriatal circuit in adolescents means they may be less able to suppress the impulse to approach appetitive stimuli, driven by the ventral striatum, even when considerable risks are involved. For example, to properly weigh the consequences of engaging in unprotected sexual activity—and choose not to do so—may require the frontostriatal circuit to exert effective suppression of activity in the ventral striatum.

To test this idea, neuroscientist Leah Somerville and colleagues assessed the performance of children, adolescents, and adults in a cued go/no-go task while their brains were being scanned by functional magnetic resonance imaging (fMRI) (Somerville, Hare, & Casey, 2011). In a cued go/no-go task, subjects are instructed to perform a response, such as pressing a button, when a stimulus is presented but to withhold that response when another stimulus is presented. This task is typically used to test participants' ability to engage in behavioral inhibition, or impulse control. The study procedure is illustrated in Figure 5.18a. The participants were instructed to press a button when they saw a calm face (go) but to withhold their response when they saw a happy face (no go).

The results are shown in Figure 5.18b. Compared to both children and adults, teens had more difficulty inhibiting their responses when they saw the happy face. This was indicated by their higher percentage of self-control failures (not being able to follow the instructions).

Figure 5.18c shows an fMRI image of activity in the ventral striatum, which signals the value of rewards, as you read earlier. The ventral striatum was significantly more activated in teens than in children or adults upon presentation of the happy face. This was taken to indicate that the reward value of stimuli is more likely to drive the behavior of teens than of children or adults. However, as shown in Figure 5.18d, both children and teens showed greater activation of the ventrolateral prefrontal cortex than adults upon presentation of the happy face. These results indicate that children and teens may exert more effort in inhibiting responses than do adults.

Taken together, these findings mean that, although the frontostriatal system of teens is significantly activated, this activation is not sufficient to override the

FIGURE 5.18

Procedure and results of the go/no-go task used in Somerville et al. (2011). (a) Participants were instructed to press a button when they saw a calm face (go) but to withhold their response when they saw a happy face (no go), while their brains were being imaged by fMRI. (b) Teens had more difficulty withholding their responses when they saw the happy face than both children and adults, indicated by a higher rate of self-control failures. (c) Activity in the striatum was higher in teens than in both children and adults, indicating that rewarding stimuli are more likely to drive behavior in teens than in children and adults. (d) Activity in the ventrolateral prefrontal cortex in children and teens was higher than in adults, indicating that both groups must exert more effort than adults to withhold responding.

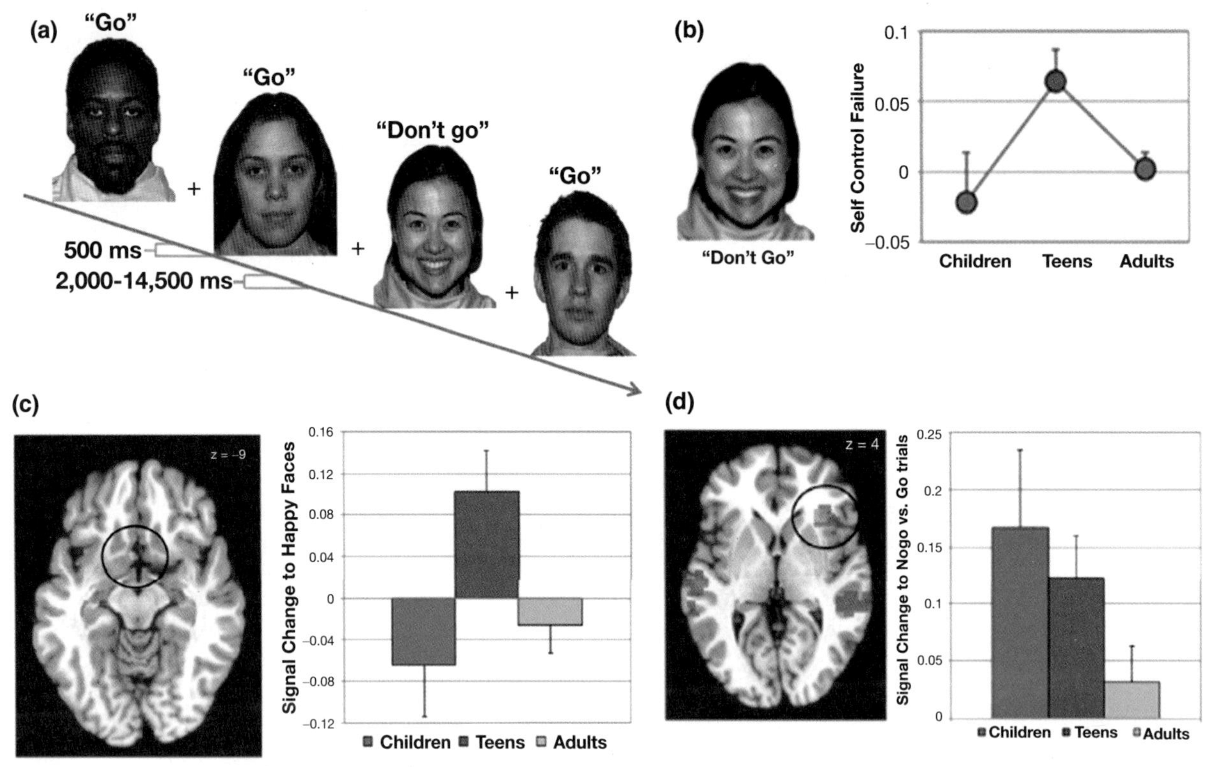

tendency for responses to be driven by the ventral striatum during no-go trials. In contrast, the activation of the ventrolateral prefrontal cortex of children was sufficient to inhibit responding. Why was the activation of the ventrolateral prefrontal cortex the lowest in adults? Since the frontostriatal system of adults is fully developed, the tendency to respond on the no-go trials may be more easily suppressed and may require less activation.

These results suggest that decision making in adolescents may be driven more by impulse than by rational decision making. But this is not all bad news. As stated earlier, the great majority of us have survived adolescence without any major issues. In fact, the propensity to take risks and to be impulsive may have evolutionary value. The very characteristics that are often viewed in a negative light drive exploration and the seeking of new experiences. Exploration and the seeking out of new experiences are at the base of learning about the world, which leads to the development of coping and adaptive strategies applied to everyday living (Jaworska & MacQueen, 2015). Another factor to consider is that adolescents take fewer risks when the consequences of their behaviors are understood (Defoe, Dubas, Figner, & van Aken, 2015). This indicates that risk-taking in adolescents may be due partly to the lack of knowledge about the consequences of their behavior. Such knowledge is acquired through accumulated life experiences.

5.3.2 NORMAL AGING OF THE BRAIN

>> LO 5.3.2 **Explain the cognitive declines that occur during normal aging of the brain.**

Key Terms

- **Fluid intelligence:** The ability to think quickly and abstractly. It includes the capacity of working memory and processing speed.
- **Processing speed:** The speed at which information can be analyzed and at which mental tasks are performed.
- **Crystallized intelligence:** Cognitive skills that depend on accumulated wisdom, knowledge, expertise, and vocabulary.
- **Disconnection hypothesis:** The hypothesis that the normal cognitive declines that occur during aging are due to the degeneration of white fiber tracts that connect the brain areas relevant to cognitive functions.

Now that you know about some of what goes on in the adolescent brain and how it impacts adolescent behavior, we turn our attention to normal aging of the brain. As you just read, research on the development of the adolescent brain focuses mainly on its relationship with risk-taking and impulse control. Research on the aging brain seeks to understand the relationships between changes in the brain and cognitive declines such as those seen in memory, attention, and executive functioning.

Normal Aging of the Brain

Normal aging of the brain is associated with a decline in cognitive abilities that begins in middle adulthood. The skills that show the highest rate of decline are the ones associated with what is known as **fluid intelligence**. Fluid intelligence refers to the ability to think quickly and abstractly. It includes working memory capacity and **processing speed**, which is the speed at which information can be analyzed and the speed at which mental tasks are performed. Slowed processing speed is considered to be the hallmark of the aging brain. Cognitive skills associated with what is known as **crystallized intelligence** depend on accumulated wisdom, knowledge, expertise, and vocabulary, and they tend not to decline with age (Figure 5.19).

Explanations for Cognitive Declines Observed During Aging

Several hypotheses have been put forward to explain the cognitive declines observed during aging. According to the **disconnection hypothesis**, cognitive decline is due to the degeneration of nerve fibers that connect the brain areas relevant to the performance of cognitive functions (Langen et al., 2017). Evidence for this hypothesis was found in a large-scale study that observed the effects of nerve fiber degeneration on executive functions and motor-speed performance. The decline in executive functions was associated with the degeneration of nerve fibers in

FIGURE 5.19

Rates of decline in crystallized and fluid intelligences during aging.

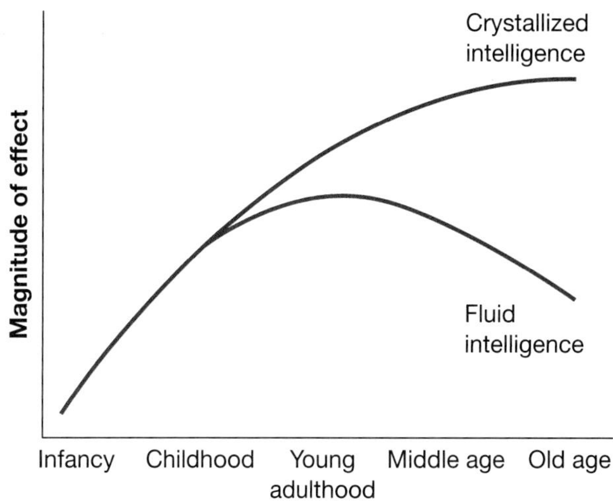

the cortico-spinal tract, and memory impairments were associated with degenerating nerve fibers in the parieto-temporal area (Lampe et al., 2017).

Aging and Neurogenesis

Could the cognitive declines observed in aging be due to a reduction in neurogenesis? Neuroscientist Maura Boldrini and colleagues set out to answer this question (Boldrini et al., 2018). They examined the hippocampi of deceased individuals who ranged in age from 14 to 79 years. They found that neurogenesis in the dentate gyrus was preserved throughout life. However, declines in angiogenesis, which is the birth of new blood vessels, and neuroplasticity were found to occur.

The authors interpreted their findings as meaning that hippocampal neurogenesis can sustain cognitive function throughout life and that cognitive impairments observed in aging may be due to a loss in cognitive-emotional resilience, which is the ability to adapt well in the face of adversity and difficult circumstances.

Other evidence points to the possibility that a decline in neurogenesis does occur. For example, in another study published at around the same time, neurogenesis was shown to be greatly reduced in the hippocampus of adults (Sorrells et al., 2018). So, the jury is still out on the issue at the time of writing this book.

5.3.3 DISEASE IN THE AGING BRAIN

>> LO 5.3.3 **Describe the cognitive declines due to a disease process (Alzheimer's) in the aged brain.**

Key Terms

- **Alzheimer's disease:** A degenerative brain disease characterized by the severe and progressive loss of memory and other thinking skills to the point where self-care is no longer possible.
- **Dementia:** An umbrella term used to designate a group of symptoms shared by several neurodegenerative diseases.
- **Mild cognitive impairment:** A condition marked by short-term memory problems that worsen over about a seven-year period. These problems are associated with a progressive degeneration of the medial temporal lobes.
- **Beta-amyloid plaques:** Plaques formed by an accumulation of the beta-amyloid peptide, which is derived from a larger protein called amyloid precursor protein.
- **Neurofibrillary tangles:** Abnormal aggregates of a protein known as tau, which is normally essential in maintaining the structural integrity of microtubules.
- **Amyloid hypothesis:** The hypothesis that Alzheimer's disease results from an accumulation of the peptide beta-amyloid, which forms plaques that cause synaptic dysfunction, inflammation, and neuronal death.
- **Amyloid precursor protein:** A transmembrane protein that is a precursor to beta-amyloid.
- **Tau hypothesis:** A hypothesis based on the observation that the progression of Alzheimer's disease is related more to the effects of changes in tau than to the formation of beta-amyloid plaques and that the formation of neurofibrillary tangles precedes the formation of beta-amyloid plaques.
- **Metabolism hypothesis:** The hypothesis that Alzheimer's disease and type-2 diabetes share common characteristics.

In the preceding unit, you learned about the declines in cognitive abilities associated with the normally aging brain. However, much more severe declines in cognitive abilities are observed when a disease process is involved. The disease most associated with such declines is known as **Alzheimer's disease**. Alzheimer's disease affects 1 in 10 individuals aged 65 years and older, and it is the most common form of **dementia** (Alzheimer's Association, 2018). Dementia is not a disorder but, rather, is an umbrella term used to designate a group of symptoms shared by several neurodegenerative diseases. These symptoms include a severe loss of memory and other thinking skills to the point where self-care is no longer possible.

Alzheimer's disease is preceded by a condition known as **mild cognitive impairment**, which is marked by short-term memory problems that worsen over about a seven-year period. These problems are associated with a progressive degeneration of the medial temporal lobes. During the next two years, a person develops mild Alzheimer's disease. At this stage, the disease spreads to include damage to the lateral temporal and parietal lobes, which is associated with problems recognizing objects and orienting in space. The cognitive impairments then deepen to include poor judgment, impulsivity, and a short attention span, which are associated with the disease spreading to the frontal lobes. At this point, a person is considered to have moderate Alzheimer's disease. Finally, this is followed about two years later by severe Alzheimer's disease, in which neurodegeneration spreads to include the occipital lobes, which may lead to visual problems. The progression from mild cognitive impairment to severe Alzheimer's disease—as well as the progression of brain damage and associated symptoms—is illustrated in Figure 5.20.

What Goes on in the Brain During Alzheimer's Disease?

The causes of Alzheimer's disease remain largely unknown, and no cure is presently available for it. Scientists are investigating several possible causes for the disease. There is thought to be a genetic risk factor for developing Alzheimer's disease. One of these factors is having inherited a particular form of the apolipoprotein E gene (*APOE*) (Blennow, de Leon, & Zetterberg, 2006). The inheritance of this form of *APOE* is related to what is known as late-onset Alzheimer's disease. This is the most common form of the disease, in which people start developing symptoms in their mid-60s. Mutations on other genes are related to what is known as early-onset Alzheimer's disease, in which symptoms start occurring when people are between their 30s and 60s.

As mentioned in Chapter 1, genes are not solely responsible for the development of traits. This includes the development of diseases such as Alzheimer's. In other words, having inherited the *APOE* gene linked to increased risk does not guarantee that you will have Alzheimer's. Age, gender, health, environmental lifestyle, and social factors interact with genetic predispositions to cause Alzheimer's (Blennow et al., 2006; Riedel, Thompson, & Brinton, 2016).

The Amyloid Hypothesis

The hallmarks of Alzheimer's disease are the presence of **beta-amyloid plaques** and **neurofibrillary tangles**. This has led to what is known as the **amyloid hypothesis** (sometimes known as the amyloid cascade hypothesis). According to the amyloid hypothesis, Alzheimer's disease is the result of an accumulation of the peptide beta-amyloid (Aβ), which forms plaques that cause synaptic dysfunction, inflammation, and neuronal death (H. G. Lee et al., 2004). The Aβ peptide is itself derived from a precursor molecule called **amyloid precursor protein** (APP). Beta-amyloid plaques are formed when APP is cleaved (cut) by enzymes called β-secretase and presenilin, resulting in the release of Aβ into extracellular space. These plaques

FIGURE 5.20

The progression of Alzheimer's disease.

Mild cognitive impairment

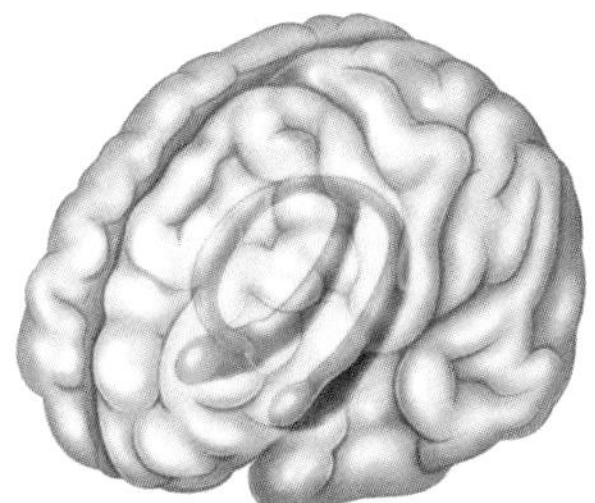

Duration: 7 years
Disease begins in medial temporal lobe
Symptoms: Short-term memory loss

Mild Alzheimer's

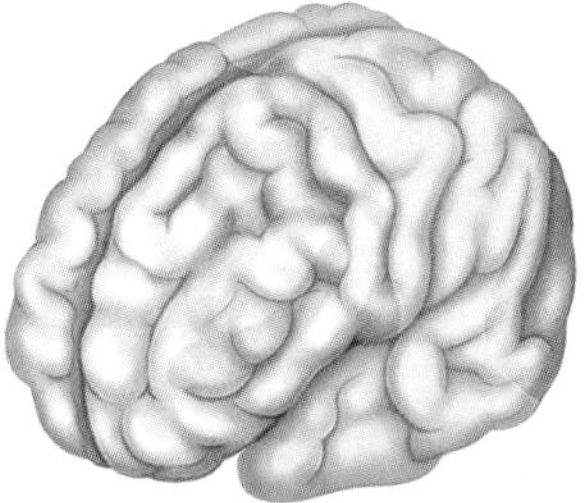

Duration: 2 years
Disease spreads to lateral temporal & parietal lobes
Symptoms: Reading problems, poor object recognition, poor direction sense

Moderate Alzheimer's

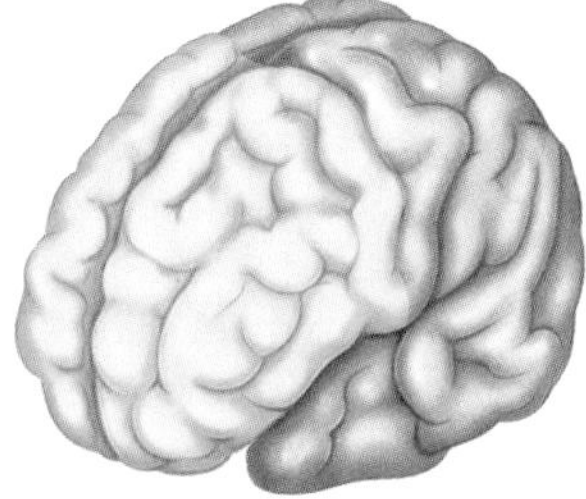

Duration: 2 years
Disease spreads to frontal lobe
Symptoms: Poor judgment, impulsivity, short attention

Severe Alzheimer's

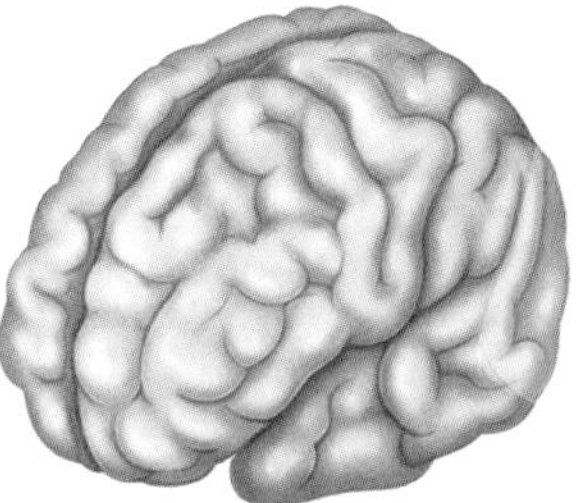

Duration: 3 years
Disease spreads to occipital lobe
Symptoms: Visual problems

Carolina Hrejsa/Body Scientific Intl.

accumulate on the axons and dendrites of neurons and prevent them from carrying out their functions.

This process, illustrated in Figure 5.21, is thought to lead to the other hallmark of Alzheimer's disease, which is the presence of neurofibrillary tangles. Neurofibrillary tangles are caused by aggregations of a protein known as tau. Tau plays an important role in stabilizing microtubules. Microtubules are essential in maintaining neurons' structural stability. They are also essential for the transport of molecules along the axons of neurons (see Chapter 2). In Alzheimer's, a chemical process called phosphorylation alters the tau protein. This change causes it to no longer be able to bind to microtubules, causing their disintegration. Devoid of microtubules, neurons lose their structural integrity and can no longer transport nutrients and carry away waste products. This process leads neurons to "commit suicide" in a process known as apoptosis, in which immune cells ensure the organized death of cells.

It had been believed that, in Alzheimer's disease, this process first occurs in the entorhinal cortex (Corder et al., 2000). However, Schmitz and colleagues recently found that the neuronal degeneration observed in Alzheimer's begins in the basal forebrain (Schmitz, Spreng, & Alzheimer's Disease Neuroimaging Initiative, 2016). The basal forebrain is an area rich in cholinergic neurons (these synthesize and release acetylcholine), which innervate the entorhinal cortex and hippocampus. As you will read in Chapter 12, these neurons are important for learning and memory. These neurons seem to be particularly sensitive to the neurodegenerative effects of neurofibrillary tangles. Therefore, the death of basal forebrain neurons interrupts an important pathway involved in processing new information (Schmitz et al., 2016).

Problems With the Amyloid Hypothesis

There are problems with the amyloid hypothesis (Makin, 2018). One of these problems is that medications developed to reduce the amount of amyloid in neurons have so far not been shown to be effective in treating the disease (Ricciarelli & Fedele, 2017). Another problem is that the progression of Alzheimer's disease is more highly related to the effects of the changes in tau than to the formation of Aβ plaques. It was also found that the formation of neurofibrillary tangles precedes the formation of Aβ plaques. This has led some researchers to propose what is known as the **tau hypothesis** (Maccioni, Farias, Morales, & Navarrete, 2010).

The Metabolism Hypothesis

In addition to the amyloid and tau hypotheses, many other hypotheses about the causes for Alzheimer's disease have been proposed (Du, Wang, & Geng, 2018). One hypothesis that has been gaining traction is known as the **metabolism hypothesis** of Alzheimer's disease. The metabolism hypothesis states that Alzheimer's disease and type-2 diabetes share common characteristics (de Nazareth, 2017). Insulin, a hormone released by the pancreas, plays an important role in the metabolism of glucose to energy. In type-2 diabetes, cells no longer respond to insulin, impairing their ability to metabolize glucose. This condition is known as insulin resistance.

Several observations support the metabolism hypothesis. For example, people with type-2 diabetes have one and a half times the risk of developing dementia compared to people without type-2 diabetes (G. Cheng, Huang, Deng, & Wang, 2012). Another study found that 81% of Alzheimer's patients had either type-2 diabetes or impaired glucose metabolism (Janson et al., 2004). In addition, an association has been found between type-2 diabetes and declines in memory and executive functions (Wrighten, Piroli, Grillo, & Reagan, 2009). Type-2

FIGURE 5.21

The amyloid hypothesis. Beta-amyloid plaques are formed when the extracellular portion of APP (blue), the precursor protein for Aβ, is cleaved by the enzymes β-secretase (red) and presenilin (green). This causes the release of Aβ strands (orange) that accumulate into plaques in extracellular space. Neurofibrillary tangles inside the neuron are caused by phosphorylated tau protein, which dissociates from microtubules, causing them to disintegrate. The tau protein then aggregates into neurofibrillary tangles.

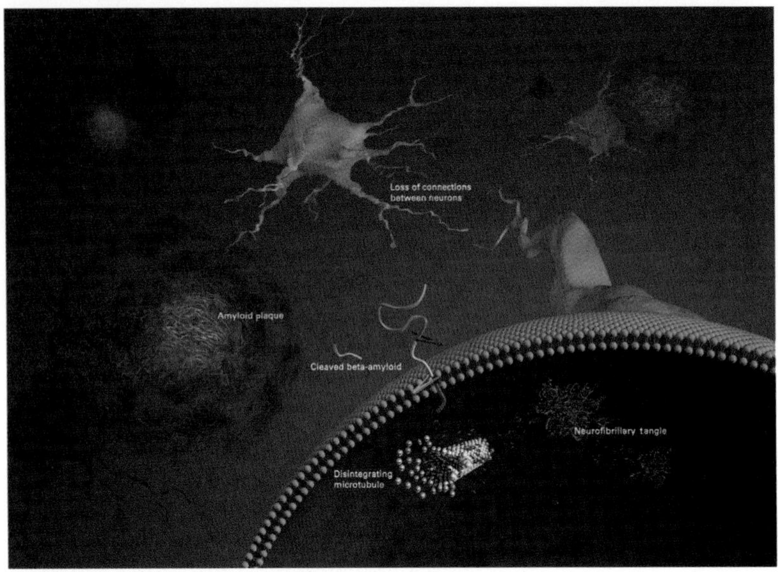

National Institute on Aging, *Progress Report on Alzheimer's Disease 2004-2005*.

diabetes was also found to be associated with phosphorylation of the tau protein and the presence of Aβ plaques (de Nazareth, 2017; Moran et al., 2015) which, as mentioned earlier, lead to the loss of neurons. In turn, phosphorylated tau may itself contribute to the development of insulin resistance (Leboucher et al., 2019).

The hippocampus, a brain area highly involved in processing memories (see Chapter 12), contains a high concentration of neurons with insulin receptors. In fact, many studies have found that the administration of insulin improved memory in both humans and animals (De Felice & Benedict, 2015). This may be because of insulin's role in synaptic plasticity (Ferrario & Reagan, 2018), which is crucial for the formation of memories. Insulin also has neurotrophic effects, meaning that it supports the growth and survival of neurons. People with type-2 diabetes, as well as people suffering from obesity, have higher than normal blood levels of free fatty acids (FFAs) and glucose. This facilitates the process by which FFAs cross the blood-brain barrier. The entry of FFAs into the brain triggers a process that causes glial cells to release inflammatory chemicals, which in turn results in insulin resistance and the death of neurons (Bagyinszky et al., 2017).

MODULE SUMMARY

Adolescents are often thought to be rebellious, irresponsible, and lacking impulse control and to frequently engage in risky behaviors. They are more at risk than any other group for depression, eating disorders, and suicide. However, most people get through adolescence without experiencing any significant problems. Risk-taking behavior and difficulties in impulse control are often taken to mean the same thing. In fact, they are different and are traced to the development of different brain areas. Risk-taking behavior refers to engaging in dangerous activities, whereas difficulties in impulse control refers to the inability to inhibit inappropriate thoughts, emotions, and actions. Risk-taking behavior is thought to be related to early-maturing and overactive dopamine-rich areas of the brain such as the ventral striatum, which processes the value of rewards. In contrast, the frontostriatal circuit—which is necessary for the control of impulses and, therefore, keeps the ventral striatum in check—is immature and less functional in adolescents.

Cognitive decline in aging occurs through a normal process. However, this normal process can be accelerated by disease. Cognitive declines that occur during normal aging include declines in skills related to fluid intelligence, which are those that include memory, attention, and processing speed. Cognitive skills related to crystallized intelligence are those that depend on accumulated wisdom, knowledge, expertise, and vocabulary, and they tend not to decline with age. The cognitive declines observed in normal aging are thought to be due, in part, to the degeneration in white fiber tracts in frontal areas, cortico-spinal tracts, and parieto-temporal areas. This is known as the disconnection hypothesis. Neurogenesis was found to persist through old age in the hippocampus.

The most common disease process that leads to accelerated degeneration of the brain is a type of dementia known as Alzheimer's disease, which leads to a wide range of cognitive deficits, including memory, attention, language, and visuospatial deficits. Significant shrinkage of the brain areas responsible for these functions is observed in people suffering from Alzheimer's disease. The hallmarks of Alzheimer's disease are beta-amyloid plaques and neurofibrillary tangles, which impede the neurons' ability to communicate with each other and lead to their death. Several other hypotheses of Alzheimer's disease exist. One that is gaining traction is the metabolism hypothesis, which states that Alzheimer's and type-2 diabetes share common characteristics.

TEST YOURSELF

5.3.1 What is the difference between risk-taking and impulsive behavior? Explain how developmental differences between brain areas can explain adolescent behavior.

5.3.2 (a) Does everybody eventually suffer from dementia? (b) Describe the differences between cognitive declines in normal aging and those associated with a disease process. (c) Describe some symptoms of Alzheimer's disease and its hallmarks.

5.3.3 Describe the amyloid hypothesis and the metabolism hypothesis of Alzheimer's disease.

APPLICATIONS

Exercise and Neurogenesis: "*Mens Sana in Corpore Sano*"

The Latin phrase *Mens sana in corpore sano* translates into "a healthy mind in a healthy body." Do you think this to be true? If you answered yes, then you have the backing of science. Exercise, which leads to a healthy body, has also been shown to lead to a healthy mind and brain. Much research has shown that regular exercise is associated with enhanced memory, learning capacity, and general cognitive functioning, and with a reduction in the decline of cognitive function in the elderly (Engeroff, Ingmann, & Banzer, 2018; Erickson et al., 2011; Kramer & Colcombe, 2018). Exercise training not only improves physical fitness and function but also leads to improvements in cognitive function and mood in people with dementia, other neurodegenerative diseases, and brain damage induced by stroke and traumatic injuries (Heyn, Abreu, & Ottenbacher, 2004; Narayanasetti & Thomas, 2017).

Exercise is associated with changes in nerve growth factor in the hippocampus, which leads to the generation of new neurons. Exercise may also play a significant role in alleviating depression by increasing the number of neurons that produce serotonin (Hong, Lee, & Kim, 2015). In fact, researchers also found that exercise leads to increased synaptic strength and plasticity (D'Arcangelo, Triossi, Buglione, Melchiorri, & Tancredi, 2017). These exercise-induced changes may explain observed enhancements in cognitive function.

How Much Exercise Is Effective?

In one study, researchers assigned 24 adults to either a six-week exercise program or a nontraining control group (Ji et al., 2017). The exercise program consisted of 30 minutes per day of a combination of yoga and aerobic, balance, and resistance exercises. Participants in the exercising group showed a significant advantage in executive functioning and memory recall for emotional events compared to the nonexercising control group. In addition, MRI scans of participants' brains showed significant changes in the brains of participants in the exercising group. These changes included increases in the volume and connectivity of the posterior cingulate cortex. Also, the striatum had increased its connectivity with the cingulate, temporal, parietal, and occipital cortices.

This frequency of exercising might seem like a lot to you, but neuroplastic changes have also been found following a single bout of moderately intense aerobic exercise (Mooney et al., 2016). For example, three 30- to 60-minute bouts of brisk walking a week or even moderate dancing once or twice a week was shown to do the job (Budde, Wegner, Soya, Voelcker-Rehage, & McMorris, 2016). Exercise was found to have even more significant effects on neuroplasticity when combined with cognitive training (Hotting & Roder, 2013). This means that studying and memorizing information in preparation for your next exam while on the treadmill may enhance the level of neuroplastic changes that occur in your brain. So, go ahead and have a great workout! ●

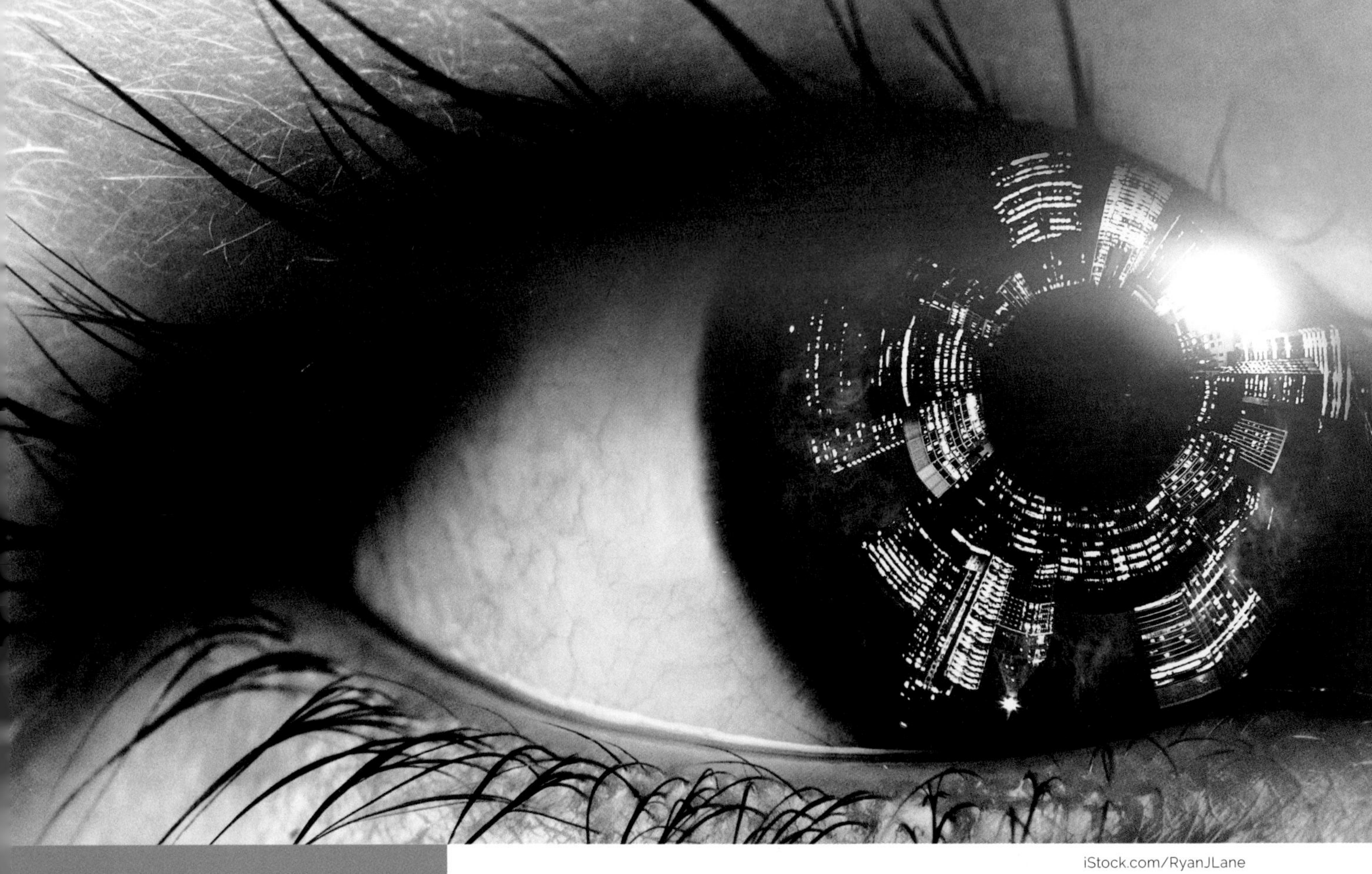

iStock.com/RyanJLane

6 Sensation and Perception 1

Vision and Hearing

Chapter Contents

Learning Objectives

6.1.1 Describe the beginnings of how information from the physical environment is transformed into a visual image.

6.1.2 Explain how light energy is transformed into the electrical signals in receptors that transmit visual information to the brain.

6.1.3 Explain the mechanisms involved in the precision of vision and the visual receptor's sensitivity to light.

6.1.4 Describe and explain how receptive fields are involved in representing the physical world.

6.1.5 Describe and explain the theories and processes involved in color vision.

6.1.6 Describe and explain the processes involved in vision in the brain.

6.2.1 Explain the difference between the physical and perceptual dimensions of sound.

6.2.2 Describe the functions of the different parts of the ear.

6.2.3 Outline the path of auditory processing from the cochlea to and within the brain.

Color-Coded Confusion

For most people, a trip to the grocery store to pick up ingredients needed for supper is a routine task. Ripe tomatoes are easily picked over unripe ones. If green olives are preferred, one easily picks them over black olives. For Geoffrey Hope-Terry, however, these are not easy tasks. Geoffrey has red-green color deficiency. This means that he confuses green and red. It's no wonder that he easily confuses unripe tomatoes with ripe ones, as they go from green to red as they ripen. Grocery shopping is not his only nightmare. In his neighborhood, as in many, sorting the trash means throwing items into color-coded bins. Regular trash goes into a green bin, biodegradable waste goes into a brown bin, glass goes into a red bin, and plastics in another green bin. Geoffrey's red-green color deficiency is known as deuteranopia. Normally, the brain makes out the colors we perceive through the inputs of three types of cells located at the back of the eyes. These cells, which capture light energy, are known as photoreceptors. Geoffrey was born without the type of photoreceptors responsible for perceiving green. This also affects the way he perceives other colors. Geoffrey's type of color deficiency is the most common, affecting approximately 8% of males and 0.5% of females. However, there are other types of color deficiencies, such as blue-yellow color deficiency. Geoffrey feels he shouldn't complain because his situation could be much worse. After all, some people cannot perceive colors at all and, instead, perceive the world in shades of gray. This indeed occurs in an extremely rare condition in which people are lacking all three types of photoreceptors needed for color vision.

Key Terms

- **Sensation:** The detection of external or internal stimuli through the stimulation of specialized receptors.
- **Perception:** What the brain makes of stimuli that activate receptors.

INTRODUCTION

In this chapter, and the next, you will learn about some of the neurobiological mechanisms underlying sensation and perception. **Sensation** refers to the detection of external or internal stimuli through the stimulation of specialized receptors. Light energy, compression and decompression of the air, airborne chemicals, and mechanical deformations of the skin are all examples of such stimuli. They are the basis of your senses of vision, hearing, smell, and touch, respectively. **Perception** is what your brain makes of these stimuli, for example, your experiences of colors, music, the fragrance of coffee in the morning, and the feeling of a bug crawling on your skin.

To appreciate the difference between sensation and perception, look at Figure 6.1 before you continue reading. What did you see? If you saw a young woman, look again. Stare at the picture until you see an old woman. If you saw an old woman, stare at the figure until you see the young woman. In class, when I put this figure up on a screen and ask students what they see, most students report seeing a young woman. The figure is known as the old lady/young lady ambiguous figure. It was first published in 1915 and later adapted by psychologist Edward Garrigues Boring (1930).

What does this ambiguous figure tell us about the difference between sensation and perception? Everyone experiences the same stimulus. That is, the same collection of lines, contours, and combination of wavelengths of light (which are perceived as colors, as you will later learn) is reflected from the screen for everyone. In other words, everyone gets the same sensation. However,

FIGURE 6.1

Young woman or old woman: Which do you see?

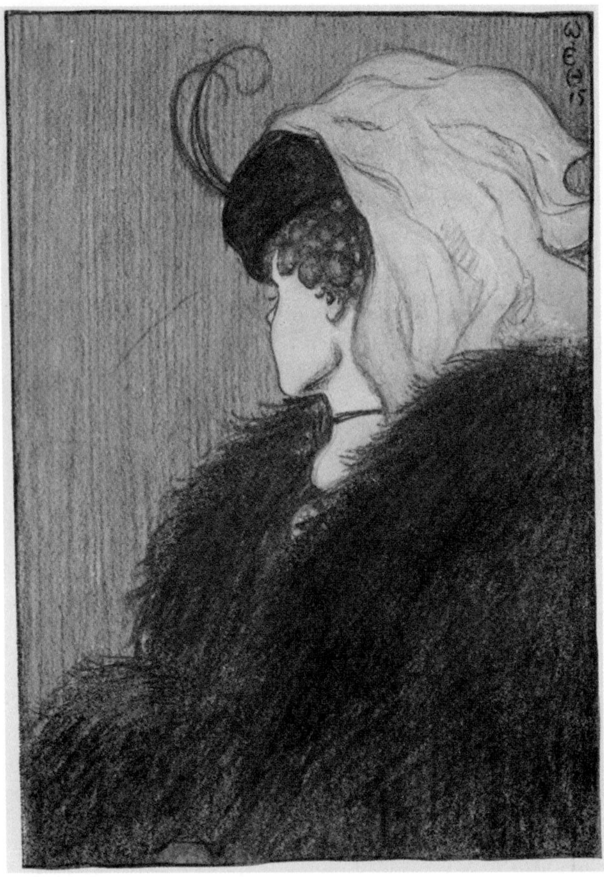

United States Library of Congress

people have a different interpretation of what they first see. That is, they differ in their perception.

What is perceived can be influenced by many factors. In the case of the old lady/young lady ambiguous figure, one's own age can influence whether one more readily perceives the old or young lady. For example, one study found that younger participants more readily perceived a young lady whereas older participants more readily perceived an old lady (Nicholls, Churches, & Loetscher, 2018). This difference between sensation and perception holds true for all your senses. In this chapter, we will cover the basic neurobiological processes that underlie vision and hearing. In Chapter 7, we will cover the chemical senses (which include taste and smell) and touch.

6.1 Vision

Module Contents

Learning Objectives

6.1.1 Describe the beginnings of how information from the physical environment is transformed into a visual image.

6.1.2 Explain how light energy is transformed into the electrical signals in receptors that transmit visual information to the brain.

6.1.3 Explain the mechanisms involved in the precision of vision and the visual receptor's sensitivity to light.

6.1.4 Describe and explain how receptive fields are involved in representing the physical world.

6.1.5 Describe and explain the theories and processes involved in color vision.

6.1.6 Describe and explain the processes involved in vision in the brain.

6.1.1 THE BEGINNINGS OF AN IMAGE

>> LO 6.1.1 Describe the beginnings of how information from the physical environment is transformed into a visual image.

Key Terms

- **Photons:** Particles that create light and travel in waves.
- **Electromagnetic energy:** Light energy.
- **Electromagnetic spectrum**: The range of all wavelengths of light.
- **Visible spectrum:** The narrow band of the electromagnetic spectrum, ranging from 400 nm to 700 nm, that can be perceived as colors.
- **Photoreceptors:** Sensory receptors that convert energy from the electromagnetic spectrum into electrical impulses.
- **Transducers:** Devices that convert one form of energy into another.
- **Retina:** The cell layer at the back of the eye that contains photoreceptors.
- **Pigment epithelium:** The layer of cells that nourishes the photoreceptors.
- **Refraction:** The change in direction of light rays as they travel from one medium to another.

- **Accommodation:** The eye's ability to keep objects in focus with changing distance.
- **Dark adaptation:** The eye's ability to adjust to low levels of light.
- **Photopigment:** A pigment that undergoes chemical changes when it absorbs light.

FIGURE 6.2

The electromagnetic spectrum. Out of this wide range, the only wavelengths that give rise to sensation and perception in humans are between 400 nm and 700 nm (visible light).

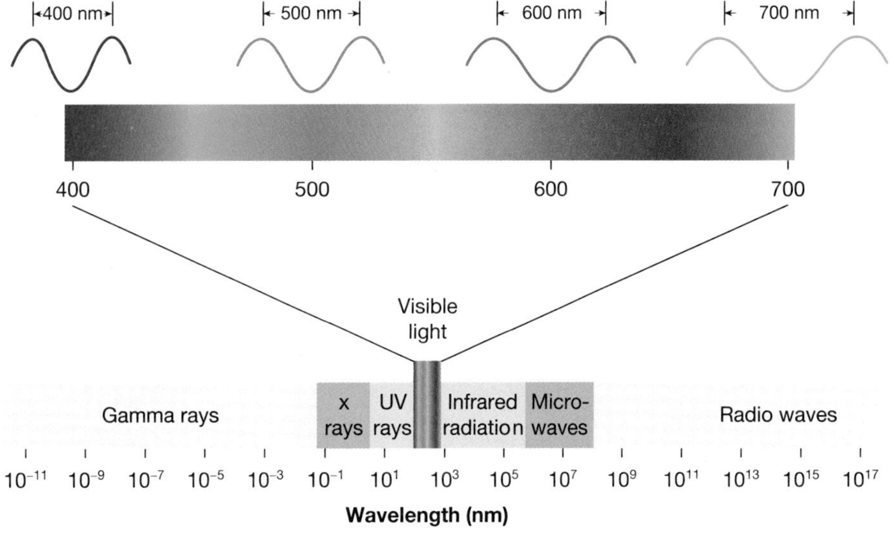

The Electromagnetic Spectrum

Many of my students are surprised to hear that colors do not exist in the physical world but, instead, are a creation of their brains. However, this fact becomes clearer to them once they understand the nature of light energy and how it interacts with the nervous system. When you turn on the lights in your room, the objects that are so familiar to you suddenly become visible. This is because flicking the light switch results in tiny particles called **photons**, which travel in waves, being emitted from the light bulb. Light energy, also known as **electromagnetic energy**, is measured in wavelengths. The range of possible wavelengths of light composes the **electromagnetic spectrum**, illustrated in Figure 6.2. Wavelengths can be measured in nanometers. One nanometer (nm) is one billionth of a meter, which is 10^{-9} meters.

As you can see from Figure 6.2, this range of frequencies along the electromagnetic spectrum is very large. It ranges from gamma rays (10^{-3} nanometers) to extremely low frequency (ELF) wavelengths, which are 10,000 kilometers wide (Barr, Jones, & Rodger, 2000) (not shown in the figure). Out of this large range of wavelengths, only a very narrow band can be perceived by humans. This band, known as the **visible spectrum**, is generally thought to consist of wavelengths ranging from approximately 400 nm to 700 nm. However, there are no agreed-upon exact limits to the visible spectrum. This is because whether light is visible depends not only on its wavelength but also on the light's intensity and on the sensitivity of the observer (Sliney, 2016).

The wavelengths that make up the visible spectrum correspond to the different colors we can perceive. However, the light waves themselves are not colored. Color perception results from the brain processing the inputs of specialized receptors, in the back of your eyes, known as **photoreceptors**. Photoreceptors, like other sensory receptors, are transducers. A **transducer** is a device that converts one form of energy into another. When activated by light, photoreceptors convert light energy from the visible spectrum into action potentials that make their way to the brain.

What about the other wavelengths? We cannot process wavelengths outside the visible spectrum because we do not have photoreceptors that can detect them. If we did, the world would probably look very different to us. However, other organisms are known to perceive wavelengths outside of the human visible spectrum. For example, certain bird species such as raptors and the common kestrel can perceive wavelengths in the ultraviolet range (Lind, Mitkus, Olsson, & Kelber, 2013, 2014), and snakes such as vipers, pythons, and boas can perceive infrared radiation (Gracheva et al., 2010). Heat is infrared radiation and, therefore, permits snakes to have a heat signature of their prey (Figure 6.3).

The Human Eye

Before learning about how photoreceptors transform light energy into trains of action potentials, ultimately resulting in the rich visual experiences that you know so well, you must first familiarize yourself with the sensory organ and network of neurons within it that begin making it possible.

Figure 6.4 depicts the main parts of the human eye. Light enters the eye through the pupil, an opening in the outer layer of the eye, surrounded by the iris, the colored area that gives eyes their characteristic color (e.g., brown, blue, green). Ciliary muscles control the zonule fibers that pull on the lens, allowing light to focus on the retina at the back of the eye. The fovea is a little pit at the center of the retina that picks up light from the point in space being looked at; it contains a high density of photoreceptors. Information leaves the eye via the optic nerve, the bundle of axons of ganglion cells that bring visual information to the brain, through a part of the eye called

FIGURE 6.3

(a) A common kestrel. (b) What we see as a yellow flower might look very different to a kestrel, which can perceive wavelengths in the ultraviolet range. (c) A viper. (d) Snakes such as the viper can perceive wavelengths in the infrared range, which permits them to have a heat signature of their prey.

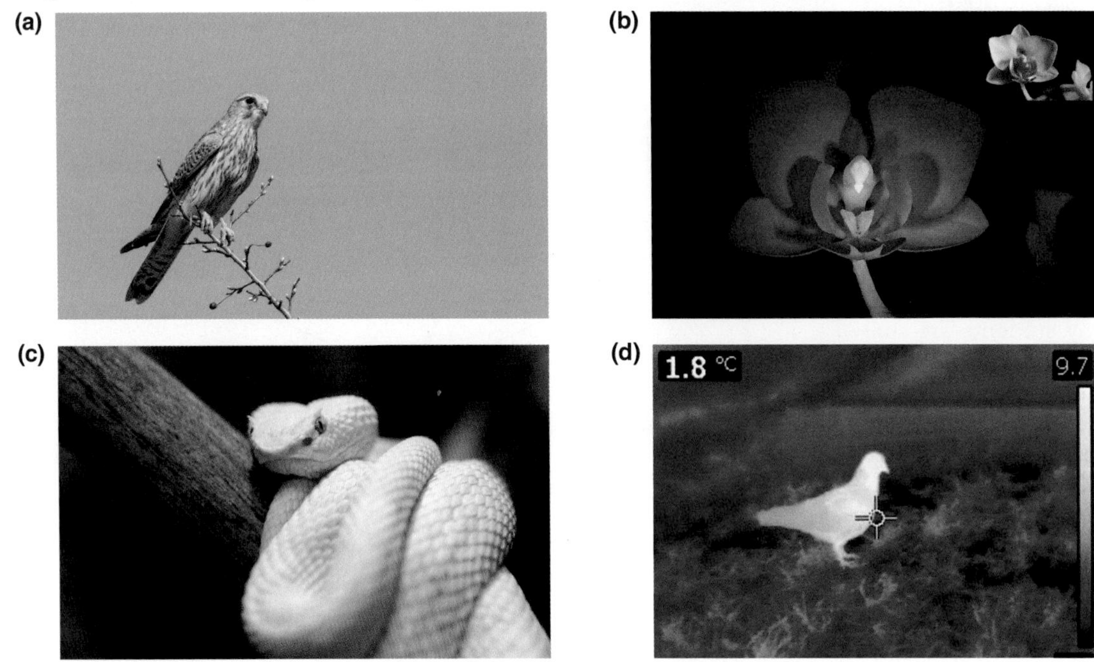

(a) iStock.com/Andyworks; (b) iStock.com/Sergey Skleznev; (c) iStock.com/hekakoskinen; (d) iStock.com/Marccophoto

FIGURE 6.4

The eye.

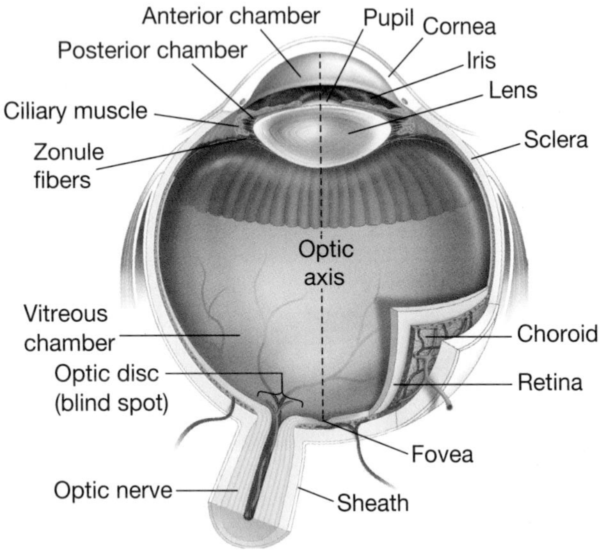

Anterior chamber
Pupil
Cornea
Posterior chamber
Iris
Lens
Ciliary muscle
Sclera
Zonule fibers
Optic axis
Vitreous chamber
Choroid
Optic disc (blind spot)
Retina
Fovea
Optic nerve
Sheath

the optic disc. Because no photoreceptors are present at the optic disc, light reflected in this area cannot be processed and therefore gives rise to a "blind spot" in the visual field. However, you do not perceive a blind spot because the visual system fills it in with information processed by receptors in the surrounding area. Other key parts of the eye are the cornea, the clear protective tissue that covers the eye; the aqueous humor, which is the watery fluid that nourishes the lens and cornea; the vitreous humor, which is the fluid that fills the space between the lens and the retina; and the sclera, the white protective layer of the eye.

For light to be focused, it must be refracted. **Refraction** refers to the change in direction of light rays as they travel from one medium to another. Light is first refracted by the cornea and then by the lens. This results in the convergence of light rays onto the middle of the retina, where it stimulates photoreceptors (Figure 6.5). Objects in our environment are visible because the light reflected from them falls onto the **retina**, which contains the photoreceptors. Part of the photoreceptors are embedded in a layer of cells called the **pigment epithelium**, from which they get their nourishment. There are different types of photoreceptors. A subset of each responds broadly to a range of wavelengths within the visible spectrum. The relative input of each type of receptor to the brain is what gives rise to color perception (discussed in Unit 6.1.5).

Accommodation

Accommodation is the ability of the eyes to keep objects in focus as they vary in distance. You may be familiar with the focusing mechanism of the lens on a camera. However, the lens of the eye does not focus light in the same way. The lens of a camera focuses

FIGURE 6.5

Refraction.

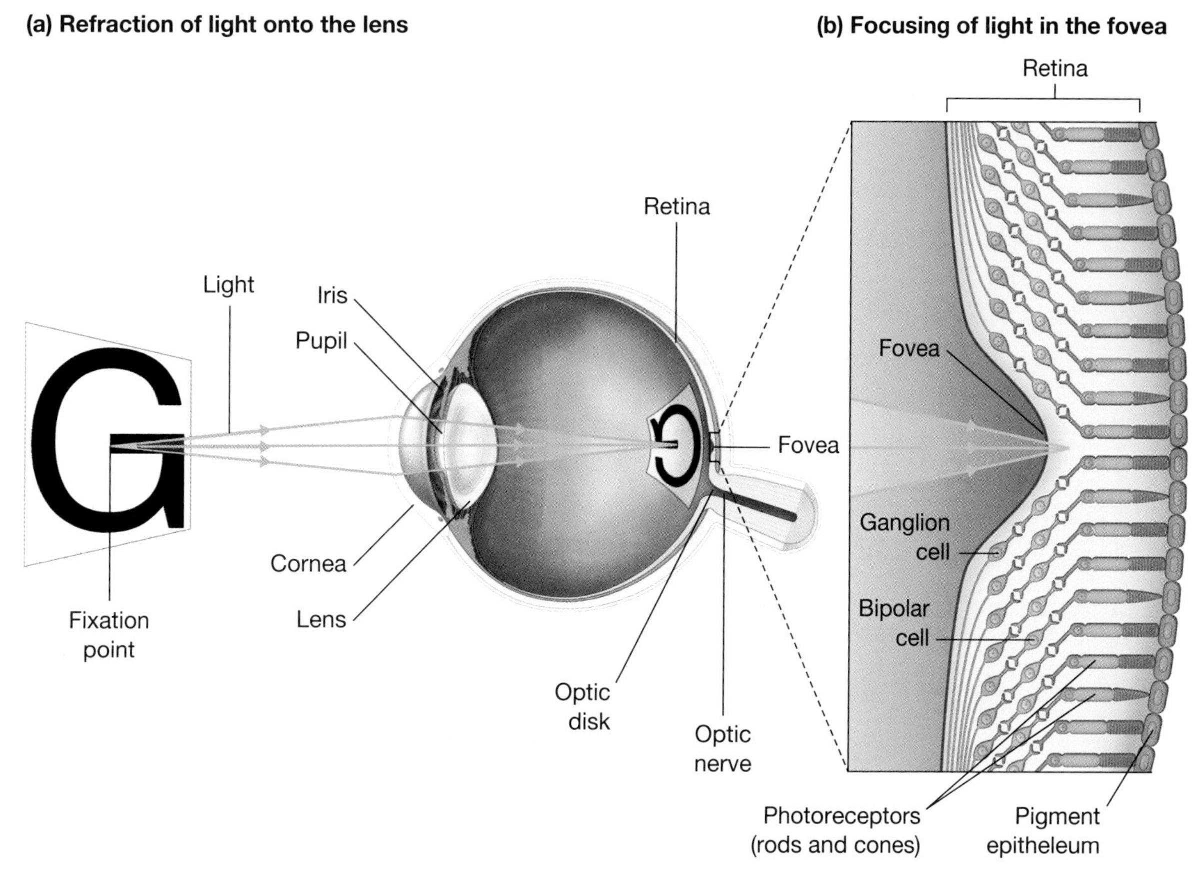

Modified from *Principles of Neural Science*, 5th Edition, Kandel, Schwartz, Jessell, Siegelbaum, Hudspeth, & Mack. The McGraw-Hill Companies, Inc. 2013.

light on film by moving in and out. The lens of the eye focuses light on the retina by changing its shape.

When tiny muscles attached to the lens, called ciliary muscles (see Figure 6.4), contract, the lens becomes more convex, increasing its focusing power. This happens as an object moves toward the eyes. When the ciliary muscles relax, the lens flattens, decreasing its focusing power. This happens as an object moves away from the eyes. When looking at an object located at least 20 feet away, the lens focuses the image of that object on the retina by remaining flat. In this case, the object is said to be at optical infinity.

Cellular Organization of the Early Visual System

As shown in Figure 6.6, the processing of visual information requires the activity of neurons within different cell layers. The flow of information in the retina begins with the activation of photoreceptors, known as rods and cones, by light. Activation of the photoreceptors activates bipolar cells, which in turn activate retinal ganglion cells. The axons of retinal ganglion cells form the optic nerve, which sends visual information to the brain. Horizontal cells, also activated by photoreceptors, are inhibitory neurons that release the neurotransmitter GABA. Their activity regulates and integrates the inputs of many photoreceptors. Another type of cell, amacrine cells, can play a similar role to that of horizontal cells except that their job is to spread activation from bipolar cells to ganglion cells. Retinal ganglion cells are of two types: midget cells and parasol cells (not shown in the figure but discussed later). Midget cells are associated with color vision. As their name suggests, they are of a relatively small size compared to parasol cells. Parasol cells do not process information about color but are sensitive to dark/light contrasts.

Rods and Cones

There are two types of photoreceptors in the retina, each having characteristic structure and function. These are the rods and cones. The structure of rods and cones as well their characteristics are illustrated in Figures 6.7a and 6.7b.

Rods. Perhaps the most obvious function of the rods that can be deduced from their position in the retina is that they are used for peripheral vision. There are no rods at the fovea (the center of the retina). Rods do

FIGURE 6.6

A close-up of the retina, showing the different types of cells it contains. The photoreceptors (the rods and cones) form the last layer of cells.

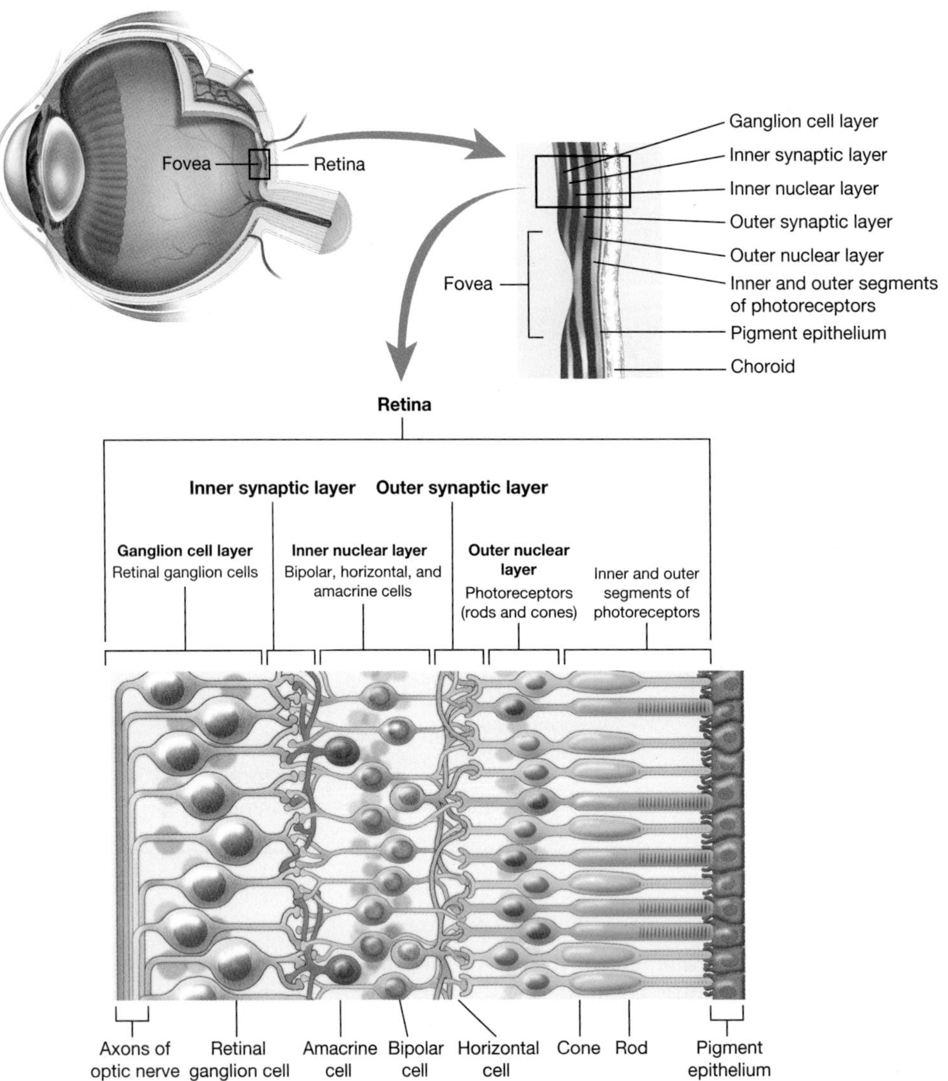

not mediate color perception but are sensitive to low levels of light. Rods are responsible for **dark adaptation**, which refers to the eye's ability to adjust to low levels of light. I am sure you experienced walking into a dark room and saw very little at first. However, after about 20 minutes you started to be able to make use of the little light available and began to distinguish features of the environment. At the same time, rods do not have much acuity. Acuity is the precision of vision, the ability to make out fine details. To see this for yourself, move your book from the center of your vision to the side, without moving your eyes, so that your text is in your peripheral vision. Can you read it? I bet that you cannot. This is because you cannot make out the fine details of individual letters using only your rods.

Cones. Cones are concentrated at the fovea. In contrast to rods, they are adapted for daytime vision and are not very effective in low-light conditions. However, they confer high acuity and are responsible for color vision. Figures 6.7a and 6.7b illustrate the differences between rods and cones. Figure 6.7c illustrates the spatial distribution of the rods and cones. Cones also show dark adaptation, but they do so at a significantly lesser degree than rods.

Photopigments. Photoreceptors contain light-absorbing molecules known as **photopigments**, which are made of the protein called opsin. Different types of photopigments are best at absorbing certain wavelengths along the visible spectrum. Humans have three types of cones: One type responds best to short wavelengths

FIGURE 6.7

Rods and cones. (a) Both rods and cones are composed of synaptic terminals, inner segments that contain the cell bodies, and outer segments that contain membranous disks that contain photopigment. (b) Characteristics of rods and cones. (c) Spatial distribution of rods and cones as a function of their numbers and distance from the fovea. Note the location of the optic disc where there are no photoreceptors due to the exit point of the optic nerve.

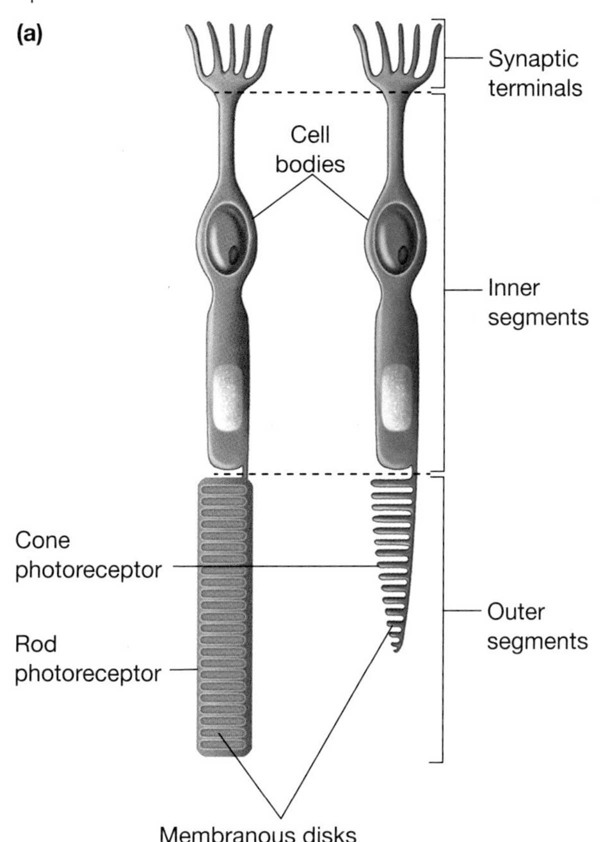

(b)

RODS	CONES
Peripheral vision	Contracted at fovea
No color vision	Color vision
Low light sensitivity (dark adaption)	Not effective in low-light conditions
Low acuity	High acuity

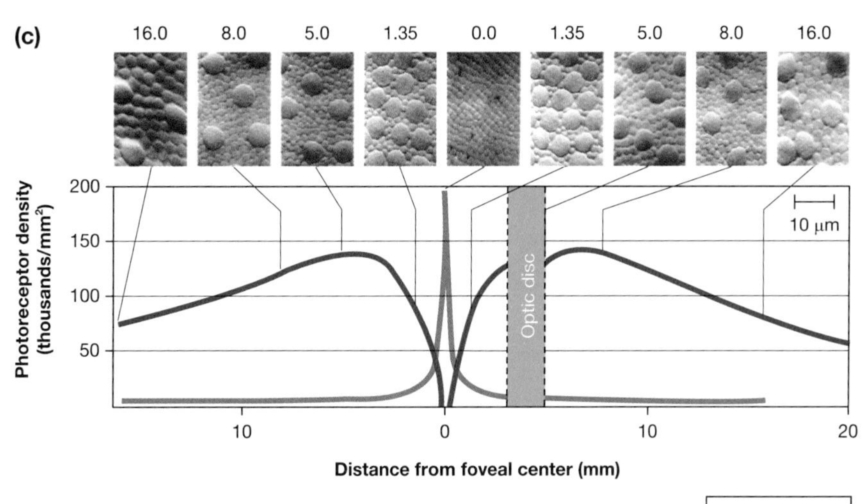

(S-cones), one to medium wavelengths (M-cones), and one to long wavelengths (L-cones). These are commonly known as blue, green, and red cones, based on the perceived colors associated with short, medium, and long wavelengths, respectively.

Although each type of cone is best at responding to a certain wavelength, it does not mean that they are not sensitive to other wavelengths. In fact, each type of cone is differentially sensitive to a range of wavelengths surrounding the one to which it best responds. This is known as spectral sensitivity.

There is only one type of rod. The photopigment contained in rods is known as rhodopsin. The spectral sensitivity of rods centers around medium wavelengths. When exposed to light, photopigments undergo a certain amount of degeneration, in a process known as bleaching. Bleaching reduces the photoreceptor's ability to transduce light to adjust to the level of illumination when moving from a brightly lighted area to a dimly lighted one. However, after some time spent in low-light conditions (about 20 minutes, as mentioned earlier), the photopigment in rods is largely regenerated compared to the photopigments in cones. This is what partly confers rods with greater ability than cones for dark adaptation. The spectral sensitivity of rods and cones is illustrated later, in Figure 6.16.

6.1.2 PHOTOTRANSDUCTION

>> LO 6.1.2 Explain how light energy is transformed into the electrical signals in receptors that transmit visual information to the brain.

Key Terms

- **Phototransduction:** The process by which light rays are converted into nerve impulses.
- **Dark current:** The process that results in rods being constantly depolarized in the dark.

For vision to occur, the energy from light rays absorbed by the photoreceptors in the retina must be transduced into nerve impulses. This process is known as **phototransduction**. This unit explains only how phototransduction occurs in rods. Phototransduction occurs in cones in a similar fashion but involves different photopigments.

The Dark Current. When rods are not stimulated by light, they are penetrated by a constant flow of Na^+ ions through cGMP-gated Na^+ channels (cGMP stands for cyclic guanosine monophosphate). This results in rods being constantly depolarized in the dark, hence, the term **dark current**. This depolarization of the photoreceptors results in the release of the neurotransmitter glutamate from their terminals. Glutamate is inhibitory for bipolar neurons. Therefore, it inhibits the firing of bipolar neurons to which rods connect.

FIGURE 6.8

Second messenger cascade induced by light absorption by the photopigment rhodopsin and the resulting closure of cGMP-dependent Na^+ channels.

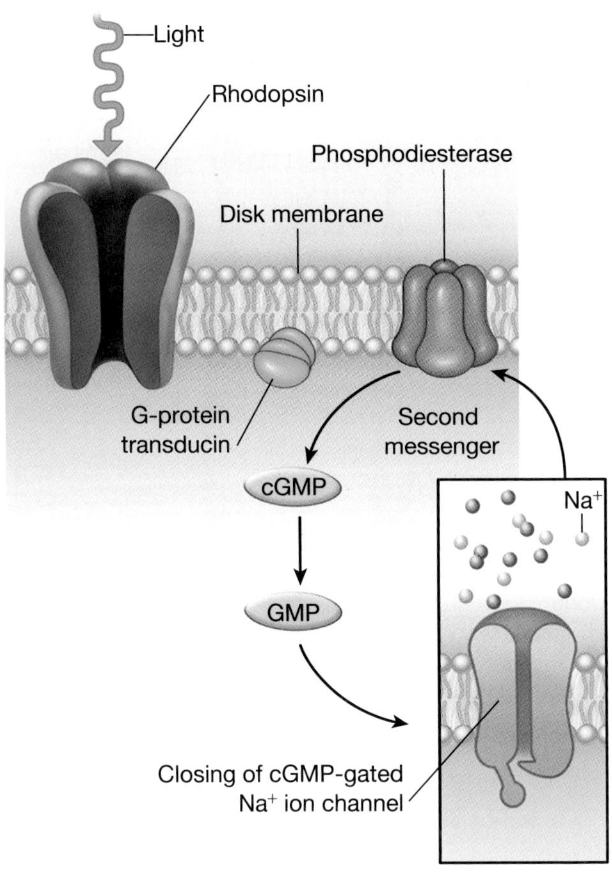

Amanda Tomasikiewicz/Body Scientific Intl.

Exposure to light reverses this situation by initiating a second messenger cascade of the type you learned about in Chapter 3. When the photopigment rhodopsin is activated by light, the G-protein transducin releases guanosine triphosphate (GTP). GTP activates the effector enzyme phosphodiesterase. Phosphodiesterase causes the second messenger cGMP to be converted to guanosine monophosphate (GMP). This results in the closing of cGMP-dependent Na^+ channels, which, in turn, results in the hyperpolarization of the photoreceptors. In response to this hyperpolarization, the photoreceptor stops releasing glutamate on bipolar neurons, thereby removing its inhibitory influence on them (Figure 6.8).

6.1.3 ACUITY AND SENSITIVITY

>> LO 6.1.3 Explain the mechanisms involved in the precision of vision and the visual receptor's sensitivity to light.

Key Term

- **Convergence:** The ratio of connectivity between photoreceptors and retinal ganglion cells.

You have just learned that rods and cones are found at different locations in the retina. Cones are found at the fovea (center) and rods on the periphery of the retina. You also learned that cones detect stimuli with more acuity than the rods and that cones are not very effective in low-light conditions, compared to the rods. But what confers on the rods and cones their different qualities, in both their levels of acuity and effectiveness under low-light conditions (other than dark adaptation)?

The answer lies in what is known as **convergence**. Convergence refers to the ratio of connectivity between photoreceptors and retinal ganglion cells. As illustrated in Figure 6.9, many more rods than cones converge onto a single retinal ganglion cell, through their connections with bipolar cells. Let's look at how these different levels of convergence can explain the differences in both acuity and sensitivity between rods and cones.

Convergence in Rods. Rods have highly convergent inputs to retinal ganglion cells. This means that a single ganglion receives the summated input of many rods, a case of spatial summation, as discussed in Chapter 3. Rods confer low acuity because the rods that converge to excite a single retinal ganglion cell come from slightly different places on the retina. Therefore, vision from the periphery of the retina lacks precision. However, rods are more sensitive to low-light conditions because the summated input from rods to retinal ganglion cells amplifies the light signal.

Convergence in Cones. Cones do not show the convergence displayed by rods onto retinal ganglion cells. This lack of convergence explains their higher levels of acuity relative to rods. Why? Because, contrary to rods, a single cone connects to a single retinal ganglion cell. This means that a retinal ganglion connected to a cone receives information from a precise location in the retina. However, the signal they receive is not amplified through spatial summation as with retinal ganglion cells connected to rods. This means that they are less sensitive to light and, therefore, less effective in low-light conditions.

FIGURE 6.9

Patterns of convergence in the periphery of the retina (left and right), which contains mostly rods, and at the fovea, which contains exclusively cones (middle). (Ganglion cells: green; bipolar cells: orange; rods: purple; cones: red, green, and blue.)

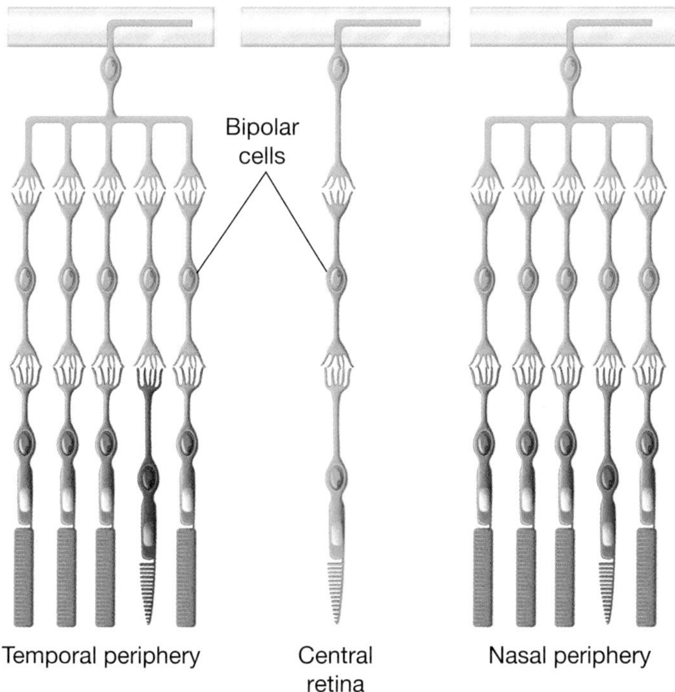

Dawn Scheuerman/Body Scientific Intl.

6.1.4 RECEPTIVE FIELDS

>> LO 6.1.4 **Describe and explain how receptive fields are involved in representing the physical world.**

Key Terms

- **Receptive field:** An area of the body where a stimulus can elicit a reflex. In vision, it is a spot on the retina, which, when illuminated, activates a single retinal ganglion cell and other cells in the visual system.
- **On-center receptive field:** A receptive field in which illumination of its center activates its associated retinal ganglion cell.
- **Off-center receptive field:** A receptive field in which illumination of its center inhibits activity in its associated retinal ganglion cell.
- **Mach bands:** An illusion that makes it easier to determine where surfaces of different brightness meet.
- **Lateral inhibition:** How receptors in the surround of on-center receptive fields have inhibitory connections with receptors located in the center of the same receptive fields.
- **Hermann grid:** An optical illusion often used to demonstrate lateral inhibition.

The term **receptive field** was coined by Charles Scott Sherrington in 1906 (Sherrington, 1906a). He used the term to refer to an area of the body where a stimulus can elicit a reflex. In the 1930s, American physiologist Haldan Keffer Hartline recorded the activity of single retinal ganglion cell axons from the optic nerves of frogs (Hartline, Wagner, & Ratliff, 1956; Ratliff, Knight, Dodge, & Hartline, 1974). He found that electrical activity in a single axon was induced when a specific spot on the retina was illuminated. He called that spot the receptive field of the retinal ganglion cell that was activated by illumination.

In this unit, you will learn about receptive fields that are activated by achromatic (noncolored) illumination, that is, by only dark and light contrasts. These receptive fields are those of parasol retinal ganglion cells. Midget cells, the other type of retinal ganglion cells, are associated with color vision and are discussed later. As illustrated in Figure 6.10, the receptive fields of retinal ganglion cells are tightly packed, resulting in their overlap.

Receptive Field Size. The receptive fields of retinal ganglion cells are not all of the same size. Two main factors are associated with the size of a receptive field: the receptive field's distance from the fovea and the type of retinal ganglion it is associated with. That is, receptive fields become progressively larger with increasing distance from the fovea, and those associated with parasol retinal ganglion cells are larger than the ones associated with midget retinal ganglion cells.

While studying how electrical signals make it from the retina to the brain, Stephen W. Kuffler (1953) discovered that not all parts of a receptive field caused the same response in its associated retinal ganglion cell when illuminated. Illuminating the center of some receptive fields increased the firing of their associated retinal ganglion cells above their spontaneous rate of firing, that is, above the firing rate observed when they are not being stimulated (remember that neurons are never completely silent). In contrast, illumination of the same receptive fields' surrounds reduced the firing of their associated retinal ganglion cells below their spontaneous firing rate. These became known as excitatory-center/inhibitory-surround receptive fields, or simply **on-center receptive fields**.

Other receptive fields induced the opposite pattern of excitation/inhibition of their associated retinal ganglion cells. Illumination of the center of those receptive fields inhibited the firing of their respective retinal ganglion cells, whereas illumination of those receptive fields' surrounds increased their firing rate. These became known as inhibitory-center/excitatory-surround receptive fields, or simply **off-center receptive fields**. Illumination of the entire receptive field resulted in the inhibition and excitation of the retinal ganglion cell canceling each other out, in which case the cell maintained its spontaneous rate of firing. The effects of different patterns of illumination of both on-center and off-center receptive fields on the firing patterns of retinal ganglion cells are illustrated in Figure 6.11.

The Functions of Receptive Fields. Receptive fields have an important role to play in perceiving contrasts. For example, can you think about which type of receptive field, on-center or off-center, is important for perceiving a dark object on a bright background or a bright object on a dark background? The answer is that the preferred stimuli for off-center receptive fields are dark objects surrounded by a light background. In contrast, the preferred stimuli for on-center receptive fields are bright objects surrounded by dark backgrounds (Figure 6.12).

FIGURE 6.10

Retinal ganglion cells are tightly packed. This results in their receptive fields overlapping onto one another.

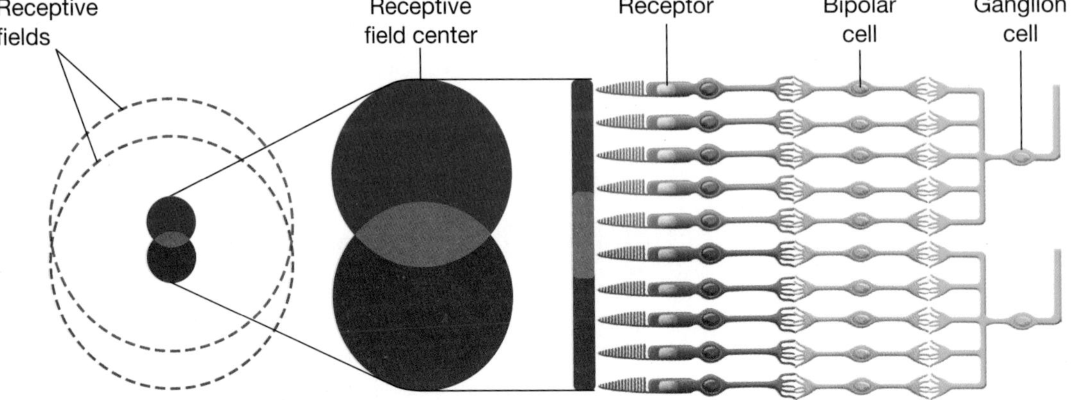

Dawn Scheuerman/Body Scientific Intl.

FIGURE 6.11

(a) Representations of on-center and off-center receptive fields, each with its associated retinal ganglion cells. (b) The amount of activity of retinal ganglion cells depends on the pattern of illumination of the center and surround of their receptive fields. For a retinal ganglion cell with an on-center receptive field to be maximally activated, its receptive field's center must be fully illuminated with no light illuminating its surround (top). Illuminating different amounts of the surround will correspondingly inhibit the retinal ganglion cell's ability to be activated (bottom). (c) For a retinal ganglion cell with an off-center receptive field, illuminating different amounts of the center will correspondingly inhibit the retinal ganglion cell's ability to be activated with no light falling on its center (top). Maximal activation occurs when its receptive field's surround is illuminated (bottom).

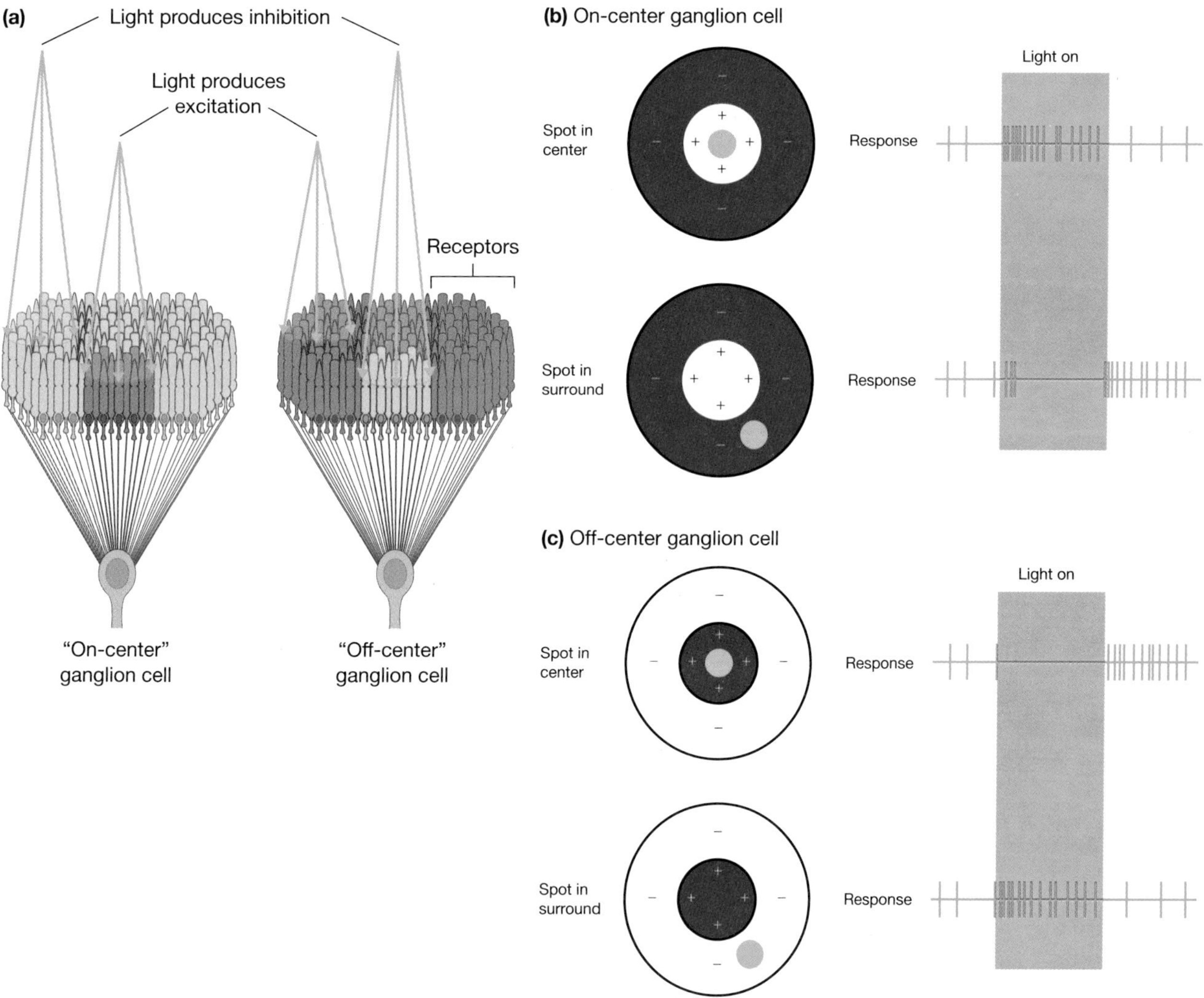

Another proposed role for receptive fields is the enhancement of edges. This role can be demonstrated in a perceptual illusion known as the **Mach bands**, named after physicist Ernst Mach (1838–1916), who described the phenomenon. Mach bands are shown in Figure 6.13a. If you look carefully at the illustration, you will notice that the leftmost edge of each band appears brighter than the rest of the band and that the rightmost edge appears darker. However, each band is a uniform shade of gray. Why such an illusion? This illusion illustrates edge enhancement. By perceiving the edges as being brighter (leftmost edge) or darker (rightmost edge), it is easier to tell where one band ends and where the other one begins. In this way, Mach bands serve an important function in determining where surfaces of different brightness meet when it may not be so obvious.

How can this illusion be explained by the function of receptive fields? One explanation is illustrated in

FIGURE 6.12

(a) The preferred stimuli for off-center receptive fields are dark objects on a bright background. (b) The preferred stimuli for on-center receptive fields are bright objects on dark backgrounds.

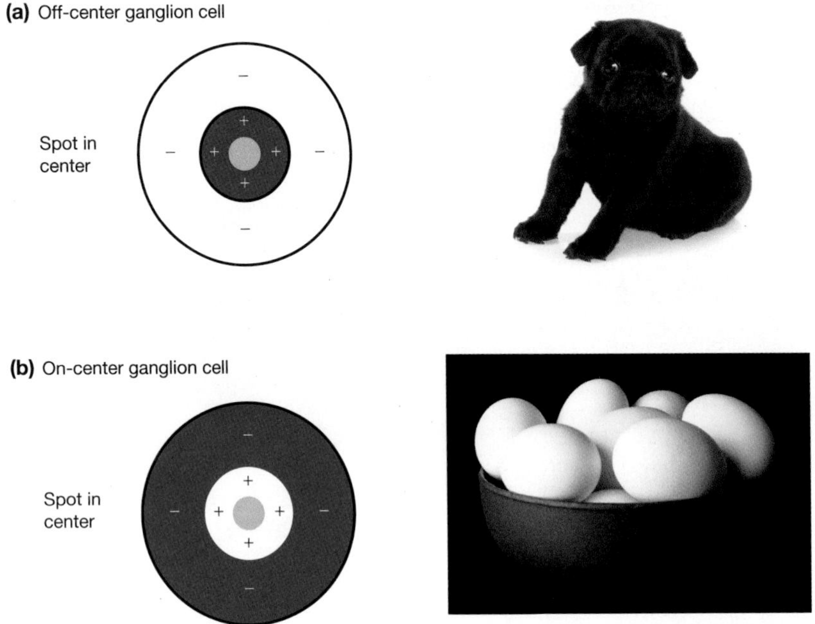

(a) iStock.com/Dixi_; (b) iStock.com/ksushachmeister

Figure 6.13b. Look at the receptive fields labeled RF4 and RF2. Both are on-center receptive fields. RF4 lies completely in the least illuminated of the two bands. In contrast, RF2 lies completely in the most brightly illuminated band. This means that the center and surround of RF4 as well as the center and surround of RF2 are equally illuminated. This causes their associated retinal ganglion cells to respond at their spontaneous firing rate.

Now look at the receptive field labeled RF1. Its center lies completely in the brightest of the two bands. However, part of its off-surround region lies in the least illuminated band. This causes its associated retinal ganglion cell to fire above its spontaneous firing rate. Because of this, the left edge of the brightest band is perceived to be brighter than the rest of it, where the retinal ganglion cells associated with the receptive fields present there (e.g., RF2) are firing at a comparatively lower rate (i.e., their spontaneous firing rate).

In contrast, RF3's off region lies partly in the most brightly illuminated band. This causes its associated retinal ganglion to fire below its spontaneous firing rate. Because of this, the right edge of the band is perceived to be darker than the rest of it, where the ganglion cells associated with the receptive fields present there (e.g., RF4) are firing at a comparatively higher rate (i.e., their spontaneous firing rate).

Lateral Inhibition

The Mach band illusion described in the preceding section can be explained by a phenomenon known as **lateral inhibition**. Lateral inhibition refers to how photoreceptors associated with the surround of on-center receptive fields form inhibitory connections with photoreceptors associated with the center of the same receptive fields. Figure 6.14 shows the organization of an on-center receptive field. This model of an on-center receptive field includes a cone photoreceptor associated with the center and two cones associated with the surround.

Each of the cones associated with the surround makes contact with a horizontal cell. However, the center cone is connected directly to a bipolar cell, which in turn connects to a retinal ganglion cell. Therefore, illumination of the receptive field's center results in hyperpolarization of its associated cone, which leads directly to the depolarization of a bipolar cell. When depolarized, the bipolar cell activates a retinal ganglion cell, which sends information to the brain via the optic nerve.

Figure 6.14 also shows what happens when an on-center receptive field's inhibitory surround is illuminated. When illuminated, horizontal cells connected to the cones in the surround send inhibitory signals to the cones associated with the center, which prevents them from exciting the bipolar cells to which they are

FIGURE 6.13

(a) Looking at the bars you should perceive the rightmost edge of each bar as being darker than the leftmost edge of the next bar, which is perceived as being brighter. (b) Mach bands can be explained by the differential activity of retinal ganglion cells, which depends on the proportion of illumination falling on the center and surround of their on-center receptive fields (RFs).

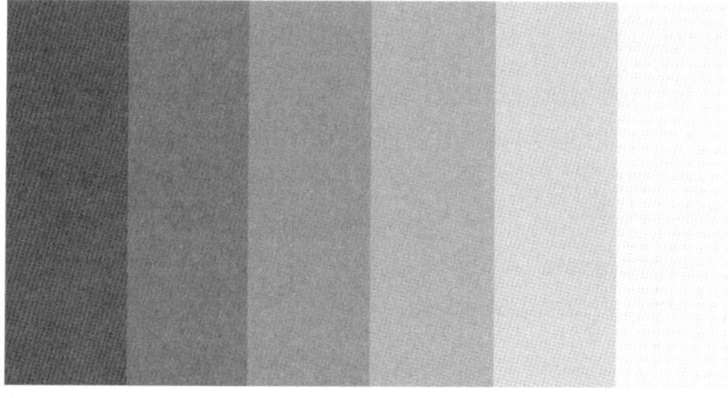

(a)

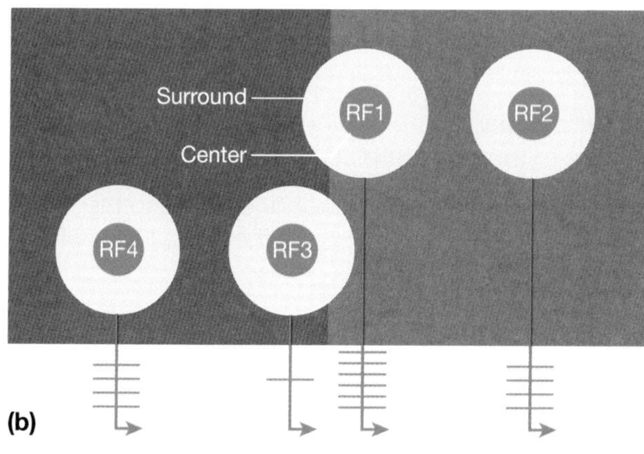

(b)

Carolina Hrejsa/Body Scientific Intl.

FIGURE 6.14

Organization of an on-center receptive field. Activity of the cones located in the surround has an inhibitory influence on the center cones' ability to activate bipolar cells, which normally cause retinal ganglion cells to fire.

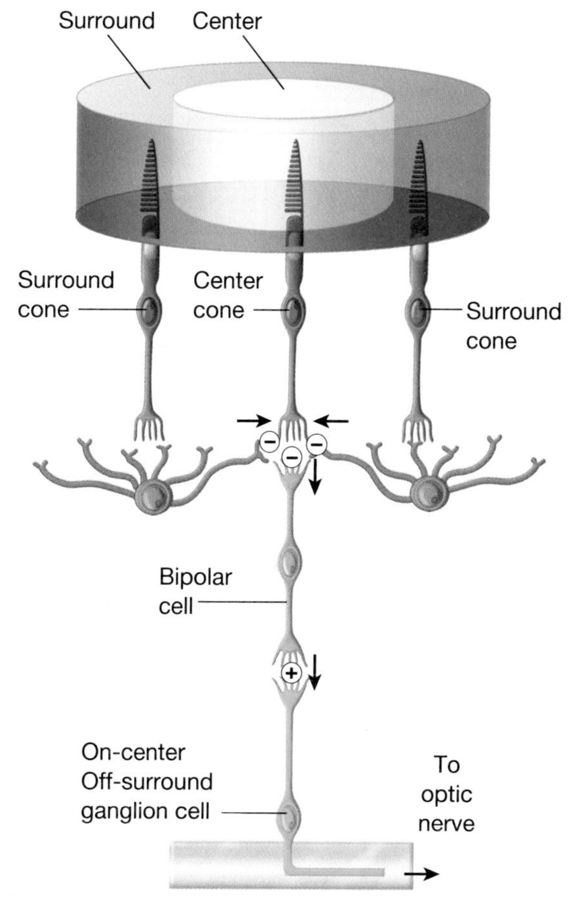

Dawn Scheuerman/Body Scientific Intl.

connected. The amount of inhibition exerted by horizontal cells is proportional to the area of the surround that is illuminated.

In addition to providing an explanation for the Mach band illusion, lateral inhibition can also explain the illusory appearance of phantom gray spots in what is known as the **Hermann grid**. Look at Figure 6.15a. Do you see anything wrong with the picture? You surely noticed the apparent existence of gray spots in the area at which two of the lines composing the corridors of the grid intersect. You will also notice that you cannot perceive a spot at an intersection that you stare at directly.

A possible explanation for this effect is illustrated in Figure 6.15b. As you can see, the large on-center receptive field on the left of the figure does not completely fit within an intersection. Its center (on-region), which lies in a bright area, is completely illuminated. However, its surround (off-region) is illuminated on four sides. This means that the retinal ganglion cells associated with this receptive field are somewhat inhibited, causing them to fire below their spontaneous rate. In contrast, the on-center receptive field on the right side of the figure is small enough to completely fit within the intersection. This means that the retinal ganglion cells associated with this receptive field are firing at their spontaneous rate.

Remember that the receptive fields on the retina increase in size with increasing distance from the fovea. When staring directly at an intersection, you are using photoreceptors located at the fovea, for which the associated retinal ganglion cells have small receptive fields. When looking away from an intersection, you are using

FIGURE 6.15

The Hermann grid. (a) While you look at the Hermann grid, gray spots appear to exist at the intersections of the alleys but disappear when you look directly at an intersection. (b) A possible explanation for the illusory gray spots is based on the concept of lateral inhibition and the fact that receptive fields in the periphery of the retina are large compared to those found at the fovea.

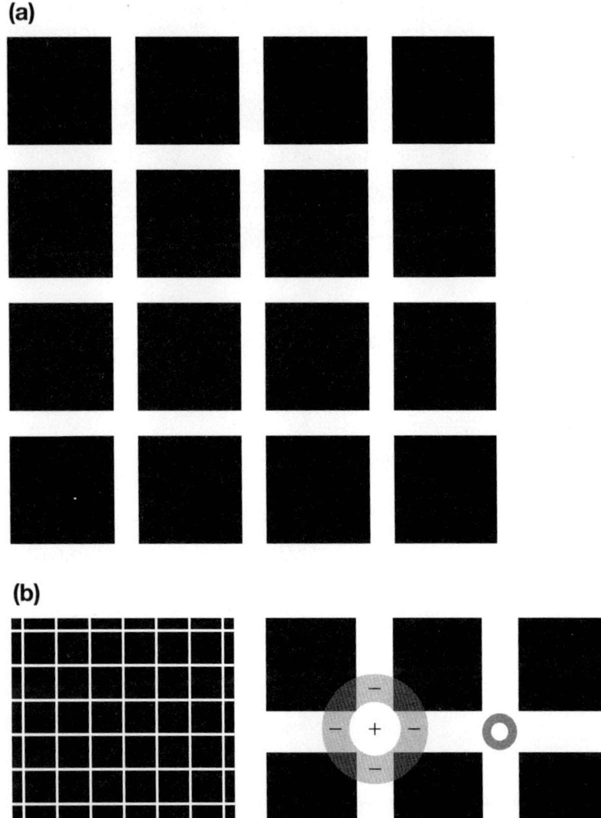

Hermann, L. (1870). Eine Erscheinung simultanen Contrastes. *Pflügers Archiv für die gesamte Physiologie, 3*, 13–15. Springer-Verlag.

photoreceptors at the periphery, which are associated with retinal ganglion cells that have comparatively large receptive fields.

Therefore, the spots appear within the intersection only when you are looking at them with your peripheral vision. This is because the off-regions of the large receptive fields located at the periphery are illuminated on four sides, causing their associated retinal ganglion cells to fire below their spontaneous firing rate. When you are looking directly at an intersection, the small receptive fields at the fovea are fully illuminated, causing their associated retinal ganglion cells to fire at their spontaneous rate.

6.1.5 COLOR VISION

>> LO 6.1.5 **Describe and explain the theories and processes involved in color vision.**

Key Terms

- **White light:** What is perceived when all the wavelengths of the visual spectrum are mixed.
- **Trichromatic theory:** The theory that the brain produces our perception of colors by reading out the combined input of three types of cones, each responding best to a specific wavelength.
- **Across-neuron response pattern theory:** The idea that precise information about stimuli is encoded not by single neurons but by the response patterns of populations of neurons.
- **Protanopia:** A type of red-green color deficiency due to the absence of L-cones.
- **Deuteranopia:** A type of red-green color deficiency due to the absence of M-cones.
- **Tritanomaly:** A type of blue-yellow color deficiency due to a limited number of functioning S-cones.
- **Tritanopia:** A type of blue-yellow color deficiency due to the complete absence of S-cones.
- **Monochromacy:** Color blindness due to the absence or failure of two of the three types of cones.
- **Rod monochromacy:** Color blindness due to the absence of cones.
- **Color afterimage:** An image of an object that persists after having stared at it for several seconds.

As mentioned earlier, colors do not exist outside your mind. As far as light is concerned, all there is out there are waves of different length, some of which we interpret as colors known as the visible spectrum. When all of the wavelengths of the visible spectrum are mixed, we perceive what is called **white light**. To demonstrate this, white light can be passed through a prism, splitting it into its constituent wavelengths. Mathematician and physicist Isaac Newton (1643–1727) described this phenomenon in 1671:

> I procured a triangular glass prism, to try therewith the celebrated phaenomena of colours. And for that purpose having darkened my chamber, and made a small hole in the window shuts, to let in a convenient quantity of the sun's light, I place my prism at his entrance, that it might be thereby refracted to the opposite wall. It was at first a very pleasing

diversion to view the vivid and intense colours produced thereby; but after a while applying myself to consider them more circumspectly, I was surprised to see them in an oblong form; which, according to the received laws of refraction, I expected would have been circular. They were terminated at the sides with strait lines, but at the ends, the decay of light was so gradual, that it was difficult to determine justly what was the figure; yet they seemed semicircular. Comparing the length of this coloured spectrum with its breadth, I found it about five times greater; a disproportion so extravagant, that it excited me to a more than ordinary curiosity of examining from whence it might proceed. (Newton, 1671, p. 682)

The Trichromatic Theory

The **trichromatic theory** of color vision, proposed by Thomas Young and Hermann Von Helmholtz in 1802, aimed to answer the question of how colors are perceived if they do not exist out in the physical world (Young, 1802). Why do you perceive the objects around you as being certain colors? For example, why should you perceive someone's T-shirt as being red and not blue or green? Part of the answer is that the materials of which objects are made reflect and absorb certain wavelengths of light along the visible spectrum. Materials that reflect short wavelengths and absorb all others are perceived as blue. Materials that reflect long wavelengths and absorb all others are perceived as red. Materials that reflect all of the wavelengths are perceived as white, and those that absorb all wavelengths along the visible spectrum are perceived as black.

Therefore, the T-shirt is perceived as being red because the dyes used to "color" it mostly reflect long wavelengths, corresponding to approximately 600 nm, and absorb the other wavelengths. However, the way in which colors are perceived is more complex. Remember that the labels of short, medium, and long wavelengths attributed to cones (blue, green, and red cones) refer to the wavelengths that each type of cone is most responsive to, not the only wavelengths each is responsive to. In other words, photoreceptors are broadly tuned, in that each type is differentially sensitive to all of the wavelengths along the visible spectrum.

As you can see in Figure 6.16, each type of cone (S-cones, M-cones, and L-cones) responds maximally to a wavelength of a particular frequency. However, each type of cone also responds to a range of other wavelengths but it does so with progressively less intensity, as the wavelengths deviate from the ones to which it is maximally sensitive. The same holds true for the short- and medium-wavelength cones (S- and M-cones, respectively). Color perception depends on the relative activity of each type of cone. This is consistent with what is known as the **across-neuron response pattern theory**, which is the idea that precise information about stimuli is encoded not by single neurons (in this case, a single type of cone) but by the response patterns of populations of neurons (G. Doetsch, 2000).

Color Deficiencies

Color deficiencies occur when an individual is lacking one or more cone photoreceptor. Color deficiencies are subdivided into three broad types: red-green, blue-yellow, and complete color blindness.

Red-green color deficiency, in which people cannot distinguish red and green, occurs due to the absence of L-cones (red), a condition known as **protanopia**, or due to the absence of M-cones (green), a condition known as **deuteranopia**, which as you may recall is the condition that Geoffrey Hope-Terry suffered (see the chapter's opening vignette).

Blue-yellow color deficiency, in which people cannot distinguish blue and yellow, occurs due to a limited number of functioning S-cones (blue) in a condition known as **tritanomaly**, or to the complete absence of S-cones, a condition known as **tritanopia**.

Complete color blindness is extremely rare. It can occur for two reasons. It may result from the failure or absence of two of the three types of cones, a condition known as **monochromacy**, or from the failure or absence of all three types of cones, a condition known as **rod monochromacy**. In this case, a person relies on only rods for vision.

FIGURE 6.16

The relative sensitivity of short (S), medium (M), and long (L) wavelength cones, corresponding to the perceptions of blue, green, and red, respectively.

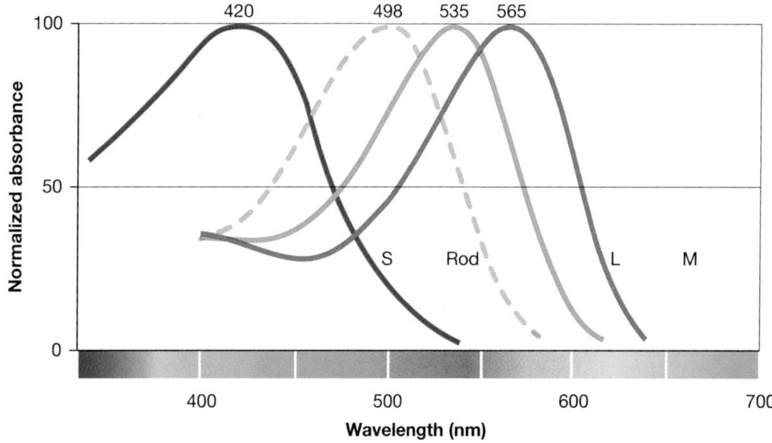

IT'S A MYTH!

Dogs See the World in Black and White

The Myth

You may have heard that dogs see the world in only black and white. This is untrue. Dogs do perceive a spectrum of colors. But they do not perceive the world as we do.

Where Does the Myth Come From?

The myth comes from the findings of early studies investigating whether dogs had color vision. Some of them concluded that dogs had limited color vision, whereas others concluded that they did not. Other researchers minimized the importance of finding out whether dogs had color vision because they believed that the detection of form and brightness was more important to dogs (P. Miller & Murphy, 1995).

The visible spectrum consists of a narrow band of wavelengths along the electromagnetic spectrum. For humans, this narrow band consists of wavelengths between 400 nm and 700 nm. It is called the visible spectrum because it comprises wavelengths for which we possess photoreceptors. The photoreceptors we use to perceive colors are known as cones and are located at the center of the retina.

Humans have three types of cones. Each of these types of cones responds optimally to different parts of the spectrum. These are known as short-, medium-, and long-wavelength cones, corresponding to the colors we perceive as blue, green, and red, respectively. The relative contribution of each type of cone, in response to the mixture of wavelengths reflected to them, determines the perceived color. The colors in which an organism perceives the world depend largely on the number of cones it has.

Why Is the Myth Wrong?

Dogs do not see the world in only black and white. It has been known since the late 1980s that dogs possess two types of cones: short- and long-wavelength cones. This permits them to sense wavelengths ranging from 429 nm to 555 nm at the peak of each cone's sensitivity (Figure 1). However, unlike humans, they lack a cone for which the response peaks at approximately 530 nm, a medium-wavelength cone (Kasparson, Badridze, & Maximov, 2013; Neitz, Geist, & Jacobs, 1989). Because dogs perceive colors based on the input of only two cones, they are referred to as dichromats. Humans, who make use of three cones, are referred to as trichromats. Figure 2 shows the spectrum of colors perceived by dichromats (like dogs) compared to trichromats (like humans). ●

FIGURE 1

Normalized spectral sensitivity functions of the dog's short-wavelength (S) and long-wavelength (L) cones and rods.

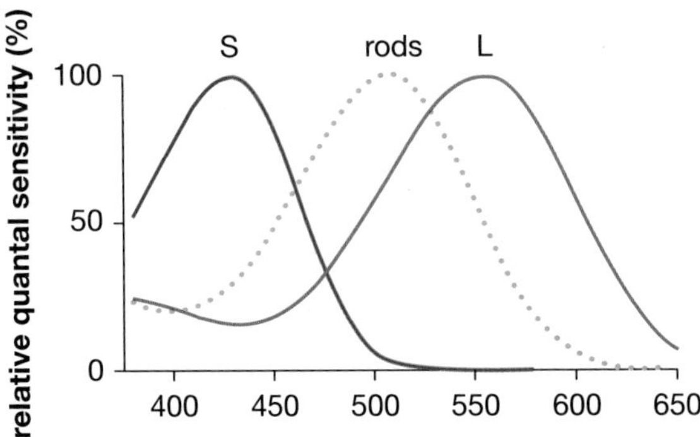

Kasparson, A. A., J. Badridze, & V.V. Maximov. (2013). Colour cues proved to be more informative for dogs than brightness. *Proceedings. Biological sciences. Proceedings of the Royal Society B. Biological Sciences, 280*(1766): 1356. With permission from The Royal Society.

FIGURE 2

Colors perceived by dichromats versus trichromats.

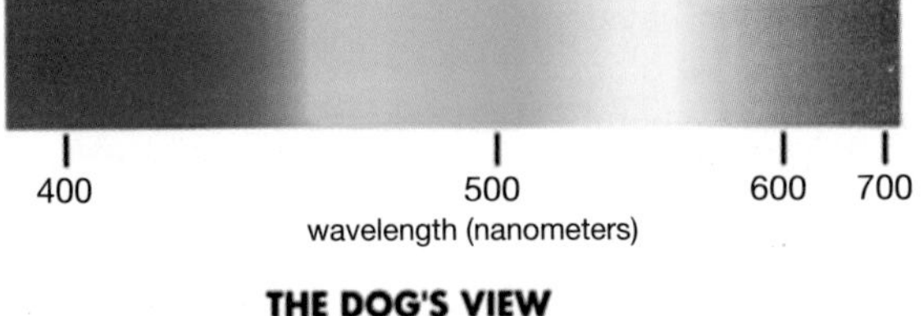

Used with permission from Mark Plonsky, Ph.D., Emeritus Professor of Psychology, University of Wisconsin.

Opponent Process Theory

Following Young and Helmholtz's proposal of the trichromatic theory, it became apparent that their theory could not explain all of the phenomena relating to color perception. In 1868, German physiologist Ewald Hering proposed the opponent-process theory of color vision to explain these other phenomena (Hering, 1964), one of which is known as **color afterimage**.

FIGURE 6.17

Color afterimage. Stare at the dot in the middle of the American flag (which is obviously in the wrong colors) for about 30 seconds, then switch your gaze to the white space to the right. What do you see?

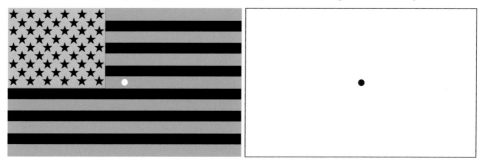

A color afterimage is an image of an object that persists after having stared at it for several seconds. The peculiarity of this afterimage is that it appears in colors that are different from the perceived color of the object itself. If you have never experienced this, try it for yourself. Before reading on, stare for at least 30 seconds at the black dot in the center of the oddly colored American flag on the left side of Figure 6.17. Then stare at the white surface to the right of the figure (or any other white surface). What do you see? How can this be?

What you should see in the white space is the American flag in its familiar red, white, and blue colors. It is this type of observation that led Hering to propose that the range of hues we perceive is not due to the relative activity of cones as suggested in the trichromatic theory. Rather, he thought that the range of hues we experience, composed of blue, yellow, red, and green, came in pairs and that the members within each pair were in opposition to each other: blue opposed to yellow (blue/yellow), red opposed to green (red/green), and a nonchromatic pair composed of black opposed to white (black/white). The mechanisms by which this is thought to operate are explained in the next unit.

6.1.6 VISUAL PROCESSING BEYOND THE RETINA

>> LO 6.1.6 **Describe and explain the processes involved in vision in the brain.**

Key Terms

- **Parvocellular (P-cells):** Cells of the LGN that receive color information from the axons of midget ganglion cells of the retina
- **Magnocellular (M-cells):** Cells of the LGN that receive contrast information from the parasol ganglion cells.
- **Koniocellular (K-cells):** Cells of the LGN that receive information from short-wavelength cones in the retina as well as from bistratified retinal ganglion cells, which convey information about spatial resolution.
- **Retinotopic mapping:** The preservation of the relative location of neurons from the retina to the cortex.
- **Orientation selectivity:** A property associated with simple cells in the primary visual cortex, which best respond when bars of a particular orientation are projected onto the retina.
- **Directional selectivity:** A property associated with complex cells in the primary visual cortex, which best respond when bars of light moving in a particular direction are projected onto the retina.
- **P-pathway:** The visual information pathway from the retina to the visual cortex that connects midget retinal ganglion cells to P-cells of the LGN.
- **M-pathway:** The visual information pathway from the retina to the visual cortex that connects parasol retinal ganglion cells to P-cells of the LGN.

As mentioned earlier, axons of the retinal ganglion cells form the optic nerve, which exits the retina through the optic disk. The primary target of visual information from the retina is a region of the thalamus known as the lateral geniculate nucleus (LGN). Although the LGN will be our primary focus of discussion, other areas that also receive information from the retina include the hypothalamus, for the regulation of circadian rhythms; the pretectum, responsible for the pupillary reflex, which controls how much light reaches the retina by constricting or dilating the pupils; and the superior colliculus, which coordinates head and eye movements.

As illustrated in Figure 6.18, the retina of each eye is divided into the nasal and temporal retina. The nasal retina refers to the portion of the retina that is nearest to the nose. The temporal retina refers to the portion of the retina that is nearest to each of the temples. The axons from the nasal retina of each eye cross over to the other side of the brain (contralateral) at the optic chiasm to form connections with the LGN. The axons from the temporal retinas remain on the same side (ipsilateral). Beyond the optic chiasm, the optic nerves are renamed *optic tract*, because, as you learned in Chapter 4, the optic nerve is one of the twelve cranial nerves (cranial nerve II) that are part of the peripheral nervous system. In the peripheral nervous system, a bundle of nerve fibers is referred to as a nerve. In the central nervous system, a bundle of nerve fibers is referred to as a tract. Once past the optic chiasm, the nerve fibers from the retinas are considered to be in the central nervous system. However, the retina and the optic nerve are technically part of the brain because they are developmentally derived from it.

The optic nerve from the nasal retina in the left eye and the temporal retina of the right eye convey information from the left visual field. Conversely, the optic nerve from the nasal retina in the right eye and the temporal retina of the left eye convey information from the right visual field. Information from the center of the visual field is conveyed by projections from the fovea of both eyes to form the foveal image. This is illustrated in Figure 6.18.

The Lateral Geniculate Nucleus

The lateral geniculate nucleus is composed of six layers. As shown in Figure 6.19, each of the six layers of the LGN, in both the right and left hemispheres, receives information either from the ipsilateral retina (i.e., right retina/right LGN) or from the retina located on the contralateral side (i.e., right retina/left LGN). Layers 2, 3, and 5 receive information from the ipsilateral eye. Layers 1, 4, and 6 receive information from the contralateral eye.

The axons of midget and parasol retinal ganglion cells each connect to different layers of the LGN. The layers of the LGN contain three different types of cells: **parvocellular (P-cells)**, **magnocellular (M-cells)**, and **koniocellular (K-cells)**. The names of the layers correspond to the types of cells they each contain: P-cell, M-cell, and K-cell layers.

P-cells make up the dorsal layers of the LGN. These consist of layers 3, 4, 5, and 6 and are known as the parvocellular layers. As mentioned earlier, P-cells receive color information from the axons of midget ganglion cells of the retina. P-cells are responsive to the same receptive fields on the retina as the midget ganglion cells. Remember that midget ganglion cells are associated with on-center and off-center receptive fields based on illumination by lights of different wavelengths.

M-cells make up the ventral layers of the LGN. These consist of layers 1 and 2 and are known as the

FIGURE 6.18

The retinas of each eye are divided into the temporal retinas (red for the left eye and blue for the right eye) and the nasal retinas (blue for the left eye and red for the right eye). The axons of retinal ganglion cells form the optic nerves. The optic nerves from the nasal retina of each eye cross over at the optic chiasm, whereas the axons from the temporal retinas remain on the same side. Axons from the temporal retina of the left eye (5, 6, 7, 8) and the nasal retina of the right eye (6, 7, 8, 9), which convey information from the right visual field, terminate in the left LGN at locations 5, 6, 7, 8, and 9 (middle left). Axons from the temporal retina of the right eye (2, 3, 4) and the nasal retina of the left eye (1, 2, 3) terminate in the right LGN at locations 1, 2, 3, 4, and 5 (middle right). Axons at the fovea of both the left (4) and right (5) eyes process information from the center of the visual field and form the foveal image. A smaller number of axons from the optic tract terminate in the superior colliculus (middle). Axons from neurons in the LGN on each side of the brain project to various areas of the visual cortex on the same side through the optic radiations.

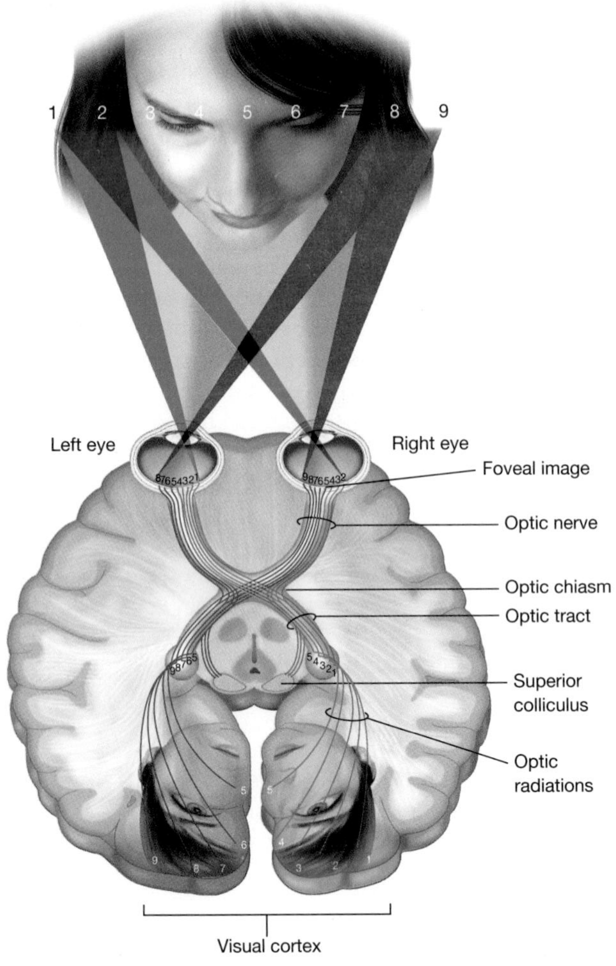

magnocellular layers. They convey information about motion and depth. Contrary to P-cells, M-cells are sensitive to contrast. They receive their information about contrast from the parasol ganglion cells. Remember that parasol ganglion cells are associated with on-center and off-center receptive fields that permit the detection of contrast.

K-cells are very small. They are located in six thin layers sandwiched in between each of the dorsal and ventral layers. These are known as the koniocellular layers. K-cells receive information from S-cones, which, as you know, are sensitive to short wavelengths. K-cells also receive information from a type of retinal ganglion cell that we have not mentioned. These are known as bistratified retinal ganglion cells, which convey information about spatial resolution.

FIGURE 6.19

Information processing in the LGN. RGCs = retinal ganglion cells.

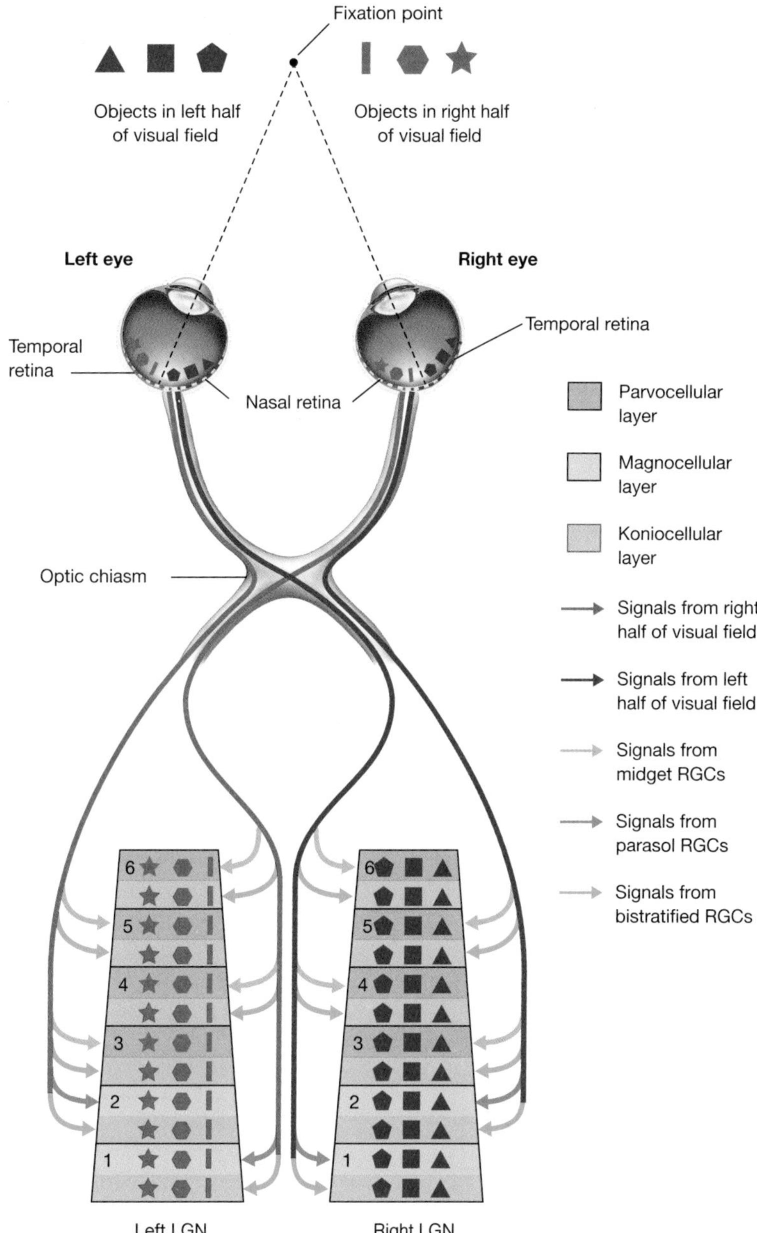

Color Opponent Cells

In the 1950s, researchers discovered retinal ganglion cells with receptive fields that respond to illumination by light of particular frequencies in the retina (Svaetichin & Macnichol, 1959) as well as in the LGN (De Valois, Smith, Kitai, & Karoly, 1958). These receptive fields work in a similar way to the on-center and off-center receptive fields of parasol cells you learned about earlier. The difference is that firing of cells located in the LGN depends on the wavelengths of light that illuminate the center or surround the receptive fields. The frequencies to which these receptive fields respond correspond to the pairs of opposing hues proposed by Hering that you learned about in the previous unit, that is, blue/yellow (B/Y) and red/green (R/G). In addition, each of the pairs was found to activate and inhibit retinal ganglion cells in the pattern of opposition that Hering proposed.

Remember that parasol retinal ganglion cells have on-center and off-center receptive fields based only on bright and dark contrasts. However, midget retinal ganglion cells process color information. The axons of parasol cells in the retina communicate with the M-cells of the LGN. Like the parasol cells in the retina, M-cells do not process color information. In contrast, midget retinal ganglion cells, which process color information, communicate with the P-cells of the LGN, which process color.

Some of the P-cells in the LGN were found to be activated when the center of the receptive field of midget retinal ganglion cells in the retina was illuminated with yellow light. The same P-cells were inhibited by illumination of retinal midget ganglion cells' surround with blue light. Those P-cells were associated with what are known as a Y+/B− receptive field. Other P-cells were associated with B+/Y−, R+/G−, and G+/R− receptive fields.

Information Processing in the Visual Cortex

Information from the LGN is conveyed to the primary visual cortex (V1) through the optic radiations (see Figure 6.18). V1 is sometimes referred to as the striate cortex because of its striped appearance when viewed under a microscope. It is situated at the back of the brain, in the occipital lobe (Figure 6.20). It is referred to as V1 because it is the first cortical destination for

FIGURE 6.20

Striate (V1) and extrastriate cortices (V2, V3, V4, and MT).

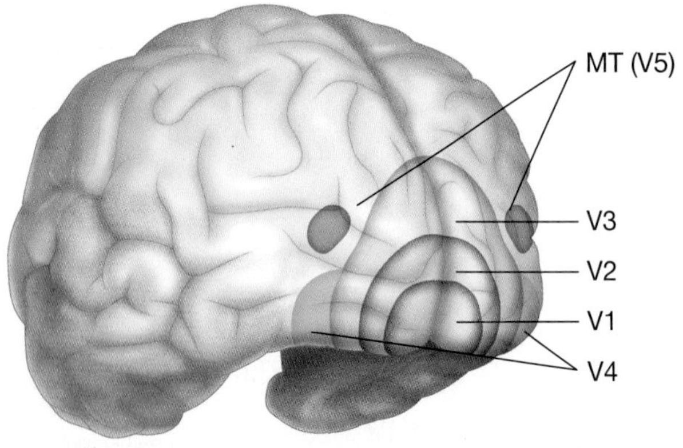

visual information after the thalamus. However, V1 is not the only cortical area that processes visual information. In fact, about 50% of the cortex was found to play some role in vision (Sheth, Sharma, Rao, & Sur, 1996). There are what are known as higher order visual areas, also referred to as extrastriate areas, which process motion, depth, form, and color. These areas are known as areas V2, V3, V4, and area MT (or V5) (DeYoe et al., 1996; Pitzalis, Fattori, & Galletti, 2015).

The striate and extrastriate cortices contain a neural map of the retina. That is, the relative positions of retinal neurons to one another is represented by neurons that have the same relative positions to one another in the striate and extrastriate cortices. This preservation of the relative location of neurons from the retina to the cortex is referred to as **retinotopic mapping**.

Until the late 1950s, great efforts were made to discover how V1 processed visual information. An important breakthrough was achieved when David Hubel and Torsten Wiesel recorded electrical activity from cells in V1 of cats as they stared at bright bars of light presented on a screen (Hubel & Wiesel, 1959, 2009).

This gave rise to the discovery of different types of cells. Two of these types of cells became known as simple cells and complex cells (Figure 6.21). The activity of simple cells was found to depend on the input of cells from the LGN. However, unlike cells in the LGN, simple cells were not found to differentially respond to illumination of center/surround receptive fields on the retina as do cells in the LGN. Rather, simple cells differentially responded best to bars of light of specific orientations illuminating a cat's retina. For this reason, simple cells are said to display **orientation selectivity**. Interestingly, the orientation selectivity of simple cells was found to depend on the combined input of sets of LGN neurons, known as concentric cells, for which the on/off receptive fields are aligned in certain directions.

Complex cells, another type of cell discovered by Hubel and Wiesel, differentially responded best to movement of a bar of light in a specific direction across a cat's retina. That is, some cells responded best when a bar of light moved from left to right, whereas others responded best when a bar moved from right to left, and so on. For this reason, complex cells are said to display **directional selectivity**. The directional selectivity of these cells was found to depend on the combined input of several simple cells with the same orientation selectivity. Complex cells are activated when their

FIGURE 6.21

Simple cells (top) and complex cells (bottom) in V1.

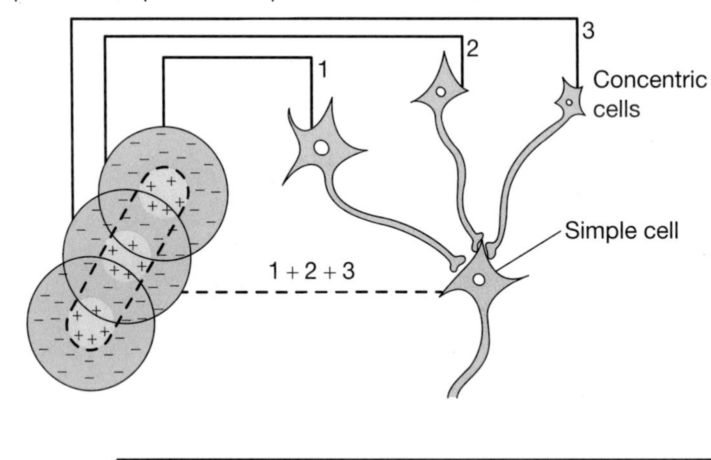

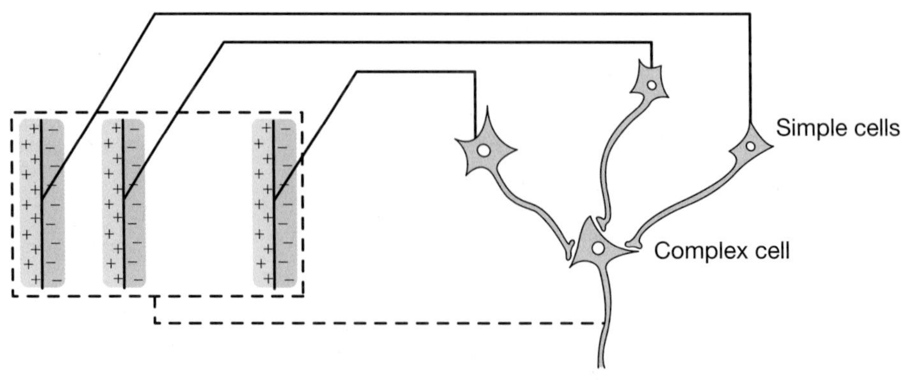

Adapted from *Principles of Neural Science*, 5th Edition, Kandel, Schwartz, Jessell, Siegelbaum, Hudspeth, & Mack. The McGraw-Hill Companies, Inc. 2013.

associated simple cells are sequentially activated as a stimulus moves from the receptive field of one simple cell to another in a particular direction.

The detection of orientation and movement by simple and complex cells, respectively, in V1 are but two examples of the complexity of visual information processing in the cortex. Remember from the previous unit that axons of three types of ganglion cells exit the retina to connect to different layers of the LGN. These connections form pathways that remain segregated all the way from the retina to V1 and extrastriate cortices. These pathways are referred to as the **P-pathway**, which connects midget retinal ganglion cells to P-cells in the LGN and the **M-pathway**, which connects parasol ganglion cells to M-cells in the LGN.

In V1, the P-pathway processes information about form and color. However, in extrastriate areas such as V2, the P-pathway processes information about depth and form but not color. In V4, the P-pathway processes information about form and color.

The M-pathway splits in two and runs dorsally, where one branch of it ends up in V2, which processes motion, depth, and form. The M-pathway then projects to area MT, where information about depth and motion is processed.

The "What" and "Where" of Vision

Since the 1960s, scientists have known that visual information from V1 follows two pathways throughout the brain, one specialized in the identification of objects and the other specialized in processing their locations (Schneider, 1969). This became known as the two-stream hypothesis of vision. In the 1980s, neuroscientists Leslie G. Ungerleider and Mortimer Mishkin found that monkeys with damage to the visual pathway that leads to the temporal lobe were impaired in the identification of objects, whereas those that had damage to the pathway leading to the parietal lobes were impaired in assessing the positions of objects in space (Mishkin & Ungerleider, 1982). It then became evident that the same pattern of impairments existed in humans with brain damage. The dorsal and ventral streams for visual perception (Figure 6.22) became known as the "what" and "where" pathways (Goodale & Milner, 1992).

FIGURE 6.22

The dorsal ("what") and ventral ("where") streams of vision.

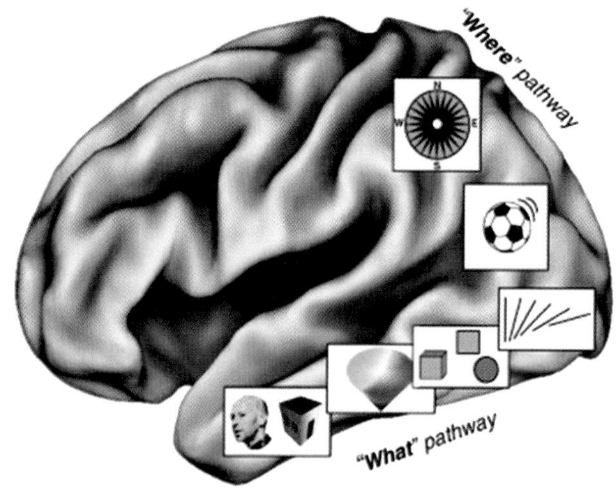

Freud, E., Plaut, D., & Behrmann, M. (2016). What is happening in the dorsal visual pathway. *Trends in Cognitive Sciences, 20*(10), 773–784.

MODULE SUMMARY

Light energy is classified into bands of wavelengths along the electromagnetic spectrum. Visible light corresponds to wavelengths ranging from approximately 400 nm to 700 nm, which are interpreted as colors. Color perception results from the brain's interpretation of messages from photoreceptors. Photoreceptors convert physical light energy into nerve impulses through the process of transduction. Light is focused to the center of the retina (fovea) by the lens. Objects are kept in focus on the fovea through accommodation. Activation of photoreceptors ultimately activates retinal ganglion cells. The axons of the ganglion cells form the optic nerve, which sends visual information to the brain.

There are two types of photoreceptors: rods and cones. Rods are sensitive to low levels of light and are responsible for dark adaptation but do not produce color vision. They confer low acuity and are found in the retina's periphery. Cones confer the ability to perceive colors. They come in three types: short-, medium-, and long-wavelength cones. They are less sensitive to low levels of light but have high acuity and are found at the fovea. Absorption of light by the photopigments inside photoreceptors hyperpolarizes photoreceptors, resulting in the depolarization of ganglion cells. Rods and cones differ in their degree of convergence onto retinal ganglion cells, which accounts for their differences in acuity and sensitivity. Rods are highly convergent, whereas cones show lower levels of convergence. A spot on the retina, which when illuminated triggers the activity or inhibition of a single retinal ganglion cell, is called a receptive field. The receptive fields of ganglion cells can either be on-center/off-surround or off-center/on-surround. Receptive fields are contrast detectors. The inhibition of retinal ganglion cells by illumination of their receptive field's surround can be explained by the process of lateral inhibition.

Two theories exist to explain color vision. The trichromatic theory states that color vision results from the combined activity of short-, medium-, and long-wavelength cones. The opponent process theory proposes that colors are processed in opposing pairs (blue/yellow, red/green, and black/white).

Beyond the retina, visual information is processed in an area of the thalamus called the lateral geniculate nucleus (LGN), in which neurons have receptive fields based on retinal ganglion cells. The receptive fields of cells in the primary visual cortex (V1) are associated with two types of neurons: Simple cells have receptive fields that detect line orientation, whereas complex cells have receptive fields that detect movement direction. Visual information from the retina to the visual cortex follows two pathways: the P-pathway and the M-pathway. The P-pathway processes information about color and form. The M-pathway processes information about depth, motion, and form. Information from V1 also follows two pathways. The "what" pathway projects to the ventral inferior temporal cortex, which is involved in the processing of color and form. The "where" pathway projects to the dorsal parietal cortex, which is involved in the processing of depth and motion.

TEST YOURSELF

6.1.1 Describe the beginnings of how wavelengths of light are converted into a visual image.

6.1.2 How is light energy transformed into electrical signals in receptors?

6.1.3 What mechanisms are involved in the differences in acuity and sensitivity between rods and cones?

6.1.4 In what ways are receptive fields involved in representing visual information?

6.1.5 Describe and explain the trichromatic and opponent process theories of color vision.

6.1.6 Discuss how the processing of visual information in the brain differs from how it is processed in the retina.

6.2 Hearing

Module Contents

Learning Objectives

6.2.1 Explain the difference between the physical and perceptual dimensions of sound.

6.2.2 Describe the functions of the different parts of the ear.

6.2.3 Outline the path of auditory processing from the cochlea to and within the brain.

6.2.1 PHYSICAL AND PERCEPTUAL DIMENSIONS OF SOUND

>> LO 6.2.1 Explain the difference between the physical and perceptual dimensions of sound.

Key Terms

- **Cycle:** One complete oscillation of a wave.
- **Hertz:** The number of cycles per second.
- **Decibels:** A measure of the intensity of sound.
- **Sensorineural hearing loss:** A type of deafness caused by damage to hair cells within the inner ear.

Physical Dimensions of Sound

In the previous module, you learned that the visual experience depends on the ability of your photoreceptors (the rods and cones) to transduce electromagnetic energy (light) into what ultimately amounts to patterns of electrical impulses. These impulses make their way to the brain, where they are interpreted to produce the visual world as you experience it. In addition to electromagnetic energy, your environment also contains energy that comes from patterns of compression and decompression of the air. These are commonly referred to as sound waves. You learned at the beginning of the previous module that light waves have no color and that your experience of color is produced by your brain. The same is true for auditory perception. If you remove the front cover of a speaker box while music is playing, you will see the subwoofer (usually the speaker at the bottom) move in and out with the patterns of bass sounds that you hear, for example, with the beat of the bass drum or bass guitar. The energy causing the speaker to move outward compresses the air in front of it. When the speaker moves back, the air is decompressed (or rarified). It is this pattern of compression and rarefaction of the air that is called sound waves. These patterns are transmitted through the air and reach your ears.

As you can see in Figure 6.23a, the wave rises as the air is compressed (increased air pressure) and dips when the air is rarefied (decreased air pressure). This refers to the sound wave's amplitude, that is, the height of the wave. The wave also has a frequency, which refers to the number of cycles per second the wave has (Figure 6.23b). One **cycle** of a wave is one complete oscillation of the wave, that is, from one peak to the next. The number of cycles per second is measured in **Hertz** (Hz). On average, humans can perceive sound waves that range between 20 and 20,000 Hz. However, we can perceive lower-frequency sounds if they are loud enough. Figure 6.23d shows the range of human hearing compared to the range of hearing for other mammals.

Amplitude is measured in **decibels** (dB). Decibels are a mathematical way to convert the extremely large range of sound pressure levels, from what you can barely hear to what is unbearable, in one manageable number. For example, the launch of a rocket creates a sound pressure change that is 10 million times that of the drop of a pin. However, the sound intensity produced by the drop of a pin is about 10 dB, whereas that produced by a rocket launch is 170 dB, a comparatively small difference. This is because every increase of 3 dB is equal to a doubling of sound intensity. Sound intensities above 130 dB can induce pain. Exposure to sounds of 85 dB or higher for a prolonged period poses a danger to your hearing. Being near a sound above

FIGURE 6.23

The physical and perceptual dimensions of sound and range of human hearing. (a) Graphic representation of a sound wave's amplitude. (b) Graphic representation of a sound wave's frequency, which is expressed in Hz, and how it relates to the psychological dimension of pitch. (c) Graphic representation of a sound wave's amplitude and how it relates to the psychological dimension of loudness. (d) The range of human hearing (20 Hz to 20,000 Hz) compared to the range of hearing for other mammals.

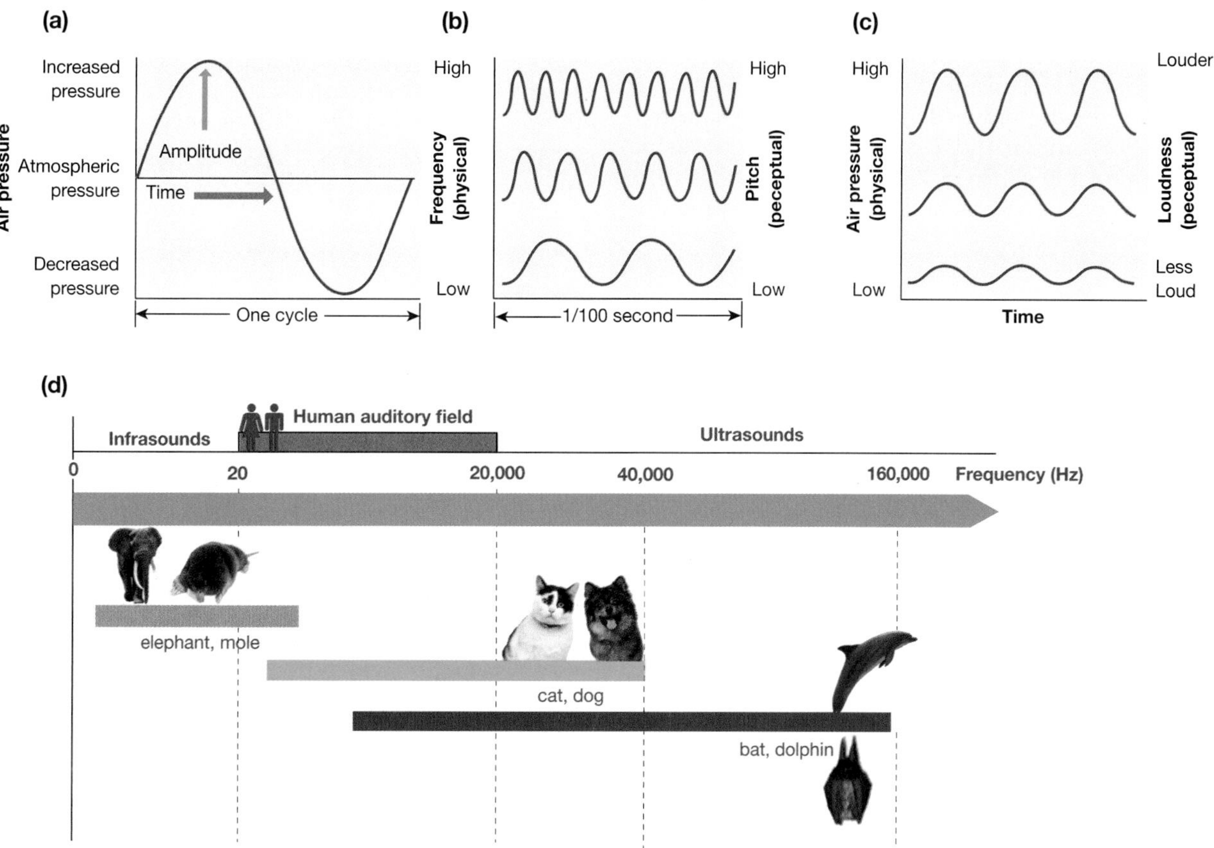

(elephant) iStock.com/DaveThomasNZ; (mole) iStock.com/step2626; (cat & dog) iStock.com/feedough, iStock.com/MirasWonderland; (dolphin) iStock.com/PhotographerOlympus

120 dB can cause immediate hearing loss. High-decibel sounds can produce a type of deafness called **sensorineural hearing loss**, which can result from damage to the hair cells of the inner ear, discussed in the "Applications" feature at the end of the chapter.

Perceptual Dimensions of Sound

How are amplitude and frequency perceived? Amplitude is the physical dimension of sound perceived as loudness (Figure 6.23c), which is its psychological dimension. For example, when you crank up the volume on your phone, you are increasing the waves' amplitude (the physical dimension), which you experience as an increase in loudness (the psychological dimension). Frequency is another physical dimension. It is perceived as pitch (Figure 6.23b), which is its psychological dimension.

Note that frequency and amplitude are independent. You can change the frequency of a sound wave without affecting its amplitude. That is, you can perceive the same pitch for a sound independently of volume and vice versa. Another psychological dimension of sound is timber. Almost all the sounds we hear come from complex sound waves. That is, they are produced by the combination of many wavelengths. However, the lowest frequency that produces these sounds can differ. The lowest frequency of many of the wavelengths that compose a complex sound is called the fundamental frequency. Different sound sources can be perceived as having the same pitch but differ in quality. This is obvious in the sounds produced by different musical instruments. Both a guitar and a trumpet can emit the same notes, producing sounds of the same perceived pitch, but you would never mistake the sound of a guitar for the sound of a trumpet. This is because the sounds of different musical instruments differ in their fundamental frequencies.

6.2.2 THE EAR

>> LO 6.2.2 Describe the functions of the different parts of the ear.

Key Terms

- **Ossicles:** Three tiny bones that connect the tympanic membrane to the inner ear.
- **Cochlea**: The snail-shaped and fluid-filled organ of the inner ear.
- **Organ of Corti:** The organ within the cochlea that contains the necessary components for hearing.
- **Hair cells:** Receptor cells responsible for hearing.
- **Basilar membrane:** The membrane within the organ of Corti on which hair cells are situated.

Figure 6.24 illustrates the different parts of the human ear. The ear has three compartments: the outer ear, the middle ear, and the inner ear. The outer ear includes the pinna and the auditory canal. The pinna is the visible part of the ear. The pinna plays an important role in collecting sounds from your environment. It is also important for localizing sounds on the vertical axis (from above to below the horizon). The auditory canal conducts sound energy from the outer ear to the middle ear. At the end of the auditory canal is the tympanic membrane (eardrum). Connected to the tympanic membrane are three tiny bones called the **ossicles**, the smallest bones in your body. These are the malleus, incus, and stapes, as they are known by their Latin names (in English: *hammer, anvil,* and *stirrup*). The tympanic membrane and the ossicles are part of the middle ear. The stapes connects to the inner ear at the oval window, which connects to the cochlea. The cochlea includes the semicircular canals, which play an important role in balance.

The cochlea is fluid filled and contains the receptors that are responsible for transducing energy from sound waves into electrical impulses, which ultimately leads to the perception of sound. However, for this to happen, sound energy must make its way to the cochlea with adequate power. Once sound waves have made their way through the auditory canal, their energy causes the tympanic membrane to vibrate. This vibration is passed on to the ossicles, which in turn pass it on to the cochlea, where its fluid is set into motion and where specialized receptors are excited.

FIGURE 6.24

The human ear.

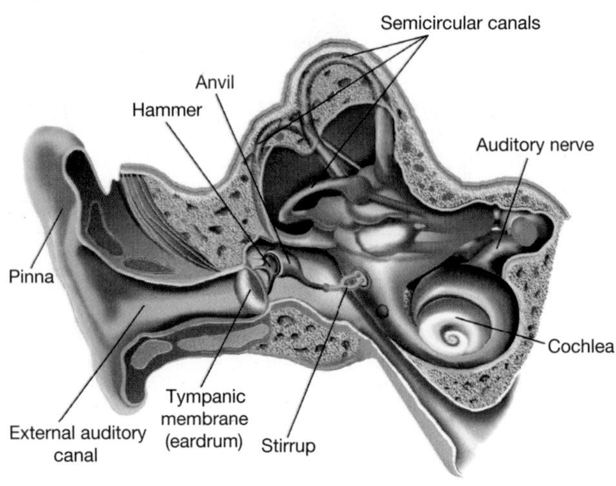

You may be wondering why there are three ossicles linking the tympanic membrane to the cochlea. The answer lies in the fact that sound waves initially travel through the air but then through the fluid inside the cochlea. Sound waves travel well through water but do not do so well when they travel from air to water. You may have experienced this if you tried to focus on what was going on outside a pool while your head was under water. For sound waves to effectively go from air to water, they need to be amplified. The ossicles act as levers that transmit the pressure exerted on the tympanic membrane by the sound waves to the oval window, situated at the base of the cochlea, which has a much smaller surface area than the tympanic membrane. This results in the pressure at the oval window being much greater than it is at the tympanic membrane (Hill, Wyse, & Anderson, 2012).

The Cochlea

The **cochlea** (Figure 6.25, top) is snail shaped and fluid filled. It coils around a bony pillar called the modiolus. Figure 6.25 (bottom) shows a cross-section of an uncoiled cochlea. The cochlea has three chambers: scala timpani, scala media, and scala vestibuli. Two types of fluids fill these chambers, endolymph and perilymph.

The scala tympani and scala vestibuli contain perilymph, whereas the scala media contains endolymph, which is rich in K^+. For our purposes, the most interesting of these chambers is the scala media. It contains what can be conceived as the equivalent of the retina for vision, the **organ of Corti**.

The organ of Corti includes the basilar membrane on which are situated the cells responsible for sound perception. These are known as **hair cells**. If we again draw an analogy to vision, hair cells are to hearing as rods and cones are to vision. The organ of Corti also includes the tectorial membrane, which extends from the modiolus. As you can see in Figure 6.25 (bottom), the hair cells are sandwiched between the basilar membrane and the tectorial membrane. You can also see how they got their name. They are ciliated, simply meaning that they have hairlike structures, called stereocilia, on top. The stereocilia of hair cells are embedded in the tectorial membrane, which is made of a gelatinous substance not unlike Jell-O. Hair cells connect to ganglion cells, which carry auditory information to the brain, through the auditory nerve. You can also see that there are inner and outer hair cells for which the functions are explained below.

The Basilar Membrane

The basilar membrane, on which the hair cells are located, is illustrated in Figure 6.26 as if the cochlea had been unrolled. As you can see, it is thick and narrow at the base and thin and wide at the apex.

FIGURE 6.25

The cochlea. Top: Cross-section of the cochlea showing its different parts along with the stapes, the smallest of three ossicles that transmit sound waves to the cochlea. Bottom: A coronal section of the cochlea showing the location of the organ of Corti, within the scala media, which is situated between the scala vestibule and scala timpani. The insert he components of the organ of Corti, which includes the basilar membrane on which the inner and outer hair cells are located. The cilia of hair cells embedded in the tectorial membrane, as well as the auditory nerve fibers that bring auditory information to the brain, are also shown.

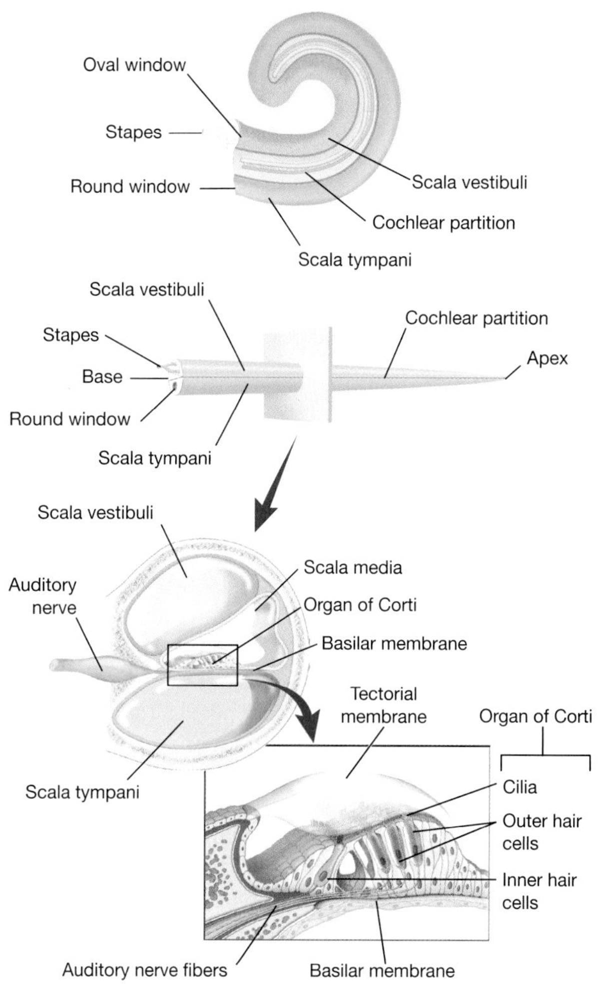

Liana Bauman/Body Scientific Intl.

The basilar membrane is flexible and is set into a wavelike motion by the energy and pressure changes that create sound waves. The peak of the wave occurs at

FIGURE 6.26

The basilar membrane with the positions where frequencies are processed.

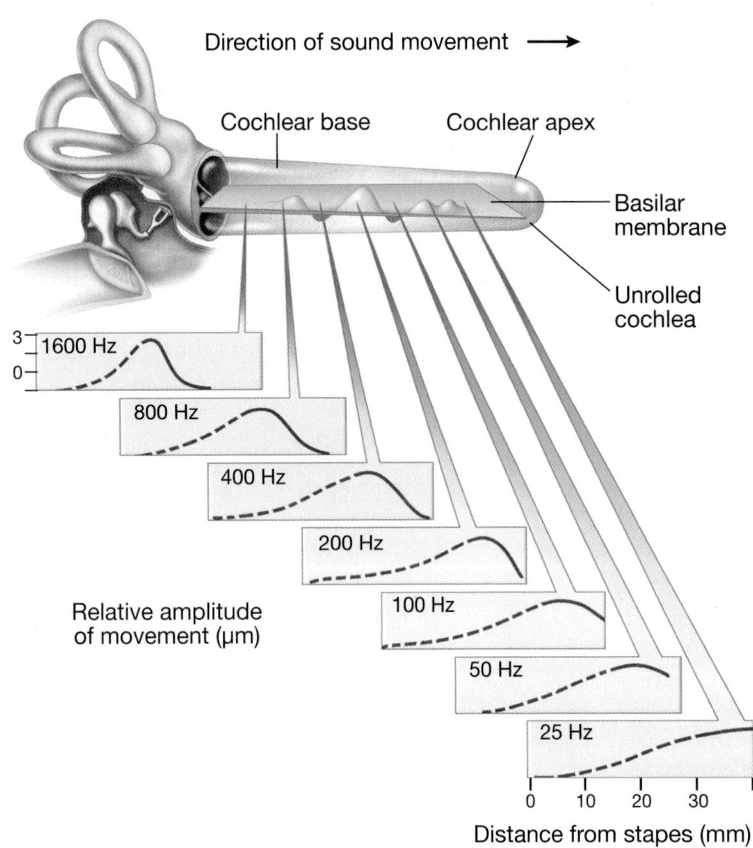

Liana Bauman/Body Scientific Intl.

different places on the basilar membrane depending on the frequency of the sound wave. Figure 6.26 shows how the basilar membrane is affected by sound waves of high, low, and middle frequencies. High-frequency sound waves create a ripple of waves that peak at the base of the basilar membrane, whereas low-frequency sounds create a ripple of waves that peak at the apex. Middle frequencies create ripples that peak around the center of the basilar membrane (Von Békésy & Wever, 1960).

How is the basilar membrane differentially affected by the different wavelengths of sounds? The answer lies in its peculiar shape. The short answer is that because it is thick at the base, high-frequency wavelengths cannot move past the beginning of the basilar membrane. Therefore, the peaks of the waves are observed early on. In contrast, low-frequency wavelengths are less affected by the thickness of the membrane at the base. Therefore, they tend to peak further down near the apex. The extra energy it takes for the wave to move further down the basilar membrane through the endolymph is compensated by the thinness of the membrane at the apex.

Hair Cells

Let's take a closer look at hair cells. Figure 6.27 shows a typical hair cell. Hair cells are mechanoreceptors. This means that they are activated when subjected to deformation. The most striking feature of hair cells is their stereocilia. In addition to stereocilia, hair cells have a cilium (referred to as true cilium) called a kinocilium. Stereocilia are flexible. They easily bend toward or away from the kinocilium. Together, the stereocilia and kinocilium form the hair bundle. As discussed earlier, hair cells send information toward the brain through afferent sensory neurons and receive information from the brain through efferent synapses.

When the basilar membrane is sent into a wavelike motion due to the energy created by changes in air pressure, the stereocilia of the hair cells bend. This happens because they are embedded in the tectorial membrane. When hair cells bend toward the kinocilium (positive direction), as occurs during the peak of a wave, the cell is depolarized and gives rise to action potentials in afferent fibers that bring auditory information to the brain. When the stereocilia bend away from the kinocilium (negative direction), as in a wave's trough, the cell hyperpolarizes and action potentials generated by the hair cell cease to occur. Another interesting feature of hair cells is that they neither have dendrites nor axons. A neurotransmitter is released from the cell body itself onto the afferent fibers and receives information from the brain through efferent fibers that make direct contact with the cell body.

Activation of hair cells is due to entry of K^+ ions. Recall that in most neurons action potentials are generated by the entry of Na^+ ions. When the stereocilia bend in the positive direction, gates that permit the entry of K^+, situated on each one of the stereocilia, are opened. This causes the cell to depolarize. Due to this depolarization, Ca^{2+} channels on the cell body open, permitting entry of Ca^{2+} into the cell. This in turn causes the synaptic vesicle to fuse with the membrane of the cell and to release neurotransmitter molecules onto afferent sensory neurons (Fettiplace & Hackney, 2006; Kozlov, Risler, & Hudspeth, 2007).

Different frequencies are perceived as pitch because the brain processes the patterns of firing of hair cells located at different places along the basilar membrane. This is known as the place theory of pitch perception.

As illustrated in Figure 6.28, there are both outer and inner hair cells. Each type plays its own role and has a different pattern of connectivity. Inner hair cells relay information related to the frequency of sound waves to the brain, though afferent fibers, whereas outer hair cells play a role in the amplification of sounds and receive information related to the location of sounds from the brain (superior olivary nucleus) through efferent fibers. There are many more outer hair cells (approximately 12,000) than there are inner hair cells (approximately 3,500). There are three rows of outer hair cells and only one row of inner hair cells. However, 95% of the auditory information relayed to the brain (cochlear nucleus) comes from inner hair cells. This is because 90% of cells known as spiral ganglion cells innervate inner hair cells. In addition, each inner hair cell connects with several spiral ganglion cells, but each ganglion cell receives information from a single inner hair cell (the cochlear nucleus and superior olivary nucleus are discussed in the next unit).

FIGURE 6.28

Patterns of connectivity of inner and outer hair cells.

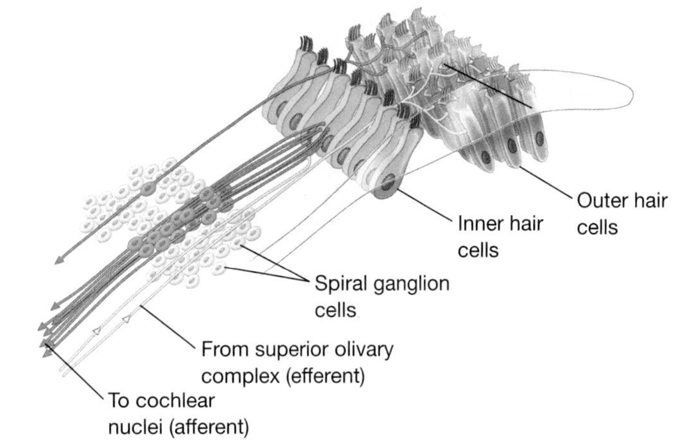

Graven, S.N. & J. Browne. (2008). Auditory Development in the Fetus and Infant. *Newborn and Infant Nursing Reviews* 8(4): 187–193. With permission from Elsevier.

FIGURE 6.27

A typical hair cell.

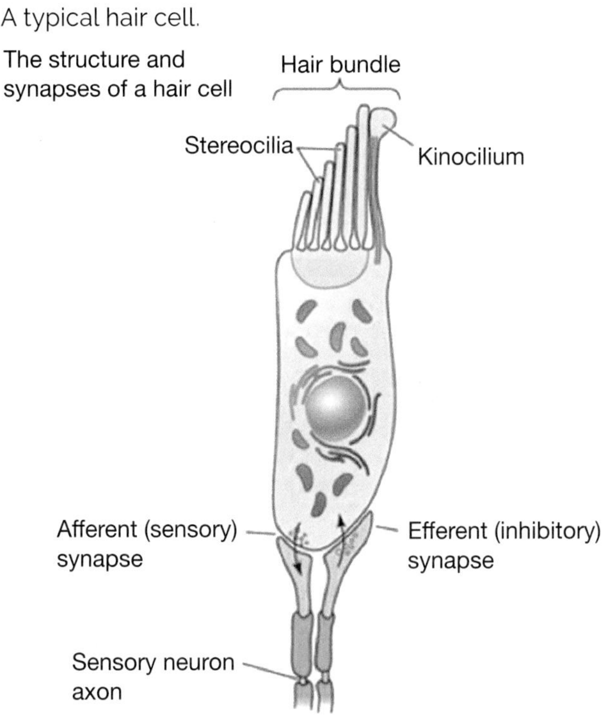

From *Animal Physiology*, 2nd Revised Edition, Hill, Wyse and Anderson, Sinauer Associates, Inc., 2003.

6.2.3 AUDITORY PROCESSING BEYOND THE BASILAR MEMBRANE

>> LO 6.2.3 **Outline the path of auditory processing from the cochlea to and within the brain.**

Key Terms

- **Spiral ganglion cells:** Cells that contact hair cells to bring auditory information to the brain.
- **Auditory nerve:** Axons of ganglion cells (also called the vestibulocochlear nerve or cranial nerve VIII).
- **Tonotopic mapping:** The preservation of the relative spatial organization of frequency processing on the basilar membrane and within the cortex.

Now that you know how sound waves are converted into action potentials that carry auditory information to the brain, in this unit you will learn about the paths that this information follows into the brain, focusing on the output of inner hair cells. These hair cells account for 90% of the connectivity with **spiral ganglion cells**, which bring information about the frequency of sound waves to the brain. The axons of spiral ganglion cells form the **auditory nerve** (also called the vestibulocochlear nerve or cranial nerve VIII). As shown in Figure 6.29, information about sound waves, carried through the ascending auditory pathways, ultimately ends up in the primary auditory cortex (A1) in the temporal

FIGURE 6.29

The ascending auditory pathways.

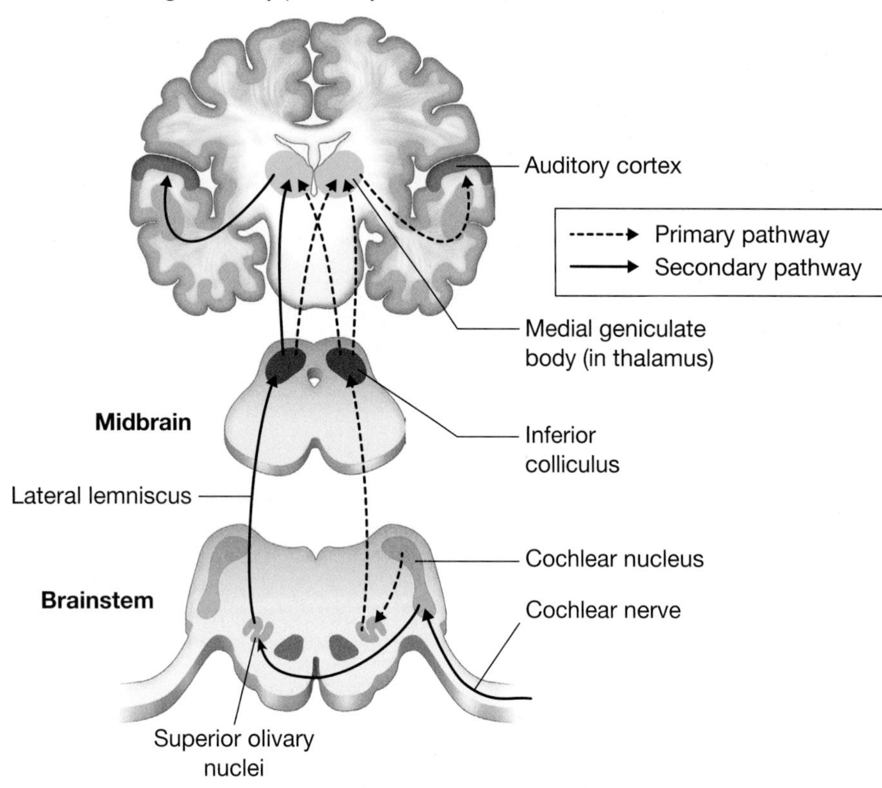

lobes, where it is processed and sent out to other brain areas for further analysis.

From their contact point with hair cells, the axons of ganglion cells that form the auditory nerve split and project to three cochlear nuclei situated in the medulla, within the brainstem. The cochlear nuclei include the dorsal, anteroventral, and posteroventral nuclei. The basilar membrane is **tonotopically mapped** onto these nuclei along their ventral to dorsal axis. This means that high-frequency sounds processed at the base of the basilar membrane are processed ventrally, whereas mid- and low-frequency sounds are processed at progressively more dorsal positions along the axis.

From the cochlear nuclei, most of the auditory information flows through the brainstem to the contralateral superior olivary nucleus. This the primary pathway for auditory information. The cochlear nuclei also send auditory information to the ipsilateral superior olivary nucleus. This is part of the secondary pathway. From the superior olivary nucleus, auditory information then flows, ipsilaterally, through the inferior colliculus of the midbrain, to both the contralateral and ipsilateral medial geniculate nucleus (MGN) of the thalamus, and finally to A1. The cochlear nucleus on each side of the brain receives information from the ear on the same side of your head. However, the cochlear nucleus sends information from that ear to both the left and right superior olivary nuclei, which means that the inferior colliculus, MGN, and A1 receive information from both ears (Pickles, 2015).

The "What" and "Where" of Hearing

Recall that visual information can be separated into the "what" and "where" of things and that this information is processed in areas beyond V1. Remember that "what" information from V1 follows a ventral stream and is processed in the ventral inferior temporal cortex and that "where" information follows a dorsal stream and is processed in the dorsal parietal cortex. Similar "what" and "where" pathways exist for hearing. The posterior part of A1 projects to the parietal lobes, which constitute the "where" pathway. The anterior part of A1 projects to the superior temporal lobes (Poremba et al., 2003). For both vision and hearing, information from the parietal and temporal lobes is transmitted to the dorsolateral prefrontal cortex (DLPC) and ventromedial prefrontal cortex (VMPC), respectively. Both visual and auditory streams are illustrated in Figure 6.30 (Rauschecker & Scott, 2009).

FIGURE 6.30

The "what" and "where" pathways (ventral and dorsal stream) for vision and hearing, starting in the primary visual cortex (V1) and primary auditory cortex (A1).

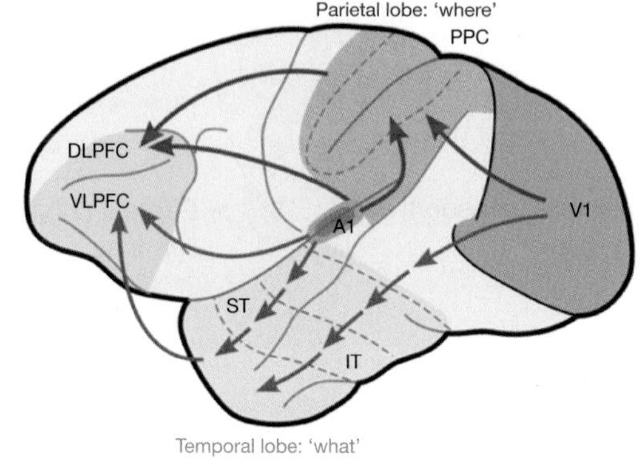

Rauschecker, J.P. & S.K. Scott. (2009). Maps and streams in the auditory cortex: nonhuman primates illuminate human speech processing, *Nature Neuroscience* 12: 718–724. With permission from Springer Nature.

MODULE SUMMARY

A sound wave has both amplitude and frequency. Amplitude refers to the height of the wave. Frequency refers to the number of cycles per second the wave has. Frequency is measured in Hertz (Hz), which refers to the number of cycles of waves per second, whereas amplitude is measured in decibels (dB). Different sound sources can be perceived as having the same pitch but differ in quality because of a difference in timber.

The ear has three compartments: the outer ear, the middle ear, and the inner ear. The middle ear contains the tympanic membrane and the ossicles: the malleus, the incus, and the stapes. The inner ear contains the cochlea, which contains the organ of Corti, in which the basilar membrane and hair cells are located. Sound waves are amplified by the ossicles that act as levers that transmit the pressure exerted on the tympanic membrane to the inner ear. The basilar membrane moves in waves. The location of the peak of these waves is determined by the frequency of the incoming sound wave.

High-frequency sound waves are processed at the base and low-frequency sound waves are processed at the apex of the basilar membrane. Mid-frequency sound waves are processed at the center of the basilar membrane. Different frequencies are perceived as pitch because the brain processes the patterns of firing of hair cells at different places on the basilar membrane. This is known as the place theory of pitch perception.

The output of inner hair cells accounts for 90% of the connectivity with spiral ganglion cells, which bring information about the frequency of sound waves to the brain. The axons of ganglion cells form the auditory nerve. The basilar membrane is tonotopically mapped onto the cochlear nuclei along their ventral to dorsal axis. "What" and "where" pathways exist for hearing. The posterior part of the primary auditory cortex (A1) projects to the parietal lobes, which constitutes the "where" pathway. The anterior part of A1 projects to the anterior parts of the temporal lobes.

TEST YOURSELF

6.2.1 Explain why sounds do not exist outside of your brain.

6.2.2 Name and describe the parts of the ear and describe their functions.

6.2.3 How are patterns of compression and decompression of air processed into what we perceive as sounds?

APPLICATIONS

The Cochlear Implant

What Is a Cochlear Implant?

A cochlear implant, as shown in Figure 6.31, is a device that provides sound and speech perception to individuals with sensorineural hearing loss (hearing loss due to damage to hair cells within the cochlea). This type of hearing loss can be caused by aging, exposure to loud noise, infections, genetic conditions, among other causes.

A cochlear implant consists of external and internal components. The implant contains a speech processor and a transmitter, both located outside the ear. The speech processor encodes sounds picked up by a microphone into a pattern of electrical stimulation. The electrical-stimulation code is sent to the transmitter, which passes on the code, by radio frequency, to a receiver located under the skin. The receiver conveys the code to an electrode array inserted in the cochlea (Macherey & Carlyon, 2014).

How Does That Translate Into Sound Perception?

In normal hearing, pitch perception is due partly to the pattern of activity of hair cells within the cochlea. When activated, hair cells send sound information to the brain through the auditory nerve. However, hair cells located at the base of the cochlea respond mostly to high-frequency sounds, whereas hair cells at the apex respond mostly to low-frequency sounds. This is known as the place theory of pitch perception.

The cochlear implant mimics this process by sending sound frequency information to the appropriate location in the cochlea, so that high-frequency sounds excite the auditory nerve fibers at the base of the cochlea and low-frequency sounds excite the fibers at the apex.

(Continued)

(Continued)

Limitations of the Cochlear Implant

Cochlear implants have major limitations when it comes to mimicking the biological process of pitch perception. For example, the normal cochlea contains approximately 3,500 hair cells and humans can perceive frequencies ranging from 20 Hz to 20,000 Hz. In contrast, a cochlear implant contains about 22 electrodes in place of the thousands of hair cells in a natural cochlea and can only process frequencies from approximately 200 Hz to 8,500 Hz. Therefore, cochlear implants do not restore normal hearing. However, they can provide people with useful representations of sounds and the ability to understand speech.

Who Gets Cochlear Implants?

Cochlear implants can be fitted for both adults and children. Children can receive implants beginning at 12 months of age. The best results in children are for those under 18 months of age, while they are still in the sensitive period for language acquisition. ●

FIGURE 6.31

Cochlear implants.

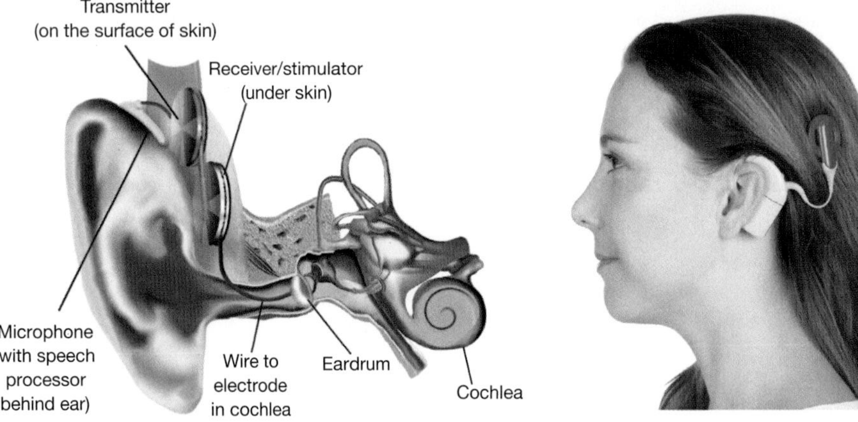

iStock.com/ELizabethHoffmann>

iStock.com/RyanJLane

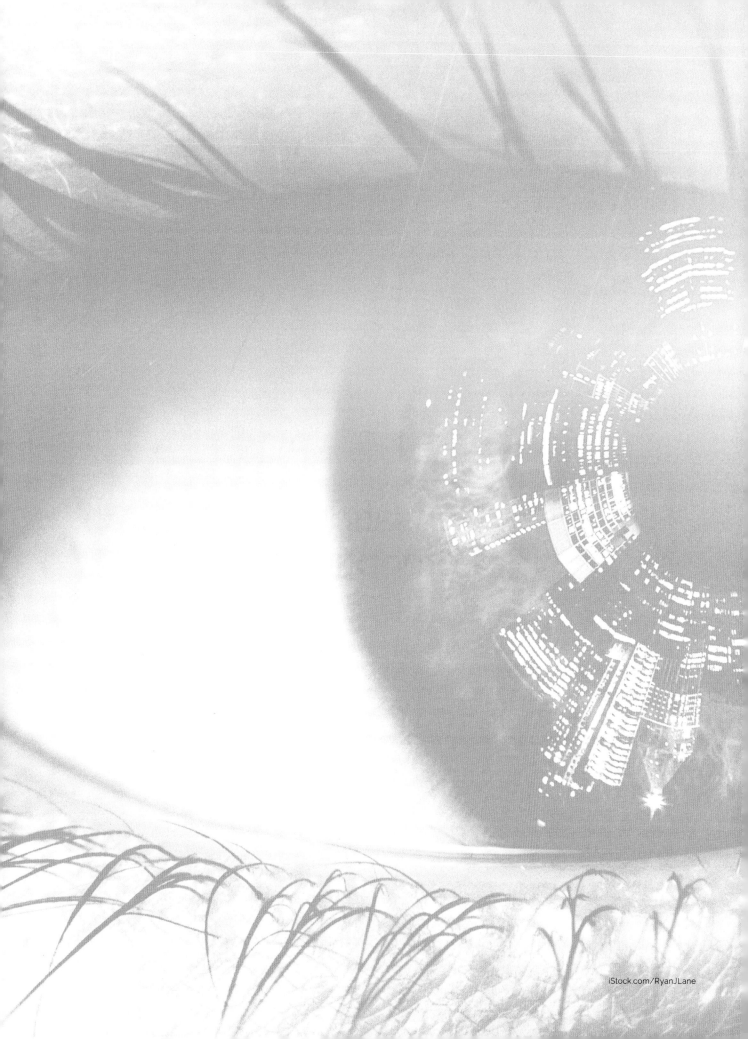

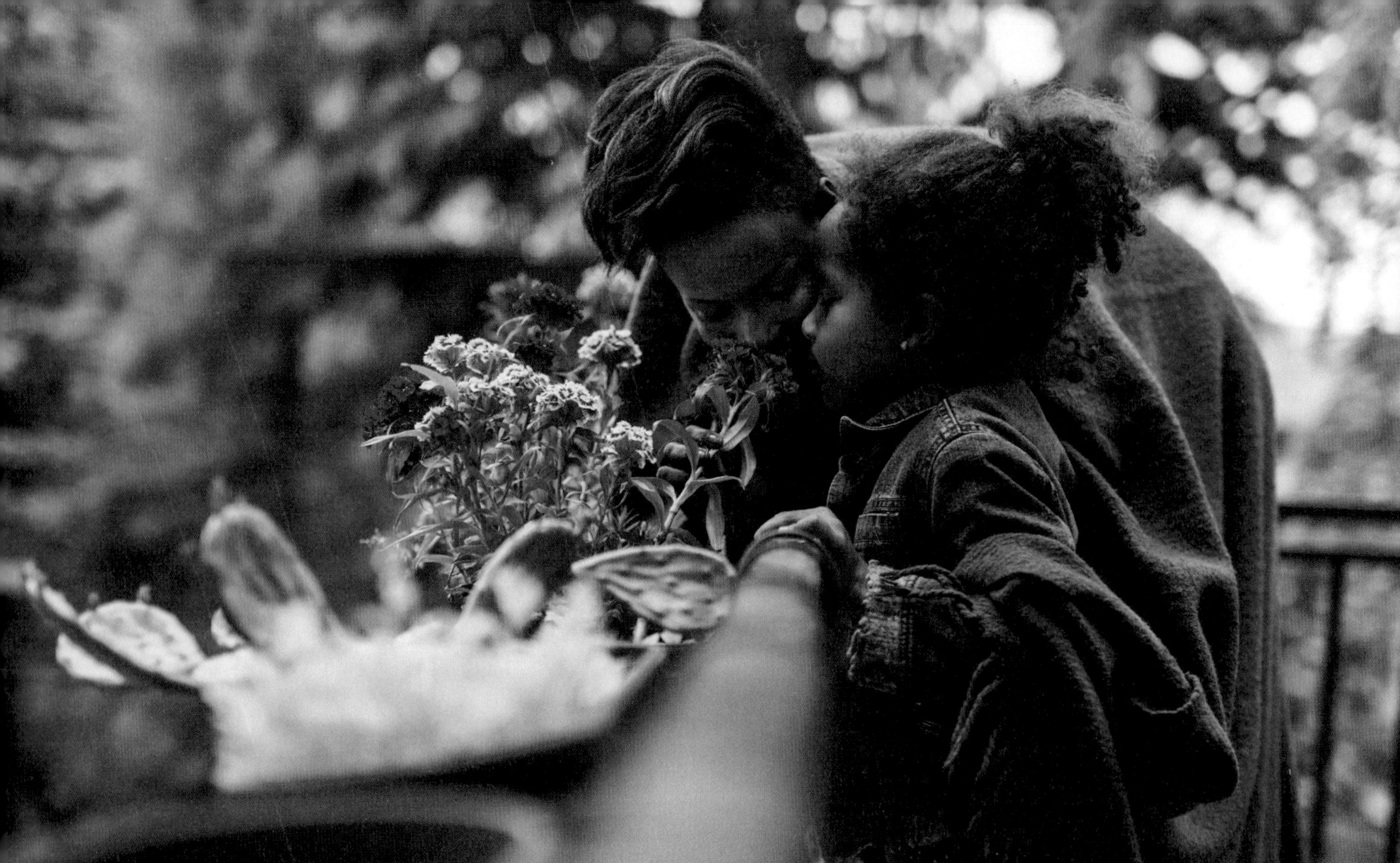

iStock.com/BraunS

7 Sensation and Perception 2

Taste, Smell, and Touch

Chapter Contents

Learning Objectives

7.1.1 Explain what makes up the experience of taste.

7.1.2 Describe the structure and functioning of taste receptors.

7.1.3 Describe each of the taste receptor cells and explain how they convey the basic tastes.

7.1.4 Explain how and where in the brain the experience of taste arises.

7.2.1 Explain what makes up the experience of smell.

7.2.2 Describe the structure and functioning of olfactory receptor neurons.

7.2.3 Explain how and where in the brain the experience of smell arises.

7.2.4 Explain what pheromones are as well as their functions and the mechanisms by which they affect behavior.

7.3.1 Explain what makes up the sense of touch.

7.3.2 Describe and differentiate between the various types of mechanoreceptors and their functions.

7.3.3 Explain how nerve impulses are triggered by mechanoreceptors.

7.3.4 Explain how touch information is conveyed from mechanoreceptors to the brain.

7.3.5 Describe the mechanism by which pain is perceived as well as how pain can be controlled.

A Sommelier's Nightmare

Pamela was a sommelier. She made a living as a wine consultant. Working in fine restaurants, she consulted in the development of wine lists and was an expert in food-wine pairings. For Pamela, her senses of taste and smell were crucial to her livelihood, which was also her life's passion. One day, while ice skating with her husband, Pamela slipped, fell backward, and hit her head on the ice. Although she was shaken up, she felt fine and the fall seemed to be of no consequence. However, the next day, while at a wine-tasting event, she noticed that something was going horribly wrong. She could no longer perceive the smells nor the tastes of the wines she was sampling. Pamela had lost her sense of smell. Her world came crashing down. As she could no longer pursue her passion, she felt desperate and depressed. Without her sense of smell, food and drink taste very bland. This is because smell contributes a great deal to the enjoyment of food. Indeed, smell and taste combine to create what is known as flavor. Other contributors to flavor include the food's texture, such as crispiness and crunchiness; its temperature; and its spiciness. Pamela tries to compensate for not being able to smell her food by choosing food that provides her with varied experiences with respect to textures. But none are satisfying substitutes.

INTRODUCTION

In Chapter 6, you studied vision and hearing. Both of these senses process information that exists in waves. You learned that vision comes from processing a narrow band of wavelengths along the electromagnetic spectrum called the visible spectrum. By contrast, hearing involves the processing of patterns of compression and decompression of the air, which are known as pressure waves.

However, the physical environment also contains a wide variety of chemicals. Some of these chemicals are part of the foods we eat and activate receptors within the mouth. Other chemicals are volatile. They bind to and activate receptors situated deep within the nasal cavity. The information provided through the activation of these receptors by chemicals is processed by the senses of taste and smell, respectively. For this reason, taste and smell are known as the chemical senses.

In nature, the main role of the chemical senses is to evaluate potential food sources. Both poisons and safe sources of nutrients must reliably be detected and discriminated. Chemoreceptors are also used as part of a communication system that can alter the physiology and behaviors of conspecifics (members of the same species), to signal alarm, provide food trails, and signal sexual receptivity.

Another way in which we perceive the world is through touch. Touch occurs through the sensing of mechanical deformations of the skin. Touch can be innocuous, or it can warn about potentially harmful stimuli. We now turn to the senses of taste, smell, and touch.

7.1 Taste

Module Contents

Learning Objectives

7.1.1 Explain what makes up the experience of taste.

7.1.2 Describe the structure and functioning of taste receptors.

7.1.3 Describe each of the taste receptor cells and explain how they convey the basic tastes.

7.1.4 Explain how and where in the brain the experience of taste arises.

7.1.1 WHAT IS TASTE AND WHAT IS IT MADE OF?

>> **LO 7.1.1 Explain what makes up the experience of taste.**

Key Terms

- **Taste:** The perception generated when chemicals are dissolved in saliva and bind to gustatory chemoreceptors.
- **Gustatory chemoreceptors:** Taste receptor cells.
- **Gustatory cortex:** The area of the brain that processes taste.
- **Flavor:** The total perceptual experience you get from food.
- **Mouth-feel:** What the food feels like in your mouth.
- **Hedonics of food:** Whether a food is perceived to be pleasant or unpleasant.

Taste (gustatory perception) is the perception generated when chemical molecules from food are dissolved in saliva within the mouth and then bind to and stimulate **gustatory chemoreceptors**, also known as taste receptor cells. Stimulation of taste receptor cells ultimately activates neurons in the **gustatory cortex**, which is the area of the brain that processes information about taste.

You surely learned while growing up that there are four basic tastes: sweet, salty, bitter, and sour. We now know, however, that there are others. For example, umami conveys the perception of a meaty or brothy taste, and oleogustus is the taste of fat (Running, Craig, & Mattes, 2015). In addition, scientists will likely discover several other basic tastes with advances in molecular biology (Hartley, Liem, & Keast, 2019). See this chapter's "It's a Myth!" feature for more on the basic tastes.

The stimulation of taste receptor cells alone is not enough to give rise to the wide range of perceptual qualities that we assign to all of the foods we eat. The total perceptual experience you get from food is known as **flavor**. As illustrated in Figure 7.1, a food's flavor depends on many factors in addition to taste, such as what the food feels like in your mouth, that is, the food's **mouth-feel** (Gawel, Smith, Cicerale, & Keast, 2018; Nederkoorn, Houben, & Havermans, 2019). Mouth-feel includes factors such as texture, temperature, coolness (such as produced by a minty candy), dryness, and even pain, such as that induced by spices such as red pepper.

Other factors such as your state of hunger, the area of the mouth most stimulated, the timing of taste onset, aftertaste, intensity, what the food looks like, and even what it sounds like when you bite into it are also important. The **hedonics of food**—that is, whether you judge it to be pleasant or unpleasant—are of utmost importance for most people (Epstein, Truesdale,

FIGURE 7.1

Factors involved in the total perceptual experience of taste. Flavor includes taste as well as several other perceptual factors.

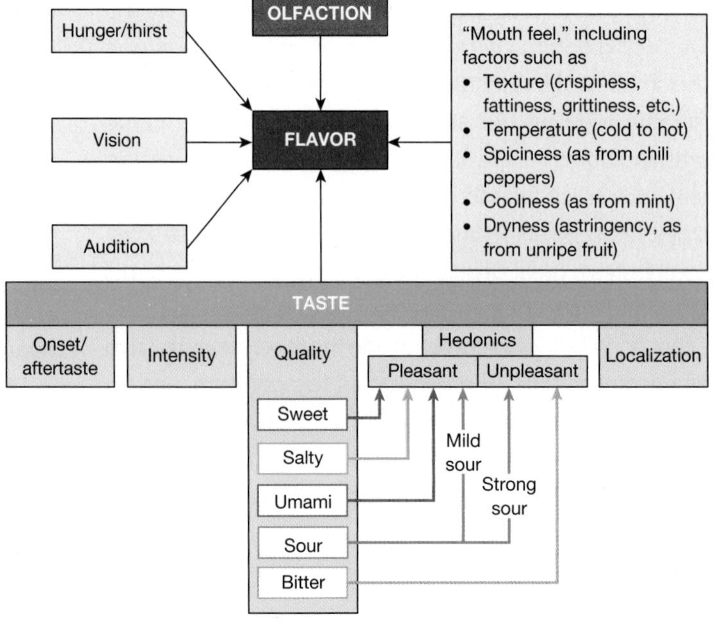

Wojcik, Paluch, & Raynor, 2003; Wisniewski, Epstein, & Caggiula, 1992). Other than the stimulation of taste chemoreceptors, smell is the greatest contributor to taste (Spence, 2015), which is why Pamela, in the opening vignette, was so devastated. You can easily demonstrate this to yourself by putting a fruity-tasting candy in your mouth while pinching your nostrils closed and then releasing them.

7.1.2 GUSTATORY CHEMORECEPTORS

>> LO 7.1.2 **Describe the structure and functioning of taste receptors.**

Key Terms

- **Taste buds:** Structures that contain taste receptor cells.
- **Papillae:** Small rounded structures that contain the taste buds.
- **Fungiform papillae:** The papillae located on the anterior surface of the tongue.
- **Foliate papillae:** The papillae located along the edges in the back of the tongue.
- **Vallate papillae:** The papillae forming a "V" in the center of the back of the tongue.
- **Basal cells:** Cells that remain undifferentiated and that can be incorporated into papillae to take the form of taste receptor cells when they need to be replenished.

Gustatory chemoreceptors (taste receptor cells) are located mainly on the tongue. Taste receptor cells are also found in the esophagus and stomach lining. However, these are not thought to contribute to taste perception. Taste receptor cells are contained within **taste buds**, which themselves are located inside small rounded structures called **papillae**.

Papillae

The papillae involved in taste perception are of three types, each located on different parts of the tongue and containing a different number of taste buds. The types and location of papillae are illustrated in Figure 7.2a. The papillae located on the anterior surface of the tongue are called **fungiform papillae**. They contain approximately eight taste buds and also contain touch and temperature receptors. The back of the tongue is covered by two types of papillae: **foliate papillae** and **vallate papillae** (sometimes called circumvallate papillae). Foliate papillae are located along the edges in the back of the tongue. Foliate papillae contain approximately 1,300 taste buds. Vallate papillae form a "V" in the center of the back of the tongue. Vallate papillae contain approximately 250 taste buds.

FIGURE 7.2

(a) Location of the three types of papillae involved in taste perception. (b) The location of taste buds inside a single papilla. (c) A taste bud with its taste cells, a taste pore, and microvilli.

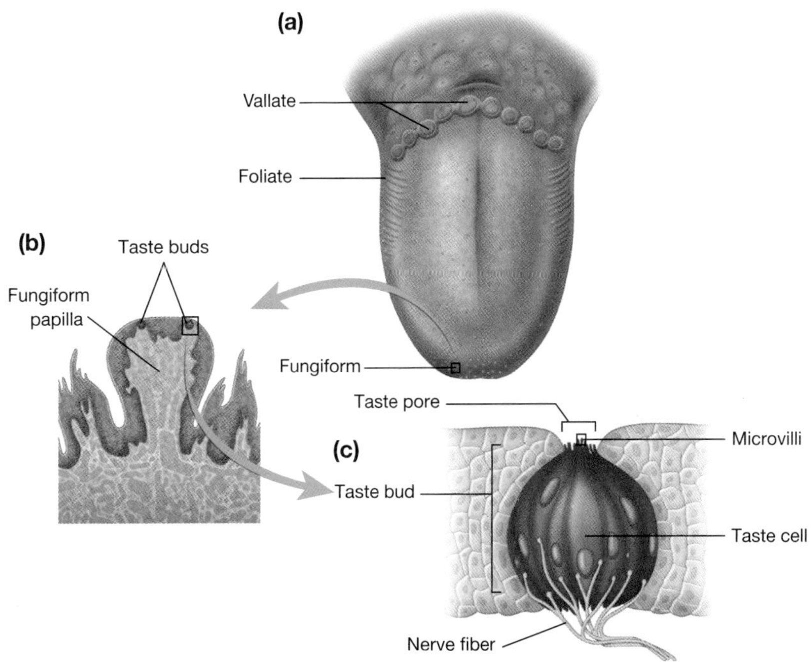

Taste Buds

Taste receptor cells are contained within the taste buds (Figure 7.2b). Each taste bud contains 20–50 taste receptor cells. Taste buds have a small opening, called a taste pore, through which small hairlike structures called microvilli protrude. The microvilli play an important role, as they capture the chemicals from food dissolved in saliva to bring them into contact with the taste receptor cells through the taste pore.

Taste buds also contain **basal cells**. The half-life of taste receptor cells is about 8–12 days. Therefore, they need to be regenerated constantly. Basal cells remain undifferentiated, meaning that they can be incorporated into papillae and take the form of taste receptor cells when they need to be replenished.

7.1.3 TASTE RECEPTOR CELLS AND THEIR MECHANISMS

>> LO 7.1.3 **Describe each of the taste receptor cells and explain how they convey the basic tastes.**

Key Terms

- **Amelioride-sensitive Na⁺ channels:** Sodium channels that are blocked by the drug amelioride.
- **Broadly tuned:** Refers to how neurons can respond to different types of stimuli.

Taste Receptor Cells

There are three types of taste receptor cells. They are known as type I, type II, and type III receptor cells. Figure 7.3 shows each type of cell, the relationships that exist between them, and their mechanisms.

Type I cells account for half the number of receptor cells in taste buds. They have glia-like function, in that they eliminate the surplus of neurotransmitter outside the cells. They are also responsible for the spatial buffering of K^+, by which they regulate the levels of extracellular potassium released by type II and type III cells, through what are known as renal outer medullar K (ROMK) channels. Type I cells convey the perception of saltiness. They are believed to do so through the entry of Na^+ through Na^+ channels. However, questions still remain about whether this is truly the case (Chandrashekar et al., 2010).

Type II cells account for one-third of the taste cells within taste buds and are larger than type I cells. Type II cells convey the tastes of sweet, umami, and bitter.

Type III cells convey sourness. They are believed to do so through the entry of H^+ ions through Na^+ channels, which causes the opening of Ca^{2+} channels. Type III cells also integrate taste information from type II cells with their own information to convey it to the brain through sensory afferent fibers. This means that type III cells are **broadly tuned**, in that they process information from different taste molecules.

FIGURE 7.3

The three types of taste receptor cells: type 1 (blue), type II (yellow), and type III (green).

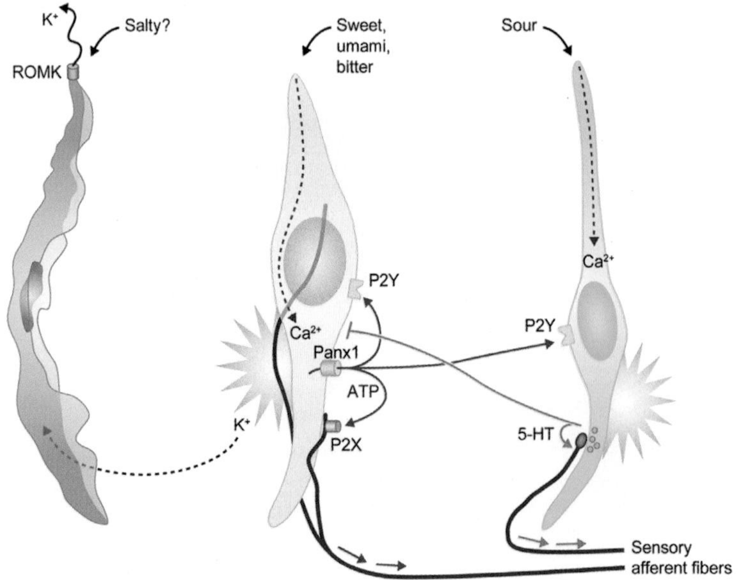

Chaudhari, N. and S. D. Roper (2010). The cell biology of taste. *Journal of Cell Biology 190*(3): 285–296. With permission from Rockefeller University Press.

The way in which type III cells integrate information from different tastes is also shown in Figure 7.3. Type II cells release adenosine triphosphate (ATP) through what are known as pannexin channels (Panx 1) when activated by food molecules. Some of the ATP binds to receptors known as P2Y, which are located on the cells that release it. This acts as a positive feedback mechanism that signals these cells to release more ATP. The ATP released by type II cells also activates what are known as P2X receptors located on sensory afferent nerve fibers originating from that cell, which conveys taste information to the brain.

In addition, the ATP released by type II cells binds to P2Y receptors located on type III cells. This causes type III cells to release the neurotransmitter serotonin (5-HT), which is also dependent on the influx of Ca^{2+}. In turn, the release of 5-HT from type III cells is believed to stimulate sensory afferent nerve fibers that send taste information to the brain. Another role for the release of 5-HT from type III cells is to provide negative feedback to type II cells to regulate their release of ATP.

Mechanisms for Sweet, Umami, and Bitter Taste Perceptions

The perceptions of sweet and umami are conveyed through different types of G-protein-coupled receptor (GPCR), which are activated when bound to by a tastant. These comprise what are known as T1R1, T1R2, and T1R3 receptors. Each of these receptors is expressed by different genes. The perception of sweetness depends on activation of T1R2 and T1R3 GPCRs. The perception of umami depends on the activation of T1R1 and T1R3 GPCRs, which are responsive to the amino acids glutamate and aspartate, found in fish, cheese, and vegetables (Chaudhari, Pereira, & Roper, 2009).

For both sweet and umami, activated G-proteins trigger the activity of the enzyme phospholipase C beta-2 ($PLC_{\beta 2}$). This results in the opening of transient receptor potential cation channel subfamily M member 5 ($TRPM_5$), by the molecule inositol triphosphate (IP_3). The opening of $TRPM_5$ permits the influx of Ca^{2+} ions into the cell, leading to its depolarization. The perception of bitter taste depends on the activation of the same GPCRs as the perception of sweetness, that is, the T1R2 and T1R3 GPCRs. The perception of sweetness and bitter are not confused because these GPCRs are found in different taste cells that each send their own taste information to the brain. The GPCR mechanisms for sweet and umami are illustrated in Figure 7.4.

Mechanisms for Salty and Sour Taste Perceptions

The perceptions of saltiness and sourness are conveyed through the entry of, respectively, Na^+ and H^+ into what are known as **amelioride-sensitive Na+ channels** (so-called because these channels are blocked by the drug amelioride).

Entry of H^+ or Na^+ depolarizes the taste cells, which leads to the opening of voltage-gated Na^+ and Ca^{2+} channels. For sourness-detecting cells, this also causes K^+ to exit the cell. In both cases, this leads to the release of neurotransmitter molecules (possibly 5-HT) into the synaptic cleft, stimulating sensory afferent fibers. These processes are illustrated in Figure 7.5.

FIGURE 7.4

The G-protein-coupled receptor mechanisms associated with the perception of (a) sweet and (b) umami.

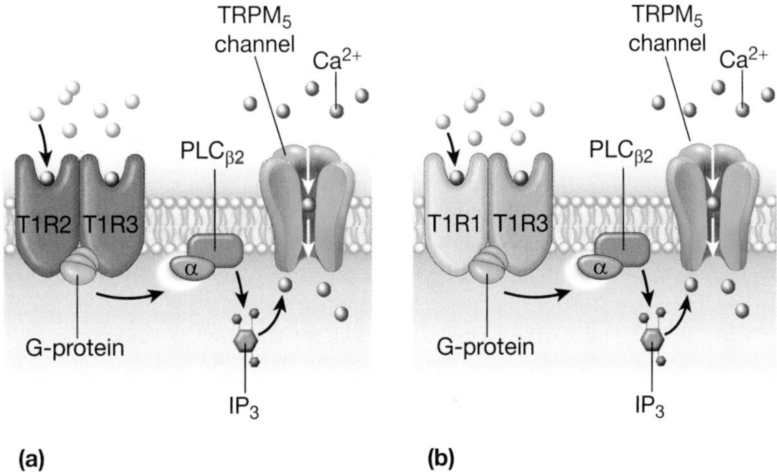

Amanda Tomasikiewicz/Body Scientific Intl.

FIGURE 7.5

Mechanisms for both (left) salty and (right) sour tastes. In both cases, the entry of ions (Na^+ and H^+) into the taste cell leads to depolarization, which causes voltage-gated Na^+ and Ca^{2+} channels to open (also K^+ channels for sourness-detecting cells), leading to the release of neurotransmitter molecules.

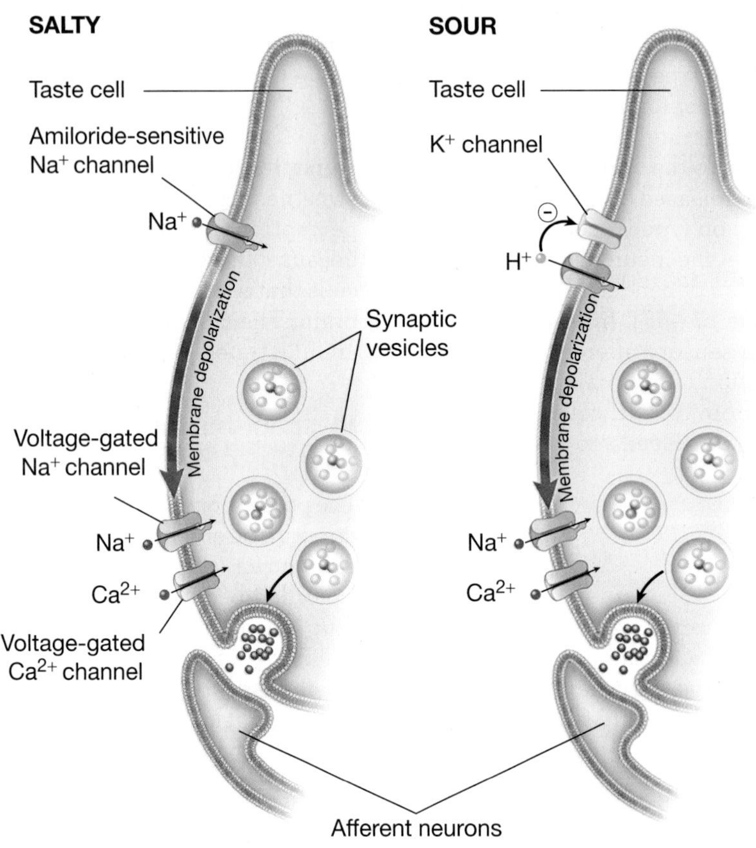

Amanda Tomasikiewicz/Body Scientific Intl.

IT'S A MYTH!

The Tongue Map

The Myth

You may have learned, growing up, that there are four basic tastes—sweet, salty, sour, and bitter—and more recently that there is a fifth taste called umami. Another thing that you may have learned is that each of the four basic tastes is sensed by a specific area of the tongue. That is, sweet is sensed in the front, salty a little further back and to the sides, bitter at the back, and sour on the central edges, as shown in Figure 1. This is known as the tongue map. Although this has been taken for a fact, it does not correspond to experience and is a myth.

Where Does This Myth Come From?

This myth has been around since the early 1900s and has even made its way into textbooks, misleading schoolchildren and adults alike. It comes from a study conducted by German psychologist D. P. Hanig, who asked people to rate the intensity of the taste they experienced when he applied the different taste qualities to different parts of their tongues. What he found was that people showed minute differences in sensitivity for the four basic tastes in different parts of the tongue, not that different parts of the tongue were

FIGURE 1

The tongue map.

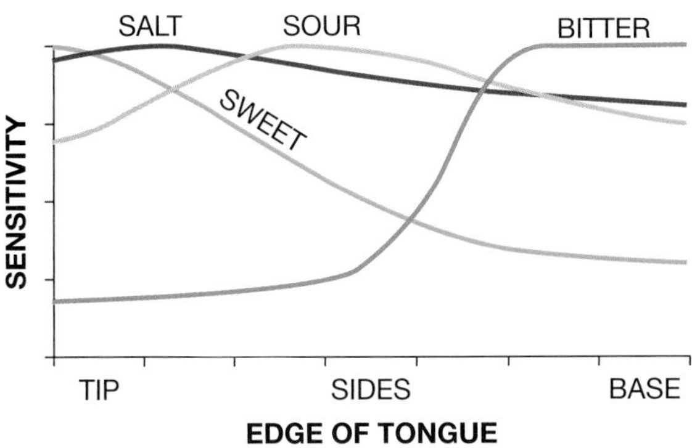

istock.com/ PeterHermesFurian

solely dedicated to processing a single taste (Hanig, 1901). However, Hanig graphed the sensitivities in a confusing way that led to misinterpretation (Figure 2). We owe the famous tongue map to Harvard University psychologist E. G. Boring (Boring, 1942), who quantified Hanig's findings and sketched a map of sensitivities to different tastes on a tongue (see Figure 1).

Why Is the Myth Wrong?

The fact is that taste buds are spread out within papillae all over the tongue and that each taste bud contains taste receptor cells that are responsive to each of the taste qualities. This was investigated in 1974 by Virginia B. Collings and confirmed that all parts of the tongue are responsive to each one of the basic tastes (Collings, 1974). Another myth that the tongue map has helped to perpetuate is the belief that we perceive *four* basic tastes. A fifth taste called *umami*, which is a Japanese word for "tasty," was proposed by Japanese chemist Kikunae Ikeda in 1908. Umami is a brothy and savory

FIGURE 2

Hanig's graph of taste sensitivities.

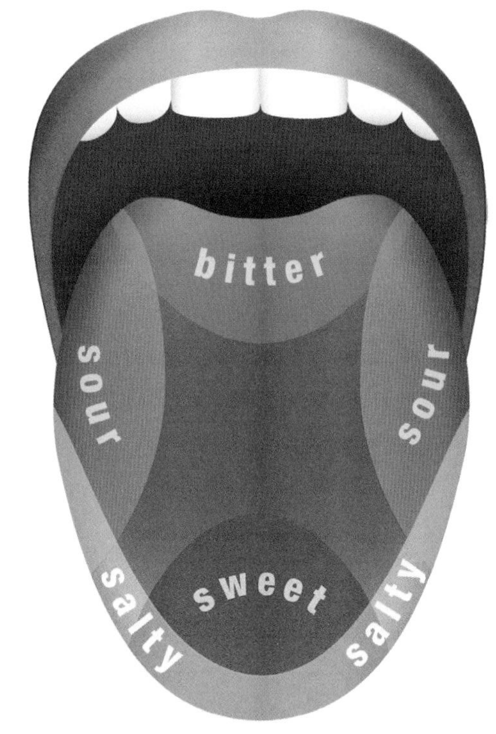

Drawing by Hanig 1901.

taste in foods such as cheese, meat, and fish. Nirupta Chaudari and colleagues confirmed that umami is indeed another basic taste and is conveyed through receptor cells that respond to glutamate (Chaudhari, Landin, & Roper, 2000). Today, there are several other candidates for qualification as one of the basic tastes. For example, a proposed sixth taste is *kokumi*, Japanese for "heartiness," which enhances sweet, salty, and umami (Ohsu et al., 2010). ●

7.1.4 TASTE PERCEPTION: BEYOND TASTE RECEPTOR CELLS

>> LO 7.1.4 Explain how and where in the brain the experience of taste arises.

Key Terms

- **Gustatory pathway:** The pattern of neuronal connections from taste receptor cells to the gustatory cortex.
- **Solitary nucleus**: A collection of cell bodies located in the medulla oblongata within the brainstem.
- **Ventral-posterior medial nucleus:** The area of the thalamus that processes gustatory information.
- **Chemotopic organization:** The concept that different areas within the gustatory cortex are dedicated to the perception of each taste.

The pattern of neuronal connections that lead to taste perception, from the activation of taste receptor cells to

FIGURE 7.6

The gustatory pathway. The flow of information from the activation of taste receptor cells to the gustatory cortex. CN = cranial nerve.

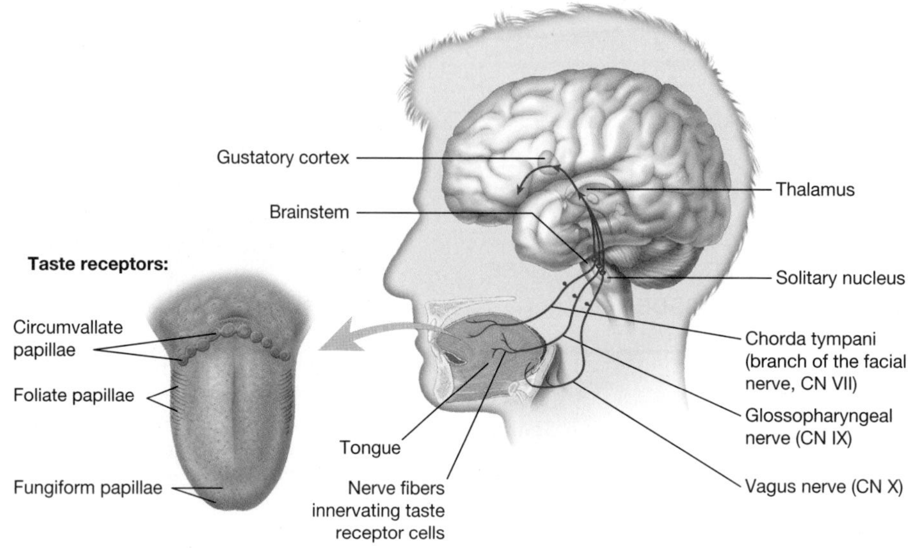

the gustatory cortex, is known as the **gustatory pathway**, illustrated in Figure 7.6. Following the activation of taste receptor cells, taste information is transferred to the **solitary nucleus**, a collection of cell bodies located in the medulla oblongata within the brainstem, via cranial nerves. Information from the anterior two-thirds of the tongue is carried along what is known as the chorda timpani branch of the facial nerve (cranial nerve VII), whereas information from the posterior one-third of the tongue is conveyed through the glossopharyngeal nerve (cranial nerve IX). The vagus nerve (cranial nerve X) conveys information from taste buds on the epiglottis situated at the very back of the mouth. From the nucleus of the solitary tract, information is relayed to the **ventral-posterior medial nucleus** of the thalamus before arriving at the gustatory cortex, also known as the primary taste cortex, which includes the insula.

Different areas within the gustatory cortex are dedicated to the perception of each taste. This is known as **chemotopic organization**. However, researcher Mircea A. Schoenfeld and colleagues (2004) found that, although the location for each taste is stable within an individual's gustatory cortex, the locations vary across individuals. This means that you and I may represent different tastes in different areas of our respective gustatory cortices. In Schoenfeld and colleagues' study, subjects were presented with different taste stimuli while their brains were scanned by functional magnetic resonance imaging (fMRI). The results for six participants are illustrated in Figure 7.7.

FIGURE 7.7

Chemotopic organization of taste perception in six participants as measured by fMRI. Note the differences in organization across the participants. MSG = monosodium glutamate.

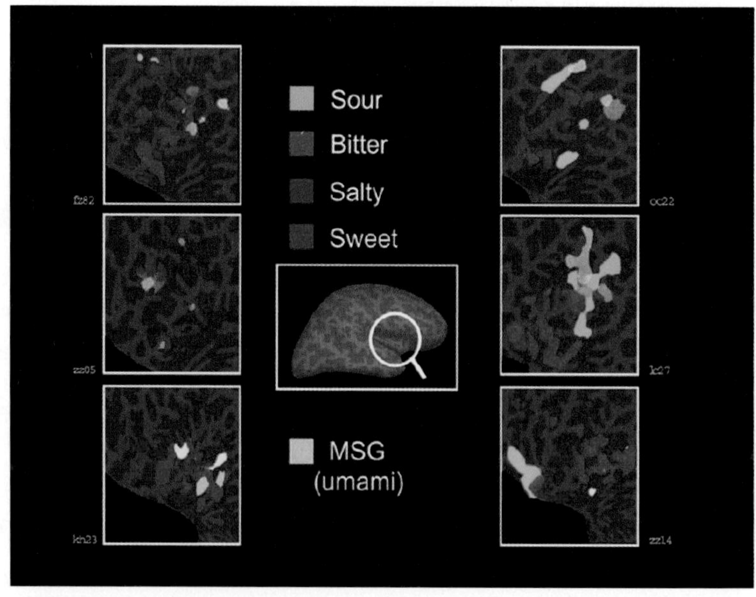

MODULE SUMMARY

Taste (gustatory perception) is generated when chemical molecules dissolved in saliva bind to and stimulate gustatory receptors. Stimulation of gustatory receptors is not enough to give rise to all the perceptual qualities of foods. Flavor is the total perceptual experience provided by food. It also includes mouth-feel, which includes a food's texture, temperature, and coolness. The hedonics of food refers to a person's perception of the pleasantness of a food when ingested. Smell also plays an important role in a food's flavor. Gustatory receptors are contained within taste buds, which are located inside papillae located on the tongue. There are three types of papillae: fungiform, foliate, and vallate (or circumvallate). There are three types of receptor cells: type I, type II, and type III. Type I cells are responsible for saltiness. Type II cells are responsible for the tastes of sweet, sour, bitter, and umami. The sweet and umami tastes are conveyed through G-protein-coupled receptors. Salty and sour tastes are transduced directly through the entry of Na^+ through Na^+ channels. The pattern of connections that lead from gustatory receptors to the gustatory cortex is called the gustatory pathway. Different areas within the gustatory cortex are dedicated to the perception of each taste. This is known as gustatory perception.

TEST YOURSELF

7.1.1 What makes up the experience of taste?

7.1.2 Describe the structure and functioning of taste receptors.

7.1.3 How do taste receptors transmit taste information to the brain?

7.1.4 Where in the brain does the experience of taste arise? How is the experience of taste generated?

7.2 Smell

Module Contents

Learning Objectives

7.2.1 Explain what makes up the experience of smell.

7.2.2 Describe the structure and functioning of olfactory receptor neurons.

7.2.3 Explain how and where in the brain the experience of smell arises.

7.2.4 Explain what pheromones are as well as their functions and the mechanisms by which they affect behavior.

7.2.1 WHAT IS SMELL AND WHAT IS IT MADE OF?

>> LO 7.2.1 Explain what makes up the experience of smell.

Key Terms

- **Odorants:** Chemical molecules from the air that bind to specialized receptors within the nasal cavity, ultimately giving rise to the perception of odors.
- **Olfactory receptor neurons (ORNs):** Cells on which olfactory sensory receptors are located.
- **Orthonasal route:** The pathway to the olfactory bulb followed by airborne molecules that have entered the nostrils.
- **Retronasal route:** The pathway to the olfactory bulb followed by molecules that have entered the mouth.

Smell (olfactory perception) is the perception generated when airborne molecules (called **odorants**) bind to specialized receptors within the nasal cavity. These receptors are embedded in **olfactory receptor neurons (ORNs)**. When bound to by odorants, these receptors trigger ORNs to send olfactory information to the brain, in the form of action potentials, where they are interpreted as odors.

The smell of any single stimulus is made up of a mixture of odorants. For example, the smell of a rose is made up of a mixture of 257 molecules (Ohloff, 1994).

The number of smells that humans can potentially discriminate is astronomical. It was once believed that humans can discriminate approximately 10,000 smells (Gilbert, 2008; Kandel, 2013). However, it was recently estimated that humans have the capacity to discriminate among more than 1 trillion smells (Bushdid, Magnasco, Vosshall, & Keller, 2014).

Odorants make it to ORNs not only through the nose but also through the back of your throat. The pathway that airborne molecules follow to the olfactory bulb is known as the **orthonasal route**, whereas the pathway that molecules follow through the inside of your mouth is called the **retronasal route** (Bojanowski & Hummel, 2012). Molecules that follow the retronasal route contribute to flavor (E. Goldberg, Wang, Goldberg, & Aliani, 2018). However, researchers also found that the perception of odors may depend on whether airborne molecules follow the orthonasal or retronasal route (Hannum, Stegman, Fryer, & Simons, 2018).

7.2.2 OLFACTORY RECEPTOR NEURONS

>> LO 7.2.2 Describe the structure and functioning of olfactory receptor neurons.

Key Terms

- **Cilia:** Hairlike projections on which olfactory receptors are located.
- **Olfactory epithelium:** Layer of cells deep inside the nostrils made up of olfactory receptor neurons and supporting cells.
- **Glomeruli:** Structures that contain different types of neurons.
- **Mitral/tuft cells:** The first neurons contacted by olfactory receptor neurons within glomeruli.
- **Lateral olfactory tract:** Formed by the axons of mitral/tuft cells, which transmit olfactory information to the cortex.
- **Odotopic mapping:** The mapping of odors in the olfactory bulb.

The sensory receptor cells to which odorants bind are located on hairlike projections referred to as **cilia**. Along with supporting cells, ORNs form the **olfactory epithelium** situated deep inside each of your nostrils (Figure 7.8). Humans possess approximately 5 million ORNs, which are subdivided into about 350 types. This contrasts greatly with other species. For example, dogs have more than 220 million ORNs. This partly accounts for their greatly enhanced sense of smell compared to humans (Niimura & Nei, 2007). Each type of ORN is responsive to only one odorant molecule. However, one odorant molecule can bind to more than one ORN.

The binding of odorant molecules to ORNs causes them to depolarize and to send olfactory information to structures called **glomeruli** (singular: *glomerulus*) located within the olfactory bulb. The olfactory bulb contains approximately 2,000 glomeruli. As shown in Figure 7.9a, ORNs that respond to the same odorant molecule send their axons to the same glomerulus. Within glomeruli, ORNs synapse with **mitral** and **tuft cells (M/T cells)**. The axons of the M/T cells form the **lateral olfactory tract**, which transmits olfactory information to the cortex.

The patterns of glomeruli activated by these neurons in response to the binding of an odorant are mapped within the olfactory bulb. The mapping of an odor within the olfactory bulb is known as **odotopic mapping** (Figure 7.9b).

The relationship between odorant molecules and receptors is that of a lock-and-key like the one between neurotransmitters and their receptors (Figure 7.10a). As illustrated in Figure 7.10b, each of the odors you can perceive results from a combination of odorant molecules, each binding to a particular combination of receptors.

FIGURE 7.8

An olfactory receptor neuron. Odorants bind to sensory receptors on cilia found on ORNs.

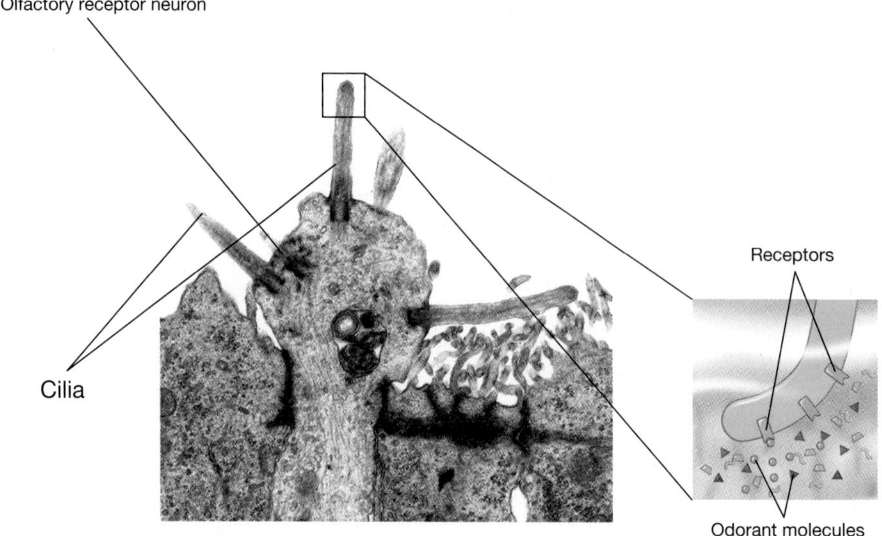

Steve Gschmeissner/Science Source

FIGURE 7.9

(a) Path followed by olfactory information from the binding of odorant molecules to receptors to the transfer of olfactory information from the olfactory bulb to the cortex. (b) Odotopic mapping of an odorant in the olfactory bulb.

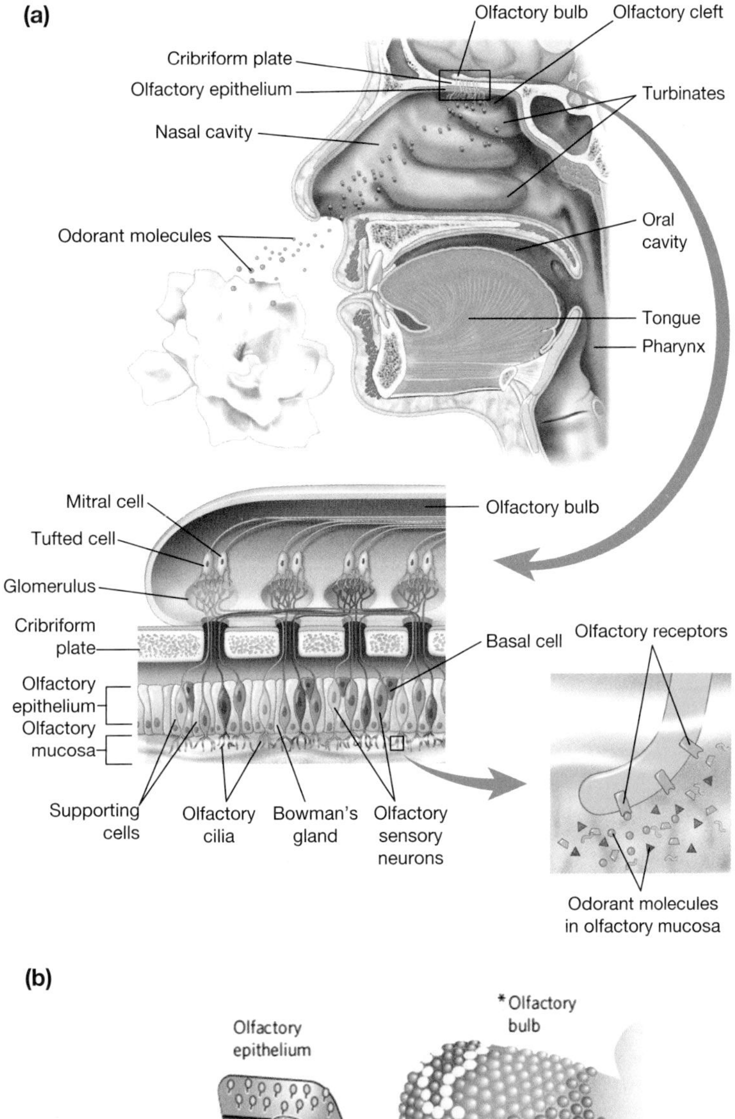

Transduction Mechanism in Olfactory Receptor Neurons

Transduction in ORNs occurs through activation of metabotropic receptors, which are bound to by the specific odorant molecules that fit them. This process is illustrated in Figure 7.11. The binding of an odorant to a G-protein-coupled receptor results in the conversion of adenosine triphosphate (ATP) to cyclic

FIGURE 7.10

(a) The same odorant molecule fits several olfactory receptors. (b) Perceived odors depend on odorant molecules binding to a particular combination of receptors.

(a) Odorant molecules

Receptors

(b)

Odorant receptors / Odorants	1	2	3	4	5	6	7	8	9	10	11	12	13	14	Description
A					●										rancid, sour, goat-like
B		●				●									sweet, herbal, woody
C	●			●	●		●			●	●				rancid, sour, sweaty
D		●			●	●									violet, sweet, woody
E	●			●	●		●	●		●	●	●			rancid, sour, repulsive
F				●	●		●			●					sweet, orange, rose
G	●			●	●		●	●		●		●		●	waxy, cheese, nut-like
H				●	●		●			●		●			fresh, rose, oily floral

(a) Adapted from *Physiology and Behavior*, 11th Edition, Carlson, Pearson Education Limited, 2014.

FIGURE 7.11

Transduction in ORNs occurs when odorant molecules bind to G-protein-coupled receptors.

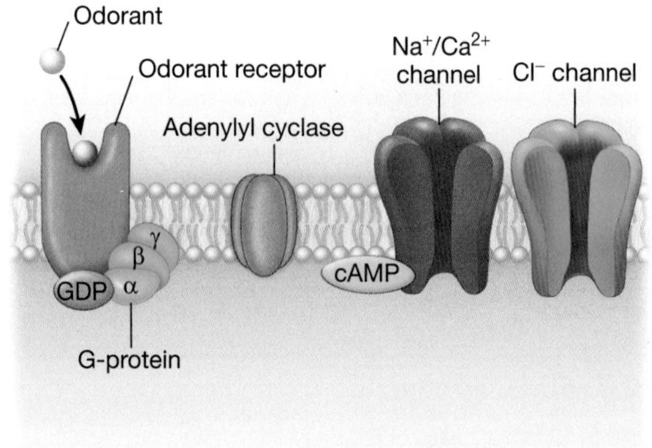

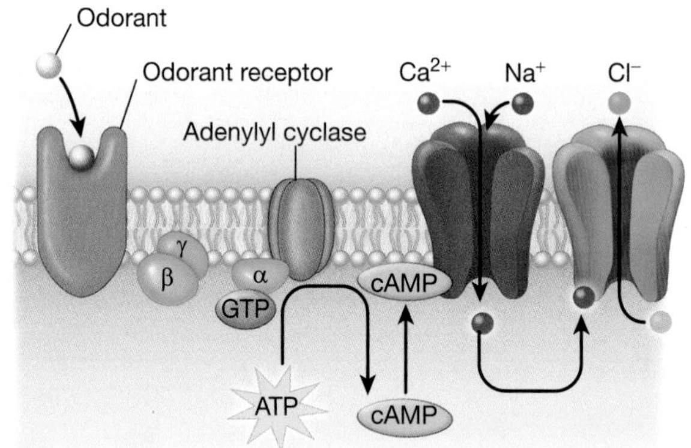

Amanda Tomasikiewicz/Body Scientific Intl.

adenosine monophosphate (cAMP), as described in Chapter 3.

Action potentials are initiated when cAMP induces the opening of Na^+/Ca^{2+} channels. The influx of these ions causes the cell to depolarize, triggering action potentials that travel up to the axon terminals of olfactory receptor cells, which synapse on the dendrites of M/T cells in the olfactory bulb. Note that Ca^{2+} also binds to receptors on Cl^- channels. The binding of Ca^{2+} to these receptors causes Cl^- channels to open, resulting in the outflow of Cl^- from the ORN, facilitating its depolarization.

7.2.3 BEYOND THE OLFACTORY BULB

>> LO 7.2.3 **Explain how and where in the brain the experience of smell arises.**

Key Terms

- **Anosmia:** The loss of the sense of smell.

- **Accessory olfactory bulb:** The part of the olfactory bulb that receives projections from the vomeronasal organ.

Figure 7.12 shows the pattern of projections of M/T cells, through the lateral olfactory tract, to the olfactory bulb. Unlike every other sense, olfactory information does not travel from sensory receptors directly to a dedicated site in the thalamus. Rather, information from the olfactory bulb is conveyed directly to a set of brain areas for further processing. The loss of the sense of smell is a condition known as **anosmia**. In Pamela's case (see opening vignette), the cause of her anosmia was unclear. However, anosmia may result from damage to olfactory sensory neurons, the olfactory bulb, or the lateral olfactory tract, or it may be due to aging (Doty, 2018; Li & Lui, 2019).

Mitral cells transmit information to the anterior olfactory nucleus, olfactory tubercle, piriform cortex (also known as the primary olfactory cortex), amygdala, and entorhinal cortex. Tuft cells project to only two of these areas: the anterior olfactory nucleus and the olfactory tubercle. Another projection arises from the **accessory olfactory bulb**, which projects to the amygdala and receives information from the vomeronasal organ, discussed in the next unit.

The anterior olfactory nucleus projects to the contralateral olfactory bulb (the olfactory bulb on the other side of the brain). The olfactory tubercle, piriform cortex, amygdala, and entorhinal cortex all send information directly to the frontal cortex and indirectly to the orbitofrontal cortex through the thalamus.

Both the amygdala and the accessory olfactory bulb send projections to the hypothalamus. In addition to the entorhinal cortex's projections to the

FIGURE 7.12

(a) Projections from M/T cells to various brain areas along the lateral olfactory tract. Also shown is the projection from the vomeronasal organ to the accessory olfactory bulb. (b) Midsagittal view of the flow of olfactory information from the activation of an ORN to various brain areas.

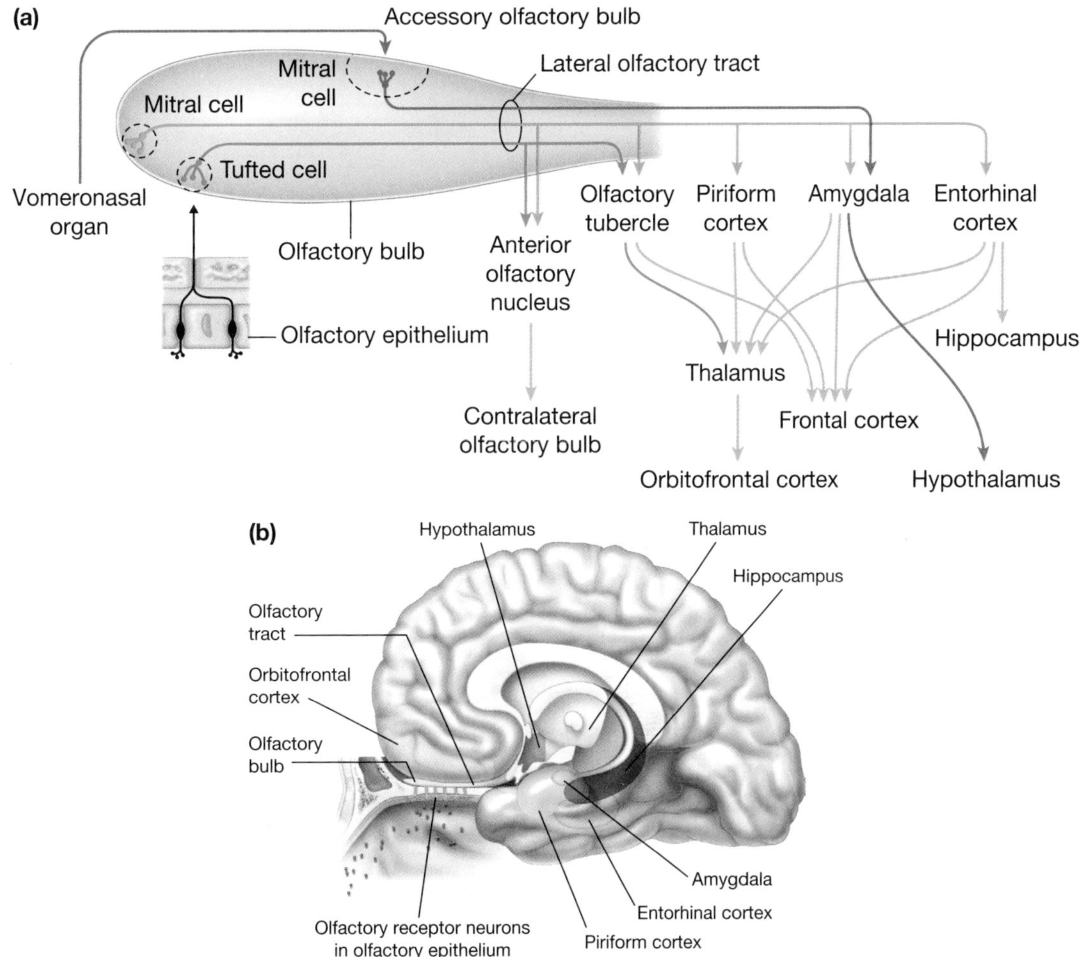

(a) Amanda Tomasikiewicz/Body Scientific Intl.

frontal cortex and thalamus, it sends information to the hippocampus.

Processing of Olfactory Information in the Cortex

As described earlier, the processing of olfactory information begins with the binding of odorant molecules to ORNs in the olfactory epithelium. As shown in Figure 7.13, each type of ORN that responds to only one odorant molecule converges on a single glomerulus in the olfactory bulb, where they synapse with M/T neurons. In turn, M/T neurons convey information to the piriform cortex (Bekkers & Suzuki, 2013). Because odors are composed of a combination of odorant molecules, each gives rise to a pattern of activation of glomeruli, known as an odotopic map.

As you learned in Chapter 6, the locations of photoreceptors in the retina, as well as the locations of hair cells in the basilar membrane, are mapped within the corresponding sensory cortices. This is known as retinotopic and tonotopic mapping, respectively.

In contrast, the olfactory system does not map odors in the same way. This is made obvious in Figure 7.13. The different-colored shapes represent the synapses formed by the axons of M/T cells with neurons in the piriform cortex. Notice how the mapping of ORNs in specific glomeruli is completely undone in the piriform cortex.

Researchers found that information from each ORN is mapped onto neurons located at seemingly random sites within the piriform cortex (Stettler & Axel, 2009). In addition, information from different olfactory neurons can converge on the same site in the piriform cortex and single neurons in the piriform cortex can receive information from several ORNs. So how does the piriform cortex convey the identity of odors? In one study, a method called optical imaging was used to identify patterns of neuronal activity induced by several odors in the piriform cortex of mice. Optical imaging uses a fluorescent dye that changes in its fluorescence intensity depending on the activity of neurons, which can be detected with a fluorescence microscope.

The results of this study are shown in Figure 7.14. The sniffing of octanol, a fruity smell commonly used in perfumes, by mice resulted in the activity of a particular set of neurons in the piriform cortex.

The image of this activity was then superimposed onto the image of the activity produced by other odorants such as ionone (the smell of violets), ethyl butyrate (the smell of apples and bananas), citronellal (the smell of lemon), butyric acid (the smell of sweat or spoiled cheese or milk), and pinene (the smell of pine). Although these smells gave rise to different patterns of activity, there was considerable overlap in their representations.

This organization of olfactory input in the piriform cortex is the same, or similar, in different individuals. This may be why we can usually agree on what something smells like. Input to the piriform cortex from the olfactory bulb occurs in two main areas of the piriform cortex: the anterior piriform and the posterior piriform. The anterior piriform conveys the identity of an odor, whereas the posterior piriform conveys the quality of an odor.

The Entorhinal Cortex

The entorhinal cortex, with its extensive connections with the hippocampus, is important for odor memory (Otto & Eichenbaum, 1992; Petrulis, Alvarez, & Eichenbaum, 2005). As you will read in Chapter 12, the hippocampus is important for episodic memories,

FIGURE 7.13

The molecules of an odorant bind to a combination of olfactory receptors in the olfactory epithelium. This, in turn, activates glomeruli in a particular pattern in the olfactory bulb, in what is known as odotopic mapping. However, this pattern of activity is not obviously mapped by neurons in the piriform cortex (primary olfactory area).

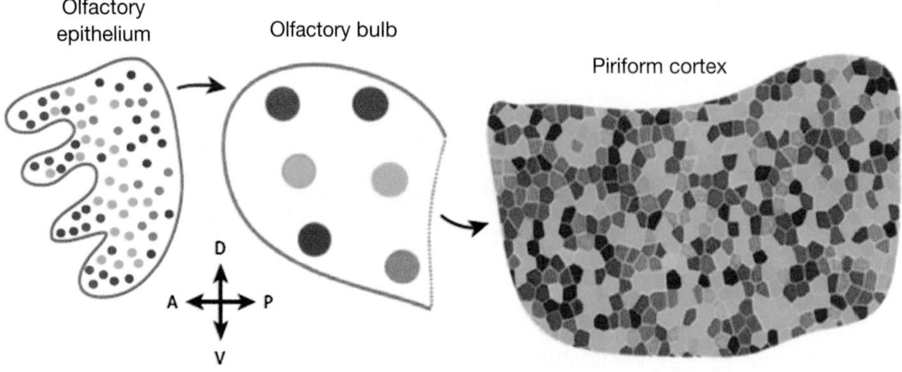

Bekkers, J. M. and N. Suzuki (2013). Neurons and circuits for odor processing in the piriform cortex. *Trends in Neurosciences 36*(7): 429–438. With permission from Elsevier.

FIGURE 7.14

The sniffing of odors by mice gave rise to particular patterns of electrical activity in neurons of the piriform cortex.

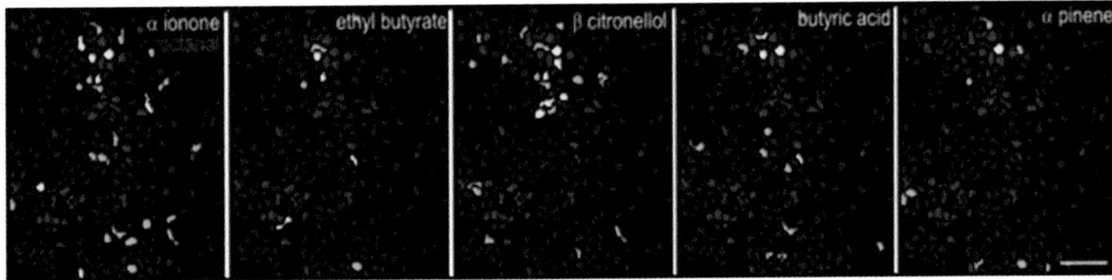

Stettler, D. D. and R. Axel (2009). Representations of odor in the piriform cortex. *Neuron 63*(6): 854–864. With permission from Elsevier.

which are memories for specific episodes of your life. Now you know why certain smells can serve as powerful reminders of your past.

The Orbitofrontal Cortex, the Amygdala, and the Hypothalamus

The orbitofrontal cortex is the site in which information from the gustatory and olfactory systems converges (Small & Prescott, 2005). This convergence of information combines taste and smell in what is known as flavor. Projections to the orbitofrontal cortex are also important for odor discrimination.

The functions of the orbitofrontal cortex combine with those of the amygdala to give odors their emotional significance (Kadohisa, 2013; Soudry, Lemogne, Malinvaud, Consoli, & Bonfils, 2011). The orbitofrontal cortex also processes the valence of smells, that is, whether you perceive an odor as being pleasant or unpleasant. The amygdala processes the intensity of odors. Because odors that are aversive to us are generally intense, it is the amygdala that produces the emotion of disgust in response to foul odors.

The hypothalamus is also involved in linking odors with food intake. I am sure you have experienced becoming hungry when smelling the odor of certain foods. In many species, the hypothalamus also links odors with mate selection and reproductive behaviors.

7.2.4 PHEROMONES

>> LO 7.2.4 Explain what pheromones are as well as their functions and the mechanisms by which they affect behavior.

Key Terms

- **Pheromones:** Chemicals (hormones) that are secreted outside of an individual's body, which can trigger specific reactions in other individuals of the same species.
- **Releaser effects**: Effects that trigger stereotypic behaviors, such as emotional responses or anxiety in other individuals as well as the attraction of females by males.
- **Primer effects:** Effects that affect development, such as the acceleration of puberty in young females.
- **Vomeronasal organ:** Also known as Jacobson's organ; part of the accessory olfactory system that sends information about pheromones to the accessory olfactory bulb.
- **Grueneberg ganglion:** An organ involved in detecting alarm signals from conspecifics.
- **Septal organ of Masera:** An organ for which the function is still a mystery, but it is suspected to serve alerting functions.

What Are Pheromones?

Pheromones are chemicals (hormones) that are secreted outside of an individual's body, which can trigger specific reactions in other individuals of the same species (Fleischer & Krieger, 2018; Gaston, Shorey, & Saario, 1967). Pheromones can have two types of effects: releaser effects and primer effects. **Releaser effects** are those that trigger stereotypic behaviors. They can elicit emotional responses such as aggression or anxiety in other individuals. They can also be used by males to attract females. **Primer effects** are those that affect development, such as the acceleration of puberty in young females. Some of the known sources of pheromones are urine, saliva, sweat, and glands located around the anus (perianal region) (Wyatt, 2003).

Pheromones are detected by receptors located in the **vomeronasal organ** (also called Jacobson's organ). The vomeronasal organ is part of the accessory olfactory system. The vomeronasal organ sends information about pheromones to the accessory olfactory bulb (see Figure 7.12). This information is then transmitted to the amygdala, where emotional responses are orchestrated. In addition, we now know that other organs responsive to pheromones exist in some species. One of these is the **Grueneberg ganglion**, which is involved in detecting alarm signals from conspecifics and the **septal organ of Masera**, whose function remains largely unknown (Ma et al., 2003).

In fact, some pheromones have been shown to act in combination and produce their effects by interacting with more than one system. For example, Inagaki and colleagues (2014) identified a mixture of two chemicals (hexanal and 4-methylpentanal) released from the perianal region of rats when stressed. They also conducted an experiment to find out if rats exposed to the chemicals became more anxious than rats not exposed to the chemicals when placed in a stressful situation. To do this, they used a risk assessment behavior test.

For the test, rats were placed in an open field, a situation known to make them anxious. A piece of absorbent paper, laden with the chemical mixture or a control substance, was placed in one corner of the open field. A hiding box, in which the rats could seek refuge, was placed in the corner opposite to where the chemical mixture was located. The hiding box had a hole through which rats could stick out their heads to assess the environment.

The procedure used in the study as well as the results are illustrated in Figure 7.15. Three behaviors were assessed in rats exposed to the chemicals or

FIGURE 7.15

Experiment by Inagaki et al. (2014). (a) Mice placed inside a box were exposed to either a mixture of pheromones (hexanal and 4-methylpentanal) or a control substance. (b) Three behaviors were assessed in the mice in response to detecting either the mixture or the control substance: head-out and concealment (indicators of anxiety) and time spent outside the box (an indicator of low anxiety). Mice exposed to the pheromone mixture spent significantly more time displaying head-out behavior and concealment than mice exposed to the control substance. (c) Pheromones released from the perianal glands of mice activate different pathways that lead to the basal nucleus of the stria terminalis (BNST), which creates anxiety-related behavioral responses such as risk assessment behavior and the acoustic startle reflex. Both hexanal and 4-methylpentanal produced anxiety by activating the BNST. However, hexanal did so by activating the main olfactory bulb (MOB) through the main olfactory system (MOS), whereas 4-methylpentanal did so by activating the accessory olfactory bulb (AOB) through the vomeronasal system (VNS).

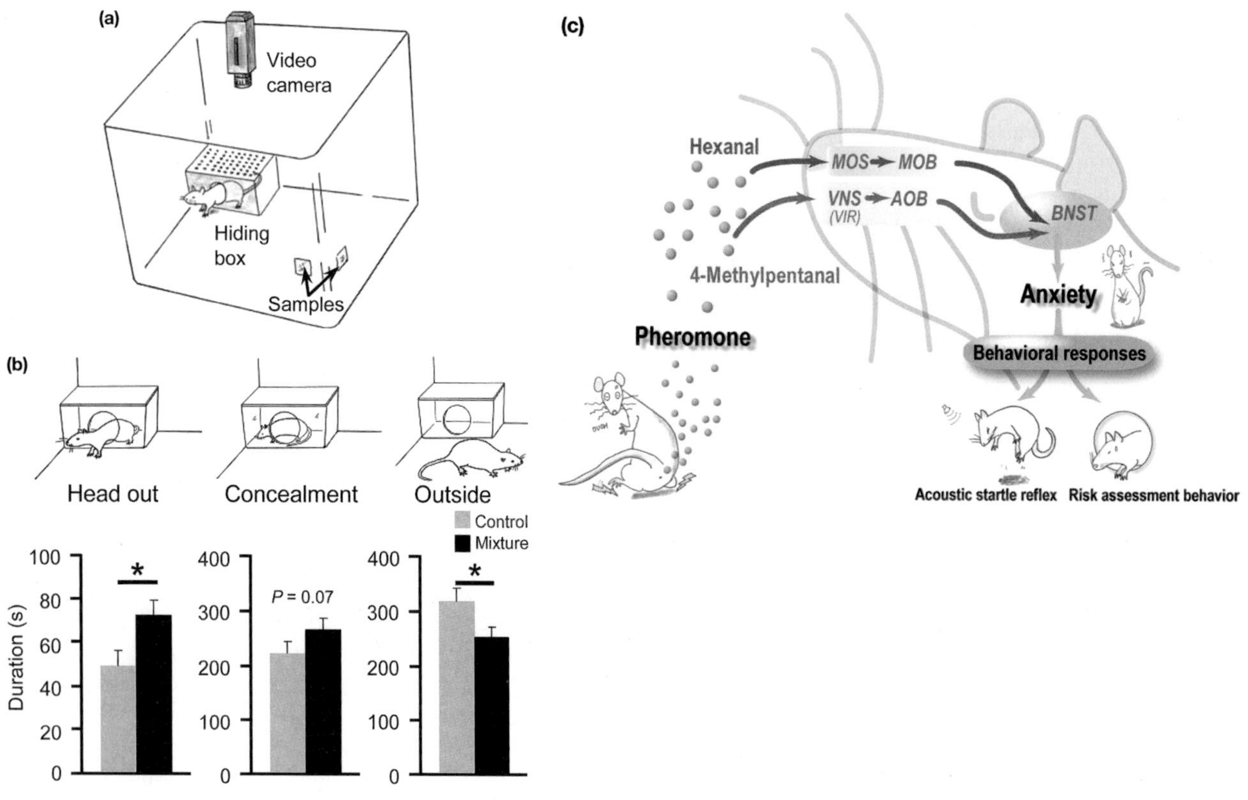

control substance: head out, concealment, and time spent outside the box. Head-out behavior and concealment were associated with high levels of anxiety, whereas the time the rats spent outside the box was associated with lower levels of anxiety. What they found was that rats exposed to the mixture of pheromones spent significantly more time displaying both head-out behavior and concealment relative to control rats. In addition, rats exposed to the mixture of pheromones spent less time outside the box. These rats were also more easily startled by a tone (acoustic startle reflex). These results indicated that the mixture of chemicals induced significant anxiety in the rats.

As mentioned earlier, pheromones may exert their effects by interacting with more than one system. Inagaki and colleagues discovered not only that a mixture of the two hormones was required to increase anxiety responses in rats but also that activation of both the main olfactory system and the vomeronasal system was required. They found that hexanal activated the main olfactory bulb through the main olfactory system but that 4-methylpentanal activated the accessory olfactory bulb through its detection by the vomeronasal system. Activity in both of these systems increased anxiety levels by activating the basal nucleus of the stria terminalis, an area related to the amygdala, which is implicated in emotional responses.

Do Humans Use Pheromones?

It is difficult to make the case for the use of pheromones by humans. First, the vomeronasal organ is not functional in humans. In addition, adult humans do not have an accessory olfactory bulb, which is the input structure for the vomeronasal organ in nonhuman animals. Second, the detection of pheromones by nonhuman animals triggers stereotypic responses such as sexual and reproductive behavior, and animals use pheromones to signal danger. In contrast, humans do not rely on stereotypic and instinctual reactions to engage in courtship or to assess potentially threatening situations; rather, they make use of higher cognitive abilities.

MODULE SUMMARY

Smell (olfactory perception) is the perception generated when molecules called odorants bind to specialized receptors within the nasal cavity. These receptors are located on the cilia of olfactory receptor neurons (ORNs). Humans can possibly discriminate among 1 trillion smells. Odorants make their way to olfactory receptors in two ways. Airborne molecules make their way to the olfactory bulb through the orthonasal route. Molecules can also make their way to the olfactory bulb through the retronasal route, which is through the mouth. When molecules bind to the receptors, their associated ORNs fire action potentials and transmit olfactory information to structures called glomeruli within the olfactory bulb. ORNs that respond to the same molecules send information to the same glomeruli. Within these glomeruli, ORNs synapse with two types of cells: mitral and tuft cells (M/T cells), which send information to the cortex through the lateral olfactory tract.

The pattern of activated ORNs is replicated in the pattern of activated glomeruli. This is called odotopic mapping. Odorant molecules fit the receptors on ORNs in a lock-and-key fashion. Each perceived odor is the result of a particular combination of odorant molecules binding to receptors. The binding of molecules to receptors triggers a response in ORNs through G-protein-coupled receptors. The axons of the M/T cells form the lateral olfactory tract, through which they send olfactory information to the cortex. Information sent to the cortex also stems from the accessory olfactory tract, which receives information from the vomeronasal organ. The targets of the tuft-cell projections are the anterior olfactory nucleus and the olfactory tubercle. The targets of the mitral cells are the piriform cortex, the amygdala, and the entorhinal cortex. Each of these areas communicates with the thalamus, with the exception of the anterior olfactory nucleus, which sends information to the contralateral olfactory bulb. The olfactory tubercle, piriform cortex, amygdala, and entorhinal cortex also communicate directly with the frontal cortex, and the thalamus with the orbitofrontal cortex. The entorhinal cortex also communicates with the hippocampus. The odotopic map formed by the pattern of activated glomeruli in the olfactory bulb seems to be undone in the piriform cortex, in which odors trigger activity in particular patterns of activation of neurons.

Pheromones are hormones that are secreted outside an individual's body. They are known to have two kinds of effects: releaser effects and primer effects. Releaser effects trigger stereotypic behaviors, whereas primer effects affect development. Pheromones are detected by receptors in the vomeronasal organ and, in some species, the Grueneberg ganglion and septal organ of Masera. Researchers have shown that some pheromones act in combination to produce their effects by acting on more than one system. For example, pheromones can work in combination to increase anxiety in animals that detect them by being processed through both the main olfactory system and the vomeronasal system.

TEST YOURSELF

7.2.1 What makes up the experience of smell?

7.2.2 Describe the structure and functioning of olfactory receptor neurons.

7.2.3 How is the experience of smell generated? Where in the brain does the experience of smell arise?

7.2.4 What are pheromones? How do they function? Through what mechanisms do they affect behavior?

7.3 Touch

Module Contents

Learning Objectives

7.3.1 Explain what makes up the sense of touch.

7.3.2 Describe and differentiate between the various types of mechanoreceptors and their functions.

7.3.3 Explain how nerve impulses are triggered by mechanoreceptors.

7.3.4 Explain how touch information is conveyed from mechanoreceptors to the brain.

7.3.5 Describe the mechanism by which pain is perceived as well as how pain can be controlled.

7.3.1 WHAT IS TOUCH AND WHAT IS IT MADE OF?

>> LO 7.3.1 Explain what makes up the sense of touch.

Key Terms

- **Interoception:** The sensing of the body's physiological condition, such as hunger and thirst.
- **Exteroception:** The sensing of innocuous touch, pain, and itch.
- **Innocuous touch:** A type of touch that does not include harmful stimulation such as pain or itch.

The sense of touch is part of a broader number of senses that are centered on the body. These senses are part of what is known as the somatosensory system. The somatosensory system comprises proprioception, interoception, and exteroception. Proprioception is the sensing of the relative position of one's own body parts and the sensing of the tension placed on muscles and joints. **Interoception** is the sensing of the body's physiological condition. For example, hunger and thirst result from the interoceptive process of detecting low glucose levels and low blood volume, respectively. These types of somatosensations are covered in Chapter 8. The focus of this chapter is **exteroception**, which includes the perceptions of pain, itch, and innocuous touch. **Innocuous touch** is touch that is not associated with pain or itch. The perception of touch arises when a stimulus comes into contact with the skin. A stimulus may stroke, stretch, apply pressure to, heat, or cool the skin. A stimulus may also vibrate the skin. Pain and itch occur when a potentially harmful stimulus is applied to the skin. As with all the other senses, innocuous touch, pain, and itch are mediated by specialized receptors.

7.3.2 MECHANORECEPTORS

>> LO 7.3.2 Describe and differentiate between the various types of mechanoreceptors and their functions.

Key Terms

- **Mechanoreceptors:** Sensory receptors that detect mechanical deformations of the skin.
- **Glabrous skin:** Hairless skin.
- **Low-threshold mechanoreceptors (LTMRs):** Mechanoreceptors for innocuous touch. These are activated by stimuli of minimal intensity.
- **High-threshold mechanoreceptors (HTMRs):** Mechanoreceptors that respond to harmful stimulation such as pain.
- **Nonneuronal capsules:** Receptors that are not neurons.
- **Afferent nerve fiber:** Sensory nerve fibers that are associated with and stimulated by nonneuronal capsules.
- **Slowly adapting fibers:** Sensory nerve fibers that keep responding to continuous contact with a stimulus.
- **Rapidly adapting fibers:** Sensory nerve fibers that respond at the initial contact with a stimulus, as well as with its removal, but will quickly stop responding with continuous stimulation.
- **Two-point discrimination test:** Test that assesses a person's ability to discriminate between two contact points on the skin.

Mechanical deformations of the skin give rise to the perception that one is in contact with a stimulus. These deformations are detected by receptors known as **mechanoreceptors**. Mechanoreceptors are found in both hairless skin, known as **glabrous skin**, and hairy skin. However, we will focus our attention only on receptors of glabrous skin. Glabrous skin is found on the palms of the hands, tips of the fingers, and soles of the feet. Note that these are the parts of the body that are often used to touch objects. Hairy skin is mainly the recipient of stimulation, such as when your skin is being stroked or massaged by another person.

Mechanoreceptors for innocuous touch have a low threshold of activation, which means they are activated by stimuli of minimal intensity. They are therefore referred to as **low-threshold mechanoreceptors (LTMRs)**. This differentiates them from **high-threshold mechanoreceptors (HTMRs)**, which respond to potentially harmful stimulation, such as stimuli associated with pain (Abraira & Ginty, 2013).

There are four types of LTMRs within glabrous skin, each one being better at detecting certain types of deformations of the skin than others. The four known mechanoreceptors are Merkel cells, Ruffini endings, Meissner corpuscles, and Pacinian corpuscles. These receptors are nonneuronal cells, meaning they are not neurons, and are sometimes referred to as **nonneuronal capsules**. Each of them is associated with a type of **afferent nerve fiber** that responds to certain types of stimulation. Out of these nonneuronal cells, only Merkel cells are found in hairy skin.

In addition to being preferentially responsive to certain types of stimulation, afferent nerve fibers can be distinguished in a variety of ways. For example, they can be distinguished by their conduction velocity, which is the speed at which action potentials travel through axons. These are Aα (A-alpha), Aβ (A-beta), Aδ (A-delta), and C fibers.

They can also be differentiated by how quickly they adapt to being in contact with a stimulus. Some are **slowly adapting fibers** (SAs), which keep responding to continuous contact with a stimulus. Slowly adapting fibers are subdivided further into SA1 fibers and SA2 fibers. The difference between SA1 and SA2 fibers lies in the pattern by which they fire action potentials. For example, the timing between action potentials is more irregular in SA1 fibers than in SA2 fibers.

There are also **rapidly adapting fibers** (RAs), which respond at the initial contact with a stimulus, as well as with its removal, but will quickly stop responding with continuous stimulation. Rapidly adapting fibers are subdivided into RA1 and RA2 fibers. The four types of mechanoreceptors of the glabrous skin, along with the types of nerve fibers associated with them, are illustrated in Figure 7.16.

RA1 fibers respond mainly to low-frequency vibration and have small receptive fields, which means they respond to stimulation of a relatively small patch of skin that surrounds them. In contrast, RA2 fibers respond mainly to high-frequency vibration and have larger receptive fields than RA1 fibers. As you can see in Figure 7.16, all mechanoreceptors have Aβ nerve fibers, which conduct action potentials at a velocity of 40–70 m/s. You can also see that each type of LTMR has a different structure and is located at different depths within the dermis. The location, type of nerve fiber, structure, function, firing patterns, and receptive fields of each LTMR are summarized in Table 7.1.

FIGURE 7.16

The types and locations of mechanoreceptors of the glabrous skin as well as the afferent nerve fibers they are associated with. The SA fibers are the Merkel cells and Ruffini endings, whereas the RA fibers are the Meissner corpuscles and Pacinian corpuscles. (SC, SL, SG, SS, and SB refer to layers of the epidermis.)

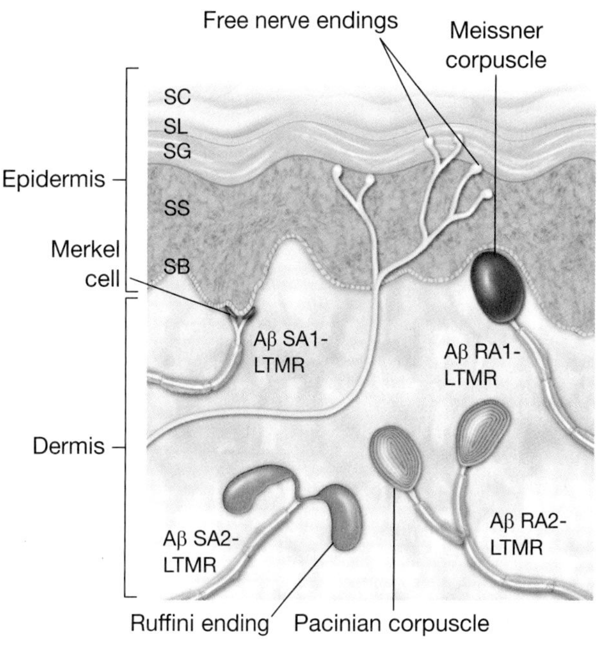

Amanda Tomasikiewicz/Body Scientific Intl.

Referring to Table 7.1, you can now think about how each LTMR is involved in exploring an object like the surface of your laptop with the tip of one of your fingers. By looking at the firing pattern of each LTMR, you can deduce the following: Merkel cells are mostly activated as you pass the tip of one of your fingers along the sides of your laptop, as you feel the sharp edges of its sides and pointy corners.

Ruffini endings are now stimulated as you press down onto one of its surfaces, while simultaneously moving your hand sideways, stretching the skin at the tip of your finger. Because these LTMRs are slowly adapting, you do not lose the feeling that you are touching the keyboard. However, the rapidly adapting LTMRs, Meissner and Pacinian corpuscles, became activated only with your initial touch of the laptop's surface and quickly stopped firing. They fired again only with the stimulation induced by lifting your finger from the surface of the laptop.

TABLE 7.1

Characteristics of Mechanoreceptors

MECHANORECEPTOR	LOCATION	NERVE FIBER	STRUCTURE	FUNCTION	FIRING PATTERN	RECEPTIVE FIELD
Merkel cells	Deepest layer of the epidermis	Aβ SA1	Oval in shape, single nerve fiber that can innervate several cells	Respond to static indentations of the skin		
Ruffini endings	Deep within the dermis	Aβ SA2	Collagen fibers encircled by unmyelinated Aβ SA2 nerve fibers	Mostly sensitive to stretching of the skin		
Meissner corpuscles	Within dermal papillae	Aβ RA1	Lamellar cells, joined together by collagen fibers	Mostly sensitive to low-frequency vibrations and motion across the skin		
Pacinian corpuscles	Deep within the dermis	Aβ RA2	End of fibers surrounded with concentric lamella	Mostly sensitive to high-frequency vibrations and motion across the skin		

If you now slowly pass your finger across the keyboard, bumping into the edges of each one of the keys simulates a low-frequency vibration, stimulating Meissner corpuscles. Increasing the speed at which you stroke the keyboard will activate Pacinian corpuscles.

You can also think about how LTMRs are involved when you have been holding an object under your arm, such as a textbook, for a while and forgot it was there, resulting in its falling to the ground as you reach out for something. Here all of your LTMRs were likely activated: (1) Merkel cells were activated by the edges and corners of the book contacting your skin, (2) Ruffini endings were activated by the stretching of your skin caused by the weight of the book pulling it downward, and (3) Meissner and Pacinian corpuscles were also activated with the initial contact of the book on your skin.

So why did you forget the book was there? You felt the book for a while after you placed it under your arm because the SA fibers of Merkel cells and Ruffini endings were active until they slowly adapted and stopped firing (this is when you stopped feeling the presence of the book). Your Meissner and Pacinian corpuscles were active only when you placed the book under your arm and then they quickly stopped firing, only to become active again when the book slipped out from under your arm.

Receptor Resolution

You learned that different mechanoreceptors have receptive fields of different sizes (see Table 7.1). Mechanoreceptors with large receptive fields collect information from wide areas of the skin but have low spatial resolution, meaning they cannot make fine discrimination about what part of the skin is being touched. Other mechanoreceptors have small receptive fields. Therefore, they collect information from a relatively small area of the skin. Mechanoreceptors with small receptive fields have high resolution, meaning they are better at making out details.

Two-Point Discrimination Test

One way to measure the resolution of the receptors in different parts of the skin is by using the **two-point discrimination test**. This test assesses a person's ability to discriminate between two contact points on the skin. Using a protractor, or other devices, the clinician or experimenter measures the distance between contact points at which a person perceives the two points as being separate. This differs significantly depending on where on the skin the test is applied.

The results of two-point discrimination tests performed on different parts of the skin are shown in Figure 7.17. Note that the minimal distance needed for a person to discriminate between two points being stimulated on the skin is much smaller at the tip of the fingers than in the middle of the back.

Why is this so? The answer has to do with the relative density and size of the receptive fields of receptors in different areas of the body. At the tip of the fingers,

FIGURE 7.17

The two-point discrimination test. (a) A protractor, or similar device, is used to stimulate the surface of the skin. When the protractor is applied to the fingertips, a person can easily tell the skin is being stimulated by two separate points. This is because receptors in the fingertips have small receptive fields, which means the two points likely each stimulate a different receptor. In contrast, receptors in the middle of the back are large. It is therefore likely that both points of the protractor stimulate the same receptor. (b) Graph showing the relationship between the part of the skin stimulated in the two-point discrimination test and the mean distance required between the two points (or threshold) of a protractor to be perceived as such. For example, when applied to the middle of the back, the two points have to be separated by at least 40 mm, versus only 5 mm or less for the tip of the fingers.

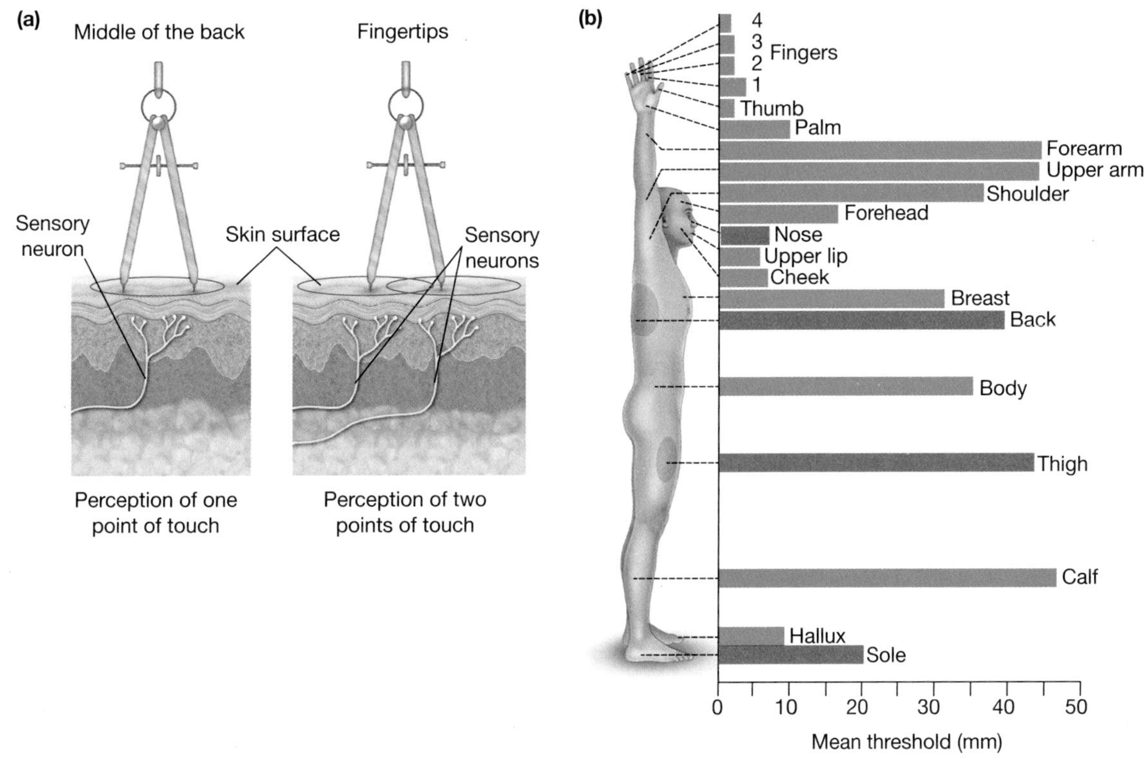

Amanda Tomasikiewicz/Body Scientific Intl.

receptors are densely packed and have small receptive fields. In contrast, the receptors in the middle of the back are less densely packed and relatively large. This means that at the tips of the fingers, the two points of the protractor stimulate patches of skin belonging to different receptive fields, telling the brain that two spots are being touched. In contrast, the same distance between the two points of the protractor fall within the same receptive field in the middle of the back, telling the brain that the same spot is being touched.

7.3.3 CONDUCTION AND MECHANORECEPTORS

>> LO 7.3.3 **Explain how nerve impulses are triggered by mechanoreceptors.**

Key Term

- **Stretch-sensitive channels:** Ion channels that open in response to indentation, stretch, or vibration of the skin.

The deformation of mechanoreceptors causes the opening of **stretch-sensitive channels** that admit Na^+ and Ca^{2+} into afferent nerve fibers, leading to their depolarization. Removal of the stimuli relieves the stretch and causes the channels to close. Three mechanisms have been proposed to explain how mechanical deformations induce the opening of stretch-sensitive channels. Two of these mechanisms lead to mechanical forces directly inducing the opening of channels. In the first of these ways, the tension caused by the stretch of the skin causes Na^+ and Ca^{2+} channels in the receptors below the stretch to open. These are known as stretch-activated channels. The Na^+ and Ca^{2+} channels in the receptors of surrounding skin may also open. These are known as tethered channels. Mechanical deformations can also trigger the opening of Na^+ and Ca^{2+} channels indirectly. That is, mechanical deformations may also be processed using second messenger pathways through what are known as indirectly gated channels.

7.3.4 BEYOND MECHANORECEPTORS

>> LO 7.3.4 **Explain how touch information is conveyed from mechanoreceptors to the brain.**

Key Terms

- **Sensory homunculus:** Map of the entire body in the somatosensory cortex.
- **Dorsal column–medial lemniscus system (DCML):** The pathway followed by afferent neurons that conduct information from mechanoreceptors to the somatosensory cortex.
- **First-order neurons:** Afferent neurons associated with mechanoreceptors.
- **Second-order neurons:** Neurons located in the medulla in the brainstem to which first-order neurons synapse.
- **Third-order neurons:** Neurons located in the thalamus to which second-order neurons synapse and that send sensory information to the somatosensory cortex.
- **Dermatome:** An area of the skin innervated by a segment of the spinal cord.

The Somatosensory Cortex

For you to feel something when a stimulus comes into contact with your skin, information conveyed through

FIGURE 7.18

Location of the somatosensory cortex (left). Somatotopic mapping of areas of the body along the somatosensory cortex (right).

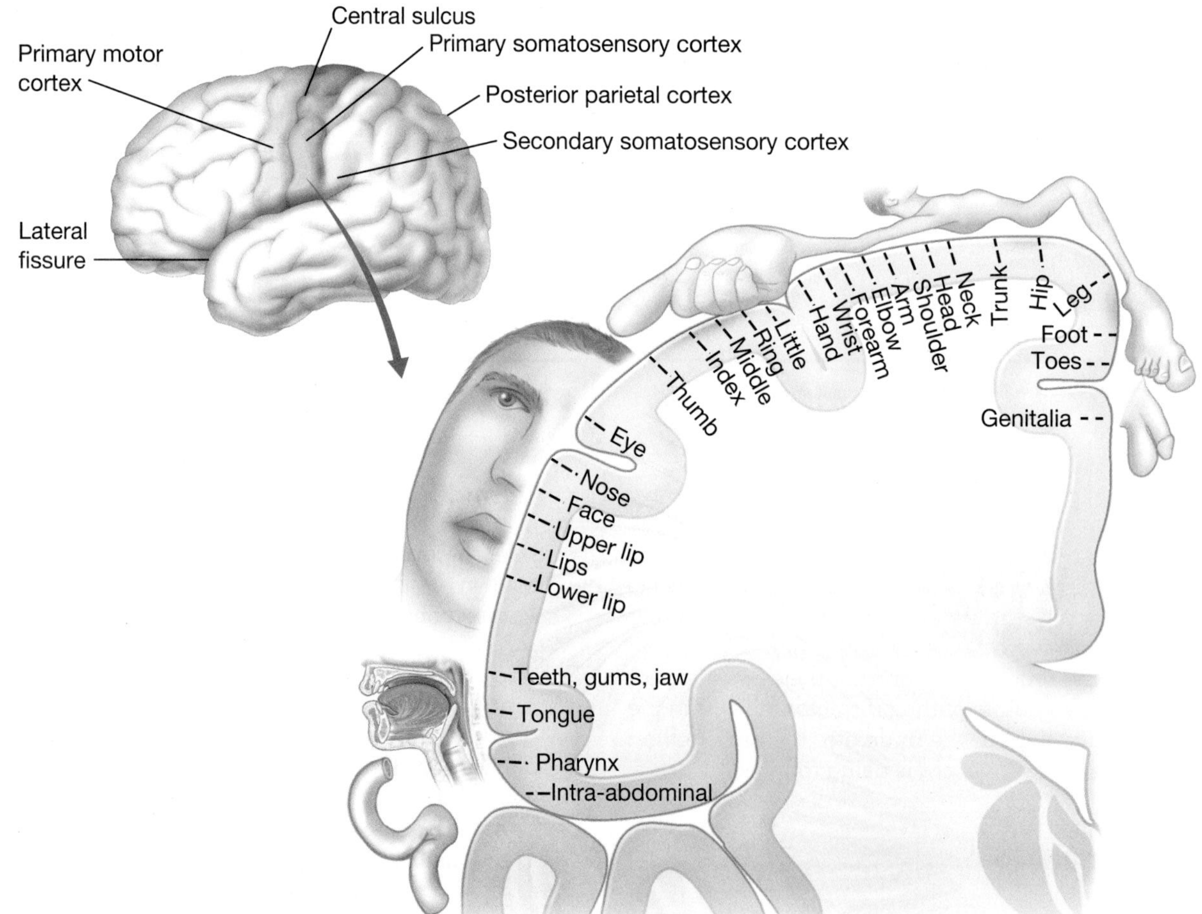

Adapted from *The Cerebral Cortex of Man*, Penfield and Rasmussen. © 1950 Gale, a part of Cengage Learning, Inc.

trains of action potential has to make it to your brain. The main brain area that processes touch is the primary somatosensory cortex, situated in the rostral-most part of the parietal lobe, just behind the primary motor cortex, which is in the frontal lobe. Because the primary somatosensory cortex lies just behind the central sulcus, it is sometimes referred to as the postcentral gyrus, as opposed to the precentral gyrus for the primary motor cortex.

As shown in Figure 7.18, the somatosensory cortex contains a map of the entire body. This map was discovered in the 1930s by Wilder Penfield, a neurosurgeon at the Montreal Neurological Institute. He discovered it by noting the part of the body in which subjects reported sensations while various areas of the cortex were stimulated.

This map of the body is represented as a homunculus (or little man), which became known as the **sensory homunculus**. Note how the size of the body parts of the homunculus are disproportionate relative to a real body. This is because, as you can see in Figure 7.18, different amounts of the somatosensory cortex are dedicated to a given body part. The amount of cortex allotted to each area of the body is proportional to the sensitivity of the given area. For example, the lips are allotted a larger area than the trunk, even if they take up considerably less space on a real body. The sensory homunculus is a representation of the sensitivity of each body part, rather than of a real body.

FIGURE 7.19

The dorsal column–medial lemniscus system (blue) carries innocuous touch information. The anterolateral system (more precisely the spinothalamic pathway [red]) carries information about pain, temperature, and crude touch.

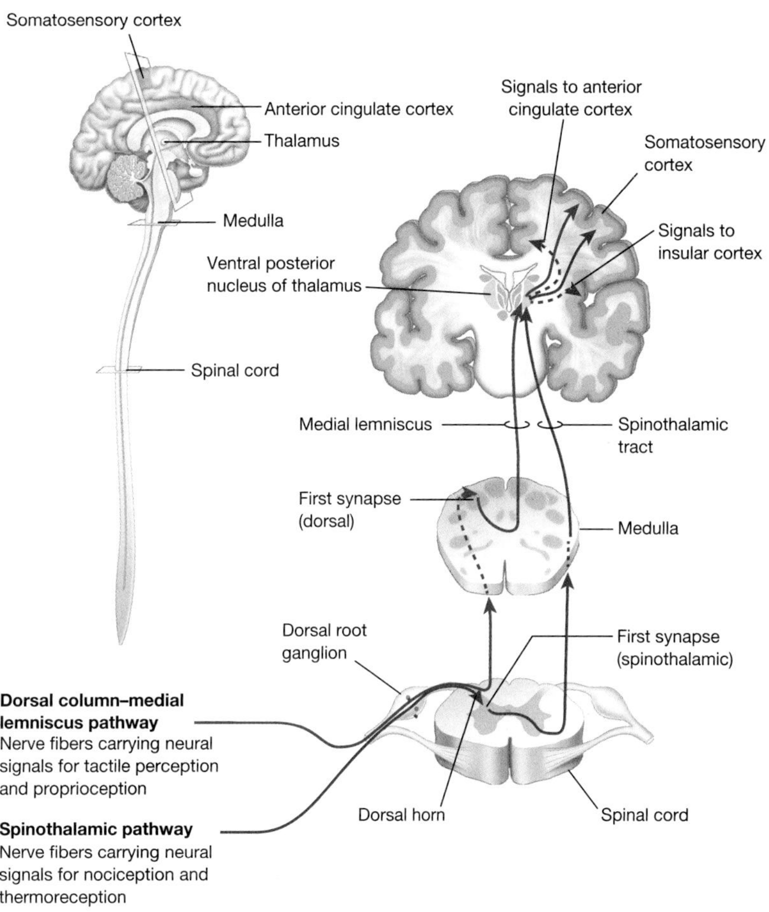

The Ascending Tracts

How does information from mechanoreceptors make it to the cortex where touch information is processed? The afferent fibers from all mechanoreceptors enter the spinal cord through the dorsal roots. From there, afferent fibers carry the information from mechanoreceptors all the way up to the brain through what are known as ascending tracts. The ascending tracts, illustrated in Figure 7.19, consist of two distinct pathways. One of these pathways is known as the **dorsal column–medial lemniscus system (DCML)**. The other pathway is known as the anterolateral system. The DCML carries information about innocuous touch (fine touch, vibration, and proprioception). The anterolateral system—more specifically, the lateral spinothalamic tract—carries information about pain (nociception), temperature (thermoception), and crude touch.

For both systems, information is first relayed by the fibers associated with the mechanoreceptors. These are referred to as **first-order neurons**. In the DCML, these terminate in the medulla, where they synapse with what are known as **second-order neurons**, which form the medial lemniscus. These second-order neurons then decussate (cross over to the other side of the spinal cord) to terminate in the ventral-posterior lateral nucleus of the thalamus, where they form synapses with **third-order neurons**. In turn, third-order neurons innervate the somatosensory cortex.

In the anterolateral system, first-order neurons terminate in the substantia gelatinosa. Second-order neurons immediately decussate to terminate in the ventral-posterior lateral nucleus of the thalamus, where they form synapses with third-order neurons. Third-order neurons innervate the somatosensory cortex, the dorsal anterior insular cortex, and the anterior cingulate cortex.

Dermatomes

You may have already guessed that afferent fibers from the different areas of the body do not all enter the DCML at the same level of the spinal cord. Indeed, they do not. The spinal cord is divided into 30 segments. Each segment has protrusions through which afferent fibers

FIGURE 7.20

(a) The 30 segments of the spinal cord through which afferent fibers enter. The areas of the skin innervated by the afferent fibers in a segment of the spinal cord are referred to as dermatomes. (b) Sensory information from areas on the face makes its way to the brain through the trigeminal and facial nerves.

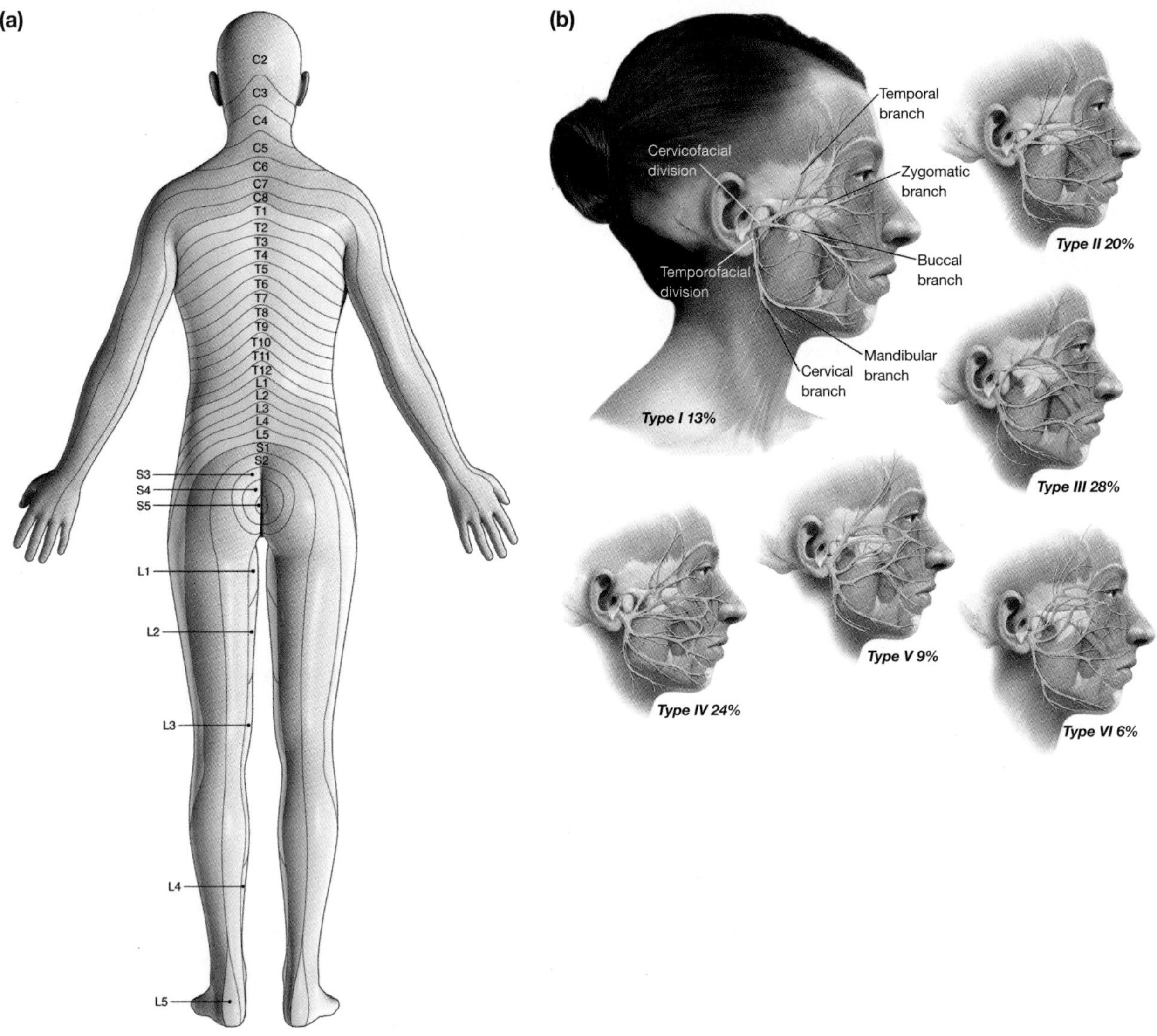

(a) Evan Oto/Science Source; (b) DNA Illustrations/Science Source

enter. These 30 segments are subdivided according to the regions of the body from which they receive afferent fibers. An area of the skin innervated by a segment of the spinal cord is known as a **dermatome** (Figure 7.20a). However, sensory information from the face is sent to the brain through the trigeminal and facial nerves, which are cranial nerves V and VII, respectively (Figure 7.20b). See Chapter 4 to review the cranial nerves.

7.3.5 PAIN

>> LO 7.3.5 **Describe the mechanism by which pain is perceived as well as how pain can be controlled.**

Key Terms

- **Nociception:** The neurobiological process that leads to the perception of pain.
- **Polymodal nociceptors:** Nociceptors, such as C nerve fibers, that respond to intense thermal, mechanical, and chemical stimulation.
- **Gate control theory:** The theory by which the transmission of nociceptive information to the brain can be inhibited by the activity of mechanoreceptors.
- **Transcutaneous electrical nerve stimulation (TENS):** A device that reduces pain through electrical stimulation.

FIGURE 7.21

The innocuous touch pathway (orange) and nociceptive pathway (blue).

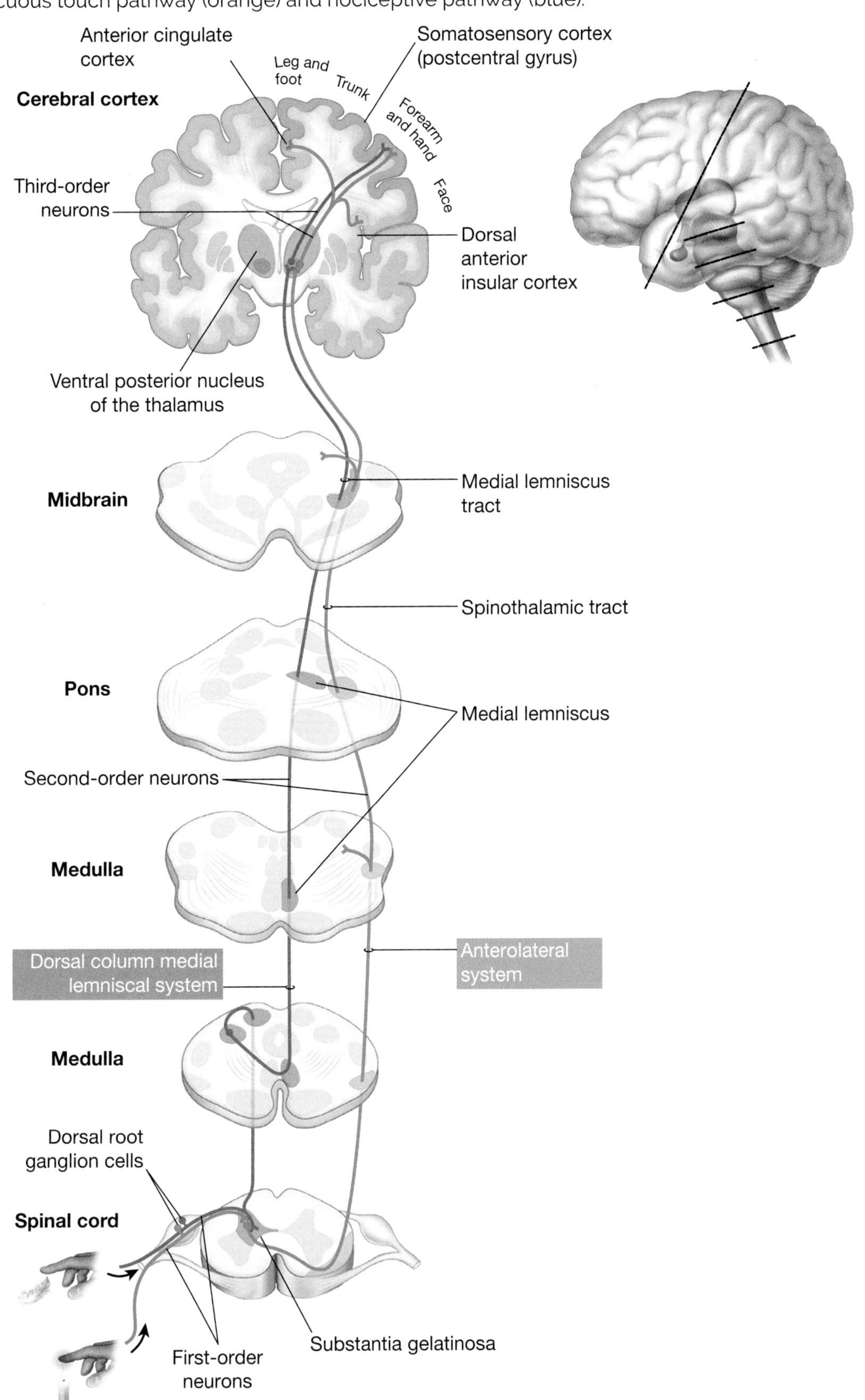

Carolina Hrejsa/Body Scientific Intl.

Pain is an unpleasant perceptual and emotional experience. Pain can be experienced in many ways. You have surely described it as throbbing, irritating, or aching. People who are in pain also often report feeling miserable or depressed. The neurobiological process that leads to the perception of pain is called **nociception**. Note, however, that pain can emerge from sources both external and internal to the body. As you know, you can feel pain from stubbing your little toe on a bedpost or from a stomachache.

Nociception requires the stimulation of receptors known as nociceptors. There are two main types of nociceptors: C fibers and Aδ fibers. Both types of nerve fibers are small when compared to those associated with the mechanoreceptors that process innocuous touch. Aδ fibers are also thinly myelinated. Both types of fibers have free nerve endings, meaning they are not encapsulated like mechanoreceptors. Because they are myelinated, Aδ fibers transmit nerve impulses faster than the unmyelinated C fibers.

Aδ fibers give rise to the perception of immediate sharp pain, like the pain you feel immediately upon stubbing your little toe. They are also thermal and mechanical nociceptors. They are activated by temperatures above 45°C (113°F) and below 5°C (41°F), which are perceived as pain. Aδ fibers also respond to intense mechanical pressure.

In contrast, C fibers are responsible for the dull aching pain you might feel in the toe you stubbed in the following hours or days. C fibers are **polymodal nociceptors**, meaning they respond to intense thermal, mechanical, and chemical stimulation.

Beyond Nociceptors: The Nociceptive Pathway

Figure 7.21 illustrates the pathway taken by information conveyed by nociceptors. The pathway for nociception differs from that of innocuous touch. It is part of what is known as the anterolateral system. In the anterolateral system, information from nociceptors crosses over to the contralateral side of the body earlier than in the DCML. It does so within the spinal cord rather than in the medulla. Note also the connection to the insula, which is known to be involved in the intensity and perceptual experience of pain (Wiech et al., 2010).

Gate Control Theory of Pain

As pain perception can be modulated by descending signals from the brain, it can also be modulated by the control of nociceptive information that comes from afferent nerve fibers in the spinal cord. Remember that non-nociceptive information from innocuous touch is carried by different nerve fibers than the ones that carry nociceptive information. Non-nociceptive information is carried by mechanoreceptors, which have large myelinated nerve fibers, whereas nociceptive information is carried by relatively small unmyelinated C fibers and thinly myelinated Aδ fibers.

In the 1960s, Patrick Wall and Ronald Melzack proposed the **gate control theory** (Melzack & Wall, 1965; Wall, 1978). The gate control theory states that nociceptive messages sent to the brain by the C and Aδ fibers can be blocked by messages sent by the comparatively large afferent fibers associated with mechanoreceptors that process innocuous touch. Figure 7.22 illustrates how this works. On their way to synapsing with second-order neurons, which bring information to the brain, fibers from both nociceptors and mechanoreceptors synapse onto inhibitory interneurons, which act as a "gate." With nerve impulses coming from only nociceptors, inhibitory interneurons are themselves inhibited, permitting nociceptive information to be passed on to the second-order neurons. However, nerve impulses from mechanoreceptors activate the inhibitory interneurons, which in turn inhibit the second-order neurons onto which C and Aδ fibers synapse. This closes the gate through which nociceptive information gets to the brain.

Can you now think about why vigorously rubbing your little toe after stubbing it against a piece of furniture helps alleviate the pain? You can thank your mechanoreceptors. This knowledge led to the development of pain management strategies and is the basis for **transcutaneous electrical nerve stimulation (TENS)**, in which small electrical currents stimulate painful areas of the body. These small nonpainful currents activate mechanoreceptors, closing the gate to nociceptors.

FIGURE 7.22

The gate control theory of pain.

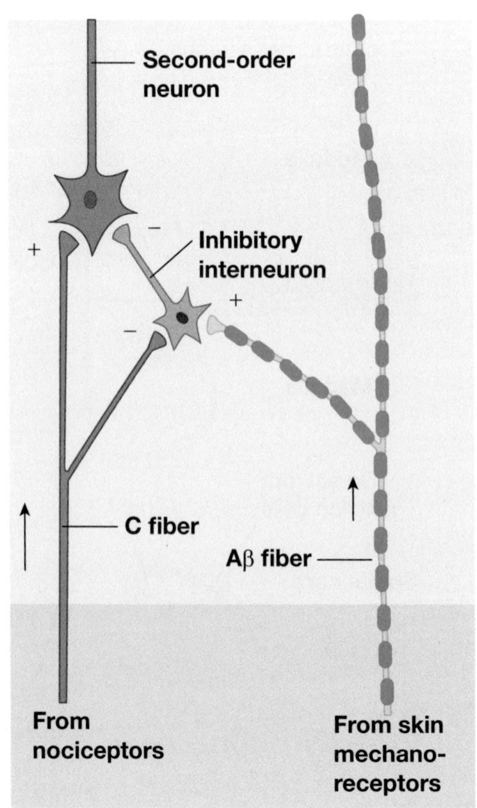

MODULE SUMMARY

Touch is part of a broader number of senses that comprise the somatosensory system, which includes proprioception, interoception, and exteroception. Exteroception includes innocuous touch, which is the result of mechanical deformations of the skin that do not arise from harmful stimuli. The receptors of innocuous touch are known as mechanoreceptors. Mechanoreceptors have a low threshold for activation and are therefore referred to as low-threshold mechanoreceptors (LTMRs). There are four types of mechanoreceptors for innocuous touch, each more sensitive to one kind of stimulation than another. These are Merkel cells, Ruffini endings, Meissner corpuscles, and Pacinian corpuscles. Activation of these receptors triggers a response, in the form of action potentials, in sensory neurons that are associated with them. This response is triggered by the opening of Na^+ and Ca^{2+} channels. These channels can be made to open in three ways. They can be stretch activated, tethered, or indirectly gated.

Touch information is processed in the primary somatosensory cortex where a map of the body called the homunculus exists. Touch information from sensory neurons is transmitted to the somatosensory cortex through the dorsal column–medial lemniscus system (DCML). Sensory neurons that carry information from different areas of the body enter the spinal cord at different segments. These segments are known as dermatomes. However, touch information from the face is carried by cranial nerves.

Pain is an unpleasant and emotional perceptual experience. The neurobiological process that leads to the perception of pain is called nociception. The receptors that respond to stimuli that provoke pain are called nociceptors. Pain can be controlled by changing the nociceptive information coming from nociceptors. In the 1960s, Ronald Melzack and colleagues found that nociceptive messages, which come from small nociceptive nerve fibers, can be blocked by the activity in the relatively large nerve fibers of innocuous touch. This became known as the gate control theory.

TEST YOURSELF

7.3.1 What is the sense of touch? Differentiate between innocuous touch and other types of touch in terms of the types of receptors and sensory nerves involved.

7.3.2 Describe each of the mechanoreceptors. How do they differ in the way they function and in their location within the skin?

7.3.3 Describe the three proposed processes by which nerve impulses are generated in somatosensory neurons.

7.3.4 Trace the journey of a nerve impulse from the stimulation of a mechanoreceptor to the brain.

7.3.5 Describe the mechanism by which pain is perceived as well as how pain can be controlled.

APPLICATIONS

Electronic Taste Stimulation

Imagine watching a cooking show on television or on your computer. Now imagine not only salivating to the sight of the wonderful dish being prepared but also being able to taste it and send your friends the corresponding taste messages through social media. We are not quite there yet, but researchers at the University of Singapore are getting close to making this possible, using what they call electronic taste stimulation (Ranasinghe, Cheok, Fernando, Nii, & Gopalakrishnakone, 2011).

What Is Electronic Taste Stimulation?

Electronic taste stimulation refers to a system that electrically stimulates taste receptor cells to simulate the sense of taste. The system consists of two submodules: a stimulator and a tongue interface. The tongue is stimulated by constant current through two pure silver electrodes. Using this method, the researchers found that they could best simulate the tastes of sourness and bitterness. The felt intensity of the tastes depended on the magnitude of the current (Figure 7.23).

What Can Electronic Taste Stimulation Be Used For?

The researchers propose that electronic taste stimulation can eventually be used for the marketing of online food products (Figure 7.24a). They also believe that it could be used for the sharing of taste experiences through social media (Ranasinghe, Cheok, & Nakatsu, 2012). For example, you can have one of your friends share the taste of the chocolate cake you're having, through a "taste message" (Figure 7.24b). ●

(Continued)

(Continued)

FIGURE 7.23

Responses to the taste strengths were related to the magnitude of the current. Sweet, bitter, and salty were the most intensely experienced tastes.

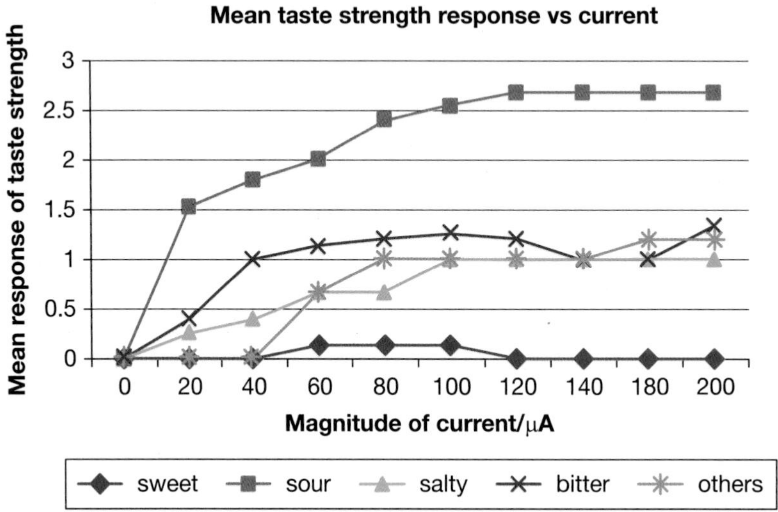

Reprinted with permission from Dr. Nimesha Ranasinghe, University of Maine, USA.

FIGURE 7.24

Researchers believe that electronic taste stimulation could eventually be used (a) to market online food products and (b) to send taste messages through social media.

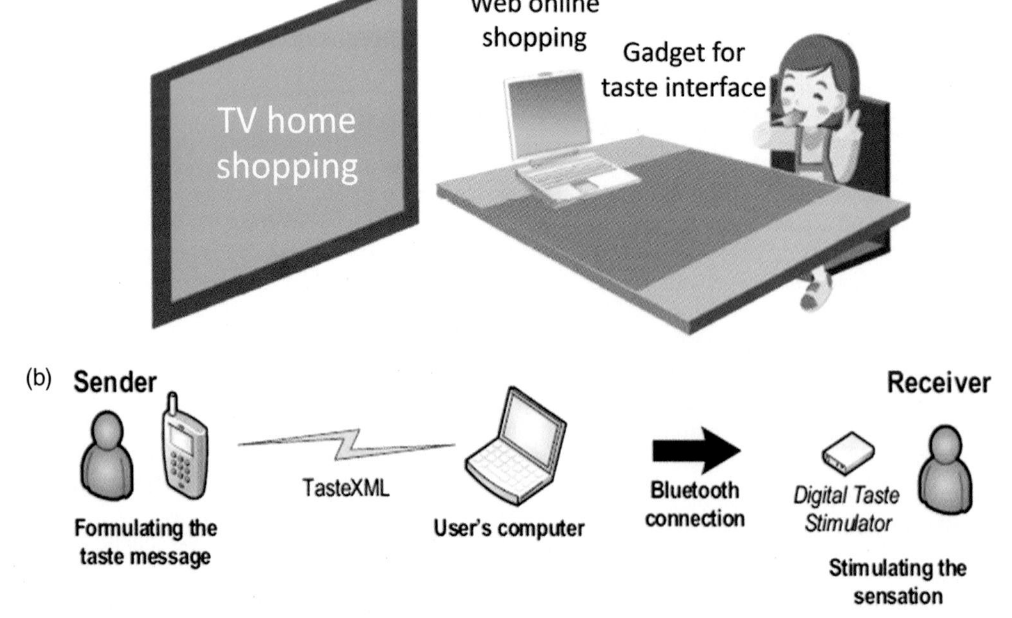

Ranasinghe N., A.D. Cheok, O.N.N. Fernando, H. Nii, P. Gopalakrishnakone. (2011). Digital Taste: Electronic Stimulation of Taste Sensations. In Keyson D.V. et al. (eds.) Ambient Intelligence. AmI 2011. Lecture Notes in Computer Science, Vol 7040. Springer, Berlin, Heidelberg. Reprinted with permission.

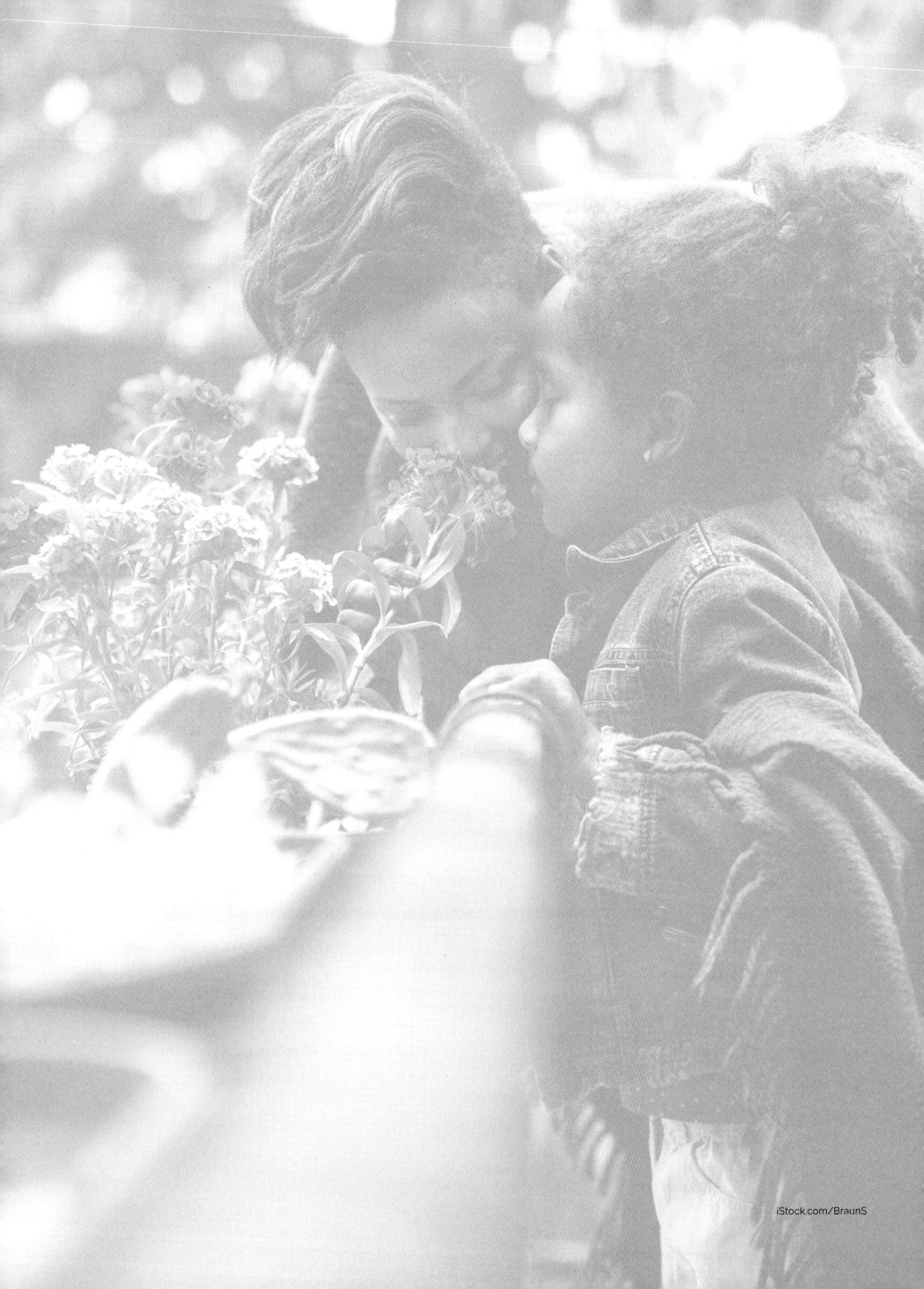

iStock.com/BraunS

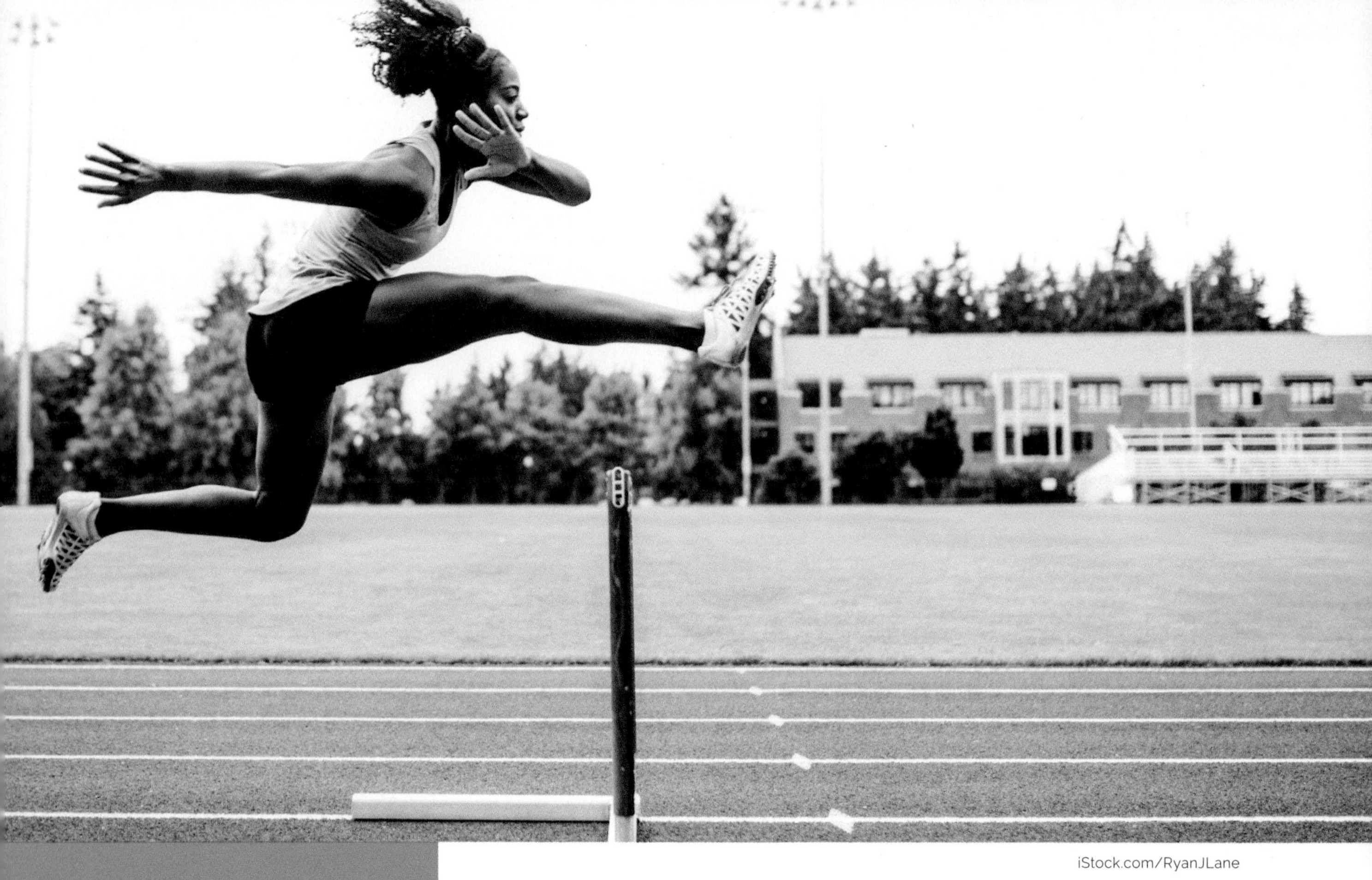

iStock.com/RyanJLane

8 Sensorimotor Systems

Chapter Contents

Learning Objectives

8.1.1 Describe the different types of muscles and how they move the body.

8.1.2 Explain how neurons innervate muscles.

8.1.3 Explain how muscles contract.

8.2.1 Know what a spinal reflex is and explain how one is generated.

8.2.2 Explain what motor programs are and describe their functions.

8.3.1 Describe what proprioception is and what it is used for.

8.3.2 Explain what the descending pathways are and describe the functions of each one.

8.3.3 Describe how different brain areas are responsible for voluntary movements.

8.3.4 Describe how various brain areas work together to produce voluntary movement.

Ian Waterman's Sensory Neuropathy

When Ian Waterman was 19 years old, he accidentally cut himself with a knife while working as a butcher. Several days later, he found himself in a hospital bed feeling that he was unable to move, with no sense of touch or of the position of his limbs. Gripped with fear, he became extremely depressed about his condition, to the point where he wished he died. It was unclear what caused Ian's condition but suspicion was that his sensory nerves were affected by a virus when he cut himself. His motor neurons, which send movement commands to the muscles, were unaffected. This meant that he was not paralyzed. So why was he not able to move? To issue effective motor commands, the motor cortex needs information about limb position through the sense known as proprioception. Without proprioception, it seemed like Ian would be confined to a wheelchair for the rest of his life. However, one day, Ian came to an amazing realization. He imagined that he could compensate for his brain being deprived of proprioceptive information by visualizing movements before he performed them. With much practice, he managed to sit up in bed. Next, he reasoned that if information about the position of his limbs could not be processed automatically through proprioception, he could give his brain this information through visual feedback. This required Ian to constantly look at his limbs as he was moving them. After four months of practice, Ian could put on his socks, and after a year he could finally stand and walk. Over the years, Ian continued to perfect his ability to move to the point where his impairment was virtually imperceptible to others. Ian's condition is extremely rare and was given the name of sensory neuropathy. It is thought to be an autoimmune disease, in which the immune system mistakenly attacks sensory nerve fibers while fighting a virus.

INTRODUCTION

The performance of mundane everyday movements, such as picking up a cup of coffee or clicking a mouse button to select an icon on a computer screen, is probably the most taken-for-granted of our abilities. However, we are capable of much more than these relatively simple behaviors. Think of the complex and highly coordinated muscle movements performed by a gymnast, baseball player, or pianist. Even the most complex motor actions become automatized with practice. For example, when learning to drive a car with a manual transmission, one must think about every action. This includes shifting into the right gears with the hand, while coordinating pressing the clutch with the foot. At the same time, one must steer the car in the right direction and be able to switch the position of the foot from the clutch to the brake. After some practice, one no longer has to think about these actions to drive the car. Such "automatization" of behavior is important as it frees up other cognitive resources, which are important for performing the task at hand. In the driving example, this includes paying attention to the road to avoid hitting pedestrians or crashing the car. Movement also requires guidance. This guidance involves the participation of sensory systems. As you just read in Ian's Waterman's story, loss of proprioception can have devastating effects on one's ability to move, even with an intact motor system. Think about what must occur to accurately throw a piece of trash in a garbage can. Information from the visual system is used to judge the distance between your hand and the garbage can. Proprioception is used to assess the starting position of the hand and the weight of the object being held before the throw. This information is integrated and communicated to the motor system so that the throw is in the right direction and executed with the proper amount of force. In addition, the vestibular system, which controls balance, is recruited to keep the visual field and the body stable while the throw is executed. If you miss, adjustments are made on every subsequent try until you can perform the feat, with little or no thought at all. These adjustments can, with practice, lead to the performance of behaviors requiring remarkable accuracy, for example, hitting a baseball no more than about 3 inches in diameter that is thrown at more than 90 miles per hour with a bat no larger than 2.61 inches in diameter.

8.1 This Is What Makes You Move

Module Contents

Learning Objectives

8.1.1 Describe the different types of muscles and how they move the body.

8.1.2 Explain how neurons innervate muscles.

8.1.3 Explain how muscles contract.

8.1.1 MUSCLES AND MUSCLE CONTRACTION

>> LO 8.1.1 Describe the different types of muscles and how they move the body.

Key Terms

- **Flexors:** Muscles that bring two body parts closer together, such as the biceps that bring together forearm and upper arm.
- **Extensors:** Muscles that move two body parts away from each other, such as the triceps, which move the forearm and upper arm away from each other.
- **Abductors:** Muscles that move body parts away from the midline of the body.
- **Adductors:** Muscles that bring body parts closer to the midline of the body.
- **Antagonistic muscle:** A muscle that directly counteracts the actions of another muscle.
- **Fast-twitch muscle fibers:** Muscle fibers that are strong but fatigue easily; important for brief, unsustained efforts.
- **Slow-twitch muscle fibers:** Muscle fibers that do not fatigue easily; effective in long, sustained efforts, such as in long-distance running.

Figure 8.1 shows microscopic images of cells from the three different types of muscle: striated (or skeletal), cardiac, and smooth. Striated muscles are the ones

FIGURE 8.1

The different types of muscles. Photomicrographs of (a) striated (skeletal) muscle cells, (b) cardiac muscle cells, and (c) smooth muscle cells.

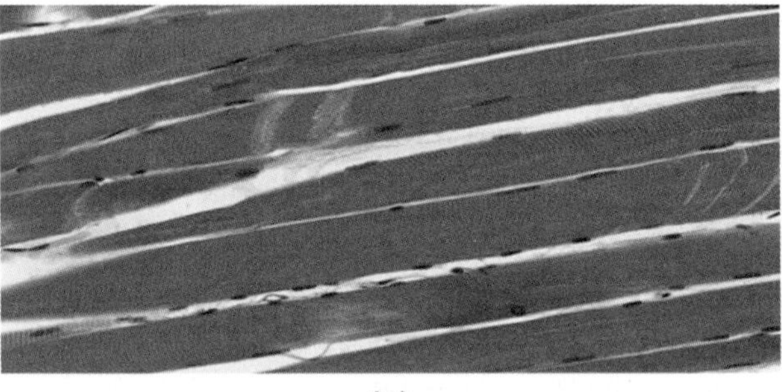

(a)

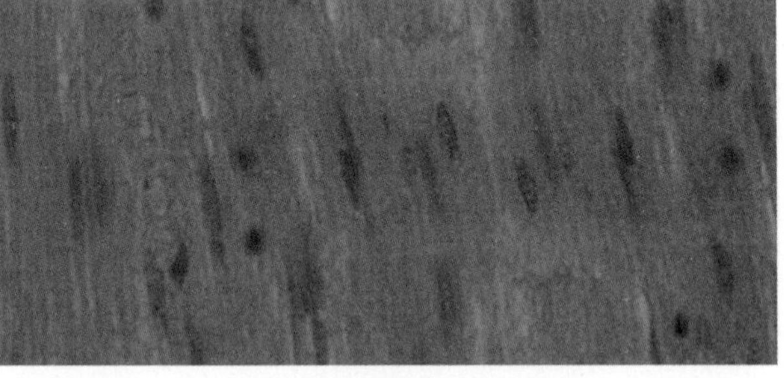

(b)

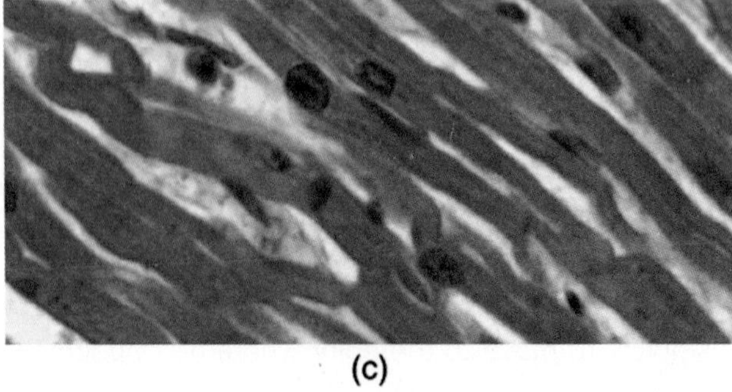

(c)

that move your body. They contract during voluntary movements (i.e., when you decide to move) and reflexive movements (i.e., pulling your hand away from a hot stove). Cardiac muscles form the heart. Their regular contractions (heartbeat), throughout life, pump blood into the general circulation. Smooth muscles line the walls of organs and intestines. Their contraction moves food through the intestines. Smooth muscles in the bladder relax as it fills with urine and then contract to empty it. Both cardiac and smooth muscle contraction is involuntary. These muscles can contract without nerve stimulation. How then, you may wonder, can we voluntarily "hold it in" when we need to go to the restroom? The answer is that the muscle that we contract to do so, the external urethral sphincter, is a striated muscle. Its contraction is, therefore, voluntary.

In this chapter, we will focus on striated muscles, which directly control the movement of your body in response to conscious commands and reflexes. Figure 8.2 shows a prototypical skeletal muscle. Muscles are composed of muscle fibers. Each muscle fiber is a muscle cell (or myocyte). The membrane surrounding each muscle fiber is called a sarcolemma. The cytoplasm of muscle cells is known as the sarcoplasm.

Muscle fibers are multinucleated, that is, they possess several nuclei. This is due to muscle cells developing from the fusion of many myoblasts, each of which contains a nucleus. Myoblasts are the precursors of muscle cells during development (Demonbreun, Biersmith, & McNally, 2015). Muscle fibers are held together in groups, called fascicles, by a membrane called the perimysium. In turn, each one of the muscle cells is wrapped in a membrane known as the endomysium. Muscle cells are composed of myofibrils, which are themselves composed of sarcomeres. Sarcomeres are responsible for the light and dark bands (striations) that characterize striated muscles. Sarcomeres are made up of thin and thick filaments made of actin and myosin proteins, respectively. Muscles also contain many nerves and blood vessels. The multiple groups of muscle cells that make up the entire muscle are kept together by the epimysium.

FIGURE 8.2

Striated muscles are composed of bundles of muscle cells, called fascicles, wrapped in perimysium.

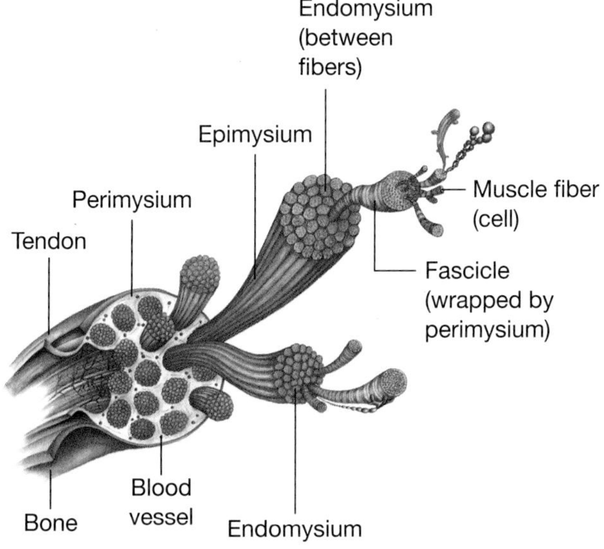

BSIP/Universal Images Group/Getty Images

Flexors, Extensors, Abductors, and Adductors

Different muscles move your limbs in different ways relative to your joints. For example, Figure 8.3a shows how muscles move the forearm at the elbow joint. You can see that when the biceps contract, the forearm (which includes two main bones, the radius and the ulna) moves upward toward the humerus, the major bone of the upper arm. The biceps are therefore **flexors**, as they bring two body parts (forearm and upper arm) closer together. In contrast, when the triceps contract, the forearm is drawn away from the upper arm. The triceps are therefore **extensors**.

Muscles move body parts in two other ways: abduction and adduction. An **abductor** such as the deltoid brings body parts away from the midline of the body. An **adductor**, such as the teres major, brings body parts closer to the midline of the body. Figure 8.3b shows an example of each.

FIGURE 8.3

Flexor, extensor, abductor, and adductor. (a) Biceps and triceps. Biceps are flexors, and triceps are extensors. They are antagonistic. The triceps relax as the biceps contract (and vice versa). (b) The deltoid is an abductor, and the teres major is an adductor. They also are antagonistic. When the deltoid contracts, the teres major relaxes (and vice versa).

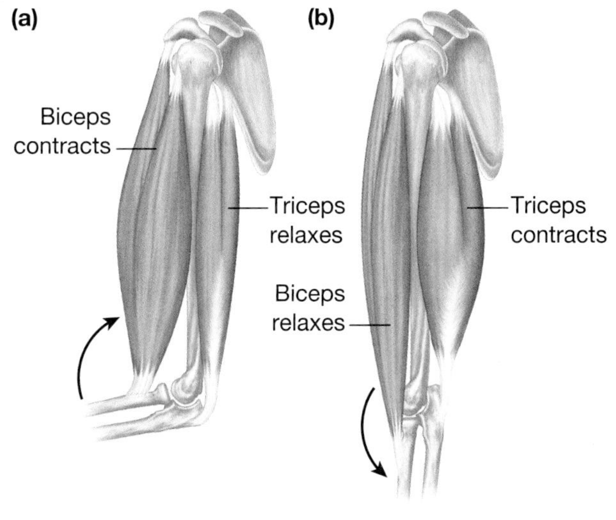

Adapted from Starr, C., & Taggart, R. (1989). *Biology: The unity and diversity of life*. Pacific Grove, CA: Brooks/Cole.

Figure 8.3 also shows that some muscles pull in opposite directions. For example, when the biceps contract, the triceps relax. In contrast, the biceps relax when the triceps contract. The same can be said about abductor and adductor muscles. A muscle that directly and reciprocally counteracts the action of another muscle is called an **antagonistic muscle**.

Another difference lies in the types of muscle fibers contained in a muscle. There are **fast-twitch muscle fibers** and **slow-twitch muscle fibers**. Fast-twitch muscle fibers are strong but fatigue easily. They are important for brief, unsustained efforts, such as lifting heavy weights. In contrast, slow-twitch muscle fibers are effective in long, sustained efforts, such as in long-distance running, as they do not fatigue easily. Fast-twitch muscle fibers appear dark, and slow-twitch muscle fibers appear white. Now you know why chicken has dark meat and white meat!

8.1.2 INNERVATION OF MUSCLE CELLS

>> LO 8.1.2 **Explain how neurons innervate muscles.**

Key Terms

- **Motor unit:** A single motor neuron as well as all the muscle cells it innervates.
- **Motor neuron pool:** All the motor neurons that innervate a single muscle.
- **Motor end plate:** The area where acetylcholine receptors are located on a muscle cell.

Muscle cells receive direct connections from lower motor neurons, whose axons exit the ventral roots of the spinal cord. Note that these contrast with upper motor neurons, which originate in the motor cortex (discussed later in the chapter). Each muscle cell receives connections from a single motor neuron, but a single motor neuron can connect with several muscle cells. A single motor neuron as well as all the muscle cells it innervates are together called a **motor unit** (Figure 8.4a, left). A single muscle can also receive input from many motor neurons. The collection of all the motor neurons that innervate a single muscle is called a **motor neuron pool** (Figure 8.4b). The location where the axon terminals of motor neurons communicate with muscle cells is known as the neuromuscular junction (Figure 8.4a, right). The number of motor units used by the muscle depends on the force of muscle contraction. For example, a strong contraction, such as is necessary for lifting a heavy weight, is related to the recruitment of more motor units compared to a relatively weaker contraction related to the lifting of a relatively light weight.

FIGURE 8.4

Motor units, neuromuscular junctions, and a motor neuron pool. (a) Left: Motor neurons exit the ventral root of the spinal cord. The axons of each motor neuron branch off and connect with multiple muscle fibers, to form a motor unit. Several branches of the same motor neurons connecting to the muscle cells' motor end plates and various neuromuscular junctions. (b) A motor neuron pool, which consists of all the motor neurons that innervate a single muscle.

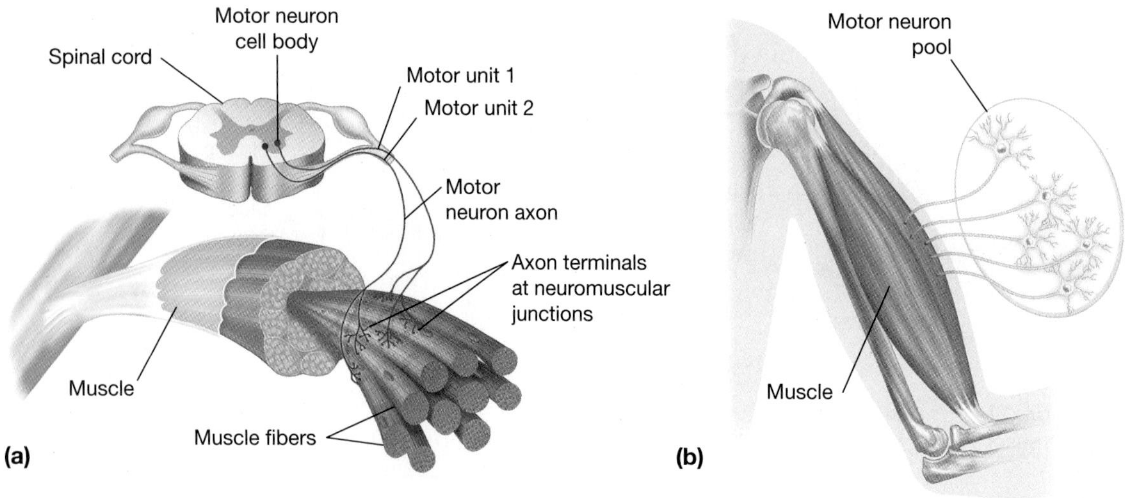

Liana Bauman/Body Scientific Intl.

Motor neurons communicate with muscle cells via the neurotransmitter acetylcholine. Acetylcholine receptors are located on the muscle cells in an area called the **motor end plate**.

8.1.3 HOW MUSCLES CONTRACT

>> LO 8.1.3 **Explain how muscles contract.**

Key Term

- **Sliding filament model:** A model proposed to explain how muscles contract.

Muscles contract when acetylcholine is released from motor neurons onto cholinergic receptors of motor end plates at neuromuscular junctions (Figure 8.5). As you already know from studying Chapter 3, the arrival of action potentials at axon terminals (or synaptic end bulbs) triggers the entry of Ca^{2+} into the cell. The entry of Ca^{2+} triggers the binding of synaptic vesicles to the membrane, and neurotransmitters are released into the synaptic cleft. In the case of motor neurons, acetylcholine molecules make their way across the synaptic cleft and bind to the receptors of a target cell, which in the present case are muscle cells.

Acetylcholine receptors are located inside indentations, called junctional folds, in the motor end plate. For this reason, the response of muscle cells to the binding of acetylcholine is extremely reliable, as the neurotransmitter is trapped inside the folds. As you learned in Chapter 3, the binding of the neurotransmitter (in this case, acetylcholine) to its receptors results in the opening of the Na^+ channels that each receptor is associated with. This results in the depolarization of the muscle cells, which leads to muscle contraction.

The Sliding Filament Model of Muscle Contraction

The mechanism by which muscles contract was discovered in the early 1950s by Andrew F. Huxley and colleagues. The name should sound familiar to you. He was one of the co-discoverers of the "ins and outs" of the action potential (Chapter 3). They described what became known as the **sliding filament model** of muscle contraction (A. F. Huxley & Niedergerke, 1954; H. Huxley & Hanson, 1954). To recap from earlier, muscle cells are composed of myofibrils, which are themselves composed of sarcomeres, which consist of a combination of thin and thick filaments of protein called myosin and actin, respectively (Figure 8.6a).

Figure 8.6b illustrates the sliding filament model of muscle contraction. Successive sarcomeres are bound on each side by another kind of filament called Z-discs (or Z-lines), to which the thin actin filaments are attached. The thick myosin filaments are situated on either side of the thin actin filaments. The regions

FIGURE 8.5

The neuromuscular junction.

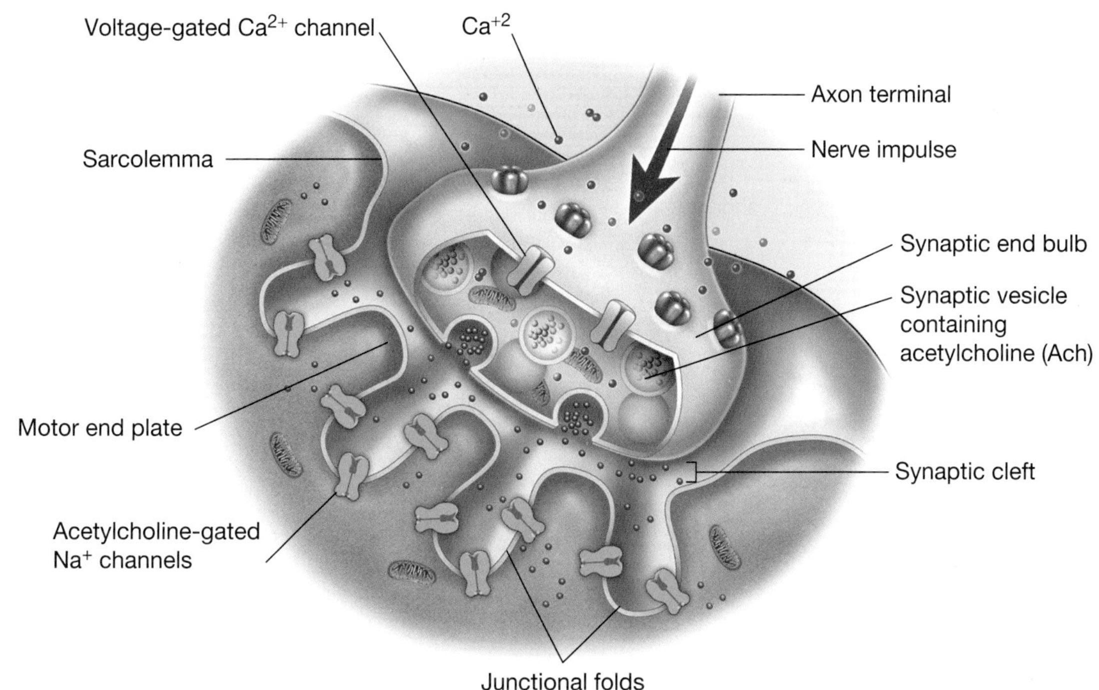

Amanda Tomasikiewicz/Body Scientific Intl.

FIGURE 8.6

The sliding filament model of muscle contraction. (a) A myofibril of a muscle cell showing a sarcomere as well as the relative locations of the Z-discs, H-zone, I-bands, and A-bands. (b) Top: A sarcomere while in a relaxed state showing the relative positions of the Z-discs, H-zone, I-bands, and A-bands. Bottom: The relative locations of the Z-discs, H-zone, I-bands, and A-bands during muscle contraction. The I-bands and H-zone shorten while the length of the A-bands remains constant. The Z-discs are pulled closer together. (c) Myosin filaments extend bulbous heads that attach to sections of the actin filaments. Contraction of the heads causes the actin filaments to slide along the myosin filaments in 10-nm steps, in a process known as actin-myosin cycling.

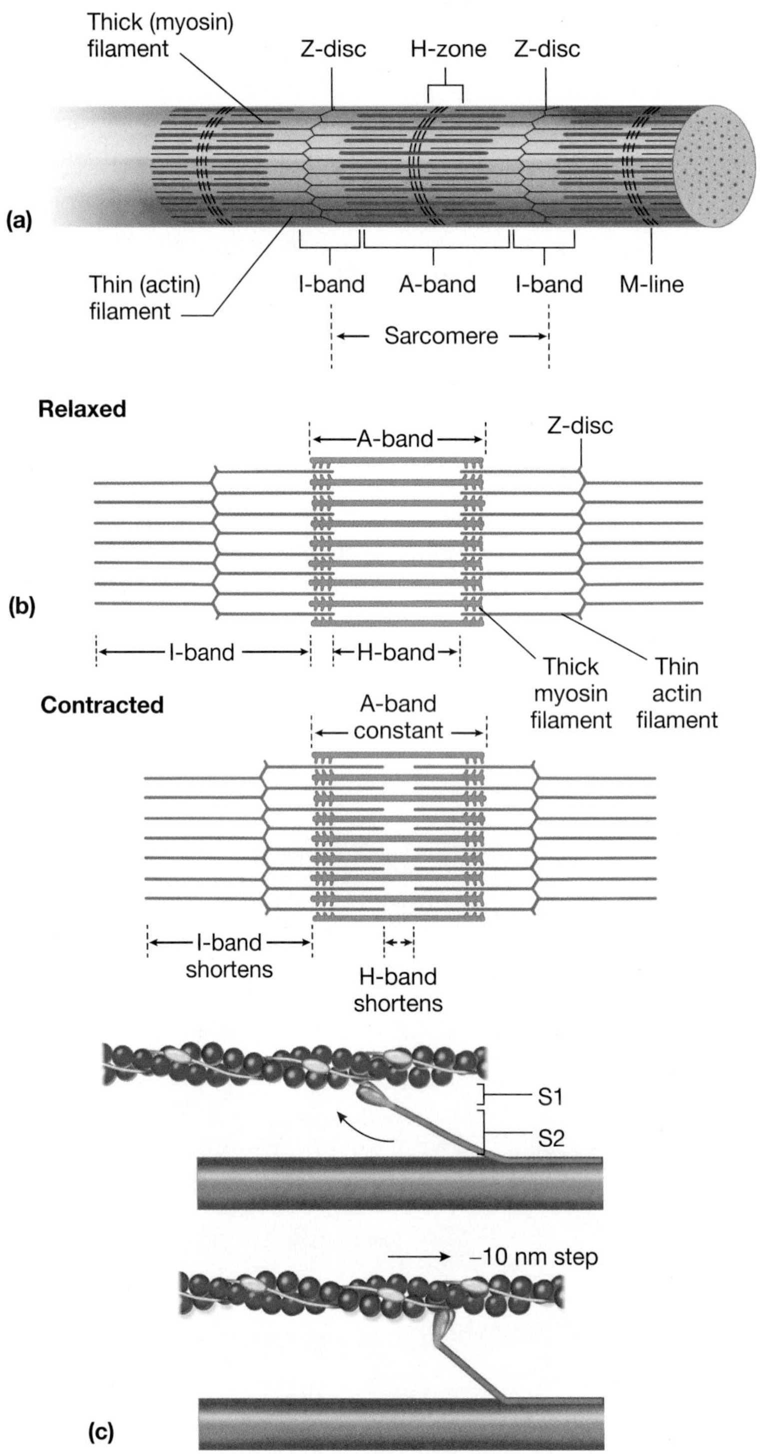

of the sarcomere in which the myosin filaments partly overlap with the actin filaments are called the A-bands. The regions of the sarcomere where the actin filaments that do not overlap with myosin filaments are situated are called the I-bands. This leaves another region, where only the myosin filaments are visible, called the H-zone, which contains the H-bands (Figure 8.6b, top).

Muscle contraction occurs when the thick myosin filaments pull on the actin filaments, causing the actin filaments to slide along the myosin filaments. This causes the I-bands on each side of the H-zone and the H-zone itself to shorten. The Z-discs are consequently pulled closer together. Note that the lengths of the A-bands remain constant (Figure 8.6b, bottom).

The sliding filament model was refined in the 1980s to better explain the mechanism by which the myosin filaments pull on the actin filaments (Hynes, Block, White, & Spudich, 1987; Spudich, 2001). The thick myosin filaments extend bulbous heads (called the S1 region) from sections of the myosin filament (called the S2 region), which reaches ahead and binds to the actin filament. The heads contract, pulling the actin filament along in steps of 10 nm. The myosin heads then release the actin filament and the process repeats itself. This process is known as actin-myosin cycling and is illustrated in Figure 8.6c.

MODULE SUMMARY

Muscles are of three main types: skeletal, cardiac, and smooth muscles. Muscle cells are called myocytes. Skeletal muscles move the limbs relative to the joint. They come in opposing pairs. Flexors bring body parts together, whereas extensors move body parts away from each other. Muscles also include abductors and adductors. A muscle that directly counteracts another is called antagonistic. There are both fast-twitch and slow-twitch muscle fibers. Fast-twitch muscle fibers are strong but tire quickly, whereas slow-twitch fibers are not as strong but do not fatigue easily.

Muscle cells receive direct connections from lower motor neurons that exit the spinal cord. Upper motor neurons are the neurons that send movement-related information from the motor cortex to the spinal cord. A motor neuron pool includes all the motor neurons that innervate a muscle. Axons contact muscle cells at what is known as the neuromuscular junction. The neurotransmitter used at the neuromuscular junction is acetylcholine. An area on a muscle cell that contains acetylcholine receptors is called a motor end plate. Muscles contract when acetylcholine binds to its receptors located inside indentations called junctional folds. The mechanism by which muscles contract is known as the sliding filament model.

TEST YOURSELF

8.1.1 What are the different types of muscles? How is each type used?

8.1.2 How do neurons innervate neuron muscle cells?

8.1.3 How does the sliding filament model account for muscle contraction?

8.2 Spinal Control of Movement

Module Contents

Learning Objectives

8.2.1 Know what a spinal reflex is and explain how one is generated.

8.2.2 Explain what motor programs are and describe their functions.

8.2.1 SPINAL REFLEXES

>> LO 8.2.1 Know what a spinal reflex is and explain how one is generated.

Key Terms

- **Stretch reflex:** A contraction initiated in response to the stretch of a muscle to prevent it from tearing.
- **Muscle spindles:** Bundles of tiny muscle fibers encircled by sensory axons inside a capsule; responsible for the stretch reflex.
- **Autogenic inhibition reflex:** A reflex that relaxes the muscle by inhibiting motor neurons in response to an overly strong muscle contraction.

- **Golgi tendon organ:** A structure located in tendons that senses changes in muscle tension; responsible for the autogenic inhibition reflex.

The Stretch Reflex

The **stretch reflex** (also called the myotatic reflex) is a muscle contraction initiated in response to the stretch of a muscle to prevent it from tearing. The stretch of the muscle is detected by **muscle spindles**, which are bundles of tiny muscle fibers (called intrafusal fibers) encircled by sensory axons inside a capsule. Muscle spindles are embedded deep inside muscles, which are composed of extrafusal fibers (Figure 8.7). The sensory axons surrounding these fibers synapse directly with motor neurons within the spinal cord. These motor neurons synapse onto the extrafusal fibers of the muscle being stretched, resulting in its contraction.

Autogenic Inhibition Reflex

The **autogenic inhibition reflex** (also called the inverse myotatic reflex) is not initiated by the stretch of a muscle as in the stretch reflex. The autogenic inhibition reflex relaxes the muscle by inhibiting motor neurons in response to an overly strong muscle contraction. This is either to prevent damage to a muscle or to coordinate muscle contractions to manipulate objects with just the right amount of force. For example, it is the autogenic inhibition reflex that permits you to pick up a cardboard cup of coffee without crushing it. You just read that the muscle spindle is the structure involved in the stretch reflex. The autogenic inhibition reflex depends on another structure called the **Golgi tendon organ**, which is found in tendons and senses changes in muscle tension.

8.2.2 MOTOR PROGRAMS

>> LO 8.2.2 Explain what motor programs are and describe their functions.

Key Term

- **Motor programs:** Neural networks situated in the brainstem that initiate automatic and rhythmic movements such as walking; also known as central pattern generators.

Many of the movements that we routinely perform without thought are the result of **motor programs** (also called central pattern generators). Motor programs are neural networks located in the brainstem that initiate automatic and rhythmic movements. The prototypical example of a motor program is walking. The only thing you need to think about when you want to get somewhere is when to start walking and when to stop. Rhythmic movements such as walking movements are initiated by the brainstem and maintained by the spinal cord. Other rhythmic behaviors maintained by motor programs include chewing and breathing. A motor program can also be reflexive, such as the withdrawal reflex described earlier, or can be activated in response to an irritant, resulting in sneezing, coughing, or scratching.

A motor program for walking was discovered in the early 1900s by Charles Scott Sherrington and Graham Brown (Sherrington, 1911). Sherrington found that rhythmic leg movements could be elicited in cats that have recovered from a transection of the spinal cord. Graham Brown extended this finding by showing that muscle contraction of the legs could also be induced

FIGURE 8.7

Muscle spindle and two types of spinal reflexes: (a) a muscle spindle, (b) a stretch reflex, (c) a withdrawal reflex.

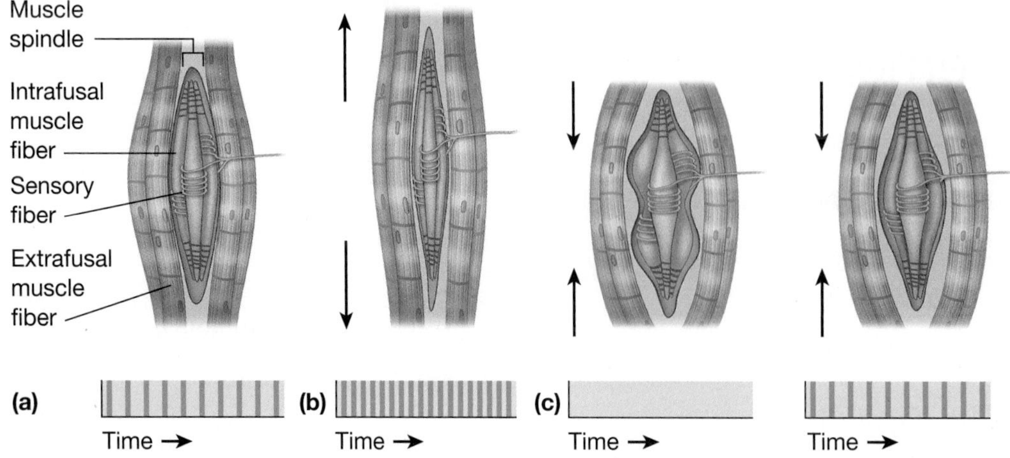

Carolina Hrejsa/Body Scientific Intl.

FIGURE 8.8

(a) Experimental set-up used by Shik, Severin, and Orlovsky. (b) Location of the cuts performed by Sherrington and Brown (B'-B) and by Shik, Severin, and Orlovsky (A'-A).

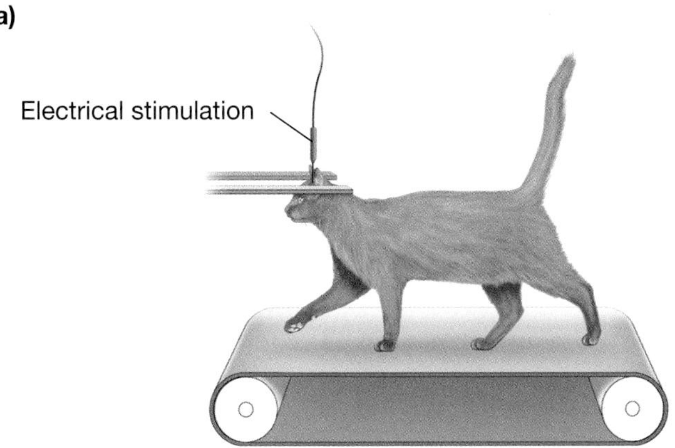

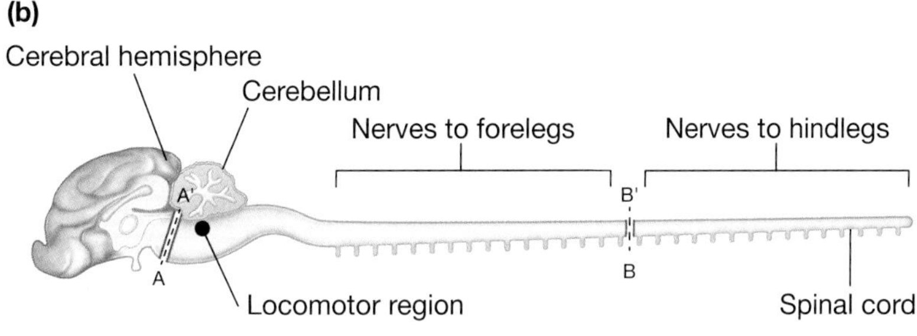

Amanda Tomasikiewicz/Body Scientific Intl.

by electrical stimulation of networks of neurons situated in the brainstem in cats in which the brainstem had been separated from the cortex (G. T. Brown, 1911).

In 1965, Russian physiologists M. L. Shik, F. V. Severin, and G. N. Orlovsky (1969) cut through the middle of the brainstems of cats, which cut off the brain from the spinal cord. Despite this disconnection, the cats could still be made to walk on a treadmill by electrically stimulating the remaining part of the brainstem (the part that remained attached to the spinal cord but not to the brain). This meant that the spinal cord can by itself generate motor activity. The set-up for such an experiment is shown in Figure 8.8a. Figure 8.8b shows the location of the transections of the spinal cord performed by Sherrington and Brown (B'-B) and where the brainstem was separated from the spinal cord by Shik, Severin, and Orlovsky (A'-A).

MODULE SUMMARY

The stretch reflex is a muscle contraction in response to the stretch of a muscle to prevent it from tearing. The stretch of a muscle is detected by muscle spindles located in sensory axons. In a stretch reflex, sensory axons synapse directly with a motor neuron in the spinal cord. This differs from a reflex arc, in which the connection between the sensory and motor neurons is mediated by an interneuron. Another type of reflex, the inhibition reflex, occurs in response to an overly strong muscle contraction. The autogenic inhibition reflex depends on a structure called the Golgi tendon organ. Movements that we routinely perform in an automatic way, such as walking, are initiated in the brainstem and spinal cord. These movements are the result of motor programs, also called central pattern generators.

TEST YOURSELF

8.2.1 What is a spinal reflex? How is one generated?

8.2.2 What are motor programs? What are they used for?

8.3 Cortical Control of Movement and Sensorimotor Integration

Module Contents

Learning Objectives

- **8.3.1** Describe what proprioception is and what it is used for.
- **8.3.2** Explain what the descending pathways are and describe the functions of each one.
- **8.3.3** Describe how different brain areas are responsible for voluntary movements.
- **8.3.4** Describe how various brain areas work together to produce voluntary movement.

8.3.1 PROPRIOCEPTION

>> LO 8.3.1 Describe what proprioception is and what it is used for.

As defined in Chapter 7, proprioception is the sense of the position of the different parts of the body relative to each other. As with the sense of touch, information about the position of body parts is conveyed through mechanoreceptors. There are two types of proprioceptors: the muscle spindles and Golgi tendon organs. Both have already been discussed because of the role they play in reflexes.

Action potentials are generated in the nerve fibers of muscle spindles in response to the stretching muscles and in the nerve fibers in Golgi tendon organs in response to muscle contraction. Proprioceptors are responsible for the perceptions of force, pressure, and weight. This information is needed to adjust the force and momentum that is applied not only to reflexes (as described earlier) but also in voluntary motor acts. For example, when you first meet someone, and want to convey how self-assured you are, you need to consciously adjust the force in your handshake so that it is firm but not so firm that you crush the person's hand. The same idea applies when giving someone a hug. As you will learn later in this chapter, information from proprioceptors is also used without your conscious awareness to adjust ongoing movements and to encode the starting point of your limbs before moving them toward target objects.

Conscious information from proprioceptors reaches the somatosensory cortex through an ascending tract known as the dorsal column–medial lemniscus pathway (DCML), shown in Figure 8.9. It is also important to note that proprioceptive information and innocuous touch innervate neurons in different areas of the somatosensory cortex (not shown in the figure). See Chapter 7 if you need to review the details of the ascending tracts.

8.3.2 THE DESCENDING PATHWAYS

>> LO 8.3.2 Explain what the descending pathways are and describe the functions of each one.

Key Terms

- **Direct pathway (motor):** Composed of the axons of neurons located in the motor cortex.
- **Indirect pathway (motor):** Composed of the axons of neurons originating in subcortical motor nuclei.
- **Pyramidal tracts:** Tracts of the direct pathway.
- **Lateral and ventral corticospinal tracts:** The individual tracts of the direct pathway.
- **Extrapyramidal tracts:** Tracts of the indirect pathway.
- **Tectospinal, vestibulospinal, rubrospinal, and reticulospinal tracts:** The individual tracts of the indirect pathway.

The descending pathways carry information from the brain to the spinal cord to produce movement (voluntary and involuntary) and for the maintenance of posture. The descending pathways can be either direct or indirect. The **direct pathway** is composed of the axons of neurons located in the motor cortex. Neurons in the direct pathway directly connect with neurons in the spinal cord. The **indirect pathway** is composed of

FIGURE 8.9

The dorsal column–medial lemniscus pathway.

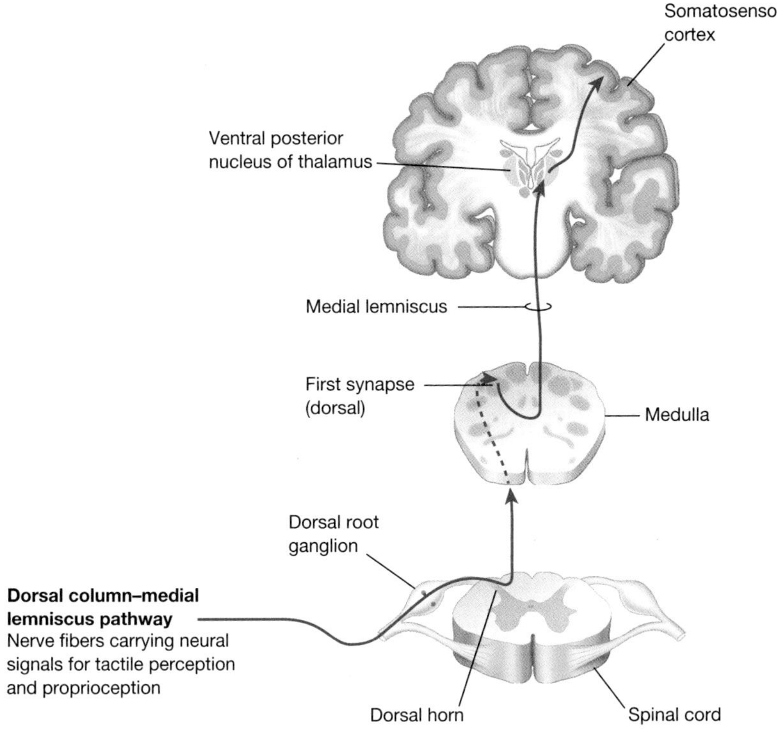

the axons of neurons originating in subcortical motor nuclei, such as the superior colliculus, vestibular nuclei, red nucleus, and reticular formation. It is called the indirect pathway because the neurons it contains do not directly connect to neurons in the spinal cord but, instead, form synapses with other sets of neurons in between.

The neurons of the descending pathways are referred to as upper motor neurons and lower motor neurons. Upper motor neurons are the neurons whose cell bodies are in the motor cortex and subcortical motor nuclei. They carry information to the lower motor neurons (discussed previously), which are situated in the spinal cord and brainstem, and synapse directly onto muscle cells.

The Direct Pathway

As mentioned earlier, the direct pathway originates from pyramidal cells in the primary motor cortex and premotor cortex. The direct pathway consists of two tracts, known as the **pyramidal tracts**. These are the **lateral corticospinal tract** and the **ventral corticospinal tract** (Figure 8.10). Neurons from both tracts carry motor messages to lower motor neurons of the spinal cord to produce voluntary movement. Axons of the corticospinal tracts decussate (cross over) in what are known as the medullary pyramids.

The Indirect Pathways

As mentioned earlier, the indirect pathways include neurons that originate in the subcortical motor nuclei, not from pyramidal cells in the motor and premotor cortices. For this reason, they are also called the **extrapyramidal tracts**. The indirect pathways consist of the **tectospinal tract**, **vestibulospinal tract**, **rubrospinal tract**, and **reticulospinal tract**. Activity in the indirect pathway mostly involves reflexive movements, such as automatically adjusting posture or following moving objects with the eyes. The indirect pathways are illustrated in Figure 8.11. Keep in mind that neurons from the subcortical motor nuclei in these tracts do not directly connect with lower motor neurons but communicate, instead, with neurons in the ventral horns of the spinal cord.

The Tectospinal Tract

The tectospinal tract originates in the superior colliculus, which is in the tectum of the midbrain (hence, the prefix *tecto-*). Its axons decussate. Its function is to automatically turn the neck so that a moving object can be followed with the eyes.

The Vestibulospinal Tract

The vestibulospinal tract originates in the vestibular nuclei in the medulla (hence, the prefix *vestibulo-*). Its axons do not decussate. Its function is to maintain balance while standing and moving around. It does so by controlling the muscles of the trunk and those that move the head.

The Rubrospinal Tract

The rubrospinal tract originates in the red nucleus of the midbrain (hence, the prefix *rubro-*). Its axons decussate. Its axons terminate in the upper part of the spinal cord and control movement of the upper limbs.

The Reticulospinal Tract

The reticulospinal tract originates in the reticular formation of the brainstem (hence, the prefix *reticulo-*). It has fibers that decussate but also some that remain on the same side. Its function is to maintain muscle tone and motor functions of the internal organs.

FIGURE 8.10

The direct pathways (pyramidal tracts): the lateral corticospinal tract (left) and the ventral corticospinal tract (right).

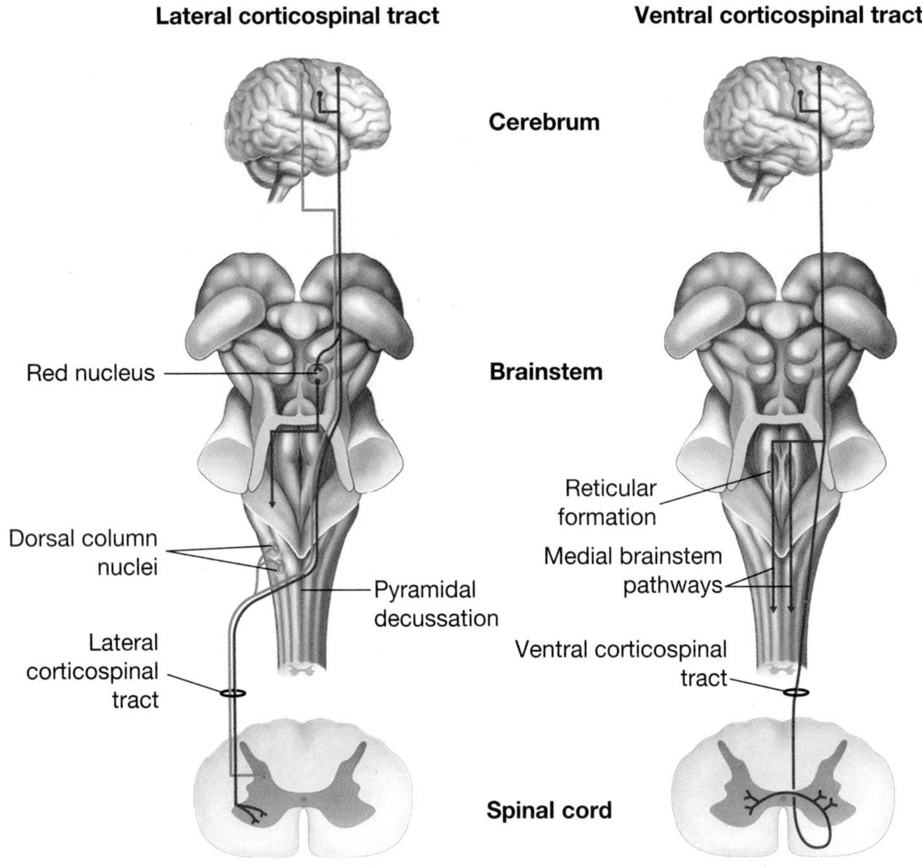

Amanda Tomasikiewicz/Body Scientific Intl

8.3.3 ANATOMY OF VOLUNTARY MOVEMENT

>> LO 8.3.3 Describe how different brain areas are responsible for voluntary movements.

Key Terms

- **Motor homunculus:** A representation of the body mapped onto the primary motor cortex.
- **Efferent copy:** A copy of a motor command sent by the primary motor cortex to another brain area.

The following are some of the things that need to happen for you to perform the simple task of picking up your cup of coffee. First, the cup itself must be identified as being a goal. Next, its spatial location must be determined, both in relation to the other objects within its space and relative to your own body parts. The proper sequence of movements and choice of muscles to contract must then be selected for your arm to move toward the cup and for you to grip the cup appropriately. The force of your grip must also be adjusted depending on whether it is a hard cup or one made of paper so that you don't crush it. You then lift the cup to your lips, taste the coffee, and determine if your actions were rewarded by a good-tasting coffee and are worth repeating.

Performance of this sequence of movements depends on several interacting brain areas, each playing its own role. In this unit, we look at these areas and the contributions they make to voluntary movement. Figure 8.12 shows the locations of some of the areas we are going to discuss, so you may want to refer to it as you read through the text.

Prefrontal Cortex

The prefrontal cortex is highly involved in decision making and action selection. Sitting at your desk, you are probably confronted with many possible actions to take. For example, you may pick up a book to start studying or turn on your laptop to work on a paper that

FIGURE 8.11

Comparison between the pyramidal tracts (direct pathways), which consist of the corticospinal tracts (only the lateral corticospinal tract is shown) (left), and the extrapyramidal tracts (indirect pathways), which consist of the rubrospinal, tectospinal, vestibulospinal, and reticulospinal tracts (right).

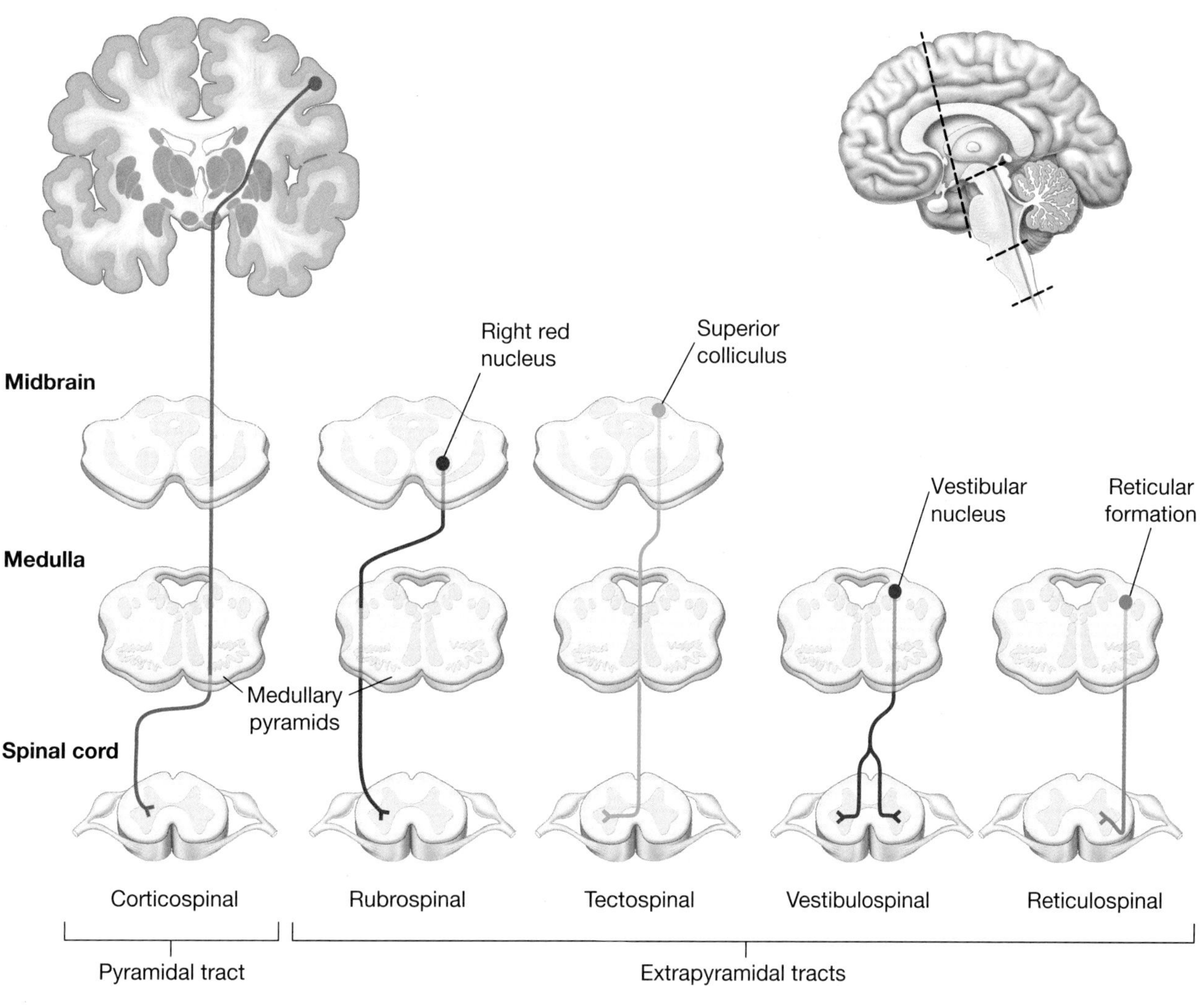

Carolina Hrejsa/Body Scientific Intl.

is due next week. You may also decide to get yourself a snack from the refrigerator. Engaging in any of these activities requires visual targets to be identified and your attention to be focused on them.

What you finally decide to do depends on many factors, for example, your memory of the consequences of engaging in one or another behavior, the payoffs associated with one of the behaviors, and whether the payoff will be immediate or delayed. The prefrontal cortex is the brain area responsible for these functions.

For visually guided movements, contributions from the primary visual cortex in the occipital lobes is also required. The recognition of the object you are about to act upon requires activity in the "what" pathway you learned about in Chapter 6. Remember that this is the pathway that runs from the visual cortex to the temporal lobe, also known as the ventral stream of vision.

Primary Motor Cortex

The primary motor cortex is at the back of the frontal lobes (see Figure 8.12). It lies just in front of the central sulcus, in what is known as the precentral gyrus, within area 4. Interest in this region goes far back in time (see Chapter 1). Electrical stimulation of this area was found to result in muscle contractions that cause the movement of body parts in both humans and animals. It was then proposed that the primary motor cortex contained

FIGURE 8.12

The anatomy of voluntary movement.

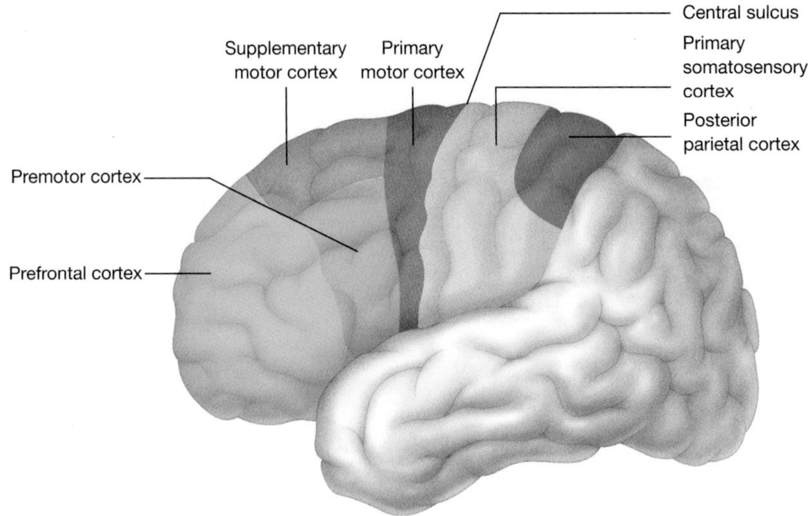

a somatotopic map, that is, a map of the body that became known as the **motor homunculus**.

This map was discovered by Wilder Penfield of the Montreal Neurological Institute (Penfield & Rasmussen, 1968). He did so by electrically stimulating the primary motor cortex in patients undergoing brain surgery and found that different parts of the body were allocated amounts of space relative to their innervation. That is, body parts with more complex connectivity are represented by a greater amount of cortex (Figure 8.13a). This is represented by a disproportionate homunculus (little man) with disproportionate body parts (Figure 8.13b). Notice also that the map is inverted relative to the actual body with feet and legs up on top and face at the bottom. This constitutes only a rough map of the body: Although it accurately represents large areas such as the legs and feet, smaller areas within these parts are much less accurately represented with a lot of overlap.

An Ethological Action Map

Although the finding that the primary motor cortex contains a somatotopic map is fascinating, the research that led to this discovery suffered from an important shortcoming. The duration of electrical stimulation used to evoke the muscle twitches, which led to the mapping of the body onto the cortex, was 20–50 milliseconds. Such brief bursts of stimulation were used to avoid the spreading of activity in nearby networks of neurons, leading to the activation of other parts of the map. This would, in turn, blur the distinction of the boundaries between the representations of specific body parts.

However, in the early 2000s, Michael Graziano and colleagues suggested that such brief stimulation times were not ethologically relevant. That is, they did not represent real-life motor activity, such as reaching out for a book on a bookshelf or bringing a cup of iced cappuccino to your lips. To test this idea, Graziano and colleagues stimulated neurons in the motor cortex of monkeys for up to 0.5 seconds (Graziano, Aflalo, & Cooke, 2005).

What they discovered was remarkable. Depending on the area they stimulated, the monkeys performed ethologically relevant behaviors, such as reaching out as if to grasp an object or lifting a hand to the mouth to eat a piece of food (Figure 8.14). The movement continued as long as the stimulus was on but stopped when the stimulus was interrupted. Also, the movement occurred independently of the limb's starting position. Movements involving upper limbs and the face responded to stimulation of the more ventral areas of cortex, whereas movements of lower limbs resulted from stimulation of the more dorsal areas, in agreement with the somatotopic map proposed by Penfield.

An Ethological Action Map in the Human Primary Cortex

There is evidence that ethological action maps also exist in the human primary motor cortex. Neuropsychologist Angela Sirugu and colleagues discovered regions of the primary motor cortex of baby humans and adults that, when electrically stimulated, produced a hand-to-mouth movement like what had been observed in monkeys (Desmurget et al., 2014). The sites that produced the movements were more sparsely distributed than in the monkey. The reason for this difference is not known, but it may be that the organization of complex movements differs between the two species.

FIGURE 8.13

Somatotopic organization of the primary motor cortex. (a) Somatotopic map proposed by Penfield. (b) The amount of cortex dedicated to a given body part is relative to the complexity of its connectivity. This results in a disproportionate representation of the body.

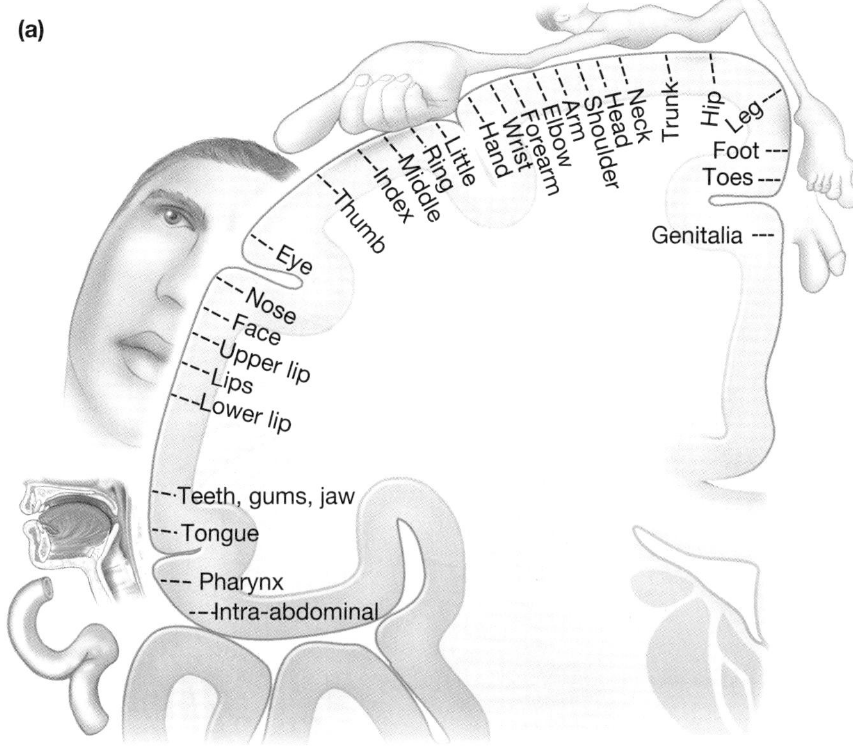

(b)

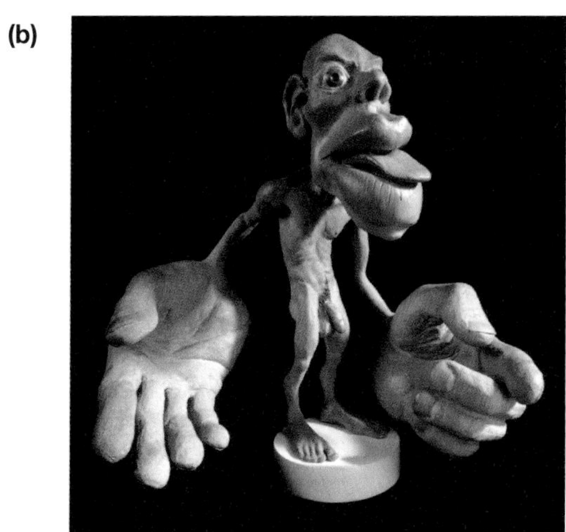

(a) Adapted from *The Cerebral Cortex of Man*, Penfield and Rasmussen. © 1950 Gale, a part of Cengage Learning, Inc.; (b) The Natural History Museum, London/Science Source.

Evidence From Electrophysiological Recordings

Further evidence for the role of the motor cortex in voluntary movement came not only from electrical stimulation but also from recording the electrical activity of individual neurons. For example, in the 1960s, Edward Evarts showed that individual neurons on one side of the motor cortex of monkeys fired a train of action potentials with the voluntary movement of a part of the body on the contralateral side (remember from the previous unit that the axons of the corticospinal tract decussate).

In a classic experiment, Evarts recorded the electrical activity of neurons in the wrist region of the primary motor cortex of monkeys while they rotated a bar attached to a load by flexing their wrists (Figure 8.15a). He found that, with training, the neurons he recorded from started firing slightly before the wrist flexion (but not wrist extension) and remained active throughout the movement. This meant that the motor cortex is involved not only in initiating and maintaining movement but also in anticipating it (Figure 8.15b). He also found that other neurons fired with the extension of the wrist but remained silent during flexion (Evarts, 1966).

In another classic experiment, Apostolos Georgopoulos found that some neurons in the primary motor cortex responded preferentially to the direction of arm movements (Georgopoulos, Kettner, & Schwartz, 1988). In that experiment, monkeys were trained to move their arm in different directions while Georgopoulos recorded from different neurons in the arm region of the primary motor cortex. He found that the firing of neurons changed in relation to the direction of the monkey's arm movement. Each neuron fired in its preferred direction. The neuron fired progressively less with movement away from its preferred direction. As in Evarts's experiment, Georgopoulos found that these cells also fired in anticipation of the movement.

Premotor Cortex and Supplementary Motor Area

Just anterior to area 4, where the precentral gyrus houses the primary motor cortex, lies area 6, which contains two

FIGURE 8.14

Some of the ethologically relevant behaviors elicited by stimulation of specific motor-cortex areas.

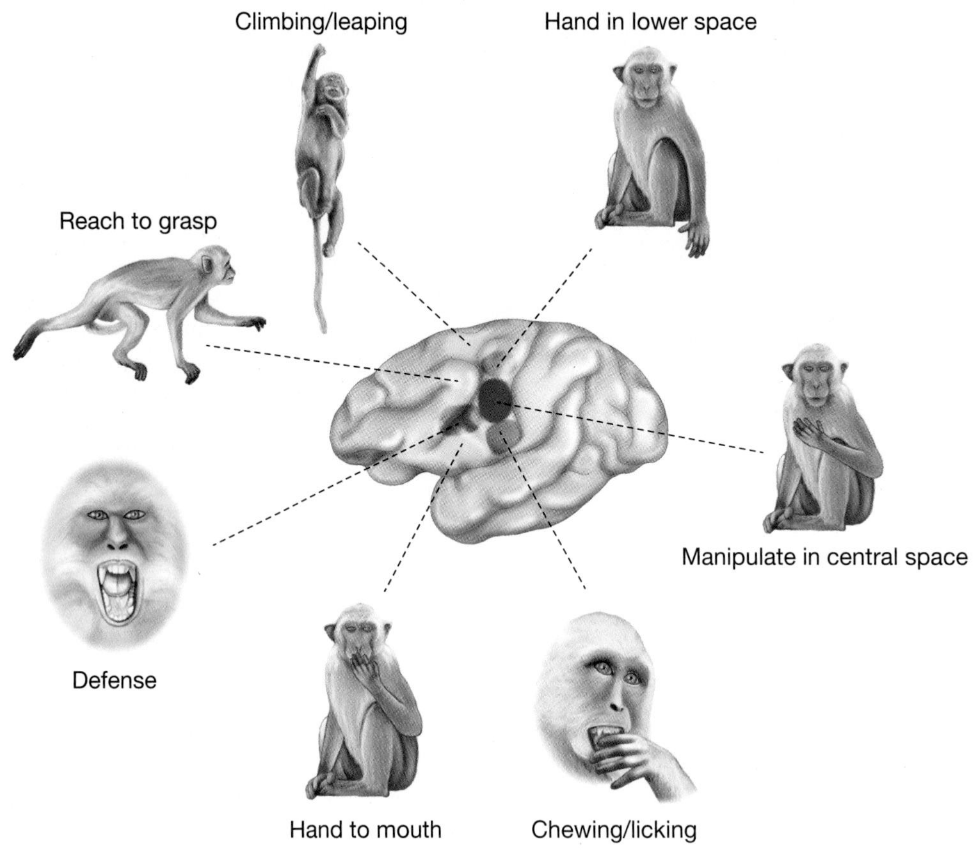

Amanda Tomasikiewicz/Body Scientific Intl.

other regions, shown in Figure 8.12, that are important for voluntary movement. These are the premotor cortex and the supplementary motor area (SMA), sometimes known as the supplementary cortex. These regions are responsible not for the generation of voluntary movements itself, as is the primary motor cortex, but for their planning and preparation. They do so by selecting the sequence of movements that will be necessary to deal with the task at hand. However, whether the premotor cortex or the SMA is involved in movements depends on whether a movement is made in response to an environmental cue, such as a traffic light turning red, or in response to an internally generated event, such as the decision to open a drawer to look for your pencil case. The following experiment dissociated the functions of these areas.

In the 1990s, Hajime Mushiake and colleagues recorded the electrical activity of single cells in the primary motor cortex, premotor cortex, and SMA of monkeys while they performed a motor task (Mushiake, Inase, & Tanji, 1991). In one condition, the monkeys were trained to reach and touch a sequence of three pads by following lights that illuminated the pads. In another condition, they were trained to remember the sequence of pads to be touched without any visual cues. Mushiake and colleagues found that the primary motor cortex was active during the performance of the sequence of movements whether it was cued by the lights or depended on memory, which is what was expected from the primary motor cortex, since it is directly involved in generating movement.

The main finding was that cells in the premotor cortex were active only when the sequence of movements was cued by the lights (visual) but not when the performance of the sequence of movements depended on memory (internal). The opposite pattern of results was observed for the SMA, which was active when movements were generated internally by memory but not when visually guided.

Mirror Neurons: Linking Perception With Action

During the 1990s, neuroscientist Giacomo Rizzolatti and colleagues were recording the electrical activity in the brains of monkeys while they were engaged in various motor acts. One day, the researchers noticed that neurons in the premotor cortex of the monkeys fired when they saw one of the researchers reach for a cup of gelato ice cream. Following this serendipitous finding, they found that the same neurons of the

FIGURE 8.15

(a) Evarts's experimental set-up. (b) Electrical activity in a motor cortex neuron was shown to increase slightly before and during wrist flexion.

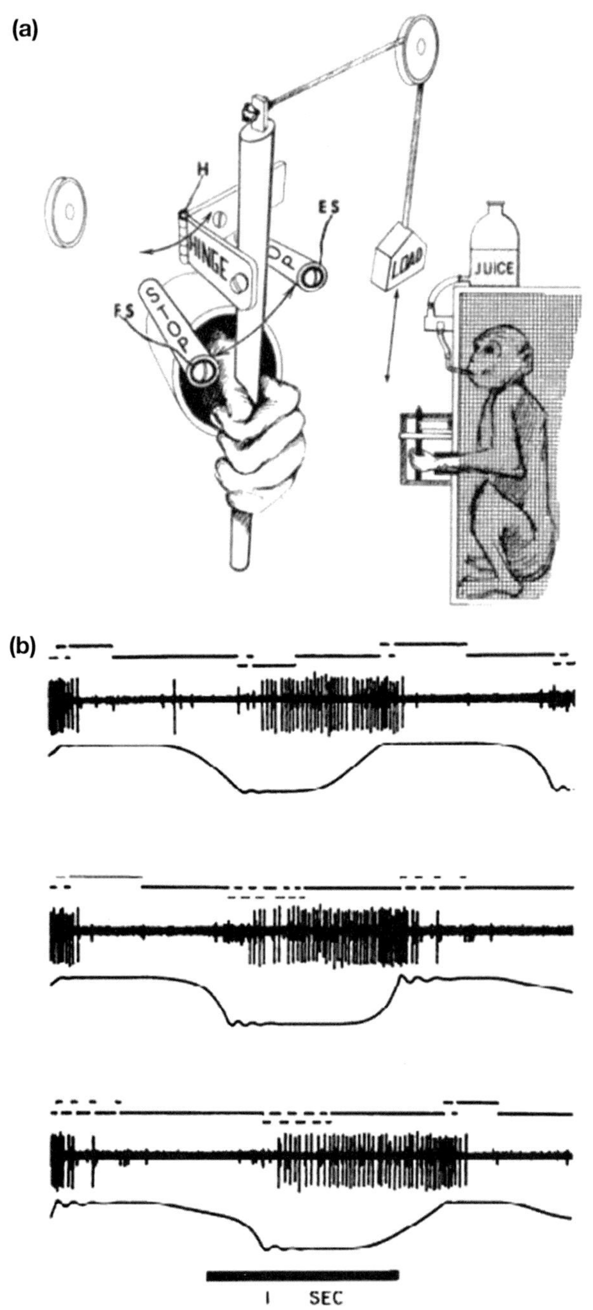

Evarts E.V. (1968). Relation of pyramidal tract activity to force exerted during voluntary movement. *Journal of Neurophysiology 31*(1):14–27. With permission from the American Physiology Society.

premotor cortex (area F5) fired either when monkeys watched another monkey (or human) perform a motor act or when they performed the same action themselves (Rizzolatti, Fadiga, Gallese, & Fogassi, 1996). For this reason, the researchers called these neurons mirror neurons, which have also been found to exist in the inferior parietal lobule (IPL) of monkeys.

Soon after, Rizzolatti and colleagues hypothesized that mirror neurons may play an important role in understanding and predicting the intentions of others. To test this hypothesis, they designed experiments to find out whether mirror neurons also fired when the result of an incomplete action could only be imagined and when the actions of others could reflect different intentions. In one experiment, they first had a monkey watch someone reach out to pick up an object, while recording from a mirror neuron in the premotor cortex. As expected, this triggered the neuron to fire. The same neuron did not fire as intensely when the monkey observed the same action but with no object present, indicating that mirror neurons also encode the *goal* of a motor act.

Next, the researchers had a monkey watch someone reaching behind an opaque screen, where the monkey knew an object was located. Again, the mirror neuron fired intensely, indicating that it responded to the intention of the action even if the monkey could not see the complete act. Finally, the mirror neuron did not fire intensely when the monkey watched someone reaching behind the opaque screen if it knew no object was located there.

In another experiment, a neuron in the IPL of a monkey fired when the monkey grasped a piece of fruit to bring it to its mouth but not when it grasped it to put it in a container. The same neuron also fired when watching a human picking up a piece of food to bring it to her mouth but not when picking it up to put it in a container. This indicated that mirror neurons fire in response to the specific intentions of a motor act, not only to the intentions of the monkey itself but also to the specific intentions of others (Fogassi et al., 2005).

Mirror Neurons in Humans

Mirror neurons have also been found to exist in the human brain. The human mirror neuron system, known as the frontoparietal mirror neuron system, comprises the superior temporal sulcus, the IPL (equivalent to the PF and PFG areas in monkeys), the ventral premotor cortex, and the inferior frontal gyrus (Iacoboni & Dapretto, 2006).

In the preceding section, you learned about studies in monkeys in which mirror neurons were shown to be involved in action understanding and in predicting the intentions of others. However, an important way by which we can decipher the intentions of others is through the context in which an action takes place. Marco Iacoboni and colleagues (2005) found that mirror neurons in humans can do just that. They showed human participants video clips of a hand grasping a cup within two different scenes, while their brains were being imaged by functional magnetic resonance imaging (fMRI) (Iacoboni et al., 2005). In one of the scenes, the context indicated that the intention of grasping the cup was for drinking tea. In the other scene, the context suggested that the cup was being grasped for cleaning up (intention). They also showed the participants clips in which the contexts of the scenes suggested arrangements of objects as they were before and after tea (context) as well as clips that showed only context-free scenes of the hand of a person grasping a cup (action). In the "intention scenes," the expected grips on the cups are the opposite of what you would expect, that is, a precision grip for cleaning up and a full-hand grip for drinking. This was to ensure that neurons responded to the intention based on the context and not the type of grip.

The inferior frontal gyrus, which is part of the mirror neuron system, was found to be significantly more active during the intention/drinking clip than in all other conditions. This showed that a subset of mirror neurons does indeed code for the intentions of others. Why was the inferior frontal gyrus not as activated during the intention/cleaning clip? The authors suggested that it is because the intention to drink when presented with such a context is much more ingrained in human behavior than is the intention to clean, which is more culturally acquired. Other functions attributed to mirror neurons include empathy, self-awareness, learning, and imitation. We discuss these properties of mirror neurons as well as their significance in social behavior in Chapter 15.

Parietal Cortex

The parietal cortex includes the primary somatosensory area, which as discussed earlier also contains a somatotopic map of the body. It lies caudally adjacent to the primary motor cortex, on the other side of the central sulcus. Therefore, it is also referred to as the postcentral gyrus. However, the parietal cortex is also subdivided in many other areas. The area of focus in this section is the posterior parietal cortex (PPC). It is situated just caudal to the somatosensory cortex, in the dorsal-most part of the cortex.

The PPC is subdivided further into several other areas. Figure 8.16a shows the location of the PPC and its main subdivisions in the monkey brain. The largest subdivision is between the superior parietal lobule (SPL) and the inferior parietal lobule (IPL). The regions are separated by the intraparietal sulcus. Other regions have been identified in both the SPL and the IPL. The IPL is subdivided into the lateral intraparietal area (LIP) and the anterior intraparietal area (AIP). The SPL contains the parietal reach region (PRR) (Figure 8.16b).

The PPC is active during the anticipation, preparation, or intention to move your hand toward a target. It encodes the position, in coordinates, of targets for movements, for example, the location of a pen on a tabletop. What is fascinating about the PPC is that it does so from different frames of reference. What does this mean? When you need to reach for something, such as the pen on a tabletop, the coordinates for its location must be computed. The coordinates for the location of the pen are computed relative to the position of your eyes, head, body, and limbs. That is, in eye-centered, head-centered, body-centered, and limb-centered coordinates. For example, the pen may lie directly in front of you, relative to your eyes. However, relative to your right arm, it is to the right. So, if all you want to do is visually describe the pen, you only need to know where it is in eye-centered coordinates. However, reaching for it requires that you know the pen's location relative to your arm, that is, in arm-centered coordinates.

This holds true for sensory modalities other than vision. For example, as I write this section, I hear music being played through a speaker in the café I am sitting in. In head-centered coordinates, I can perceive the music as coming from above my head. However, if asked to point

FIGURE 8.16

Subdivisions of the posterior parietal cortex. (a) The intraparietal sulcus divides the posterior parietal cortex (PPC) into the superior parietal lobule (SPL) and the inferior parietal lobule (IPL). (b) The IPL is subdivided further into the lateral intraparietal area (LIP) and the anterior intraparietal area (AIP). The SPL contains the parietal reach region (PRR).

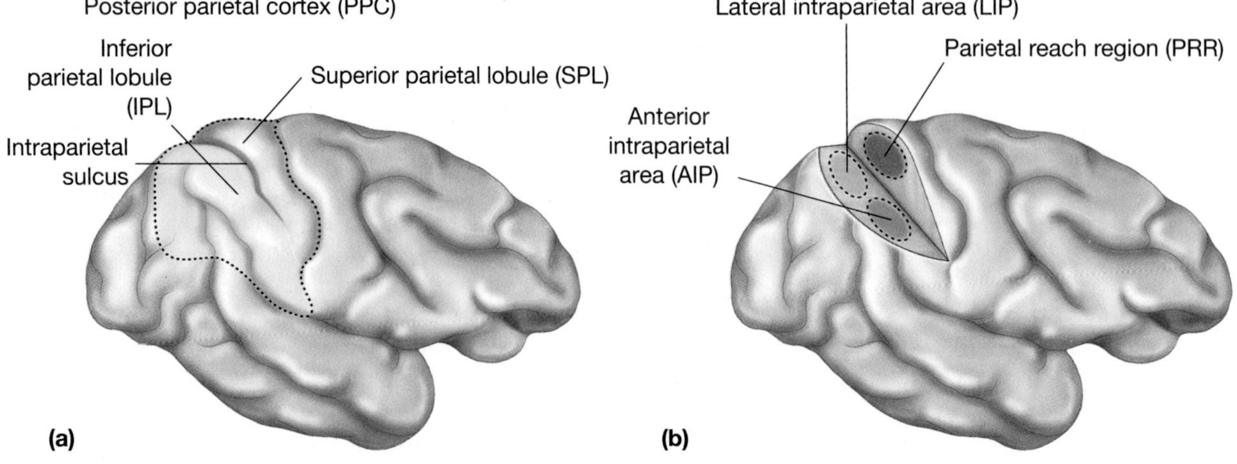

Amanda Tomasikiewicz/Body Scientific Intl.

FIGURE 8.17

Roles of the lateral intraparietal cortex (LIP) and parietal reach area (PRR). (a) Monkeys were trained to keep touching a button located directly in front of them. While the monkeys kept a hand on the button, either a green or a red light was lit to their right. The monkeys were rewarded to shift their gaze toward the light when it was red (saccade) and to reach and touch it when it was green. After training, (b) neurons in the LIP were activated when the red light came on, indicating that the LIP was activated when the monkeys anticipated making a saccade and (c) neurons in the PRR were activated when the green light came on, indicating that the monkeys anticipated reaching for the target.

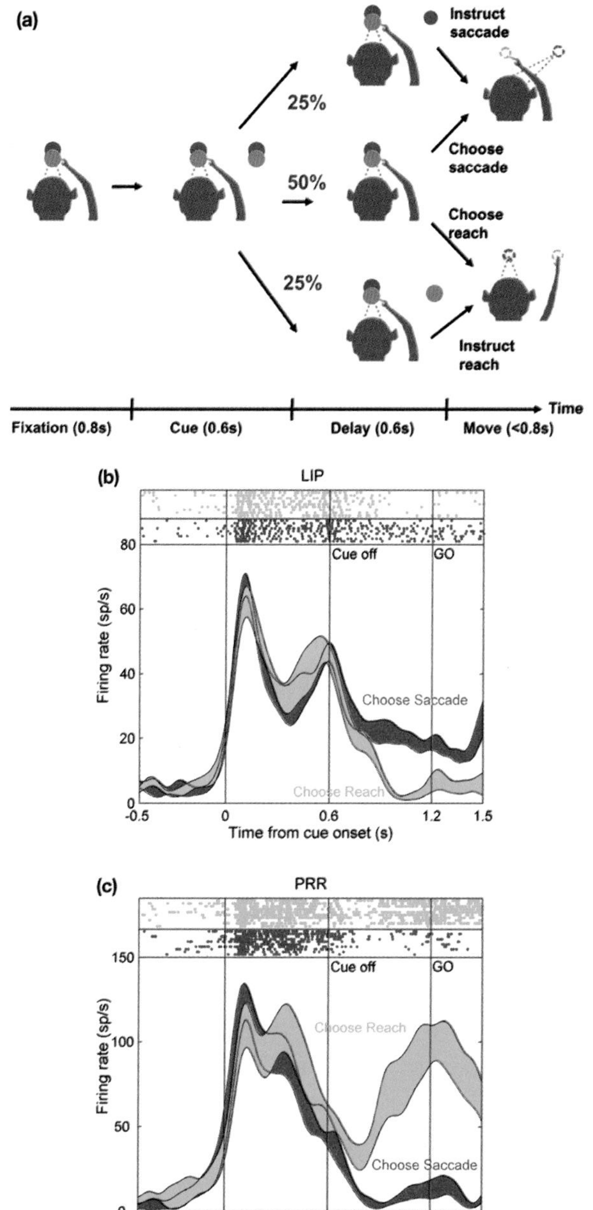

Cui, H. & R.A. Andersen. (2007). Posterior parietal cortex encodes autonomously selected motor plans. *Neuron 56*(3): 552–9. With permission from Elsevier.

to the source of the music, I would have to know the location of the speaker relative to my hand, that is, in hand-centered coordinates.

We now shift our focus to the PPC areas illustrated in Figure 8.17. Each of these plays a different role in the intention of moving. The LIP region is involved in the intention of moving the eyes toward a target, whereas the PRR is active when intending to reach for an object. The anterior intraparietal area region is necessary to shape the hand in a way that is appropriate for grasping an object.

This means that when I feel like sipping my coffee, I shift my gaze from the computer screen to visually locate the cup, involving the LIP region. As I reach for the cup, which involves the PRR, I shape my hand so that I can effectively grasp the cup, which involves the AIP region. The roles of the LIP and PRR were investigated by recording the electrical activity in the neurons of both regions. For example, as illustrated in Figure 8.17a, Cui and Andersen (2007) trained monkeys to keep touching a button located directly in front of them, in which both a green and a red light were lit. Then, while the monkeys kept a hand on the button, either a green or a red light was lit to their right. The monkeys were rewarded to shift their gaze toward the light when it was red (saccade) and to reach and touch it when it was green. After training, the researchers found that neurons in the LIP were activated when the red light came on and that neurons in the PRR were activated when the green light came on. This indicated that the LIP was activated when the monkeys anticipated making a saccade and that the PRR was activated when the monkeys anticipated reaching for the target. The results are shown in Figures 8.17b and 8.17c.

The Basal Ganglia and the Cerebellum

The Basal Ganglia

The basal ganglia are collections of interconnected nuclei involved in regulating movement. They do so by striking a balance between generating and inhibiting movement. For example, movement needs to be generated to reach for your phone, but it also needs to be inhibited so that you do not unnecessarily reach for it with both hands. Also, movements are often prioritized. For example, movement is generated so that you can reach for your phone, but it also has to be inhibited if you are holding a cup of hot coffee in the hand with which you usually reach for it.

FIGURE 8.18

The basal ganglia.

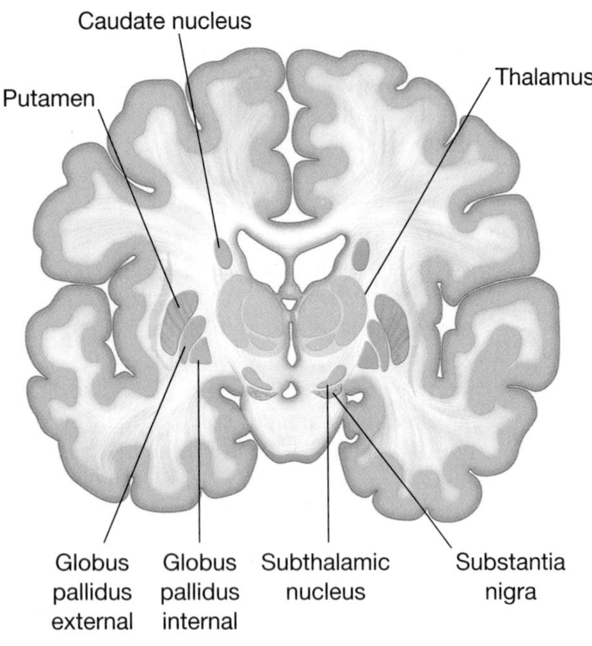

Carolina Hrejsa/Body Scientific Intl.

FIGURE 8.19

The direct pathway. See text for details. Blue and green arrows represent excitatory connections, and red arrows represent inhibitory connections.

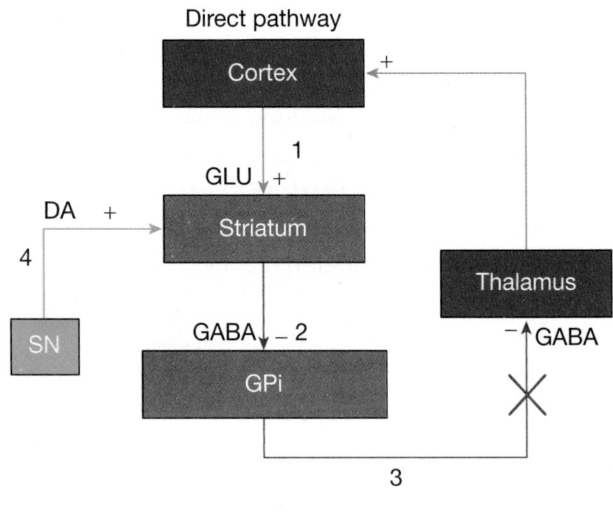

Adapted from The Basal Ganglia. What-when-how: In Depth Tutorials and Information. The-Crankshaft Publishing.

The location of the basal ganglia is shown in Figure 8.18. They comprise the putamen, the caudate nucleus, the globus pallidus internal (GPi), the globus pallidus external (GPe), the substantia nigra (SN), and the subthalamic nucleus (STN). Together, the putamen and caudate are known as the striatum.

Inputs to the basal ganglia include cortical areas related to movement, sensory areas, and association areas. The striatum is the primary recipient of these inputs. The basal ganglia process the information from these inputs and generate responses that are fed back to the cortex through the thalamus.

Information flows through the basal ganglia and back to the cortex along distinct pathways. As you will read in the sections that follow, the aim of the direct pathway is to generate movement, whereas the aim of the indirect pathway is to inhibit movement.

The Direct Pathway. The direct pathway is named as such because the striatum has direct connections to the GPi. The aim of the direct pathway, illustrated in Figure 8.19, is to facilitate movement, which is ultimately created when the motor cortex sends excitatory messages to your muscles. The role of the thalamus, which is the major output structure of the basal ganglia, is to excite the motor cortex. However, the motor cortex cannot constantly be under the excitatory influence of the thalamus, because if it did movements would go unchecked. This would make the simple task of accurately reaching out for your cup of iced cappuccino an extremely difficult one.

For this reason, some level of inhibition has to be exerted on the thalamus. The structure of the basal ganglia that inhibits the thalamus is the GPi. Therefore, for movement to occur, the inhibitory influence of the GPi on the thalamus has to be removed. This occurs as an outcome of the flow of information through the direct pathway of the basal ganglia in the following way:

1. When you want to move, the motor cortex sends excitatory messages, using the neurotransmitter glutamate (GLU), to neurons in the striatum.
2. These striatal neurons are inhibitory and use GABA as a neurotransmitter. When activated, these neurons form inhibitory synapses with neurons of the GPi.
3. Since the thalamus is normally inhibited by the GPi, through GABAergic projections, inhibition of the GPi by the striatum removes its inhibitory influence on the thalamus (as indicated by the X on the inhibitory connection in Figure 8.19), leaving it free to excite the motor cortex.
4. Neurons in the SN, which use dopamine (DA) as a neurotransmitter, participate in regulating the activity of the GPi by further activating GABAergic neurons in the striatum.
5. The STN sends excitatory messages to the SN, using GLU, increasing its activity. Its own activity is regulated by negative feedback via inhibitory connections from the SN (not shown in the figure).

The Indirect Pathway. To continue with our example from the preceding section, reaching for your iced cappuccino requires you to generate movements. The generation of these movements is made possible by the information that flows within the basal ganglia in the direct pathway. However, as you reach for the cup, unintended movements have to be inhibited, such as moving both your hands toward the cup or other irrelevant movements. You can probably guess that, if generating movement involves loosening the GPi's inhibitory influence on the thalamus, then inhibiting movement involves increasing the amount of inhibition that the GPi has on the thalamus. This occurs through activity within the indirect pathway of the basal ganglia. The indirect pathway is named as such because within this pathway the striatum connects to the GPi only indirectly by way of the GPe and the STN. The flow of information within the indirect pathway is described by the steps outlined here and illustrated in Figure 8.20:

1. To inhibit unintended movement, excitatory messages are transmitted from the motor cortex to the striatum using GLU.
2. The excitatory messages from the motor cortex trigger the striatum to send inhibitory projections to the GPe using GABA.
3. The GPe sends inhibitory GABAergic projections to the STN.
4. The STN has excitatory connections with the GPi using GLU.
5. The GPi is then permitted to inhibit the thalamus though its GABAergic projections, which results in a reduction of excitation of the motor cortex.

FIGURE 8.20

The indirect pathway. See text for details. Blue and green arrows represent excitatory connections, and red arrows represent inhibitory connections.

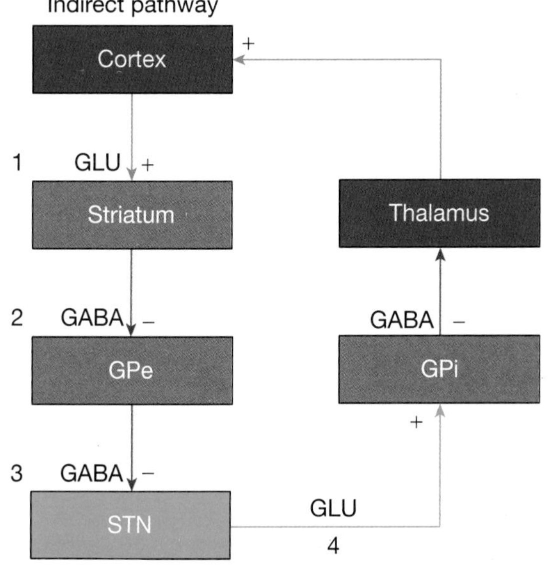

Adapted from The Basal Ganglia, What-when-how: In Depth Tutorials and Information, The-Crankshaft Publishing.

Disorders of the Basal Ganglia. After reading the preceding section, I am sure you can imagine that disruptions of the pathways within the basal ganglia could lead to a progressive loss in the ability to execute voluntary, smooth, and controlled movements. Two of these disorders are Parkinson's disease and Huntington's disease. The psychological disorder known as obsessive-compulsive disorder (OCD) is also believed to involve dysfunctions within the basal ganglia, and is discussed in Chapter 14.

Parkinson's Disease

Parkinson's disease is characterized by three main symptoms: bradykinesia, which refers to slowness in movements; rhythmic involuntary muscle contractions, known as tremors (shaking), at rest; and muscular rigidity. The symptoms of Parkinson's are due, at least in part, to the depletion of dopamine neurons in the SN.

The lack of dopaminergic input to the striatum results in an increase in the inhibitory effect the striatum has on the GPe within the indirect pathway. Increased inhibition of the GPe leads to disinhibition of the STN, leaving it free to excite the GPi, which inhibits the thalamus. This increased activity in the indirect pathway, induced by the loss of dopamine neurons in the SN, is coupled with decreased activity in the direct pathway. This results in an inappropriate decrease in the amount of inhibition exerted on the GPi, leading it to overly inhibit the thalamus (DeLong & Wichmann, 2007).

Huntington's Disease

Huntington's disease is characterized by what are known as choreiform movements. These include involuntary twitches and jerky movements, which worsen over the years. These motor symptoms are accompanied by a progressive loss of cognitive ability. The symptoms of Huntington's are due in part to the loss of GABAergic neurons in the striatum within the indirect pathway. Remember that in the indirect pathway the striatum normally has an inhibitory effect on the GPe, which ultimately results in the inhibition of the thalamus, limiting its ability to excite the motor cortex. Therefore, in Huntington's disease, the direct pathway is inappropriately freed from the inhibitory influence of the indirect pathway, leading to overexcitation of the motor cortex (C. A. Ross & Tabrizi, 2011).

The Cerebellum

Figure 8.21a illustrates the location of the cerebellum. The cerebellum is a structure of the hindbrain. It sits

IT'S A MYTH!

Muscle Memory

Think of an action that you perform without having to give it any thought. This could be when you type text messages to your friends without even having to look at the letters. If you learned to drive a car with a standard transmission, you know how at the beginning you had to think of every action, such as switching into the correct gears and coordinating the actions of your feet to press the clutch, the gas pedal, and the brake at the right times. However, soon enough these highly coordinated motor acts became automatic and you no longer needed to give them conscious thought.

The Myth

It is not uncommon to hear that automatic actions such as these are due to "muscle memory." Once learned, these actions are retained forever, like riding a bike. To call this "muscle memory" is misleading, though, because muscles do not store memories. Memories can only be stored in the brain.

Where Does the Myth Come From?

The origins of this myth are from early definitions of skills, which did not include mental abilities but only motor skills. The most influential of these definitions was that of British psychologist Tom Hatherley Pear, who said, "Skill is the integration of well-adjusted muscular performances" (Adams, 1987; Pear, 1948). Also contributing to the myth is the fact that people associate with the brain actions that require thoughtful reflection, not seemingly mindless acts, such as reflexes, highly practiced routines, and habits.

Why Is the Myth Wrong?

Behaviors that have been repeated so often that they have become automatic are a function of procedural memory, which is itself a type of implicit memory, or memories that can be expressed without conscious awareness. Procedural memory, not muscle memory, is produced through the strengthening of synapses between neurons throughout the motor system, which includes the cerebral cortex, basal ganglia, thalamus, and cerebellum (Squire, 2004). ●

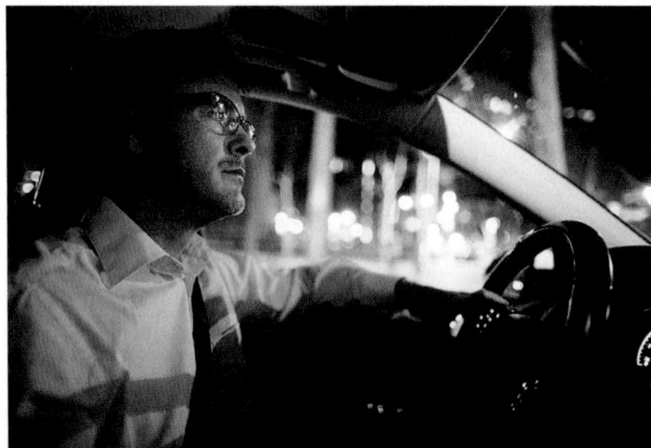

iStock.com/aluxum

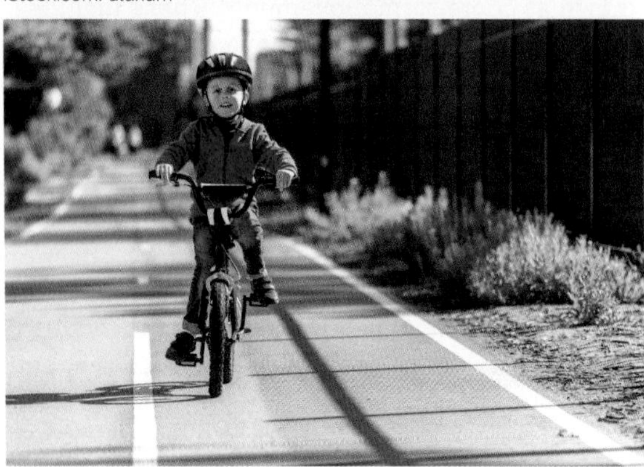

iStock.com/Andrey Moisseyev

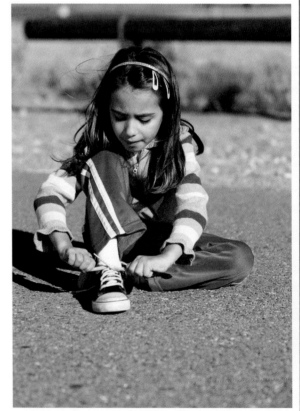

iStock.com/nicolesy

FIGURE 8.21

(a) The location of the cerebellum with the brain. (b) The types of cells in the cerebellum as well as how they are interconnected.

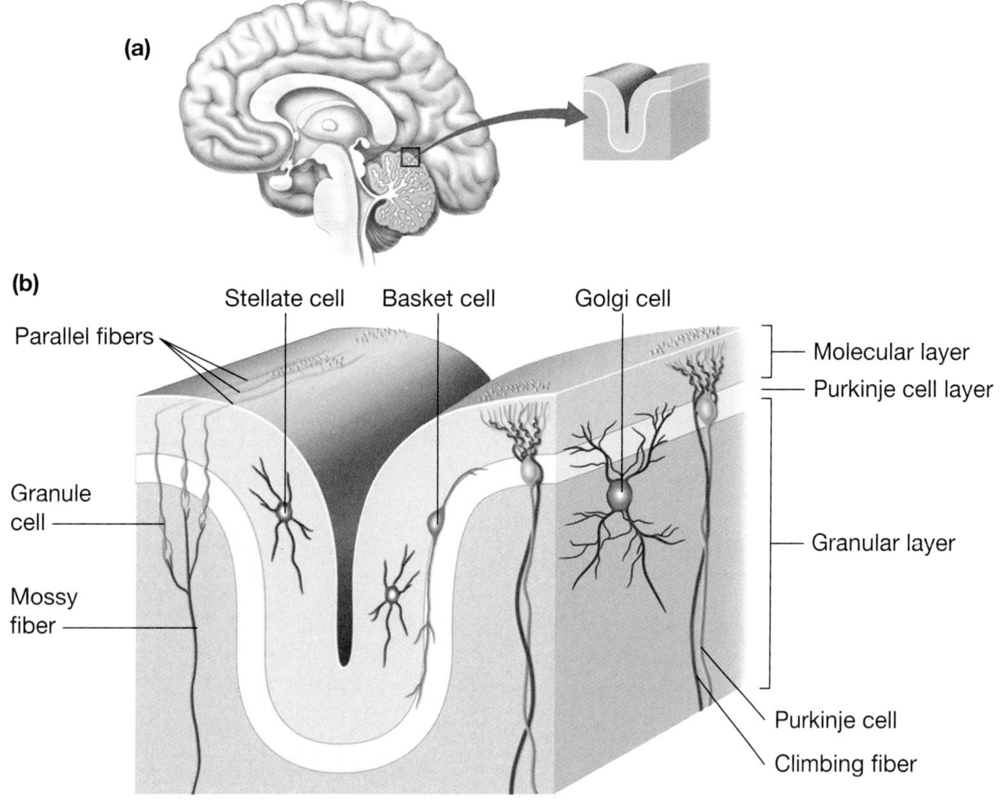

Amanda Tomasikiewicz/Body Scientific Intl.

in the back of the brainstem, at the level of the pons. The cerebellum plays an important role in motor coordination and motor learning. The cerebellum also plays an important role in cognition (Noroozian, 2014; Rapoport, van Reekum, & Mayberg, 2000; Thach, 1998). In this section, we will focus on the cerebellum's role in motor coordination and motor learning.

The cerebellum is interconnected with the brain areas important for movement, namely, the primary motor cortex, the premotor cortex, the parietal cortex, and the prefrontal cortex. However, the cerebellum's connections with the primary motor cortex are the most important for voluntary movement of the limbs. For this reason, we will focus only on these connections. When you issue a motor command to reach for your cup of iced cappuccino, your primary motor cortex sends a copy of that command to the cerebellum. This copy of the motor command is called an **efferent copy**. In addition, the cerebellum receives afferent information about the current state of the body. In this situation, the cerebellum enables you to accurately reach for the cup by providing the primary motor cortex with information to correct the trajectory of the movement if necessary.

The cerebellum contains two main types of cells: Purkinje cells and granule cells. Each type is located within its own layer of the cerebellum. Purkinje cells are the recipients of the sensory information coming from the body through what are known as climbing fibers. They are called that because of how they wrap themselves around the dendrites of Purkinje cells. A climbing fiber synapses on only one Purkinje cells, but a single Purkinje cells receives afferent connections from many climbing fibers. The arrangement of these cells as well as their fibers is illustrated in Figure 8.21b.

The efferent copy of the motor command from the primary motor cortex is conveyed through the cortico-ponto-cerebellar pathway, illustrated in Figure 8.22. This arrangement enables the cerebellum to predict the intended position of a limb through the efferent copy of the motor command it receives from the primary motor cortex through the pons, which takes less than 10 milliseconds.

This error-correction mechanism is very important for motor learning. When you perform a new motor act, as when you learn a new skill or sport, your cerebellum

FIGURE 8.22

The cortico-ponto-cerebellar pathway.

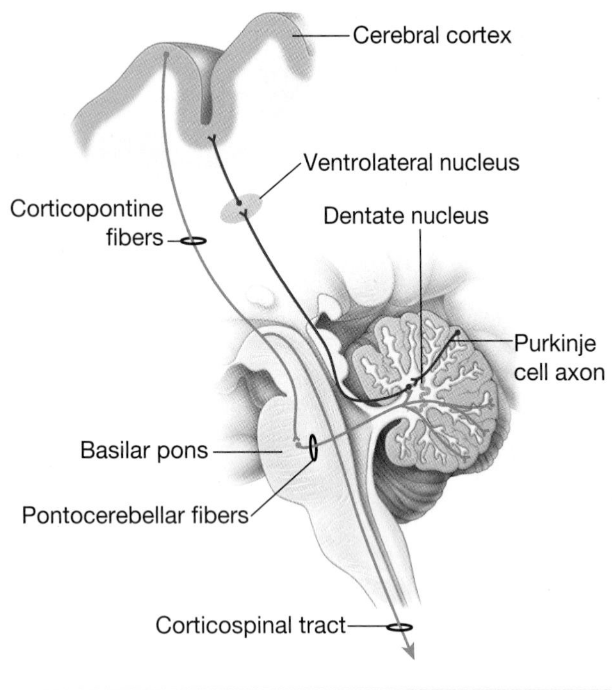

Amanda Tomasikiewicz/Body Scientific Intl.

works very hard to try to match the goal of your movements with the proper trajectories for you to be able to reach them. As you practice, this mismatch becomes progressively less pronounced.

The Basal Ganglia and the Cerebellum: Putting It All Together

Smooth and precise movements require the participation of both the basal ganglia and the cerebellum. As you can see in Figure 8.23, the motor commands sent to the primary motor cortex are sent to both. Think of the basal ganglia as the gatekeeper for movement and the cerebellum as an error-correction system. Note how both send information back to the primary motor cortex through the thalamus. The primary motor cortex then sends the revised motor commands to the brainstem and spinal cord for their execution. It is as though the basal ganglia "tell" the thalamus to "tell" the primary motor cortex whether it can or cannot create a movement and the cerebellum "tells" the thalamus to "tell" the primary motor cortex that if the movement is going to be accurate it will have to adjust it.

8.3.4 PUTTING IT ALL TOGETHER

>> LO 8.3.4 Describe how various brain areas work together to produce voluntary movement.

Now that you have learned about the major components of sensorimotor integration, it is time to summarize all you learned by putting it together. Figure 8.24 will help you do this. We could not fit all the finer details of what each area does, so you will have to go back and read the appropriate sections.

To summarize, voluntary movement involves deciding (decision making) which of several targets to

FIGURE 8.23

Interaction between basal ganglia and the cerebellum in the production of smooth movements.

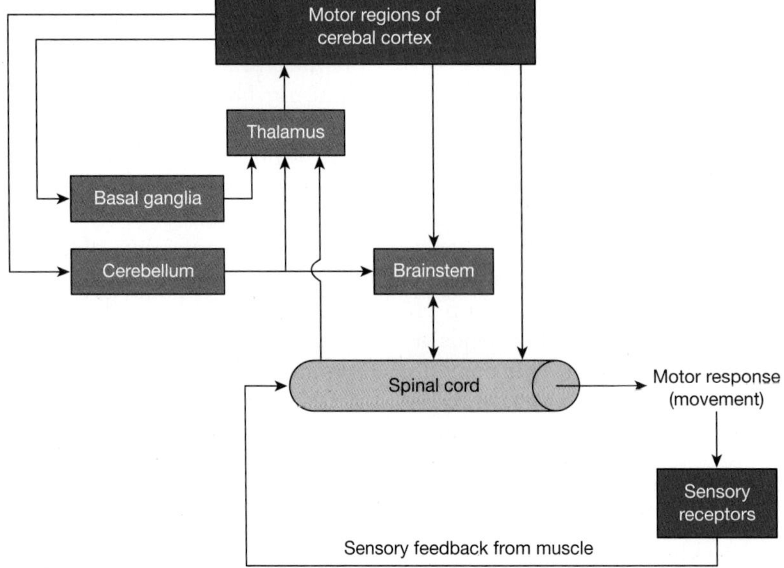

FIGURE 8.24

Visual summary of how sensory-motor integration is achieved in the brain.

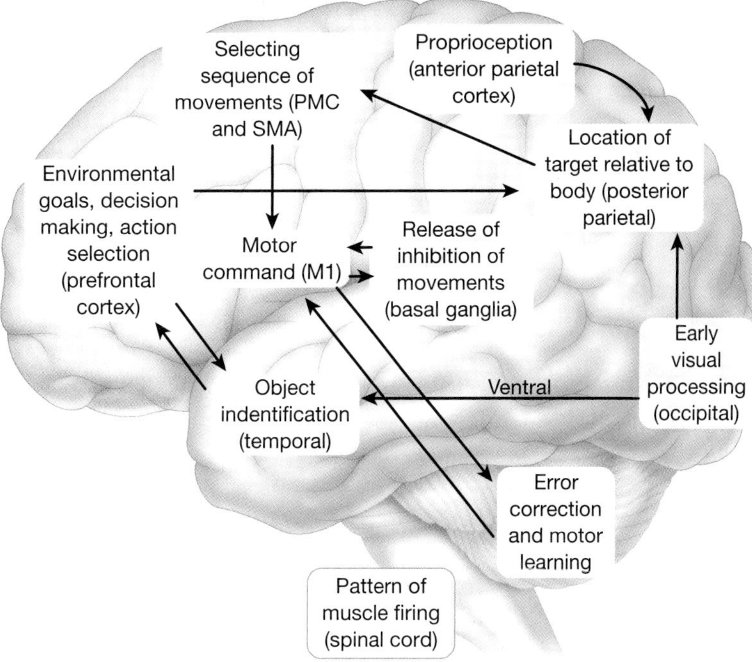

Amanda Tomasikiewicz/Body Scientific Intl.

act upon and which specific motor acts you will perform on them (action selection). This is done by the prefrontal cortex. If these are visual targets, the prefrontal cortex requires input from the primary visual cortex, in the occipital lobe. Objects also need to be recognized and identified, a function of the temporal cortex, which is part of the ventral stream of visual processing.

To be acted upon, targets for movement also need to be located in relation to the body. This function is carried out by the posterior parietal cortex, which requires proprioceptive information from the body, provided by the anterior parietal cortex. To appropriately act upon objects, a proper sequence of movements must be selected. This is done by the premotor cortex and supplementary motor area. Based on this information, the primary motor cortex issues movement commands to the spinal cord, where a pattern of muscle firing is selected. However, before the final movement commands are issued by the primary motor cortex, they are filtered out by the basal ganglia, which can inhibit certain movements and release others. Finally, the cerebellum receives an efferent copy of motor commands from the primary cortex and monitors the current position of the limbs through proprioceptive inputs. This information is used by the cerebellum to provide the primary motor cortex with feedback about the accuracy of the movement so that it can apply corrections to it and learn.

MODULE SUMMARY

Proprioception is the sense of position of different parts of the body. Proprioceptive information is conveyed through proprioceptors, which are muscle spindles and Golgi tendon organs. This information is conveyed to the somatosensory cortex through the dorsal column–medial lemniscus pathway. Movement commands from the brain are carried to the spinal cord through the descending pathways. These are the direct pathway and the indirect pathway. Neurons of the descending pathways are the upper and lower motor neurons. Upper motor neurons originate in the motor cortex and carry information to lower motor neurons in the spinal cord. Lower motor neurons synapse directly with muscle cells. The direct pathway has two separate tracts: the lateral corticospinal tract and the ventral corticospinal tract, which crosses over to the opposite side of the body at the medullary pyramids. The direct pathway is responsible for voluntary movements. Neurons of the indirect pathway originate in subcortical motor nuclei. The indirect pathway has four tracts: the tectospinal, vestibulospinal, rubrospinal, and reticulospinal tracts. The indirect pathway is responsible for reflexive movements.

The performance of movements depends on the activity of many brain areas. The prefrontal cortex is involved in action selection. The primary motor cortex directly controls movement. It is the site of a somatotopic map known as the motor homunculus. Evidence for the role in the primary motor cortex comes from electrical stimulation and electrophysiological recordings. The premotor cortex is active if a planned sequence of movements is cued, but not if drawn from memory, whereas the supplementary motor area is active in planning movements when drawn from memory but not when cued.

The premotor cortex is also the site of mirror neurons. Mirror neurons are active when an individual performs an action or when one watches another individual performing the same action. Mirror neurons were found to form a network spanning several brain areas. They became known as the frontoparietal mirror neuron system. The parietal cortex is active during the anticipation, preparation, and intention to move and when reaching for objects. The basal ganglia are involved in initiating wanted movements and in inhibiting unwanted movements. The cerebellum is important for motor coordination and motor learning.

TEST YOURSELF

8.3.1 How is proprioception involved in movement?

8.3.2 What is meant by "descending pathways"? Describe and explain the function of each one.

8.3.3 Name the different brain areas involved in movement and describe their functions.

8.3.4 How do various brain areas work together to produce movement?

APPLICATIONS

Brain-Machine Interface

What Is a Brain-Machine Interface?

A brain-machine interface is a reciprocal link between an animal or human brain and a virtual or robotic limb. A brain-machine interface can be used as a device to permit people with damage to the nervous system, such as spinal cord injury, to regain the use of a paralyzed limb. This is achieved by enabling patients to use their own self-generated electrical brain activity to control the movements of such a limb.

How Does a Brain-Machine Interface Work?

Figure 8.25 illustrates the process involved in the generation of the movement in a robotic arm. A brain-machine interface works by recording the electrical activity from hundreds of neurons located in brain areas involved in motor control through multiple channels, while a person tries to "will" the movement of a paralyzed limb. The electrical signals generated by the neurons are processed and analyzed. Movement parameters are decoded and transmitted by telemetry (wirelessly) to a receiver, which transmits the information into the circuitry of the robotic arm, which executes the movement commands. The patients can then receive proprioceptive feedback, through electrical stimulation of the somatosensory cortex, and visual feedback by observing movement of the arm (Lebedev & Nicolelis, 2017).

Who Is Doing the Research?

Leigh R. Hochberg and colleagues at Brown University reported on two patients who became tetraplegic, meaning they lost the use of all four limbs, resulting from a brainstem stroke. Both were fitted with brain-machine interfaces, which permitted them to successfully reach for and grasp objects (Hochberg et al., 2012). One of these patients is shown using the brain-machine interface in Figure 8.26. ●

FIGURE 8.25

The general plan of a brain-machine interface.

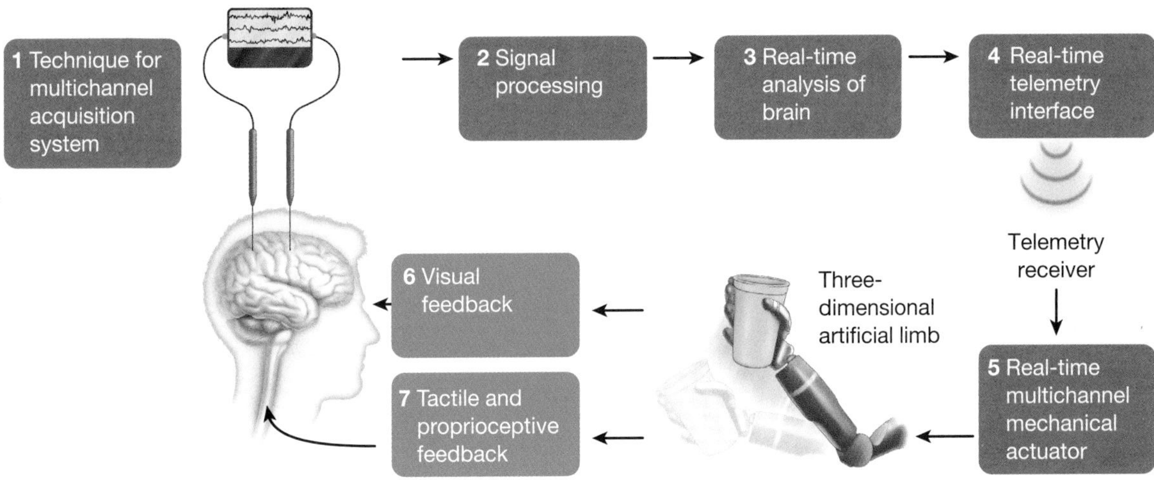

Amanda Tomasikiewicz/Body Scientific Intl.

FIGURE 8.26

Patient using a brain-machine interface to bring a drink container to her mouth with a robotic arm.

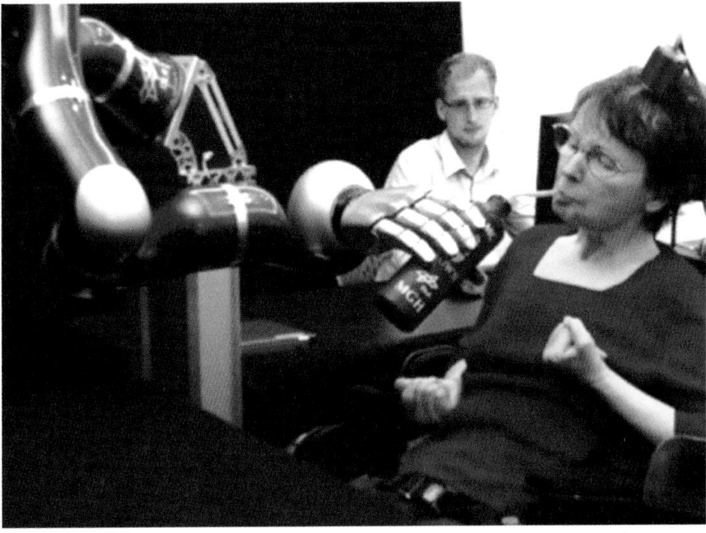

Hochberg, L.R., et al. Reach and Grasp by People With Tetraplegia Using a Neurally Controlled Robotic Arm. *Nature 485(7398)*: 372–377. With permission from Springer Nature.

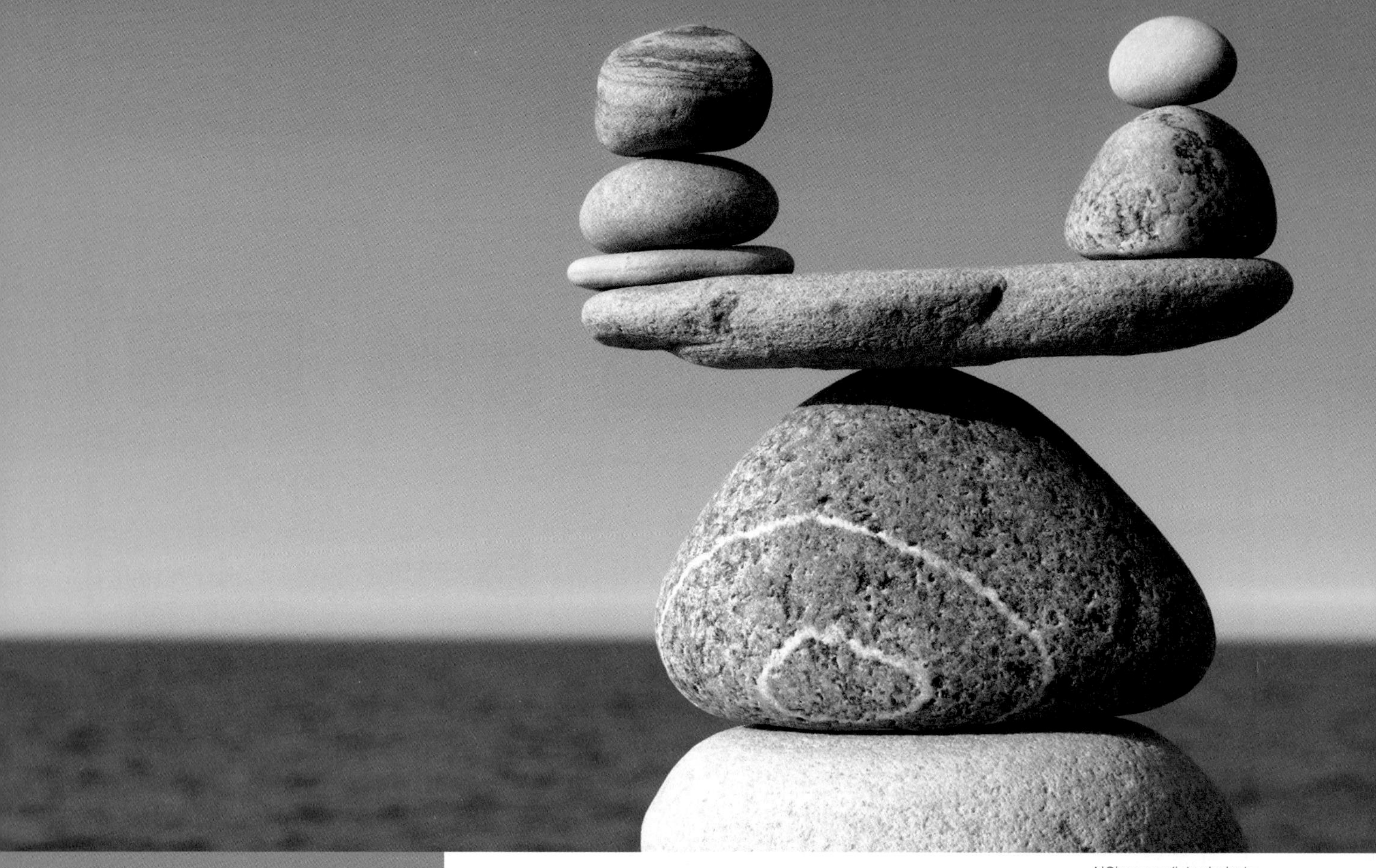

AlSimonov/istockphoto

9 Motivation

Theories, Temperature Regulation, Energy Balance, and Sleep

Chapter Contents

Learning Objectives

- **9.1.1** Define and explain motivation.
- **9.1.2** Describe need reduction theory and how it involves homeostasis.
- **9.1.3** Describe arousal theory and how it is related to personality and performance.
- **9.1.4** Describe the different theories aimed at explaining the neurobiological basis of reward.
- **9.2.1** Explain how organisms regulate their body temperatures.
- **9.2.2** Explain the mechanisms that underlie hunger and satiety.
- **9.3.1** Know how sleep is studied as well as how it is subdivided into stages.
- **9.3.2** Explain how sleep is regulated by homeostatic and circadian processes.
- **9.3.3** Explain how brain areas and neurotransmitters interact in wakefulness and sleep.

Fatal Familial Insomnia

People can sometimes have difficulty falling or staying asleep. This condition is known as insomnia. When severe, insomnia can cause significant impairments in the lives of people who suffer from it. We all have bouts of insomnia every now and then. However, imagine not ever being able to fall asleep again. Such is the fate of people with fatal familial insomnia (FFI). Fatal familial insomnia is a rare neurodegenerative disease caused by prions. Prions are proteins that can become infectious due to a mutated gene. As is implied by its name, FFI is invariably fatal. In FFI, neurons in the thalamus, which is important for the regulation of sleep, die. The course of FFI follows specific stages, beginning with disturbances in attention and memory, followed by a state of confusion, dementia, and death, all within a duration averaging 18 months. Fatal familial insomnia is a genetic disease. It is not transmissible from person to person. If one parent has FFI, the offspring each have a 50% chance of being afflicted. In his book *The Family That Couldn't Sleep*, science writer D. T. Max (2007) writes about a Venetian family that has been plagued by the disease for more than 200 years.

INTRODUCTION

The science of motivation attempts to explain why organisms behave the way they do. This includes behaviors that are necessary for survival and tightly regulated by biological mechanisms, such as eating, drinking, sleeping, and the regulation of body temperature. It also includes behaviors that are not required for survival such as eating for pleasure, athletic sport performances, various hobbies, the consumption of drugs, and a whole range of other behaviors. Motivation also affects your life choices, for example, the schools you would like to attend, the career you pursue, and who you choose to be friends with. In this chapter, you will first learn about how psychologists define motivation. You will then learn about some of the theories of motivation and the different perspectives from which it can be viewed. More specifically, you will learn that behavior can be geared toward the reduction of biological needs, finding the right levels of stimulation, or seeking pleasure. We will then take a closer look at how survival needs such as for food, temperature regulation, and sleep are satisfied.

9.1 Theories of Motivation

Module Contents

Learning Objectives

- **9.1.1** Define and explain motivation.
- **9.1.2** Describe need reduction theory and how it involves homeostasis.
- **9.1.3** Describe arousal theory and how it is related to personality and performance.
- **9.1.4** Describe the different theories aimed at explaining the neurobiological basis of reward.

9.1.1 WHAT IS MOTIVATION?

>> LO 9.1.1 **Define and explain motivation.**

Key Term

- **Motivation:** The processes that determine the initiation, maintenance, direction, and termination of behavior.

Motivation refers to the processes that determine the initiation, maintenance, direction, and termination of behavior. For example, if you go to the gym regularly, you can probably think of the reasons why you started (initiation). This may have been the desire to get back in shape, lose some weight, or simply feel better about yourself. Now that you are an avid gym-goer, think about the factors that keep you going (maintenance). This may be the feeling of satisfaction you get after a good workout or your enhanced stamina. When you joined the gym, you may have had a specific goal in mind: losing so many pounds or gaining muscular strength. Whatever the goal, you may choose a specific program that will help you achieve it (direction). There are also factors that will make you terminate your workouts. This could be completing all the exercises in your program, feeling exhausted, or quitting going to the gym altogether due to the perception that all of your efforts are in vain.

9.1.2 NEED REDUCTION THEORY

>> LO 9.1.2 **Describe need reduction theory and how it involves homeostasis.**

Key Terms

- **Primary motive:** An innate need that must be fulfilled to ensure survival.
- **Drive:** An internal state that pushes an organism to fulfill a deficiency.
- **Need reduction theory:** The theory that states that organisms are motivated by the fulfillment of needs.
- **Set point:** The desired target value of a system.
- **Nonhomeostatic drive:** A drive that is not aimed at fulfilling a physiological need.

The psychologist Clark Hull (1884–1952) believed that animals were motivated by physiological needs, for example, the needs for warmth, food, and water. These needs that are so basic to survival are referred to as **primary motives**. A deficiency in any one of those needs gives rise to a **drive**. A drive is an internal state that pushes an animal to fulfill a deficiency (Hull, 1943).

Hull believed that animals are motivated to fulfill those needs through what is known as homeostasis. Homeostasis refers to the tendency of biological systems to maintain a stable internal environment. For example, to maintain basic physiological functions, animals must store a minimal amount of food energy. A deficiency in food energy gives rise to the drive of hunger. Hunger pushes an animal to behavioral responses targeted at finding food, reducing its hunger drive. Soon enough, the animal will deplete its stores of food energy, again creating the physiological need for food. This cycle consisting of a physiological need → drive → behavioral response → need reduction is part of what is known as **need reduction theory** (Figure 9.1).

Homeostatic mechanisms are reminiscent of the functioning of a thermostat. A thermostat is a device that senses the temperature of a system so that it can be maintained at a desired target value, known as a **set point**. Most homes, schools, and office buildings are equipped with thermostats.

In the case of a thermostat, the set point refers to the temperature at which you would like a room to remain. You would enter this temperature, say, 74°F (23°C), into the thermostat. The thermostat will sense the temperature in the room and adjust the heating or air conditioning accordingly. For example, if the temperature drops below 74°F, it will turn on the heating

FIGURE 9.1

An illustration of need reduction theory.

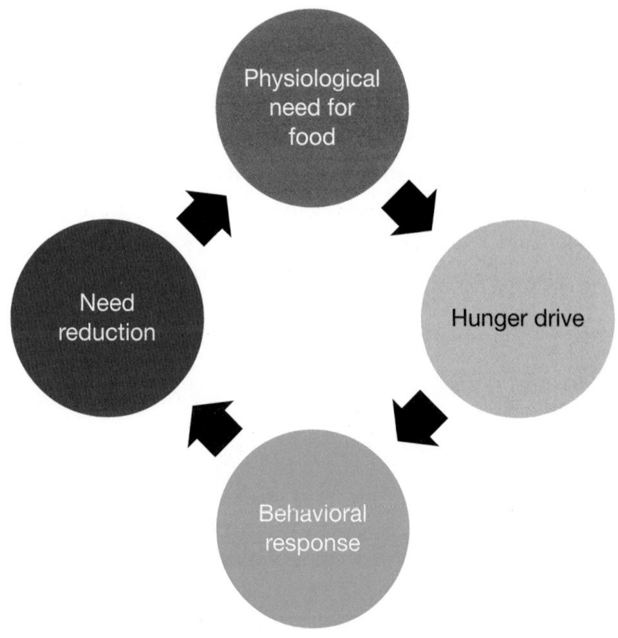

FIGURE 9.2

Location of the hypothalamus within the brain.

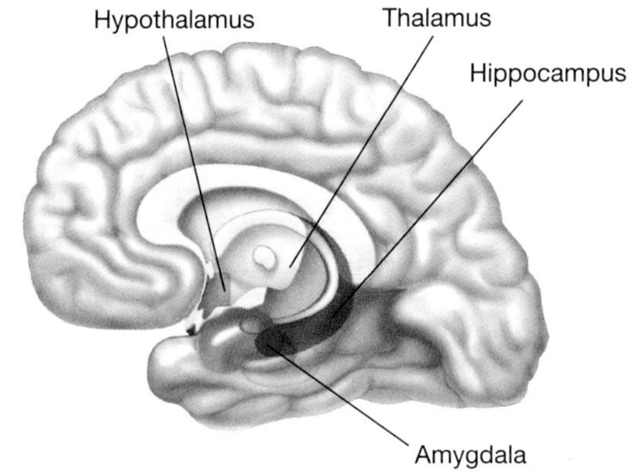

until the desired temperature is restored. In contrast, if it is hot out, and the temperature rises above 74°F, then the air conditioning will be turned on.

Similarly, the brain controls systems that keep the body's internal environment constant. The key structure in the performance of this function is the hypothalamus. Its location within the brain is illustrated in Figure 9.2.

Need reduction theory does a good job of explaining the motivation to fulfill physiological needs. However, not all behaviors can be explained by it. After all, many of the things we are motivated to do are not aimed at fulfilling physiological needs. In fact, many of our behaviors are motivated by **nonhomeostatic drives**. For example, going out to have fun with your friends, feeling like enjoying a good movie, or wanting to get onto a rollercoaster have nothing to do with fulfilling physiological needs. You may also be motivated to make changes in your life because things are not going the way you like, or because you simply need a change.

9.1.3 AROUSAL THEORY

>> LO 9.1.3 **Describe arousal theory and how it is related to personality and performance.**

Key Terms

- **Arousal theory (activation theory):** The theory proposing that an organism's motivation to act is based on the organism's state of physiological activity.
- **Arousal:** The state of physiological activity of an organism.
- **Arousal continuum:** The continuum of arousal states, associated with various activities, ranging from low to high.
- **Yerkes-Dodson law:** The relationship between performance and levels of arousal.
- **Reward deficiency syndrome:** A proposed syndrome in which high sensation seekers have inherited a low number of a type of dopamine receptors in the striatum and prefrontal cortex.

Arousal theory, also known as activation theory, was proposed by psychologist Donald B. Lindsley (1952). It explains how the motivation of organisms to act is based on their level of **arousal**, which is defined as the state of physiological activity of an organism. States of arousal range from low to high and are associated with corresponding amounts of behavioral activation, which range from deep sleep to extreme excitement. This is illustrated by the **arousal continuum** (Figure 9.3).

When it comes to performance, researchers have found that more arousal is not always better. For example, if you are too relaxed about an upcoming exam, you may not be motivated to study much, possibly resulting in your not doing well on it. At the other end of the spectrum, if you are extremely nervous about it, you may be anxious to the point of not being able to focus, resulting in poor performance on the exam. Your best performance on the exam would be related to a level of anxiety that falls somewhere between these two extremes. The relationship between performance and levels of arousal is known as the **Yerkes-Dodson law**, developed by psychologists Robert M. Yerkes and John D. Dodson (Yerkes & Dodson, 1908). The Yerkes-Dodson law is illustrated by the inverted-U function in Figure 9.4.

Although the inverted-U function of the Yerkes-Dodson law serves us well in understanding the role of arousal in motivation, it does not necessarily hold for every task. That is, when a task is simple, moderate levels of arousal are conducive to efficient performance (Figure 9.5a); however, when a task is complex, lower

FIGURE 9.3

The arousal continuum. Arousal levels range from low to high. Very low levels of arousal are associated with sleep, whereas high levels of arousal are associated with extreme excitement.

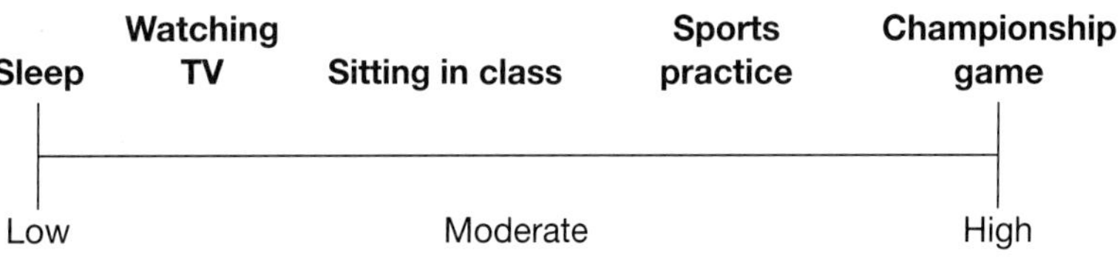

FIGURE 9.4

The Yerkes-Dodson law. Performance is related to levels of arousal in an inverted-U function, with both extremely low and extremely high levels of arousal being detrimental to efficient performance.

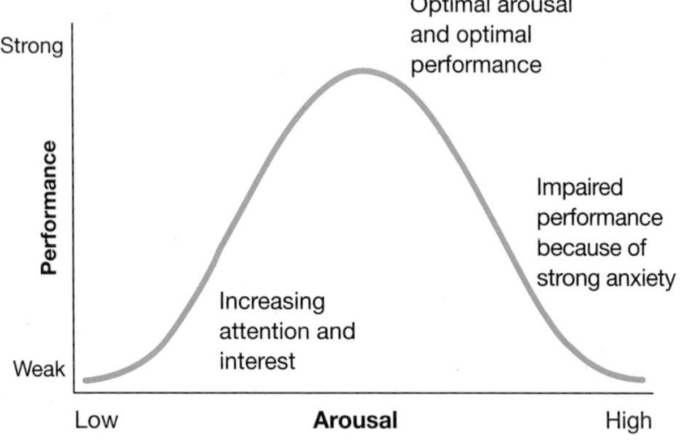

Diamond, D.M., et al. (2007). The Temporal Dynamics Model of Emotional Memory Processing. *Neural Plasticity*. Volume 2007, pp. 1–33.

levels of arousal are ideal (Figure 9.5b). For example, tasks that require fine motor coordination like performing a perfect stroke in golfing will be impaired by high levels of physiological arousal. That is why you see golfers calming down and focusing before a shot. In contrast, other tasks require that one raises arousal levels as they rely less on fine motor skills. That is why you see weightlifters "psyching up" before a lift by slapping their chest or even slapping themselves in the face.

Arousal Levels and Personality

People differ in their basal levels of physiological arousal. Some people have inherited levels of arousal that are higher than others. You may have heard that some people are high sensation seekers. These are the people who are constantly looking to raise their arousal levels. For example, you probably know people who always want to do things that are exciting, such as riding rollercoasters or jumping out of perfectly well-functioning airplanes with a parachute. By contrast, others are low sensation seeking. That is, while some of their friends are out bungee jumping, they would rather stay home reading a book (Zuckerman, 1979; Zuckerman & Neeb, 1979).

Understanding High Sensation Seeking

Over the years, much of the research aimed at understanding high sensation seeking focused on the neurotransmitter dopamine, which as you learned previously, is associated with sensations of pleasure. It was found that high sensation seekers have inherited a low number of a type of dopamine receptors (D2) in the striatum and prefrontal cortex. This leaves sensation seekers with a deficit in experiencing positive moods and the rewards provided by

FIGURE 9.5

Relationship between arousal levels and the performance of simple and complex tasks. (a) When a task is simple, moderate levels of arousal are conducive to efficient performance. (b) When a task is complex, lower levels of arousal are ideal.

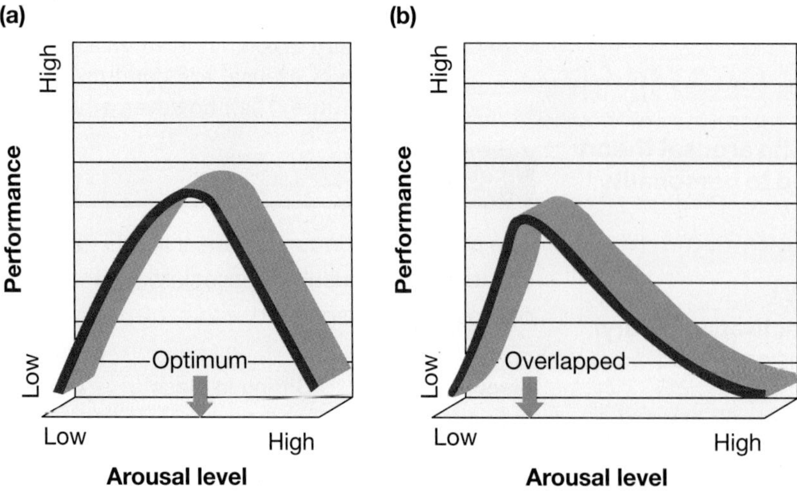

Adapted from *Psychology: A Journey*, 3rd Edition, Coon and Mitterer. Wadsworth Publishing Company, 2007.

events most people perceive as being pleasurable (Blum et al., 1996).

This became known as the **reward deficiency syndrome**, proposed by pharmacologist Kenneth Blum in the 1990s. Blum proposed that sensation seekers, because of their lower numbers of inherited D2 receptors, are constantly motivated by the search for more intense sources of rewards. On a more negative note, high sensation seekers are more prone to having problems with self-control, drug abuse, risky sexual behavior, and aggressive behavior (Charnigo et al., 2013; Heidinger, Gorgens, & Morgenstern, 2015; Kalichman, Heckman, & Kelly, 1996).

9.1.4 PLEASURE SEEKING AND REWARD

>> LO 9.1.4 **Describe the different theories aimed at explaining the neurobiological basis of reward.**

Key Terms

- **Pimozide:** A dopamine receptor antagonist used as an antipsychotic.
- **Prediction error:** The extent to which the conditioned stimulus predicts the presence of the unconditioned stimulus.
- **Dopamine ramping:** The way in which dopamine is released in increasing amounts as the steps required to obtain a reward are completed.
- **Hedonic hotspots:** Brain areas that enhance "liking" reactions when stimulated with opioids.
- **Hedonic coldspots:** Brain areas that enhance disgust reactions when stimulated with opioids.

You just learned that two primary factors that move people to act are the need for the body to maintain homeostasis and the need to maintain a certain degree of psychological and physiological arousal. However, people often seek activities that they know will provide them with pleasure. People are also motivated to act to avoid pain. We now focus on the neurobiological mechanism associated with pleasure.

In the early 1950s, psychologists James Olds and Peter Milner noticed that rats would return to an area of a desktop where they received electrical stimulation of the brain. Olds and Milner then wanted to know if the same rats would learn to press a lever to receive the same stimulation in a box, like the one in Figure 9.6. Lo and behold, the rats did so repeatedly (Olds & Milner, 1954).

FIGURE 9.6

Similar setup to that used by Olds and Milner for electrical self-stimulation in rats.

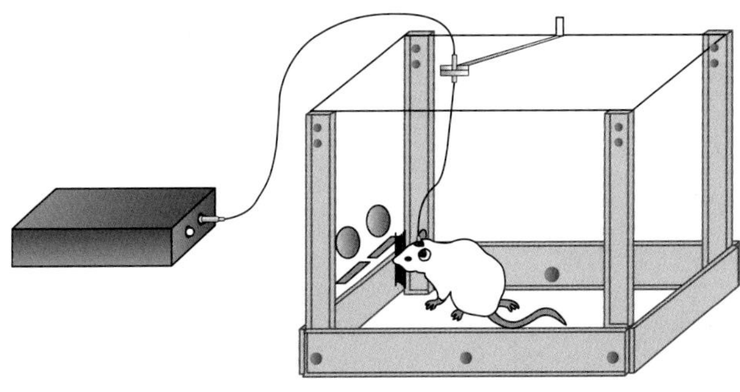

Watterson, L.R. & M.F. Olive. (2014). Synthetic Cathinones and Their Rewarding and Reinforcing Effects in Rodents. *Advances in Neuroscience* Volume 2014, pp. 1–9.

The next step was to identify the brain area that, when stimulated, reinforced the rats' lever presses. Olds and Milner found this area to be the ventral-tegmental area (VTA), from which dopamine neurons project to the nucleus accumbens (NAc) and widespread areas of the forebrain, including the prefrontal cortex. Figure 9.7 shows the location of the VTA in the rat as well as its projections to the NAc and cortex.

It was later suggested that the neurochemical basis of reward was the release of the neurotransmitter dopamine. It is well accepted that all drugs of abuse and natural reinforcers such as food and sex activate the dopamine system. In fact, it was found that rats' lever presses for access to these reinforcers is greatly

FIGURE 9.7

Location of the VTA and its projections to the NAc and cortex of the rat.

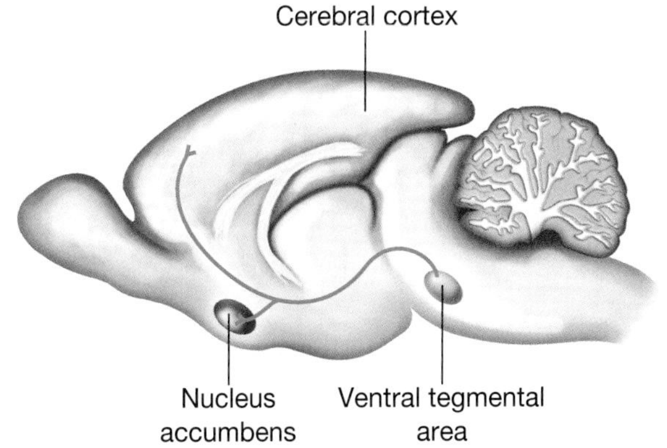

Amanda Tomasikiewicz/Body Scientific Intl.

reduced when injected with drugs that block dopamine receptors.

In the 1970s, neuroscientist Roy Wise showed that dopamine receptor antagonists, such as the antipsychotic drug **pimozide**, reduced the amount of work rats would do to receive a food reward. Figure 9.8 shows the effects of two doses of the dopamine receptor antagonist pimozide on the number of lever presses performed to obtain a food reward (De Wit & Wise, 1977). Note that the suppression of lever pressing for food was higher when the dose of the drug was increased.

Prediction Error

In the 1980s, Wolfram Schultz recorded the electrical activity of dopamine neurons in the mesolimbic dopamine system (e.g., VTA and substantia nigra [see Chapter 3 to review neurotransmitter systems]) during a task in which monkeys learned the association between the presentation of a visual stimulus and a juice reward. Eventually, monkeys learned that the visual stimulus, which became a conditioned stimulus (CS), predicted the delivery of juice, the unconditioned stimulus (US). Schultz called the extent to which the CS predicts the presence of the US **prediction error** (PE) (Schultz, Dayan, & Montague, 1997). A large PE occurs when the CS does not reliably predict the US and gradually falls to "0" as the learning of the association between the CS and the US progresses. The PE is negative when the US is omitted. Schultz (1986) reported four main findings about the activity of dopamine neurons while monkeys were performing this task (Figure 9.9):

1. During initial training on the task, dopamine neurons showed heightened activity after monkeys received the US by itself.
2. The same dopamine neurons gradually stopped responding to the US as the monkeys learned that the CS reliably predicted the US.
3. As dopamine neurons lost their response to the US, the same neurons started to respond to the reward-predicting CS.
4. Omission of the US (creating a negative PE), after the presentation of the CS, resulted in a dip in the response of dopamine neurons.

Neuroscientist Mark W. Howe and colleagues found that dopamine works in another way as well. Dopamine levels increased gradually in the striatum (another area associated with reward) of rats, as they came closer to achieving the goal of obtaining a food reward while navigating a maze (Howe, Tierney, Sandberg, Phillips, & Graybiel, 2013). Howe and colleagues called this process **dopamine ramping**. In other words, dopamine is released in increasing amounts as the steps required to get rewarded are completed. For example, imagine the steps required for

FIGURE 9.8

The effects of pimozide (a dopamine receptor antagonist) on lever pressing for access to food in rats across four days of testing. (a) Number of lever presses before the administration of pimozide. (b–c) Pimozide-induced reduction in the number of lever presses at 0.5 and 1.0 mg/kg, respectively.

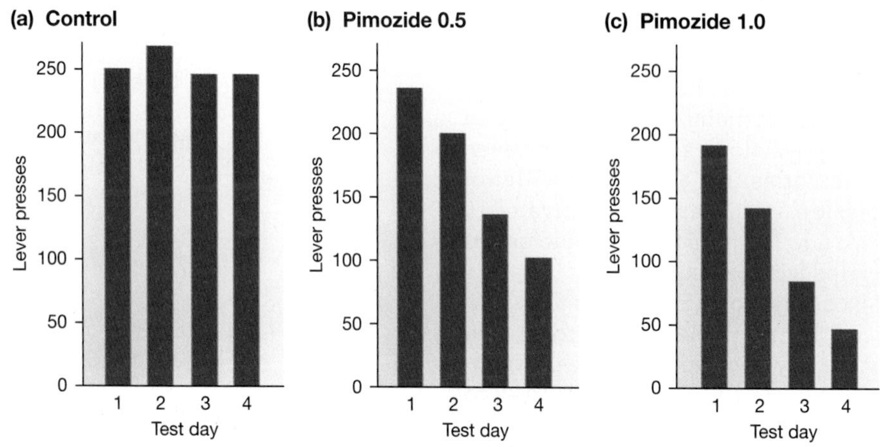

FIGURE 9.9

Patterns of responses of dopamine neurons to the presentation of the US (reinforcer [R]) and the CS. During initial training on the task, dopamine neurons showed heightened activity after monkeys received the US by itself (top). The same dopamine neurons gradually stopped responding to the US as the monkeys learned that the CS reliably predicted the US. Also, as dopamine neurons lost their response to the US, the same neurons started to respond to the reward-predicting CS (middle). Omission of the US (creating a negative PE) after the presentation of the CS resulted in a dip in the response of dopamine neurons (bottom).

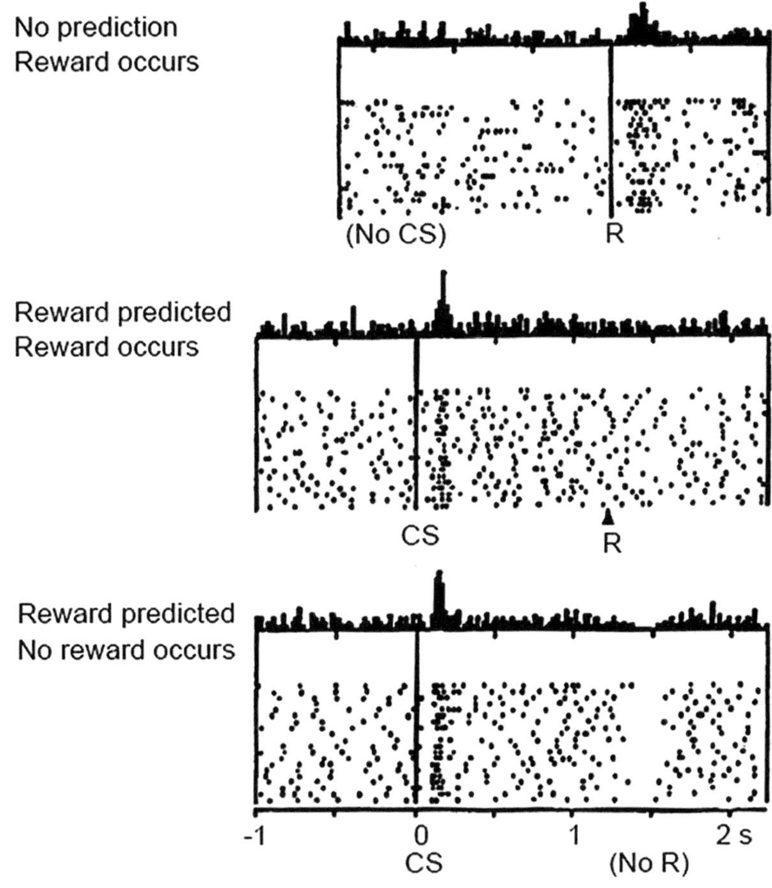

Schultz, W. et al. (1997). A neural substrate of prediction and reward. *Science 275*(5306):1593–1599. With permission from AAAS.

the person portrayed in Figure 9.10 to finally pour herself a cup of coffee. In this case, you would be making a positive reward prediction. However, dopamine levels would drop suddenly should she sip the coffee and realize that it tasted sour.

Incentive-Salience Theory

As you have been reading, the idea that dopamine is involved in reinforced behavior has been modified since the original discovery that the administration of dopamine antagonists reduced lever pressing for food in rats. In another example, researchers found that rats given a dopamine antagonist continued to like foods but were not motivated to perform work, such as pressing a lever, to obtain food (Dickinson, Smith, & Mirenowicz, 2000). Also, remember Schultz's findings (described earlier) that the activity of dopamine neurons switched from being triggered by the delivery of a reward (the US) to the anticipation of reward created by presence of a stimulus that predicted its delivery (the CS).

These findings, as well as others, led neuroscientists Terry Robinson and Kent Berridge to propose the

FIGURE 9.10

(a) Location of the striatum and dopaminergic neurons. (b) Dopamine concentrations are high when a rewarding goal has been reached. (c) Dopamine levels fall off if achieving the goal is not rewarded. (d) Dopamine levels in the striatum gradually increase as the steps toward the delivery of a reward are completed.

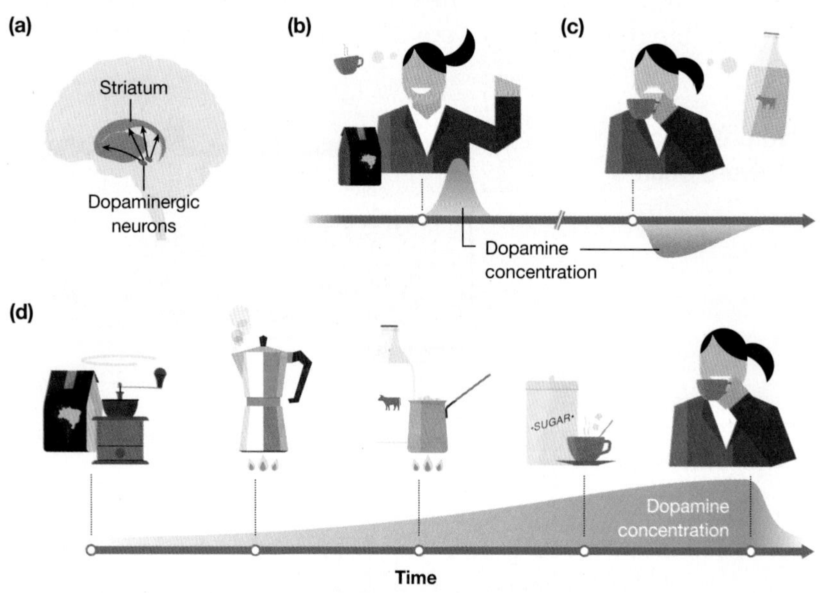

Niv, Y. (2013). Neuroscience. Dopamine ramps up. *Nature 500*: 533–535. With permission from AAAS.

incentive-salience theory of motivation, as mentioned in Chapter 3 in the context of drug addiction (Berridge & Robinson, 1998, 2016; Robinson & Berridge, 2008). To recap, Robinson and Berridge proposed that the conditioned stimuli associated with a reward act as powerful cues to its delivery and that exposure to those cues creates a state of "wanting." For individuals suffering from drug addiction, this state of wanting, after being exposed to cues they have associated with taking a drug, is characterized by intense cravings that may lead to seeking behaviors. You may have also experienced the state of wanting when driving by your favorite fast food restaurant or from the smell of your favorite cake being baked. According to the incentive-salience theory, it is this state of wanting that is generated by activity in the mesolimbic dopamine system.

When the addicted person gets the drug, the enjoyment of the drug—or in many cases the relief that is felt after having ingested the drug—creates the state Robinson and Berridge referred to as "liking." You also experience the state of liking once you have bitten in to your favorite burger or sunken your teeth into the cake.

Robinson and Berridge found that liking is associated with specific facial expressions in reactions to sweet tastes in rats, monkeys, and human babies. In contrast, bitter-tasting stimuli gave rise to different facial expressions related to what is interpreted as disgust. Because these reactions are present in human babies, they are believed to be innate (Figure 9.11a).

Robinson and Berridge also observed that liking reactions were enhanced by stimulating certain brain areas with opioids, suggesting that liking is associated with the release of endorphins rather than dopamine. They designated these brain areas **hedonic hotspots**, which include subcortical areas such as the shell of the nucleus accumbens, the ventral pallidum, and the parabrachial nucleus in the pons. They also potentially include cortical areas such as the orbitofrontal cortex and the insular cortex. By contrast, different parts of the nucleus accumbens and ventral pallidum enhanced disgust reactions when stimulated with opioids. These were designated as **hedonic coldspots** (Figure 9.11b) (Berridge & Kringelbach, 2015).

FIGURE 9.11

(a) "Liking" reactions to a sweet stimulus (left) and disgust reactions to a bitter stimulus (right). (b) Midsagittal section of a rat's brain. Opioid stimulation of parts of the nucleus accumbens, ventral pallidum, and parabrachial nucleus (hedonic hotspots) enhanced liking reactions in rats. In contrast, opioid stimulation of other parts of the same areas (hedonic coldspots) enhanced disgust reactions. The orbitofrontal cortex and insular cortex are potential hotspots.

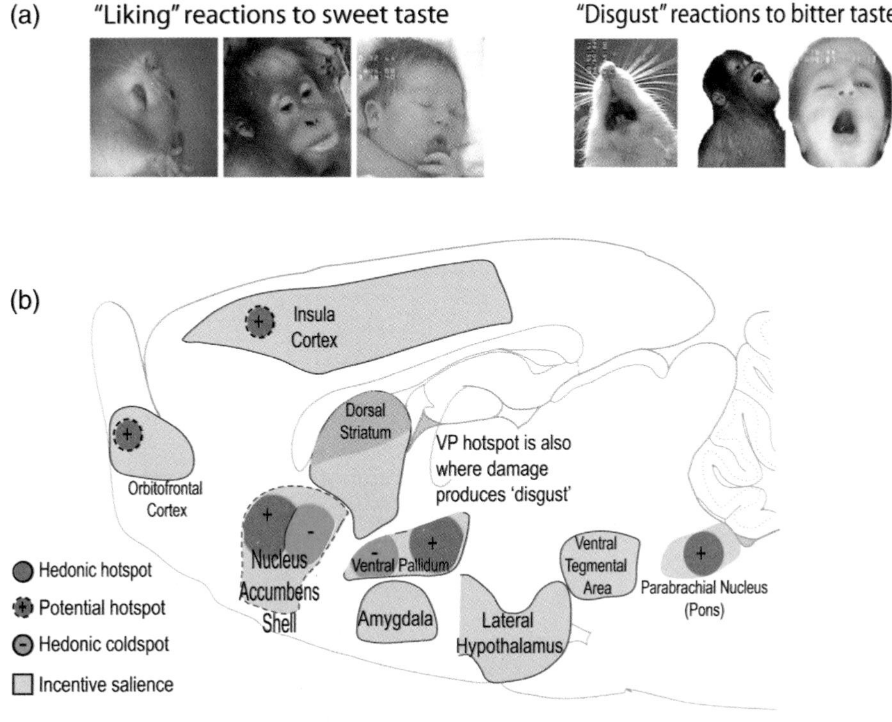

Berridge, K.C. & M.L. Kringelbach. (2015). Pleasure systems in the brain. *Neuron 86*(3): 646–664. With permission from Elsevier.

MODULE SUMMARY

Motivation is defined as the factors that determine the initiation, maintenance, direction, and termination of behavior. Theories of motivation include the need reduction theory and the arousal theory. Need reduction theory is based on the biological need to maintain homeostasis. Arousal theory is based on the idea that organisms are motivated to maintain optimal levels of arousal. However, people and other organisms are motivated not just to maintain homeostasis or optimal levels of arousal. People and other organisms are also motivated by stimuli that provide pleasure.

Dopamine was once widely thought to be associated with pleasure sensations upon the delivery of a rewarding stimulus. However, a more recent theory (prediction error) proposed that dopamine is associated not with the delivery of a reward but, rather, with learning the association between environmental cues that predict the delivery of a reward and the reward itself. It was also found that dopamine is released in progressively larger quantities as the steps toward achieving a goal are completed; this is known as dopamine ramping.

Another theory, known as incentive salience, proposes that dopamine is not necessary for "liking" a rewarding stimulus but that it generates feelings of "wanting" the rewarding stimulus when presented with cues that are associated with the reward. The delivery of a rewarding stimulus generates liking, which is inferred from observing the facial expressions of various species. Within this theory, liking is associated not with the release of dopamine but with the stimulation of various hedonic hotspots in several brain areas by endorphins.

TEST YOURSELF

9.1.1 Give an example of a motivated behavior and identify the factors that initiate, maintain, give direction to, and terminate the behavior.

9.1.2 Explain need reduction theory and homeostasis and how they are associated with each other.

9.1.3 Explain the ideas within arousal theory, such as optimal arousal, and how it is related to personality and performance.

9.1.4 Trace the evolution of how dopamine was thought to be directly implicated in reward and how more recent theories have caused scientists to revise this concept.

9.2 Physiological Mechanisms

Module Contents

Learning Objectives

9.2.1 Explain how organisms regulate their body temperatures.

9.2.2 Explain the mechanisms that underlie hunger and satiety.

9.2.1 TEMPERATURE REGULATION

>> LO 9.2.1 Explain how organisms regulate their body temperatures.

Key Terms

- **Preoptic area (POA):** The region of the hypothalamus involved in temperature regulation.
- **Endotherms:** Animals that can regulate their body temperature through internal mechanisms.
- **Ectotherms:** Animals that have no internal mechanisms to regulate their body temperature.
- **Negative feedback:** A mechanism by which a stimulus input causes a system to react by causing an opposite output to maintain a desired set point.
- **Cold defense:** Output from the hypothalamus in response to potentially threatening cooling of the body.
- **Heat defense:** Output from the hypothalamus in response to potentially threatening heating of the body.
- **Shivering:** Shaking of skeletal muscles that generate heat through the expenditure of energy.
- **Spinothalamocortical pathway (STC pathway):** The pathway through which body temperature is conveyed to the somatosensory cortex for the perception of temperature.
- **Lateral parabrachial nucleus (LBN):** The region of the brainstem involved in temperature regulation.
- **LBN-POA pathway:** The pathway through which body temperature is conveyed to the LBP and POA for temperature regulation.

One of the roles of the hypothalamus, more precisely the **preoptic area (POA)**, is to regulate body temperature. Only mammals and birds can regulate their body temperature through internal mechanisms. These are known as **endotherms**, also called warm-blooded animals. Animals like lizards, snakes, and some fish are known as **ectotherms**, also called cold-blooded animals. Ectotherms have no internal mechanisms to regulate their body temperature. Therefore, they do so by external means. For example, snakes and lizards warm their bodies by basking in the sun and cool off by moving into the shade (Figure 9.12). Fish regulate their temperatures by moving to warmer or cooler waters.

Maintaining constant body temperature is vital to the function of enzymes, which catalyze chemical reactions in the body. The proper functioning of the nervous system, such as the activity of ion channels, also depends on an optimal set point for body temperature (Guler et al., 2002; Hodgkin & Katz, 1949). Optimal body temperature varies from species to species. For humans, it is approximately 98.6°F (37°C).

Part of regulating body temperature occurs automatically. This is done through a thermoregulatory

FIGURE 9.12

Ectotherms such as lizards regulate their body temperatures by basking in the sun to warm up and cool their bodies by staying in the shade.

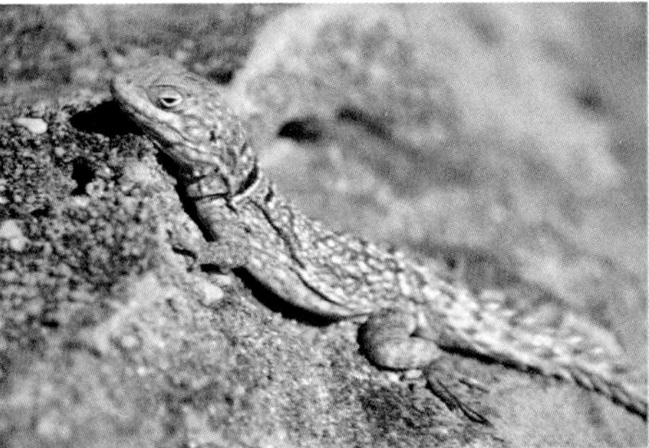

Conk_NL/ istockphoto

network of connections between the body and the brain. Thermoregulation works through **negative feedback** mechanisms. Negative feedback is a mechanism by which a stimulus input causes a system to react by causing an opposite output to maintain a desired set point. The thermostat analogy described earlier is a perfect example of a negative feedback mechanism.

In this sense, the hypothalamus can be thought of as a biological thermostat. The input to the hypothalamus comes from thermoreceptors in both the skin and organs of the body. The output from the hypothalamus is in response to potentially threatening cooling or heating of the body. These responses are known as **cold defense** and **heat defense**, respectively (Morrison, 2016).

Cold-defense responses decrease heat loss. They include the constriction of blood vessels of the skin (vasoconstriction). This results in increased blood

FIGURE 9.13

Thermoregulation is achieved through negative feedback.

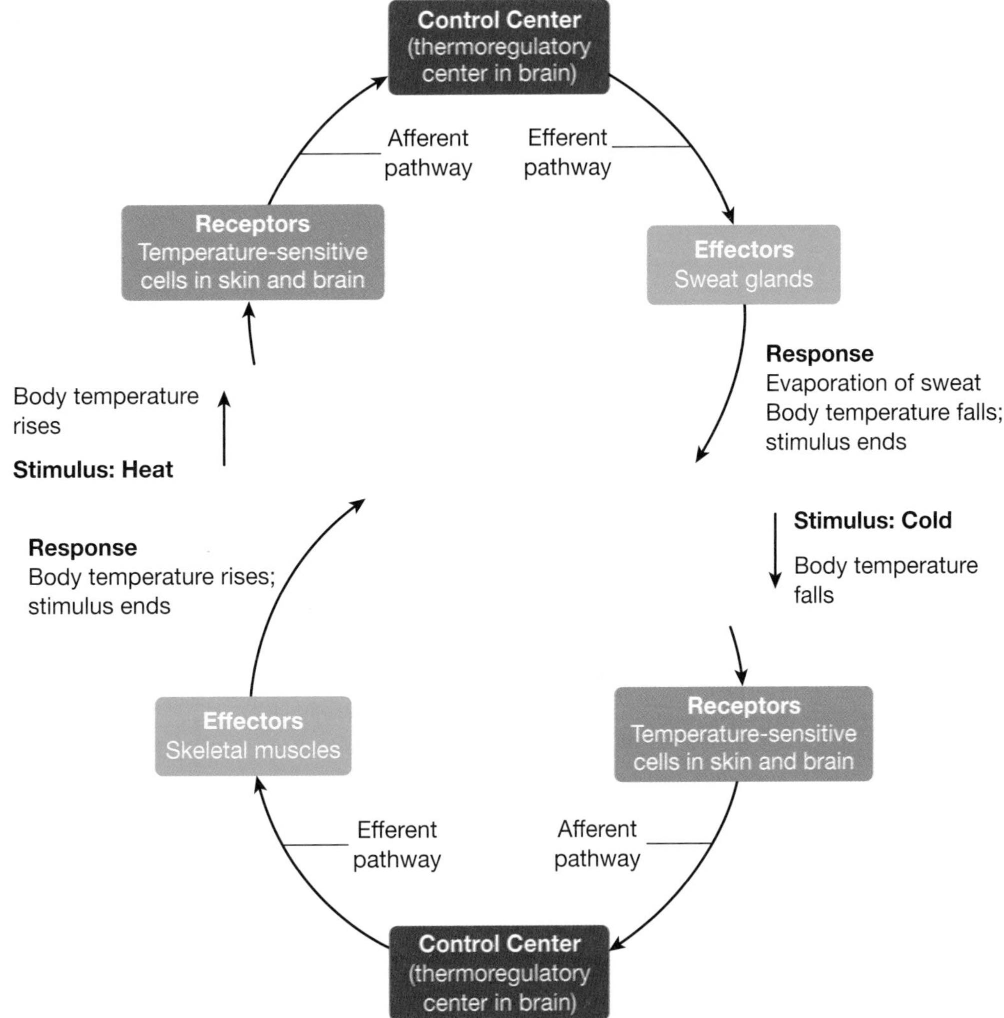

Adapted from *Human Anatomy & Physiology*, 10th Edition, Marieb and Hoehn. Pearson, 2015.

circulation to the core of the body, preventing it from losing too much heat. Another response triggers skeletal muscles to shake in what is known as **shivering**. Shivering generates heat through the expenditure of energy.

Heat-defense responses increase heat loss. They include the dilation of blood vessels in the skin (vasodilation) and vasoconstriction of the blood vessels of internal organs, both resulting in a loss of heat from the core of the body. Another way in which the body loses heat is by evaporative cooling, which you may know as "sweating." These processes are illustrated in Figure 9.13.

These reactions, automatically triggered by the hypothalamus, are combined with behavioral responses such as putting on a warm sweater or generating heat by frantically moving around while waiting for the bus on a cold winter morning. You also have a set of behavioral responses for when it gets too hot, such as taking a dip in the pool or cranking up the air conditioner.

Thermoregulatory Circuits in the Nervous System

Information about body temperature is detected by thermoreceptors deep within the body, whereas temperature of the immediate surroundings (ambient temperature) is detected by thermoreceptors near the surface of the skin. Both types of information are conveyed to the brain along two pathways:

FIGURE 9.14

Differences in the function of the STC and LPB-POA pathways in perceiving temperature and thermoregulation. Body temperature as well as environmental temperature is conveyed through thermoreceptors that send information to the brain along two pathways: the STC pathway and the LPB-POA pathway. The STC pathway leads to the perception of temperature by activating the somatosensory cortex. The LPB-POA pathway leads to the regulation of body temperature by producing heat defense and cold defense behaviors (see text for details).

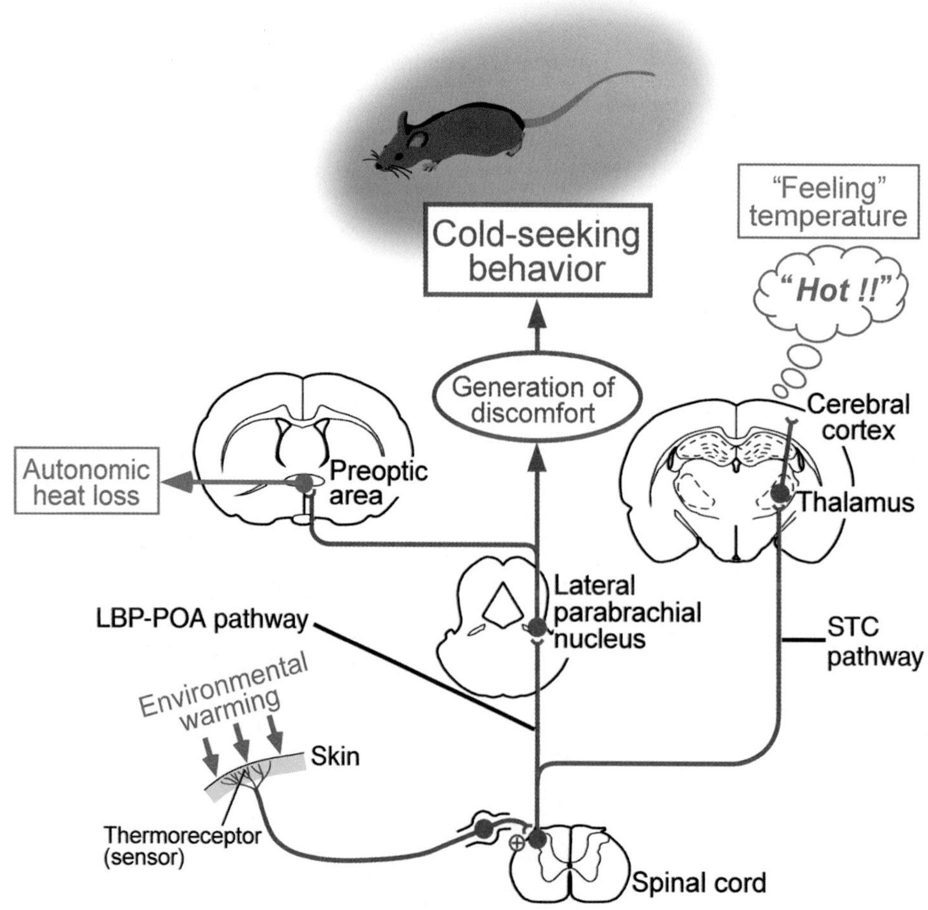

(1) the **spinothalamocortical pathway (STC pathway)**, through which information about temperature is conveyed to the somatosensory cortex via the thalamus, and (2) a pathway that runs from the **lateral parabrachial nucleus (LPB)** in the brainstem to the preoptic area (POA) of the hypothalamus, known as the **LPB-POA pathway**.

Sensory information that leads to the perception of temperature is mediated by the STC pathway. However, information about temperature leading to thermoregulation was found to be processed in the LPB-POA pathway (Morrison & Nakamura, 2011). Upon receiving information about temperature, the POA triggers the cold-defense or heat-defense mechanisms discussed earlier, as well as appropriate behaviors that result in the cooling or warming of the body. The STC and LBP-POA pathways are illustrated in Figure 9.14.

That temperature information used for thermoregulation is conveyed through a different pathway than the one that leads to the perception of temperature was demonstrated in an experiment conducted by researchers at Nagoya University in Japan (Yahiro, Kataoka, Nakamura, & Nakamura, 2017). They did so by testing the response of rats placed on floor plates of different temperatures. When given a free choice, the rats preferred to remain on floor plates kept at 28°C rather than on floor plates kept at 15°C or 38°C, which presumably felt too cold or too hot, respectively.

These researchers found that when they injected the rats with a toxin that damaged the STC pathway (which as you read earlier is responsible for perceiving temperature), the rats were able to produce behaviors aimed at regulating their body temperatures. That is, they chose to remain on the 28°C floor plate rather than the 15°C or 38°C floor plates. This was an intriguing result given that they presumably were no longer able to perceive temperature due to their damaged STC pathway. However, rats in which the researchers disabled part of the LPB-POA pathway no longer tried to avoid the cold and hot plates, which showed that they failed to produce behaviors aimed at regulating their body temperatures. The results of the study led to two conclusions: (1) Input of the STC to the somatosensory cortex, hence, the sensation of temperature, is not necessary to produce behaviors aimed at maintaining body temperature, and (2) behaviors aimed at maintaining body temperature are dependent on the LPB-POA pathway.

9.2.2 ENERGY BALANCE, HUNGER, AND EATING

>> LO 9.2.2 Explain the mechanisms that underlie hunger and satiety.

Key Terms

- **Energy homeostasis:** The process that maintains cellular metabolism.
- **Prandial state:** A state in which energy stores are replenished as nutrients are absorbed in the bloodstream and stored.
- **Postabsorptive state:** A state in which nutrients are no longer entering the bloodstream and when the body relies on the release of stored energy from the liver as glucose and from fat cells as fatty acids and ketones.
- **Orexigenic:** An agent such as a drug or a hormone that stimulates appetite.
- **Arcuate nucleus:** A region of the hypothalamus involved in the regulation of food intake.
- **Nucleus of the solitary tract (NST):** A bundle of nerve fibers that carries excitatory messages from the stomach to the hypothalamus.
- **Neuropeptides:** Molecules that can act as neurotransmitters or hormones.

Energy Homeostasis

The brain consumes 20% of the body's energy. Neurons consume twice the amount of the energy as other cells in the body. Two-thirds of the energy used by neurons is for neurotransmission, whereas the other third is for cellular maintenance. **Energy homeostasis**, which is the process that maintains cellular metabolism, depends on a continuous supply of calories and oxygen (D. Clarke & Sokoloff, 1999).

Food energy comes from macronutrients: carbohydrates, fats, and proteins. Carbohydrates are metabolized into glucose. Glucose is stored as glycogen in the liver. Fats are stored in adipose cells (fat cells) as triglycerides. Energy demands by neurons and other cells are met by (1) the release of glycogen from the liver, which is transformed back into glucose, and (2) the release of triglycerides from fat cells, which are transformed into fatty acids and ketones.

While you eat, and in the period immediately after, your energy stores are replenished, as nutrients are absorbed into the bloodstream and stored (as mentioned, carbohydrates are stored as glycogen and fats as triglycerides). This is referred to as the **prandial state** or, simply, "fed."

Later, when nutrients no longer enter the bloodstream, the body relies on the release of stored energy from the liver as glucose and from fat cells as fatty acids and ketones. This is referred to as the **postabsorptive state**, or "fasted." These two metabolic states are illustrated in Figure 9.15.

The Neurochemistry of Hunger and Satiety

In this unit, we will survey some of the molecules involved in hunger and satiety. Many of these chemicals

FIGURE 9.15

Metabolic states. (a) Prandial state and (b) postabsorptive state.

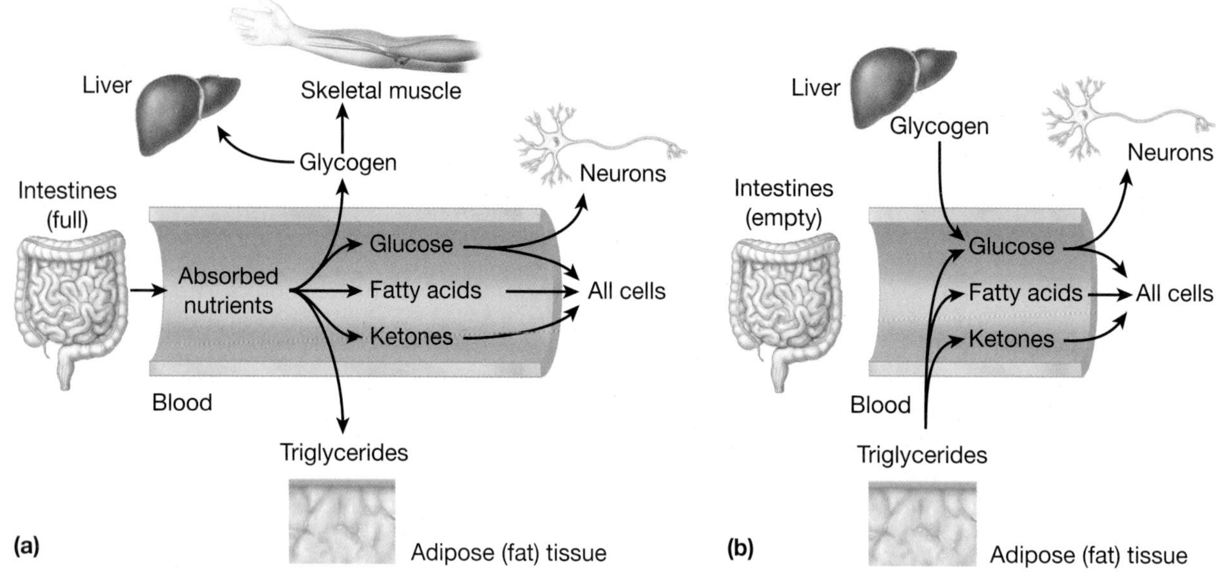

Amanda Tomasikiewicz/Body Scientific Intl.

are known as hormones. Hormones are chemical messengers. They are substances that can have effects on cells distant from the cells that released them. Hormones are discussed at greater length in Chapter 10. Other molecules, known as neuropeptides, can act as neurotransmitters or as hormones.

Hunger is the drive generated when energy stores are not sufficient to sustain energy balance. Satiety refers to the state of being fed or to the feeling of satisfaction that follows a meal. Hunger and satiety depend on the actions of hormones released from the gut, adipose cells (fat cells), and the hypothalamus. Some of these actions are described in the discussion that follows and are illustrated in Figure 9.16.

Hunger or What Makes You Start Eating

Ghrelin. Ghrelin is a hormone found mainly in the stomach. It is **orexigenic**, meaning that it promotes eating, and plays a major role in energy homeostasis. Levels of ghrelin are high approximately 20–30 minutes before meals, only when there is no food in the upper gastrointestinal tract. Levels of ghrelin drop as soon as food is ingested. Injections of ghrelin stimulate food intake and increase the frequency of meals (Erlanson-Albertsson, 2005).

Following its release, ghrelin travels through what is known as the hormonal route to a region of the hypothalamus, called the **arcuate nucleus**, where it binds to receptors on neurons that contain two peptide neurotransmitters. One is called neuropeptide-Y (NPY) and the other agouti-gene-related peptide (AgRP) (Sohn, 2015).

The binding of ghrelin to these receptors causes NPY and AgRP to be released into another region of the hypothalamus called the paraventricular nucleus (PVN). There, NPY and AgRP bind to receptors on melanin-concentrating hormone (MCH) and corticotropin-releasing factor (CRF). In ways that we do not yet understand, this results in the generation of hunger signals, which promote energy homeostasis. Ghrelin released in the stomach binds to receptors on the vagus nerve, which carries excitatory messages to the hypothalamus through the **nucleus of the solitary tract (NST)** of the brainstem.

Satiety or What Makes You Stop Eating

Leptin. Like ghrelin, the hormone leptin is produced and released from the stomach and adipose tissue (fat cells). Receptors for leptin are found on the same cells of the arcuate nucleus to which ghrelin bind, that is, cells containing NPY and AgRP.

However, contrary to ghrelin, leptin suppresses hunger. It does so by inhibiting the release of AgRP and NPY from those neurons. Leptin also suppresses hunger by having excitatory effects on neurons containing **neuropeptides**, which are molecules that can act as neurotransmitters or hormones. These

FIGURE 9.16

Hormones released from the gut and adipose cells influence the activity of the arcuate nucleus and paraventricular nucleus (PVN) of the hypothalamus through a neuronal and hormonal route. (See text for details.)

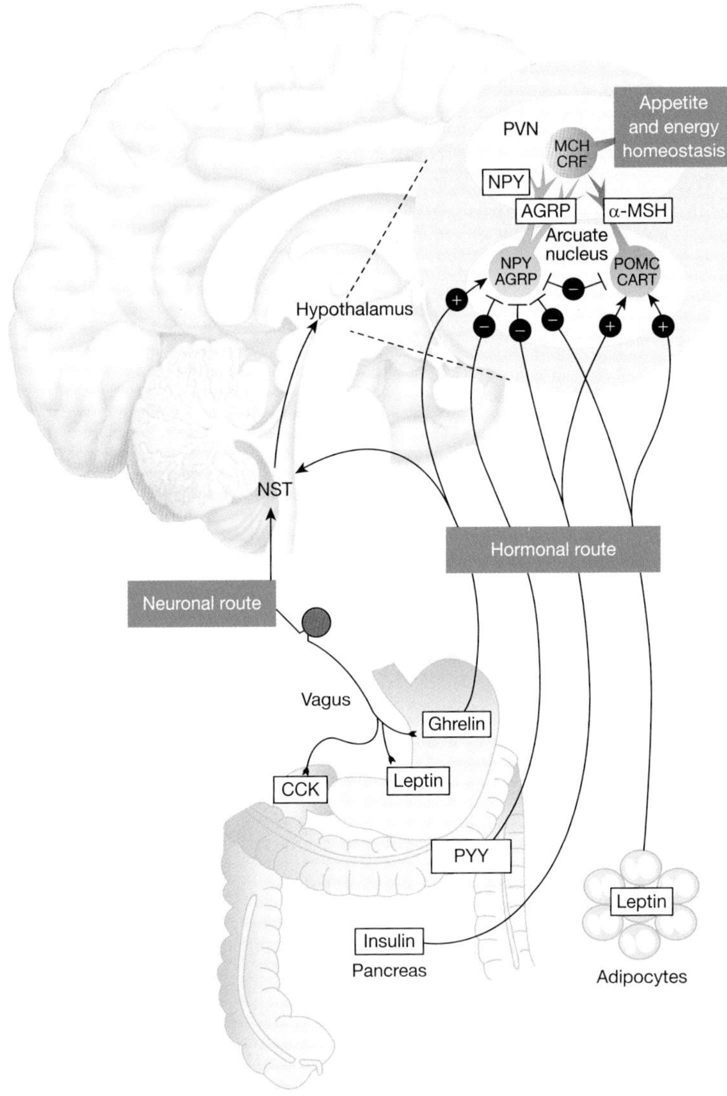

neuropeptides are known as proopiomelanocortin (POMC) and cocaine-amphetamine-relatedtranscript (CART). In turn, the release of POMC and CART in the PVN produces anorexic effects and plays an important role in feelings of satiety. Leptin is secreted in response to high levels of insulin and glucose. Leptin levels increase with body mass and with the size of fat cells. This means that leptin also plays an important role in maintaining weight in the long term. For example, after a large holiday meal, much fat has been accumulated by fat cells, resulting in the control of hunger in the following days.

Leptin is also produced and released by the stomach, where it binds to receptors on the vagus nerve, which sends inhibitory messages to the hypothalamus through the NST (Robertson, Leinninger, & Myers, 2008).

Insulin. Insulin is also anorexigenic. It is released by cells of the pancreas. The release of insulin is directly related to glucose levels. It is secreted shortly before meals and as food is ingested and nutrients are absorbed. Insulin also regulates the storage and release of glucose for energy in a manner that is appropriate for energy demands. Like leptin, insulin inhibits AgRP and NPY neurons in the arcuate nucleus and has an excitatory effect on POMC and CART neurons (Pliquett et al., 2006).

Cholecystokinin (CCK). Cholecystokinin (CCK) is released from the small intestine when the stomach is full. CCK binds to receptors on the vagus nerve, which carries inhibitory messages to the hypothalamus through the NST, to suppress appetite (Little, Horowitz, & Feinle-Bisset, 2005).

Peptide Tyrosine-Tyrosine (PYY). Peptide tyrosine-tyrosine (PYY) is also released from the large intestine. It is released in the circulation after meals and is reduced during fasting. It suppresses appetite by inhibiting AgRP and NPY neurons in the arcuate nucleus but has no effect on POMC and CART neurons (Little et al., 2005).

Homeostatic Feeding Interacts With Nonhomeostatic Feeding

Not all eating fulfills a homeostatic need. I am sure that you sometimes are not able to say "no" to a wonderful dessert after a meal that left you feeling completely full, thinking that nothing else could fit in your stomach. This is because, as you know, we also eat for pleasure. What we know about a certain food—its taste, texture, aroma, and the social context in which the food is consumed—can make us eat to an extent far beyond our homeostatic need.

This means that eating is also driven by the rewarding properties of food. In addition to a brain system involved in the homeostatic regulation of food intake, nonhomeostatic eating is regulated by a separate system. Both of these systems, however, interact to regulate eating (Cameron & Doucet, 2007). For example, the homeostatic feeding system gives rise to hunger, which in turn makes you look for something to eat. However, your choice of food will depend not only on the availability of food but also on other factors, such as what you feel like eating at the time.

Incentive-Salience Theory and Eating. Recall the incentive-salience theory discussed earlier in the chapter. According to this theory, environmental cues associated with the memory of a certain food can induce a feeling of "wanting" that food (a nonhomeostatic drive), influencing what you choose to eat when hungry (a homeostatic drive). Eating the food will make you feel sated, as your homeostatic drive for feeding is fulfilled. A feeling of "liking" the food will keep you eating, often beyond the fulfillment of your homeostatic need. However, once sated, the incentive value of the food is often reduced to the point where continuing to eat it will stop being rewarding and the craving for the food will diminish or even disappear.

Remember that wanting and liking are dependent on two distinct systems. Wanting is associated with activation of the mesolimbic dopamine system. By contrast, liking reactions are associated with the release of endorphins in hedonic hotspots within the nucleus accumbens, ventral pallidum, parabrachial nucleus, orbitofrontal cortex, insular cortex, and amygdala (Berridge, 2009).

MODULE SUMMARY

Homeostasis refers to how the balance of various factors is maintained in the body. The brain area most associated with homeostasis is the hypothalamus. Body temperature is regulated by a region of the hypothalamus called the preoptic area (POA). Organisms that cannot regulate their own body temperatures are called ectotherms; those that can are called endotherms. Ectotherms must take advantage of environmental conditions to warm or cool their bodies. The hypothalamus triggers cold-defense and heat-defense mechanisms depending on whether the environment causes the body to become too warm or too cold. Cold-defense mechanisms decrease heat loss through, among other things, constricting blood vessels and shivering. Heat-defense mechanisms increase heat loss through, among other things, the dilation of blood vessels and sweating. Body temperature is detected by thermoreceptors. The perception of temperature is conveyed to the somatosensory cortex through the spinothalamocortical pathway (STC). The detection of temperature that gives rise to homeostasis is conveyed from thermoreceptors to the parabrachial nucleus of the brainstem (LPB) and then to the POA, in what is known as the LPB-POA pathway. Rats engage in behaviors aimed at regulating their body temperatures with a damaged STC pathway, as long as their LPB-POA pathway is left intact. Homeostatic mechanisms regulate energy balance to maintain cellular function. Food energy comes from carbohydrates, fats, and proteins. The period immediately after someone eats is called the prandial state (fed), during which food energy is stored. Later, when nutrients no longer enter the bloodstream, the body relies on stored energy. This is referred to as the postabsorptive phase (fasted).

Hunger is the drive that occurs when energy stores are no longer sufficient to support energy balance. Whether hunger or satiety is felt depends on the actions of hormones released from the gut and from adipose cells. The hormone most associated with hunger is ghrelin. The hormones most associated with satiety are leptin, insulin, CCK, and PYY. These hormones activate or inhibit neurons in the arcuate nucleus of the hypothalamus, which contains neurons that contain neuropeptide-Y and AgRP. When stimulated by ghrelin, these neurons activate neurons in another region of the hypothalamus called the PVN, producing feelings of hunger; when inhibited by leptin, insulin, and PYY, these neurons produce satiety. The arcuate nucleus also has neurons that contain POMC and cocaine-amphetamine-related transcript (CART). When stimulated by leptin, these neurons inhibit neurons in the PVN, resulting in feelings of satiety. Feeding behavior is influenced by both homeostatic and nonhomeostatic mechanisms. The incentive-salience theory of motivation can explain both the craving and enjoyment of food. The rewarding value of food plays an essential role in energy homeostasis as it greatly contributes to the extent to which we will seek food or keep eating until sated. However, because food is rewarding, individuals often keep eating past the point at which they are sated.

TEST YOURSELF

9.2.1 Explain the mechanisms by which organisms regulate their body temperatures. Which brain areas are involved, and how do they interact? How were the mechanisms for the regulation of temperature and temperature perception dissociated?

9.2.2 What hormones and brain areas are associated with hunger and satiety? Explain how these brain areas and hormones interact to produce hunger and satiety.

9.3 Regulation of Sleep and Wakefulness

Module Contents

Learning Objectives

9.3.1 Know how sleep is studied as well as how it is subdivided into stages.

9.3.2 Explain how sleep is regulated by homeostatic and circadian processes.

9.3.3 Explain how brain areas and neurotransmitters interact in wakefulness and sleep.

9.3.1 WHAT IS SLEEP?

>> LO 9.3.1 Know how sleep is studied as well as how it is subdivided into stages.

Key Terms

- **Polysomnography:** A set of physiological measures that includes electroencephalography, electrooculography, and electromyography.
- **Electrooculography (EOG):** Recording of eye movements through changes in the electrical activity of eye muscles.
- **Electromyography (EMG):** Recording of movements of the body through measuring changes in the electrical activity of muscles.
- **Alpha, beta, theta, and delta:** Brain waves that differ in amplitude and/or frequency; identified by EEG.
- **NREM sleep:** Non–rapid eye movement sleep. Sleep that is subdivided into four stages of progressively deeper sleep.
- **REM sleep:** Rapid eye movement sleep. Sleep stage mostly associated with dreaming; characterized by relative muscle paralysis and eye movements.
- **Sleep spindles:** Series of high-frequency spikes of activity lasting anywhere from 0.5 to 1.0 seconds.
- **K-complexes:** Slight negative deflections in brain waves (wave movement is exaggerated downward) followed by a positive deflection (exaggerated upward).
- **Paradoxical sleep:** Another name given to REM sleep because brain activity during REM resembles that of wakefulness.

About one-third of your life is spent sleeping. During sleep, your eyes are closed and there are changes in breathing, heartbeat, and muscle tone. It was once believed that the brain shuts down during sleep. However, we now know that sleep is associated with brain activity that differs from waking but not to a shutdown. Researchers typically study what goes on during sleep using **polysomnography**.

As illustrated in Figure 9.17, polysomnography includes measures of the brain's electrical activity, eye movements, and muscle contraction. These measures are obtained through the use of electroencephalography (EEG), **electrooculography (EOG)**, and **electromyography (EMG)**, respectively. Measures of blood oxygen, airflow, and respiratory effort can also be taken.

Sleep Stages

As you learned in Chapter 2, brain waves are a result of the electrical activity of neurons and are measured by EEG. Brain waves, like any other wave (e.g., sound waves), vary in frequency and amplitude. As described in Chapter 7, frequency is measured in Hertz (Hz) or

FIGURE 9.17

Polysomnography.

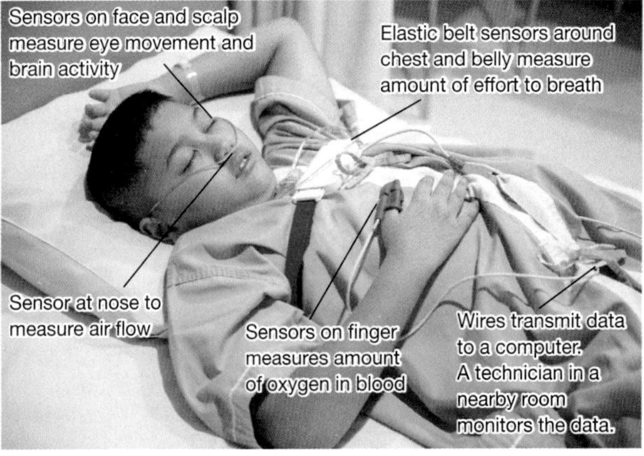

Devilkae/ istockphoto

FIGURE 9.18

The rollercoaster ride of sleep. From wakefulness, sleep moves down and back up through stages, from light sleep to deep sleep and REM sleep. As sleep goes on, progressively more time is spent in REM sleep at the expense of NREM sleep.

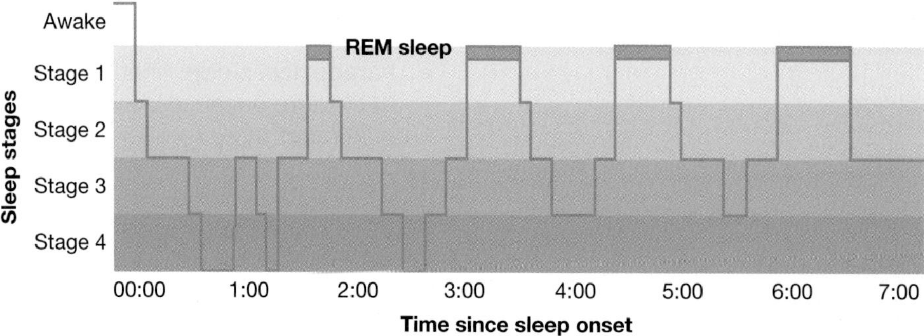

cycles per second. One cycle of a wave is one peak of a wave to the next. Amplitude refers to the height of the wave and is measured in microvolts (μV). One microvolt is one millionth of a volt.

In the 1930s, scientist Alfred Loomis discovered that the brain's patterns of electrical activity differed depending on whether an individual was awake or asleep. He did so by measuring the wavelengths emitted by the brain during waking and sleeping using EEG. He also noticed that this pattern of activity changed during sleep. Brain waves, differing in amplitude and/or frequency during sleep, were identified as **alpha, beta, theta, and delta** (Loomis & Newton, 1937).

In the 1950s, sleep researchers Eugene Aserinsky and Nathaniel Kleitman described eye movements detected only at certain periods while subjects were sleeping (Aserinsky & Kleitman, 1953). These eye movements occurred during what came to be known as rapid eye movement sleep (**REM sleep**). The sleep periods devoid of rapid eye movements were called non-REM sleep (**NREM sleep**). NREM sleep was subdivided into four stages of progressively deeper sleep (Rechtschaffen & Kales, 1968). However, stages 3 and 4 have been combined (Hori et al., 2001). About 75% of our sleep is spent in NREM sleep and about 25% in REM sleep.

When represented graphically, the sleep stages resemble peaks and valleys (Figure 9.18). From waking, the brain progresses through stages 1 to 4, then works its way back up through the stages to REM sleep, which replaces stage 1. Stage 1 sleep is a transitional state from wakefulness to sleep that occurs only once. As sleep progresses, the amount of time spent in the deeper stages of sleep is reduced and the time spent in REM sleep is increased. REM sleep is the type of sleep mostly associated with dreaming. It is characterized by relative muscle paralysis and eye movements.

Figure 9.19 shows how each sleep stage is differentiated by its characteristic EEG rhythm. The waking state is characterized by what are known as beta waves. These are low-amplitude waves of high frequency, ranging from 13 to 30 Hz. However, when a person is awake, but in a relaxed state, alpha waves, which are more regular and of lower frequency, are observed. Alpha waves range from 8 to 13 Hz. These waves become more frequent if the relaxing person's eyes are closed. Following are descriptions of what happens during the four stages of sleep:

- *Stage 1 sleep* is the transition between wakefulness and deeper stages of sleep. Stage 1 is characterized by theta waves, which are of slightly higher amplitude compared to that of beta and alpha waves but are of lower frequency (3 to 7 Hz).
- *Stage 2 sleep* is marked by what are known as **sleep spindles** and **K-complexes**. Sleep spindles are series of high-frequency spikes of activity lasting anywhere from 0.5 to 1.0 seconds. K-complexes are slightly negative deflections in a wave (the wave's movement is exaggerated downward) followed by a positive deflection (exaggerated upward). Stage 2 is a light form of sleep from which a person is easily awakened. If you wake someone up during this stage, she may or may not know that she was sleeping. If you ever feel asleep while watching a movie with your friend and denied that you were sleeping after he woke you up, you were probably in stage 2.
- *Stages 3 and 4* are the stages of deep sleep. These stages are marked by high-amplitude and low-frequency wavelengths, ranging from 1 to 4 Hz, known as delta waves. At this point, your friend would be difficult to wake up and

FIGURE 9.19

EEG rhythms associated with each of the sleep stages. Note that although stages 3 and 4 are depicted separately, they have been combined.

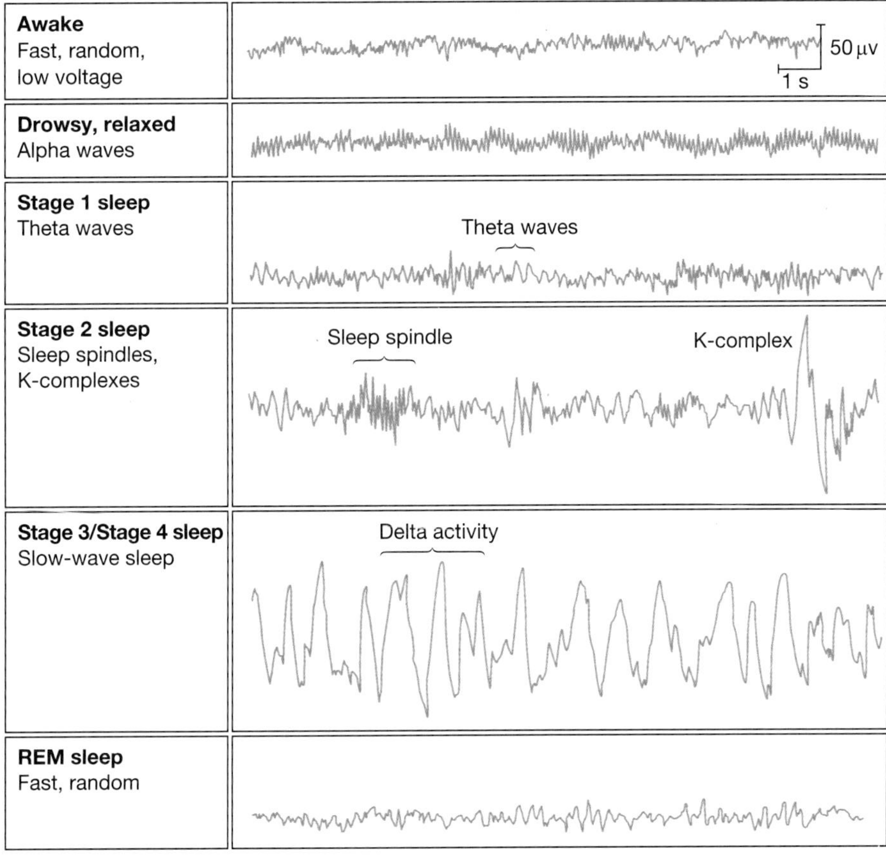

From *Current Concepts: The Sleep Disorders*, by P. Hauri, Kalamazoo, MI: Upjohn, 1982.

may be angry with you if you succeed. The appearance of delta waves is associated with stage 3. Stage 4 sleep is characterized by delta waves consisting of more than 50% of recorded brain waves. Stages 3 and 4 are also known as slow-wave sleep (SWS).

- *REM sleep* is marked by brain activity that resembles wakefulness. The rhythm observed during REM sleep is remarkably similar to that of beta waves. For this reason, REM sleep is sometimes referred to as **paradoxical sleep**. In addition, wakefulness-like brain activity on EOG can detect that the eyes are moving back and forth under the closed eyelids. At the same time, there is a significant loss of muscle tone resulting in the sleeper becoming relatively paralyzed as detected by an EMG. REM sleep is the sleep stage mostly associated with dreams. It was, therefore, hypothesized that this temporary paralysis occurs to prevent people from acting out their dreams.

9.3.2 HOMEOSTATIC AND CIRCADIAN INFLUENCES ON SLEEP AND WAKEFULNESS

>> LO 9.3.2 **Explain how sleep is regulated by homeostatic and circadian processes.**

Key Terms

- **Somnogens:** Substances in the body that produce sleep.
- **Humoral theory of sleep regulation:** The idea that sleep-inducing chemicals accumulate in the body during wakefulness.
- **"Second wind" effect:** Periods of alertness interspersed with periods of sleepiness after being sleep deprived.

- **Circadian rhythm:** Physiological, behavioral, or psychological events that occur over an approximate 24-hour cycle.
- **Melatonin:** A hormone, released by the pineal gland, that induces sleepiness.
- **Entrained rhythm:** A rhythm regulated by external cues, such as light or heat.
- **Free running rhythm:** A rhythm that is self-regulated, not requiring any external cues.
- **Suprachiasmatic nucleus (SCN):** The region of the hypothalamus thought to control circadian rhythms (sometimes called the master clock).
- **Melanopsin:** A pigment in certain photoreceptor cells of the retina, which influences the light-dark cycle through projections to the suprachiasmatic nucleus.
- **Retinohypothalamic projections:** The projections of photoreceptors containing melanopsin from the retina to the hypothalamus.
- **Zeitgebers:** Factors in the environment that influence circadian rhythms.

The mechanisms involved in wakefulness and sleep, outlined in the preceding unit, are influenced by factors that apply pressure for either going to sleep or remaining awake. Think of it as a light switch. To turn the light off, you have to apply downward pressure on the switch. If you do this slowly, the pressure will gradually build until the switch passes a critical point beyond which the lights will go out. Of course, the opposite will happen when the lights are off and you flip the switch upward to turn them on. The idea of a sleep-wake switch controlled by a variety of brain areas is discussed in the next unit. Three main factors influence this sleep-wake switch. These are homeostatic influences, circadian influences, and emotional/cognitive influences.

Homeostatic Influences

Japanese physiologist Kuniomi Ishimori was one of the first scientists to investigate the neurobiological processes involved in the homeostatic mechanisms that regulate sleep (K. Kubota, 1989). In the early 1900s, he made dogs fall asleep by giving them intracerebral injections of cerebrospinal fluid extracted from dogs that were sleep deprived.

As a result of this finding, it was hypothesized that sleep-inducing chemicals must accumulate in the body during wakefulness, to the point when an individual becomes sleepy and falls asleep. These chemicals became known as **somnogens**. This idea gave rise to the **humoral theory of sleep regulation**, which states that the degree of wakefulness is related to the accumulation of somnogens that lead to the homeostatic drive for sleep. Some of these somnogens are discussed in the next unit.

Circadian Influences

You may have noticed that your levels of alertness and wakefulness do not necessarily depend on the amount of sleep you were deprived of and on how long you have been awake. It has been shown that sleep-deprived individuals will go through cycles of increased and decreased sleepiness throughout the day. You may have experienced this yourself if you ever spent all night partying. Sorry! I meant studying. After pulling an all-nighter, people often get a "second wind" in the morning, around the time they would normally wake up after a night's sleep. Therefore, the humoral theory of sleep regulation, mentioned earlier, cannot fully explain the cycles of sleep and wakefulness.

This **"second wind" effect** is due to the influence of a **circadian rhythm**. Circadian rhythms are physiological, behavioral, or psychological events that occur over a 24-hour cycle (*circadian* is Latin for "about a day"). Some of these rhythms are illustrated in Figure 9.20. The figure includes the rhythm for **melatonin**. Melatonin is a hormone, released by the pineal gland, that induces sleepiness.

Circadian rhythms can be **entrained** or **free running**. An entrained rhythm is regulated by external cues, such as light or heat. A free-running rhythm is self-regulated, not requiring any external cues. The wake-sleep cycle of humans runs about 25 hours. However, because the earth takes 24 hours to complete

FIGURE 9.20

Circadian rhythms for body temperature, K+ excretion, melatonin, cortisol, melatonin, and growth hormone.

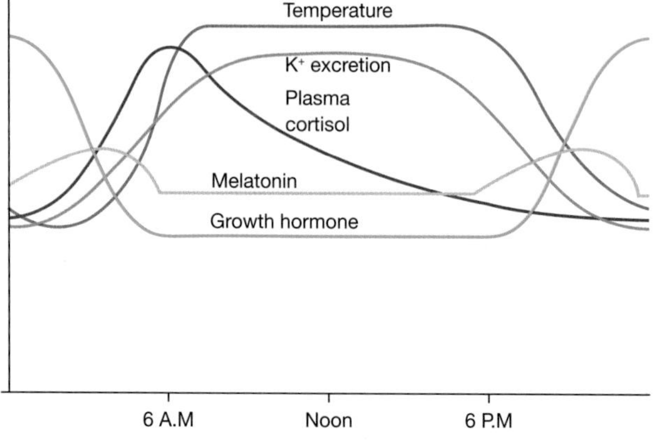

a revolution, we are forced to function with a 24-hour cycle of light and dark. Thus, the wake-sleep cycle is partly entrained by light. However, this begs a question: What would happen if people were put into a situation in which light cues were absent?

Physiologist Nathaniel Kleitman and assistant Bruce Richardson set out to answer this question in 1938, by spending over a month inside Mammoth Cave, located in Kentucky. They discovered that, although deprived of the fluctuation of light and dark cues, the rhythmicity of physiological processes such as body temperature and hormone secretion remained constant.

Later, in the 1960s, another researcher, Jurgen Aschoff, found that circadian rhythms of several physiological mechanisms were maintained while living in an underground bunker without time cues (Aschoff, 1967). In the early 1980s, sleep researcher Charles Czeisler compared the sleep-wake cycles of subjects when free to choose their own light-dark cycles (free running) to when a dark cycle was imposed (entrained) for six weeks. Figure 9.21 shows the results of this experiment. Czeisler and colleagues found that subjects on a free-running cycle displayed a sleep rhythm of about 25 hours (as mentioned earlier), compared to 24 hours when the cycle was entrained (Czeisler, Weitzman, Moore-Ede, Zimmerman, & Knauer, 1980).

FIGURE 9.21

Sleep rhythm of people on an unscheduled, free-running rhythm compared to when light-dark cycles were scheduled. With an unscheduled rhythm, the subjects' sleep cycle ran about 25 hours.

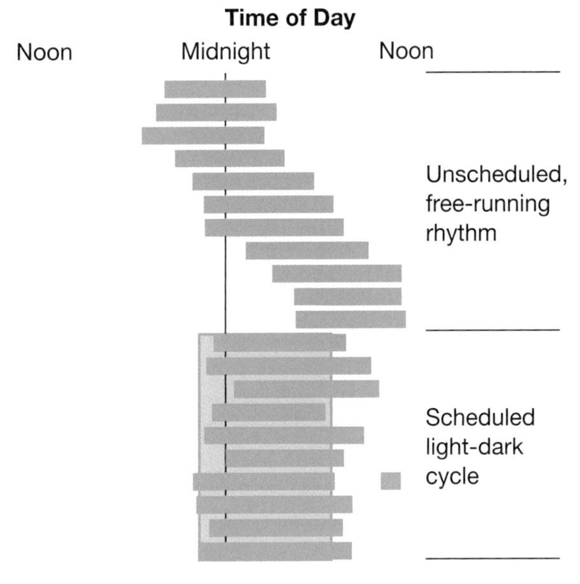

From *Introduction to Psychology, Gateways to Mind a nd Behavior* (non InfoTrac version), 9th ed., by D. Coon, Wadsworth, a division of Thomson Learning, 2001.

FIGURE 9.22

Melatonin and the retinohypothalamic tract. The process by which waking and sleeping are regulated by the interactions between the photoreceptors, the SCN, and the pineal gland. Not shown is the ventrolateral preoptic area of the hypothalamus, which is the target of inhibition by the SCN.

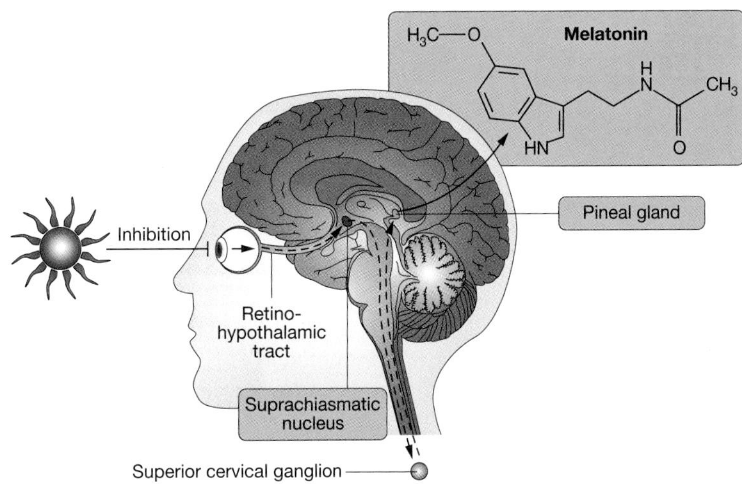

Birgit, C.P., et al. (2009). Circadian sleep-wake rhythm disturbances in end-stage renal disease. *Nature Reviews Nephrology* 5(7): 407–416. With permission from Springer Nature.

Altogether, this shows that some cycles are stable despite the absence of light-dark cues. Examples of these are body temperature and cortisol levels. Levels of alertness, memory, and speed of decision making have periodic daytime peaks that are stable during free-running conditions, which may explain the "second wind effect," described earlier. However, sleep-wake cycles can become desynchronized from stable rhythms not entrained by light-dark cues.

What Controls Circadian Rhythms?

Circadian rhythms are controlled by circadian clocks, which are present in every system of the body. However, these clocks are controlled by a master clock located in the brain. This master clock is thought to be the **suprachiasmatic nucleus (SCN)**, located in the hypothalamus. The SCN is influenced by light-dark cycles through projections from photoreceptor cells in the retina that contain the photopigment **melanopsin**. Projection from these cells form the **retinohypothalamic projections**. This ultimately leads to the release of melatonin from the pineal gland shortly before sleep. In turn, melatonin binds to receptors in the SCN, closing a feedback loop that provides the brain with a mechanism for determining circadian time. This process is illustrated in Figure 9.22.

However, light is not the only factor that entrains the wake-sleep cycle. Other factors also have an influence on biological clocks, including latitude, work schedules, social demands, and cultural traditions. Factors in the environment that influence circadian rhythms are known as **zeitgebers**.

9.3.3 THE NEUROCHEMISTRY AND PHYSIOLOGY OF WAKEFULNESS AND SLEEP

>> LO 9.3.3 Explain how brain areas and neurotransmitters interact in wakefulness and sleep.

Key Terms

- **Ascending arousal system (AAS):** A wakefulness-promoting system that includes areas of the brainstem.
- **Executive system for wakefulness:** A system that includes orexinergic neurons in the lateral hypothalamus.

The Neurochemistry of Wakefulness and Sleep

Many of the neurotransmitters you learned about in Chapter 3 as well as hormones are involved in waking and sleeping.

Wakefulness. The neurotransmitters that promote waking include norepinephrine, serotonin, histamine, glutamate, and acetylcholine. In addition to these neurotransmitters, the neuropeptide hypocretin (also known as orexin) is important for the maintenance of wakefulness.

Sleep. The neurochemicals that promote sleep include the neurotransmitters GABA, glutamate, and adenosine. In addition to these, melatonin, mentioned in the preceding unit, and melanin are also involved in promoting sleep. These chemicals, which promote sleep, also suppress the activity of the excitatory neurotransmitters that promote waking.

Knowing this should now make you aware of how stimulant and depressant drugs (discussed in Chapter 3) affect wakefulness. For example, stimulant drugs, such as amphetamine, keep people awake by increasing the release of norepinephrine. Wakefulness can also be induced by inhibiting chemicals that promote sleepiness. For example, levels of adenosine rise with prolonged periods of wakefulness and promote sleepiness. Levels of adenosine are also high in the morning. Caffeine "wakes you up" by inhibiting the binding of adenosine to its receptors. So, next time you drop by your coffee shop, instead of ordering a cup of coffee, you could say, "Please inhibit my adenosine."

Depressant drugs such as alcohol, barbiturates (sleeping pills), and benzodiazepines (e.g., anxiety-reducing drugs such as Valium) induce sleepiness by binding to GABA receptors, which suppresses excitation. As caffeine inhibits sleepiness, histamine, as mentioned earlier, is related to wakefulness. This is why antihistamines (a common ingredient in cold medicines) make you drowsy.

The Physiology of Wakefulness and Sleep

Wakefulness. Italian physiologist Giuseppe Moruzzi discovered the brain areas related to wakefulness by electrically stimulating the brains of cats (Moruzzi & Magoun, 1949). He found that wakefulness is maintained by structures within the brainstem that border the pons and in the midbrain. Together, these areas became known as the **ascending arousal system (AAS)**, illustrated in Figure 9.23. The AAS promotes wakefulness by exciting the cortex.

The AAS includes the pedunculopontine/laterodorsal tegmental nuclei (PPT/LDT), locus coeruleus (LC), raphe nucleus (RN), and tuberomammillary nucleus (TMN), which are the sources of cholinergic, noradrenergic, serotonergic, and histaminergic neurons, respectively. Cholinergic neurons also project from the basal forebrain.

Projections from the AAS excite the cortex through two distinct pathways, an indirect pathway and a direct pathway. As shown in Figure 9.23a, the indirect pathway consists of cholinergic neurons in the PPT and LDT that activate the cortex through connections in the thalamus. The direct pathway (Figure 9.23b)

FIGURE 9.23

(a) Wake-promoting areas of the AAS. Also illustrated are the indirect (blue) and direct (green) pathways to cortical stimulation. The VLPO (orange dot) contains inhibitory neurotransmitters GABA and galanin and contributes to the maintenance of sleep. (b) Orexinergic neurons in the lateral hypothalamus (red) stimulate the AAS and cortex (see text for details).

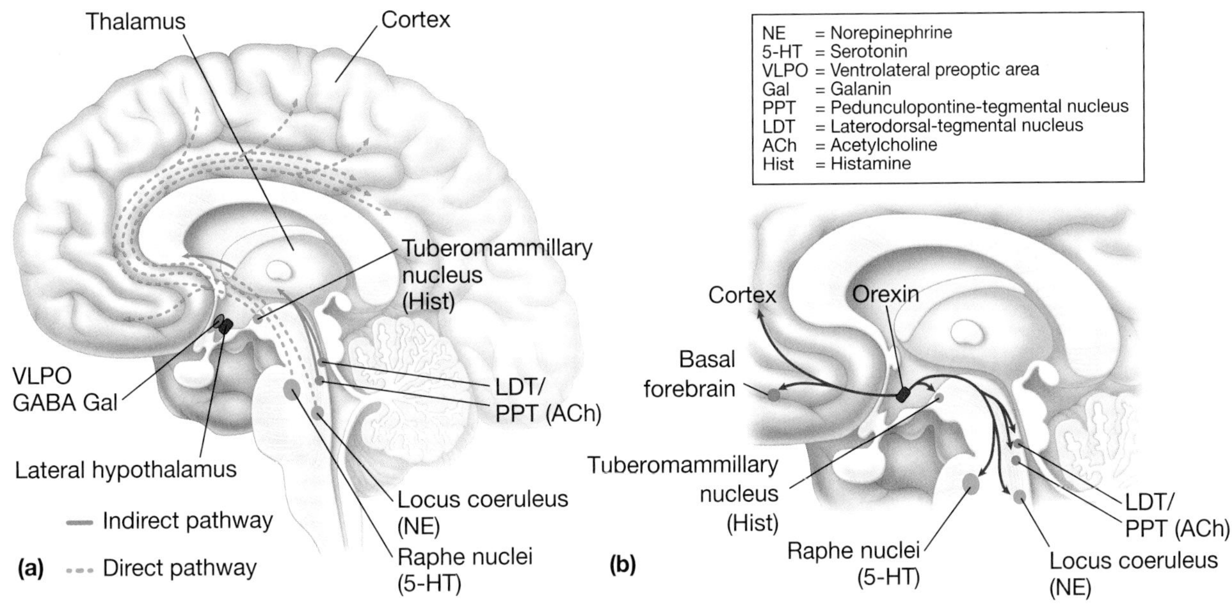

Amanda Tomasikiewicz/Body Scientific Intl.

consists of noradrenergic, serotonergic, and histaminergic neurons situated in the LC, RN, and TMN, respectively, that directly activate the cortex.

Activity in the AAS itself is stimulated by the input from orexinergic neurons in the lateral hypothalamus (LH). The lateral hypothalamus can therefore be said to be part of an **executive system for wakefulness** (Saper, Chou, & Scammell, 2001).

Sleep. Sleep is maintained by inhibitory connections to the orexinergic neurons of the LH and histaminergic neurons of the TMN from GABA and galanin neurons in the ventrolateral preoptic area of the hypothalamus (VLPO). This promotes sleepiness by inhibiting the excitatory influences of orexin and histamine on the AAS. The location of the VLPO and its inhibitory influence on the AAS are illustrated in Figure 9.24. The VLPO thus can be said to be part of an executive system for sleep (Saper et al., 2001).

The Wake-Sleep Switch. It may seem to you that falling asleep is a gradual process. After all, in the evening, for example, you might start watching television and feel increasingly sleepy as the evening moves along. You then decide that you have had enough and go to bed, where you fall asleep. In reality, falling asleep and waking up in the morning are quite abrupt transitions. Think about when you woke up this morning. Do you

FIGURE 9.24

The sleep-promoting VLPO. The VLPO (orange) promotes sleep by inhibiting the AAS (green and blue) through GABAergic and galaninergic projections.

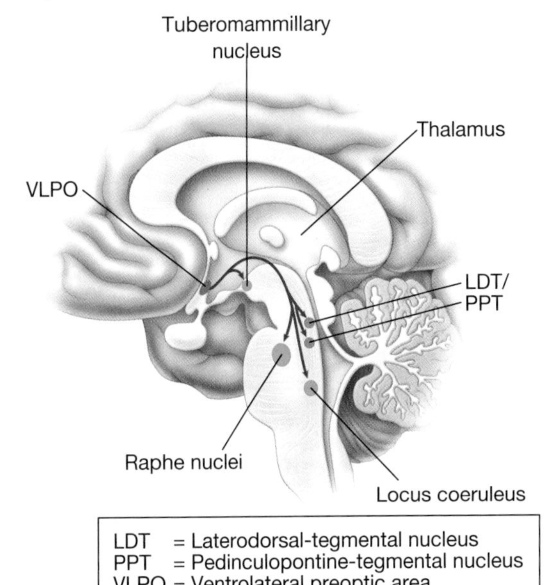

Amanda Tomasikiewicz/Body Scientific Intl.

FIGURE 9.25

The wake-sleep switch. (a) Wakefulness is promoted when the switch is in the "on" position. Orexin neurons in the LH excite neurons in the LC, TMN, and RN (AAS), which in turn inhibits the firing of neurons in the VLPO. (b) Sleep is promoted when the switch is in the "off" position. GABA and galanin neurons in the VLPO inhibit the firing of orexin neurons in the LH as well as neurons in the AAS.

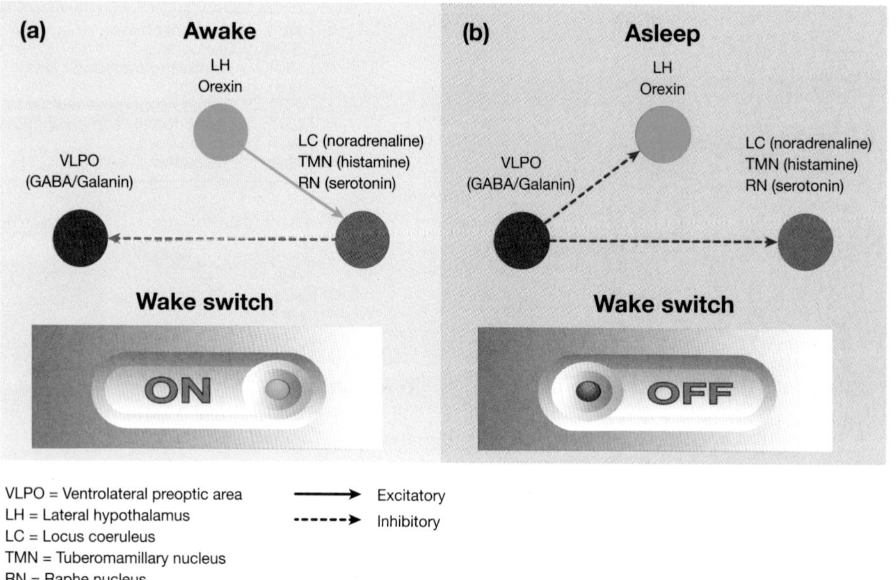

Amanda Tomasikiewicz/Body Scientific Intl.

feel that you woke up gradually or that you just did? You are awake or asleep. There is no transition stage. You may feel groggy in the morning or sleepy in the evening, but you are still awake.

In the early 2000s, neurologist Clifford B. Saper and colleagues proposed that wake-sleep transitions occur through the function of what is similar to a light switch. You can turn the light either on or off (J. Lu, Sherman, Devor, & Saper, 2006; Saper et al., 2001).

As illustrated in Figure 9.25a, GABA and galanin in the VLPO play the role of applying pressure to the switch to turn wakefulness on or off. The transition from sleep to wakefulness as well as the maintenance of wakefulness occurs when orexin neurons in the LH stimulate the LC, RN, and TMN neurons of the AAS. At the same time, neurons in the VLPO are inhibited by projections from neurons in the AAS.

Alternatively, the transition from wakefulness to sleep, as well as the maintenance of sleep, occurs when GABA and galanin neurons in the VLPO inhibit the firing of orexin neurons in the LH and in the LC, RN, and TMN neurons of the AAS (Figure 9.25b).

IT'S A MYTH!

Dreams Represent Hidden Motives and Conflicts

The Myth

The most influential figure when it comes to attempting to decipher the meaning of dreams was Sigmund Freud (1856–1939). Freud believed that dreams were "the royal way to the subconscious." By this he meant that dreams revealed unconscious desires, fears, and anxieties in a disguised manner.

He divided the content of dreams into latent content and manifest content. The manifest content, he said, is the dream as it is recounted. For example, if you dreamed that you were sitting in class surrounded by family members instead of your classmates, that would be the manifest content. By contrast, the latent content could be that you are feeling a lot of pressure from your family to get an education. You can understand from this explanation how dreams can be so strange.

A Neurobiological Theory

Sleep researchers Allan Hobson and Robert McCarley proposed what is known as the *activation-synthesis hypothesis*. They suggested that the activation-synthesis theory accounts for five aspects of dreaming:

1. Visual and motor hallucinations
2. Acceptance that the hallucinations are real
3. Bizarre spatial and temporal distortions
4. Strong emotions
5. Weak memory for dreams

According to the activation-synthesis hypothesis, visual and motor hallucinations experienced in a dream arise partly from electrical activity initiated in the brainstem and spread throughout the brain. Because of REM paralysis, this results in motor commands that cannot be carried out. The brain then tries to make sense of this activity by creating scenes using images from disparate memories. For example, a motor command to the legs may be interpreted as walking or running through a corridor.

The brain takes these experiences as reality. Temporal and spatial distortions do not matter. This is because in its sleeping state the brain cannot measure these experiences against external reality. The brain may also interpret eye movements as tracking people or objects moving in various directions. Emotions are generated through inputs from the amygdala, which is involved in emotional processing. Our relatively poor memory for dreams can be explained by the absence of cholinergic transmission (which is important for memory) during REM.

In contrasts to Freud's explanations for dreams, the activation-synthesis hypothesis takes dream events and images at face value and not as representations of hidden motives and conflicts. ●

MODULE SUMMARY

Contrary to popular belief, sleep is not a cessation of most brain activity. Sleep is thought to be important for cellular repair, brain development, and memory. Researchers study sleep using polysomnography, with which they found two types of sleep: REM sleep and non-REM (NREM) sleep. NREM sleep is subdivided into four stages. Each stage is characterized by a particular type of brainwave activity. REM sleep, also called paradoxical sleep, is the stage of sleep associated with vivid dreams. It is characterized by rapid eye movement (hence, the acronym REM), muscle paralysis, and brainwave activity that resembles the waking state.

Sleep is regulated both by a homeostatic drive and by circadian rhythm. The humoral theory of sleep regulation states that wakefulness is related to the accumulation of somnogens that lead to the homeostatic drive for sleep. Adenosine and prostaglandins induce sleepiness by inhibiting the release of neurotransmitters that promote wakefulness, such as histamine and orexin. Sleep is also regulated by a circadian rhythm. Circadian rhythms are physiological, behavioral, or psychological events that occur over an approximate 24-hour cycle. For example, levels of the hormone melatonin, which promotes sleepiness, are low during the day, rise during the evening, and remain high throughout the night. Circadian rhythms can be entrained, which means that they are regulated by external cues such as light and dark, or they can be free running, which means that they are self-regulated. The free-running wake-sleep cycle of humans runs approximately 25 hours. Wake-sleep cycles are controlled by an area of the hypothalamus called the suprachiasmatic nucleus (SCN). The SCN is activated by photoreceptor cells in the retina. Activation of the SCN in turn suppresses the inhibitory actions on the wake system. Shortly before sleep, the SCN stimulates the pineal gland, which releases melatonin. Factors in the environment that influence circadian rhythms are called zeitgebers.

Some neurotransmitters promote waking and others promote sleep. Wakefulness is maintained by excitatory neurotransmitters. Chemicals that promote sleep do so by suppressing the activity of excitatory neurotransmitters. Wakefulness is maintained by the ascending arousal system (AAS), which comprises structures within the brainstem. The projection from these areas follows two distinct pathways to the cortex, an indirect pathway that activates the cortex through the thalamus and a direct pathway that activates the cortex directly. All of the areas included in the AAS receive projections from neurons in the lateral hypothalamus. The lateral hypothalamus is part of an executive system for wakefulness. Falling asleep and waking are abrupt transitions. Wake-sleep transitions occur through the function of what is similar to a light switch, known as the wake-sleep switch. The transition from sleep to wakefulness as well as the maintenance of wakefulness occurs through the actions of orexin.

TEST YOURSELF

9.3.1 What are the characteristics that correspond to the different sleep stages? Be sure to include both REM and NREM sleep.

9.3.2 What are the two main influences on the regulation of sleep? Explain each one.

9.3.3 Describe and explain the chemical process involved in sleep as well as how various brain areas interact to produce sleep and wakefulness.

APPLICATIONS

Altering Brain-Satiety Signals for Weight Loss

In 2014, the weight-loss market was valued at $64 billion. This is not surprising given that 37.7% of the U.S. population is classified as obese (Flegal, Kruszon-Moran, Carroll, Fryar, & Ogden, 2016). Obesity is also associated with heart disease and cardiovascular disease (Garcia et al., 2016).

Through marketing and advertising campaigns, consumers are continually bombarded with weight-loss options. These include diet books and accessories for exercise. Pharmacological solutions are also available, in the form of obesity drugs. Many of these drugs target the neurobiological mechanisms that underlie feeding (Adan, Vanderschuren, & la Fleur, 2008). One recently available medication aims to reduce weight loss by controlling food cravings and by reducing hunger. This medication, known as Contrave, is a combination of two drugs: naltrexone and bupropion.

How Does It Work?

The mechanisms by which these drugs work in the context of weight loss are shown in Figure 9.26 (Christou & Kiortsis, 2015). Naltrexone is an opiate receptor antagonist, whereas bupropion is a

FIGURE 9.26

Mechanisms of action of naltrexone and bupropion in the context of weight loss.

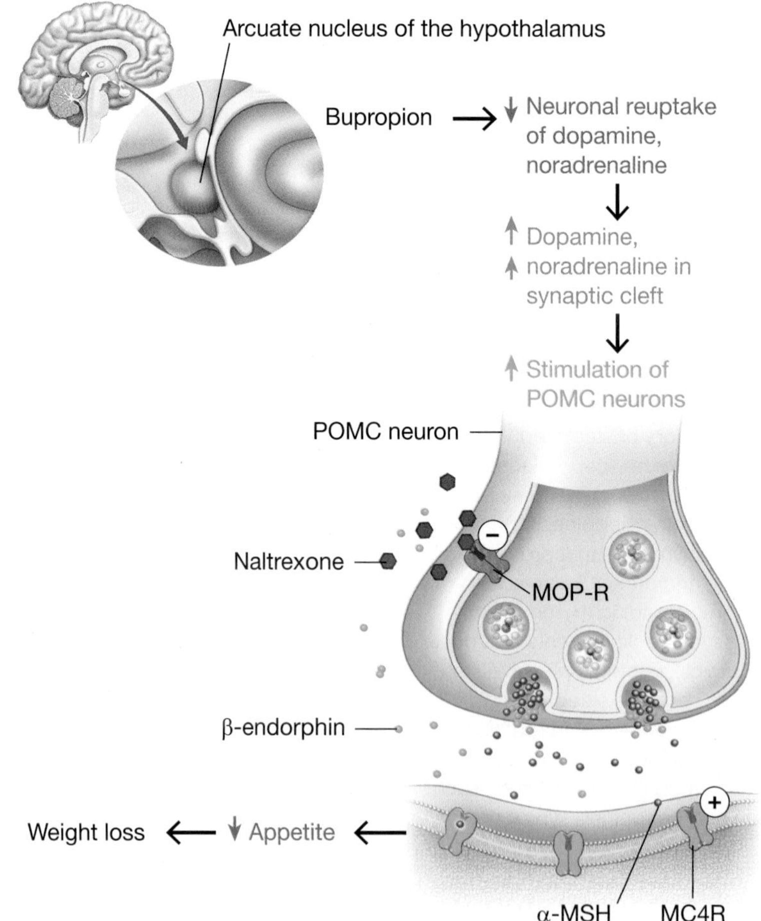

Amanda Tomasikiewicz/Body Scientific Intl.

dopamine and norepinephrine reuptake inhibitor. Why combine those two drugs? Proopiomelanocortin (POMC) is a precursor of α-melanocyte-stimulating hormone (α-MSH), which produces anorectic effects by binding to melanocortin-4 receptors (MC4R) in the paraventricular hypothalamus. That is, it produces sensations of satiety and inhibits eating. In contrast, β-endorphin released by POMC neurons plays an autoinhibitory role through binding to μ-opioid receptors (MOP-R), reducing the amount of POMC released.

Naltrexone

Naltrexone, being a MOP-R antagonist, prevents β-endorphin molecules from binding to its receptors, which in turn increases the release of POMC.

Bupropion

Bupropion, being a dopamine and norepinephrine reuptake inhibitor, increases the amount of dopamine present in the synaptic cleft, which therefore increases the stimulation of POMC neurons. ●

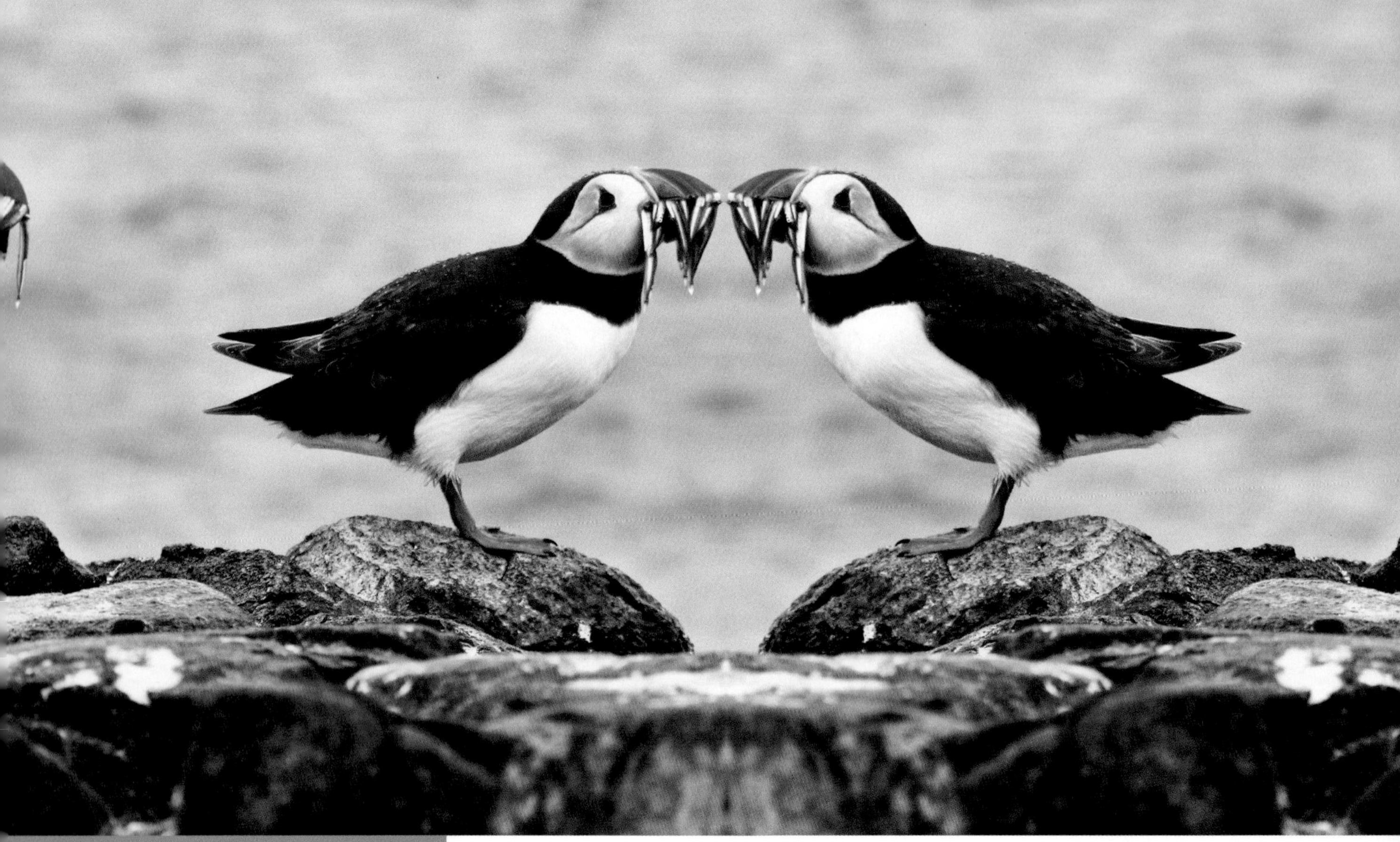

Simon11uk/istockphoto

10 Hormones

Social and Reproductive Behavior

Chapter Contents

Learning Objectives

10.1.1 Explain what hormones are and describe how they were discovered.

10.1.2 Identify the different types of hormones and explain the roles played by the hypothalamus and pituitary.

10.1.3 Differentiate steroid and nonsteroid hormones by their structure and their actions.

10.1.4 Explain the actions of specific hormones.

10.2.1 Describe the hormonal bases of social behaviors.

10.2.2 Explain the hormonal bases for and differences in female and male reproductive behavior.

10.3.1 Describe how male and female phenotypes are activated and organized.

10.3.2 Explain the role of hormones in determining sexual orientation.

Androgenic-Anabolic Steroids: What's With All the Rage?

Anabolic-androgenic steroids are synthetic drugs that mimic the effects of the hormone testosterone. The term *androgenic* refers to the masculinizing effects of the drug, and *anabolic* refers to its building effects on the body. These drugs have legitimate medical uses, but they have also been used to enhance athletic performance through increased muscularity and strength since at least the 1950s. Arguably, the most publicized and most infamous case of steroid use in athletics is that of Canadian sprinter Ben Johnson, who in 1988 was stripped of his Olympic gold medal in the 100-meter dash, after testing positive for steroids. Another widely publicized case was that of track star Marion Jones, who admitted using steroids in preparation for the 2000 Olympic games in Sydney and was subsequently stripped of her medals.

Androgenic-anabolic steroids are also used for aesthetic reasons (i.e., simply to look good), which is especially problematic in male adolescents. The use of steroids in bodybuilding is no secret, and most professional bodybuilders (men and women) admit to their use, so much so that it has become an integral part of the sport. You can easily verify this fact by simply looking up the search terms "bodybuilding and steroids" on Google or YouTube. You will have no trouble finding bodybuilders (professionals and nonprofessionals alike) speaking openly about their use of steroids and even giving advice on how to use them. Steroid use carries significant health risks that have been documented in many studies. Of great concern are multiple deaths suspected of being related to steroid abuse. Another concern is the cases of seeming steroid-induced aggression known as "roid rage." The best-known case attributed to "roid rage" is that of Canadian professional wrestler Chris Benoit, who in 2007 killed his wife, their 7-year-old son, and himself. A more recent case is that of former martial artist Jonathan "war machine" Koppenhaver, who was arrested for assault five times in a span of three years and was sentenced to life in prison for a range of violent crimes including a vicious attack on his girlfriend in 2014.

In 2018, "roid rage" was used as a defense in the case of Keith Duke, who brutally murdered his wife. However, with all the rage over "roid rage," it is important to realize that not everyone who uses steroids becomes a dangerous monster. In fact, in many of these cases, other factors were likely involved, including the use of other drugs and a history of violent behavior that preceded the individual's steroid use. Androgenic-anabolic steroids are discussed in more depth in Unit 10.1.3.

INTRODUCTION

After reading the chapter-opening vignette, you probably realized that hormones—chemicals produced within the brain and at various sites throughout the body—can have a powerful influence on behavior, emotions, and physical characteristics. In this chapter, we will explore these influences. But first, we briefly review some key historical moments in the discovery of hormones and their influence. Next, you will learn about the parts of the brain that synthesize and release hormones so that they can exert their effects and how different hormones are associated with a number of these effects. Hormones are important for the generation of social behaviors, and we will take a look at their involvement in social behaviors that are crucial for the survival of species: bonding, parenting, and sexual and reproductive behaviors. Finally, you will learn about the important role of hormones in determining gender and sexual orientation.

10.1 What Are Hormones?

Module Contents

Learning Objectives

10.1.1 Explain what hormones are and describe how they were discovered.

10.1.2 Identify the different types of hormones and explain the roles played by the hypothalamus and pituitary.

10.1.3 Differentiate steroid and nonsteroid hormones by their structure and their actions.

10.1.4 Explain the actions of specific hormones.

10.1.1 HORMONES AND THEIR DISCOVERY

>> LO 10.1.1 Explain what hormones are and describe how they were discovered.

Key Terms

- **Synaptic signaling:** Communication mediated by neurotransmitters at a local level.
- **Hormones:** Substances released into the bloodstream that have their effects by binding to receptors on cells at distant locations.
- **Endocrine glands:** Glands that produce and release hormones in various regions of the body.
- **Endocrine signaling:** Communication mediated by hormones, having their effects by binding to receptors on cells at distant locations in the body.
- **Endocrine system:** The system of glands that release hormones at various locations within the body.
- **Secretin:** Pancreatic secretions triggered by the release of an agent from the intestines in response to the applications of hydrochloric acid.

You already learned that neurons communicate with each other and with other types of cells through the release of neurotransmitters. Communication mediated by neurotransmitters occurs at a local level. This means that a neurotransmitter released at a synapse binds to receptors located only nanometers across the synaptic cleft. This is known as **synaptic signaling**. In contrast, **hormones** are produced and secreted by glands, known as **endocrine glands**, into the bloodstream and have their effects by binding to receptors on cells at distant locations in the body. This is known as **endocrine signaling**. Together, these glands, which are found in various locations within the body, form what is known as the **endocrine system** (Figure 10.1a). The difference between the signaling mediated by neurotransmitters and hormones is illustrated in Figure 10.1b.

A Bit of History

In the 19th century, physiologist Arnold Adolph Berthold (1803–1861) showed that behavioral characteristics can be influenced by a substance produced in the testes. He did so by conducting an experiment in roosters (Berthold, 1849). He assigned six roosters to three groups. Each one of the groups consisted of a pair of roosters (Figure 10.2). Berthold then castrated (removed the testes from) the pair of roosters in the first group. He observed that these roosters developed as capons, which are roosters that have been castrated (with testes removed) to improve the quality of their flesh for consumption. Exactly as he expected based on his prior observations of capons, they never fought with other males, did not crow, avoided females, and did not display mating behavior. They also had small heads, had atrophied wattles, and were pale in color. For the second group, Berthold reimplanted one of the testicles in the abdominal cavity of each rooster of the pair after they had been castrated.

Finally, for the third group, Berthold transplanted one of the testicles from each of the roosters into the other of the pair. The pair of roosters in the second and third groups (reimplanted and transplanted testicles) recovered normal male physical development and behavior. Berthold also noted that the reimplanted testicles in the second group attached themselves to the intestines and developed a shared system of blood vessels. He also observed that the reimplanted testicles produced sperm. He concluded from his experiment that a substance released in the blood from the testicles influenced physical and behavioral development.

In another experiment, physiologists William Bayliss (1860–1924) and Ernest Starling (1866–1927) discovered that infusions of hydrochloric acid in a denervated dog jejunum (a part of the small intestine) resulted in the release of secretions from the pancreas (Bayliss & Starling, 1902). They then found that the pancreatic secretions were triggered by the release of an agent from the intestines in response to

FIGURE 10.1

(a) The glands that compose the endocrine system and their location in the human body. (b) The difference between synaptic (top) and endocrine (bottom) signaling as described in the text.

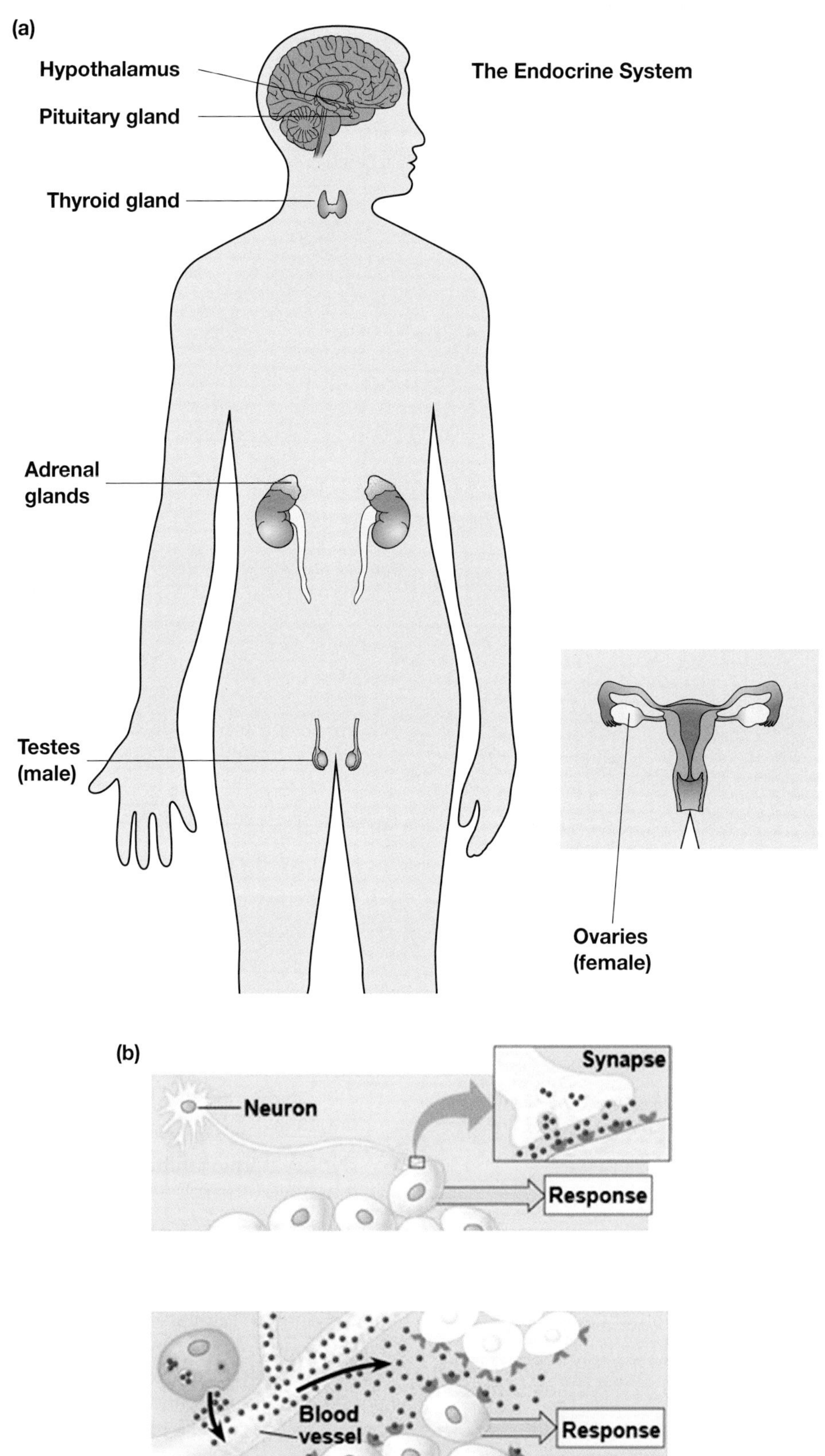

FIGURE 10.2

Berthold's experiment.

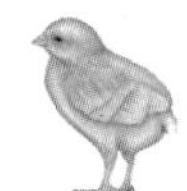
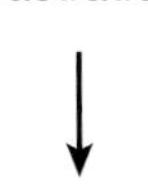
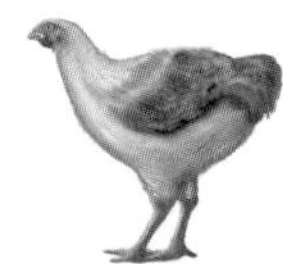
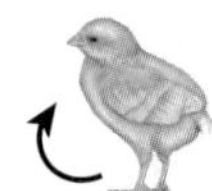
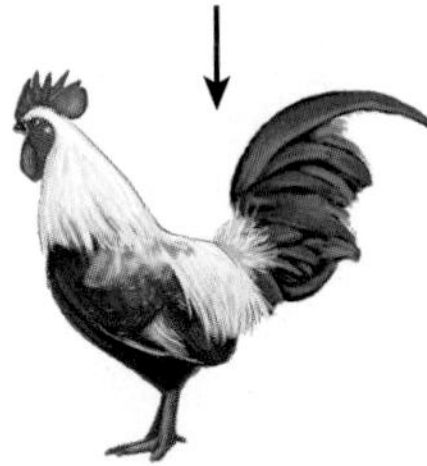
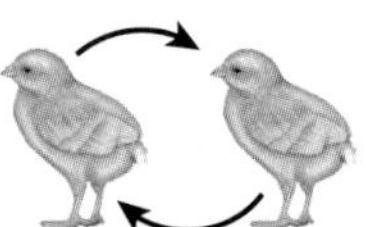
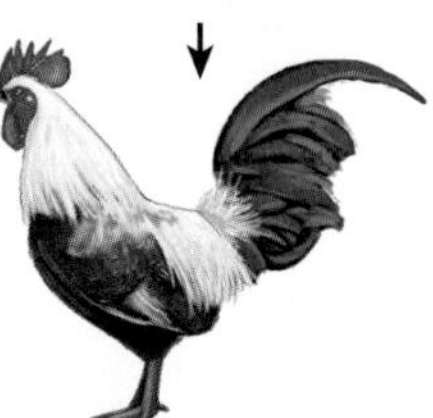
Group 1
Castration
Caponization
• Small comb and wattles
• No interest in hens
• No aggression towards other males
Group 2
Castration and reimplantation of testis
Normal male development
• Normal comb and wattles
• Normal male behavior
Group 3
Castration and transplantation of testis
Normal male development
• Normal comb and wattles
• Normal male behavior

Amanda Tomasikiewicz/Body Scientific Intl.

the applications of hydrochloric acid. They called this agent **secretin**, which they later renamed *hormone*, derived from the Greek word *hormon*, which means "to set into motion or to excite."

10.1.2 TYPES OF HORMONES AND THE ROLES OF THE HYPOTHALAMUS AND PITUITARY

>> LO 10.1.2 Identify the different types of hormones and explain the roles played by the hypothalamus and pituitary.

Key Terms

- **Chemical messengers:** A substance that mediates effects within the cell that produces it or that affects the function of other cells.
- **Intracrine hormone:** A hormone that mediates effects within the same cell that synthesized it.
- **Autocrine hormone:** A hormone that binds to receptors located on the cell that released it to regulate its function.
- **Paracrine hormone:** A hormone that affects cells in the immediate vicinity of the cell that released it.
- **Exocrine hormone:** A hormone released into an organism's external environment.
- **Endocrine hormone:** A hormone released into the bloodstream that affects the function of cells at some distance from the source of release.
- **Neurosecretory cells:** Cells of the hypothalamus that synthesize and release hormones.
- **Hypothalamic releasing hormones:** Hormones that cause the release of hormones from the pituitary.
- **Hypothalamic inhibiting hormones:** Hormones that inhibit the release of hormones from the pituitary.
- **Hypophyseal portal system:** The mesh of small blood vessels that connect the hypothalamus to the anterior pituitary.

Hormones are **chemical messengers**. A chemical messenger is a substance that mediates effects within the cell that produces it or that affects the function of other cells. Hormones can be intracrine, autocrine, paracrine, exocrine, or endocrine. The differences

FIGURE 10.3

Hormones can have intracrine, autocrine, paracrine, exocrine, or endocrine effects. That is, they can have effects within the same cell that synthesized them, bind to receptors located on the cell that released them, affect cells in their immediate vicinity, be released into an organism's external environment, or be released into the bloodstream to affect the function of cells at some distance from their source of release.

Intracrine mediation

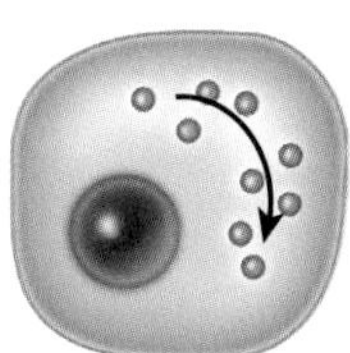

Intracrine substances regulate intracellular events

Autocrine mediation

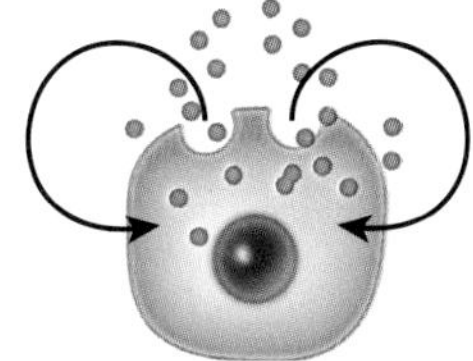

Autocrine substances feed back to influence the same cells that secreted them

Paracrine mediation

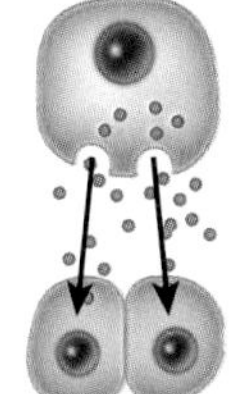

Paracrine cells secrete chemicals that affect adjacent cells

Ectocrine mediation

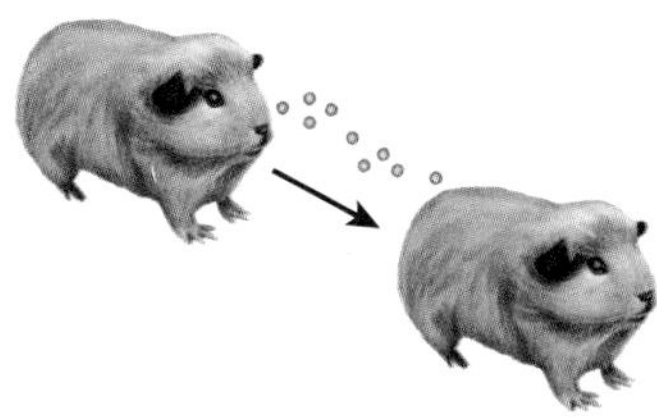

Ectocrine substances, such as pheromones, are released into the environment by individuals to communicate with others

Endocrine mediation

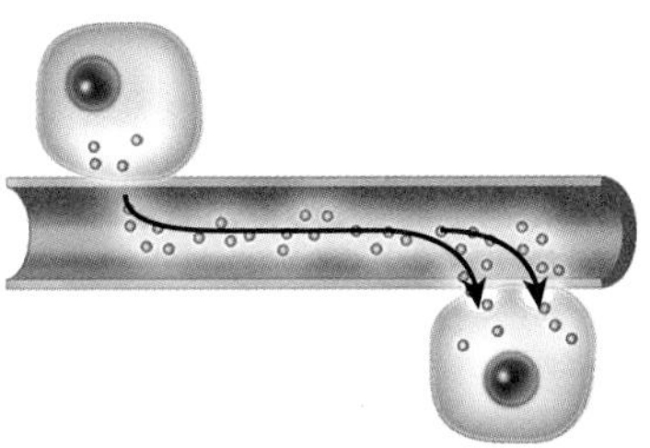

Endocrine substances released into bloodstream to affect function of cells at some distance from their source of release

Amanda Tomasikiewicz/Body Scientific Intl.

between these kinds of hormones are illustrated in Figure 10.3. An **intracrine hormone** mediates effects within the cell that synthesized it. An **autocrine hormone** is a hormone that, after its release from a cell, can bind to receptors located on that same cell that released it to regulate its function. A **paracrine hormone** affects cells in the immediate vicinity of the one that released it.

Exocrine hormones are released by glands into an organism's external environment. For example, pheromones (discussed in Chapter 7) are exocrine hormones that act on receptors located in other organisms. Once bound to receptors of another organism, the pheromone can have significant effects on that organism's behavior. Their effects are wide ranging. They can be used as an alarm system, as when released by an animal under attack by a predator, producing an escape response in conspecifics. They can also be used to attract potential mates from a distance or to mark territory. In addition, they can be used to lay down chemical trails marking the direction to food sources.

Endocrine hormones fit the description of hormones given at the beginning of the chapter. To reiterate, endocrine hormones are substances released into the bloodstream that affect the function of cells at some distance from the source of release. It is to these hormones that we now turn our attention.

The Pituitary Gland and the Hypothalamus

The pituitary gland is often referred to as the "master gland." This is because it releases several hormones that regulate a wide array of biological functions. However, the pituitary does not act by itself. Some of these hormones are synthesized by what are known as **neurosecretory cells** in the hypothalamus. These are oxytocin and antidiuretic hormone (ADH, also known as vasopressin). Other neurosecretory cells in the hypothalamus produce what are known as **hypothalamic releasing hormones** and **hypothalamic inhibiting hormones**. These hormones, respectively, cause or inhibit the release of hormones from the pituitary.

FIGURE 10.4

(a) Location of the hypothalamus and pituitary glands in the brain. (b) Oxytocin and vasopressin are produced by neurosecretory cells in the hypothalamus and move down to the posterior pituitary, from which they are released into the general circulation. Neurosecretory cells also synthesize releasing and inhibiting hormones, which are released into the hypophyseal portal system, which connects the hypothalamus to the anterior pituitary. In response to these releasing and inhibiting hormones, the anterior pituitary releases or withholds the release of the corresponding hormones.

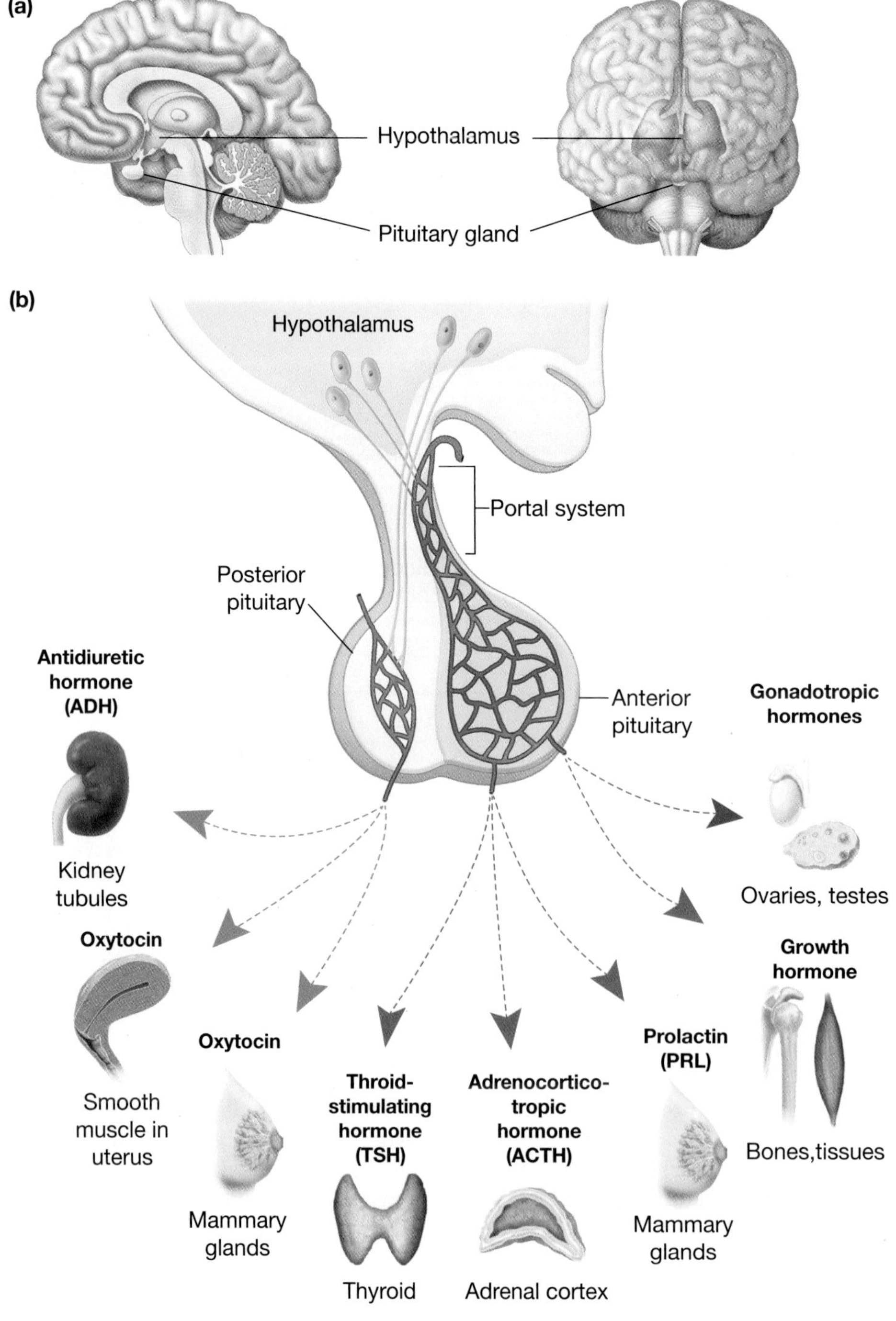

Liana Bauman/Body Scientific Intl.

As shown in Figure 10.4, the main hypothalamic releasing hormones are thyrotropin-releasing hormone (TRH), growth hormone–releasing hormone (GHRH, also known as somatocrinin), gonadotropin-releasing hormone (GnRH), and corticotropin-releasing hormone (CRH). The main inhibiting hormones are growth hormone–inhibiting hormone (GHIH, also known as somatostatin) and gonadotropin-inhibiting hormone (GnIH). Dopamine, the well-known monoamine neurotransmitter, also acts as an inhibitory hormone. In this function, dopamine is known as prolactin-inhibiting hormone (PIH).

The pituitary is subdivided into two parts, the posterior pituitary and the anterior pituitary. Oxytocin and ADH are released into the bloodstream of the posterior pituitary from the axon terminals of neurosecretory cells. Hypothalamic releasing hormones and hypothalamic inhibiting hormones are released from the axon terminals of other neurosecretory cells into the **hypophyseal portal system**, a mesh of small blood vessels that connect the hypothalamus to the anterior pituitary. This results in the release or inhibition of hormones of the anterior pituitary. The hormones released by the anterior pituitary are thyroid-stimulating hormone (TSH), adrenocorticotropic hormone (ACTH), prolactin (PRL), growth hormone (GH), and gonadotropic hormone (Figure 10.4). Figure 10.5 matches the hypothalamic releasing and inhibitory hormones with the corresponding anterior-pituitary hormones they release or inhibit.

10.1.3 STEROID AND NONSTEROID HORMONES

>> LO 10.1.3 Differentiate steroid and nonsteroid hormones by their structure and their actions.

Key Terms

- **Steroid hormones:** Hormones synthesized from cholesterol; produced in the adrenal glands, ovaries (in women), and testes (in men). Steroid hormones can cross the cell membrane and can cause DNA to synthesize proteins.
- **Nonsteroid hormones:** Also known as peptide or protein-like hormones; short chains of amino acids. Nonsteroid hormones cannot cross the cell membrane; they act through second messenger cascades.

FIGURE 10.5

Hypothalamic releasing hormones (top left) and hypothalamic inhibiting hormones (bottom left) and the anterior-pituitary hormones they release (top right) and inhibit (bottom right). Oxytocin and vasopressin are released by the posterior pituitary and are synthesized by neurosecretory cells of the hypothalamus (see Figure 10.4b).

Hypothalamic releasing hormones	Hormones released from the anterior pituitary
Thyrotropin-releasing hormone (TRH) →	Thyroid-stimulating hormone (TSH)
Growth hormone–releasing hormone (GHRH [somatocrinin]) →	Growth hormone (GH)
Gonadotropin-releasing hormone (GnRH) →	Gonadotropic hormones
Corticotropin-releasing hormone (CRH) →	Adrenocorticotropic hormone (ACTH)
Hypothalamic inhibiting hormones	**Inhibited anterior-pituitary hormones**
Growth hormone–inhibiting hormone (GHIH [somatostatin]) →	Growth hormone (GH)
Gonadotropin-inhibiting hormone (GnIH) →	Gonadotropic hormone
Dopamine (prolactin-inhibiting hormone [PIH]) →	Prolactin (PRL)

- **Anabolic-androgenic steroids:** Drugs designed to mimic the muscle-building (anabolic) and masculinizing (androgenic) effects of male steroids.
- **Roid rage:** A condition associated with users of anabolic-androgenic steroids, characterized by the loss of impulse control and overreaction to stimuli that do not usually provoke a reaction.

Hormones are further subdivided into two broad categories: steroid hormones and nonsteroid hormones (also known as peptide hormones or protein-like hormones). Hormones of each category have different structures and achieve their effects through different mechanisms. **Steroid hormones** are synthesized from cholesterol, which is a type of fat. Steroid hormones are produced in the adrenal glands, ovaries (in women), and testes (in men). Steroids produced in the adrenal glands include aldosterone and cortisol. Steroids produced in the ovaries and testes include progesterone and testosterone, respectively. **Nonsteroid hormones** are peptides, which are short chains of amino acids, the building blocks of proteins. Nonsteroid hormones include norepinephrine, insulin, leptin, and ghrelin (discussed in Chapter 9).

As mentioned earlier, steroid and nonsteroid hormones differ not only in their structure but also in the mechanism by which they have their effects. As shown in Figure 10.6, steroid hormones trigger the synthesis of new proteins by DNA. They do so by (1) diffusing through cell membranes, (2) binding receptors within cells, and (3) entering the cell nucleus and binding to the DNA, which contains the code to synthesize proteins.

In contrast, nonsteroid hormones do not have the ability to enter the cell. They have their effects by binding to receptors located on the cell membrane, which stimulates a second messenger within the cell (see Chapter 3). This triggers a cascade of events, which activates enzymes within the cell.

Anabolic-Androgenic Steroids

Anabolic-androgenic steroids are drugs designed to mimic the muscle building (anabolic) and masculinizing (androgenic) effects of male steroids (see the

FIGURE 10.6

Steroid and nonsteroid hormones produce their actions through different mechanisms. Steroid hormones diffuse through cell membranes and cause DNA to synthesize proteins (left). Nonsteroid hormones do not enter the cell but produce their effects through second messenger cascades, which ultimately activate enzymes within the cell (right).

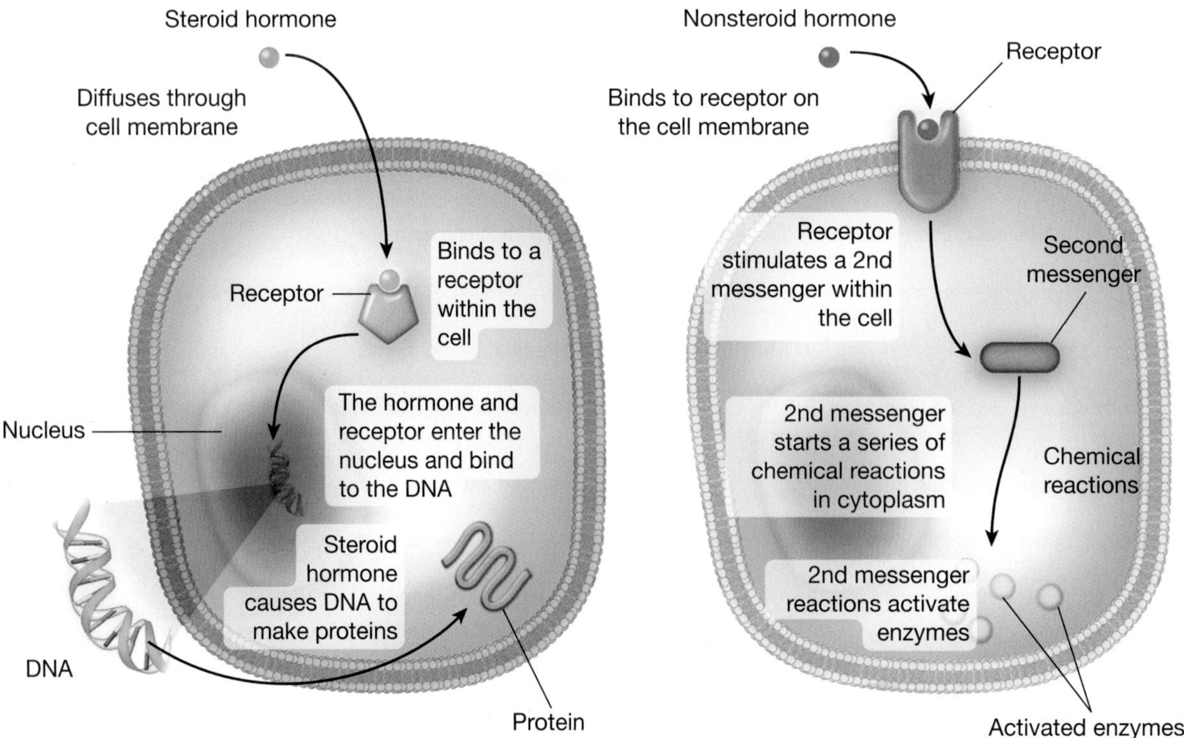

Amanda Tomasikiewicz/Body Scientific Intl.

chapter-opening vignette). In his book *Juiced*, Jose Canseco (2005) recounted his experiences using steroids as a Major League Baseball (MLB) player and named several other players who also used steroids. *The Mitchell Report* shed further light on the widespread use of steroids by MLB players (G. Mitchell, 2007). Steroids are banned in most amateur and professional sports competition, but their use is nevertheless often detected. Many weightlifters and bodybuilders, such as the one seen in Figure 10.7, freely admit to steroid use, attesting to the efficacy of these drugs in enhancing one's ability to build muscle (P. Perry, Lund, Deninger, Kutscher, & Schneider, 2005). In addition, both men and women use anabolic-androgenic steroids for cosmetic purposes.

Unfortunately, the prolonged use of anabolic-androgenic steroids is associated with many side effects, some of which may be dangerous. These include acne, balding, reduced sexual desire, atrophy of the testes, decline in sperm count, and gynecomastia (the enlargement of breast tissue in males). Women who take steroids experience masculinizing effects such as the growth of facial hair, baldness, deepening of the voice, breast shrinkage, and clitoral enlargement. On the more dangerous side, these steroids are associated with cardiac dysfunctions and multiorgan failure (Flo, Kanu, Teleb, Chen, & Siddiqui, 2018; Frati, Busardo, Cipolloni, Dominicis, & Fineschi, 2015; J. Rasmussen et al., 2018).

The use of anabolic-androgenic steroids is also associated with psychological side effects such as depression, mania, extreme mood swings, and a history of illicit drug use (Ip et al., 2012). The most publicized possible psychological side effect of their use is increased aggression, in the so-called **roid rage**. Roid rage is associated with the loss of impulse control and overreaction to stimuli that do not usually provoke a reaction. You may have heard stories, like the ones presented in the opening vignette, in which consumption of steroids is implicated in violent crimes committed by athletes. However, although anabolic-androgenic steroid use increases aggressive behavior in rodents (McGinnis, 2004; Ricci, Morrison, & Melloni, 2013), there is little evidence that steroid use by itself leads to aggressive behavior in humans. Lundholm and colleagues found a strong association between committing violent crimes and anabolic-androgenic steroid use; however, they also found that users who committed violent crimes also abused other drugs, such as amphetamine and cocaine (Lundholm, Frisell, Lichtenstein, & Langstrom, 2015). In the case of Chris Benoit, the professional wrestler mentioned in the opening vignette, it is also important to know that he was found to suffer from chronic traumatic encephalopathy, a neurodegenerative disease caused by multiple brain injuries (Garber, 2009; Trotta, 2007). It was therefore suggested that his behavior may have been better explained by brain damage.

FIGURE 10.7

Many bodybuilders develop their extremely muscular bodies with the help of anabolic-androgenic steroids.

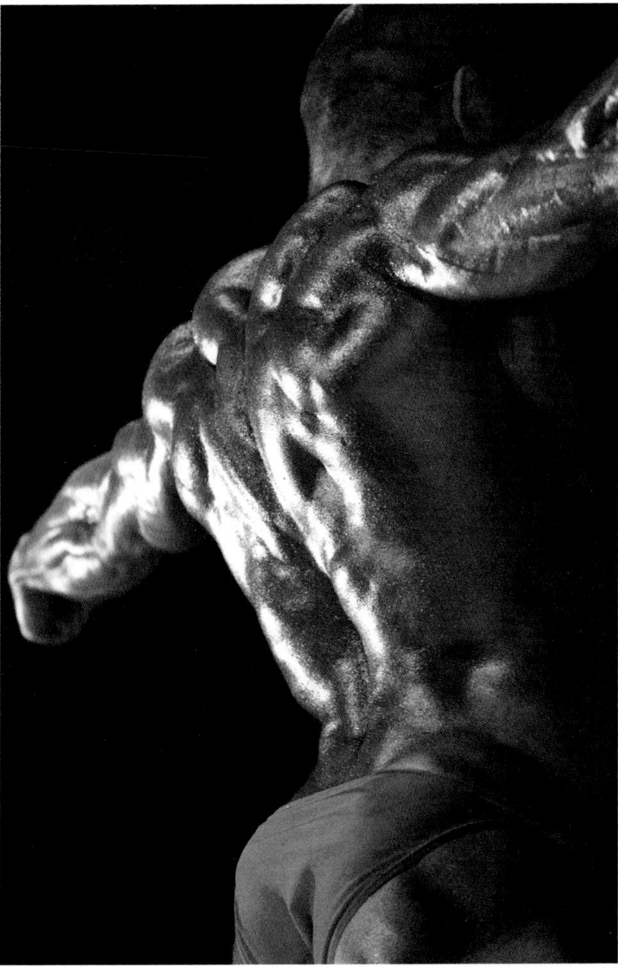

vuk8691/ istockphoto

10.1.4 THE ACTIONS OF SPECIFIC PITUITARY HORMONES

>> LO 10.1.4 **Explain the actions of specific hormones.**

Key Terms

- **Hypertonic:** When salt is overly concentrated relative to water inside blood cells.
- **Thyroxine:** A hormone released by the thyroid gland that is important for maintaining the body's metabolic rate, muscle control, and brain development.
- **Hypothyroidism:** A condition in which the thyroid gland does not produce enough thyroxine.

- **Hyperthyroidism:** A condition in which the thyroid gland produces too much thyroxine.
- **Hypothalamic-pituitary-adrenal (HPA) axis:** The hormonal link between the hypothalamus and the adrenal glands via the pituitary. The HPA axis is activated in the presence of environmental stressors.
- **Cortisol:** A hormone released by the adrenal glands in response to stress.
- **Adult growth hormone deficiency (AGHD):** Abnormally low levels of growth hormone in adults with disease or trauma that affects the hypothalamus or pituitary.
- **GH therapy:** The therapeutic administration of growth hormone in individuals with abnormally low levels of the hormone.

Hormones of the Posterior Pituitary

ADH (Vasopressin). Antidiuretic hormone (also called vasopressin), as its name suggests, prevents the loss of water (from the Greek *diouretikos,* which means "prompting urine"; therefore, the prefix *anti-* means that ADH prevents urination). When salt is overly concentrated in blood plasma, which is the part of the blood that carries water, salt, and enzymes, relative to its concentration inside blood cells. In this condition, the plasma is said to be **hypertonic**, a condition in which cells lose water. This triggers the synthesis of ADH by the hypothalamus, which is released into the posterior pituitary. In turn, the posterior pituitary releases ADH into the general circulation. This induces the kidneys to retain more water and to decrease perspiration through sweat glands. It also acts to increase blood pressure by constricting blood vessels during severe blood loss (its other name, vasopressin, from the Latin *vasopressor,* literally means "constriction of blood vessels").

Oxytocin. Oxytocin, by contrast, is involved in reproductive functions. Its release causes contraction of the uterus during birth. Oxytocin is also responsible for the "letdown" reflex in mothers. It is released in response to stimulation of the nipple, causing a milk letdown. The reflex can become conditioned to environmental stimuli, leading to the release of oxytocin in response to the sight of a baby or the sound of a crying baby.

As you will learn in the next module, vasopressin and oxytocin are also involved in social behaviors such as pair bonding and parenting.

Hormones of the Anterior Pituitary

Thyroid-Stimulating Hormone (TSH). Thyroid-stimulating hormone induces the thyroid gland to release the hormone **thyroxine**. Thyroxine is important for, among other things, maintaining the body's metabolic rate, muscle control, and brain development. Infants born with insufficient levels of thyroxine will suffer intellectual deficiency unless it is administered to them shortly after birth. In a condition called **hypothyroidism**, the thyroid gland does not produce enough thyroxine. Among a whole range of symptoms, hypothyroidism can lead to depression, fatigue, and memory impairments. The opposite condition, known as **hyperthyroidism**, also exists. In hyperthyroidism, the thyroid produces too much thyroxine. An excess of thyroxine increases the body's metabolic rate, also leading to a range of symptoms. These include weight loss, anxiety, irritability, fatigue, and muscle weakness.

Adrenocorticotropic Hormone (ACTH). ACTH is at the center of what is known as the stress response. The stress response can be triggered by anything from a mildly stressful situation, such as getting up in the morning, to extremely stressful experiences, such as witnessing or being the victim of a car accident or being in the middle of a natural disaster. The stress response is activated by activity in the **hypothalamic-pituitary-adrenal (HPA) axis** (Figure 10.8).

In the presence of a stressor, the hypothalamus releases corticotropin-releasing hormone (CRH) into the anterior pituitary. In response to CRH, the anterior

FIGURE 10.8

The hypothalamic-pituitary-adrenal axis (HPA).

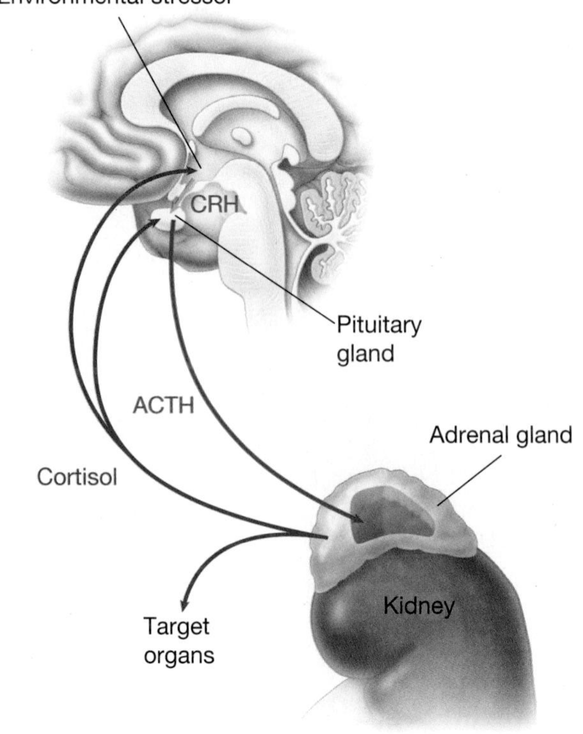

pituitary releases ACTH in the general circulation. ACTH binds to receptors in the adrenal glands located on top of the kidneys. The binding of ACTH to these receptors stimulates the release of the hormone **cortisol**. It is involved in triggering the "fight or flight" response of the sympathetic nervous system (see Chapter 4). It also provides the body with a burst of energy by preventing glucose from being stored, thus making more of it available to the muscles, while shutting down processes that are not essential for immediate survival.

Prolactin. You read earlier that oxytocin is released in response to stimulation of the nipple in mothers, causing a milk letdown. However, in order to have a milk letdown, milk has to be produced. Prolactin, which is released in response to the release of prolactin-releasing peptide from the hypothalamus, is the hormone that stimulates the production of milk (Figure 10.9).

Growth Hormone. Growth hormone is released from the anterior pituitary in response to the release of GHRH from the hypothalamus. Growth hormone is responsible for the growth of all tissues of the body. Children deficient in GH must be treated through supplementation. If they are not, they will achieve a mature height of only 4 to 4½ feet. During puberty, a surge of GH accounts for the significant increase in body size. A gradual drop in GH occurs during aging. This drop results in loss of muscle and body mass, increased body fat, thinning of the skin, and decreased cardiovascular functioning.

Abnormally low levels of growth hormone in adults, who have a condition known as **adult growth hormone deficiency (AGHD)**, can be treated with GH supplementation. This is commonly known as **GH therapy**. Candidates for GH therapy are those with disease or trauma that affects the hypothalamus or pituitary. It is therefore not administered to people with normal declines in GH due to aging. Successful treatment results in increased lean body mass, increased bone mass, and an increase in the ability to exercise as well as general improvement in life satisfaction (Boguszewski, 2017). It is widely believed that taking GH increases athletic performance. However, only limited evidence supports that belief. Improvement in athletic performance in athletes following the administration of GH can be confounded with the use of other drugs, such as androgenic-anabolic steroids or various training regimens (Franke & Berendonk, 1997).

Gonadotropic Hormones. Gonadotropic hormones play a crucial role in reproduction. They are released from the anterior pituitary in response to GnRH from

FIGURE 10.9

Stimulation of a mother's nipple results in the release of oxytocin from the posterior pituitary, causing a milk letdown. Milk production is stimulated by the release of prolactin from the anterior pituitary.

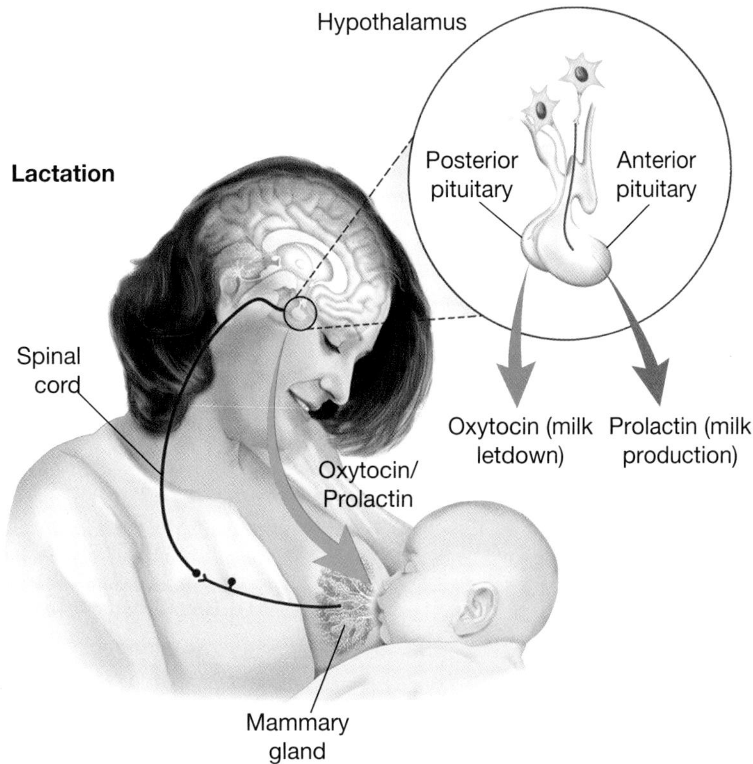

Liana Bauman/Body Scientific Intl.

the hypothalamus. The gonadotropic hormones include luteinizing hormone (LH) and follicle-stimulating hormone (FSH). In women, LH stimulates the production of estradiol (an estrogen) from the ovaries and FSH stimulates the growth of ovarian follicles, the fluid-filled sacs that contain immature eggs. In men, LH stimulates the production of testosterone from the testes and FSH stimulates sperm production.

MODULE SUMMARY

Hormones are substances released by endocrine glands into the bloodstream that have effects on cells distant from their site of release. This is known as endocrine signaling. This differentiates them from neurotransmitters, which have a local effect, in what is called synaptic signaling. In the 19th century, Arnold Adolph Berthold conducted an experiment with roosters that showed that behavioral and physical characteristics can be mediated by a substance produced in the testes. Bayliss and Starling discovered that an agent from the intestines was released in response to the application of hydrochloric acid. They called this substance secretin, which was later renamed "hormone."

There are different types of hormones. They can be intracrine, autocrine, paracrine, exocrine, or endocrine. The pituitary gland was once known as the master gland. However, it releases hormones in response to other hormones released by neurosecretory cells in the hypothalamus. The hypothalamus releases releasing and inhibiting hormones, which cause or inhibit the release of hormones from the pituitary. These are released into a small mesh of blood vessels known as the hypophyseal portal system, which links the hypothalamus to the pituitary. Endocrine hormones can also be classified as steroid and nonsteroid hormones. Steroid hormones are synthesized by the ovaries in females and in the testes in males. They can cross the cell membrane and affect protein synthesis. Nonsteroid hormones, also known as peptide or protein-like hormones, are chains of amino acids that cannot cross the cell membrane and have their effects through second messenger systems. Anabolic-androgenic steroids are synthetic versions of steroid hormones. They are used medically to treat conditions in which there is a significant loss of muscle. They are also used by certain athletes as performance-enhancing drugs, due to their muscle-building properties.

The pituitary gland is subdivided into two main parts: the posterior and anterior pituitary. The two hormones of the posterior pituitary are vasopressin and oxytocin. The main hormones of the anterior pituitary are thyroid-stimulating hormone, which maintains metabolic rate and brain development; adrenocorticotropic hormone, which plays an important role in the stress response; prolactin, which stimulates milk production; growth hormone, which is responsible for the growth of all tissues in the body; and gonadotropin hormones, which include luteinizing hormone, which stimulates the production of estrogen in women and the production of testosterone in men, and follicle-stimulating hormone, which stimulates the growth of follicles in women and the production of sperm in men.

TEST YOURSELF

10.1.1 Contrast hormones with neurotransmitters. Describe the landmark experiment that led to their discovery.

10.1.2 Describe the roles of the hypothalamus and the anterior pituitary and the hormones they produce.

10.1.3 Differentiate between steroid and nonsteroid hormones by their mechanisms. What uses are made of them and why?

10.1.4 Name the main hormones of the posterior and anterior pituitary and briefly discuss their functions.

10.2 Hormones and Behavior

Module Contents

10.2.1 Social Behavior

10.2.2 Sexual and Reproductive Behavior

Learning Objectives

10.2.1 Describe the hormonal bases of social behaviors.

10.2.2 Explain the hormonal bases for and differences in female and male reproductive behavior.

10.2.1 SOCIAL BEHAVIOR

>> LO 10.2.1 Describe the hormonal bases of social behaviors.

Key Terms

- **Social behavior:** Behavioral interactions between individuals of the same species that are beneficial to one or more individuals of the species.
- **Social behavior neural network:** A network of interconnected brain areas that are thought to underlie the neurobiological basis of social behaviors.
- **Social recognition:** The ability to recognize individuals to determine how to act with them.
- **Pair bonding:** A monogamous relationship between a male and a female (sometimes between individuals of the same sex) of the same species that leads to reproduction and a lifelong bond.
- **Parenting:** The process that promotes and supports the development of offspring through caregiving. Depending on the species, this may include physical, emotional, behavioral, intellectual, and social development.
- **Network of parental care:** A network of brain areas known to be involved in generating and maintaining parental behavior, which consists of the median preoptic area, the amygdala, and the dopamine reward pathway.

The hormones most associated with social behavior are oxytocin and vasopressin. **Social behavior** can be defined as behavioral interactions between individuals of a species that are beneficial to one or more individuals of the same species. Some social behaviors, such as copulatory behaviors and parenting, are meant to bring animals together. Other behaviors, such as aggression, are meant to ward off other individuals.

Social behaviors are mediated by the outputs of the **social behavior neural network** (SBNN), which is a network of interconnected brain areas thought to underlie the neurobiological basis of social behaviors (Newman, 1999). These areas are thought to include the extended amygdala, the preoptic area, the anterior hypothalamus, the ventromedial hypothalamus, the periaqueductal gray matter, and the lateral septum. The hormones oxytocin and vasopressin have receptors in each of the areas of the SBNN. Myriad social behaviors exist, including cooperation, competition, social recognition, and pair bonding (Caldwell, 2017). We focus on only two of them: social recognition and pair bonding. Newman (1999) suggested that different types of social behaviors were associated with different patterns of activation of neurons in the SBNN, for example, aggression, sexual behavior, and paternal care. This is illustrated in Figure 10.10.

Social Recognition

Social recognition refers to the ability to recognize individuals to determine how to act with them. For example, some individuals are to be avoided whereas others are to be interacted with. The hippocampus,

FIGURE 10.10

The social behavior neural network. Bottom: Depiction of the interconnected brain areas of the SBNN suggested by Newman (1999), which includes the extended amygdala (extAMY), the preoptic area (PO), the anterior hypothalamus (AH), the ventromedial hypothalamus (VMH), the periaqueductal gray matter (PAG), and the lateral septum (LS). Top: The peaks in the topographic maps indicate the differences in the intensity of firing of the neurons within each area for each type of behavior.

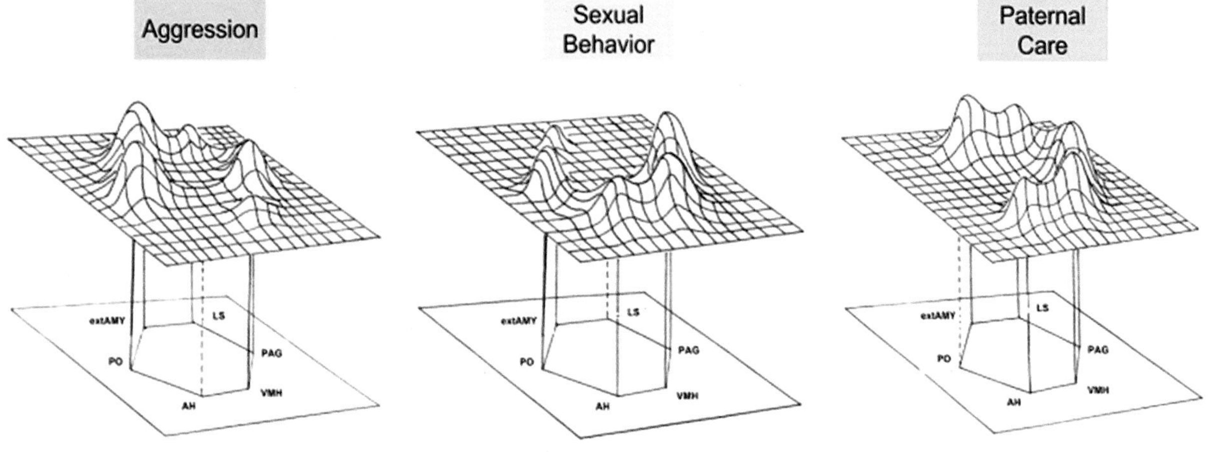

Newman, S. W. (1999). The medial extended amygdala in male reproductive behavior. A node in the mammalian social behavior network. *Annals of the New York Academy of Sciences 877*(1): 242–257. With permission from John Wiley & Sons.

FIGURE 10.11

Social recognition test in mice. T1–T3 (familiarization): A mouse is exposed to another mouse during several familiarization trials (in the figure, three 5-minute trials). Test: The mouse is then given a trial in which both the familiar mouse and one it has seen before (novel) are present. Normal mice will spend more time in the area containing the novel mouse, indicating that it can remember the mouse to which it has been rendered familiar.

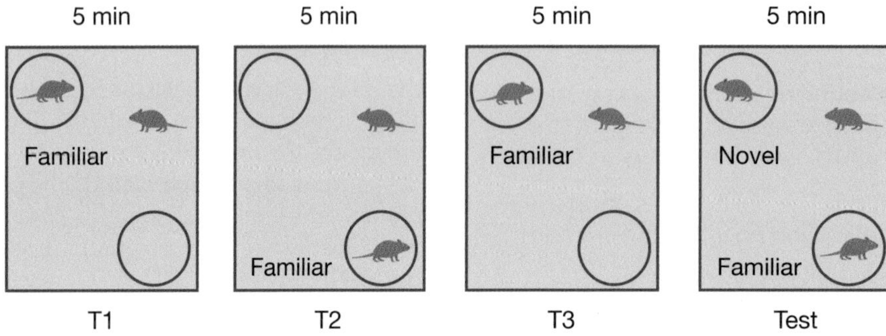

Vladyslav Severyn/istockphoto

which lies within the medial temporal lobes, has for a long time been implicated in the formation of memories (see Chapter 12). More recently, parts of the hippocampus were found to be rich in both oxytocin and vasopressin receptors. Studies have shown that inhibiting those receptors impairs social recognition. In contrast, enhancing the function of these receptors facilitates social recognition (Cilz, Cymerblit-Sabba, & Young, 2019; Raam, McAvoy, Besnard, Veenema, & Sahay, 2017; A. S. Smith, Williams Avram, Cymerblit-Sabba, Song, & Young, 2016). Figure 10.11 shows how social recognition can be tested in mice. A mouse is given multiple exposures to another mouse, rendering it familiar. Following these exposures, the mouse is presented with the familiar mouse along with one it has never encountered. Normal mice will spend more time in the area containing the novel mouse. This indicates that it can remember the mouse to which it has been rendered familiar.

Pair Bonding

Pair bonding defines a monogamous relationship between a male and a female (sometimes between individuals of the same sex) of the same species that leads to reproduction and a lifelong bond. Although it is generally used in reference to animal bonds, it is also sometimes used to characterize human relationships. Only about 3%–5% of mammals are monogamous (Kleiman, 1977), meaning that each member of the pair bond is selective to a single partner for copulation and sharing a nest. Members of the pair bond also show biparental care of offspring.

Since the 1970s, scientists have been using the prairie vole (Figure 10.12) to study pair bonding in mammals. Prairie voles show the typical traits of monogamous pair bonding. That is, males and females form lifelong associations with one another in the defense of their nest and territory as well as to care for their young together. In contrast, other varieties of voles such as the meadow and montane vole are nonmonogamous. For this reason, the prairie vole is ideal to study the neurobiological underpinnings of pair bonding (Carter & Getz, 1993).

FIGURE 10.12

Prairie voles are selective to a single partner for copulation and sharing a nest.

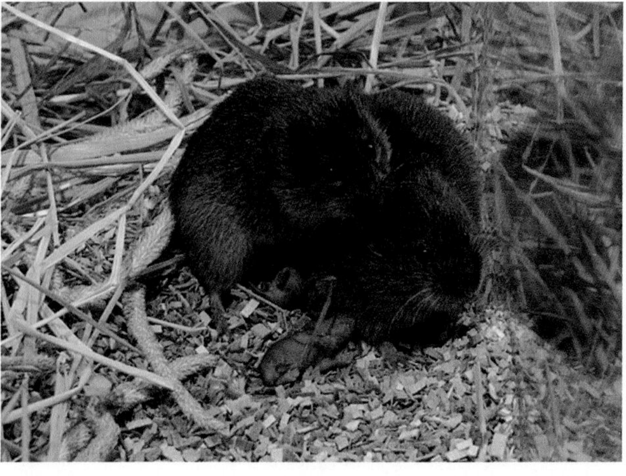

Cormier, Z. (2013). Gene switches make prairie voles fall in love: Epigenetic changes affect neurotransmitters that lead to pair-bond formation. *Nature*, June 2, 2013. Photo attributed to Zuoxin Wang. With permission from Springer Nature.

Over the years, studies have shown that both oxytocin and vasopressin are important for the development of pair bonding. The first clue pointing to the possibility that oxytocin is involved in pair bonding was provided when biologist Peter H. Klopfer (1971) observed that its release was associated with the development of social bonds between the mothers and offspring in goats. Other researchers found that stimulation of the vagina as well as intracerebroventricular infusions of oxytocin (directly into the ventricles) facilitated social bonds in sheep (Kendrick, Keverne, & Baldwin, 1987; Keverne & Kendrick, 1992). Oxytocin has also been shown to be released by social touching, mating, and cohabitation (Okabe, Yoshida, Takayanagi, & Onaka, 2015).

In a landmark study, the effects of intracerebroventricular infusions (directly into the brain's ventricles)

FIGURE 10.13

Partner-preference test for prairie voles. (a) Experimental setup. (b) Intracerebroventricular infusions of oxytocin, 10 ng or 100 ng, facilitated the preference for the familiar male (dark blue bars) over the unfamiliar one (light blue bars), as measured by the mean number of minutes spent in side-by-side contact, compared to voles that received only cerebrospinal fluid (CSF). In contrast, oxytocin did not result in a significant partner preference in female prairie voles in which the gene encoding oxytocin receptors (OTA) in the brain was inhibited (OTA\OT). (c) Peripheral infusions of oxytocin at a dose that was effective when administered centrally had no effect (ng = nanograms which is 10^{-9} grams).

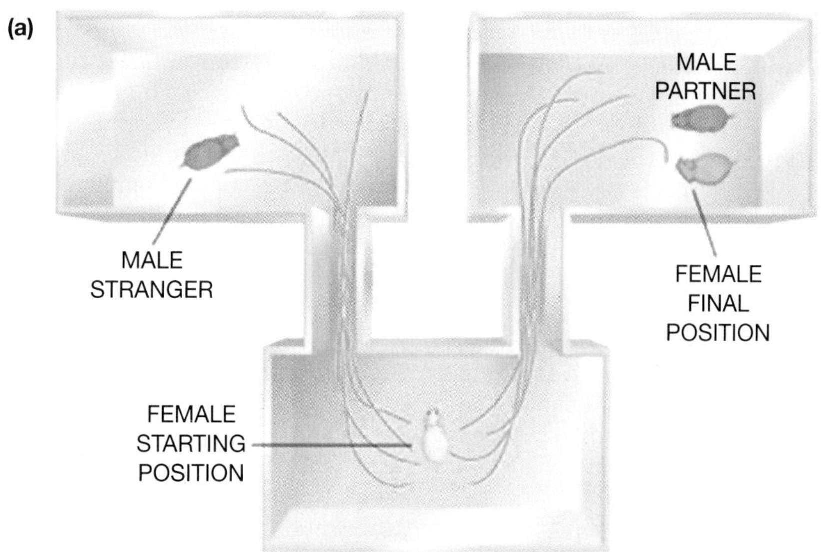

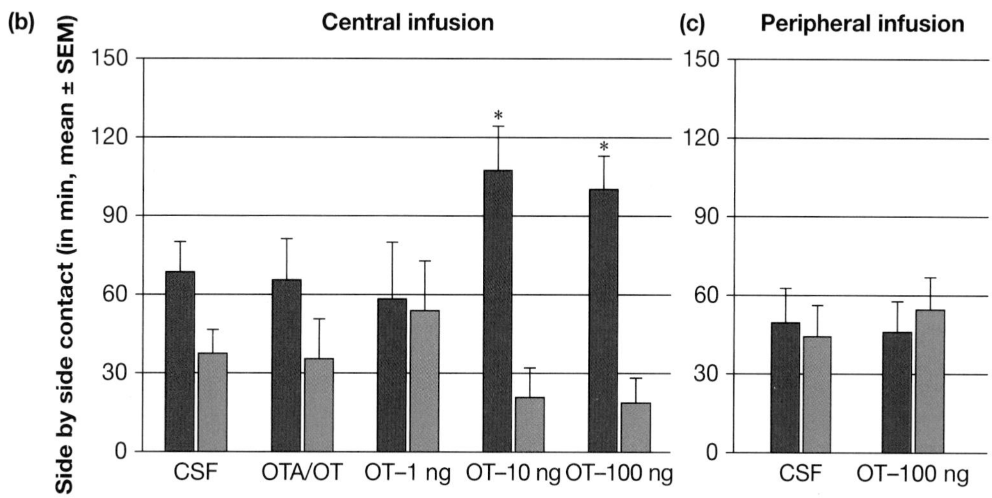

of different doses of oxytocin on the development of a preference for a male partner (as measured by the number of minutes spent in side-by-side contact) were tested on female prairie voles (Williams, Insel, Harbaugh, & Carter, 1994). In this test, a female prairie vole is placed in one compartment of a three-compartment apparatus. From this compartment, the female vole has access to a compartment that contains either an unfamiliar male or a male that is familiar (Figure 10.13a).

The results of the experiment are illustrated in Figures 10.13b and 10.13c. Intracerebroventricular infusions of oxytocin facilitated the preference for the familiar male over the unfamiliar male compared to the infusions of only cerebrospinal fluid. In contrast, infusions of oxytocin did not result in significant partner preference in female prairie voles in which the gene encoding oxytocin receptors in the brain was inhibited (Keebaugh, Barrett, Laprairie, Jenkins, & Young, 2015). Only infusions within the brains of the voles resulted in a facilitated preference. Peripheral infusions (throughout the body) had no effect. This means that the infused oxytocin exerted its effects by acting on cells within the brain.

In another study, increased partner preference was found in prairie voles in which oxytocin receptors were overexpressed. However, overexpression of oxytocin receptors did not result in increased partner preference in the nonmonogamous meadow vole (H. E. Ross et al., 2009).

What about vasopressin? Vasopressin may play a role that is opposite to that of oxytocin. Remember that pair bonding also includes defending the nest and territory. This requires the voles to act aggressively. Male voles also attack novel male intruders during mating. These types of behaviors in voles have been shown to be regulated by vasopressin. Mating males showed no signs of aggression toward an intruder when injected with a vasopressin-receptor antagonist (Winslow, Hastings, Carter, Harbaugh, & Insel, 1993).

The differences in social behavior between monogamous and nonmonogamous varieties of voles may be explained by differences in the distribution of oxytocin and vasopressin receptors in their respective brains. For example, in the nonmonogamous montane vole, oxytocin receptors were found to be highly concentrated in the lateral septum, ventromedial hypothalamus, and cortical nucleus of the amygdala. In contrast, the density of oxytocin receptors in the prairie vole was highest in the nucleus accumbens, prefrontal cortex, and bed nucleus of the stria terminalis. In the nonmonogamous montane vole, the density of vasopressin receptors was highest in the medial prefrontal cortex and lateral septum. In the prairie vole, the density of vasopressin receptors was highest in the lateral and medial amygdala, accessory olfactory bulb, diagonal band, thalamus, and ventral pallidum (H. E. Ross et al., 2009; Smeltzer, Curtis, Aragona, & Wang, 2006).

How does this pattern of results explain greater pair bonding in monogamous than nonmonogamous voles? The answer may lie in the observation that, in the monogamous prairie vole, oxytocin receptors are highly concentrated in areas associated with reward, such as the nucleus accumbens, which is also rich in dopamine receptors, and that their activation by oxytocin may become conditioned to the presence of their partner.

Parenting

Parenting is often defined as a process that promotes and supports the development of offspring through caregiving. Depending on the species, this may include physical, emotional, behavioral, intellectual, and social development. Parenting also involves the transmission of morals and values of the parents' respective cultures.

The process of parenting begins during pregnancy. In fact, parental behavior is primed by the hormones of pregnancy. These are the steroid hormones progesterone and estrogen. As shown in Figure 10.14, levels of progesterone and estrogen rise gradually during pregnancy, peak at childbirth, and then drop sharply. After childbirth (postpartum), the hormones associated with lactation—prolactin and oxytocin—are released. During childbirth, oxytocin induces uterine contractions. As mentioned earlier, suckling of the baby on the mother's breasts triggers the hypothalamus to release oxytocin into the posterior pituitary, resulting in the contraction of the cells of the mammary glands, which in turn cause the release of milk. Prolactin triggers milk production and prepares breast tissue for its release. As progesterone and estrogen prime parental behavior, prolactin and oxytocin form its trigger.

The Neurobiology of Parental Behavior. Much of our knowledge of the neurobiological basis of parenting was acquired through the use of animal models. A pioneer in the use of animal models to study the biology of maternal behavior was psychologist Jay S. Rosenblatt (1923–2014). He and others of his generation believed that parenting could only be understood by defining its underlying physiological systems. In rodents, parental behavior largely consists of hardwired automatic responses to (1) stimuli from the pup (which can be auditory, visual, or tactile), (2) external cues from the environment (such as the presence of predators), and (3) the animal's internal state (such as its reproductive state). Parental behaviors in rodents include nest building, licking and grooming, retrieval and transport of the pups, nursing, guarding, and call vocalizations.

The brain area considered to be central in the regulation of parenting behavior is the median preoptic area (MPOA) of the hypothalamus. The activity of neurons of the MPOA is thought to be regulated by the hormones of pregnancy—estrogen and progesterone—as well as oxytocin and prolactin, which, as you learned earlier, are present in high levels during the period surrounding childbirth (Dobolyi, Grattan, & Stolzenberg, 2014). The MPOA also has a high number of receptors for these hormones.

FIGURE 10.14

Levels of progesterone and estrogen rise gradually during pregnancy, peak at childbirth, and drop sharply after childbirth (postpartum), when the hormones associated with lactation—prolactin and oxytocin—are released.

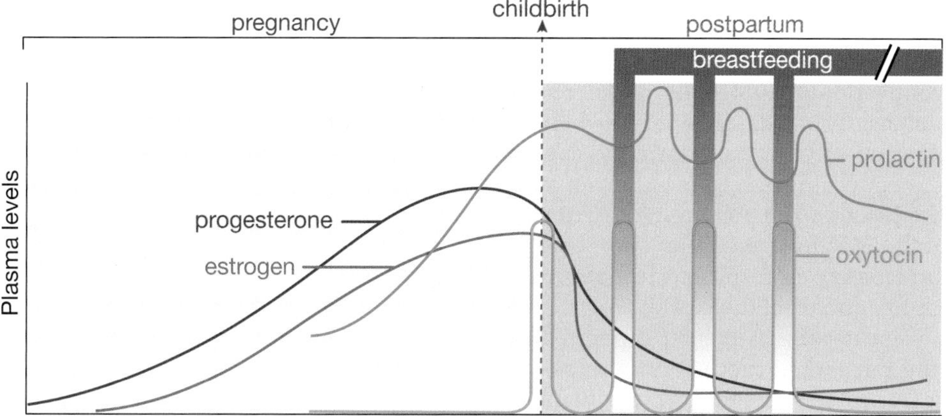

A strong indicator that the MPOA is important for parental behavior is that when the area is lesioned, parental behavior is disrupted. In contrast, direct stimulation of the MPOA with estrogen facilitates parental behavior. However, the MPOA does not function by itself in the generation of parental behavior. Rather, it acts in concert with an array of other brain areas in the generation of the various behaviors involved in parenting. In fact, the MPOA is interconnected with at least 20 other brain areas. These areas include the amygdala, which is involved in emotional responses, and the brain's dopamine reward pathway, which includes areas such as the nucleus accumbens (NAc), the ventral-tegmental area (VTA), and the striatum.

Why would the MPOA project to the amygdala and the brain's dopamine reward pathway? In rodents, the MPOA, amygdala, and dopamine reward pathway are part of what is known as the **network of parental care**. The projections to the dopamine reward pathway place incentive on stimuli from offspring, which may otherwise be ignored. The projections to the amygdala increase maternal vigilance, which facilitates behaviors that promote the safety of offspring.

A specific set of MPOA neurons in mice was recently found to be responsible for generating parental behavior in mice (Kohl et al., 2018). These neurons release the neuropeptide galanin (MPOA^{GAL}). MPAO^{GAL} neurons are interconnected with at least 20 different brain areas in both males and females. MPOA^{GAL} neurons are thought to integrate the inputs consisting of stimuli from pups, environmental stimuli, and the internal state of the animals to then excite the brain areas responsible for the output of appropriate parental behaviors. As illustrated in Figure 10.15, these include pup grooming, nest building, or the motivation to interact with pups. In addition, behaviors that compete with parenting, such as mating, aggressive behaviors, and eating, are suppressed (Kohl & Dulac, 2018).

FIGURE 10.15

MPOA^{GAL} neurons process inputs from pups, the animal's internal state, and environmental stimuli and integrate these stimuli to produce outputs that generate appropriate behaviors while suppressing behaviors that compete with parenting.

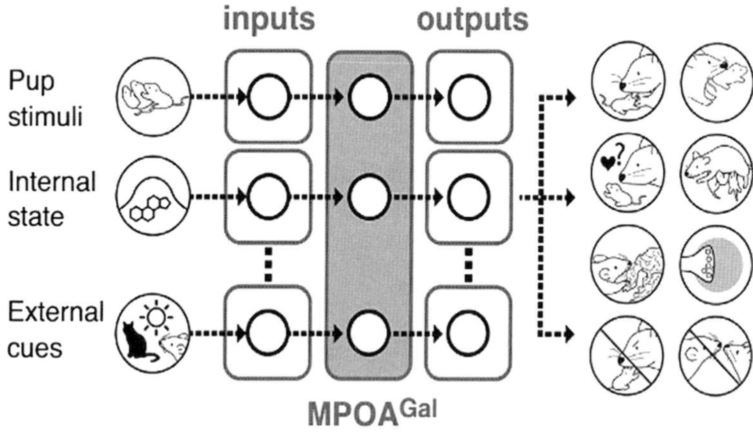

Kohl, J., & C. Dulac. (2018). Neural control of parental behaviors. *Current Opinions in Neurobiology 49*: 116–122. With permission from Elsevier.

In addition to the connections with the amygdala and the dopamine reward pathway (which includes the NAc, VTA, and striatum), MPOA^{GAL} neurons project to other areas known to be part of the network of parental care. These include the paraventricular nucleus (PVN), anteroventral paraventricular nucleus (AVPe), periaqueductal gray matter (PAG), and medial amygdala (MeA).

Distinct parental behaviors in mice were associated with connections of MPOA^{GAL} neurons to specific brain areas. This was discovered when the connections between MPOA^{GAL} neurons and specific connections to other brain areas were either activated or inhibited (Kohl et al., 2018). Activating the connections between the MPOA^{GAL} neurons and the PAG increased pup grooming and sniffing in both males and females but did not affect the motivation to interact with pups. That is, when a barrier separated the parents from the pups, their motivation to cross the barrier was not affected. In addition, virgin males who usually attack and kill pups did so to a lesser degree. Activating the connections from MPOA^{GAL} neurons to the VTA increased the number of times parents crossed a barrier to reach the pups, but they did not interact with the pups more and virgin males remained aggressive. Activating the connections between MPOA^{GAL} neurons and the MeA decreased the time spent by females in their nest but not the motivation to interact with pups.

Inhibiting the connections between MPOA^{GAL} neurons and the PAG reduced pup grooming and sniffing but did not affect other behaviors. Inhibiting connections between MPOA^{GAL} neurons and the VTA reduced barrier crossings to reach pups but did not affect time spent in the nest. Finally, inhibiting connections between MPOA^{GAL} neurons and the MeA did not affect interactions with intruders or other behaviors. The results of activating and inhibiting connections between MPOA^{GAL} neurons and these other areas are summarized in Table 10.1.

Human Parental Caregiving Network. After reading the previous section, you may wonder if the parental care provided by humans to their offspring relies on the same mechanisms as in rodents. Part of the answer is that the basic caregiving network that you learned about is conserved in humans.

However, as mentioned earlier, parental care in rodents and other animals is largely dependent on automatic hardwired behaviors in response to stimuli from the pups, the environment, and the animal's internal state. Thus, parental behaviors in nonhumans are largely driven by bottom-up processes, which means they are driven by the stimuli. In humans, parental care is driven by both bottom-up and top-down processes, which means that parental behaviors are also generated by conscious thought, based on information from the senses. These nonautomatic behaviors are more flexible and rely on cortical rather than subcortical brain areas.

For example, human parents can respond to a child based on the perception of a child's emotional state or that the child is in pain (Bornstein et al., 2017). A human parent may also develop an affinity for recognizing a child's nonverbal signals and intentions (Bernhardt & Singer, 2012). A human parent is also able to consciously regulate his or her own emotions in order to act appropriately in a given situation or according to a child's emotional state (Samuelson, Krueger, & Wilson, 2012). Human parental caregiving also depends on cultural norms and practices as well as short- and long-term family goals. These behaviors, which are generated by top-down processes, require the participation of cortical areas.

TABLE 10.1

Effects of activation and inhibition of connections between MPOA^{GAL} neurons to three different brain areas: the periaqueductal gray matter (PAG), the ventral-tegmental area (VTA), and the medial amygdala (MeA).

CONNECTION	ACTIVATION	INHIBITION
MPOA^{GAL} PAG	• Increased pup grooming and sniffing in both males and females • Did not affect the motivation to interact with pups	• Reduced pup grooming and sniffing • Did not affect other behaviors
MPOA^{GAL} VTA	• Increased the number of times parents crossed a barrier to reach the pups • Did not interact with pups more • Virgin males remained aggressive	• Reduced barrier crossings to reach pups • Did not affect time spent in the nest
MPOA^{GAL} MeA	• Decreased the time spent by females in their nest • Did not affect the motivation to interact with pups	• Did not affect interactions with intruders or other behaviors

10.2.2 SEXUAL AND REPRODUCTIVE BEHAVIOR

>> LO 10.2.2 Explain the hormonal bases for and differences in female and male reproductive behavior.

Key Terms

- **Reproductive behavior:** Any behavioral pattern that results in sperm and egg being brought together to produce offspring.
- **Sexual behavior**: A component of reproductive behavior that includes responses directly associated with genital stimulation and copulation.
- **Behavioral estrus:** The period during which female animals mate, corresponding to vaginal proestrus, which is coordinated to occur just before ovulation when a mature egg is released from the ovary, ready to be fertilized.
- **Receptivity:** Actions performed by a female that are necessary for copulation.
- **Lordosis:** The position observed when a female animal crouches so that the vagina is brought into a horizontal position with the tail deflected to the side.
- **Lordosis pathway:** A set of neuroanatomical regions that, when activated, result in contraction of the appropriate set of muscles to result in lordosis.
- **Menstrual cycle:** The regular changes that occur in the female reproductive system that make pregnancy possible.
- **Attractivity:** A female's stimulus value in evoking a sexual response in a male.

Reproductive behavior refers to any behavioral pattern that results in sperm and egg being brought together to produce offspring. **Sexual behavior** is a component of reproductive behavior that includes responses directly associated with genital stimulation and copulation. In this section, we first explore some of what is known about the reproductive behavior of rodents, since much of what we know about reproductive behavior comes from studying rodents, and then we look at what we know about reproductive behavior in humans.

The Female Reproductive Cycle and Behavior

The female reproductive cycle, which lasts four to five days in rodents, is subdivided into four distinct stages: vaginal estrus, diestrus I, diestrus II, and vaginal proestrus. These stages correspond to changes in the cells of the vagina, which are themselves correlated with the activity of the ovaries. Unlike males, which can mate at any time (discussed in the next section), females mate only during what is known as **behavioral estrus**. Behavioral estrus corresponds to vaginal proestrus, which is coordinated to occur just before ovulation, which is when a mature egg is released from the ovary, ready to be fertilized.

For mating to occur, the female has to be receptive. **Receptivity** is defined by the actions performed by a female that are necessary for copulation. These actions vary between species. In most mammals, receptive females display what is known as **lordosis** (or the lordotic reflex). Lordosis is observed when the female crouches so that the vagina is brought into a horizontal position with the tail deflected to the side. Finally, successful reproduction also must include the drive to copulate.

The coordination of ovulation, receptivity, and the desire to mate is achieved by the estrogen hormone estradiol. Ovulation is controlled by the hypothalamic-pituitary-gonadal (HPG) axis. As illustrated in Figure 10.16a, the hypothalamus releases GnRH into the anterior pituitary. This causes the anterior pituitary to release the gonadotropic hormones LH and FSH. This in turn stimulates the ovaries to release the steroid hormones estrogen and progesterone. The release of GnRH and gonadotropic hormones is regulated by a negative feedback loop, which reduces the amounts of GnRH released from the hypothalamus and gonadotropic hormones released from the anterior pituitary.

However, during the female reproductive cycle, rising levels of estrogen lead to a surge in the release of GnRH from the hypothalamus, which in turn results in a surge in the release of gonadotropic hormones. This stimulates the gonads to cause ovulation. The rising levels of estrogen and progesterone also activate the **lordosis pathway** (Figure 10.16b). The lordosis pathway comprises a set of neuroanatomical regions that when activated result in contraction of the appropriate set of muscles to result in lordosis. The brain areas that are part of the lordosis pathway include the amygdala, the bed nucleus of the stria terminalis (BNST), the preoptic area (POA), the ventromedial nucleus of the hypothalamus (VMN), the periaqueductal gray matter (PAG), and the medullary reticular formation (MRF). Receptors for progesterone are found on neurons in the POA and VMN. Estrogen receptors are found within the amygdala, BNST, POA, VMN, and PAG.

The muscle contractions resulting in the lordotic reflex are mediated by the MRF, situated within the hindbrain. The MRF is also a major component of the lordotic reflex arc, which is triggered by sensory input from the flank and the rump. However, stimulation of the MFG alone is not sufficient to induce the lordotic reflex; input from the PAG is also necessary. The activation of other senses such as smell (including the

FIGURE 10.16

(a) The hypothalamic-pituitary-gonadal (HPG) axis. (b) The lordosis pathway. (c) Estradiol binds to receptors on GABAergic neurons in the striatum, reducing their inhibitory effect on dopamine neurons.

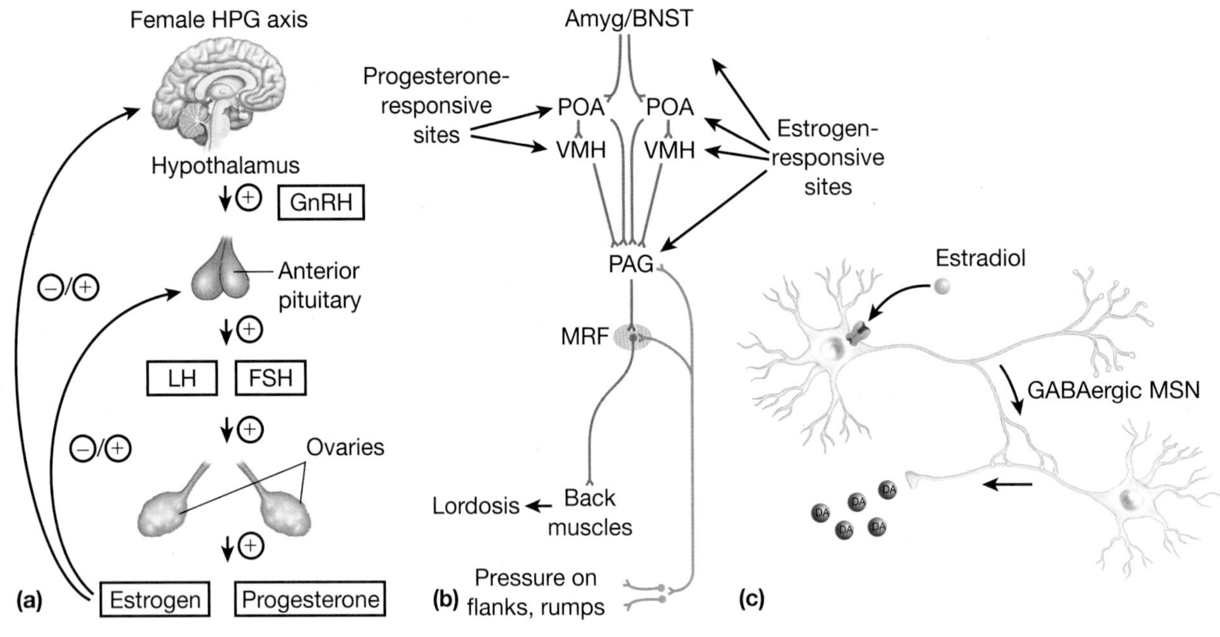

Amanda Tomasikiewicz/Body Scientific Intl.

detection of pheromones), vision, and hearing, as well as touch to parts of the body other than the flank and rump, also participate in inducing lordosis. The lordosis pathway is more complex than we have space to fully expand upon here. It also includes the participation of several other brain areas, such as the periventricular nucleus and arcuate nucleus of the hypothalamus, in which estrogen receptors are found, as well as various neurochemicals, such as neuropeptide-Y, endorphins, and neurotransmitters (Micevych & Meisel, 2017; Micevych, Mermelstein, & Sinchak, 2017).

The final component of reproductive behavior we discuss is the drive to copulate. As with any other motivated behaviors, such as eating and drug consumption, sexual activity activates the brain's dopamine reward pathway (NAc, VTA, and striatum). Dopamine levels in the NAc of female rats rise in the anticipation of mating, and estradiol binds to receptors on GABAergic neurons in the striatum, reducing their inhibitory effect on dopamine neurons (Yoest, Cummings, & Becker, 2014) (Figure 10.16c). In addition, estradiol binds to receptors in the NAc, increasing sexual motivation (Tonn Eisinger, Larson, Boulware, Thomas, & Mermelstein, 2018).

Male Reproductive Behavior

Contrary to female rats, which can mate only during a specific period in the reproductive cycle corresponding to behavioral estrus, males have the capacity to mate at any time. A typical sexual encounter between a male and a female rat begins with the male investigating the female's anogenital region. Following this investigative phase, the male reproductive behavior consists of three stages: mounting, intromission, and ejaculation. Mounting consists of the male straddling the female from behind, thrusting its hips while attempting to locate the female's vagina with its penis. Once the vagina is located, the male rat continues its thrusting motion. This stage is known as intromission. This is followed by ejaculation, in which semen is discharged from the penis.

The main stimulus for reproductive behavior in male rats is pheromones, released by a female in estrus. Pheromones activate the vomeronasal pathway (Keverne, 2004). As discussed in Chapter 7, the vomeronasal organ is part of the accessory olfactory system and sends information about pheromones to the accessory olfactory bulb.

Information about the detection of pheromones in the vomeronasal system, as well as somatosensory stimulation from the genitals, is processed in the amygdala before being sent to the MPOA, which also receives information from all sensory systems (E. Hull, Wood, & McKenna, 2006; Kondo & Arai, 1995). The motivation to engage in reproductive behavior in males is thought to occur through the release of dopamine in the MPOA. As you read earlier, the MPOA projects to many different brain areas. One of these areas is the VTA (E. Hull et al., 2006). In fact, the VTA may be the brain area most heavily involved in the motivational aspects of sexual behavior, whereas the MPOA is most heavily involved in its performance (Everitt, 1990).

Electrical stimulation of the MPOA of rats facilitated copulatory behavior by reducing the number of intromissions required for ejaculation (Malsbury, 1971). This was taken to mean that MPOA stimulation increased sexual excitement. Stimulation of MPOA with glutamate in rats activated the neural pathways that control erections (Giuliano et al., 1996). In contrast, ablating the MPOA results in impaired male sexual behavior in rats and several other animal species (Pfaff, 2009).

The major hormone involved in male reproductive behavior is testosterone. The role of testosterone is to facilitate dopamine release in the MPOA. Usually, an increase of dopamine release is observed in male rats in response to a female in estrus. However, this effect was eliminated in castrated male rats that also did not copulate with females when given a chance (E. M. Hull, Du, Lorrain, & Matuszewich, 1995). In addition, MPOA dopamine release and copulatory ability were restored in castrated rats by injections of testosterone (Putnam, Du, Sato, & Hull, 2001).

Human Reproductive Behavior

Now that you know the basics of reproductive behavior in rodents, you are probably wondering how much of that applies to human reproductive behavior. Your first reaction might be to dismiss what you just learned as not being relevant to humans. But keep in mind that humans have the same sex steroids as rodents and that these hormones are present in similar concentrations with a similar distribution of receptors within the brain.

However, you would be right to point out that human sexual behavior is not as tightly controlled by an estrus cycle in females or by the detection of pheromones by males. Human sexual behavior is much more flexible due to being influenced by social factors, learning, culture, and expectations. In addition, humans have sex for a whole range of reasons other than reproduction. Psychologists Cindy Meston and David Buss (2007) listed the top 50 reasons for why people have sex. These include stress reduction, pleasure, physical desirability, and experience seeking. Keep in mind that, in humans, these factors interact with the biological factors discussed in the preceding section.

It is still worth asking about what role hormones play in human sexual activity. First, it is important that you understand the **menstrual cycle**, which refers to the regular changes that occur in the female reproductive system that make pregnancy possible. The menstrual cycle includes the production of oocytes, which are the cells that become the eggs, and the preparation of the uterus for pregnancy (Silverthorn, Johnson, Ober, Ober, & Silverthorn, 2016). This means that the menstrual cycle can be described either by the cycle that goes on within the ovaries (ovarian cycle) or by the events that occur within the uterus (uterine cycle). The uterus is where the embryo implants and develops.

The uterine cycle refers to the changes in the endometrium, which is the tissue that lines the uterus, over a 28-day period to prepare for the possibility of a pregnancy. The uterine cycle is driven by steroid hormones produced in the ovarian cycle (Figure 10.17). The ovarian cycle consists of two phases: the follicular phase and the luteal phase. In between the two is ovulation, which is the release of an egg from the ovaries. The follicular phase is marked by the release of follicle-stimulating hormone (FSH) and luteinizing hormone (LH) from the anterior pituitary in response to the release of GnRH from the hypothalamus. The release of FSH triggers the release of estrogens from the follicles. In addition, androgens, which are released due to the actions of LH, are converted to estrogens. As you can see in the figure, the peak of estrogen levels occurs at just about the time of ovulation. However, the sharp rise in estrogen levels triggers the hypothalamus to stop releasing GnRH, which inhibits the release of FSH and LH from the pituitary. Therefore, levels of estrogen decline sharply after ovulation. At that time, a hormone-secreting structure called the corpus luteum develops in the ovary. Luteinizing hormone stimulates the corpus luteum to release progesterone. These high levels of progesterone support pregnancy should fertilization occur. However, if fertilization does not occur, LH levels fall and the corpus luteum undergoes degeneration.

As we mentioned earlier, unlike the females of other species, which can engage in reproductive behavior only during estrus, women can engage in sexual intercourse at any time. However, research has shown that sexual desire in women varies during the ovarian cycle. In fact, sexual desire in women is driven by estrogen, the levels of which peak just before ovulation (Sherwin, Gelfand, & Brender, 1985). What about the ovarian hormone progesterone and testosterone, which is produced in women by the adrenal glands? Roney and Simmons (2013) found that the amount of

FIGURE 10.17

The ovarian cycle.

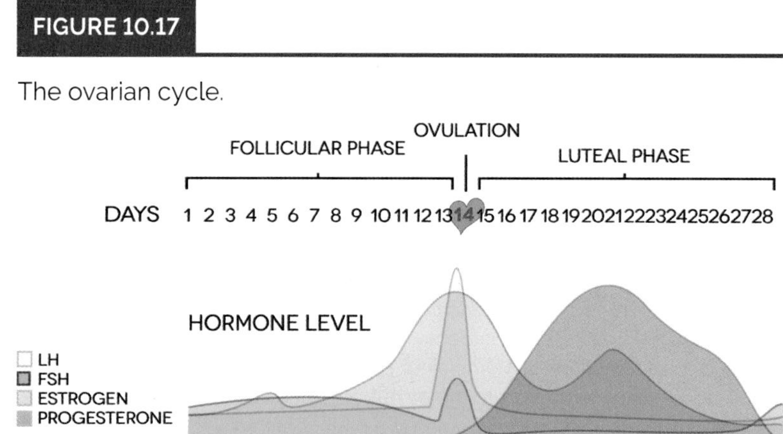

TefiM/ istockphoto

sexual desire was associated with levels of estrogen at about midcycle (close to ovulation). In addition, the amount of sexual desire was negatively correlated with the rising levels of progesterone (after ovulation).

A woman's stage in her ovarian cycle was also shown to influence her **attractivity**, defined as a female's stimulus value in evoking a sexual response in a male (Beach, 1976). This was demonstrated by a gutsy study in which female dancers in a gentleman's club made bigger tips around the time of ovulation than during any other time in the menstrual cycle (G. Miller, Tybur, & Jordan, 2007). That is, they averaged $335 during ovulation (which is when estrogen levels are at their peak), $260 during the luteal phase (when estrogen levels are low and progesterone levels high), and only $185 during menstruation (the period of vaginal bleeding early in the cycle). What about testosterone? The role of testosterone in women's sexual desire is still debated, with some studies showing minimal to no effects (Cappelletti & Wallen, 2016; Roney & Simmons, 2013). One study did show that testosterone intake increased sexual arousal in women after being shown excerpts of erotic films (Tuiten et al., 2000). The results of other studies suggest that increased testosterone levels are associated with cues linked to potential sexual partners and not desire per se. For example, one study found that women who have multiple sexual partners had higher testosterone levels than single women (van Anders, Hamilton, & Watson, 2007).

IT'S A MYTH!

All Women Get PMS

The Myth

Do all women get premenstrual syndrome (PMS)? The PMS myth is the popular belief that once a month, during the days preceding the onset of menstruation, all women become dangerous monsters not to be messed with. This stereotype continues to be propagated in films, sitcoms, magazines, greeting cards, self-help books, advertising, and many other types of media. In addition, girls learn about the specter of the onset of menstruation, and everything horrible associated with it, from mothers, sisters, and grandmothers (DeLuca, 2017). However, some commentators have argued that PMS is a culture-bound syndrome, shaped by negative expectations and attitudes toward menstruation. In fact, in societies in which women are pregnant most of their adult lives, attitudes and expectations toward menstruation are less negative and they do not as easily associate psychological symptoms, such as mood fluctuations, with the coming onset of menstruation.

Where Does the Myth Come From?

The idea that women completely "lose it" once a month has a long history. For example, descriptions of a syndrome affecting the behavior and emotional states of women in the days preceding menstruation date from the time of Hippocrates. However, a more recent history of PMS begins with clinical cases treated by American gynecologist Robert Frank in the early 1930s. He described the intense personal suffering that occurred in a large group of women shortly before menstruation. He used the term *premenstrual tension* to point to a set of symptoms that included extreme restlessness, irritability, and a range of somatic complaints. At around the same time, psychoanalyst Karen Horney publish her own set of symptoms observed in women in a paper entitled "Premenstrual Mood Swings." However, it wasn't until the 1950s that PMS was established as a disorder by British physician Katharina Dalton. Dalton coined the term *premenstrual syndrome*, describing women afflicted by this monthly malady as being more prone to having car accidents and psychiatric illnesses and as not being able to perform adequately at work. She was so convincing at promulgating the existence of the syndrome that in 1980, as an expert witness, she successfully argued for the defense of two women on the grounds that they were not responsible for their crimes due to PMS. One woman was accused of arson, assault, and threatening to kill a police officer. The other was accused of murder.

In fact, PMS started to be recognized as a real disorder in the 1980s. However, it was defined by a range of symptoms so wide that almost anyone could diagnose themselves as having it. The description of symptoms associated with PMS was so vague that between 5% and 97% of women were thought to be afflicted by it. This range is much too wide to be of any scientific value. The wide range and vagueness of symptoms previously attributed to PMS was due to poor research methodology, such as the lack of proper control groups and precise criteria for determining whether a woman had PMS. In addition, most studies included only white, middle-class women, which called into question the generalizability of results.

Why Is the Myth Wrong?

Remember that the myth is that "all" women suffer from PMS. Some percentage of women do suffer from symptoms ascribed to PMS, but the numbers are far lower than originally believed. In 1994, PMS made it into the fourth edition of the American Psychiatric Association's *Diagnostic and Statistical Manual of Mental*

Disorders (*DSM-IV*) under the category of postmenstrual dysmorphic disorder (PMDD).

Proper research methods have significantly tightened the criteria for diagnosing what is now called PMDD. With those criteria in place, the prevalence of PMDD in women ranges between 2% and 5% (Tschudin, Bertea, & Zemp, 2010). For a condition to qualify as a disorder, it has to cause significant distress and impairments in behavioral, psychological, and emotional functioning that have a significant negative impact on one's personal and professional life. This does not mean that 95%–98% of women do not experience symptoms associated with PMDD but that the symptoms experienced by most women are not that debilitating.

Several studies have debunked the idea that women are cognitively impaired during the premenstrual period. For example, no significant differences in mental abilities as measured by the performance of cognitive tasks such as visuospatial ability, verbal ability, and cognitive control were found across the menstrual cycle (Sundstrom Poromaa & Gingnell, 2014).

Culturally driven expectations and beliefs seem to account for the perpetuation of the myth that all women conform to the PMS stereotype. Researchers found that the stronger the belief in the stereotype, the more likely a woman is to recall negative aspects of her last premenstrual period (McFarland, Ross, & DeCourville, 1989). Also, one study found that women who believe that most women have PMS reported significantly worse premenstrual symptoms when asked to think about their last period, compared to women who did not believe that most women have PMS (Marvan & Cortes-Iniestra, 2001). In addition, according to a meta-analysis of 47 studies that examined the link between mood and the menstrual cycle, only 7 studies found an association between mood and the premenstrual phase (Romans, Clarkson, Einstein, Petrovic, & Stewart, 2012). ●

FIGURE 10.18

(a) Skateboarders first performed one easy and one difficult trick 10 times in front of a male experimenter (♂ blue bar left). They were then asked to repeat the tricks in front of the same experimenter for another 10 trials each (♂ orange bar left). The bars show the number of aborted tricks. In front of a male experimenter, the skateboarders aborted the same number of tricks in the second block of trials that they did in the first. However, when the second block of trials was in front of an attractive female experimenter, the skateboarders aborted a significantly lower number of tricks (♀ orange bar right) than when performing in front of a male experimenter (♂ blue bar right). (b) Saliva concentrations of testosterone were significantly higher when the skateboarders performed risky tricks in front of an attractive female than in front of a male.

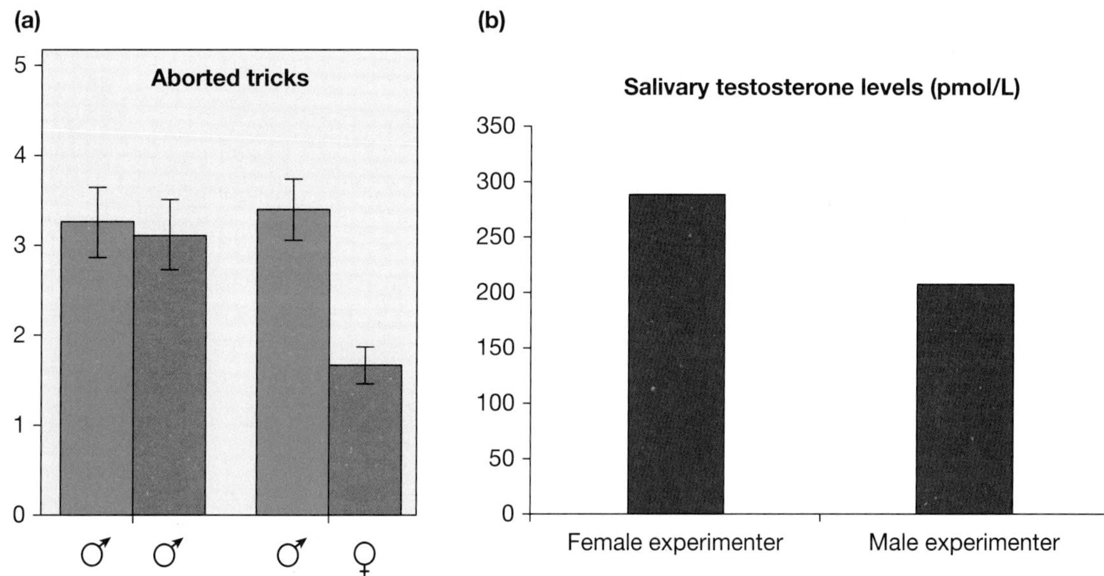

In men, there is evidence that testosterone levels rise during encounters with potential sexual partners (van der Meij, Buunk, van de Sande, & Salvador, 2008). This points to the possibility that testosterone is associated with arousal and the effort exerted to find a mate. Testosterone may also be associated with a male's risk-taking behavior to impress a female. This was demonstrated in a study involving skateboarders (Ronay & von Hippel, 2010). In that study, male skateboarders were asked to choose one easy trick with a low risk of failing and one difficult trick, which they considered to come with a high risk of failure. They were then asked to perform each trick 10 times while being recorded by a male experimenter. They were then asked to do the same but this time in front of an attractive female experimenter. The skateboarders could abort performing a trick if they considered the risk of failure was too high.

The results are shown in Figure 10.18. As the researchers expected, the skateboarders took significantly more risks, as indicated by the lower number of aborted tricks, when they knew they were being observed by a female experimenter than by a male experimenter. The finding of most interest to the researchers was that testosterone levels in the skateboarders were significantly higher when they performed in front of the female experimenter than in front of the male experimenter (Ronay & von Hippel, 2010).

As you learned for rats, dopamine plays a significant role in sexual behavior, and testosterone may facilitate the release of dopamine in the MPOA. Some of the evidence for the role of dopamine in sexual behavior comes from the observation that men treated with the drug L-dopa, a precursor of dopamine used in the treatment of Parkinson's disease, experience an increase in sexual desire (Sidi et al., 2017). In contrast, patients treated with antipsychotic medications, which are dopamine antagonists, experienced a decrease in sexual desire (Meyer, 2008).

MODULE SUMMARY

Social behavior can be defined as behavioral interactions between individuals of the same species that are beneficial to one or more individuals of the species. The hormones mostly associated with social behavior are vasopressin and oxytocin. Social behaviors are driven by a network of brain areas known as the social behavior neural network. Social behaviors include social recognition, pair bonding, and parenting. Social recognition refers to the ability to recognize individuals to determine how to act with them. The hippocampus plays an important role in social recognition. The hippocampus is rich in both vasopressin and oxytocin receptors. Inhibiting those receptors impairs social recognition, whereas activating them facilitates social recognition.

Pair bonding refers to a monogamous relationship between a male and a female of the same species (sometimes between individuals of the same sex) that lead to reproduction and a lifelong bond. Prairie voles have been the animal of choice to study pair bonding in mammals since the 1970s. Some varieties of voles are monogamous, whereas other varieties are nonmonogamous. Vasopressin and oxytocin have been shown to be important for the development of pair bonds in monogamous voles.

Parenting is often defined as a process that promotes and supports the development of offspring through caregiving. Parental behavior is primed by the hormones of pregnancy, estrogen and progesterone. Prolactin and oxytocin, which are associated with lactation, are released after childbirth. In rodents, parental behavior consists of automatic responses to stimuli from the pups, external environmental cues, and internal cues. The medial preoptic area (MPOA) is central to the generation of parental behavior. The MPOA neurons found to be involved in parental care are the ones that release the neuropeptide galanin. These neurons project to brain areas specific to different components of parenting. Human parental care is driven not only by hardwired automatic processes but also through top-down processes. This permits humans to use conscious thought to guide parental behavior.

Reproductive behavior consists of any behavioral pattern that results in sperm and egg coming together to produce offspring. Sexual behavior is a component of reproductive behavior. Much of what we know about the role of hormones in reproductive behavior comes from research in rodents. Except for humans, all female animals can mate only during behavioral estrus. To mate, a female has to be receptive. Receptivity is defined by the multiple actions performed by a female that are necessary for copulation. In most mammals, receptive females display lordosis. Receptivity is coordinated with ovulation by estrogen. The rising levels of estrogen and progesterone activate the lordosis pathway. The drive to copulate involves the activation of the brain's reward pathway. Contrary to females, males have the ability to copulate at any time. Male reproductive behavior in the rat consists of three stages: mounting, intromission, and ejaculation.

The main stimulus for reproductive behavior in male rats is pheromones, released from the receptive female and activating the vomeronasal pathway, which in turn leads to the release of dopamine in the MPOA. Testosterone was shown to facilitate the release of dopamine in the MPOA. Humans are the only species that engage in reproductive behavior for reasons other than procreation. Several researchers studied human sexual behavior. Although women can copulate at any time during the ovarian cycle, research found that they show more sexual desire and are more attractive to males during ovulation. In men, testosterone facilitates the release of dopamine in the MPOA but is also released during encounters with potential sexual partners. Testosterone is also associated with risk-taking behavior, with the goal of impressing females.

TEST YOURSELF

10.2.1 Describe the social behaviors you learned about, and explain the roles of the hormones and brain areas involved in each one.

10.2.2 Describe male and female reproductive behavior in both humans and nonhuman animals. Which hormones and brain areas are involved in each, and what are the commonalities?

10.3 Organizing Effects of Hormones and Sexual Orientation

Module Contents

Learning Objectives

10.3.1 Describe how male and female phenotypes are activated and organized.

10.3.2 Explain the role of hormones in determining sexual orientation.

10.3.1 THE ORGANIZING EFFECTS OF HORMONES

>> LO 10.3.1 Describe how male and female phenotypes are activated and organized.

Key Terms

- **Organizational-activation hypothesis:** The idea that hormones have organizing effects on the brain by acting on neuronal circuits soon after conception and that action on those circuits determines gender-typical sexual behavior.
- **Defeminization:** The loss of the ability of males to display behaviors that are characteristic of females.
- **Sex-determining region Y protein:** A protein made from the instruction of the *SRY* gene located on the Y chromosome that causes the fetus to produce male gonads and inhibits the formation of female gonads.

You have read about how hormones trigger the onset of sexual activity. Hormones have organizing effects on the brain by acting on neuronal circuits soon after conception. Action on those neuronal circuits determines gender-typical sexual behavior. This is known as the **organizational-activation hypothesis** (Phoenix, 2009; Phoenix, Goy, Gerall, & Young, 1959). Early exposure to testosterone gives rise to a male phenotype with all of its behavioral characteristics. At the same time, the ability of males to display behaviors that are characteristic of females is lost. This is known as **defeminization**. In contrast, the female phenotype develops in the absence of the action of hormones or in the presence of low levels of estrogen. That early exposure to testosterone determines sex-specific phenotypes is supported by studies in which castrated males behave like females and females treated with testosterone or its metabolite estradiol behave like males (Phoenix, 2009; Phoenix et al., 1959) (Figure 10.19).

Hormones are not the only factors involved in determining differences in sexual characteristics between males and females. Hormones interact with the expression of genes that are present on the X and Y chromosomes. For example, researchers found that the *SRY* gene located on the Y chromosome provides the instructions to make a protein known as the **sex-determining region Y protein**. It is this protein that causes the fetus to produce male gonads and inhibits the formation of female gonads (Choudhury, Uddin, & Chakraborty, 2018; Waters, Wallis, & Marshall Graves, 2007).

Organizing Effects of Hormones in the Developing Brain

Several differences exist between the brain structures of males and females (Sacher, Neumann, Okon-Singer, Gotowiec, & Villringer, 2013). The most

FIGURE 10.19

Early exposure to testosterone produces a male phenotype (typical male sexual behavior). However, castrated males (CX), which are therefore not exposed to testosterone, develop a female phenotype (typical female sexual behavior). Early exposure to testosterone (+T) or its metabolite estradiol (E_2) produces a male phenotype (typical male sexual behavior). Females not exposed to hormones develop a female phenotype (typical female sexual behavior).

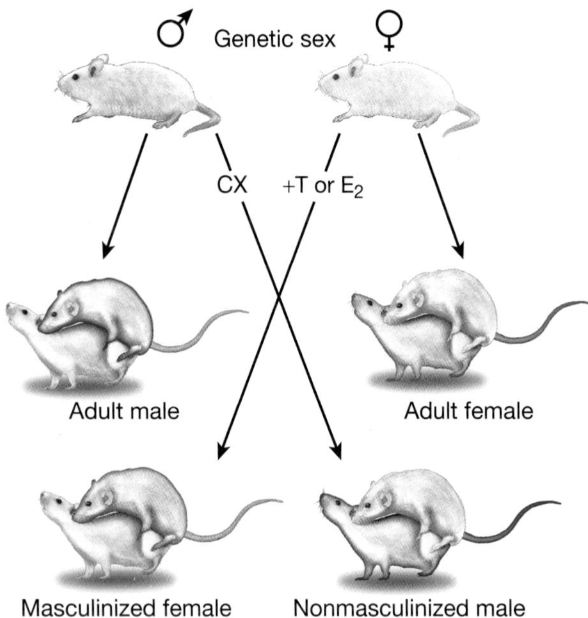

Amanda Tomasikiewicz/Body Scientific Intl.

obvious difference is in the size of the sexually dimorphic nucleus of the preoptic area (SDN-POA) of the hypothalamus, discovered in rats in the 1970s (Gorski, Gordon, Shryne, & Southam, 1978). This difference has also been found in humans (Hofman & Swaab, 1989). The SDN-POA is critically involved in male-typical sexual behavior. In fact, the SDN-POA is three times larger in males than in females. A known reason for this difference is that cells in the SDN-POA of females die from the lack of estradiol stimulation (E. Davis, Popper, & Gorski, 1996). Therefore, this difference in size between the male and female SDN-POA is thought to be due to the action of testosterone. This difference is maintained through adulthood and cannot be reversed.

Another difference in size between brain areas of males and females is that of the interstitial nucleus of the anterior hypothalamic area (INAH), in which one group of cells (INAH-3) is 2.8 times larger in males than in females (L. S. Allen, Hines, Shryne, & Gorski, 1989).

10.3.2 SEXUAL ORIENTATION

>> LO 10.3.2 Explain the role of hormones in determining sexual orientation.

Key Terms

- **Sexual orientation:** The term used to define sexual identity, attraction, and behavior.
- **Congenital adrenal hyperplasia (CAH):** A genetic disorder in which people lack one of the enzymes used by the adrenal glands to produce cortisol and melanocorticoids and have higher than normal levels of testosterone.
- **Fraternal birth order effect:** Derived from the observation that gay men have a greater number of older brothers than heterosexual men.
- **Maternal immune hypothesis (MIH):** A hypothesis aimed at explaining the fraternal birth order effect, which states that some mothers develop an immune response to a specific substance, important for determining sexual orientation, on the Y chromosome of the male fetus.

Sexual orientation is the term used to define sexual identity, attraction, and behavior. However, sexual orientation has been conceptualized in several ways (Wolff, Wells, Ventura-DiPersia, Renson, & Grov, 2017). In a national survey, 86% of women and 92% of men said that they were attracted exclusively to members of the opposite sex (traditionally known as heterosexuality). In the same survey, about 4% of men and 14% of women reported having had at least one same-gender sexual experience (traditionally known as homosexuality) (Chandra, Mosher, Copen, & Sionean, 2011).

This raises the question of what accounts for the development of sexual orientation. Scientists agree that the development of sexual orientation depends on social factors, such as learning, education, and expectation, but that these factors interact with biological differences already present at birth. As you read in the preceding unit, gender-specific sexual behaviors are organized during early life by the presence or absence of testosterone. Knowing this should lead you to ask an obvious question: Is sexual orientation also organized by exposure to steroid hormones early in life? The answer to this question is a resounding yes.

The main line of evidence that supports this idea is that many behavioral, physiological, and morphological traits differ between homosexuals and heterosexuals. These differences have been attributed to homosexuals being exposed to atypical amounts of testosterone during development. For ethical reasons, it is impossible to manipulate hormonal levels in humans in early life to see whether this correlates with heterosexuality or homosexuality later in life. However, conditions in which people have been exposed to abnormal levels of hormones early in life exist. In the sections that follow, we review evidence that the effects of early differences in the exposure to sex hormones are related to sexual orientation.

Differences in Brain Structures

Differences in brain structures between homosexual and heterosexual men have been found. For example, the suprachiasmatic nucleus was found to be 1.7 times larger in homosexual men than in heterosexual men (Swaab & Hofman, 1990). Also, INAH-3, which you read about in the preceding unit, is twice as large in heterosexual men as it is in homosexual men (LeVay, 1991).

Congenital Adrenal Hyperplasia (CAH). **Congenital adrenal hyperplasia (CAH)** is a genetic disorder in which people are deficient in the production of a range of hormones. One of these hormones is melanocorticoid. Melanocorticoid, which regulates sodium and potassium levels, also regulates levels of androgens such as testosterone. Therefore, females with CAH display masculinized genitals and behavior (Bhimji & Sinha, 2018). Women with CAH are less likely to be heterosexual than women in the general population (Hines, 2011; Meyer-Bahlburg, Dolezal, Baker, & New, 2008).

Fraternal Birth Order Effect. Interestingly, birth order is associated with the chances of being homosexual. This is a fact supported by several studies. In the 1990s, sexologist Ray Blanchard and psychologist Anthony Bogaert found that the chances that a male will be gay is related to the number of older brothers he has (Blanchard, 1997; Blanchard & Bogaert, 1996). That is, gay men have a greater number of older brothers than do heterosexual men. This is known as the **fraternal birth order effect**. Each older male sibling increases the chances of being homosexual by 28% to 48%, depending on the study (Blanchard & Bogaert, 1996; Blanchard, Zucker, Siegelman, Dickey, & Klassen, 1998; Ellis & Blanchard, 2001).

What accounts for the fraternal birth order effect? Blanchard and Bogaert (1996) proposed that some mothers develop an immune response to a specific substance on the Y chromosome of the male fetus (only males have a Y chromosome) that is important for determining sexual orientation. The intensity of this response is accentuated with every male pregnancy, such that later-born males are more affected, depending on the number of male siblings that preceded them. This is known as the **maternal immune hypothesis**.

MODULE SUMMARY

The organizational-activation hypothesis is the idea that hormones have organizing effects on the brain soon after conception and that activation of brain circuits by those hormones determines sex-specific traits and behaviors. The male phenotype and all of its behavioral characteristics are determined by testosterone. Testosterone also suppresses the emergence of female characteristics in what is known as defeminization. Hormones interact with the expression of genes on the Y and X chromosomes in determining the differences between males and females. The sex-determining region Y protein causes the fetus to produce male gonads and to inhibit the formation of female gonads. The most obvious difference in brain structures between males and females is the size of the sexually dimorphic nucleus of the preoptic area (SDN-POA) of the hypothalamus. Another notable difference in humans is the size of the interstitial nucleus of the anterior hypothalamic area (INAH).

Sexual orientation is the term used to define sexual identity, attraction, and behavior. Sexual orientation develops via interactions between social factors and biological differences already present at birth. Many behavioral, physiological, and morphological traits differ between homosexuals and heterosexuals. The suprachiasmatic nucleus was found to be 1.7 times larger in homosexual men than in heterosexual men. Women with a genetic disorder called congenital adrenal hyperplasia are less likely to be heterosexual than women in the general population. Also, the chances that a male will be gay are related to the number of older brothers he has. This is known as the fraternal birth order effect.

TEST YOURSELF

10.3.1 (a) Define the organizational-activation hypothesis. (b) What is the most obvious structural difference that was found between males and females and what can account for this difference?

10.3.2 (a) How can hormones account for sexual orientation? (b) Name and describe some of the differences in brain structure that were found between homosexuals and heterosexuals. (c) How can a disorder like congenital adrenal hyperplasia explain some differences of sexual orientation in women? (d) How is fraternal birth order associated with homosexuality in men?

APPLICATIONS

Hormone Replacement Therapy

What Is Hormone Replacement Therapy?

Hormone replacement therapy (HRT) is used to replace hormones that women lose during menopause. Menopause marks the period in a woman's life associated with the cessation of the menstrual cycle and the ability to become pregnant. This is in itself due to the loss of function of the ovaries and the hormones they produce, namely, estrogen. The average age at menopause is 51 years, but it can vary widely between women, with some experiencing it as early as in their 30s and others as late as in their 60s. The symptoms of menopause are wide ranging. They may include vaginal dryness, hot flashes, chills, night sweats, sleep problems, mood changes, weight gain and slowed metabolism, thinning hair and dry skin, and loss of breast fullness. Many women seek to resolve these symptoms by resorting to HRT.

Hormone replacement can be achieved through several different routes of administration. Estrogen may be taken orally or transdermally (through the skin) via creams, patches, or vaginal inserts (Harper-Harrison & Shanahan, 2018).

Prevention of Depressive Symptoms During the Perimenopausal Period

The perimenopausal period is the period of transition to menopause when the ovaries gradually produce less estrogen. The lifetime prevalence of depression in women is 21%. Interestingly, the incidence of depression in woman increases around reproductive events, for example, postpartum depression, which follows childbirth; premenstrual dysphoric disorder (PMDD); and depression that occurs during the transition to menopause. Perimenopausal women have two to four times the risk of depression. What do all of these events have in common? A shift in the balance of the reproductive hormones estrogen and progesterone.

This finding has motivated researchers to explore the possibility that HRT may be used in the prevention of depression in perimenopausal women. In a recent study, 172 women were given transdermal estradiol or micronized progesterone (progesterone taken in pill form) for 12 months (Gordon et al., 2018). The researchers found that 32.3% of women receiving a placebo developed clinically significant symptoms of depression versus only 17.3% of the women receiving treatment.

Not all women experience depressive symptoms during perimenopause. The risk is significantly higher in women who have a history of depression or who have had PMDD. Also, severe depressive symptoms such as those observed in major depressive disorders are better treated with antidepressant medication. HRT may be more appropriate to treat mild symptoms and is not recommended as a first-line treatment. When seeking treatment for perimenopausal depression, women should also consider psychotherapy, which works more gradually than HRT but may have longer lasting benefits (Soares, 2017). ●

FIGURE 10.20

Hormone replacement therapy can be administered through a transdermal patch in combination with capsules of progesterone taken orally.

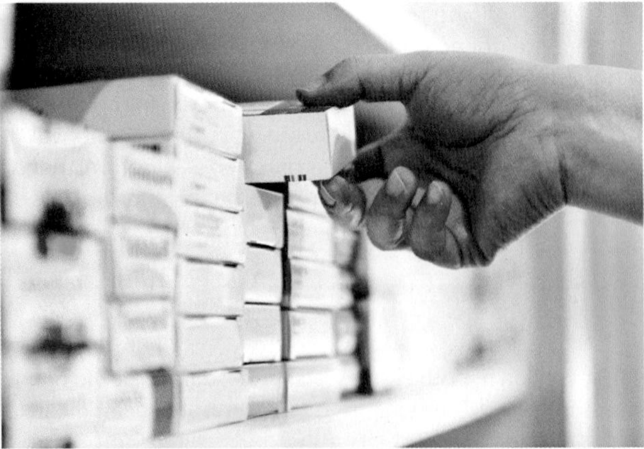

MJ_Prototype/istockphoto

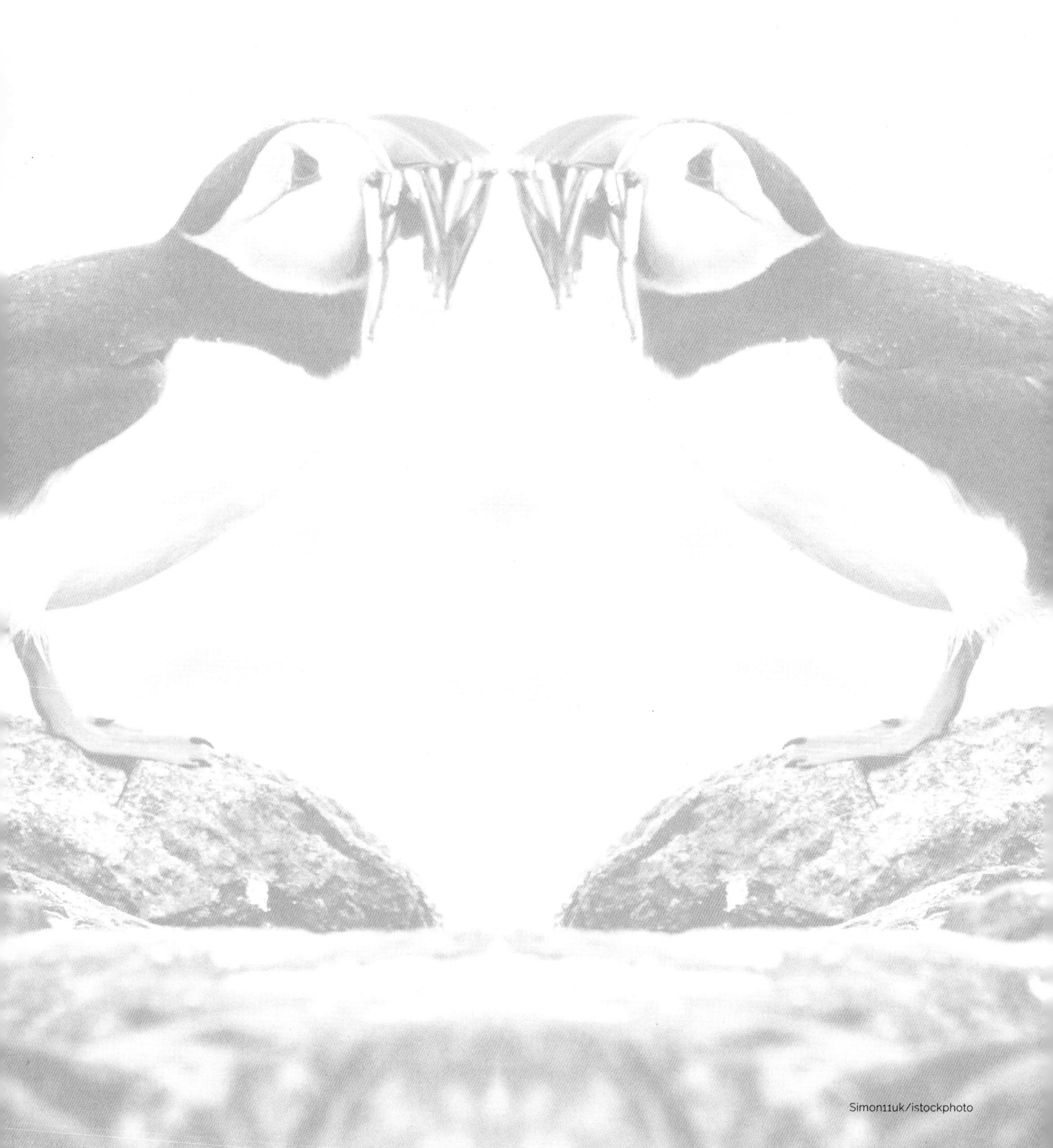

Simon11uk/istockphoto

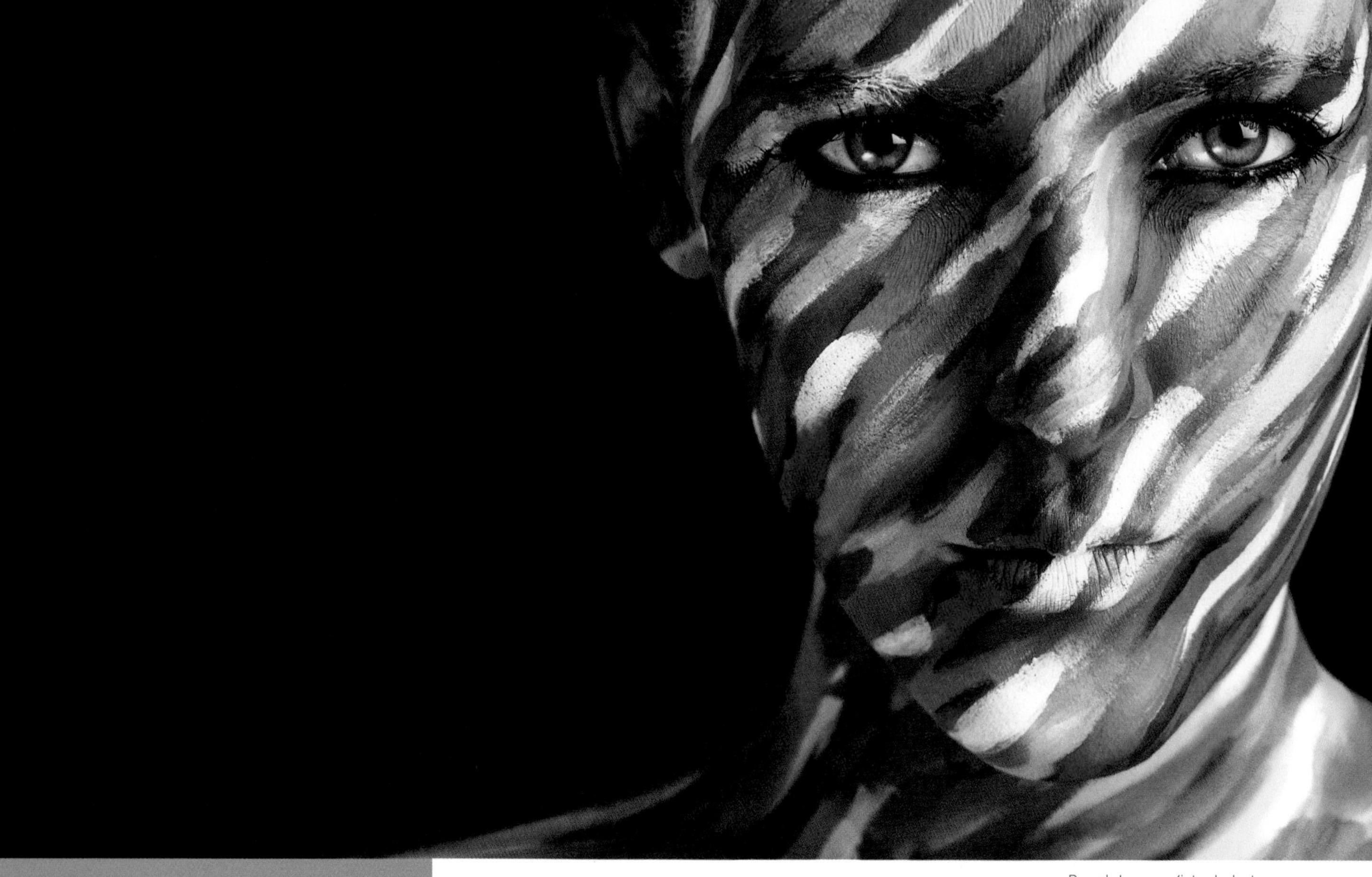

PeopleImages/istockphoto

11 Emotions

Chapter Contents

Learning Objectives

11.1.1 Define emotion, and differentiate between emotional experience and emotional expression.

11.1.2 Describe the theories of emotions.

11.2.1 Identify the networks of brain areas involved in emotions.

11.2.2 Describe how the amygdala is involved in processing emotions.

11.2.3 Explain how the amygdala is involved in the emotions of humans.

11.3.1 Describe some of the functions of the prefrontal cortex in emotions.

11.3.2 Explain the somatic-marker hypothesis.

11.4.1 Define aggression as well as its different types.

11.4.2 Identify some of the neurobiological bases of aggression.

11.4.3 Explain how hormones and neurotransmitters may be involved in aggressive behavior.

Murder, the Brain, and the Law

On July 22, 2011, Anders Breivik cold-bloodedly murdered 77 people in Norway. He killed the first eight with a bomb he exploded just outside a government building in Oslo. He then went on to shoot 69 people where a youth organization was holding an island retreat. This was the worst mass murder in Norwegian history. No one knows exactly what was going on in Breivik's brain at the time of these horrible events.

However, some neuroscientists are hard at work trying to find out what can go wrong in someone's brain to lead to such devastating acts of aggression. One of these neuroscientists is Kent Kiehl from the University of New Mexico in Albuquerque. In 2010, Kiehl sought to explain the acts of convicted murderer Brian Dugan, who killed two people in the 1980s and was sentenced to the death penalty for previous killings.

The results of a psychiatric interview revealed that Dugan fit the profile of a psychopath, which is characterized by the use of manipulation, intimidation, and violence to control others in order to satisfy one's needs. Psychopaths are also capable of impulsive and violent crimes without feeling any remorse or regrets.

In 2010, Kiehl performed a functional magnetic resonance imaging (fMRI) scan of Dugan's brain to find out if it showed abnormalities that would support this profile. Kiehl found abnormalities in areas of Dugan's brain that are involved in regulating emotions (V. Hughes, 2010).

At the request of Dugan's lawyers, Kiehl presented his findings at Dugan's trial, in an effort to provide mitigating circumstances for the crimes. This was the first court case in the world in which fMRI evidence was presented. Kiehl showed the court the abnormalities in Dugan's brain but did not convince the jurors that they explained Dugan's actions. He was sentenced to death. Even though Kiehl's findings didn't exonerate Dugan, the bulk of Kiehl's research and the research of others shows that human aggression can be explained at least in part by brain abnormalities.

INTRODUCTION

The term *emotion* comes from the Latin word *emovere*, which means "to move or to excite." It is not surprising that this term came to signify the feelings associated with the perception of objects or events as being either a threat to one's survival or the source of pleasure and enjoyment. These objects or events are perceived to create "movement" within the body. This perception is made evident in everyday expressions such as when one says, "I was moved by the words of the speaker," "I felt a chill running down my spine," or "That was a stomach-churning experience."

In this chapter, you will learn about what is meant by the term *emotion* and some of the theories proposed to explain how emotions are experienced and expressed, as well as how they are related to the activity of networks of brain areas. You will also learn that, contrary to popular belief, emotions sometimes help us make the right decisions by biasing our choices away from those that can potentially bring us harm or that can be disadvantageous to us. Finally, you will learn about aggression and how it is believed to be generated in the brain through changes in brain chemistry.

11.1 What Are Emotions?

Module Contents

Learning Objectives

11.1.1 Define emotion, and differentiate between emotional experience and emotional expression.

11.1.2 Describe the theories of emotions.

11.1.1 EMOTIONS, EMOTIONAL EXPERIENCE, AND EMOTIONAL EXPRESSION

>> LO 11.1.1 **Define emotion, and differentiate between emotional experience and emotional expression.**

Key Terms

- **Emotion:** An automatic physiological, behavioral, and cognitive reaction to external or internal events.
- **Emotional experience:** Subjective feelings that are labeled to identify particular emotions.
- **Emotional expression:** The covert and overt behaviors that accompany emotions.

An **emotion** can be defined as an automatic physiological, behavioral, and cognitive reaction to an external or internal event (Sternberg, 1998). An emotion is accompanied both by a subjective feeling, which is referred to as the **emotional experience**, as well as by covert and overt behavior, which is referred to as the **emotional expression**. When I ask students to define emotion, I often get answers that resemble the following: "It's a feeling that you get . . . you know, when you feel sad, scared, or angry." When answering in this way, the students are referring to the emotional experience, in other words, the "feeling." *Sad* and *angry* are labels that serve to identify the experience of particular emotions. These labels make sense to us relative to the context in which an emotion occurs. You rarely hear people say that they feel sad or angry at a joyous event like their graduation or joyful at a funeral.

If you asked a friend who just witnessed a horrible accident how she felt when it happened, she would probably tell you: "I got really scared" or "It was frightening." This would define her emotional experience. She may also tell you that she was frozen in fear or that she ran away (Figure 11.1a). The fact that she was afraid was also probably made obvious by her facial expression. What may not have been so obvious was her accelerated heartbeat, increased rate of respiration, dilated pupils, slowed digestion, and increased muscle tension. These behaviors would define her emotional expression. Emotions are experienced in part through our interpretation of those bodily changes based on situational factors and past experiences. That is, the patterns of bodily changes that occur when you are greeted by family and friends at a birthday party (Figure 11.1b) are similar to the ones that occur when you have just received a failing grade on a final exam. In the former case, the interpretation of why those changes are occurring is associated with a joyful event, whereas in the latter case, the interpretation of why the changes are happening is associated with the angering event.

11.1.2 THEORIES OF EMOTIONS

>> LO 11.1.2 **Describe the theories of emotions.**

Key Terms

- **James-Lange theory:** A theory of emotions in which the sensory stimuli that compose certain sensory events directly result in bodily changes and emotions are the brain's interpretation of these changes.
- **Cannon-Bard theory:** A theory of emotions in which physiological arousal and emotional experience can occur at the same time and are independent of each other.
- **Schachter and Singer's two-factor theory:** A theory of emotions in which physiological changes triggered by stimuli are accompanied by an interpretation of what these changes mean.
- **Discrete theories of emotions:** Theories in which a small set of emotions can be distinguished from one another and represented by particular response patterns in the brain, physiological processes, and facial expressions.

FIGURE 11.1

(a) Witnessing an accident can elicit a strong physical reaction. (b) Bodily changes are also be associated with a joyful event such as a birthday party.

(a)

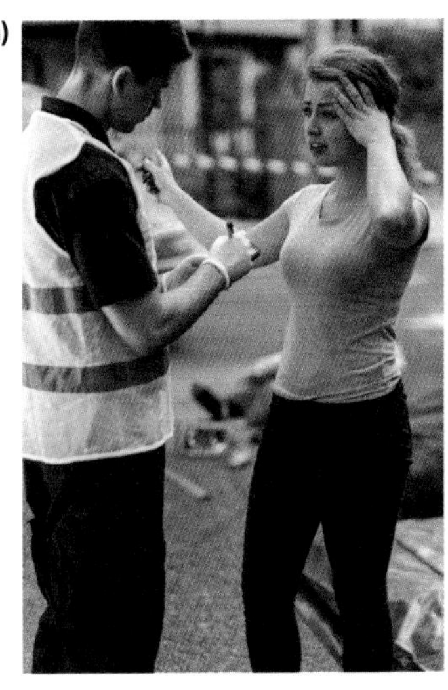

(b)

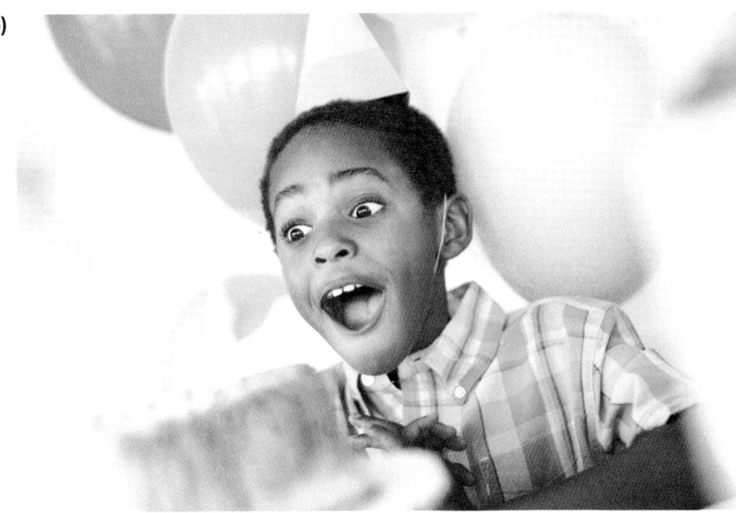

(a) KatarzynaBialasiewicz/istockphoto; (b) GlobalStock/istockphoto

- **Basic emotions:** A subset of discrete emotions thought to be universal across cultures.
- **Dimensional theories of emotions:** Theories in which emotions can be broken down into basic elements and individual differences exist in the way people experience emotions.
- **Theory of constructed emotions:** The theory that emotions are not hardwired entities but emerge into consciousness from interoception and categorization.
- **Categorization:** The process by which signals from the body are labeled using knowledge about emotions, past experiences, and the current situation.

Evolutionary Theory

British naturalist Charles Darwin (1809–1882) thought that emotions were important for the survival of species and that they serve adaptive functions and are universal across cultures (Darwin, 1873). After all, feelings of love and affection compel parents to take care of their children, ensuring their survival. The same feelings also lead people to mate and to produce offspring, ensuring the survival of the species. In contrast, fear and anxiety are important in that they permit us to flee potentially dangerous situations and to avoid them in the future. It is also important to recognize emotions in others so that we can respond appropriately. For example, approaching someone who is displaying obvious expressions of extreme anger might be dangerous.

The James-Lange Theory

In the 1880s, American psychologist William James (1842–1910) and Danish physiologist Carl Lange (1834–1900) independently came up with one of the most articulated theories of emotions. This theory became known as the **James-Lange theory**. According to this theory, the sensory stimuli that compose experiential events are processed by sensory areas of the brain. In response, the brain triggers increased activity in the autonomic and somatic nervous systems, giving rise to an increase in physiological arousal and muscle tension, respectively. According to the James-Lange theory, this process is not accompanied by emotional experience. The emotion arises from the brain's interpretation of these changes (James & Richardson, 2010).

To illustrate, imagine feeling sad and crying while watching an emotional movie. Common sense would tell you that your crying results from feeling sad (Figure 11.2a). However, the James-Lange theory states that the opposite is true. That is, the sensory stimuli within the movie, after being processed by sensory areas of the brain, triggered the physiological arousal that consisted of crying. The emotional experience of feeling sad came from the brain's interpretation of the crying (Figure 11.2b).

The Cannon-Bard Theory

In the early 1920s, American physiologist Walter Cannon (1871–1945) and his student Philip Bard (1898–1977) proposed an alternative to the James-Lange theory, which became known as the **Cannon-Bard theory** (Cannon, 1987). They pointed out that the James-Lange theory could not be correct because the same patterns of physiological responses can be caused by a variety of stimuli. As a result, the theory could not explain how the brain would determine what emotion should be felt in response to the wide range of possible stimuli. Instead, the Cannon-Bard theory proposed that physiological arousal and emotional experience can occur at the same time and that they are independent from each other. According to the Cannon-Bard theory, different stimuli create different patterns of activity in the thalamus. It is these different patterns of activity that give rise to the wide range of emotions that can be experienced (Figure 11.2c).

Schachter and Singer's Two-Factor Theory

In the early 1960s, psychologists Stanley Schachter (1922–1977) and Jerome Singer (1934–2010) proposed what became known as **Schachter and Singer's two-factor theory** (Schachter & Singer, 1962). This theory proposed that sensory events directly trigger physiological arousal and that emotions are differentiated on the basis of a cognitive label applied to these physiological reactions. This cognitive label is consistent with the situational context in which the physiological arousal occurs. It is this combination (physiological arousal + cognitive label) that dictates the type of emotion experienced (Figure 11.2d).

To illustrate this theory, imagine hearing the fire alarm going off in your school. This would likely trigger the emotional experience of fear, which would accompany significant levels of physiological arousal. However, if you interpreted the alarm as being part of a fire drill (the cognitive label), your fear would soon subside. In contrast, if you smelled smoke or saw students running in the corridor, you would likely interpret the situation as involving real danger, accentuating your fear.

FIGURE 11.2

Three theories of emotions: James-Lange, Cannon-Bard, and Schachter-Singer.

(a) Common sense

"I tremble because I feel afraid"

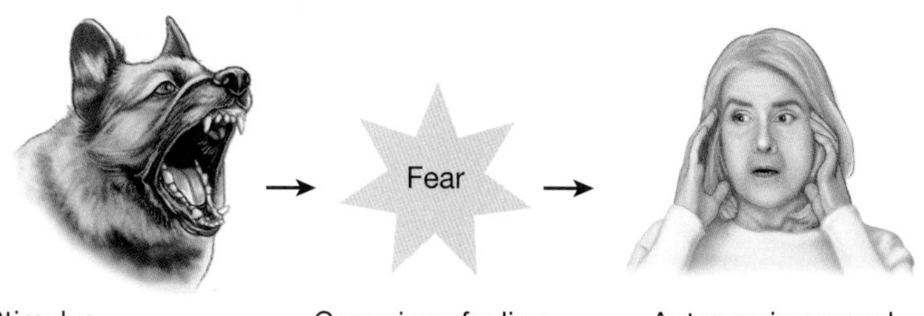

(b) James-Lange

"I feel afraid because I tremble"

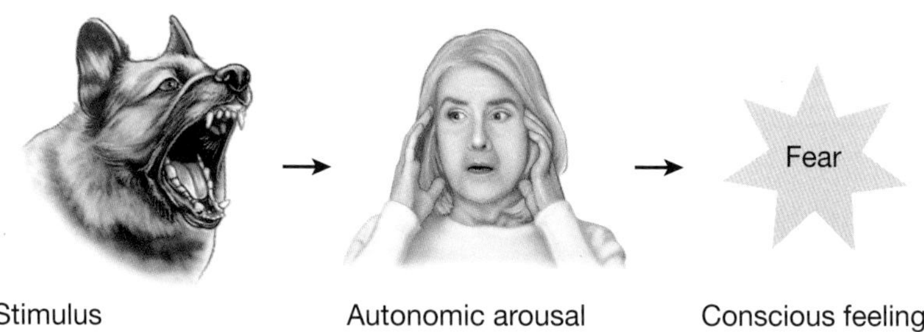

(c) Cannon-Bard

"The dog makes me tremble and feel afraid"

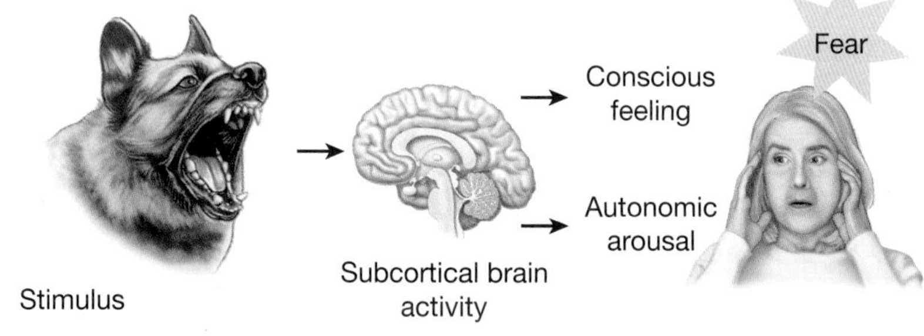

(d) Schachter-Singer

"I label my trembling as fear because I appraise the situation as dangerous"

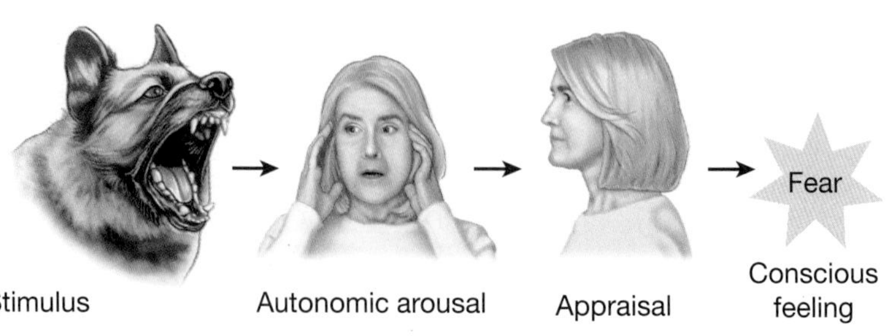

Amanda Tomasikiewicz/Body Scientific Intl.

Emotions Are Induced Partly by Patterns of Bodily Change

Remember that Cannon and Bard's criticism of the James-Lange theory was that emotions could not be differentiated by patterns of emotional arousal. In the Schacter-Singer theory, the experienced emotion depends on the cognitive label applied to the physiological arousal. However, researchers have found more recently that emotions can be differentiated by the patterns of bodily changes to which they give rise. For example, in one study (Nummenmaa, Glerean, Hari, & Hietanen, 2014), participants were exposed to words, movies, and stories meant to arouse emotions. The same participants were also shown blank silhouettes on which they were asked to color in the parts of the body where they experienced increased activity when exposed to the stimuli. The results of the study are shown in Figure 11.3. The stimuli triggered a variety of emotions in the participants. Each of these emotions was accompanied by different patterns of bodily responses. Warmer colors that pull toward red show areas in which participants experienced increased activity, whereas colors that pull toward blue show areas in which participants reported experiencing low levels of activity.

Discrete and Dimensional Theories of Emotions

Discrete Theories. **Discrete theories of emotions** propose that a small set of emotions exist that can be distinguished from one another. Each of these emotions is believed to be represented by particular response patterns in the brain, physiological processes, and facial expressions. According to psychologist Paul Ekman, a subset of discrete emotions, which became known as **basic emotions**, are universal across cultures, evolved through adaptions to the environment, and are shaped by social learning (Ekman, 1982, 1992; Tomkins, 2008). It is also believed that the universality of basic emotions arose in response to common human

FIGURE 11.3

Areas of the body in which participants reported activity in response to the emotions they felt when exposed to emotional words, movies, or stories.

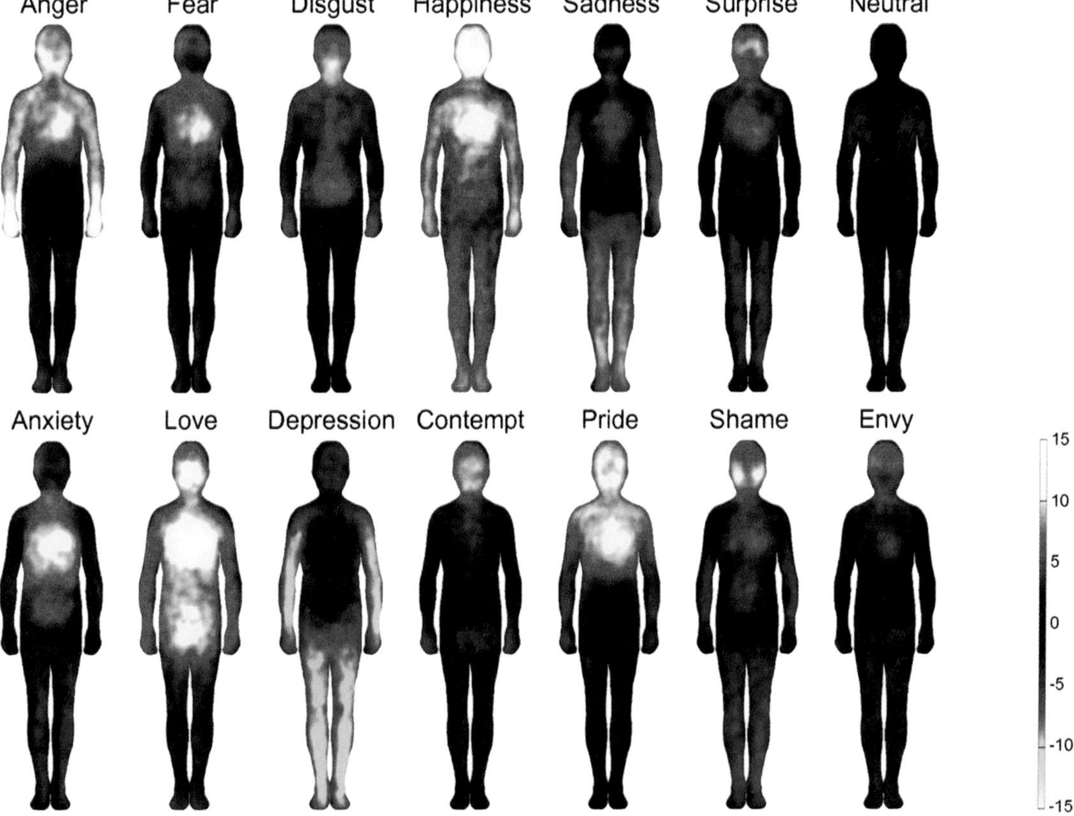

From Nummenmaa, L. et al. (2014). Bodily maps of emotions. *Proceedings of the National Academy of Sciences U S A, 111*(2): 646–651. With permission from The National Academy of Sciences.

experiences such as losses, frustrations, and successes (Ekman & Cordaro, 2011).

Originally, the proposed basic emotions were anger, fear, disgust, happiness, sadness, and surprise. The choice of these emotions was prompted by Ekman's discovery that each of these basic emotions was associated with particular facial expressions, which could be recognized across cultures (Ekman, 1982). The list of basic emotions has since grown to 22 (Cordaro et al., 2018).

Dimensional Theories. **Dimensional theories of emotions** were born out of the perceived lack of psychophysiological evidence that emotions can be grouped in discrete categories (Barrett, 2006a; Lindquist, Siegel, Quigley, & Barrett, 2013). In contrast to discrete theories, the proponents of dimensional theories argue that emotions do not fit neatly into categories. They believe that emotions can be broken down into basic elements and that individual differences exist in the way people experience emotions (L. A. Feldman, 1995).

These basic elements include the (1) emotional valence, which is the perception of whether an emotion is pleasant (positive) or unpleasant (negative); (2) arousal, which refers to how strongly an emotion is felt; (3) potency, which refers to feelings of power or weakness; and (4) unpredictability, which is an appraisal of novelty (Fontaine, Scherer, Roesch, & Ellsworth, 2007). Figure 11.4 shows how Ekman's original basic emotions, triggered by various stimuli, can be represented along the dimensions of valence and arousal.

The Theory of Constructed Emotions

The **theory of constructed emotions**, which is a type of dimensional theory proposed by psychologist Lisa Feldman Barrett (2006b), states that emotions are not hardwired entities but emerge into consciousness by the way of interoception and categorization. Interoception refers to the process by which the brain senses and integrates signals from the body. **Categorization** refers to the process by which a person gives meaning to these signals using knowledge about emotions, past experiences, and the current situation.

According to the theory of constructed emotions, emotional experiences arise from a process analogous to that of color perception. That is, people perceive colors as discrete entities such as blue, green, red, etc. However, out in the world, all that exist, relating to color perception, are wavelengths along the electromagnetic spectrum (see Chapter 6). The perception of color is the result of the brain's analysis of the pattern

FIGURE 11.4

Basic emotions triggered by various stimuli are represented along the dimensions of valence and arousal. For example, a smiling baby (top right) triggers happiness, which can be construed as an emotion made up of high levels of positive valence and moderately high levels of arousal. In contrast, a funeral is associated with high negative valence and moderately low levels of arousal.

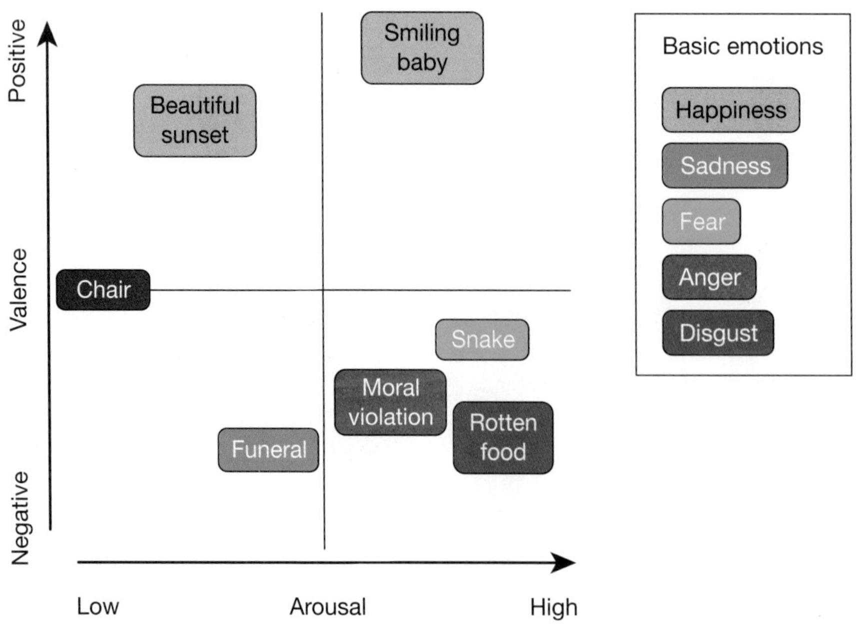

Hamann, S. (2012). Mapping discrete and dimensional emotions onto the brain: controversies and consensus. *Trends in Cognitive Science 16*(9): 458–66. With permission from Elsevier.

of excitation of photoreceptors on the retina, in the same way that emotional experiences result from the brain's analysis of signals from the body, the current situation, and personal experiences.

MODULE SUMMARY

An emotion can be defined as an automatic physiological, behavioral, and cognitive reaction to an external or internal event. Several theories of emotion exist. These include the James-Lange theory, in which the emotional expression precedes emotional experience; the Cannon-Bard theory, in which the emotional experience and physiological arousal occur at the same time; and the Schacter-Singer two-factor theory, in which a cognitive label is applied to physiological arousal. Different emotions give rise to particular patterns of bodily sensations. Emotions can be thought of as discrete entities or as being continuous along different dimensions. A popular idea, based on the idea that emotions are discrete entities, is that humans possess a number of basic emotions, which are inborn and universal across cultures. Proponents of dimensional theories believe that emotions can be categorized along different dimensions, such as their valence and the amount of physiological arousal with which they are associated. The theory of constructed emotions suggests that emotions are made from interoception, which is the perception and integration of bodily signals, and categorization, a process by which bodily sensations are given meaning, based on knowledge about emotions, past experiences, and the current situation.

TEST YOURSELF

11.1.1 Define emotion, and differentiate between emotional experience and emotional expression.

11.1.2 Name and define the different theories of emotions. Discuss the differences between discrete and dimensional theories of emotions.

11.2 Emotions: Where in the Brain?

Module Contents

11.2.1 Emotional Networks in the Brain

11.2.2 Emotions and the Amygdala

11.2.3 Emotions and the Amygdala in Humans

Learning Objectives

11.2.1 Identify the networks of brain areas involved in emotions.

11.2.2 Describe how the amygdala is involved in processing emotions.

11.2.3 Explain how the amygdala is involved in the emotions of humans.

11.2.1 EMOTIONAL NETWORKS IN THE BRAIN

>> LO 11.2.1 **Identify the networks of brain areas involved in emotions.**

Key Terms

- **Papez circuit:** The circuit of brain areas once thought to be dedicated to processing emotions.
- **Limbic system:** A revised version of the Papez circuit that includes the amygdala, septum, and prefrontal cortex.

The Papez Circuit

American neuroanatomist James Papez (1883–1958) believed that a system dedicated to processing emotions existed in the brain. This system became known as the **Papez circuit** (Papez, 1995). Within this circuit, the hypothalamus is responsible for the behavioral responses that are part of emotional expression. Emotional experience is thought to be produced by the cingulate cortex. The hypothalamus and the cingulate cortex are linked to each other through a loop that

FIGURE 11.5

The limbic system.

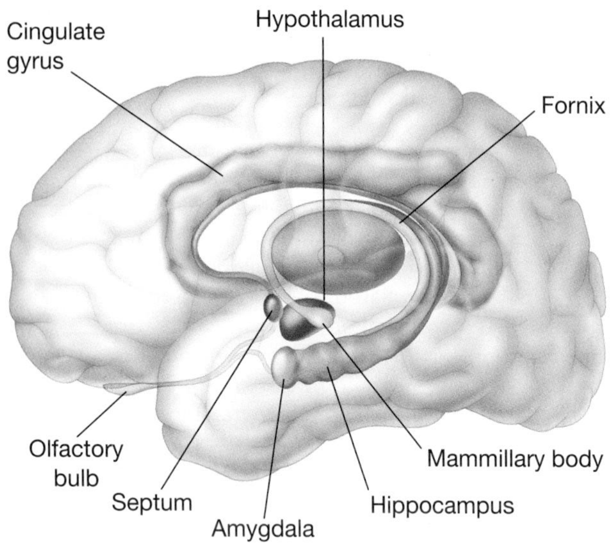

Carolina Hrejsa/Body Scientific Intl.

includes the hippocampus and the anterior thalamic nuclei. This arrangement suggested a way in which emotional expression and emotional experience could be integrated.

Another psychologist, Paul McLean (1913–2007), later added the amygdala, septum, and prefrontal cortex to the list of structures proposed by Papez. He named the set of structures involved in emotional processing the **limbic system** (Rajmohan & Mohandas, 2007), illustrated in Figure 11.5. Over the years, the idea that emotions are regulated by a single system in the brain was abandoned. We now know that emotions are processed in several networks of brain areas.

You learned in the preceding unit that discrete theories of emotion suggest that emotions are discrete entities that can be distinguished by particular patterns of brain activity, physiological processes, and facial expressions. Evidence that discrete emotions can be distinguished by patterns of brain activity can be found in a meta-analysis performed by psychologists Katherine Vytal and Stephan Hamann (2010). They included in their analysis studies in which five of the proposed basic emotions (happiness, sadness, anger, fear, and disgust) were induced by presenting participants with emotionally arousing stimuli such as emotional pictures or emotional facial expressions while their brains were being scanned by either fMRI or positron emission tomography (PET).

The results of their analysis are shown in Figure 11.6. They found that happiness was associated mainly with activity in the right superior temporal gyrus, sadness was associated mostly with activity in the left medial frontal gyrus, anger was associated mainly with activity in the left inferior frontal gyrus, fear was associated mostly with activity in the left amygdala, and disgust

FIGURE 11.6

Patterns of activity associated with five of the proposed basic emotions.

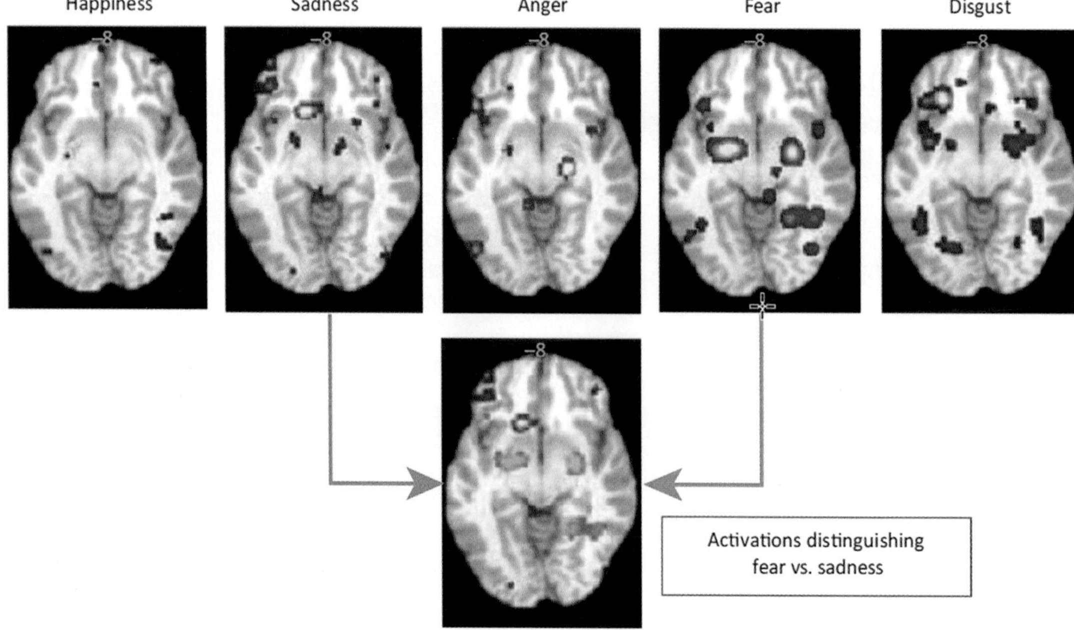

Hamann, S. (2012). Mapping discrete and dimensional emotions onto the brain: controversies and consensus. *Trends in Cognitive Science 16*(9): 458–66. With permission from Elsevier.

was associated mostly with activity in the right insula and inferior frontal gyrus. Also shown in Figure 11.6 (bottom) are the patterns of activation that distinguish fear from sadness. Areas in blue indicate areas of activity that are more likely to be activated for fear than for sadness, that is, areas clustered around the amygdala. Areas in red are areas that are less likely to be activated for sadness than for fear.

Although each emotion seems to be associated with activity located mostly in a single brain area, many researchers believe that emotions are not likely to be dependent on any single area but on functional networks consisting of several areas (Barrett & Satpute, 2013). In fact, a close look at Vytal and Hamann's (2010) results, shown in Figure 11.6, revealed that the same brain areas were activated for more than one emotion. This has led some observers to interpret the results as being consistent with the theory of constructed emotions (described in the preceding unit), according to which emotions are constructed from basic

FIGURE 11.7

Results of a logistic regression that shows the odds that an emotional experience, expression, or component of an emotion, such as arousal level and perception, could predict activity in a brain area of interest. The rectangles contain the names of brain areas (amygdala, insula, dorsolateral prefrontal cortex [DLPFC], anterior temporal lobe [ATL], ventrolateral prefrontal cortex [VLPFC], dorsomedial prefrontal cortex [DMPFC], anterior medial cingulate cortex [aMCC], subgenual anterior cingulate cortex [sACC], and orbitofrontal cortex [OFC]). The blue lines represent the left hemisphere and the green lines represent the right hemisphere. Different emotions and components of emotions are written across the rings. The percentages represent the odds that an emotion or a component of emotions would trigger activity in a given brain area (lines going toward the periphery) or that it would not trigger activity in a given brain area (lines going toward the center). Points above zero represented odds of 100% that an area would be activated, whereas points below zero represented odds of 100% that an area would not be activated (see text for examples).

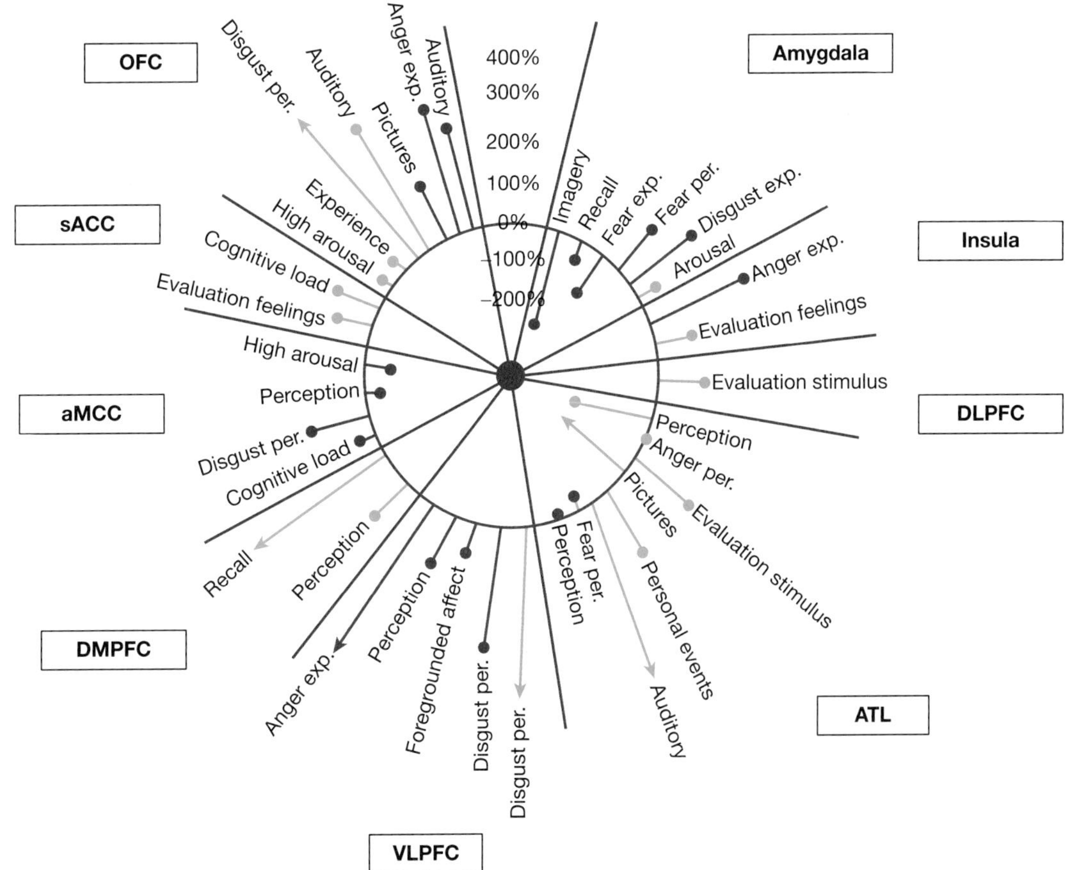

Lindquist, K. A., et al. (2012). The brain basis of emotion: a meta-analytic review. *Behavioral and Brain Sciences 35*(3): 121–143. With permission from Cambridge University Press.

components, which could be represented by each of the areas activated during an emotion (Kober et al., 2008).

Remember, from the preceding unit, that the theory of constructed emotions proposes that emotions consist of signals such as valence and arousal and a categorization process. The categorization process gives meaning to the signals using knowledge about emotions, past experiences, and the current situation. Support for the theory of constructed emotions comes from studies in which the contribution of several brain areas to a range of emotions was assessed (Barrett, Mesquita, Ochsner, & Gross, 2007; Kober et al., 2008). In a meta-analysis, a method that compiles the results of many studies (Lindquist, Wager, Kober, Bliss-Moreau, & Barrett, 2012), it was hypothesized that, contrary to what would be predicted by a basic emotions approach, the same brain areas could be activated across a range of components that comprise different emotions. This is exactly what was found. Lindquist and colleagues (2012) obtained their results by using a statistical procedure known as logistic regression. This procedure permitted the researchers to measure the probability that a particular emotion or component of an emotion would predict activity in a given brain area.

The results of the study are shown in Figure 11.7. The rectangles surrounding the figure contain the names of brain areas. The blue lines represent the left hemisphere and the red lines represent the right hemisphere. Different emotions and components of emotions are written across the rings. The percentages represent the odds that an emotion or a component of emotions would trigger activity in a given brain area. Any value above zero meant that the odds that an emotion or a component of emotions would trigger activity in the corresponding brain were 100%. Any value below zero meant that the odds that activity in a given brain area would *not* be triggered by an emotion or a component of emotions were 100%.

For example, by looking at the colored lines that project outward from zero toward the periphery, the odds that the experience of anger predicted activity in the left orbital frontal cortex (OFC), left insula, and left ventrolateral prefrontal cortex (VLPFC) were 100%. You can also see that the odds that the evaluation of feelings predicted activity in the right insula and that the evaluation of stimuli predicted activity in the right dorsolateral prefrontal cortex (DLPFC) were also 100%. In contrast, by looking at the lines that project from zero toward the middle, you can see that the odds that pictures and perception would *not* trigger activity in the right anterior temporal lobe (ATL) were 100%.

11.2.2 EMOTIONS AND THE AMYGDALA

>> LO 11.2.2 Describe how the amygdala is involved in processing emotions.

Key Terms

- **Klüver-Bucy syndrome:** A set of symptoms, including a loss of fear and flattened emotions, that follow the removal of the temporal lobes.
- **Fear conditioning:** A procedure in which animals (typically rats) are exposed to a mild foot shock simultaneously to hearing a tone, resulting in the conditioning of a fear response.
- **Direct pathway (to the amygdala):** Also known as the low road and "quick and dirty road"; brings sensory information from the thalamus directly to the amygdala.
- **Indirect pathway (to the amygdala):** Also known as the high road and "slow but accurate road"; brings sensory information from the thalamus indirectly through the cortex.

In the late 1930s, psychologist Heinrich Klüver (1897–1979) and neurosurgeon Paul Bucy (1904–1992) surgically removed the temporal lobes of monkeys in their investigation to discover how mescaline produced its hallucinogenic effects. The surgeries included the removal of the hippocampus and amygdala. Independently of whether the monkeys received mescaline, Klüver and Bucy observed that the monkeys subjected to the removals engaged in strange behaviors. For example, they could no longer recognize objects by sight (psychic blindness), had persistent visual responses to objects (hypermetamorphosis), had a tendency to explore objects with their mouths (oral tendencies), and showed an increase in sexual behavior. In addition, the monkeys, which usually acted quite wildly, became tame and fearless and had flattened emotions. This set of symptoms that followed temporal lobe removal became known as the **Klüver-Bucy syndrome** (Lanska, 2018). A particular aspect of the brain damage sustained by the monkeys could explain each of these symptoms. Later it was suggested that the effect on the monkeys' emotions was due to damage to the amygdala.

As shown in Figure 11.5, the amygdala is buried deep within the medial temporal lobes. Much of what we know about the role of the amygdala and emotions comes from studies involving a procedure known as **fear conditioning** (Maren, 2001). In this procedure, animals (typically rats) are exposed to a mild foot shock simultaneously to hearing a tone (Figure 11.8a, middle). This results in the tone becoming a conditioned stimulus (CS) that predicts the delivery of the shock, an unconditioned stimulus (US). Subsequently, the tone causes the rats to freeze in place, a conditioned response (CR) when they hear the tone (Figure 11.8a, left). This reaction is taken to be a display of fear. You may have guessed that we learn about potentially threatening stimuli in our environment in essentially the same way. For example, objects, places, situations, and people can all be conditioned to aversive events to

FIGURE 11.8

(a) Top: The fear conditioning procedure. Bottom: Blood pressure measurements and the percentage of time the rats spent freezing at each stage of the procedure. (b) Example of how an aversive stimulus triggers activity along two pathways that each end up stimulating the amygdala. Along one pathway, the direct pathway, the thalamus connects directly with the amygdala. Along the other pathway, the indirect pathway, sensory information is routed to the amygdala through the cortex. (c) The amygdala is subdivided into several nuclei. The input to the amygdala is through the lateral nucleus. Its outputs, which give rise to responses associated with fear, are through the central nucleus. Also shown are the direct and indirect routes.

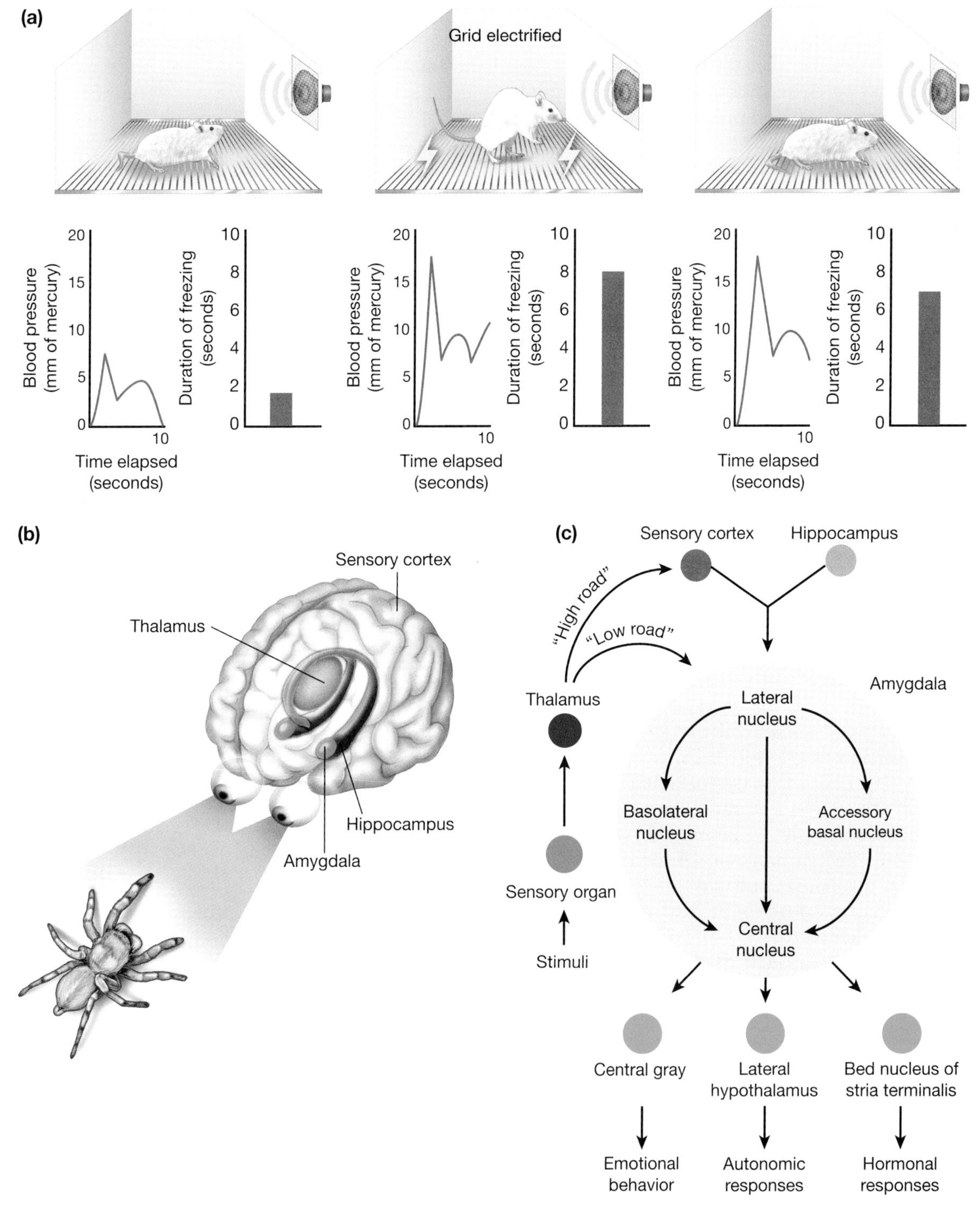

Amanda Tomasikiewicz/Body Scientific Intl.

create a fear response. For example, one may feel fear while stepping back into a place where something horrible was experienced. Conditioned fears can also be expressed in exaggerated ways, resulting in psychological disorders such as phobias and posttraumatic stress disorder (both discussed in Chapter 14).

Graphs that show changes in blood pressure as well as the duration of freezing at each phase of fear conditioning are also shown in Figure 11.8. You can see that before conditioning (left), with presentation of only the tone, a small rise in blood pressure is observed and the percentage of time the rat spends freezing is minimal. However, when the rat receives a shock, its blood pressure rises significantly, and it spends a significantly greater percentage of time freezing (middle). Subsequently, the rat's blood pressure and percentage of time spent freezing when hearing the tone by itself (without the shock) are equal to when the rat received the shock.

Evidence for the importance of the amygdala in this type of fear learning comes from studies in which rats with lesions of the amygdala failed to show a conditioned fear response to a tone after it was paired with a shock (Kim & Jung, 2006). The amygdala is subdivided into several areas that consist of particular cell nuclei. These include the lateral nucleus, the accessory basal nucleus, the central nucleus, and the basolateral nucleus. Sensory information from the thalamus is relayed to the lateral nucleus. The lateral nucleus sends projections to the central nucleus, both directly and by way of the accessory basal and basolateral nuclei. Activation of the central nucleus leads to emotional responses such as freezing, increased autonomic system activity, and the release of cortisol through the central nucleus's connections with the central gray matter, lateral hypothalamus, and basal nucleus of the stria terminalis, respectively (Figure 11.8c).

Sensory information that represents a potentially dangerous stimulus, such as the sight of a scorpion (Figure 11.8b), triggers activity in the amygdala, which results in the behavioral and physiological activation just described. Sensory information makes it to the amygdala along two pathways (LeDoux, 1996, 2002). Along one pathway, sensory information about a potentially dangerous stimulus is sent first to the thalamus. From the thalamus, information about the stimulus flows directly to the amygdala. This is known as the **direct pathway**, also referred to as the low road. Along the other pathway, information about the stimulus also flows to the thalamus but is directed toward the cortex before arriving in the amygdala. This is known as the **indirect pathway**, also referred to as the high road (Figure 11.8c). Note the involvement of the hippocampus as part of the indirect pathway. The hippocampus is thought to further process the information along the indirect pathway by analyzing whether the information matches anything stored in memory so that a proper response can be prepared. For example, this could mean remembering how to deal with the danger or drawing on past experiences to determine that the stimulus is not a threat after all.

Information in the direct pathway gives rise to a quick and reflexive response to potential threats. However, because information along this pathway is not analyzed by the cortex, the direct pathway cannot discriminate between a real threat (a snake) and an innocuous situation (a branch sticking out of the ground). Nevertheless, this response is adaptive. It has tremendous survival value as it permits one to get out of danger quickly.

Whether activation of the amygdala was really worth it is assessed moments later along the indirect route, in which information is sent to the sensory cortices where it is analyzed and discriminated. The outcome

FIGURE 11.9

The low road along which sensory information is processed by the thalamus and sent directly to the amygdala. The low road is the direct pathway, also known as the "quick and dirty road." Along the high road, information is sent from the sensory thalamus to the amygdala only after having been processed by the cortex. The high road, which is the indirect pathway, is also known as the "slow but accurate road."

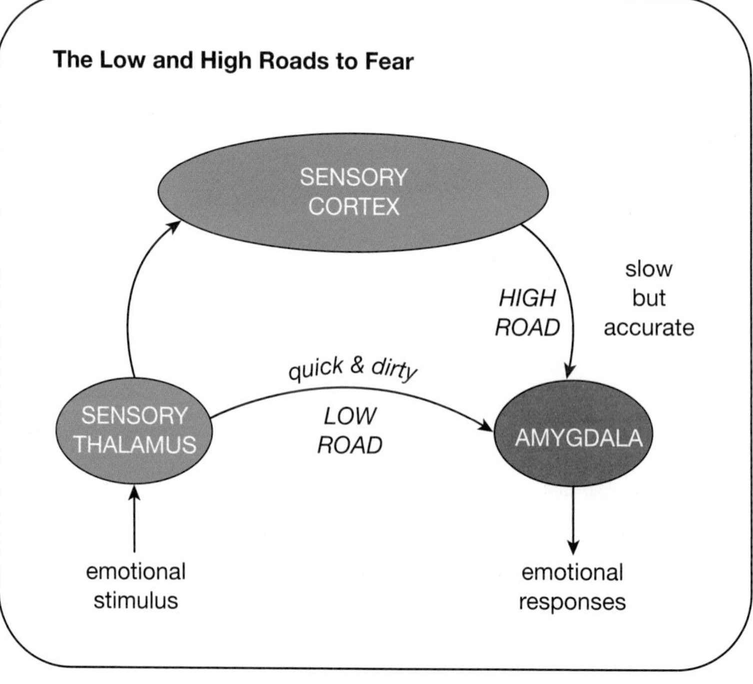

Adapted from *The Emotional Brain: The Mysterious Underpinnings of Emotional Life*. LeDoux, J. E. Simon & Schuster, 1996.

of this analysis is then transmitted to the amygdala. If a stimulus indeed presents a danger, the amygdala's response is accentuated. If it does not present a danger, the amygdala's response is attenuated.

In the 1980s, psychologist Joseph LeDoux demonstrated how the direct pathway triggers emotional reactions, independent from the conscious analysis that takes place along the indirect pathway. To do this, LeDoux and colleagues subjected rats, rendered deaf by lesions of the auditory cortex, to the fear conditioning procedure described previously. The deaf rats responded to the tone in the same way as normal rats (LeDoux, Sakaguchi, & Reis, 1984).

How can fear be conditioned to a tone in deaf rats? As shown in Figure 11.9, along the direct pathway information flows from the thalamus directly to the amygdala. In the indirect pathway, sensory information flows to the amygdala by way of the cortex. However, stimulation of both of these pathways ends up in the outputs from the central amygdala, which through its connections gives rise to emotional behaviors, activation of the autonomic nervous system, and the release of cortisol. Since lesions of the auditory cortex do not interfere with the direct pathway, the stimulus itself triggers a response in the amygdala by way of the thalamus. Because information along the direct pathway (low road) quickly reaches the amygdala but is not discriminated by processing in the cortex, it has been dubbed the "quick and dirty road." In contrast, information along the indirect pathway (high road) is slower to get to the amygdala, but stimuli can be discriminated. For this reason, it has been dubbed the "slow but accurate road."

IT'S A MYTH!

The Amygdala Is Dedicated to Fear

The Myth

It happens all the time. Ask someone what part of the brain he or she believes is dedicated to fear, and the reply will be "the amygdala." This is the answer you will get from many laypeople, psychology students, and experts alike.

Where Does the Myth Come From?

A major source of the myth is another myth, that of the triune brain proposed by neuroscientist Paul MacLean in the 1960s (Figure 1). In his book *The Triune Brain in Evolution*, McLean (1990) divided the brain into the reptilian complex (reptilian brain), the paleomammalian complex (mammalian brain), and the neomammalian complex (the neocortex). According to McLean, these structures have developed sequentially in the course of evolution, a proposal that most evolutionary biologists have rejected. McLean believed that the reptilian brain, which consists of regions within the basal ganglia, was responsible for species-typical and instinctual behavior. McLean believed that behavior of birds and reptiles was under the strict control of the reptilian brain and that the other two complexes were subservient to it. The mammalian brain consists of the limbic system, which includes the septum, amygdala, hypothalamus, hippocampal, and cingulate cortex, which he believed was responsible for processing emotions. Finally, the crowning achievement of humans was the development of the neocortex, which consists of the cerebral cortex, which he believed was responsible for language, perception, and the ability to plan for the future.

FIGURE 1

The triune brain.

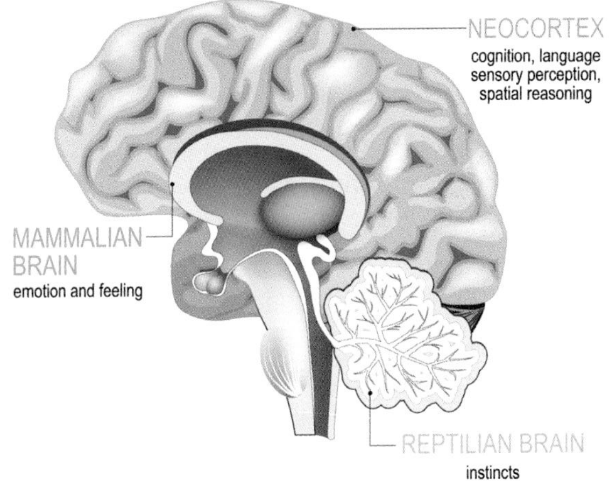

iStock.com/ttsz

Also propagating the myth were early studies in which monkeys with damage to the amygdala had drastically flattened emotions and failed to display typical fear responses when in the presence of potentially dangerous stimuli, such as snakes (Lanska, 2018). The myth was perpetuated further by the enormous number of studies that investigated the amygdala's role in processing aversive stimuli, such as shock avoidance

(Continued)

(Continued)

and fear conditioning (Maren, 2001). The results of human case studies in which impaired emotional processing was found after damage to the amygdala also propagated the idea that the amygdala is dedicated to processing fear. The most popular of such case studies is that of patient SM, who suffered damage to the amygdala due to Urbach-Wiethe disease (Tranel et al., 2006). The popular media have also contributed to the propagation of this myth. For example, a quick Internet search done by entering the terms "SM" and "fear" returns links to newspapers, magazines, and television documentary websites, practically all of which emphasize the amygdala's role in fear (Sanders, 2010; Yong, 2010).

Why Is the Myth Wrong?

There is no doubt that the amygdala plays an important role in the expression of fear. However, the amygdala is also important in processing pleasant emotional information. In fact, some neurons in the amygdala are involved in learned fears as other neurons mediate learning about rewards (Janak & Tye, 2015) or learning about cues that are predictive of reward (Watanabe, Sakagami, & Haruno, 2013). The amygdala is also important for evaluating rewards and for directing attention to potentially important events in the environment (Holland & Gallagher, 1999). Overall, focusing on the myth of the amygdala as the fear brain area obscures its extremely important role in general survival. In fact, the amygdala responds to environmental stimuli to coordinate the corresponding behavioral, autonomic, and hormonal responses. These include those necessary for feeding, fighting, mating, maternal care, and responding to environmental stressors (Kandel, 2013). ●

11.2.3 EMOTIONS AND THE AMYGDALA IN HUMANS

>> LO 11.2.3 Explain how the amygdala is involved in the emotions of humans.

Key Terms

- **Urbach-Wiethe disease:** A disease that causes the temporal lobes to degenerate because of a calcium build-up in the brain.
- **Subliminal stimuli:** Stimuli that are not consciously perceived but that can nevertheless influence behavior.
- **Implicit racial prejudice:** Prejudice shown in people who do not endorse any form of prejudice toward other groups but who demonstrate a negative bias on evaluation.

Unlike with animals, it is not possible, for obvious ethical reasons, to purposefully damage the amygdala in humans so that they can be put through fear conditioning. However, neuroscientists can study cases in which patients with a damaged amygdala respond to situations designed to induce fear. One such case is that of a patient known as SM (Tranel et al., 2006). SM suffers from **Urbach-Wiethe disease**, which causes the temporal lobes to degenerate because of a calcium build-up in the brain. The disease has disintegrated SM's amygdala on both sides of the brain. The study of SM revealed that she cannot be conditioned to fear stimuli and shows a remarkable absence of fear when exposed to a variety of stimuli that usually provoke fear in other people, such as snakes, spiders, and visiting supposedly haunted houses (Feinstein, Adolphs, Damasio, & Tranel, 2011). Interestingly, SM is also unable to recognize emotional facial expressions, especially fearful ones. In fact, when SM was asked to draw facial expressions of different emotions, she did so without difficulty with the exception of drawing a face expressing fear. She said she did not know what a fearful expression looked like (Aggleton, 1992). Similar results have been found in other patients suffering from the same condition (Becker et al., 2012). Figure 11.10 compares MRI scans of a normal brain and the brains of SM and two other patients (AM and BG) suffering from the same condition. The location of the amygdala in the comparison brain and where it should be located in the brains of SM, AM, and BG is circled in red (Feinstein et al., 2013).

As mentioned earlier, some people, like SM, who have damage to the amygdala are impaired in recognizing emotions in other people's facial expressions (Adolphs, Tranel, Damasio, & Damasio, 1994; Anderson, Spencer, Fulbright, & Phelps, 2000). Evidence for the involvement of the amygdala in processing emotional facial expressions was found in a study in which participants were presented with emotional facial expressions while their brains were being imaged by fMRI. The amygdalas of participants responded to a significantly higher degree when facial expressions such as those depicting fear, anger, and disgust were shown, compared to those depicting happiness, neutral faces, and pictures of buildings (Mattavelli et al., 2014). These findings are consistent with the idea that one of the amygdala's roles is to process potential threats in the environment.

FIGURE 11.10

MRI scans of the brains of patient SM and two other cases (AM and BG) suffering from the same condition. The red circle indicates the location of the amygdala in the comparison brain and where it should be located in the patients.

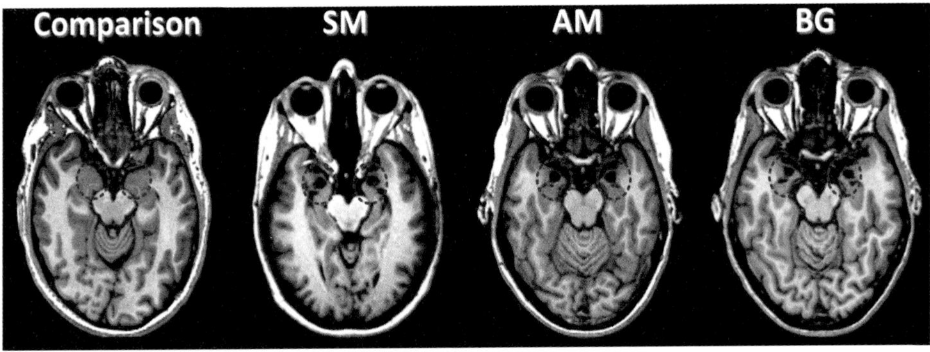

Feinstein, J.S., et al. (2013). Fear and panic in humans with bilateral amygdala damage. *Nature Neuroscience 16*(3): 270–272. With permission from Springer Nature.

A seminal study conducted by psychologist Arne Öhman and colleagues showed that the amygdala can even learn to respond to potential threats without conscious awareness of the stimuli provoking the response (J. S. Morris, Öhman, & Dolan, 1998). In the first phase of the study, participants were shown pictures of expressionless and angry faces. Some of the angry faces were presented along with an unpleasant sound while the others were not. Pictures of expressionless faces did not increase autonomic activity in participants as measured by skin conductance (which measures the extent to which sweating influences the skin's electrical conductivity). However, angry faces presented along with an unpleasant sound did increase autonomic activity.

In the second phase of the study, angry faces were then presented for a very brief period (30 milliseconds) followed by a masking stimulus, which consisted of an expressionless face. The participants indicated that they saw the expressionless face but not the angry face. The participants who previously had been exposed to angry faces followed by the aversive sound showed a significantly higher degree of skin conduction than participants whose presentations of the angry faces were not followed by the aversive sound. In addition, the same participants also showed increased activity in the amygdala. Remember that this is despite the fact that the participants reported not having consciously perceived the angry faces.

These results show that emotional expressions can be triggered by stimuli that are not consciously perceived, also known as **subliminal stimuli**. Note the similarity between the results of this study and the results found by Joseph LeDoux in which rats, rendered deaf by lesions of the auditory cortex, were nevertheless conditioned to associate a tone with a shock. The explanation for that result was that the conditioned stimulus, which consisted of a tone, was processed along the direct pathway, which carries sensory information from the thalamus directly to the amygdala. An emotional response was produced in the rats, without the participation of the indirect pathway, in which sensory information would have been analyzed by the cortex. In the Öhman study, the angry faces also likely triggered an emotional response through the direct pathway, which does not depend on conscious experience to activate the amygdala. These findings may also explain the neurobiological processes behind **implicit racial prejudice** (Izuma, Aoki, Shibata, & Nakahara, 2019; Öhman, 2005). Implicit racial prejudice is shown in people who do not consciously endorse any form of prejudice toward other groups but who show a negative bias on evaluation (see the "Applications" box at the end of this chapter).

MODULE SUMMARY

The brain was once thought to possess a network of brain areas dedicated to processing emotions. This became known as the limbic system. It is now known that emotions are not processed in a single system of brain areas but that emotions are made up of different components processed in widespread brain areas. Evidence for discrete emotions was believed to be found in brain imaging studies. However, the results of these studies could be interpreted as different brain areas being involved in different aspects of emotions, providing evidence for the theory of constructed emotions. Emotions in animals can be studied using fear conditioning, in which a tone is associated with a shock.

The amygdala is thought to play a central role in fear. Stimuli can trigger the expression of emotions without its conscious perception. This has been found in rats rendered deaf by lesions of the auditory cortex and subjected to fear conditioning. This is possible because information from an environmental stimulus follows two pathways to the amygdala. These pathways are known as the high road and the low road. Along the high road, information from the stimulus travels from the sensory receptors to the thalamus, the cortex, and then to the amygdala, which triggers autonomic and musculoskeletal responses. Information along the low road travels from the sensory receptors, to the thalamus, and then directly to the amygdala. The role played by the amygdala in fear has been studied in patients with Urbach-Wiethe disease, which leads to degeneration of the amygdala. These patients have an inability to experience fear. Emotions can also be triggered without conscious awareness. This has been shown in a classic study in which participants responded with fear to angry faces, presented subliminally, that had been conditioned to an aversive stimulus.

TEST YOURSELF

11.2.1 Describe the Papez circuit and the limbic system. What is the neurobiological evidence for discrete emotions and for the theory of constructed emotions?

11.2.2 Describe the role of the amygdala in fear. Describe what is meant by the high road and the low road.

11.2.3 How can the role of the amygdala in fear be studied in humans? Describe an experiment that shows that emotions can be triggered in an unconscious manner.

11.3 Emotions and Decision Making: Beyond the Amygdala

Module Contents

Learning Objectives

11.3.1 Describe some of the functions of the prefrontal cortex in emotions.

11.3.2 Explain the somatic-marker hypothesis.

11.3.1 THE PREFRONTAL CORTEX

>> LO 11.3.1 Describe some of the functions of the prefrontal cortex in emotions.

Key Terms

- **Phineas Gage:** A historical and prototypical case of prefrontal cortex function.
- **Ventromedial prefrontal cortex:** A part of the prefrontal cortex important for planning and judgment.

As you just learned, the amygdala is highly involved in processing fear. However, you also learned that emotions are thought to be created through the activation of entire networks of brain areas that include the amygdala. Another brain area known to be involved in processing emotions is the prefrontal cortex. The prototype of emotional disturbances after damage to the prefrontal cortex is that of **Phineas Gage**, a railroad worker for the Rutland and Burlington Railroad Company (Fleischman, 2002).

In 1848, Gage was preparing an explosive charge in order to blast through large rocks blocking the intended path for a railway to be laid through the state of Vermont. This was done by first drilling a hole into a rock and filling it halfway with explosive powder. A fuse was then inserted, and the powder was covered with sand. The sand was then tightly tamped down against the powder with an iron rod so that the explosion was directed inward into the rock. However, on that day, Gage drilled the hole, poured in the explosive powder, and inserted the fuse but asked one of his coworkers to cover the powder with sand. He then proceeded to tamp into the hole with the iron rod, not realizing that his coworker never covered the powder with sand. The iron rod created a spark against the rock that fell directly onto the uncovered powder, resulting in a terrible explosion. The explosion was directed outward and propelled the iron rod into the direction of Gage's head. The rod entered his left cheek, pierced the base of his skull, and went through the front of his brain. The rod came out of the top of his head, flew through the air and landed

25 meters away. A reconstruction of Gage's injury is shown in Figure 11.11.

Miraculously, Gage survived. He was carried in an ox cart to a nearby hotel, where physician John Martyn Harlow examined and treated him (Macmillan, 2001). Gage made a full recovery. All of his senses were intact. He suffered no paralysis or deficits in his speech or language comprehension. However, something seemed to be wrong with his personality. Before the accident, Gage had been a well-mannered and balanced man. He was of good character and temperate habits. He had many plans, which he always executed. After the accident, Gage is reported to have become irreverent, often indulging in profanities. He could make plans but could not carry them out. He was also impaired in making decisions that were advantageous for his survival (J. M. Harlow, 1999).

FIGURE 11.11

(A) The skull of Phineas Gage, showing the hole created by the iron rod. (B–D) Computer reconstructions of the passage of the iron rod through Gage's head.

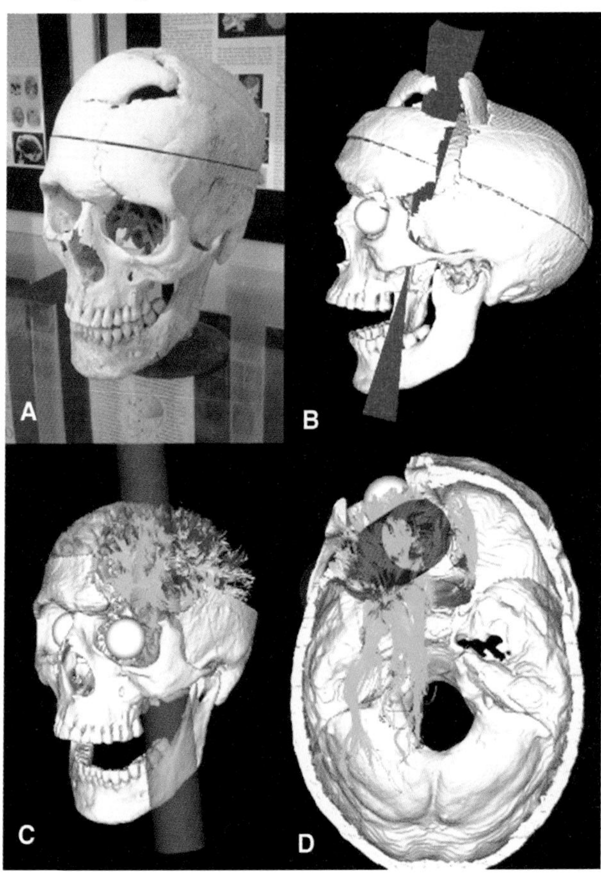

Van Horn, J.D., et al. (2012). Mapping connectivity damage in the case of Phineas Gage. *PLoS One, 7*(5), e37454.

In his book *Descartes' Error*, Antonio Damasio (1994) describes the case of Elliot, who suffered damage to the frontal lobes as a result of the surgical removal of a tumor. In many ways, the changes observed in Elliot after his surgery were similar to the ones observed in Phineas Gage following his accident. Like Gage, Elliot had no changes in speech, language, or motor skills. All of his senses were also preserved. His ability to do arithmetic was intact, and he retained good short-term and long-term memory. However, his ability to make decisions was greatly impaired, in striking similarity to what was observed in Gage. His emotions were also affected. For example, he told the story of his life in an emotionally detached way.

In short, both Gage and Elliot suffered severe disruptions in decision making and in the ability to regulate their emotions, both of which depend on the **ventromedial prefrontal cortex** (VMPFC) (Bechara, Tranel, & Damasio, 2000; Fellows & Farah, 2007). In fact, it is thought that the VMPFC plays a role in emotional regulation by dampening the activity of the amygdala (Motzkin, Philippi, Wolf, Baskaya, & Koenigs, 2015).

11.3.2 THE SOMATIC-MARKER HYPOTHESIS

>> LO 11.3.2 **Explain the somatic-marker hypothesis.**

Key Terms

- **Somatic-marker hypothesis**: The hypothesis that the unconscious activation of past emotional experiences informs decision making.
- **Somatic marker:** The perception of physiological changes that act as a biasing mechanism in decision making.
- **Iowa gambling task:** A task used to assess the role played by emotions in decision-making processes in brain-damaged patients.

When having to make a decision, we are often confronted with a variety of options from which to choose. And sometimes we have to decide on one of these options quickly, with no time to engage in a rational analysis of potential costs and benefits associated with each option. When we are uncertain which option constitutes the rational and logical choice, we often rely on gut feeling, which biases our choice toward one option versus another.

To explain this phenomenon, neuroscientist Antonio Damasio proposed what became known as the **somatic-marker hypothesis** (SMH). According to the SMH, rational analysis is not enough to make decisions that are personally beneficial, especially under conditions of uncertainty. In fact, according to Damasio, the role of emotions in decision making is greatly underestimated (Bechara & Damasio, 2005). The hypothesis was developed in response to the observation that people with damage to the VMPFC (such as Elliot, whose case was described in the previous unit) are severely impaired in personal and social decision making, leaving other intellectual abilities intact (Damasio, 1996). The decision making impairments in these patients is thought to reflect their inability to use their emotions or gut feelings to help them make choices. Instead, they engage in an endless deliberative process, weighing the possible costs and benefits of every option presented to them. Think about a situation when you had difficulty deciding among several equivalent options. This could be about choosing between restaurants, brands of cereal, or classes. How did you finally decide? Chances are that you had a gut feeling about what the best option was.

According to the SMH, bodily changes induced by autonomic nervous system activity, as well as changes in posture and muscle tension that result from emotionally arousing stimuli, are stored within the brain as **somatic markers**. These somatic markers and the events they were associated with are stored in the VMPFC, for example, the association between encountering a mountain lion and the bodily changes that compose the emotion one felt when encountering it. This may cause one to later experience a similar pattern of bodily changes and the emotions associated with them when encountering a house cat.

You may be wondering what this has to do with decision making. Well, the perception of somatic markers is thought to act as a biasing signal that constrains the decision-making process toward choosing one option over another. For example, a company manager decided to buy from supplier A rather than from supplier B. When asked to explain her choice, she simply stated that she didn't really know, but that she had a hunch that supplier B could not be trusted. She later realized that company B's logo resembled the logo of a company that had previously defrauded her company of a considerable sum of money. According to the SMH, the manager's choice to shy away from choosing company B was due to the reactivation of the somatic marker created when her company was defrauded.

The Iowa Gambling Task

Support for the SMH comes from experimental findings based on the performance of patients with damage to the VMPFC in what is known as the **Iowa gambling task** (Bechara, Damasio, Damasio, & Anderson, 1994). In this task, subjects are given a sum of play money, say $2,000, to gamble with. The participants are then made to choose from four decks of cards, labeled A, B, C, and D, on a computer screen (Figure 11.12). Choosing from two of the decks, for example, A and B, results in consistently low monetary payoffs combined with small losses. However, choosing from the other two decks, C and D, results in higher monetary payoffs but is associated with larger losses. After a certain number of choices, the participants are told that the game is over

FIGURE 11.12

The Iowa gambling task.

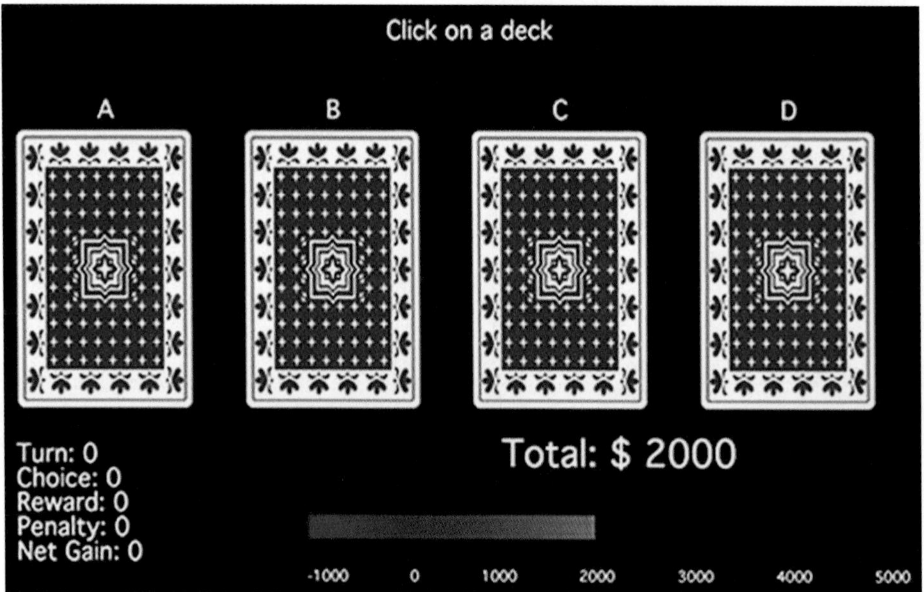

Iowa gambling task: Parenting and ADD, Jessica Borelli and Warren Szewczyk, and Todd Shimoda. Pomona EdTech.

and that they could no longer continue picking cards from the decks. The goal of the game is to end up with more money than one started with.

Normal participants quickly learned to avoid choosing from the decks associated with higher monetary gains but that also carried larger losses, namely, decks C and D. They instead tended to consistently choose from the decks associated with lower monetary payoffs but smaller losses, decks A and B, which made them winners in the long run. In contrast, patients with damage to the VMPFC consistently failed to learn to avoid decks C and D, which resulted in higher losses in the long run. Importantly, the task is designed so that it is not possible to consciously keep track of which decks to choose from in order to come out a winner. This means that the learning that takes place must be done in an implicit manner, that is, without conscious awareness.

So how is this happening? In one study, participants' autonomic nervous system activity was monitored using **skin conduction response** (SCR, described earlier) while subjected to the task (Bechara, Tranel, Damasio, & Damasio, 1996). In normal subjects, choosing from the bad decks, C and D, presumably resulted in the creation of somatic markers, biasing their choices away from those decks in the future. This was observed by an increased SCR in the moments before choosing from the bad decks. In contrast, patients with damage to the VMPFC showed no such increase in SCR. These results suggest that, when uncertain about one's choices, making decisions that lead to personally advantageous situations involves the activation of somatic markers, as measured by increased SCR. In the Iowa gambling task, these somatic markers biased participants' choices away from the bad decks.

MODULE SUMMARY

The ventromedial prefrontal cortex (VMPFC) is involved in emotions and decision making. People with damage to the VMPFC have trouble regulating their emotions and have problems in planning, judgment, and decision making. The first evidence for this comes from the study of brain-damaged patients. The most famous of these cases is that of Phineas Gage, whose frontal lobes were damaged when an iron rod went through his skull. Neuroscientist Antonio Damasio thinks that, contrary to popular belief, emotions help in making good decisions. To explain the role of emotions in decision making, Damasio proposed the somatic-marker hypothesis, according to which emotions triggered by the similarity between a current situation and a past experience bias decisions toward choosing one option over another. The performance and lack of emotional reactivity in people with damage to the VMPFC in the Iowa gambling task is taken as evidence for the somatic-marker hypothesis.

TEST YOURSELF

11.3.1 Describe some of the functions of the prefrontal cortex in emotions.

11.3.2 Explain the somatic-marker hypothesis.

11.4 Aggression

Module Contents

11.4.1 What Is Aggression?

11.4.2 Aggression in the Brain

11.4.3 Aggression: Testosterone, Cortisol, and Serotonin

Learning Objectives

11.4.1 Define aggression as well as its different types.

11.4.2 Identify some of the neurobiological bases of aggression.

11.4.3 Explain how hormones and neurotransmitters may be involved in aggressive behavior.

11.4.1 WHAT IS AGGRESSION?

>> LO 11.4.1 **Define aggression as well as its different types.**

Key Terms

- **Aggression:** A type of hostile social behavior aimed at inflicting damage or harm on others.
- **Instrumental aggression:** Also known as predatory aggression; cold-blooded (unemotional), often premeditated actions directed toward others.
- **Impulsive aggression:** Also known as defensive or affective aggression; occurs in response to perceived threats.

Aggression can be defined as a type of hostile social behavior aimed at inflicting damage or harm on others (Miczek, Fish, De Bold, & De Almeida, 2002). But aggression is not a unitary trait. It is likely built up of several cognitive, behavioral, and genetic factors. Therefore, this definition does not encapsulate all of the complexities involved in aggressive behaviors. We know that, in nature, aggressive behavior is adaptive, as it provides a means for species to protect their young and their territory as well as to fight over food or mates and to maintain social hierarchies. Aggressive behaviors can be subdivided into two categories: instrumental aggression and impulsive aggression (Wrangham, 2018).

Instrumental aggression, also known as predatory aggression, refers to cold-blooded (unemotional), often premeditated actions directed toward others. Instrumental aggression is not associated with high levels of physiological arousal (Dodge & Coie, 1987). In humans, instrumental aggression includes actions such as bullying, stalking, and premeditated murder. In extreme cases, instrumental aggression can take the form of mass or serial killings perpetrated by individuals such as Anders Breivik, whose murdering spree was described briefly in this chapter's opening vignette. **Impulsive aggression**, also known as defensive or affective aggression, occurs in response to perceived threats. Impulsive aggression is often accompanied by fear or anger. In contrast to instrumental aggression, impulsive aggression is emotion driven and associated with high levels of physiological arousal (Barratt & Slaughter, 1998). Examples of impulsive aggression in humans include reacting defensively to being provoked, threatened, or attacked.

Categorizing aggression into two subtypes may be too simplistic if we are to understand its full nature. Aggressive behavior may also include several other subtypes (Daly, 2018).

11.4.2 AGGRESSION IN THE BRAIN

>> **LO 11.4.2 Identify some of the neurobiological bases of aggression.**

Key Terms

- **Decortication:** A procedure in which the cortex is removed to varying degrees.
- **Sham rage:** A range of autonomic and motor reactions associated with rage devoid of accompanying subjective feelings.

Investigations into the neurobiological bases of aggression began in the 1920s, when physiologist Philip Bard (you should remember his name from reading about the Cannon-Bard theory) studied the behavior of cats who had been subjected to **decortication**, a procedure in which the cortex is removed to varying degrees (Bard, 1928). Bard's cats displayed what became known as **sham rage**. Sham rage consists of a range of autonomic and motor reactions associated with rage. These include increased heart-rate and blood pressure, arching of the back, extended claws, and lashing of the tail. This display of rage was

FIGURE 11.13

(a) Sham rage was not displayed by cats from which the entire hypothalamus was removed along with the decortication. (b) Sham rage was displayed only when the posterior hypothalamus was left intact. Also shown are the midbrain, medulla, and pons.

(a) No "sham rage"

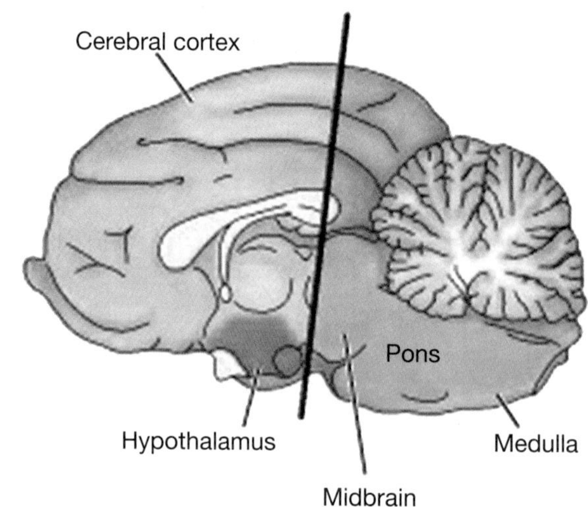

(b) "Sham rage" remains

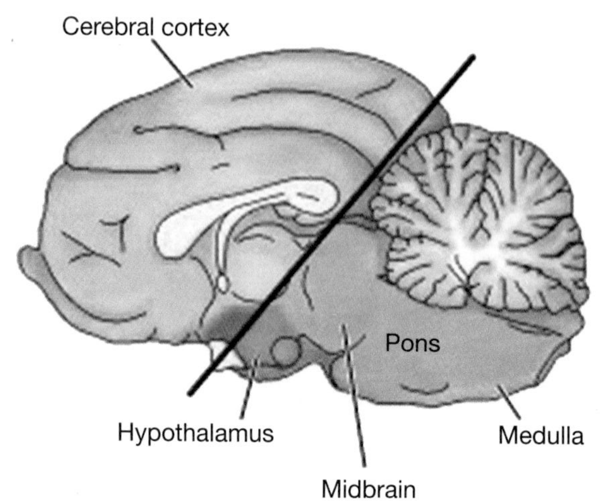

given the name of sham rage because it occurred without inner subjective feelings of rage. Remember that the cats were decorticated. Bard also found that no sham rage occurred if the decortication involved the removal of the posterior hypothalamus (Figure 11.13a). The cats displayed sham rage only if the posterior hypothalamus was left intact (Figure 11.13b). These results indicated that the rage induced by the posterior hypothalamus was kept in check by the anterior hypothalamus and the cortex.

Physiologist Walter R. Hess (1932) later found that electrically stimulating the hypothalamus in a particular area resulted in the autonomic nervous system reactions we associate with fear, whereas stimulating another region attenuated these reactions. This was followed by the discovery by John P. Flynn and colleagues that instrumental (predatory) and impulsive (affective) aggression can be triggered in cats by electrically stimulating different parts of the hypothalamus (Wasman & Flynn, 1962). Flynn found that instrumental aggression can be triggered by stimulating the lateral hypothalamus but that impulsive aggression resulted from stimulation of the medial hypothalamus.

11.4.3 AGGRESSION: TESTOSTERONE, CORTISOL, AND SEROTONIN

>> LO 11.4.3 **Explain how hormones and neurotransmitters may be involved in aggressive behavior.**

Key Terms

- **T/CRT ratio:** The ratio of testosterone to cortisol.
- **Dual hormone/serotonergic hypothesis:** The hypothesis that impulsive aggression is related to high levels of testosterone in the presence of low cortisol and low serotonin.

Today we know that the neurobiological basis for aggressive behavior involves complex interactions at several levels of analysis. These include interactions between hormonal and neurotransmitter systems. For example, in the 1990s, it was found that levels of the hormone cortisol and the androgen hormone testosterone were related to aggression (Montoya, Terburg, Bos, & van Honk, 2012). However, testosterone levels were associated with aggression only in the presence of low levels of cortisol. The measure of the ratio of testosterone to cortisol is known as the **T/CRT ratio** (Terburg, Morgan, & van Honk, 2009). In contrast, high levels of cortisol combined with low levels of testosterone result in fear and withdrawal. These opposite effects are thought to result because testosterone and cortisol inhibit each other's actions.

It was also found that testosterone facilitates aggressive approach behavior by stimulating increased levels of the hormone vasopressin in the amygdala and periaqueductal gray matter. Cortisol results in fear and withdrawal behavior through stimulating increased levels of corticotropin-releasing hormone in the amygdala. Interestingly, the type of aggression observed depends on levels of the neurotransmitter serotonin. In what is known as the **dual hormone/serotonergic hypothesis**, impulsive aggression depends not only on a high T/CRT ratio but also on low levels of serotonin (Montoya et al., 2012). Why serotonin? Low levels of serotonin are associated with impulsive behavior (Cardinal, 2006). Therefore, serotonin is thought to be involved in the inhibition of impulsive behavior through its actions in the prefrontal cortex (Frankle et al., 2005).

MODULE SUMMARY

Aggression can be defined as a type of hostile social behavior aimed at inflicting damage or harm on others. Aggression can be subdivided into two subtypes: instrumental aggression and impulsive aggression. Instrumental aggression is unemotional, premeditated, and considered a means to an end. Instrumental aggression is not associated with increased autonomic system activity. Impulsive aggression occurs in response to a threat or provocation. Impulsive aggression is associated with heightened autonomic nervous system activity.

The hypothalamus was found to be important for aggressive behaviors. Decorticated cats in which the posterior hypothalamus was left intact exhibited sham rage, in which the physiological and somatic signs of anger are expressed without their associated subjective feelings. The medial hypothalamus is associated with impulsive aggression, and the lateral hypothalamus is associated with instrumental aggression.

The androgen hormone testosterone and the stress hormone cortisol are related to aggression. However, testosterone leads to aggression only when levels of cortisol are low. Fear and withdrawal are observed when levels of cortisol are high in relation to testosterone. Testosterone leads to impulsive aggression in the presence of low cortisol levels when the levels of the neurotransmitter serotonin are low. This became known as dual hormone/serotonergic hypothesis.

TEST YOURSELF

11.4.1 Define aggression and its different subtypes.

11.4.2 What parts of the brain were first thought to be involved in aggression and why?

11.4.3 (a) Define T/CRT ratio. How is it related to aggression? (b) Define the dual hormone/serotonergic hypothesis.

APPLICATIONS

Implicit Bias

Implicit bias refers to attitudes or stereotypes that affect our understanding, actions, or decisions in an unconscious manner. That is, an implicit bias is activated involuntarily, without intentional control. An implicit bias can be positive or negative, and no one is immune to them. Implicit bias results from being exposed to information about groups of people. The content of this information is triggered automatically when thinking about or interacting with members of the group. The expression of an implicit bias occurs when one's understanding or thoughts about a group reflect this information. Importantly, an implicit bias may also influence one's actions and decision-making process directed toward the group.

In psychology and neuroscience, the term *implicit* refers to brain processes that can influence one's thought process, behavior, and emotions in an unconscious and effortless manner. For example, the same unpleasant emotions that were felt in the presence of a certain object or situation can automatically be triggered when one encounters a similar object or situation. The term *explicit* refers to information that is retrieved in a conscious and deliberate manner, such as when you purposefully recall the items you need to purchase from the grocery store.

This means that one's social perceptions, impression formation, judgment, and motivations toward certain groups may not always be under conscious control because of implicit attitudes and stereotypes (Greenwald & Krieger, 2006). For example, one might exert caution, fear, or a high level of preparedness toward a person from a group that is in line with an implicit racial stereotype. These implicit attitudes or stereotypes can be held even if they do not reflect what one consciously endorses. This phenomenon is known as dissociation.

Implicit bias can be studied in the laboratory using what is known as the race implicit association test (race IAT) (Greenwald, McGhee, & Schwartz, 1998). In this test, participants first practice distinguishing faces of people of different races, presented on a computer screen, by pressing either a right or a left key on a keyboard. For example, the participants may be asked to press the right key when they see a picture of an African American (AA) face and the left key when they see the face of a European American (EA). The participants are then made to distinguish words with a pleasant meaning from words with an unpleasant meaning. Next, the participants learn to respond to one key when they see either an AA face or a pleasant word and to press another key when they see an EA face or an unpleasant word. Finally, the participants are required to do the opposite, that is, press one key when they see either an AA face or an unpleasant word and another key when they see an EA face or a pleasant word. The critical measure in this task is the speed with which participants respond to the presentations of the members of the different categories (i.e., faces versus types of words). Americans respond more quickly when EA faces are paired with pleasant words. This means that for Americans EA faces form a stronger association with pleasant words than do AA faces. These findings are taken to mean that EA faces are preferred to AA faces. The results of the race IAT given to registered voters was found to predict the results of the 2008 U.S. presidential election between Barack Obama and John McCain (Greenwald, Smith, Sriram, Bar-Anan, & Nosek, 2009).

Implicit Bias and the Brain

The brain areas most often implicated in the study of race are the amygdala, the anterior cingulate cortex (aACC), the fusiform face area (FFA), and the dorsolateral prefrontal cortex (DLPFC) (Kubota et al., 2012). For example, several studies have shown that the amygdala, which is involved in processing fear, is significantly more activated when research participants viewed outgroup faces versus ingroup faces (D. A. Stanley et al., 2012). Other studies have shown that implicit biases are also associated with activation of the aACC, which is thought to be involved in detecting conflict (Richeson et al., 2003). Increased activity of the aACC is thought to be due to the conflict produced by implicitly held negative beliefs and attitudes, on the one hand, and the explicitly held conscious effort not to hold such negative beliefs and attitudes, on the other (i.e., dissociation, described earlier). The aACC is often coactivated along with the DLPFC (D. Stanley, Phelps, & Banaji, 2008). The role of the DLPFC in implicit bias is thought to be to keep implicit biases under control. Finally, the FFA, which is activated when seeing faces, was more strongly activated when seeing faces from ingroup members versus faces from outgroup members (Golby, Gabrieli, Chiao, & Eberhardt, 2001).

Putting It All Together

These findings suggest that implicit bias involves activity in a network of areas. As shown in Figure 11.14, these include the amygdala, aACC, DLPFC, and FFA (Kubota, Banaji, & Phelps, 2012). The amygdala is involved in the automatic race-based evaluation of faces detected as being from ingroup or outgroup members. The conflict that arises between the implicit negative evaluation of outgroup members and the explicit desire to act without such bias is detected by the aACC. The DLPFC receives information about the conflict from the aACC and acts to keep implicit biases in check while in an interracial context.

Taken together, these findings show evidence for the existence of racial implicit bias at both the behavioral and neurobiological levels. This is important, given that a deeper understanding of how negative stereotypes and attitudes are acquired and generated is required in the hopes of eliminating racial prejudice.

FIGURE 11.14

The network implicated in racial implicit bias.

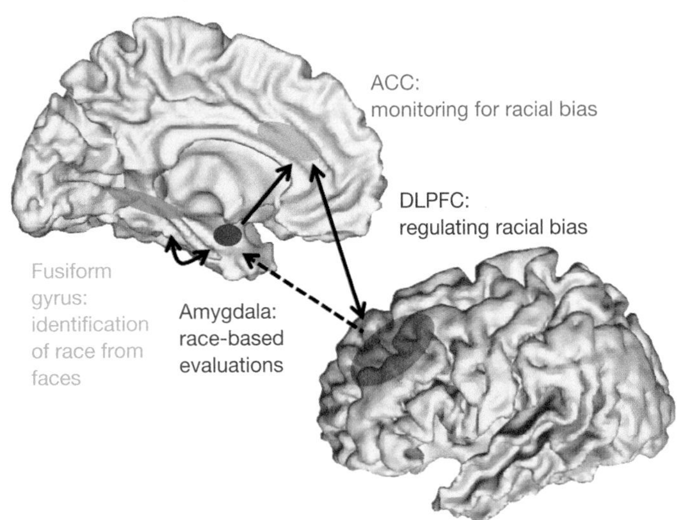

Kubota, J. T., M.R. Banaji & E.A. Phelps. (2012). The neuroscience of race. *Nature Neuroscience 15*(7): 940–948. With permission from Springer Nature.

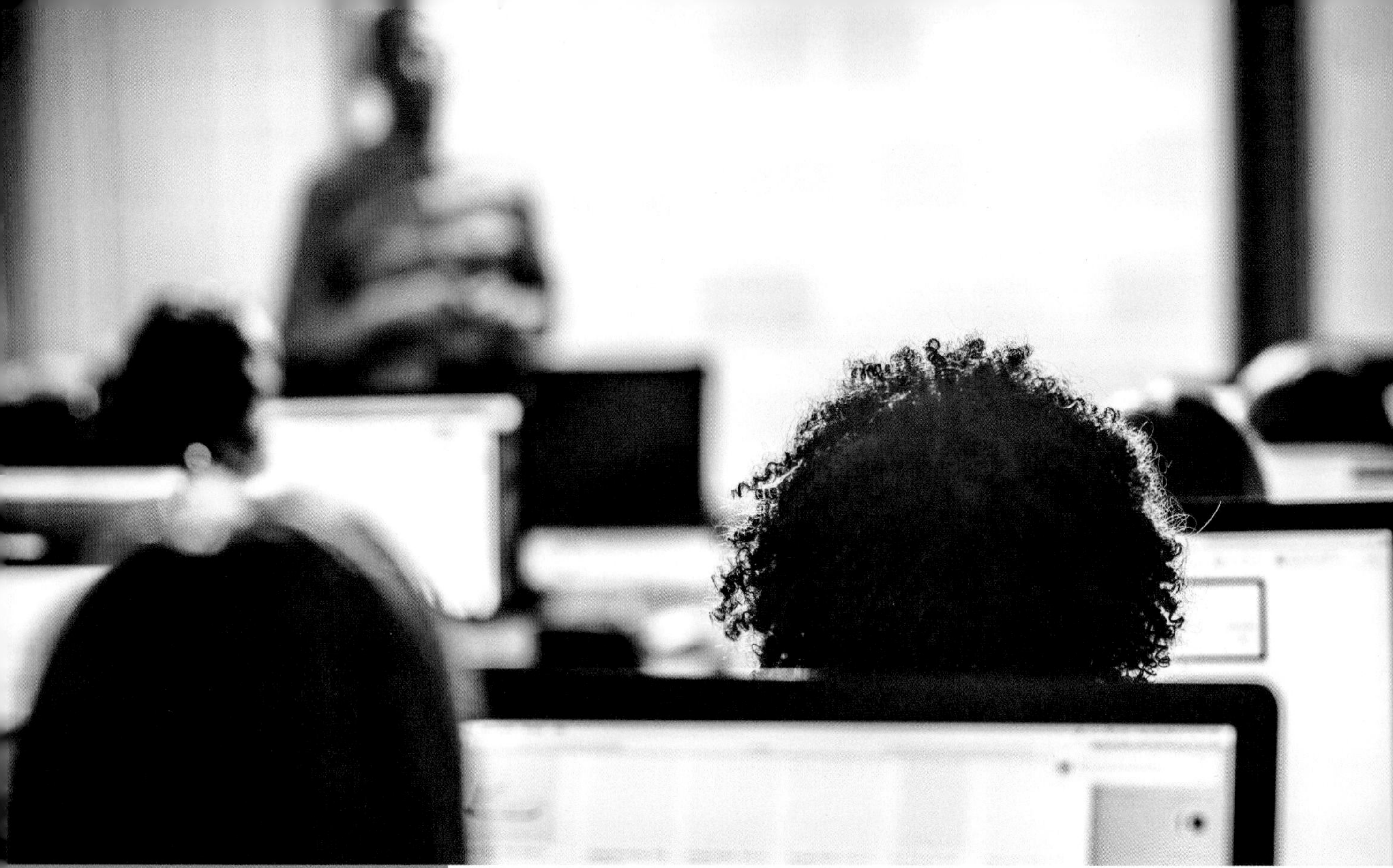

skynesher/istockphoto

12 Memory and Memory Systems

Chapter Contents

Learning Objectives

12.1.1 Define memory and its functions.

12.1.2 Describe the stages of memory.

12.1.3 Name and describe the registers of memory.

12.1.4 Identify the brain area thought to be most involved in working memory as well as a task used to assess it.

12.2.1 Describe and differentiate between the forms of long-term memory.

12.2.2 Identify the brain areas associated with different types of long-term memory.

12.3.1 Define memory consolidation and describe its proposed neurobiological mechanisms.

12.3.2 Describe the main theories of memory consolidation and differentiate between them.

12.4.1 Define spatial memory and explain how the hippocampus is involved in processing spatial information.

12.4.2 Describe the different types of cells involved in processing spatial information.

12.4.3 Explain how the role of the hippocampus and associated areas in spatial and nonspatial memory can be differentiated.

12.5.1 Define learning and explain the different ways in which learning can occur.

12.5.2 Describe nonassociative learning and its neurobiological basis.

12.5.3 Describe associative learning and its neurobiological basis.

12.5.4 Describe synaptic plasticity and its relevance to learning.

A Prodigious Memory: The Case of AJ

In 2006, memory researcher James McGaugh and his colleagues at the University of California in Irvine reported on the case of a 34-year-old woman known by the initials AJ, who possesses a significantly higher than normal capacity to remember facts about her personal life and public events. For example, given a date, AJ can recall with uncanny accuracy the day of the week, the public events that occurred on that day, and details of her personal life. For AJ, these memories come to her without effort and without the use of mnemonics (tricks that aid memory). Bewildered, McGaugh mentioned that similar unusual memory ability is sometimes observed in autistic savants, who are children or adults who have autism, a neurodevelopmental disorder characterized by significant social and communicative impairments. However, AJ's ability differs drastically from what is observed in people with autism, who tend to recall information specific to a precise domain.

In 2012, McGaugh and colleagues reported the results of a study in which they tested 10 additional individuals with memory abilities equivalent to those of AJ. Although the subjects scored normally on a set of standard laboratory memory tests, their memory for public and personal life events was astounding. The researchers' goal was also to find out whether these individuals' brains differed significantly from the brains of people with normal memory. Brain images obtained by MRI revealed that these individuals' medial temporal lobes, the area in which the hippocampus is located, had greater amounts of gray and white matter than the medial temporal lobes of control subjects. This finding provided evidence not only that the hippocampus is important for memory but also that differences in specific behaviors or abilities between individuals can be traced back to differences in the brain.

INTRODUCTION

Learning and memory are the processes by which we acquire, store, and use information so that we can reminisce, inform our current behaviors, and plan for the future. In this chapter, you will learn what psychologists and neuroscientists have discovered about these processes at the behavioral, systems, and molecular levels of analysis (see Chapter 1 to review the levels of analysis). This chapter covers both memory and learning. First you will learn about memory and the different types of memories that exist, including those that you consciously make an effort to acquire, and later to retrieve, such as when you pay attention in class so that you can remember the information during the next exam. Memories also include those that are recalled in an automatic way, such as when you automatically reach for your phone when it rings or when you automatically turn one way or the other when exiting the classroom to get to your next class. You will then learn about the brain areas thought to be involved in processing these different types of memories. The last module in this chapter is focused on learning, which can be defined as the processes by which memories are acquired. You will explore simple forms of learning and their neurobiological mechanisms by studying a well-known animal model.

12.1 Memory and Memory Systems

Module Contents

Learning Objectives

12.1.1 Define memory and its functions.

12.1.2 Describe the stages of memory.

12.1.3 Name and describe the registers of memory.

12.1.4 Identify the brain area thought to be most involved in working memory as well as a task used to assess it.

12.1.1 WHAT IS MEMORY?

>> LO 12.1.1 **Define memory and its functions.**

Key Term

- **Memory:** The processes by which information is encoded, stored, and retrieved for the purposes of remembering the past, informing current behavior, and planning the future.

Memory is often defined as the faculty that acquires, encodes, stores, and retrieves information. However, this simple definition does not do justice to the important functions and complex neurobiological processes required to realize them. If you haven't given this much thought, you may think of memory as being only about the past. In reality, memory is about the past, present, and future. There are several reasons for our ability to remember the past. For example, you may think about that pleasant daytrip you went on with your best friend last weekend. Doing so, you mentally travel back in time, replaying the events as if they were occurring again. Remembering these events puts a smile on your face as you start feeling the same positive emotions you did on that day. You enjoyed the time spent with your friend so much that you are already planning another trip. However, on another occasion, you remember what your professor said at the beginning of the term about assignments being handed in late, which is making you nervous because you have not yet started on the one due next week. Not wanting to be late handing it in, you immediately get to it.

These simple examples of everyday life should quickly make you realize that memory is not just about remembering the past. In both examples, remembering past events triggered an emotional experience, joy in the first and panic in the second, which were both experienced in the present. In both cases, remembering the past ultimately led to planning the future, another trip in the first case and writing a paper in the second. For this reason, we must update the incomplete definition of memory offered at the beginning of the chapter. Let's instead propose the following: Memory refers to the processes by which information is encoded, stored, and retrieved for the purposes of remembering the past, informing current behavior, and planning the future.

You also probably realized that we have different types of memories. For example, you may remember the name of one of your grade-school teachers, which is a fact, but not remember much about the activities you did in her class, which are entire episodes of your life. You also remember how to brush your teeth but probably not the events that surrounded the first times you did it by yourself. When you hear the ring of your cellphone, your hand automatically reaches for it without giving it much thought. You can hold information in mind just long enough to perform a task, or you can make sure to remember important information for a long period. These examples, and many others, demonstrate that memory takes on many forms. Different forms of memories are processed by different memory systems in the brain. In the remainder of this module, you will learn about the different types of memories that exist, as well as the brain systems responsible for them.

12.1.2 THE STAGES OF MEMORY

>> LO 12.1.2 **Describe the stages of memory.**

Key Terms

- **Encoding:** Converting the information acquired by your senses into patterns of activity within groups of neurons within the brain.

- **Storage:** The retention of information acquired by your senses.
- **Retrieval:** The recollection of information stored in memory.
- **"Tip of the tongue" phenomenon:** A type of retrieval failure accompanied by the strong feeling that temporarily forgotten information is on the verge of being recalled.

According to the definition at the beginning of this chapter, memory is a process that includes three stages: **encoding**, **storage**, and **retrieval** (Figure 12.1). This view of memory is derived by using the computer as an analogy and applying an information-processing approach to psychology (D. E. Broadbent, 1958). It is based on the idea that, similarly to how the words you type into your computer have to be encoded into computer language so that they can be stored and retrieved as a recognizable term paper, sensory and emotional information has to be encoded into patterns of activity within groups of neurons throughout the brain.

It follows that a lapse in memory can occur due to a failure in the stages of encoding, storage, or retrieval. For example, not remembering that the exam was postponed can be due to your not paying enough attention to the teacher, resulting in the information not being well encoded. It could also be due to a failure in the storing of the information. For example, you may have remembered the information shortly after your teacher mentioned it but eventually forgot it. It could also be that you do not remember whether she said that the exam was postponed or canceled. In this case, you might be having a problem with retrieval. An obvious case of retrieval failure is commonly known as the **"tip of the tongue" phenomenon**, which has been studied for decades (A. S. Brown, 1991; S. R. Brown, 2000; Marco et al., 1989). This occurs when you have temporarily forgotten information that you are certain of knowing, such as someone's name or that of a good restaurant, accompanied by the strong feeling that you are on the verge of recalling it. In this case, being reminded of part of the information is often enough to come up with the name and end your horrible bout of frustration. Evidence of a retrieval failure is that a cue that reminds you of the information often leads to instant recall, showing that it was encoded and stored.

FIGURE 12.1

The stages of memory.

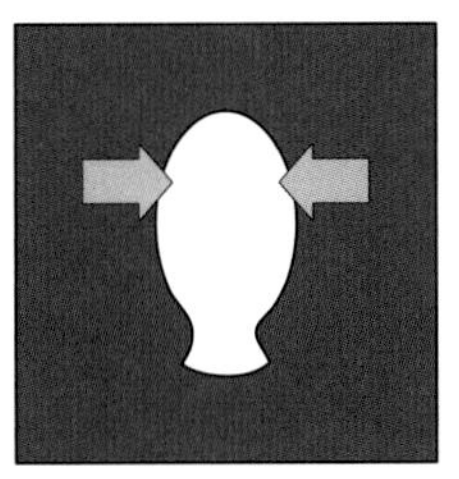

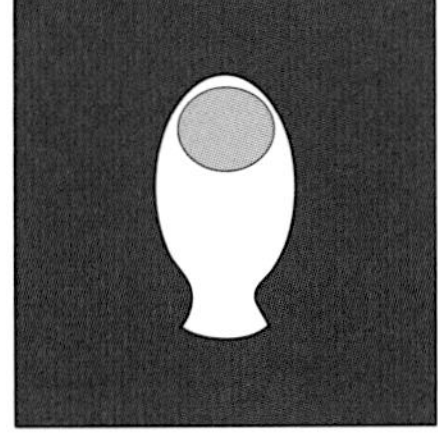

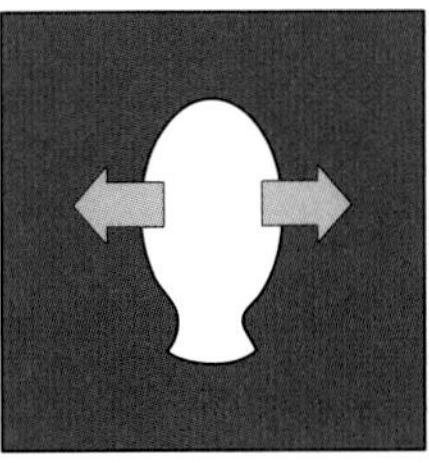

Adapted from Sense and Sensation: Writing on Education, Creativity, and Cognitive Science.

12.1.3 THE REGISTERS OF MEMORY

>> LO 12.1.3 **Name and describe the registers of memory.**

Key Terms

- **Sensory memory:** The persisting representation of a sensory stimulus for a brief period after it is no longer physically present.
- **Working memory:** A memory register of limited capacity for both the amount of information it can store and the time for which information is retained.
- **Long-term memory:** A memory register of potentially unlimited capacity for both the amount of information it can store and the time for which information is retained.
- **Multicomponent working memory model:** A model in which working memory is thought to depend on the operations of several components: a visuospatial sketch pad, a phonological loop, an episodic buffer, and a central executive.

Now that you know that memory is thought to consist of a process comprising three stages (encoding, storage, and retrieval), you should also know that memories are processed within three registers. These consist of sensory memory, working memory, and long-term memory. Each register has different capacities for storing information, in terms of both the amount of information it can store and the period for which the information can be stored. We will now explore sensory memory and working memory. Because of the details involved in our discussion of long-term memory, I have given it its own module.

Sensory Memory

Sensory memory refers to the persisting representation of a sensory stimulus for a brief period after it is no longer physically present. However, only a subset of this information is remembered if it becomes the focus of attention (Sperling, 1960). Sensory memories for visual, auditory, and tactile information are known, respectively, as iconic, echoic, and haptic memory. Each type of memory is processed by the sensory cortex associated with each one of the senses, that is, the visual cortex for iconic memory (Sligte, Scholte, & Lamme, 2009), the auditory cortex for echoic memory (Alain, Woods, & Knight, 1998), and the somatosensory cortex for haptic memory (Zhou & Fuster, 1996). However, sensory memories are processed in networks of cortical areas beyond their respective primary sensory areas (Gallace & Spence, 2009; Keysers, Xiao, Földiák, & Perrett, 2005; Saneyoshi, Niimi, Suetsugu, Kaminaga, & Yokosawa, 2011). In addition, each type of sensory memory can combine to form more complex representations (Zhou & Fuster, 1997).

Iconic Memories. Iconic memories are persisting representations of visual information after it has faded. These representations are stored for less than 500 milliseconds (Rensink, 2014). Iconic memory is important for detecting changes in the environment such as the perception of movement. You have experienced iconic memory in action if you have ever written your name in the air with a sparkler. This experience is known as the sparkler's trail effect (Figure 12.2).

Echoic Memories. Echoic memories are persisting representations of sounds after they have faded. These representations were found to persist for up to 10 seconds (N. Cowan, 1984; Lu, Williamson, & Kaufman, 1992). Echoic memory is important for keeping track of speech during a conversation. You have experienced echoic memory if you ever asked someone to repeat a question but were able to answer it before the person finished repeating. This occurred because you processed the persisting representation (or "echo") of the auditory information.

FIGURE 12.2

The sparkler's trail effect occurs because the light of the sparkles is retained in iconic memory for a brief period after it has faded.

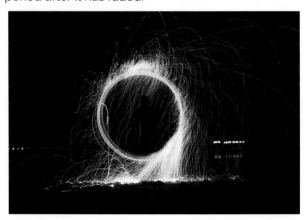

seyfettinozel/istockphoto

Haptic Memories. Haptic memories are persisting representations for tactile information after it has faded. The duration of haptic memory is approximately 2 seconds (Shih et al., 2009). Haptic memory is important for manipulating and recognizing objects by touch.

Working Memory

Short-term memory refers to the retention of small amounts of information for a short period. Within short-term memory, a system exists that maintains and manipulates this information. This system is known as **working memory**. Manipulating information in working memory includes rehearsing information in your mind, such as what you are supposed to buy at the grocery store; keeping track of the words being said in a conversation; or being able to get back to where you were studying in your textbook before you were interrupted by a text message from your friend.

One of the major characteristics of working memory is its vulnerability to disruption. Items in working memory are easily forgotten if they cease being the focus of attention or if other processes interfere with the rehearsal of information. For example, you may have been well on your way to memorizing a list of concepts until you became hungry and could no longer focus enough attention on them. After your meal, you realize that you cannot remember any of them. Or you thought you remembered what you were supposed to get at the grocery store until you bumped into one of your friends and spoke for an hour.

There are several models of working memory. The best known is the **multicomponent working memory model** developed and later updated by British psychologists Alan Baddeley and Graham Hitch (Baddeley & Hitch, 1974, 2007). The model proposes that working memory depends on the operations of several components, as illustrated in Figure 12.3. The top part of the figure shows the components of working memory. Working memory is considered to be a fluid system because its components are activated only temporarily. The components of working memory consist of (1) a visuospatial sketch pad, in which visual images are stored; (2) a phonological loop, in which verbal information is rehearsed by subvocalization and visual images are converted into a phonological code; (3) an episodic buffer, which integrates information from the visuospatial sketch pad and the phonological loop with a sense of time, so that memories can be experienced as sequences of events; and (4) a central executive. Four important roles have been attributed to the central executive: to focus attention, to divide attention, to permit switching from task to task, and to interface with long-term memory. The bottom part of the figure illustrates how **long-term memory**, which is discussed in the next module, is viewed as a memory register of potentially unlimited capacity for both the amount of information it can store and the time for which information is retained.

FIGURE 12.3

The multicomponent working memory model. LTM = long-term memory.

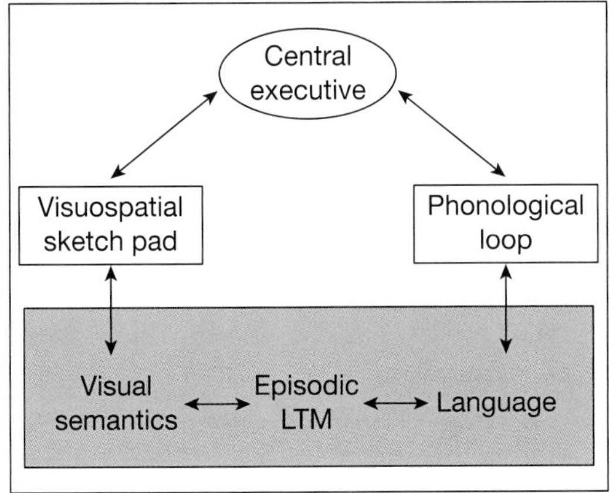

Baddeley, A. (2012). Working memory: theories, models, and controversies. *Annual Review of Psychology* 63: 1–29. With permission from Annual Reviews, Inc.

Working memory interacts with long-term memory in two ways. First, a subset of the information stored in working memory may eventually be stored in long-term memory. Second, as mentioned earlier, information in working memory comes from focusing on incoming sensory information and/or information stored in long-term memory.

12.1.4 WORKING MEMORY AND THE BRAIN

>> LO 12.1.4 **Identify the brain area thought to be most involved in working memory as well as a task used to assess it.**

Key Terms

- **Delayed-response task:** A behavioral task that requires holding a stimulus in working memory, after it has disappeared from view, to later make a correct choice.
- **Oculomotor delayed-response task:** A delayed-response task in which the location of a stimulus on a screen has to be held in short-term memory to later perform a correct response, as demonstrated by moving the eyes toward the area in which the stimulus previously appeared.

The prefrontal cortex is known to play a major role in executive functions (also referred to as cognitive control). These functions involve the control of attention, planning, goal setting, judgment, self-control, and working memory. Suspicions that the prefrontal cortex was important for executive functioning came from observing the behavior of people who sustained damage to the frontal lobes (Szczepanski & Knight, 2014), the most famous example being that of Phineas Gage (see Chapter 11).

As illustrated in Figure 12.4, the prefrontal cortex is subdivided into the orbitofrontal, rostral, dorsolateral, ventrolateral, dorsomedial, and ventromedial areas. Each area is implicated in some aspects of executive functioning (Narayanan & Laubach, 2006; Tranel, Bechara, & Denburg, 2002; Wallis, 2011).

The areas of the prefrontal cortex mostly associated with working memory are the dorsolateral and ventrolateral prefrontal cortices. The first experimental evidence that pointed to the involvement of the dorsolateral prefrontal cortex (DLPFC) in working memory came from early studies in which monkeys with damage to this area were impaired on what is known as a **delayed-response task** (Jacobsen & Nissen, 1937; Levy & Goldman-Rakic, 1999), which is designed to assess working memory. This task is divided into three phases. In the first phase (the cue phase), food is randomly placed in one of two food wells visible to the monkey. In the second phase (the delay phase), the food wells are covered, and a screen is lowered to obstruct the monkey's view for a predetermined period. In the third phase (the response phase), the screen is raised, and the monkey reaches for the food. It is thought that to be able to reach for the food at the correct location, the monkey has to keep a representation of the location of the food in working memory during the delay.

In the 1970s, neuroscientists Joaquin Fuster and Garrett Alexander (1971) recorded the electrical activity of single neurons in the DLPFC of monkeys engaged in a similar delayed-response task. Neurons in the DLPFC of the monkeys remained active through the delay period of the task. This suggested that these neurons actively maintained the memory of the cue throughout the delay phase.

FIGURE 12.4

The subdivisions of the prefrontal cortex.

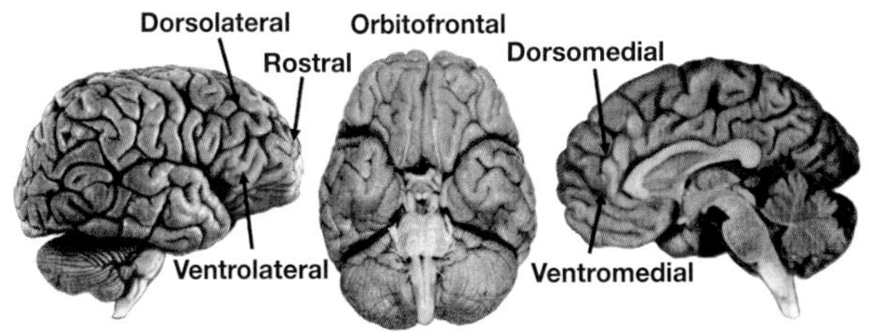

Szczepanski, S.M., & R.T. Knight. (2014). Insights into human behavior from lesions to the prefrontal cortex. *Neuron* 83(5): 1002–1018. With permission from Elsevier.

In another study, the delayed-response task just described was taken to the video screen by neuroscientist Patricia Goldman-Rakic (1937–2003), in what became known as an **oculomotor delayed-response task**. The procedure of the task is illustrated in Figure 12.5 (top row). During the cue phase, a monkey stares at a fixation point on a screen (cross) while a cue (black square) is presented at one of several locations in the periphery of the screen (the monkey was previously trained to stare at the center of the screen). During the delay phase, the cue disappears as the monkey keeps staring at the center of the screen. This signals the response phase, during which the monkey learns to shift its gaze from the center of the screen to the location where the cue was previously visible. The results of the study are shown in Figure 12.5 (middle row). As you can see, some of the neurons in the DLPFC fired during the cue and response phases of the task. However, most striking is the predominance of activity in neurons during the delay phase (Funahashi, Bruce, & Goldman-Rakic, 1989). This supported previous findings that the prefrontal cortex was important for maintaining information in working memory.

FIGURE 12.5

Oculomotor delayed-response task. Top row: The phases of the task consist of cue, delay, and response phases (see text). Middle row: The response of neurons in the DLPFC. Neurons fired at significantly higher rates during the delay phase, indicating that they may be maintaining a trace of the memory for the location of the cue. Bottom row: A monkey's gaze.

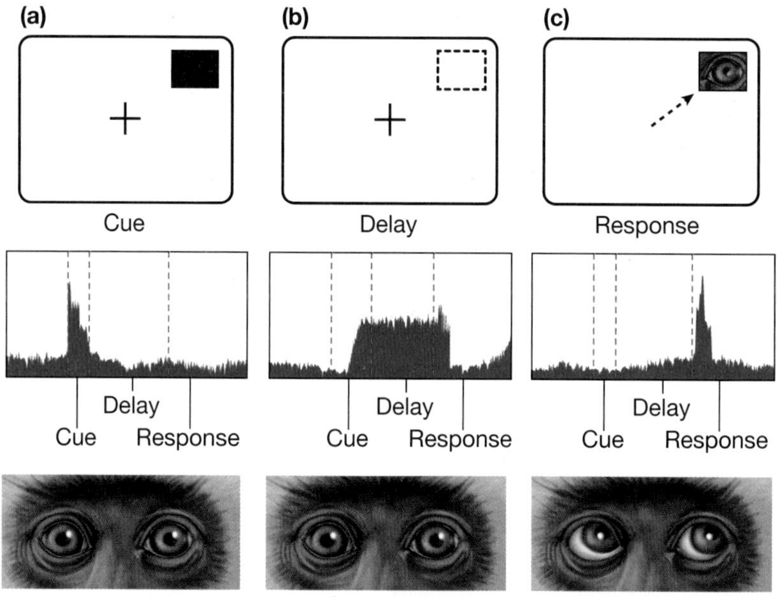

Amanda Tomasikiewicz/Body Scientific Intl.

MODULE SUMMARY

Memory refers to the processes by which information is encoded, stored, and retrieved for the purposes of remembering the past, informing current behavior, and planning the future. Memory is thought to comprise three phases: encoding, storage, and retrieval. Attention plays an important role in the encoding of information as it results in the neurons in the relevant brain areas firing simultaneously. However, not the same level of attention is required for all types of memories. Memory is thought to be encoded and stored in three registers: sensory memory, working memory, and long-term memory. Working memory is a type of memory in which a limited amount of information is stored for a limited amount of time. Working memory is vulnerable to disruption. Information in working memory is easily forgotten if it stops being the focus of attention. The best-known model of working memory is the multicomponent working memory model, which consists of a visuospatial sketch pad, a phonological loop, an episodic buffer, and a central executive. The brain area most associated with working memory is the prefrontal cortex. This was found by subjecting monkeys with lesions of the dorsolateral prefrontal cortex to delayed-response tasks.

TEST YOURSELF

12.1.1 Define memory and describe its functions.

12.1.2 What are the stages of memory? In what ways can memory fail?

12.1.3 What are the registers of memory? Name the characteristics of the registers discussed in this unit.

12.1.4 Which cortical area is thought to be important for working memory and why?

12.2 Long-Term Memory

Module Contents

Learning Objectives

12.2.1 Describe and differentiate between the forms of long-term memory.

12.2.2 Identify the brain areas associated with different types of long-term memory.

12.2.1 WHAT IS LONG-TERM MEMORY?

>> LO 12.2.1 Describe and differentiate between the forms of long-term memory.

Key Terms

- **Declarative memories:** Long-term memories that require the conscious recollection of information.
- **Nondeclarative memories:** Memories that are expressed only through the performance of tasks and habits, without the need for conscious recollection of information.
- **Semantic memories:** Declarative memories that comprise learned facts and life events.
- **Episodic memories:** Declarative memories that comprise life events; rich in contextual details including the time and place in which an event occurred.
- **Mental time travel:** The ability to travel back in time, in your mind's eye, to reexperience an event.
- **Chronesthesia:** The awareness of the passage of subjective time.
- **Autonoetic consciousness:** The ability to reflect upon past events while being aware that those are your own memories.
- **Priming:** A type of nondeclarative memory, in which exposure to a stimulus influences response to a later stimulus.
- **Procedural memories**: A type of nondeclarative memory that leads to the performance of skills and habit without the need for conscious recollection of information.

In the previous module, you learned about sensory and working memories as well as some of their neurobiological bases. You also learned that models of working memory suggest that it interacts with long-term memory. However, we have not defined, in detail, what constitutes long-term memories. That is the subject of the present module. Before we go on, it may be useful to get an overview of the different types of long-term memories. Figure 12.6 presents a classification scheme for types of long-term memories (Squire, 2004). With the exception of nonassociative learning, which is discussed in the final module of the chapter, the rest of the present module is dedicated to describing these types of memories. You will also learn about the brain areas involved in processing each type.

As mentioned in the preceding module, long-term memory refers to a memory register of potentially unlimited capacity for both the amount of information it can store and the time for which information is retained. Information in long-term memory is widely believed to be stored in a permanent and stable form. However, before we delve into this topic, it is important for you to know that there are different types of long-term memories. A crucial distinction to make regarding the different types of long-term memories is between those that require conscious and deliberate recollection and those whose recollection is made evident only through the performance of a task and that do not depend on the conscious recollection of information (Schacter, 1987; Squire & Zola, 1996). Long-term memories that require the conscious recollection of information are known as **declarative memories**. Declarative memories are also referred to as explicit memories, because they make explicit reference to specific knowledge. Other types of memories are expressed only through the performance of tasks and habits, without the need for conscious recollection of information. These types of long-term memories are known as **nondeclarative memories**. Nondeclarative memories are also known as implicit memories, because the source of their influence on behavior seems to come from within (Schachter, 1987).

Declarative memories are memories for learned facts and life events. Memories for learned facts are known as **semantic memories**. The retrieval of semantic memories does not require you to mentally travel back in time to reexperience the event in which the fact was learned. For example, remembering a fact such as "the Alamo is in Texas" does not require you to remember the context in which the fact was learned (i.e., where you were, who was with you, who told you, and when). Memories for life events are known as **episodic memories**. Episodic memories are rich in contextual details including the time and place in which an

FIGURE 12.6

Classification scheme for different types of long-term memories.

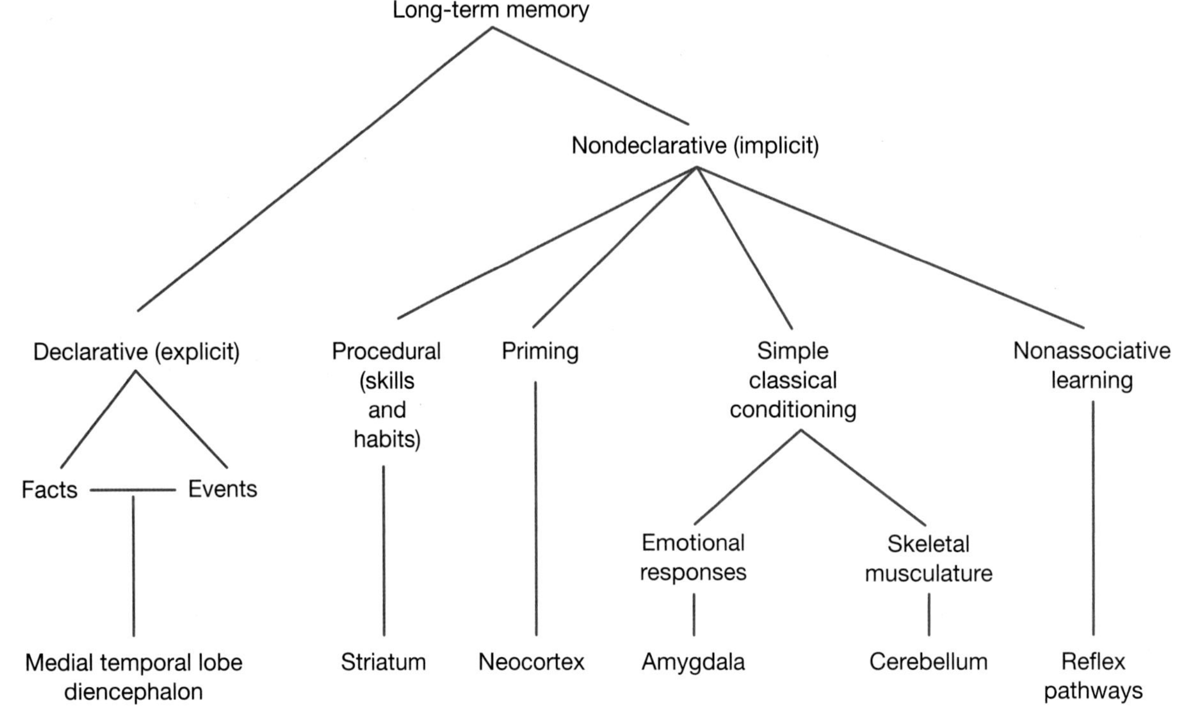

event occurred, hence, the "when," "where," and "what" of experiences (Nyberg, McIntosh, & Tulving, 1998; Tulving, 1983).

To psychologist and prominent memory researcher Endel Tulving, the defining characteristic of episodic memories is that their retrieval requires **mental time travel**, which enables you to travel back in time, in your mind's eye, to reexperience an event. Tulving believes that episodic memories include the awareness of the passage of subjective time, an ability known as **chronesthesia**. He also believes that episodic memories require **autonoetic consciousness**, which is the ability to reflect on past events while being aware that those are your own memories (Tulving, 1983).

The following example should help to clarify the difference between a semantic and an episodic memory. If you were asked where the Statue of Liberty is located, you would most likely remember that it is in New York City. Retrieving this fact from your memory did not require you to mentally travel back in time to the moment you learned it. By contrast, if your friend asks what you did during your summer vacation, you may answer by describing the time you spent in New York City, whom you went with, what you saw, the restaurants you ate at, and what your visit to the Statue of Liberty was like. Your memory of the trip will also include how the events during your vacation unfolded in time (chronesthesia), and you will be aware that the memory of those events represents your own experience (autonoetic consciousness) (Figure 12.7).

Nondeclarative Memory

In the preceding section, you learned about the two types of declarative memories, semantic and episodic memories, and that both types are retrieved through conscious recollection. In this section, we explore different types of nondeclarative memories. These include those acquired through the processes known as classical conditioning, priming, and procedural learning.

Classical Conditioning. We discuss classical conditioning in more detail in Unit 12.4. The conditioning of fear responses is also discussed in Chapter 11.

Classical Conditioning of Emotional Responses

The conditioning of emotional responses usually involves exposing a person or an animal to a stimulus likely to trigger an emotional reaction, such as a shock or other aversive stimuli, along with a neutral stimulus such as a tone or specific environmental context. For example, exposure to a previously neutral stimulus by itself can give rise to the same emotional response experienced when the aversive stimulus was present. Conditioned emotional responses are thought to be a way in which people acquire phobias (discussed in Chapter 14).

Classical Conditioning of Motor Responses

Classical conditioning of motor responses involves exposing a person or an animal to a stimulus likely to

FIGURE 12.7

Which of these thought bubbles represents a semantic memory? Which represents an episodic memory?

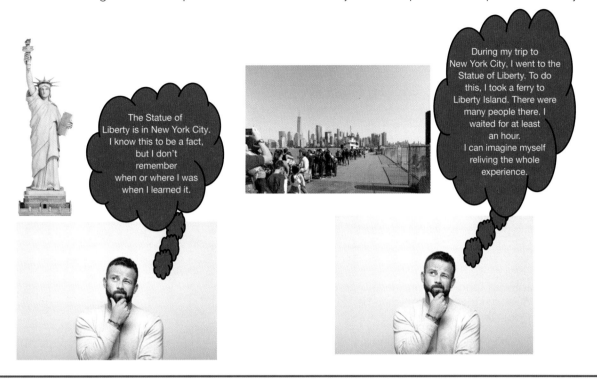

(clockwise from top left) izusek/ istockphoto; helen89/ istockphoto; Bet_Noire/ istockphoto

trigger a motor response, such as blinking in response to a puff of air to the eye, along with a neutral stimulus such as a tone. Later exposure to the previously neutral stimulus by itself (i.e., the tone) gives rise to the same motor response triggered by the stimulus that originally produced the response (Thompson, 1986; Yeo, 1991). For a real-life example of this, imagine going to your friend's house. You notice that she is in the backyard watering her lawn with a hose, onto which a spray nozzle is attached. She pretends not to see you, but as soon as you get close enough, she turns around and sprays a jet of water toward you, compelling you to lift your hands up in front of your face. Later that day, she picks up the hose and points the nozzle at you, again, without "firing." As soon as she does so, your hands automatically spring up in front of your face. The spray nozzle, which had previously been a neutral stimulus, became a conditioned stimulus leading to the automatic raising of your hands in front of your face, a conditioned response.

Priming. **Priming** refers to a type of nondeclarative memory in which exposure to a stimulus influences your response to a stimulus presented later (Weingarten et al., 2016). For example, if presented with the word *liberty* and later presented with the syllable *lib-*, you will be more likely to think of the word *liberty* than *library*. Similarly, if presented with the word *book*, you are more likely to notice the word *library* in a list than the word *moose*, because *book* and *library* are related in meaning. You are also more likely to notice a particular piece of clothing on someone if you own a similar one. Remember: Priming is a type of nondeclarative memory. This means that the primed words automatically come to mind and the similar piece of clothing seems to "pop out" without conscious effort (Tulving & Schachter, 1990). You have also not made any conscious effort to remember the information with the goal of influencing your response to subsequent stimuli.

Procedural Memory. **Procedural memory** is a type of nondeclarative memory that leads to the performance of skills and habit without the need for the conscious recollection of information (Cohen, Poldrack, & Eichenbaum, 1997; Lum & Conti-Ramsden, 2013). The following example provides an insightful look at procedural memory in action. The door to my office has a coded door lock. Several times a day, I get to my office door and press the code to get in. One day, a new teacher, with whom I share the office, forgot the code, so I started to tell him what it was. Out of the four digits that make up the code, I remembered only the first two. Being quite embarrassed by this,

I told him to follow me to the office door. Much to my amazement, I automatically pressed the correct combination of numbers as he watched. I am sure you have had similar kinds of experiences. Other behaviors performed through the retrieval of procedural memories include habits such as brushing your teeth or combing your hair. Complex skills such as riding a bicycle, texting, drawing, writing, playing a musical instrument, performing the complex series of movements in many sports, dancing, and many others all rely on procedural memory.

12.2.2 THE NEUROANATOMY OF LONG-TERM MEMORY

>> LO 12.2.2 Identify the brain areas associated with different types of long-term memory.

Key Terms

- **Neuroanatomy of long-term memory:** The collection of brain structures known to be involved in long-term memory.
- **Amnesia:** Memory deficits resulting from brain damage or psychological trauma.
- **Anterograde amnesia:** The inability to form new memories since brain damage has occurred.
- **Retrograde amnesia:** Memory loss for information acquired before brain damage.
- **Temporally graded retrograde amnesia:** A type of amnesia in which information acquired shortly before brain damage is lost but memories formed at a more remote period are preserved.

The **neuroanatomy of long-term memory** refers to the collection of brain structures known to be involved in long-term memory. Figure 12.8 (top), as well as Figure 12.11, shows some of these structures.

Declarative Memory

The brain areas most studied for their involvement in declarative memory are the ones contained within the medial temporal lobes. Figure 12.8 (bottom) shows a midsagittal section of the brain exposing the structures within the medial temporal lobes. These include the hippocampus and related cortical areas known as the perirhinal, entorhinal, and parahippocampal cortices as well as the amygdala.

Another region important for declarative memory is the medial diencephalon. This area includes the thalamus and the mammillary bodies of the hypothalamus (Figure 12.11). The hippocampus is connected to structures of the medial diencephalon via a bundle of nerve fibers known as the fornix. The connections between the hippocampus and the medial diencephalon need to be intact for declarative memories to be stored and retrieved normally. The fornix also links the hippocampus to the septum, which provides it with cholinergic innervation (input from neurons that use acetylcholine for neurotransmitter).

FIGURE 12.8

The medial temporal lobe. The structures of the medial temporal lobe include the hippocampus, perirhinal cortex, entorhinal cortex, parahippocampal cortex, and amygdala.

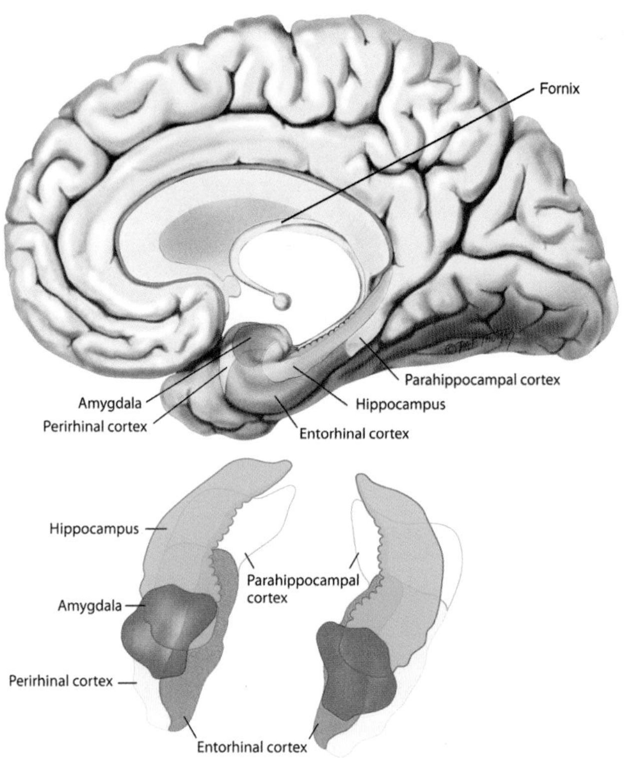

Raslau, F.D., et al. (2015). Memory Part 2: The Role of the Medial Temporal Lobe. *American Journal of Neuroradiology 36*(5): 846–849. Adapted from *Principles of Cognitive Neuroscience*, Purves et al. Sinauer Associates, 2008. With permission from the American Society of Neuroradiology and Oxford University Press.

Much of what we know about the neuroanatomy of long-term memory comes from the study of patients suffering from **amnesia**. Amnesia refers to memory deficits resulting from brain injury or psychological trauma. In this chapter, we focus on cases of amnesia that are due to brain damage. The two main types of brain injury are traumatic brain injury and anoxic/hypoxic brain injury. The brain damage observed in traumatic brain injury can be focalized to a particular brain area, which is what might happen when someone has an accident in which an object penetrates the skull, such as a gunshot wound. The brain damage may also be more diffuse (spread out), such as what happens in someone who suffers a concussion. A concussion occurs when the head undergoes sudden deceleration, causing the brain to move back and forth, hitting the inside of the cranium (Nortje & Menon, 2004). In anoxic/hypoxic brain injury, brain damage results from a total (anoxia) or partial (hypoxia) deprivation of blood to the brain. It is observed in cardiac arrest, strangulation, vascular injury, poisoning, and several other conditions (Lacerte & Mesfin, 2019).

As illustrated in Figure 12.9, two broad types of amnesia can be differentiated on the basis of whether there is memory loss for information acquired before brain damage, which is known as **retrograde amnesia**, or if there is an inability to form new memories since brain damage has occurred, which is known as **anterograde amnesia**. Most of the time, patients with amnesia have both retrograde and anterograde types and the severity of both tends to match, but it can happen that someone has more of one type than the other (Smith, Frascino, Hopkins, & Squire, 2013). In many cases, memories for information acquired shortly before the brain damage are lost, but memories from more remote times are preserved. This is a pattern of retrograde amnesia known as **temporally graded retrograde amnesia**. Whether more remote memories are affected depends on the extent of the brain damage (Rempel-Clower, Zola, Squire, & Amaral, 1996). For example, someone with limited damage may have memory loss for events that occurred three years before the brain damage was sustained but preserved memory for events that occurred longer ago. Another person with more extensive damage may have only childhood memories intact.

A Famous Case Study of Amnesia. Much of what we know about the brain areas that compose memory systems comes from case studies of brain-damaged patients. The most famous of these cases is that of Henry Molaison (1926–2008), known as patient HM. In 1953, HM, who was 27 years old at the time, underwent bilateral surgical removal of the medial temporal lobes—including the hippocampus, amygdala, and parahippocampal cortex (see Figure 12.10a)—to relieve epileptic seizures he had been suffering since the age of 10. After the surgery, the frequency of his seizures diminished greatly. However, following the surgery, neurological testing of HM revealed that he had both severe anterograde amnesia and temporally graded retrograde amnesia extending to his childhood (Scoville & Milner, 1957). This meant that he could no longer form new long-term memories and had a loss of memory for events extending from the time of his surgery back to his childhood. More recent studies, using better testing methods, showed that even his childhood memories were affected (Steinvorth, Levine, & Corkin, 2005).

However, not all types of memories were impaired in HM. He had normal short-term memory. That is, he could remember information as long as he was permitted to rehearse it. The types of memories affected in HM are the subtypes of declarative memories we discussed earlier: semantic and episodic memories. Although HM had memory impairments of both subtypes, his episodic memories were relatively more affected than his semantic memories (Augustinack et al., 2014). Also, HM recognized objects he was previously shown. However, he could only remember them as being familiar but could not recollect how he first encountered them.

The most notable aspect of HM's pattern of memory impairment was that his performance was intact on tasks that required only nondeclarative memory (that is, those retrieved without conscious awareness). These include tasks in which procedural memory, priming, and classical conditioning were tested. One of these tasks is a test of procedural memory known as the mirror tracing task (Figure 12.10b). In this task, participants are required to trace a star by looking only at their drawing hand in a mirror. Sounds easy? It's not. As you can imagine, while looking at

FIGURE 12.9

Two types of amnesia. Retrograde amnesia refers to memory loss for information acquired before brain damage. Anterograde amnesia refers to an inability to form new memories. Note that the most remote memories are preserved.

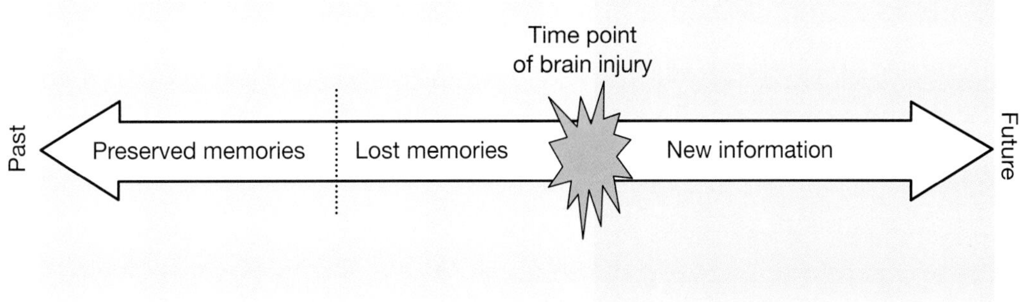

FIGURE 12.10

(a) HM's brain after his surgery (right) compared to a normal brain (left). The structures removed from HM's brain included the hippocampus, amygdala, and parahippocampal region (or gyrus). (b) The mirror tracing task. In this task, patients are required to learn to trace a star pattern by looking only at the reflection of their hand in a mirror (top). The number of errors made by HM in tracing the star pattern across three days. HM's progression in learning the task matched that of normal participants (bottom).

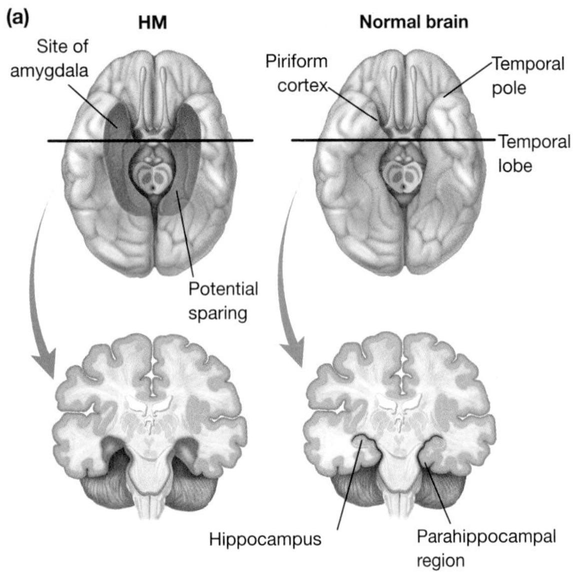

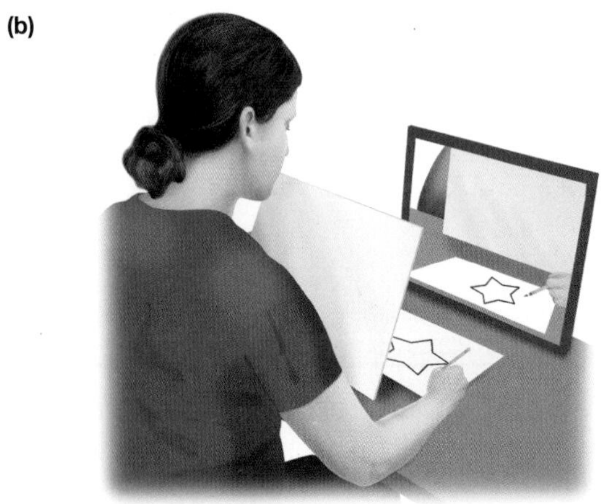

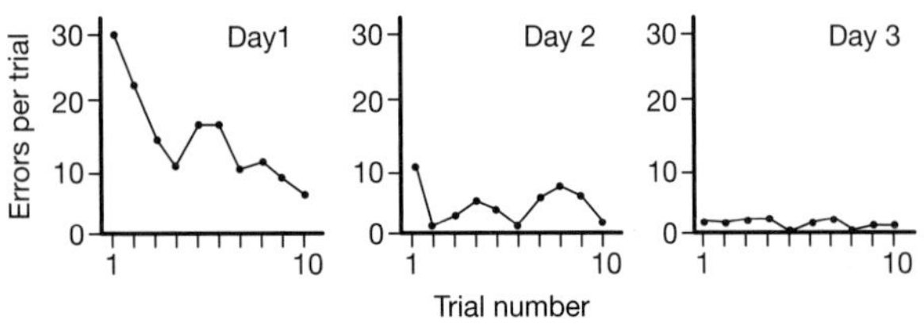

your hand in the mirror, what looks like having to trace a line toward the left has to be translated into moving your hand toward the right and vice versa. However, participants learn to do this quite efficiently with a few days of practice. As can be seen in Figure 12.10b, HM became proficient at the task after two days of practice and made virtually no mistakes on day 3 (Milner, 1972). What was striking was that HM's performance was comparable to that of normal subjects. However, because HM could not form new declarative memories, he never remembered having practiced the task.

The findings obtained from studying HM showed that the hippocampus plays an important role in declarative memory. However, the findings also showed that nondeclarative memories do not depend on the hippocampus.

The Medial Diencephalon. Other regions shown to be important for the storage of declarative memories are those that comprise the medial diencephalon, namely, the mammillary bodies and the thalamus, shown in Figure 12.11. Damage to these regions causes memory deficits similar to the ones observed in HM.

For example, neuroscientist Larry Squire and colleagues reported on a brain-damaged patient known as NA, who was accidentally stabbed by a miniature fencing foil by his friend (Squire, Amaral, Zola-Morgan, Kritchevsky, & Press, 1989; Squire & Moore, 1979). The foil penetrated one of NA's nostrils and perforated his brain. The foil damaged his left dorsomedial thalamus and the mammillary bodies on both sides. He suffered considerable anterograde amnesia as well as some retrograde amnesia. Similarly to HM, NA suffered no impairments of nondeclarative memory.

Psychologist Lawrence Weiskrantz and neuropsychologist Elizabeth Warrington studied several patients who had Korsakoff syndrome (Warrington & Weiskrantz, 1970), which results from years of chronic alcoholism. Because alcohol prevents the absorption of thiamine (vitamin B1), the primary cause of Korsakoff syndrome is thiamine deficiency. Thiamine deficiency results in the deterioration of the dorsomedial thalamus and of the mammillary bodies, the same regions damaged by the miniature fencing foil in NA. The pattern of memory impairment in these patients was similar to that observed in HM and NA, providing further evidence of the implication of the medial diencephalic structures in declarative memory.

Nondeclarative Memory

You have learned in this unit that memory impairments in HM, due to damage to his medial temporal lobes, were limited to declarative memories. You may be wondering what brain areas are

FIGURE 12.11

Regions of the medial diencephalon such as the thalamus and mammillary bodies are thought to be involved in the storage of declarative memories.

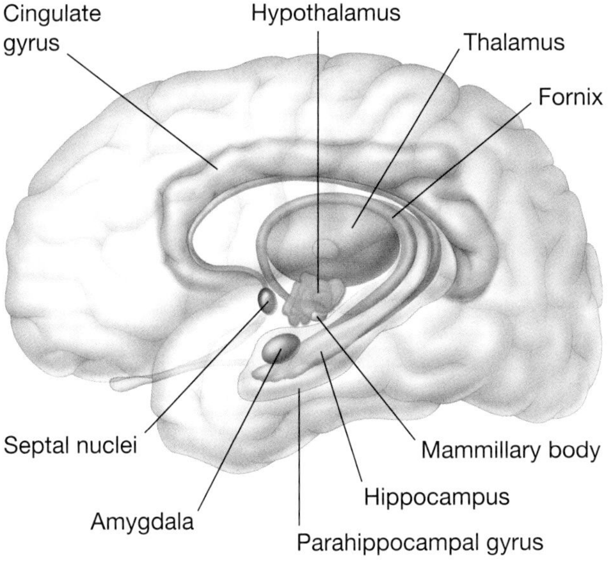

involved in processing nondeclarative memories. In the preceding unit, we briefly discussed classical conditioning, priming, and procedural memories, which are all types of nondeclarative memory. Because of limited space, we cannot engage in a discussion of nondeclarative memory equivalent to that provided for declarative memory. What you need to remember is that each of these types of nondeclarative memory depends on areas located outside of the hippocampus and diencephalon. For example, memories formed through classical conditioning of motor responses were found to depend on circuits of neurons in the cerebellum (Thompson, 1986). Classical conditioning of emotional responses was found to depend on the amygdala (D. T. Cheng, Knight, Smith, Stein, & Helmstetter, 2003; Furmark, Fischer, Wik, Larsson, & Fredrikson, 1997; Maren & Fanselow, 1996) (see Chapter 11). Evidence for the involvement of specific brain areas in priming is less clear. Nevertheless, the brain regions thought to be implicated in priming include the frontal and temporal cortices and relevant sensory cortical areas (Schott et al., 2005). Finally, procedural memories were shown to depend on the basal ganglia, more specifically, the striatum (Mayor-Dubois, Maeder, Zesiger, & Roulet-Perez, 2010; White, 1997).

MODULE SUMMARY

Long-term memory refers to the memory register in which information is stored in a relatively permanent and stable form. There are different types of long-term memories. The main type of long-term memories involves those that are subject to conscious recollection. These are known as declarative or explicit memories. Other types of memories are not retrieved to conscious recollection, but evidence for their existence is seen through the performance of some task. These are known as nondeclarative or implicit memories. Declarative memories include memories for facts, known as semantic memories, and memories for events in one's life, known as episodic memories. Nondeclarative memories include those acquired through classical conditioning, priming, and procedural learning.

The brain areas most important for declarative memories are the hippocampus and surrounding areas. This was discovered through the study of famous brain-damaged patient HM. However, areas of the diencephalon such as the mammillary bodies and the thalamus are also important for declarative memories. This was discovered by the study of patients who sustained brain damage to these regions, either through accidents, such as in patient NA, or as a result of Korsakoff syndrome, which is due to a deficiency in thiamine. Finally, the brain areas important for nondeclarative memories lie outside the hippocampus and diencephalon. Areas involved in classical conditioning include the amygdala for the conditioning of emotional responses and the cerebellum for the conditioning of motor reflexes. Priming is dependent on the frontal and temporal cortices as well as on the relevant sensory cortical areas. Procedural learning is dependent on the basal ganglia.

TEST YOURSELF

12.2.1 Define long-term memory. Name and define the types of long-term memories you learned about in this unit.

12.2.2 Which brain areas are thought to be involved in the types of memories you learned about in this unit?

12.3 Memory Consolidation

Module Contents

Learning Objectives

12.3.1 Define memory consolidation and describe its proposed neurobiological mechanisms.

12.3.2 Describe the main theories of memory consolidation and differentiate between them.

12.3.1 WHAT IS MEMORY CONSOLIDATION?

>> LO 12.3.1 Define memory consolidation and describe its proposed neurobiological mechanisms.

Key Terms

- **Memory consolidation:** The process by which memories go from a temporary and fragile state to a more stable and long-lasting form.
- **Cell assembly:** A group of neurons that fire together in response to a stimulus.
- **Reverberating activity:** The continuous firing of the neurons in a cell assembly.
- **Hebbian modification:** The process by which reverberating activity strengthens the connections between the neurons in a cell assembly.
- **Engram:** The stable representation of the stimuli in the cell assembly.
- **Cellular consolidation:** The early and local (within the same brain area) molecular processes that occur shortly after learning.
- **Systems consolidation:** The reorganization in systems throughout the brain that are involved in the storage of memories.

Memory consolidation refers to the process by which memories go from being in an unstable and fragile state to a more stable and long-lasting form (Squire, Genzel, Wixted, & Morris, 2015). In the first experimental demonstration of memory consolidation, Elias Muller and Alfons Pilzecker, of the University of Gottingen in Germany, had participants learn a list of nonsense syllables. The subjects were then made to learn a second list. Learning the second list interfered with the subjects' memory of the first list; however, learning the second list had no effect on the subjects' memory of the first list if they learned it more than six minutes later. Muller and Pilzecker reasoned that learning the second list too soon after learning the first list interfered with a process that solidified the memory of the syllables on the first list. Once this process was completed, memory for the syllables on the first list was no longer as vulnerable to disruption. They called this process memory consolidation (Muller & Pilzecker, 1900).

Neurobiological Mechanisms of Memory Consolidation

In his book *The Organization of Behavior: A Neuropsychological Theory*, Canadian psychologist Donald Hebb (1949) proposed a way in which short-term memory could be consolidated into long-term memory. He suggested that stimuli excite groups of neurons that fire together, in what he called a **cell assembly** (Figure 12.12a). He called the continuous firing of the neurons within the cell assembly **reverberating activity**. According to Hebb, reverberating activity continues after the stimulus is gone and strengthens the connections between the neurons in the cell assembly. This process became known as **Hebbian modification**, which he suggested formed the basis for short-term memory.

The connections between neurons within the cell assembly are initially fragile and vulnerable to disruption. However, with continued reverberation, the representation of the stimuli in the cell assembly stabilizes in a relatively permanent state he called an **engram**, which Hebb proposed forms the basis for long-term memory (Figure 12.12b). Once information is stored in long-term memory, partial activation of the assembly reactivates the engram that represents the entire stimulus (Figure 12.12c).

Evidence of Memory Consolidation in Animals

In 1949, Carl Duncan published the results of the first experimental demonstration of memory consolidation in animals (Duncan, 1949). To do this, he trained rats to avoid an electrical grid. The rats then received an electroconvulsive shock at different intervals after training. One group of rats received the electroshock 20 seconds after training. Other groups received the electroshock 40 seconds, 1 minute, 4 minutes, or 15 minutes after training. Memory for how to avoid the shock was most affected in the 20-second group and progressively less affected

FIGURE 12.12

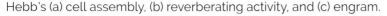

Hebb's (a) cell assembly, (b) reverberating activity, and (c) engram.

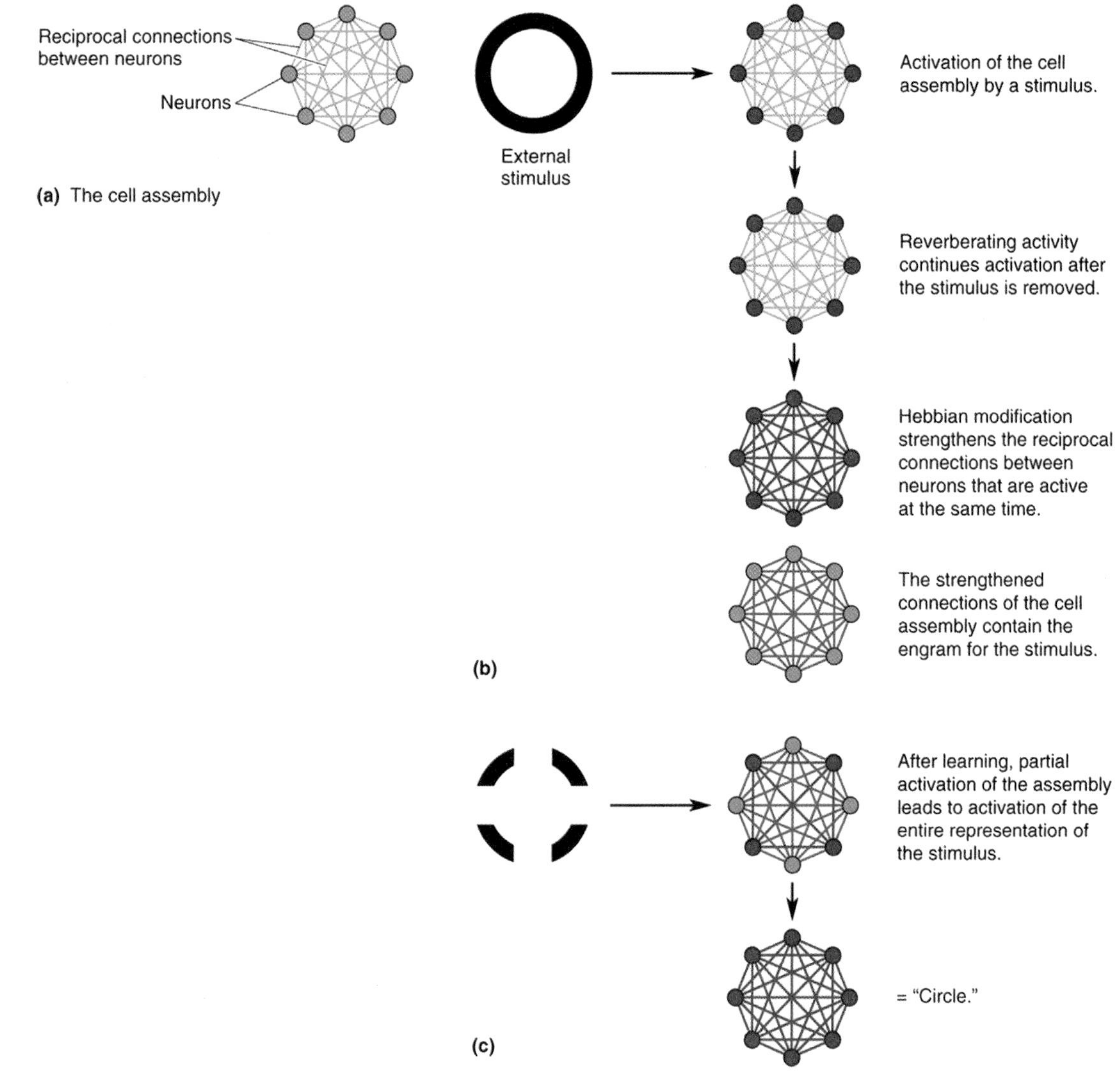
Reciprocal connections between neurons
Neurons
(a) The cell assembly
External stimulus
Activation of the cell assembly by a stimulus.
Reverberating activity continues activation after the stimulus is removed.
Hebbian modification strengthens the reciprocal connections between neurons that are active at the same time.
The strengthened connections of the cell assembly contain the engram for the stimulus.
(b)
After learning, partial activation of the assembly leads to activation of the entire representation of the stimulus.
= "Circle."
(c)

Adapted from *Neuroscience: Exploring the Brain* 4th Edition, Bear, Connors, and Paradiso, 2016..

in the others. The memory for how to avoid the shock in rats that received the electroshock 1 hour, 4 hours, or 14 hours after training was not at all affected. These results confirmed Muller and Pilzecker's observation that new memories require a period of consolidation before being stored in a more permanent form. It also supported Hebb's idea that an initially fragile cell assembly is eventually stored in a relatively permanent engram.

Cellular and Systems Consolidation

Memory consolidation is thought to take place at the cellular and systems levels. **Cellular consolidation** reflects Hebb's idea that short-term memories are represented in the reverberating activity within ensembles of neurons, to then be stabilized as long-term memories in what he called the engram. Accordingly, cellular consolidation refers to the early and local (within the same brain area) molecular processes that occur within hours after learning. At the cellular level, representations of stimuli are first stored in short-term changes at synapses, at which point interfering with the consolidation process is possible. However, over a short period of time, molecular processes, such as the synthesis of new proteins, stabilize memory representations and render them less vulnerable to disruption. Interfering with these processes, by the administration of drugs that inhibit the synthesis of proteins or by other types of manipulation, interferes with cellular consolidation (H. P. Davis & Squire, 1984; Ozawa, Yamada, & Ichitani, 2017). In fact, because of the time frames used in Duncan's experiment, the memory impairments he observed were due to a disruption of cellular consolidation.

Systems consolidation refers to the reorganization in systems that are involved in the storage of memories throughout the brain. In contrast to cellular consolidation, which occurs within minutes and hours after learning, systems consolidation takes place over days, weeks, months, or even years (Squire et al., 2015). The idea that memories undergo systems consolidation to be stored in long-term memory is based on observations that individuals with brain damage sometimes show a gradient of memory loss, in which memories for events that recently preceded the brain damage are lost but those from the more distant past are preserved. As you learned earlier, this pattern of memory loss is known as temporally graded retrograde amnesia (see Figure 12.9). Remember that this is the type of amnesia suffered by brain-damaged patient HM. You also learned that HM's amnesia was due to damage to the hippocampus. Correspondingly, systems consolidation is widely believed to involve interactions between the hippocampus and the cortex. However, the nature of these interactions as well as their mechanisms are still the focus of much debate and theorizing. It is to some of these theories that we turn in the next unit.

12.3.2 THEORIES OF MEMORY CONSOLIDATION

>> LO 12.3.2 Describe the main theories of memory consolidation and differentiate between them.

Key Terms

- **Standard model:** The idea that the hippocampus is needed only temporarily as the cortex gradually stores memories.
- **Multiple-trace theory:** The idea that the hippocampus is always involved in the storage and retrieval of memories.
- **Unified theory (or "C" theory):** The memory consolidation theory in which learning induces cellular consolidation in both the cortex and the hippocampus rapidly and simultaneously.
- **Engram cells:** Neurons that become active during learning and are reactivated with the presentation of cues related to the context of learning.
- **Reconsolidation:** The idea that consolidated memories return to a fragile state when reactivated and require another round of consolidation to be stabilized.

Over the years, neuroscientists have sought to discover the mechanisms by which memories consolidate, that is, how they go from an initially fragile state to be stored in a long-lasting and stable representation. After the findings in patient HM that recent but not remote memories seemed to be dependent on the hippocampus, a case of temporally graded retrograde amnesia, several theories have been put forward to explain how the hippocampus might interact with the cortex in the consolidation of memories. The two most influential of these theories are the standard model and multiple-trace theory.

The Standard Model

According to the **standard model** (Alvarez & Squire, 1994), elements of a memory—such as the cognitive, perceptual, and motor information that composes it—are encoded in groups of neurons, known as cortical modules (see Figure 12.13). These modules are located in widespread areas of the cortex. Initially, the connections between the modules are weak. Over an extended period, which can span weeks, months, or even years, the connections between the modules become stronger (Figure 12.13a) due to repeated reactivations of the memory by the hippocampus, which temporarily stores the memory within networks of neurons. At the same time, the connections between the hippocampus and the modules gradually become weaker (Figure 12.13b). A memory is consolidated once the connections between the cortical modules that represent it have become strong enough so that they can be sustained without the participation of the hippocampus (Figure 12.13c).

How does this explain temporally graded retrograde amnesia? According to the standard model, damage to the hippocampus affects only memories that

FIGURE 12.13

The standard model.

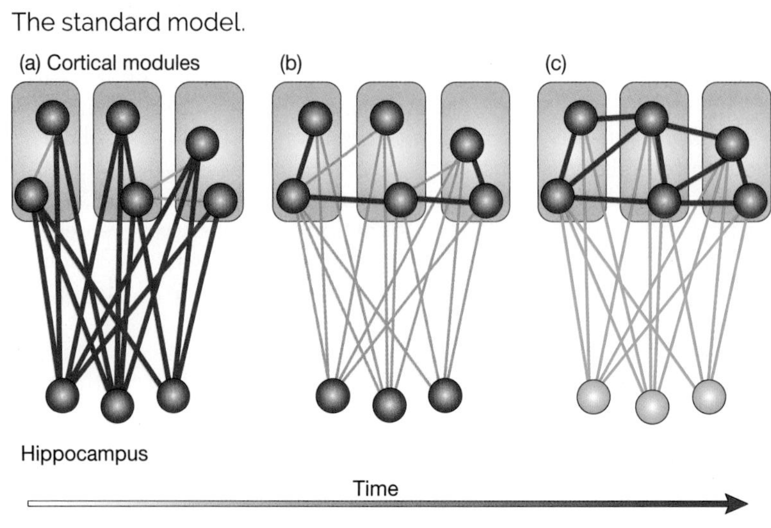

Frankland, P.W. & B. Bontempi (2005). The organization of recent and remote memories. *Nature Reviews Neuroscience* 6(2): 119–130. With permission from Springer Nature.

were acquired shortly before brain damage, because they were still in the process of being stabilized by the hippocampus through its interactions with the cortex. In contrast, remote memories, for which the connections in the cortex have already been stabilized, are spared, because they no longer require their maintenance by the hippocampus. According to the proponents of the standard model, this applies equally to semantic and episodic memories.

Multiple-Trace Theory

In contrast to the standard model, **multiple-trace theory**, illustrated in Figure 12.14, states that the hippocampus is always involved in the storage and retrieval of episodic memories, regardless of their age, that is, whether they were formed recently before brain damage or at more remote periods (Nadel & Moscovitch, 1997). According to this theory, the hippocampus is thought to process the spatial and temporal contexts in which memories are formed.

As in the standard model, the proponents of multiple-trace theory believe that the elements of memories are represented in cortical modules and that these modules are bound through repeated reactivations by the hippocampus. However, in multiple-trace theory, each reactivation of a memory, through its retrieval, creates a new trace of the memory that contains the spatial and temporal contexts in which the memory was reactivated, a process thought to depend on the hippocampus. For example, if I am reminded of a trip to Arizona while sitting at a restaurant, a new trace to the memory of the trip is created that also includes the memory of the restaurant. Therefore, the next time I am in that restaurant or even think about it, I may be reminded of my trip to Arizona.

According to multiple-trace theory, the temporary involvement of the hippocampus in the consolidation of memories proposed by the standard model applies only to semantic memories. This is because semantic memories can be retrieved devoid of the spatial and temporal contexts in which they were acquired (see Unit 12.2.1 to review the difference between episodic and semantic memories).

How does multiple-trace theory account for temporally graded retrograde amnesia? The answer is that remote memories are preserved because it is likely that many more traces have been associated with them through their reactivation over time than is the case for recent memories. This renders remote memories more resistant than recent memories to hippocampal damage. For remote memories to be affected, more extensive damage to the hippocampus is necessary. For example, with destruction of the entire hippocampus, both recent and remote episodic memories are lost, resulting in what is known as a flat gradient of memory loss.

More Recent Consolidation Theories

Although the standard model and multiple-trace theory have influenced memory research for decades, other theories have since been put forward (Dash, Hebert, & Runyan, 2004; Maguire, 2014; Runyan, Moore, & Dash, 2019; Teyler & Rudy, 2007; Tse et al., 2007). Some researchers have found that the standard model and multiple-trace theory do not account for some aspects of experimental findings. In a theory known as the **unified theory (or "C" theory)** (Dash et al., 2004), the storage of explicit memories (memories for facts and events) occurs simultaneously in both the hippocampus and the cortex through rapid cellular consolidation within networks of neurons known as **engram cells**. In contrast to the standard model, this is believed to occur over a period of hours or days, rather than weeks, months, or years.

Within this framework, the hippocampus is initially important for memory retrieval by sending and receiving input to and from the cortex to reactivate engram cells within which the components of memories are stored. However, once engram cells in the cortex have grown stable connections, the reactivation of the networks they formed occurs through the presentation of cues related to the context of learning.

Kitamura et al. (2017) found evidence for the unified theory. In this study, mice were subjected to contextual fear conditioning (see Chapter 11). During learning, or encoding (Figure 12.15a), engram

FIGURE 12.14

Multiple-trace theory. (a) The retrieval of semantic memories, which are devoid of spatial context, becomes independent of the hippocampus over time. (b) The retrieval of episodic memories, which include the spatial and temporal contexts in which they are retrieved, remains dependent on the hippocampus.

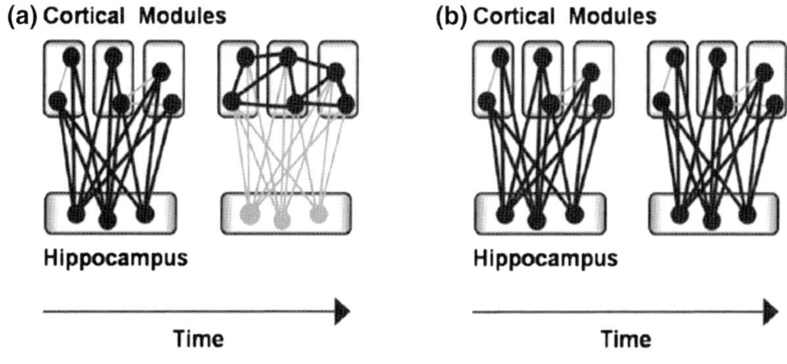

Akers, K.G. & P.W. Frankland. (2008). Grading Gradients: Evaluating Evidence for Time-dependent Memory Reorganization in Experimental Animals. *Journal of Experimental Neuroscience 2009*(2). With permission from SAGE.

FIGURE 12.15

Evidence for the unified theory (or "C" theory) of memory consolidation. BLA = basolateral amygdala; HPC = hippocampus; MEC = medial entorhinal cortex; PFC = prefrontal cortex.

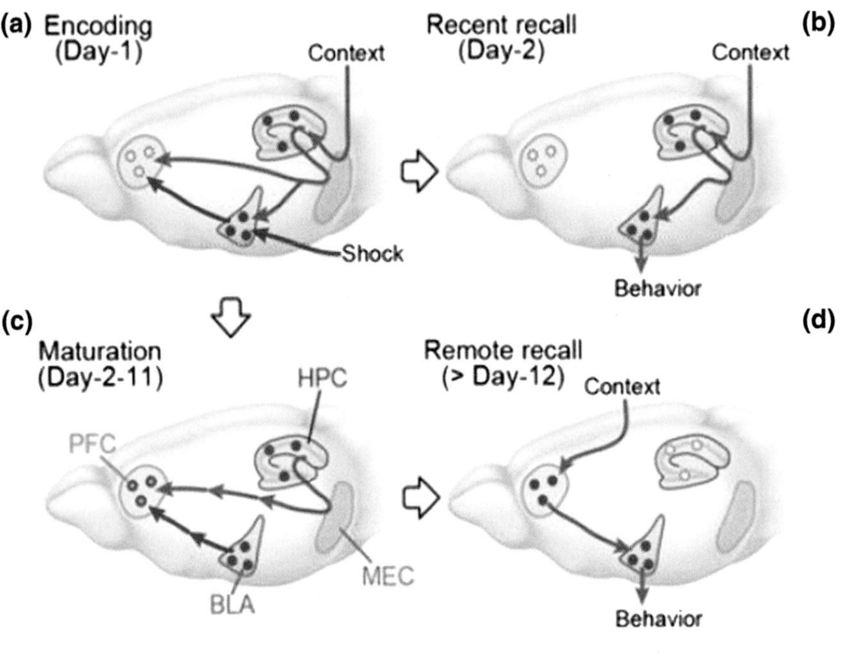

Kitamura, T., et al. (2017). Engrams and circuits crucial for systems consolidation of a memory. *Science 356*(6333): 73–78. With permission from AAAS.

cells became activated in the hippocampus, medial prefrontal cortex, and basolateral amygdala over approximately the same amount of time. At first (recent recall), cortical engram cells were not activated by cues associated with the context of learning (Figure 12.15b). However, they became progressively more involved in the retrieval of the context over the next 2–11 days (maturation). Their activity was still being coordinated by input from the hippocampus, through its connections with the entorhinal cortex (Figure 12.15c). Finally, from day 12 onward (remote recall), engram cells in the cortex became activated by exposure to the context of learning without input from the hippocampus (Figure 12.15d).

Reconsolidation

Reconsolidation refers to the idea that when consolidated memories are retrieved, they can return to the fragile and unstable state they were in before consolidation. This means that when memories are retrieved, they need to go through the consolidation process again, hence, the term *reconsolidation*. This phenomenon was demonstrated in studies performed in the 1960s. In one study (Misanin, Miller, & Lewis, 1968), different groups of rats were placed in a chamber, equipped with a water spout, in which they learned to associate a white noise, which served as a conditioned stimulus (CS), with a foot shock (the unconditioned stimulus). Rats demonstrated that they learned this association by showing a fear reaction—diminishing the rate at which they licked the spout—when exposed again to the CS (the conditioned response). One group of rats received an electroconvulsive shock (ECS) through metal ear clips immediately after the white noise–foot shock pairing. This treatment was meant to induce retrograde amnesia. Indeed, rats that received ECS immediately after the pairing did not significantly reduce their lick rate when exposed to the CS, showing that they did not remember the association between the CS and the foot shock. However, rats that received the ECS 24 hours after the white noise–foot shock pairing diminished their lick rate significantly, showing that the memory for the pairing had been consolidated (i.e., it was no longer fragile or vulnerable to disruption). Another group of rats also received ECS 24 hours after the pairing. However, these rats were exposed to the CS shortly before they received the ECS. The purpose of this manipulation was to reactivate the memory that they received a foot shock shortly after hearing the CS.

The most important finding was that the rats in which the memory of the shock was reactivated by the CS briefly before the ECS did not diminish their lick rate when exposed again to the CS. This showed that the reactivation of the memory of receiving a foot shock by the exposure to the CS returned it to the same fragile state as it was in the rats that received the ECS immediately after the foot shock. This suggested that even consolidated memories can be vulnerable to disruption if reactivated just before receiving an amnestic treatment such as ECS. This finding has been replicated in many studies with various types of memories and amnestic treatments in both humans and animals (Haubrich & Nader, 2018; Sara, 2010). For example, the reconsolidation of a conditioned fear in rats has also been blocked by the administration, after reactivation, of drugs that block the synthesis of protein (protein synthesis inhibitors), which is necessary for the long-lasting synaptic changes that lead to the formation of long-term memories (Nader, Schafe, & Le Doux, 2000). In humans, the amnestic treatments often comprised various behavioral tasks that interfered with the reconsolidation of previously learned information. For example, in one study, the consolidated memory for a list of objects was reactivated and blocked from reconsolidation by the learning of a new list (Hupbach,

Gomez, Hardt, & Nadel, 2007). In another study, the consolidated memory for a finger-tapping pattern was blocked from reconsolidation by the learning of a new pattern (Walker, Brakefield, Hobson, & Stickgold, 2003).

The updating of memories through memory reconsolidation occurs on a daily basis. For example, imagine that, from what you can remember, your professor said it was not necessary to include references at the end of your paper. However, while in conversation with one of your classmates, you are reminded of the paper being due. Next, your friend mentions that a reference list at the end of the paper is, in fact, mandatory. Because the memory of the paper being due was reactivated, you now reconsolidate the memory, updated with the fact that references are mandatory. To use a computer analogy, reactivation is similar to clicking on the icon that opens the file containing one of your assignments. This allows you to update the file by making changes to it. Once you click "save," the file is stored again containing the new information.

MODULE SUMMARY

Memory consolidation refers to the process by which memories go from a temporary and fragile state to a more stable and long-lasting form. The first experimental demonstration of memory consolidation was from Muller and Pilzecker in the early 1900s. A cellular mechanism for memory consolidation was proposed by psychologist Donald Hebb. He thought that neurons fired together with the presentation of a stimulus in what he called a cell assembly. He called continuous firing of the cells reverberating activity, which formed the basis of short-term memory. He also thought that this reverberating activity eventually settled into what he called an engram, which he thought formed the basis for long-term memory.

Memory consolidation takes place at two levels: at the cellular level, in what is called cellular consolidation, and at the systems levels, which is known as systems consolidation. Consistent with Hebb's idea, information is first stored as local changes at synapses and is then stored by more lasting changes that require protein synthesis over a short period. In contrast, systems consolidation occurs over a comparatively long period and involves interactions between the hippocampus and the cortex.

Different theories exist to explain how these interactions occur. The two most influential theories are the standard model, according to which the hippocampus is involved only temporarily in the retrieval of declarative memories, both semantic and episodic, and multiple-trace theory, according to which the hippocampus is always involved in the retrieval of episodic but not semantic memories regardless of their age. According to a newer theory, the unified theory (or "C" theory), changes in the hippocampus and in the cortex occur rapidly and simultaneously until contextual memories can eventually be retrieved without the participation of the hippocampus. Another idea is that even consolidated memories can become fragile and vulnerable to disruption if reactivated shortly before an amnestic treatment. This means that after reactivation, memories have to undergo consolidation again, in what is known as reconsolidation.

TEST YOURSELF

12.3.1 (a) Explain the concept of memory consolidation and the first experiment demonstrating it. (b) Explain cellular and systems consolidation by outlining the differences between them.

12.3.2 Describe the main memory consolidation theories. Explain how each accounts for the consolidation of memories.

12.4 Navigating Through Space: Spatial Memory

Module Contents

Learning Objectives

12.4.1 Define spatial memory and explain how the hippocampus is involved in processing spatial information.

12.4.2 Describe the different types of cells involved in processing spatial information.

12.4.3 Explain how the role of the hippocampus and associated areas in spatial and nonspatial memory can be differentiated.

12.4.1 WHAT IS SPATIAL MEMORY? THE HIPPOCAMPUS AS A NAVIGATIONAL DEVICE

>> LO 12.4.1 Define spatial memory and explain how the hippocampus is involved in processing spatial information.

Key Terms

- **Spatial memory:** The encoding, storage, and retrieval of spatial information that results in successful navigation toward goals in the environment.
- **Cognitive map:** A map within the brains of animals that stores associations among environmental cues.
- **Eight-arm radial maze:** A maze consisting of an octagonal central platform with an arm radiating from each side.
- **Morris water maze:** A pool of water in which animals search for a submerged platform.

Spatial memory refers to the encoding, storage, and retrieval of spatial information that results in successful navigation toward goals in the environment, using a combination of spatial cues. In the 1940s, Edward C. Tolman proposed that place is not defined by single environmental cues but by a **cognitive map** within the brains of animals, which stores the association of cues to one another (Tolman, 1948). In a classic demonstration of cognitive mapping, Tolman trained rats to reach a goal box by following a specific path. Then the original path was blocked and a set of 18 arms radiating from the start position replaced the original maze. Remarkably, the rats chose the arm that led most directly to the original location of the goal box significantly more often than any other arm. This showed that the rats had information about the location of the goal box in the spatial environment because they never learned to get to the food that way. This is similar to what happens when someone comes to a roadblock while driving around town. With good knowledge of the general layout of the neighborhood (a cognitive map), the driver can find a way around the roadblock that will

FIGURE 12.16

Top left: A rat in a radial maze. radial maze. Top right: The Morris water maze. A wading pool, placed in a room, contains several spatial cues. Bottom left: rat (or mouse) is placed in the water from various starting locations and eventually finds the submerged platform, which is hidden from view. For the first few trials, the rat follows a circuitous path toward the platform. Bottom right: After several training trials, the rat follows a straight path to the platform, showing that it has learned the location of the platform relative to the spatial cues present in the room.

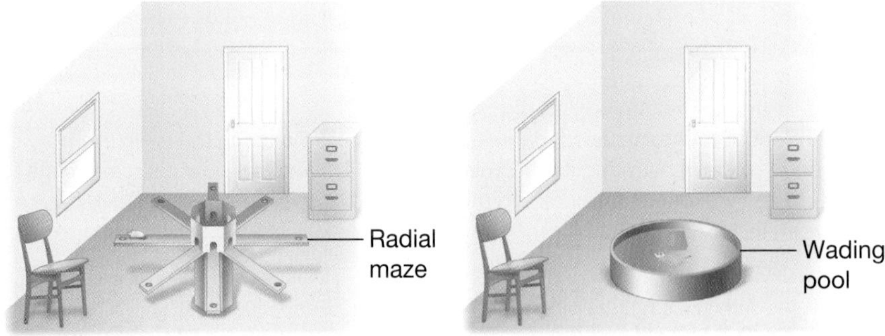

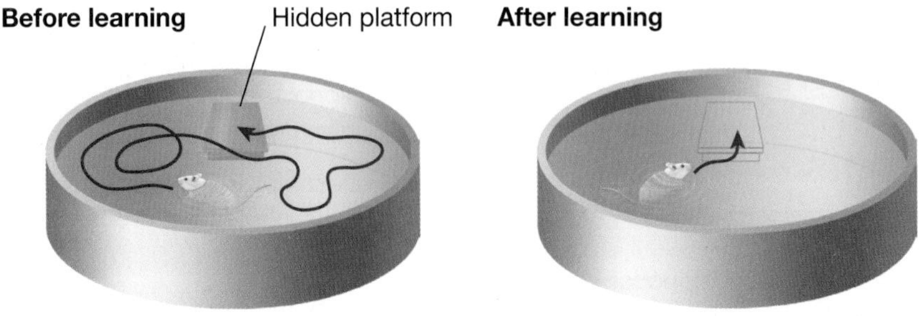

Carolina Hrejsa/Body Scientific Intl.

lead to the proper destination. Over the years, it became widely accepted that the formation of a cognitive map of space involves the hippocampus.

Much of the evidence for the role played by the hippocampus in memory comes from studies of the effects of damage to the hippocampus on spatial memory. To do this, researchers devised a wide range of tasks to test spatial memory in rats. Two of the most widely used tasks to assess spatial memory in rodents are the radial maze and the Morris water maze (Figure 12.16 [top left and top right, respectively]).

In the 1970s, David Olton devised an **eight-arm radial maze** consisting of an octagonal central platform with an arm radiating from each side. The maze was placed in the center of a room, which contained an array of spatial cues. A food pellet was placed at the end of each arm and a hungry rat was placed at the center of the maze and given free access to all arms. Rats learned to retrieve all of the food pellets on the maze without returning to an arm they had already visited (Olton & Samuelson, 1976). This presumably occurred because the rats had learned the spatial location the arms relative to the cues in the room.

In the 1980s, neuroscientist Richard Morris (1984) and Canadian researchers Ian Whishaw, Bryan Kolb, and Robert Sutherland (Sutherland, Kolb, & Whishaw, 1982) devised a task in which rats (or other animals) can be trained to use spatial cues to find a platform submerged in a pool of water. The task devised by Morris became known as the **Morris water maze**. In the Morris water maze task, rats (or mice) are placed in a wading pool that contains a hidden platform. The platform is hidden because the water is made opaque with nontoxic paint or powdered milk. The pool is located in a room that contains several cues (Figure 12.16, right a). When placed in the pool, rats swim around in a circuitous path until they accidentally bump into the platform and get a reprieve from being in the water by standing on it (Figure 12.16, right b). After several trials, the rats are able to reach the platform in a straight path, indicating that they have learned the location of the platform (Figure 12.16, right c). The rats can do this regardless of their starting position. This means they could not learn to get to the platform by making a habitual turn to the left or to the right. Instead, the rats have to learn the location of the platform relative to spatial cues in the room.

As mentioned earlier, rats with experimentally induced hippocampal damage are significantly impaired in the performance of these tasks. In the eight-arm radial maze, rats with hippocampal damage repeatedly return to arms they have already visited and gotten the food from, showing that they have difficulty remembering the location of the arms relative to spatial cues (Olton & Papas, 1979). In a water maze, rats with hippocampal lesions have difficulty finding the platform in a wading pool, showing that they cannot locate it relative to the cues present in the room (R. Morris, 1984; Sutherland, Kolb, & Whishaw, 1982). The importance of the hippocampus in spatial learning has been replicated in many different studies, using different types of tasks (R. E. Clark, Broadbent, & Squire, 2005; Gaskin, Tardif, & Mumby, 2011; Mumby, Gaskin, Glenn, Schramek, & Lehmann, 2002).

12.4.2 CELLS FOR SPACE: AN INTERNAL GPS

>> LO 12.4.2 Describe the different types of cells involved in processing spatial information.

Key Terms

- **Place cells:** Cells located in the hippocampus that indicate a rat's position in its environment.
- **Head-direction cells:** Cells located in the subiculum and other brain areas that indicate the orientation of the rat's head.
- **Grid cells:** Cells located in the entorhinal cortex that record the metrics of space.
- **Border cells:** Cells that record the location of boundaries in the rats' environment.

In their book *The Hippocampus as a Cognitive Map*, John O'Keefe and Lynn Nadel (1978) proposed that the hippocampus is necessary for the formation of cognitive maps that result from learning about spatial relationships among cues in the environment. These learned relationships may then be used to locate important stimuli such as food.

The initial evidence for the role of the hippocampus in spatial learning comes from electrical recordings made of its cells (Figure 12.17a). These cells, originally discovered by O'Keefe and Nadel, are known as **place cells**. In addition to place cells, researchers have discovered other types of cells located in areas related to the hippocampus that process various features of the spatial environment. These different types of cells and their locations are illustrated in Figure 12.17 and briefly discussed in the sections that follow.

Place Cells

The most striking evidence that rats possess a cognitive map of space is the presence of place cells in the hippocampus (Figure 12.17b). A subset of these cells increase their firing rate (shown as red squares that represent spikes in the figure) when a rat finds itself in a familiar area within an environment, showing that place cells contribute to a sense of location. The areas in which the cells become active are known as place fields.

Head-Direction Cells

Head-direction cells provide rats with information about heading and orientation. They fire according to the orientation of the rat's head. A subset of those

FIGURE 12.17

(a) Set-up for recording the activity of cells in the brain of a rat. (b–e) The pattern of activity in each type of cell (see text for details).

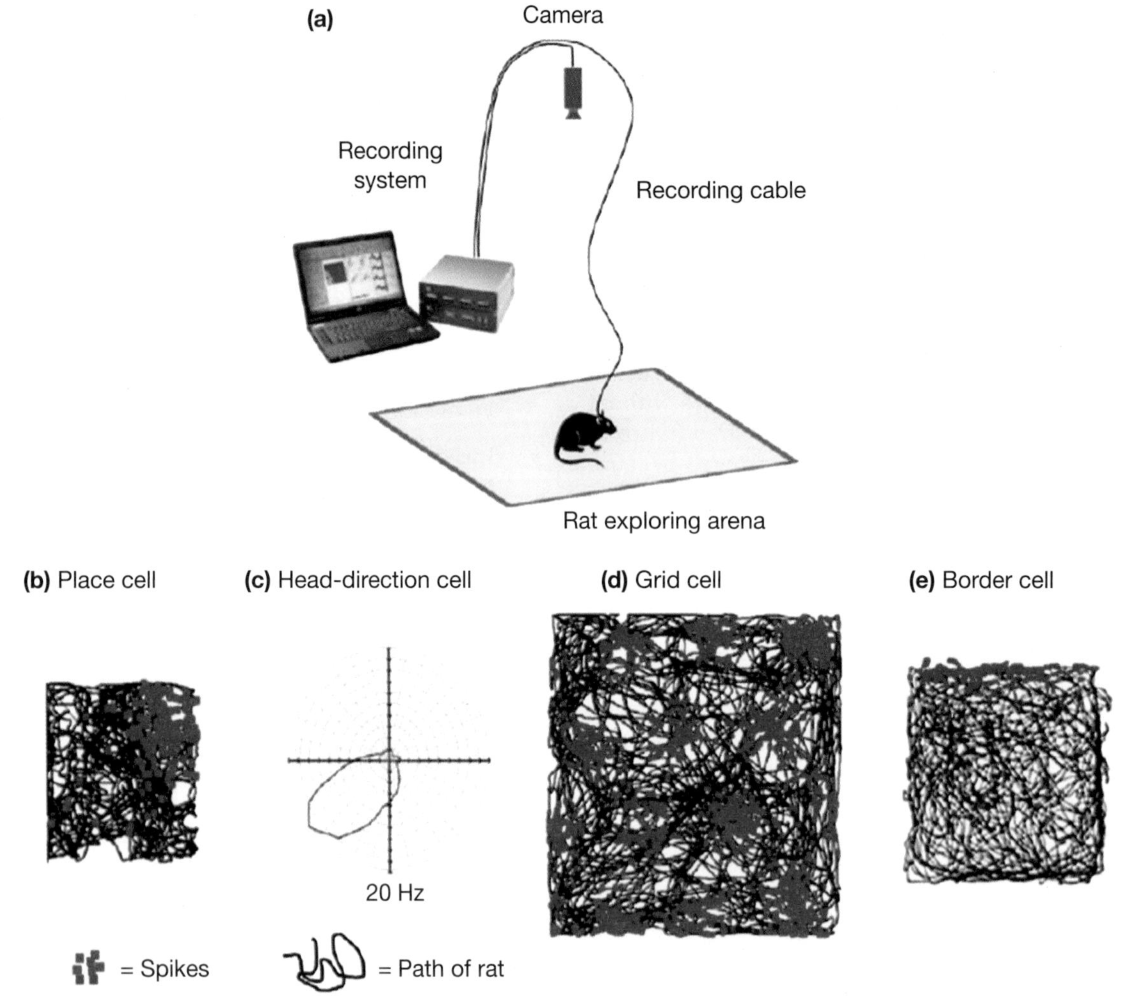

Marozzi, E. & K.J. Jeffery. (2012). Place, space and memory cells. *Current Biology 22*(22): R939–R942. With permission from Elsevier.

cells fire only when the rat's head is pointed in a specific direction independent of the rat's location. Figure 12.17c shows their frequency of firing in relation to the direction in which the rat's head is pointed. These cells are located mainly in the subiculum but are also present in other areas such as the thalamus and the striatum (Taube, Muller, & Ranck, 1990; Wiener & Taube, 2005).

Grid Cells

Grid cells fire at equal intervals as a rat moves through space. These cells record distance as rats traverse the cells' place fields that tile the floor at equal intervals not unlike the squares on graph paper (Figure 12.17d). Grid cells are located in the entorhinal cortex (Hafting, Fyhn, Molden, Moser, & Moser, 2005; Moser, Kropff, & Moser, 2008; Solstad, Moser, & Einevoll, 2006).

Border Cells

Border cells record the location of boundaries in the rats' environment (Figure 12.17e). These boundaries include walls, ridges, and various objects. Like head-direction cells, border cells are recorded in the subiculum (Barry et al., 2006; Lever, Burton, Jeewajee, O'Keefe, & Burgess, 2009; Zhang, Schonfeld, Wiskott, & Manahan-Vaughan, 2014).

Putting It All Together

Taken together, the existence of place cells, head-direction cells, grid cells, and border cells shows that the brain has an efficient system to represent location, direction and orientation, distance, and enclosure, respectively. This also means that the brain really does, in some way, contain a cognitive map of space as suggested by O'Keefe and Nadel. As an analogy, the brain

FIGURE 12.18

(a) MRI image of the right posterior hippocampus of a taxi driver. (b) Correlation between gray matter volume and years of experience driving a taxi in London.

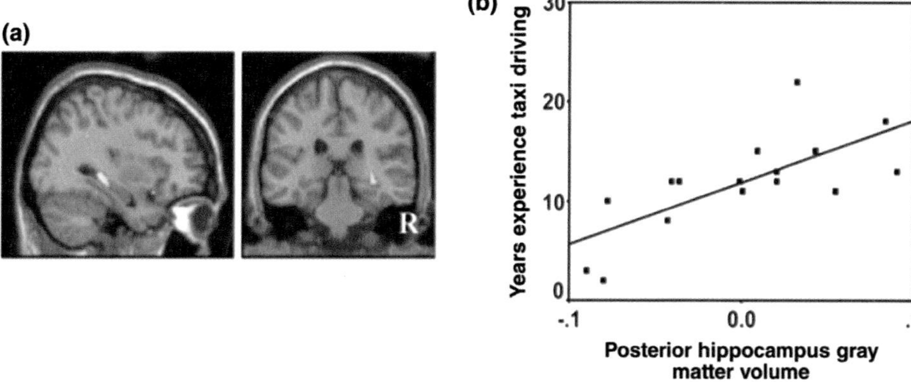

Maguire, E. A., K. Woollett & H.J. Spiers. (2006). London taxi drivers and bus drivers: a structural MRI and neuropsychological analysis. *Hippocampus, 16*(12): 1091–1101. With permission from John Wiley & Sons.

can be said to have its very own global positioning system (GPS). The discovery of this navigational system of the brain earned John O'Keefe, May-Britt Moser, and Edvard Moser the 2014 Nobel Prize in Physiology or Medicine (Burgess, 2014).

Spatial Memory and the Hippocampus in Humans

You may be wondering if humans also use their hippocampi for spatial memory. The answer is a resounding yes. Psychologist Eleanor Maguire and colleagues studied the brains of London taxi drivers to find out whether their hippocampi differed in some way from those of people who do not drive taxis (Maguire, Woollett, & Spiers, 2006).

Why London taxi drivers? To become a London taxi driver, candidates must pass stringent tests. They have to become experts at the spatial layout of London streets, which is extremely complex. They also have to know the locations of thousands of landmarks. Therefore, they made excellent subjects in which to investigate the role of the hippocampus in spatial memory. As shown in Figure 12.18, Maguire and colleagues found that the volume of gray matter in the posterior hippocampi of London taxi drivers increased with the number of years spent driving a taxi. This was not found in bus drivers, who follow predetermined routes and, thus, do not require input from the hippocampus.

What about place cells? Using functional magnetic resonance imaging (fMRI) especially tuned to analyze activity in the hippocampus, the same researchers were able to tell in which of four rooms subjects were situated just by looking at the patterns of activity in their hippocampal neurons (O'Keefe, Burgess, Donnett, Jeffery, & Maguire, 1998). This suggests that, just like in rats, we have cells that are specialized for encoding our spatial locations. However, it is not yet known if these are the exact same kind of cells.

IT'S A MYTH!

Cannabis Is Harmless

The Myth

Possibly the most persistent myth surrounding the use of drugs is that cannabis is harmless.

Why Is the Myth Wrong?

The idea that cannabis is harmless is completely bogus. Scientific evidence shows that the frequent use of cannabis can lead to a variety of health problems, including cognitive dysfunctions such as impaired judgment, memory deficits, and slowed reaction time (Bossong, Jager, Bhattacharyya, & Allen, 2014; Schoeler & Bhattacharyya, 2013). These cognitive dysfunctions can lead to poor decision making, poor academic performance (Phillips, Phillips, Lalonde, & Tormohlen, 2015), and impaired driving (Busardo, Pellegrini, Klein, &

(Continued)

(Continued)

di Luca, 2017). In fact, cannabis use doubles the chances of being involved in a vehicular accident (Asbridge, Hayden, & Cartwright, 2012). Cannabis use during adolescence may, in combination with genetic and environmental factors, increase the risk of developing schizophrenia and other mental health problems (Chadwick, Miller, & Hurd, 2013). The consumption of cannabis can also lead to various other health problems (Meier et al., 2016; Subbaraman & Kerr, 2018). Also, contrary to popular belief, cannabis is indeed addictive (Volkow, Baler, Compton, & Weiss, 2014). One of the most concerning aspects of frequent cannabis use is that the adolescent brain, which is still in a period of development, is particularly vulnerable to the neurotoxic effects of cannabis (Meruelo, Castro, Cota, & Tapert, 2017). In addition, a pregnant woman's cannabis use can significantly affect the health of her fetus; this includes low birth weight and long-term physical and mental health problems (Gunn et al., 2016).

Cannabis and Memory

The effects of cannabis on memory have been studied for decades (Deahl, 1991). The kinds of memories that have mostly been associated with the effects of cannabis are declarative memories (i.e., memories for facts and events of one's life). More specifically, researchers have focused on working memory. To investigate the effects of cannabis on memory and the brain, researchers have tested its effects using a range of memory tasks and brain scans. Frequent users of cannabis have been found to have various degrees of memory impairments. However, the extent to which memory impairments are observed depends on the age at which the subject started to use cannabis. For example, in one study, students who started using cannabis when approaching or during adulthood did not experience as noticeable memory deficits as students who started using cannabis at a younger age (e.g., at age 14 or 15), in which memory impairments were significant. This means that the earlier one starts using cannabis, the worse the outcome on memory performance. This can of course result in a significant negative impact on academic performance (Schuster, Hoeppner, Evins, & Gilman, 2016). The good news, however, is that the impact of cannabis on learning is reduced greatly after one has quit using it (Schuster et al., 2018).

In another study, researchers used fMRI to investigate the effects of cannabis on adolescent brain development. Adolescents who used cannabis had reduced functional connectivity in frontal brain areas such as the anterior cingulate cortex (ACC) and frontal gyrus as well as between the ACC and the dorsolateral prefrontal cortex over time compared to control participants. Cannabis users also had lower IQ scores and slowed cognitive function (Camchong, Lim, & Kumra, 2017). ●

12.4.3 THE HIPPOCAMPUS AND NONSPATIAL MEMORY

>> LO 12.4.3 Explain how the role of the hippocampus and associated areas in spatial and nonspatial memory can be differentiated.

Key Terms

- **Delayed nonmatching-to-sample (DNMS) task:** A test used to assess object-recognition memory.
- **Delayed nonmatching-to-place (DNMP) task:** A test used to assess spatial memory.
- **Novel-object-preference (NOP) paradigm:** Object-recognition memory test that takes advantage of an animal's preference for novelty.

The medial temporal lobes comprise several areas: the hippocampus (including the CA-cell fields, dentate gyrus, and subiculum), the entorhinal cortex, the perirhinal cortex, and the parahippocampal gyrus. There is some question as to whether these regions, which are closely associated with the hippocampus, play different roles in memory. In the 1990s, neuroscientist Elizabeth Murray and colleagues set out to answer this question (Meunier, Bachevalier, Mishkin, & Murray, 1993). To do so, they studied the performance of monkeys with damage to either the hippocampus or the perirhinal cortex on different types of tasks: one that assesses object-recognition memory and the other that assesses spatial memory. To assess object-recognition memory, they tested monkeys in what is known as the **delayed nonmatching-to-sample (DNMS) task**, which consists of three phases (Figure 12.19). In the first phase, the monkey is presented with an object, which covers one of two food wells (Figure 12.19a [the sample object, which on this trial is a key]). Displacing the object reveals a food reward located at the bottom of the well it covers. The wells and the object are then hidden from view for a delay period.

Next, the monkey is again presented with the object, but this time it is accompanied by an object the monkey has never seen before (Figure 12.19b [the blue bowl]), which is now the one that covers the well that contains the food. After several trials, in which new pairs of objects are used, the monkey learns to displace the new object (the blue bowl) to get the food reward. This is taken as evidence for object recognition because, to learn the nonmatching rule (i.e., always pick the object that does not match the sample), the monkey has to recognize the sample object. Murray found that damage to the hippocampus did not impair the monkey's performance in this

FIGURE 12.19

The delayed nonmatching-to-sample task.

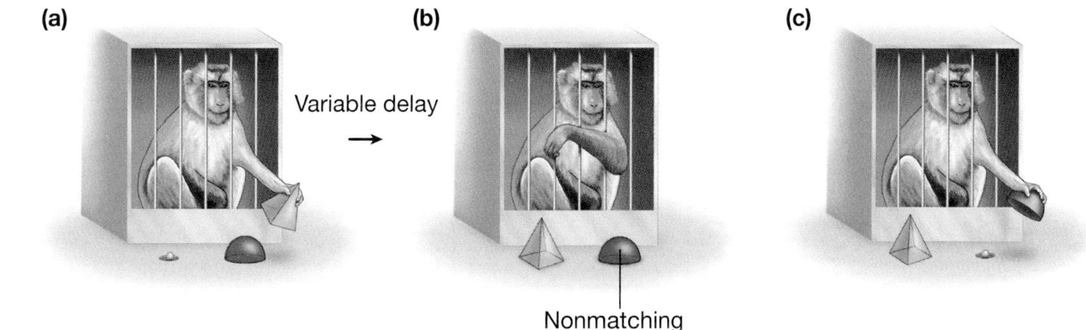

Amanda Tomasikiewicz/Body Scientific Intl.

task. However, monkeys with damage to the perirhinal cortex were impaired.

Spatial memory in the monkeys was assessed in a similar task known as the **delayed nonmatching-to-place task (DNMP)**. In this task, monkeys are rewarded for choosing an identical copy of the sample object that is now covering a different food well, indicating that the monkeys could remember where the sample object was located. In this version of the task, Murray observed the opposite set of results. Monkeys with damage to the hippocampus were impaired, whereas monkeys with damage to the perirhinal cortex performed as well as monkeys with no brain damage.

Object-recognition memory can also be tested using what is known as the **novel-object-preference (NOP) paradigm**, sometimes known as the visual paired-comparison (VPC) test or the novel-object-recognition test. In the NOP paradigm, rats are placed in an open field and permitted to explore two identical copies of a sample object. After a delay, the rats are presented with a single copy of the sample object along with one it has never seen before (novel object). When left to freely explore, normal rats, because of their fondness for novelty, spend more time investigating the novel object than the one they have already seen. This is taken as evidence for object recognition because, to show a preference for the novel object, rats presumably have to recognize the sample object.

Rats with lesions of the hippocampus have been found to be impaired in this test, indicating that the hippocampus may be important for object-recognition memory. However, whether rats with lesions of the hippocampus are impaired in the NOP paradigm may depend on the way in which the rats are tested. That is, when lesions of the hippocampus were made before the rats were trained (i.e., before they learned about the sample objects), the impairment in object recognition was either mild or nonexistent. However, when the rats received lesions of the hippocampus in between training and testing, a more convincing impairment in objection-recognition memory was observed (N. J. Broadbent, Gaskin, Squire, & Clark, 2010; Gaskin, Tremblay, & Mumby, 2003; Mumby et al., 2002). You should be able to recognize here that lesions of the hippocampus made before the rats were trained were meant to model anterograde amnesia, whereas lesions made after training were meant to model retrograde amnesia. Can you explain why?

MODULE SUMMARY

Spatial memory refers to the encoding, storage, and retrieval of spatial information that results in successful navigation toward goals in the environment. The hippocampus is widely believed to store a cognitive map of space, which permits navigation in the environment. Several types of tasks were designed to test spatial memory in animals. Damage to the hippocampus impairs the performance of rats in these tasks, showing that the hippocampus is important for spatial learning and memory. Evidence for the role of the hippocampus in spatial memory also comes from the observation that rats have hippocampal cells (called place cells) that are activated when a rat finds itself in a familiar area.

Other types of cells that process spatial information were also found in rats in areas closely related to the hippocampus. These are head-direction cells, grid cells, and border cells. The important role played by the hippocampus in spatial memory was also found in humans, for example, London taxi drivers, who must pass a stringent test on the spatial layout of London as well as the location of many landmarks in order to get their taxi license. London taxi drivers had more gray matter in the hippocampus, compared to bus drivers, who follow predetermined routes. In monkeys, it was found that object-recognition memory is not dependent on the hippocampus. However, rats displayed either mild or no anterograde amnesia but convincing retrograde amnesia in the novel-object-preference paradigm, which is a test of object-recognition memory.

TEST YOURSELF

12.4.1 What is meant by spatial memory? What brain structure seems to be the most important for spatial memory?

12.4.2 What types of cells are involved in spatial memory? What does each type of cell do?

12.4.3 Which two types of memories are involved in a controversy regarding the functions of the hippocampus? How are they tested, and what was done to differentiate both types?

12.5 Learning: The Acquisition of Memories

Module Contents

Learning Objectives

12.5.1 Define learning and explain the different ways in which learning can occur.

12.5.2 Describe nonassociative learning and its neurobiological basis.

12.5.3 Describe associative learning and its neurobiological basis.

12.5.4 Describe synaptic plasticity and its relevance to learning.

12.5.1 WHAT IS LEARNING?

>> LO 12.5.1 Define learning and explain the different ways in which learning can occur.

Key Term

- **Learning:** The mechanisms by which new information is acquired through experience.

Learning can be defined as the mechanisms by which new information is acquired through experience. The acquisition of new information that results in learning occurs in a variety of ways. This includes the formation of associations between stimuli, such as when a rat associates pressing a lever with obtaining a food reward or when a person associates taking a drug with the pleasurable effects it provides (see Chapter 3). Learning also includes automatically responding to a stimulus rendered significant through its association with another either pleasant or unpleasant stimulus. You already know about this if a smile comes to your face automatically when you hear the cellphone ringtone you have assigned to your best friend or if you are overwhelmed with anxiety when you hear the ringtone you assigned to your parents.

Learning can result from observing others behaving in a certain way, such as when you are instructed to watch an experienced worker while being trained at a new job or when someone fears an object or situation after observing someone else being afraid of that very same object or situation. Learning can account for no longer responding, or not responding as much, to a stimulus that once signaled something important or that startled you but no longer does, such as the sirens of emergency vehicles in the streets outside your bedroom window. Learning also accounts for an increase in the intensity or frequency of a response to a stimulus when it does signal something important.

Note that in our definition of learning and in the preceding examples, the changes in behavior are the result of experience. This is because a change in behavior can occur for reasons other than experience with the environment. Instincts, fatigue, maturation, drugs, and illness are all factors that can change behavior. However, the changes in behavior that occur due to these factors do not result from experience and are, therefore, not considered to be the result of learning (Domjan & Grau, 2015).

12.5.2 NONASSOCIATIVE LEARNING

>> LO 12.5.2 Describe nonassociative learning and its neurobiological basis.

Key Terms

- **Nonassociative learning:** A type of learning in which a change in behavior does not involve associations between stimuli or between a stimulus and any kind of reward or punishment.
- **Habituation:** A decrease in response to a stimulus with its repeated occurrence.
- **Sensitization:** An increase in response to an innocuous stimulus after being exposed to an aversive stimulus.
- **Gill-withdrawal reflex:** The reflexive withdrawal of the sea slug's gill as a defense mechanism when its siphon is touched.

Nonassociative learning refers to a type of learning in which a change in behavior does not involve associations between stimuli or between a stimulus and any kind of reward or punishment. Imagine that at the beginning of the semester, one of your professors (who goes by the name of Dr. Cruello) would hide behind the classroom door and scare each one of the students by vocalizing a loud "Boo!" every time one walked into the classroom. On the first day of class, many students would be startled in response to such stimuli. This startle response would include several reflexes including blinking of the eyes and jerking of several body parts such as the head, shoulders, and arms as well as many of the fight-or-flight responses triggered by the sympathetic nervous system (Cosic et al., 2016). However, I am sure that you can also imagine that the startle response of most students would decrease in intensity with each one of the experiences until the response might actually disappear.

The decrease in the intensity or frequency of response to a stimulus with its repeated occurrence is known as **habituation**. In habituation, an organism learns that a stimulus does not predict any event that presents a threat to its survival and that it can dispense with responding to it. In our example, the students habituated to the stimulus ("Boo!") without its being associated with any other stimulus, which is in line with our definition of nonassociative learning.

Now consider the following scenario: You are sitting in the library studying hard for an upcoming exam. Sitting next to you is a classmate who is also studying for the exam. However, this student is listening to music through earbuds. The music is quite loud, and you can overhear it. This is never enough to annoy you, and you easily tolerate it as a slight distraction. A few minutes later, you start hearing the voices of two other students conversing in a nearby aisle. Not only does this start to annoy you, but now the music coming from your classmate's earbuds is becoming such a distraction that you put your books away and leave to go study at home.

Your response to a stimulus that did not initially bother you very much started annoying you to the point where you could no longer study. In this case, constant exposure to the stimuli resulted in an increase in the intensity of your response, that is, from being a slight tolerable distraction to an outright annoyance. An increase in the intensity or frequency of a response to a stimulus is known as **sensitization**, another type of nonassociative learning. Sensitization requires a sensitizing stimulus. In our example, the sensitizing stimulus was the students conversing in the nearby aisle. Sensitization occurs because sensitizing stimuli increase levels of arousal. This increase in arousal levels lowers the threshold at which we respond to other stimuli.

Habituation and Sensitization in the Sea Slug

In the late 1960s, Nobel Prize laureate and neuroscientist Eric Kandel and colleagues discovered a network of neurons responsible for both habituation and sensitization. He did so in an elegant set of experiments

FIGURE 12.20

(a) *Aplysia californica* and (b) its basic parts.

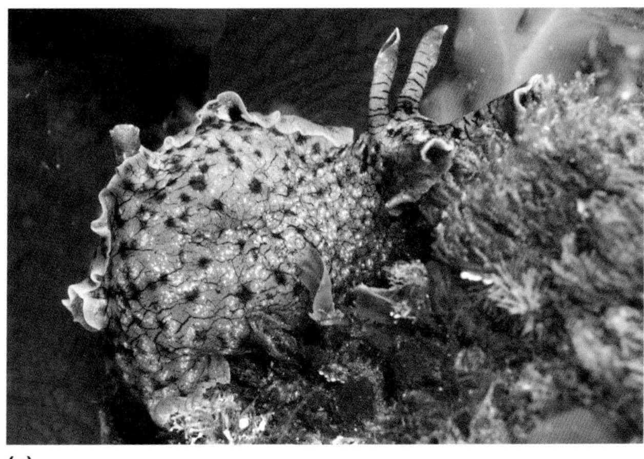

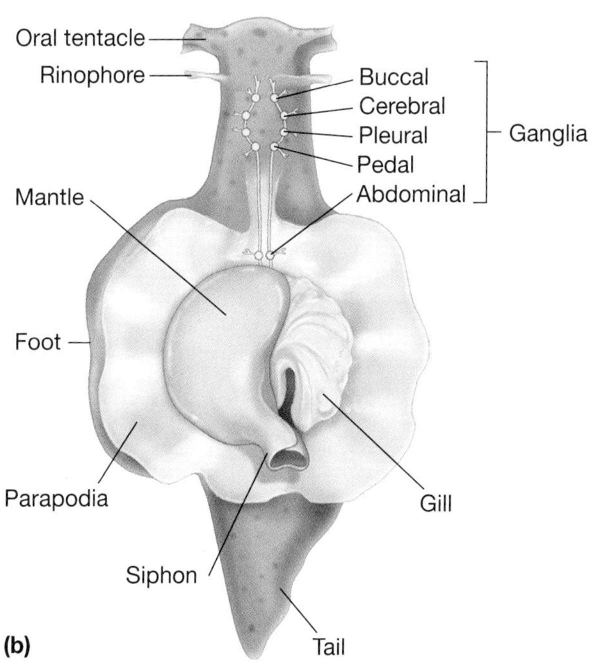

(a) iStock.com/Natalie Ruffing; (b) Liana Bauman/Body Scientific Intl.

using sea slugs known as *Aplysia californica*, shown in Figure 12.20a (Carew, Castellucci, & Kandel, 1971; Castellucci, Pinsker, Kupfermann, & Kandel, 1970; Pinsker, Kupfermann, Castellucci, & Kandel, 1970). Kandel chose to experiment on the sea slug for the following reasons: (1) It has a nervous system made of few cells, (2) its cells are collected in clusters called ganglia, (3) its cells are the largest in the animal kingdom and can be seen with the naked eye, and (4) the location of these neurons is consistent across individual sea slugs.

Figure 12.20b shows the sea slug's basic parts. The parts we will be focusing on, to understand Kandel's experiments, are the gill and the siphon. The gill is used by the sea slug to extract oxygen from its environment. It is reflexively withdrawn under the mantle as a defense mechanism when its siphon is touched. This is known as the **gill-withdrawal reflex**, illustrated in Figure 12.21. The other region to focus on is the abdominal ganglion. The abdominal ganglion is one of several ganglia within the sea slug's body, each of which control some aspects of its behavior. However, the abdominal ganglion is responsible for the sea slug's higher functions, normally attributed to a brain. For our purposes, it suffices to know that the abdominal ganglion contains the connections between sensory neurons of the siphon and the motor neurons that connect to the gill. Something else made the sea slug perfect for these studies: The abdominal ganglion can be removed and studied while keeping those connections intact.

Habituation. Figure 12.21 illustrates Kandel's habituation experiment with a sea slug. Kandel and colleagues found that when the sea slug's siphon was stimulated with a brief jet of water, the gill withdrew (Figure 12.21a). However, with repeated stimulation of the siphon, the gill withdrew with progressively less intensity as measured by the diminishing intensity of

FIGURE 12.21

The gill-withdrawal reflex. (a) Stimulation of the sea slug's siphon resulted in the reflexive withdrawal of the gill. (b) The neuronal connections, within the abdominal ganglion, that are responsible for the gill-withdrawal reflex. Control (left): Stimulation of the siphon causes glutamate to be released at the synapse between a siphon's sensory neuron and a motor neuron that in turn releases neurotransmitter on the gill muscles, causing it to retract. The siphon's sensory neuron also synapses onto excitatory and inhibitory interneurons. Habituation (right): Repeated stimulation of the siphon causes the sensory neuron to release progressively less neurotransmitter at synapses, which in turn causes the motor neuron to release less neurotransmitter on the gill muscles, causing it to contract with less intensity.

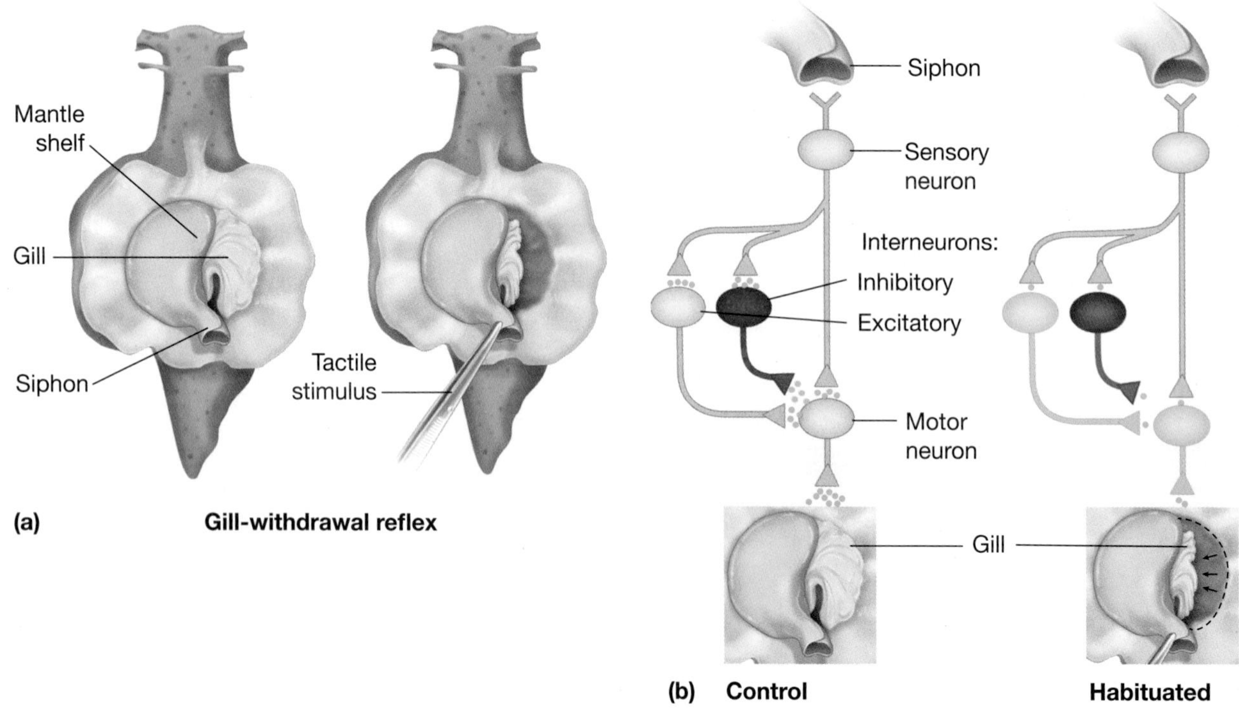

Liana Bauman/Body Scientific Intl.

the gill's contractions upon consecutive stimulations. This is similar to how, in the earlier example, the students ceased to be startled by the teacher trying to scare them as they walked into the classroom. Kandel also found that habituation occurred only if the stimulus was mild but failed to occur with a stronger stimulus (Pinsker et al., 1970), just as it would have been harder for the students' startle response to habituate if the teacher made a louder sound.

Finding out which neuronal connections, within the abdominal ganglion, were responsible for the habituation of the gill-withdrawal reflex was an important step because Kandel had to rule out that the reduction in the intensity of the reflex was not simply due to fatigue or to a decrease in the sea slug's ability to sense the stimulus. As you read earlier, this would not be considered to be learning.

Kandel did this by first recording the electrical activity of a sensory receptor in the siphon, as it was being stimulated repeatedly. He recorded no change in electrical activity. This meant that the observed decrease in the intensity of reflex did not occur because of changes in the response of sensory receptors in the siphon. He then electrically stimulated a motor neuron that attaches to the gill and found that the gill retracted normally. This meant that the decrease in intensity of the reflex did not occur because of a decrease in function of the motor neurons connected to the gill.

This left only one place at which the change could have occurred. That is, at the synapse between the sensory neurons of the siphon and the motor neurons connected to the gill. Kandel found that, with repeated stimulation, the sensory neurons of the siphon released progressively less of the neurotransmitter glutamate onto the motor neurons attached to the gill. This occurred because, with repeated stimulation, less Ca^{2+} entered the axon terminals of the siphon sensory neurons (Klein, Shapiro, & Kandel, 1980). Remember, from Chapter 3, that Ca^{2+} entry into the axon terminals is what signals synaptic vesicles to bind to the neuronal membrane, releasing neurotransmitter molecules into the synaptic cleft.

Next, Kandel found that the sensory neurons attached to the tail of the sea slug synapsed on the axon terminal of the siphon's sensory neurons. A simplified model of the experiment is illustrated in Figure 12.21b. You can see how a sensory receptor neuron innervates the siphon and makes direct synaptic contact with a motor neuron, which, when stimulated, triggers the gill to contract. The siphon sensory neuron also contacts

FIGURE 12.22

Sensitization in the sea slug. (a) A weak stimulus was applied to the siphon. This resulted in a weak withdrawal of the gill. The sea slug then received a shock to the tail, which produced a strong gill-withdrawal response. Then, a weak stimulation of the siphon, which originally produced only a weak response, now produced a strong gill-withdrawal reflex, reflected by the amount of time the gill remained withdrawn. (b) The extent to which the gill-withdrawal reflex was sensitized was related to the number of shocks to the tail received by the sea slug. The magnitude of the response was measured as the amount of time the gill remained withdrawn (duration of withdrawal as a percentage of the control). The results are shown for a single tail shock, four tail shocks, and four trains of shocks given on four consecutive days.

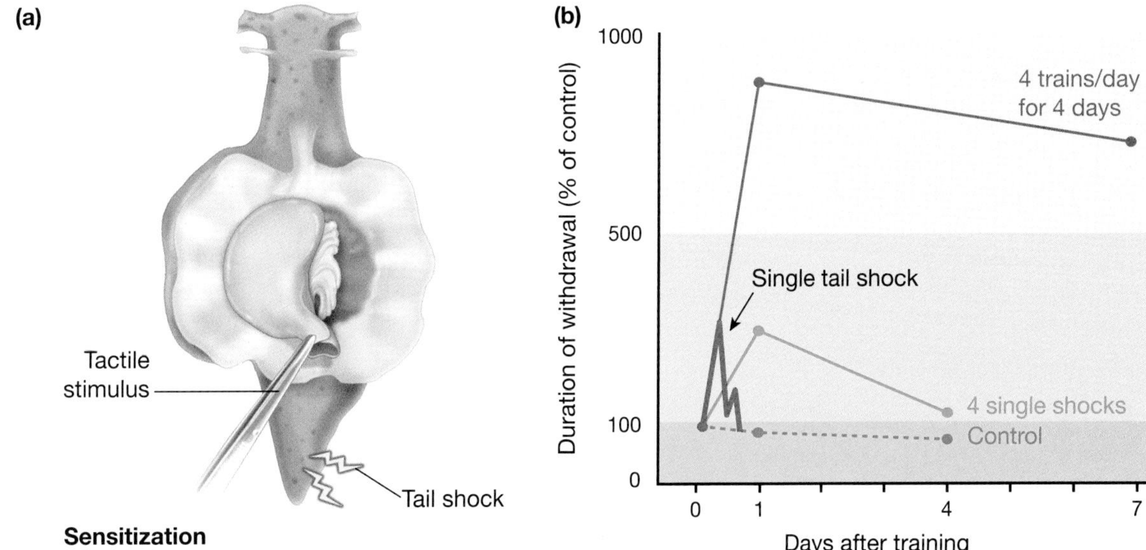

Liana Bauman/Body Scientific Intl.

the motor neuron indirectly through excitatory and inhibitory interneurons (left). With repeated stimulation, fewer neurotransmitter molecules were released at each one of these synapses (right).

Sensitization. Kandel also experimented on the sea slug to explain sensitization (Figure 12.22a). He administered a weak stimulus to the siphon, which resulted in a weak withdrawal of the gill. He then gave the sea slug a strong shock to the tail, which produced a strong gill-withdrawal response. Then he noticed that weak stimulation of the siphon, which originally produced only a weak response, now produced a strong gill-withdrawal reflex, reflected by the amount of time the gill remained withdrawn. The sensitized gill-withdrawal reflex lasted about an hour with a single strong shock to the tail but lasted several days when shocks were administered repeatedly. This is similar to how, in our earlier example of sensitization, overhearing music in the library was but a mere distraction to the student who was studying (akin to the weak stimulation of the siphon) before other students started conversing in a nearby book aisle (akin to the shock to the tail), which became a major annoyance.

Kandel found that this happened because the shock to the tail activated an interneuron that facilitated the release of the neurotransmitter serotonin, which closed K^+ channels in the siphon's sensory neurons. Therefore, the sensory neurons of the siphon produced longer-lasting action potentials, which resulted in a greater amount of glutamate being released onto the motor neuron of the gill (Figure 12.22b). This increased the magnitude of the gill's withdrawal response (Carew et al., 1971).

12.5.3 ASSOCIATIVE LEARNING

>> LO 12.5.3 Describe associative learning and its neurobiological basis.

Key Terms

- **Associative learning:** A change in behavior that results from the association between stimuli.
- **Operant conditioning:** A form of associative learning in which an association is created between a behavior and its consequence.
- **Classical conditioning:** A form of associative learning in which a neutral stimulus is associated with a meaningful stimulus to create a reflexive response.

Associative learning refers to a change in behavior that results from the association between stimuli. Associative learning includes **operant conditioning** (also known as instrumental conditioning) and classical conditioning (also known as Pavlovian conditioning). However, the focus of this unit will only be on classical conditioning. Operant conditioning is discussed in the context of the rewarding effects of drugs in Chapter 3 and in the context of motivation in general in Chapter 9.

Classical Conditioning

Classical conditioning is a form of associative learning in which a neutral stimulus is associated with a meaningful stimulus to create a reflexive response. The name most associated with classical conditioning is that of Russian physiologist Ivan Petrovich Pavlov (1849–1936). In the 1920s, Pavlov trained dogs to salivate in response to the sound of the metronome (Pavlov & Anrep, 1927). He did so by repeatedly producing the sound at the same time that the dogs received food. After several repetitions of these metronome-food pairings, the sound of the metronome, which initially did not cause salivation, came to elicit salivation even when the dogs weren't given food. The sound of the metronome, because it initially did not elicit salivation, was called a neutral stimulus (NS). The food, because it produced salivation by itself, was referred to as the unconditional stimulus (US [often referred to as the unconditioned stimulus]). Salivation to the US (the food) was called the unconditional response (UR [often referred to as the unconditioned response]). Once the metronome sound (NS) elicited salivation by itself, it became a conditional stimulus (CS [often referred to as a conditioned stimulus]). Salivation to the sound of the metronome by itself (without the food) became known as the conditional response (CR [often referred to as a conditioned response]).

Many behaviors are learned by classical conditioning. For example, if you have a dog, you know that it gets excited when you shake the box that contains its favorite treats. When you hear the cellphone ringtone you have assigned to your best friend, a smile automatically comes to your face, and on a more negative note, people who are addicted to drugs will often experience intense cravings when exposed to cues related to their consumption of drugs (see Chapter 3). In each situation, the NS, US, UR, and CR can be identified. In the first example, the sound of the treats shaking around in the box initially means nothing to your dog (NS). The treats contained in the box are "yummy to your dog" (US). Your dog already gets excited when it gets yummy treats (UR). After several pairings consisting of shaking the box and giving your dog the treats, it now gets excited by just hearing the treats shaking around in the box (CR). Can you identify the stimuli for the other two examples?

In the early 1980s, Kandel and colleagues used the sea slug to investigate the synaptic changes that occur during classical conditioning (Carew, Hawkins, & Kandel, 1983). Figure 12.23 illustrates the procedure

FIGURE 12.23

Classical conditioning procedure with the sea slug.

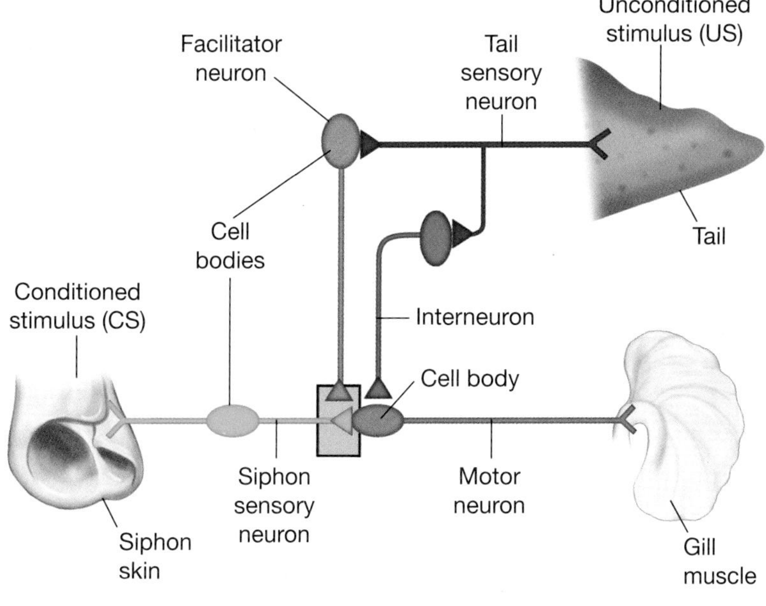

Liana Bauman/Body Scientific Intl.

they used. The CS was a light tactile stimulus to the siphon. Note here that this stimulus produced only a weak reaction in the gill, initially being an NS.

The US was a strong shock to the tail. This produced a strong withdrawal reflex of the gill, the UR. After 15 pairing trials of the CS with the US, application of the CS by itself induced a strong withdrawal of the gill.

During the paired presentations of the CS and the US, entry of Ca^{2+} in the presynaptic terminal of the siphon sensory neuron resulted in reduced amounts of K^{+} exiting the cell. This resulted in the prolongation of action potentials, contributing to the creation of a strong association between the CS and the US.

After learning about the synaptic changes that occur during sensitization and classical conditioning of the sea slug, students often say that they do not understand the difference between the two procedures. Although the procedures for both sensitization and classical conditioning are similar, there are important differences between them. First, in the procedure used for sensitization, the shocking of the tail and the stimulation of the siphon occur in an unpaired fashion. That is, the timing of siphon stimulation does not overlap that of the shock to the tail. Second, sensitization is nonspecific. This means that any other stimulus that aroused the sea slug would likely have the same effect.

In contrast, during the classical conditioning procedure, stimulation of the siphon, which becomes the CS, precedes and overlaps the delivery of the shock to the tail, the US. Also, classical conditioning is stimulus specific. This means that the increase in responding as measured by a greater amplitude of the gill-withdrawal response (the CR) occurs only when the trained CS (stimulation of the siphon) occurs. Stimulation of another part of the body could not replace the trained CS. Another difference is in the response magnitude. The classical conditioning procedure resulted in a gill-withdrawal reflex of greater magnitude than did the procedure used for sensitization.

12.5.4 SYNAPTIC PLASTICITY: NEURONS THAT WIRE TOGETHER FIRE TOGETHER

>> LO 12.5.4 Describe synaptic plasticity and its relevance to learning.

Key Terms

- **Activity-dependent synaptic plasticity:** The change in the strength of synapses that occurs as a result of repeated experience.
- **Long-term potentiation (LTP):** The increase in the efficiency of a synapse following high-frequency electrical stimulation.
- **Long-term depression (LTD):** The decrease in the efficiency of a synapse following low-frequency electrical stimulation.
- **cAMP-responsive element-binding protein (CREB):** A protein that puts into motion the transcription of DNA by messenger ribonucleic acid (mRNA).

You just learned how the neurobiological mechanisms of habituation, sensitization, and classical conditioning were discovered using a simple animal model, which involved stimulating different parts of a sea slug and observing its responses. These were groundbreaking discoveries, as they showed that these simple forms of learning could be explained by changes in the strength of synapses. The change in the strength of synapses that occurs as a result of repeated experience is known as **activity-dependent synaptic plasticity**. Neuroscientists consider activity-dependent synaptic plasticity to be the mechanism by which learning and the subsequent storage of information in memory occurs.

The idea that learning and memory depend on changes in the synaptic strength between neurons is far from new. It is often attributed to Santiago Ramón y Cajal (discussed in Chapter 2), who hypothesized it in 1913 (W. M. Cowan & Kandel, 2001; Ramón y Cajal, 1995). But, in fact, the idea predates Ramón y Cajal's hypothesis. The idea that changes in synaptic strength might account for learning was anticipated in the late 1800s by Sigmund Freud (Centonze, Siracusano, Calabresi, & Bernardi, 2004), psychologist William James (1890), and others (Berlucchi & Buchtel, 2009).

It was Canadian psychologist Donald Hebb (1949) who proposed the most influential theory of the neurobiological mechanisms of learning and memory based on changes in synaptic strength between neurons. Hebb stated that learning occurred when a neuron (neuron A) persistently activated another neuron (neuron B). He thought that this persistent activation resulted in changes occurring in both neurons, which facilitated the ability of neuron A to activate neuron B. This led to arguably the most famous quote in neuroscience, "neurons that fire together wire together," which is best explained in Hebb's own words:

> When an axon of cell A is near enough to excite cell B and repeatedly or persistently takes part in firing it, some growth process or metabolic change takes place in one or both cells such that A's efficiency, as one of the cells firing B, is increased.
>
> Hebb (1949, p. 62)

Long-Term Potentiation (LTP)

Although learning and memory had long been hypothesized to be due to changes in the strength of synapses, no experimental evidence had so far been found. This had to wait until the 1970s, when neuroscientists Timothy Bliss and Terje Lømo (1973) electrically stimulated the axons of the perforant path of live rabbits (Figure 12.24a). The perforant path is a bundle of nerve fibers that relays information from the entorhinal cortex to a part of the hippocampus called the dentate gyrus.

Bliss and Lømo (1973) found that a single pulse of electrical stimulation to the perforant path caused neurons in the dentate gyrus neurons to fire, which was not a surprise. Their major discovery was that the delivery of a high-frequency train of electrical stimulation to the perforant path enhanced the response of dentate gyrus neurons to a single pulse of electrical stimulation. They also found that the change in the response of neurons in the dentate gyrus to a single pulse, after high-frequency trains of stimulation to the perforant path, persisted for hours, days, or weeks. This phenomenon, which was first referred to as long-lasting potentiation, became known as **long-term potentiation (LTP)** (Douglas & Goddard, 1975), which is defined as the increase in the efficiency of a synapse following high-frequency electrical stimulation.

An example of LTP is illustrated in Figures 12.24b and 12.24c. It shows the effects of high-frequency trains of electrical stimulation of a bundle of fibers, known as the Schaffer collaterals, on the response of neurons they synapse with. The Schaffer collaterals have their cell bodies in an area of the hippocampus known as CA3 and synapses with neurons in the CA1 area (Figure 12.24a) (Malinow, Schulman, & Tsien, 1989). In this experiment, the Schaffer collaterals were divided into two pathways. The response of CA1 pyramidal cells in pathway 1 was recorded one minute before and one hour after the Schaffer collaterals received a high-frequency train (tetanus) of electrical stimulation (stimulus 1 in Figure 12.24b). Their response was compared to the pyramidal cells in pathway 2, in which the Schaffer collaterals did not receive a high-frequency train of stimulation.

The results of the experiment are shown in Figure 12.24c. The size of excitatory postsynaptic potentials (EPSPs) evoked by a single pulse of electrical stimulation in CA1 pyramidal cells was significantly enhanced after the high-frequency train of stimulation compared to before the high-frequency train of stimulation. In contrast, the size of EPSPs to a single electrical pulse to the Schaffer collateral in pathway 2, which did not receive a high-frequency train of stimulation, did not change.

Long-Term Depression (LTD)

The fact that the strength of synapses between neurons can be strengthened by the process of LTP begs the question as to whether the strength of synapses can also be weakened. The answer is yes. This occurs through a process known as **long-term depression (LTD)**. If you can define LTP, you can easily define LTD. Whereas LTP is the strengthening of a synapse following a high-frequency train of stimulation, LTD refers to the weakening of a synapse following a train of low-frequency stimulation.

LTD was first discovered in neuronal pathways of the cerebellum, in which it plays an important role in motor learning (Ito & Kano, 1982). However, LTD in the cerebellum involves a complex network of neurons. LTD can be explained briefly by an experiment similar to the one used to explain LTP. In that experiment, the Schaffer collaterals were given a train of low-frequency stimulation for 10–15 minutes. As can be seen in Figure 12.24d, this resulted in a reduction in the amplitude of EPSPs in CA1 neurons with subsequent stimulation relative to before the administration of the low-frequency train (Mulkey & Malenka, 1992).

Effects of LTP and LTD at the Synapse

You may be wondering how LTP and LTD result in enhancing and reducing synaptic efficacy, respectively. LTP and LTD have their effects by increasing (for LTP) and decreasing (for LTD) the number of α-amino-3-hydroxy-5-methyl-4-isoxazolepropionic acid (AMPA) receptors on the postsynaptic membrane of synapses. In Chapter 3, you learned that activation of AMPA receptors by the neurotransmitter glutamate depolarized the postsynaptic membrane, which results

FIGURE 12.24

(a) The position of stimulation and recording electrodes in the hippocampus in Bliss and Lømo's experiment. (b) Position of the stimulation and recording electrodes in a long-term potentiation (LTP) experiment. (c) Results of the LTP experiment. (d) Position of the stimulation and recording electrodes in a long-term depression (LTD) experiment (left). The results of a train of low-frequency stimulation to the Schaffer collaterals on the excitability of the pyramidal cells in the CA1 area (right). See the accompanying text for details.

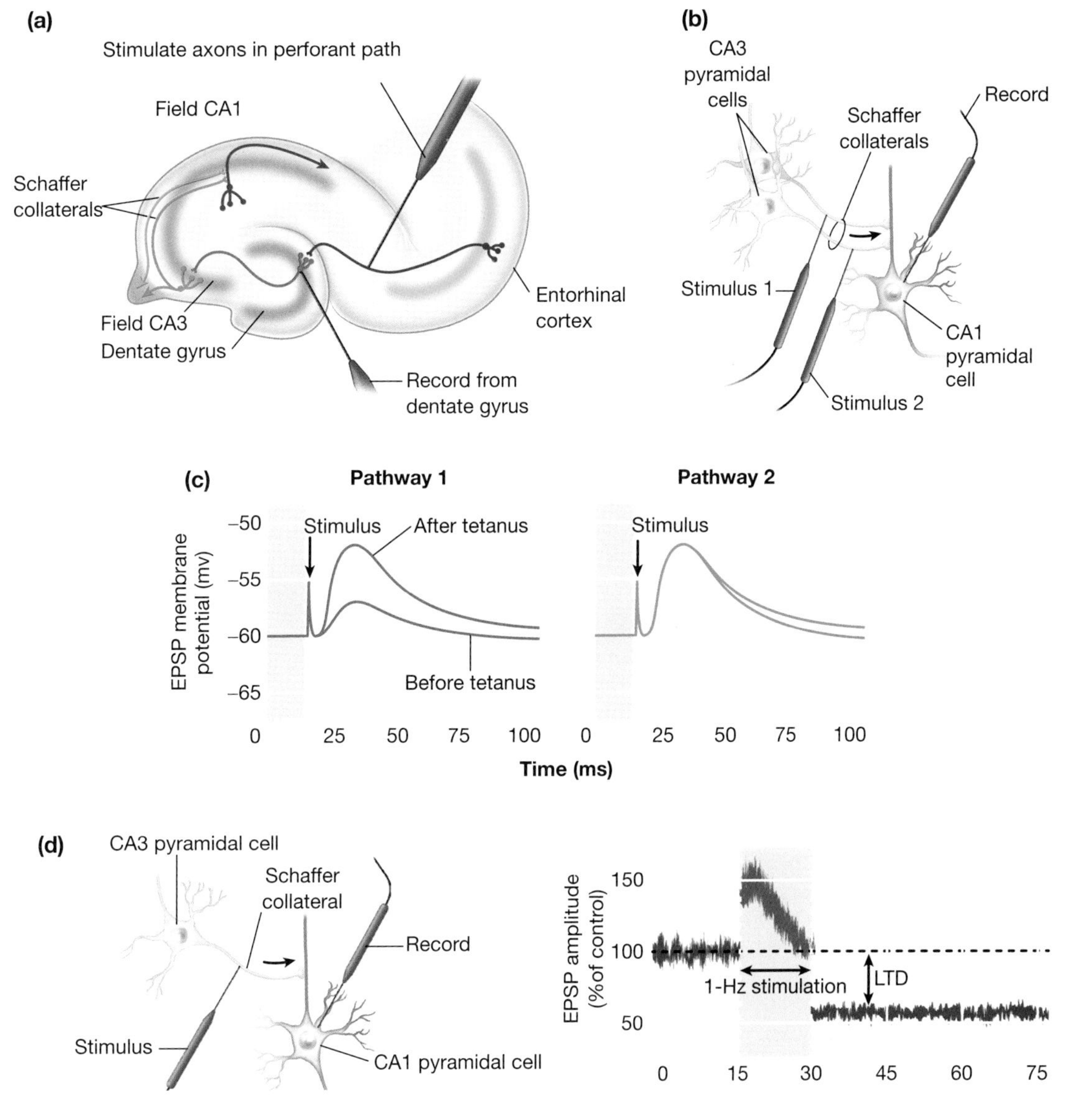

Amanda Tomasikiewicz/Body Scientific Intl.

in the removal of a magnesium (Mg^{2+}) block from N-methyl-D-aspartic acid or N-methyl-D-aspartate (NMDA) receptors. You also learned that removal of the Mg^{2+} block permits NMDA receptors to respond to the binding of glutamate, resulting in the entry of calcium ions (Ca^{2+}) into the postsynaptic neuron.

As shown in Figure 12.25, following a train of high-frequency electrical stimulation of the presynaptic neuron, Ca^{2+} activates a protein known as calcium/calmodulin-dependent protein kinase II (CaMKII). In turn, CaMKII activity causes AMPA receptors, which are stored into vesicles, to be inserted into the postsynaptic membrane, increasing the neuron's response to glutamate released by the presynaptic neuron. In LTD, low-frequency stimulation causes Ca^{2+} to activate what is known as calcineurin, which activates proton-pump inhibitors (PPIs). Activation of PPIs causes AMPA receptors from the membrane to retract into the postsynaptic neuron and be absorbed into vesicles. This decreases the neuron's ability to respond to glutamate released by the presynaptic neuron (Lisman, Yasuda, & Raghavachari, 2012).

FIGURE 12.25

Effects of LTP (left) and LTD (right) at the synapse.

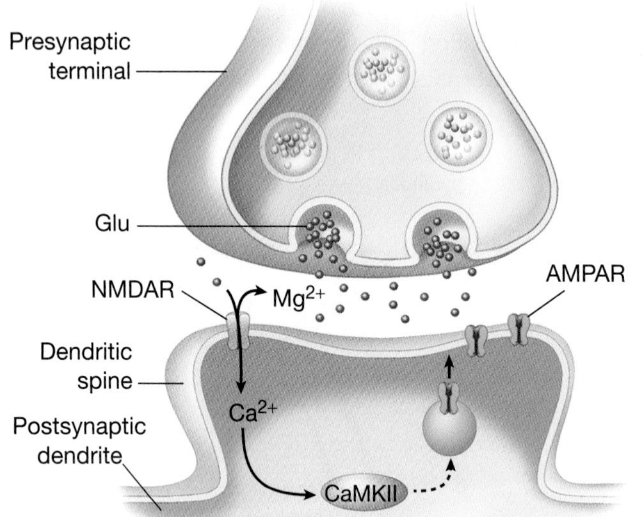

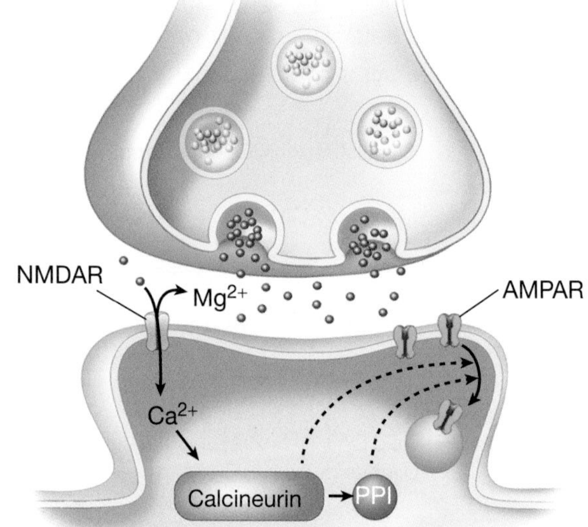

Carolina Hrejsa/Body Scientific Intl.

Two Forms of LTP

Two forms of LTP exist: short-lasting LTP (S-LTP) and long-lasting LTP (L-LTP). The form of LTP described previously corresponds to S-LTP. S-LTP is induced by weak high-frequency stimulation. The changes induced in S-LTP involve molecules that are already present within the postsynaptic neuron. In S-LTP, the changes in synaptic efficacy last only for a few minutes or a few hours. The processes of S-LTP are not stable and are easily disrupted, and the changes induced by it are rapidly reversed after stimulation has ended. Therefore, S-LTP alone is not believed to be the mechanism for the formation of long-term memories.

The long-lasting changes that result in the formation of long-term memories are induced by L-LTP, which requires strong high-frequency stimulation. L-LTP requires the synthesis of new proteins. Far too many mechanisms are involved in the generation of protein synthesis to cover all of them in this chapter. Therefore, we will cover only one.

One such mechanism involves the activation of the enzyme adenylyl cyclase, which is discussed in Chapter 3. Once activated, adenylyl cyclase activates an enzyme called protein kinase A (PKA), which in turn activates the second messenger cyclic adenosine monophosphate (cAMP). In turn, cAMP activates a protein called **cAMP-responsive element-binding protein (CREB)**. CREB is a protein known as a transcription factor, which puts into motion the molecular processes that synthesize new proteins.

The synthesis of new proteins results in the long-lasting changes believed to lead to long-term memories. This includes changes in the morphology of dendritic spines. For example, some spines become shorter but much broader, permitting a higher number of AMPA receptors to be inserted into the membrane, resulting in greater entry of Na^+ into the neuron, leading to more reliable depolarization and, therefore, greater activation of NMDA receptors. This leads to a greater entry of Ca^{2+} into the postsynaptic neuron. Another noted change that can be observed is the sprouting of new spines close to spines that are already activated. Dendritic spines can also bifurcate. That is, they can split up in a Y shape, increasing the number of possible synapses in which they can engage.

LTD: Why Would the Strength of Synapses Need to Be Weakened?

As mentioned earlier, LTD results in the weakening of synapses. This begs the question of why synapses would need to be weakened. The answer is that if synapses just kept being strengthened, they would reach a point where they would become static and no longer be able to encode new information. There are also situations in which synapses do not need to be kept functioning at maximal efficacy but nevertheless need to be maintained. Another reason is that the strength of individual synapses must be regulated in relation to the activity of the entire network of neurons of which they are a part. This process is known as homeostatic plasticity (Surmeier & Foehring, 2004; Turrigiano & Nelson, 2004).

MODULE SUMMARY

Learning can be defined as the mechanisms by which new information is acquired through experience. Two broad categories of learning are nonassociative learning and associative learning. The two types of nonassociative learning are habituation and sensitization. Habituation refers to the decrease in the intensity or frequency of the response to a stimulus with its repeated occurrence. Sensitization is the increase in the intensity or frequency of a response with repeated exposure to a stimulus. Associative learning refers to learning in which the association between stimuli is learned.

One form of associative learning is classical conditioning. The neurobiological basis of this form of learning was discovered by Eric Kandel by studying the gill-withdrawal reflex in the sea slug. Kandel found that repeatedly stimulating the gill of the sea slug led to a reduction in the intensity of the withdrawal of the gill, an example of habituation. He also found that giving a strong shock to the tail of the sea slug resulted in an increase in the intensity of the gill's withdrawal, an example of sensitization. Finally, he found that a tactile stimulus to the siphon (the CS) can be paired with a strong shock to the tail (the US) to produce a strong conditioned withdrawal of the gill (the CR).

It was found that repeated experience can induce changes in synaptic strength. This is known as activity-dependent synaptic plasticity. One known mechanism for synaptic plasticity is long-term potentiation (LTP), which was discovered by electrically stimulating the perforant path and measuring the resulting response in the dentate gyrus of the hippocampus. High-frequency trains of stimulation of the perforant path increased the efficacy of synapses in the dentate gyrus. The opposite was also found to be true. Trains of low-frequency stimulation of the Schaffer collaterals resulted in a decrease in the efficiency of synapses in the CA1 region of the hippocampus, a phenomenon known as long-term depression (LTD). Two forms of LTP were discovered: short-lasting LTP (S-LTP) and long-lasting LTP (L-LTP). S-LTP involves changes in synaptic efficacy that last only a few minutes or hours and is therefore not thought to form the basis of long-term memory. In contrast, L-LTP is thought to involve long-lasting changes, which includes the activation of the enzyme adenylyl cyclase and the second messenger cyclic adenosine monophosphate (cAMP) and the protein cAMP-responsive element-binding protein (CREB).

TEST YOURSELF

12.5.1 Define learning and the different ways in which it occurs.

12.5.2 (a) Define nonassociative learning. (b) Describe two forms of nonassociative learning and how their neurobiological mechanisms were discovered.

12.5.3 (a) Define associative learning. (b) Describe a form of associative learning and how its neurobiological mechanisms were discovered.

12.5.4 Describe the processes of LTP and LTD, how they were discovered, and how they are implicated in learning.

APPLICATIONS

Reconsolidation in the Treatment of Conditioned Fears

Consolidated memories can be made fragile and vulnerable to disruption again after being reactivated. While in an unstable state, memories can be updated with new information and integrated by being reconsolidated along with the new information (Hupbach et al., 2007; J. Lee, Nader, & Schiller, 2017). The updating of memories through reconsolidation may form the basis for the treatment of conditioned fears, such as those observed in posttraumatic stress and phobias (discussed in Chapter 14) (Lee et al., 2017). For example, someone who has been conditioned to fear dogs (Figure 12.26a) can be reminded of the experience by being shown an object that relates to it, such as a dog collar (Figure 12.26b). Within minutes following reactivation of the memory, the person's memory can be updated by extinction, counterconditioning, or interference trials (Figure 12.26c), resulting in the retrieval of the memory without the accompanying intense fear (Figure 12.26d).

(Continued)

(Continued)

FIGURE 12.26

(a) Example of a learned fear. (b) Reminder used to reactivate the fear memory, in this case, a dog collar. (c) Treatments that can affect the reconsolidation of memories: extinction, counterconditioning, and interference. (d) The retrieval test. (e) The game Tetris used as an interference task in the study by E. James et al. (2015); see text for details. (f) The main results of the James et al. (2015) study: Participants who were made to play Tetris (the intervention) reported a significantly lower frequency of intrusive thoughts than those who were not made to play Tetris.

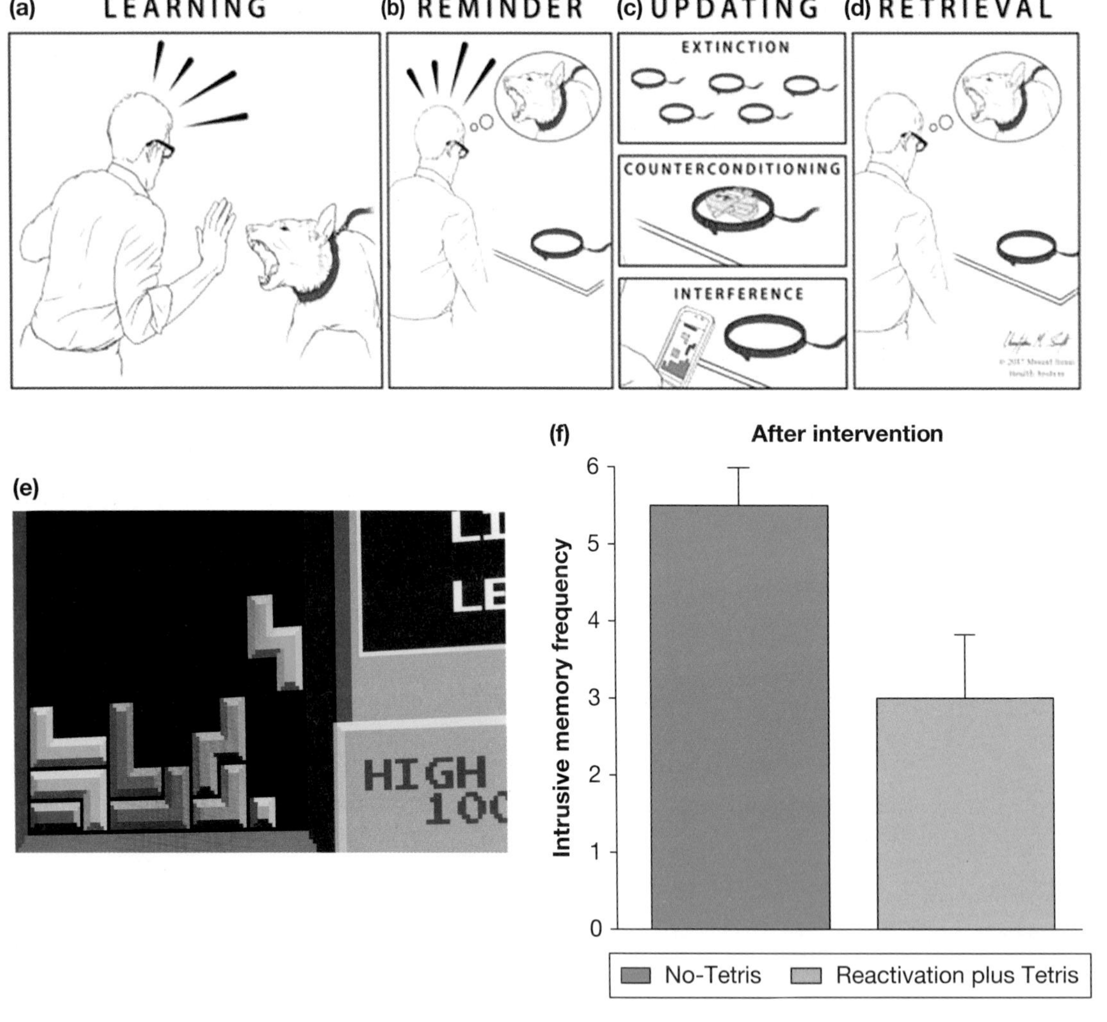

(a–d) Lee, J.L.C., K. Nader, & D. Schiller. (2017). An Update on Memory Reconsolidation Updating. *Trends in Cognitive Science 21*(7), 531–545. With permission from Elsevier; (e) ilbusca/ istockphoto; (f) Adapted from Kitamura, T., et al. (2017). Engrams and circuits crucial for systems consolidation of a memory. *Science 356*(6333), 73–78.

Extinction is the process by which exposure to the conditioned stimulus (CS) alone, without the unconditioned stimulus (US) associated with it, results in the reduction or elimination of the unconditioned response (UR). This is thought to be due to the new learning that the CS is not a reliable predictor of the US. In extinction trials, the reactivation of the fear memory is reactivated by exposing the person to a dog collar (CS) without the associated stimulus (the dog); the person is not permitted to escape the situation, the UR. The idea is that the memory of the CS will be updated and reconsolidated to include the memory that the dog collar does not reliably predict the presence of the dog. Accordingly, this results in the person being able to retrieve the memory of the collar without showing the sometimes extreme fear reactions he or she once experienced.

Counterconditioning refers to the process by which a CS, which has been associated with an aversive or appetitive US, is subsequently conditioned to signal an appetitive or aversive stimulus, respectively. For example, attenuating the fear experience by the exposure to the dog collar might also be achieved by memory reactivation followed shortly by counterconditioning trials. During these trials, the fearful person may be exposed to the dog collar paired with an appetitive stimulus, such as a stack of candy bars. The idea here is that the memory of the collar will be reconsolidated, incorporating the update that the dog collar may actually signal something pleasant.

Another way in which fear reactions can be attenuated is through *interference* with the reconsolidation of the memories that trigger them. To continue with our fear-of-dog example, the person's memory may be reactivated by the presentation of the dog collar followed immediately by a distractor. The idea here is that, after being interfered with, only a weakened version of the fear memory will be reconsolidated.

In one study, researchers used what is known as the traumatic-film paradigm, which is an experimental procedure that consists of showing participants short films known to create traumatic memories (E. L. James et al., 2015). After having seen the films, participants reported experiencing intrusive memories related to the films they had seen. The purpose of the study was to find out whether engaging in a demanding cognitive task shortly after the memory was reactivated would interfere with the reconsolidation of those intrusive memories. The experiment was divided into three sessions. In the first session, the participants watched a traumatic film alone in a darkened room and were asked to rate the emotions they felt during the film as well as the extent to which they found it distressing. They were told to keep a diary of the frequency of intrusive memories related to the film that they experienced over the next 24 hours.

In the second session, the participants were assigned to two groups. In one group, the participants' memories for the traumatic film were reactivated by presenting them with blurred still images of the film. Ten minutes later, the participants were made to play the video game Tetris for 12 minutes (Figure 12.26e), as the cognitive task that can potentially interfere with the reconsolidation of the intrusive memories. In the second group, which served as the control, the participants were not made to play Tetris after the reactivation. The participants were then sent on their way but were required to keep the diary of intrusive thoughts for the next seven days.

At the third session, the participants returned with their completed diaries. The main results of the study are shown in Figure 12.26f. Participants made to play Tetris 10 minutes after traumatic memories from the film were reactivated (the intervention in Figure 12.26f) reported a significantly lower frequency of intrusive thoughts compared to participants who did not play Tetris following reactivation.

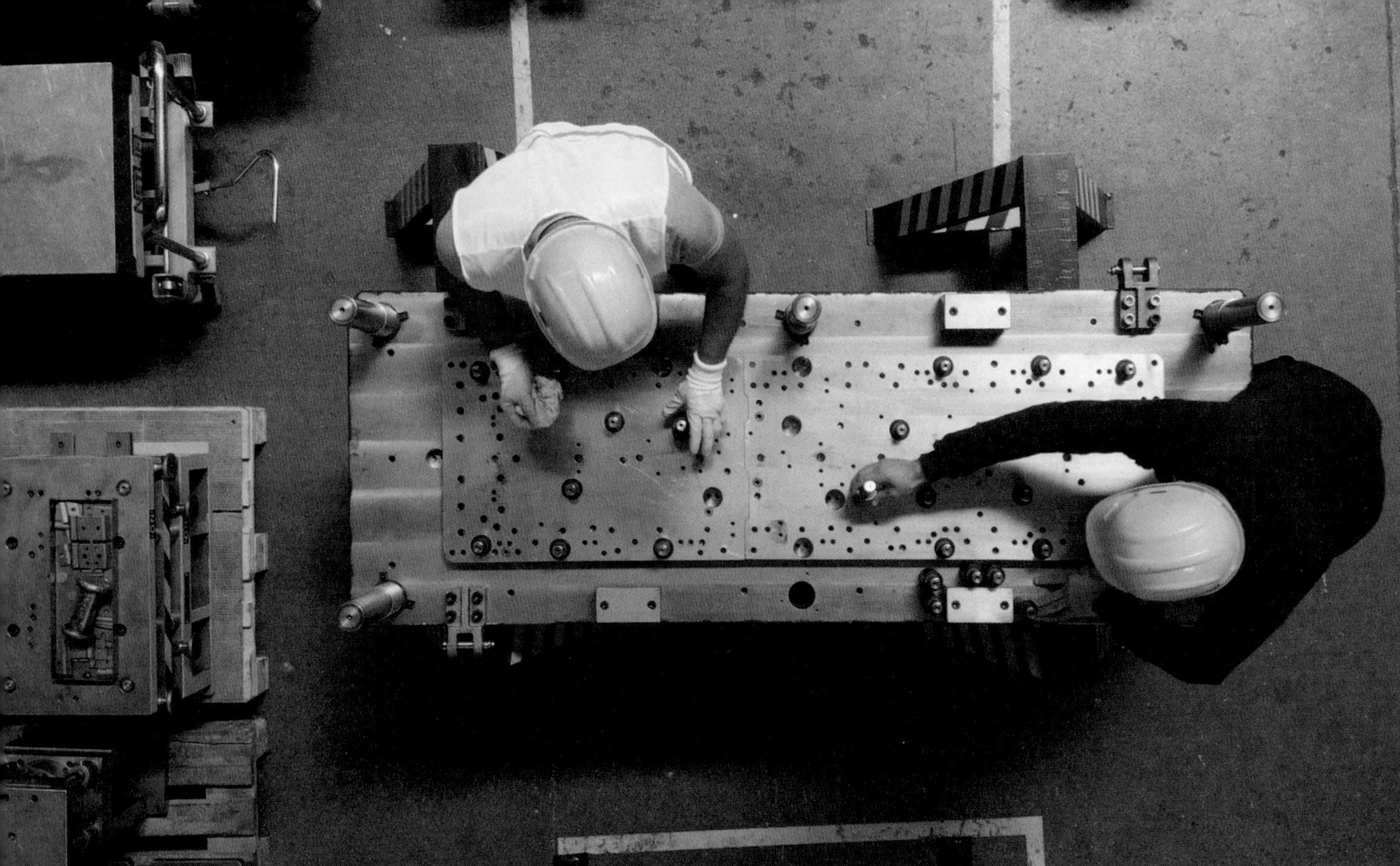

tunart/istockphoto

13 Attention and Consciousness

Chapter Contents

Learning Objectives

13.1.1 Define attention and describe some of the concepts associated with it.

13.1.2 Describe and explain the various concepts in the study of attention.

13.1.3 Describe the main brain networks of attention and how they were discovered.

13.1.4 Describe two disorders of attention due to brain damage.

13.2.1 Explain what scientists know about consciousness and describe its components.

13.2.2 Define and explain the hard and easy problems of consciousness.

13.2.3 Explain what is meant by neural correlates of consciousness.

13.2.4 Describe and explain the global workspace theory of consciousness.

13.2.5 Describe and explain some disorders of consciousness.

13.2.6 Explain how consciousness can be hidden.

13.2.7 Describe and explain experiments designed to test whether humans have free will.

Unresponsive Wakefulness: The Case of Terri Schiavo

The most taken-for-granted of our mental abilities is consciousness. Consciousness can be defined as the awareness of the constant stream of stimuli, both external and internally generated, that make up our daily lives, for example, the sight of an apple, its taste, and the emotions triggered by the warm memories of watching your grandmother baking apple pie. This ability depends on the intact functioning and integrity of the neocortex. Brain damage resulting from an accident or stroke (interruption of blood flow to a part of the brain) can potentially wipe out consciousness. Such is the case of Terri Schiavo. In 1990, at age 26, Schiavo suffered cardiac arrest and collapsed, depriving her brain of oxygen. There was much speculation about the reason for her collapse, but in the end the cause was undetermined.

Whatever the reason, the lack of oxygen caused enough brain damage to leave Schiavo in a state of unresponsive wakefulness (then called a persistent vegetative state), in which vital functions such as heartbeat and respiration, as well as a normal sleep-wake cycle, are preserved but no awareness of the environment exists. Wakefulness and vital functions are regulated by regions of the brainstem, the medulla, and the hypothalamus. These regions all remain intact in people with unresponsive wakefulness. Unable to eat, Schiavo required a feeding tube. She remained in this state for 15 years. At times, Schiavo seemed to show signs of awareness. For example, she seemed to follow commands to open and shut her eyes and could track a balloon and flashing lights with her eyes. However, doctors called these responses involuntary reflexes, which are also mediated by the brainstem. In 2005, after a long legal battle between her husband, who asserted that she would not have wanted to live this way, and her parents, who wanted her to remain alive, the decision was made to remove Schiavo's feeding tube and she died nearly two weeks later.

INTRODUCTION

You likely learned what the word *attention* means early in life. You were surely told to "pay attention" by your parents and teachers. We can assume that their wish was that you listen to what they were saying. In everyday life, the term *attention* is used in many ways. Regardless of how it is used, *attention* always refers to narrowing one's focus to something specific. This is made evident in the quotes about attention that follow:

> Pay attention to your enemies, for they are the first to discover your mistakes.
>
> Antisthenes (Greek philosopher, 445 B.C.E.–365 B.C.E.)

> You have to pay attention to details to have success in the playoffs. You can't take anyone lightly.
>
> Nicklas Lidstrom (former professional hockey player)

> Attention is psychic energy, and like physical energy, unless we allocate some part of it to the task at hand, no work gets done.
>
> Mihaly Csikszentmihalyi
> (famous psychologist)

Scientists who study attention have defined many concepts that further characterize the subject. They have also identified brain circuits that control attentional processes and how damage to these circuits lead to disorders of attention. It is to these topics that we turn in the first part of this chapter.

The second part of the chapter is dedicated to consciousness. There is no agreed-upon definition for consciousness. One definition refers to the experience of the continuous flow of your thoughts, feelings, and perceptions. Consciousness is studied by philosophers, psychologists, and neuroscientists. How the brain produces consciousness remains a mystery. In this chapter's treatment of consciousness, you will learn about some of the early ideas about consciousness held by past and contemporary philosophers. You will also learn about some of the problems that need to be addressed if we are to understand how the brain produces consciousness. We will also look at what brain areas are activated during conscious events and explore what can go wrong with a person's consciousness following brain damage.

13.1 Attention

Module Contents

Learning Objectives

13.1.1 Define attention and describe some of the concepts associated with it.

13.1.2 Describe and explain the various concepts in the study of attention.

13.1.3 Describe the main brain networks of attention and how they were discovered.

13.1.4 Describe two disorders of attention due to brain damage.

13.1.1 WHAT IS ATTENTION?

>> LO 13.1.1 Define attention and describe some of the concepts associated with it.

Key Terms

- **Attention:** The ability to select a stimulus, focus on it, sustain that focus, and shift that focus at will.
- **Overt attention:** The shifting of attention that includes the reorienting of sensory receptors.
- **Covert attention:** The ability to shift attention from stimulus to stimulus without reorienting sensory receptors.
- **Endogenous attention:** Self-directed and voluntary attention to a stimulus.
- **Exogenous attention:** Attention drawn toward a stimulus in a reflexive and involuntary manner.
- **Spatial attention:** Attention directed to the spatial location of stimuli.
- **Object attention:** Attention directed at a specific object.
- **Feature attention:** Attention directed at a specific feature of an object.

Attention is the ability to select a stimulus, focus on it, sustain that focus, and shift that focus at will. Attention can be overt or covert. For example, while studying this chapter you are choosing to focus your attention on the words you are reading. However, if you are expecting one of your friends, you may occasionally shift your gaze from the words in your textbook to a window through which you might notice your friend's arrival. In this case, it would be obvious to someone looking at your eyes that your focus of attention has changed. The shifting of attention, which includes the reorienting of sensory receptors, in this case, your eyes, is known as **overt attention**.

Now, as you stare at the center of the page you are reading, notice that, without moving your eyes, you can switch your attention to an object other than the page. In this case, someone looking at your eyes would not be able to tell what your focus of attention is. The ability to shift attention from stimulus to stimulus without reorienting sensory receptors is known as **covert attention**. Another example of covert attention would be looking at your friend straight in the eyes while she speaks to you in a café, while monitoring the more interesting conversations going on around you. Hermann von Helmholtz (1821–1894) is credited as the first scientist to provide experimental evidence for covert attention in the 1860s. He stared at the center of an array of letters on a screen in the dark. As he did this, he focused on a different part of the screen without shifting his gaze. He then lit a spark that illuminated the screen. What he noticed was that

FIGURE 13.1

Hermann von Helmholtz's covert attention experiment.

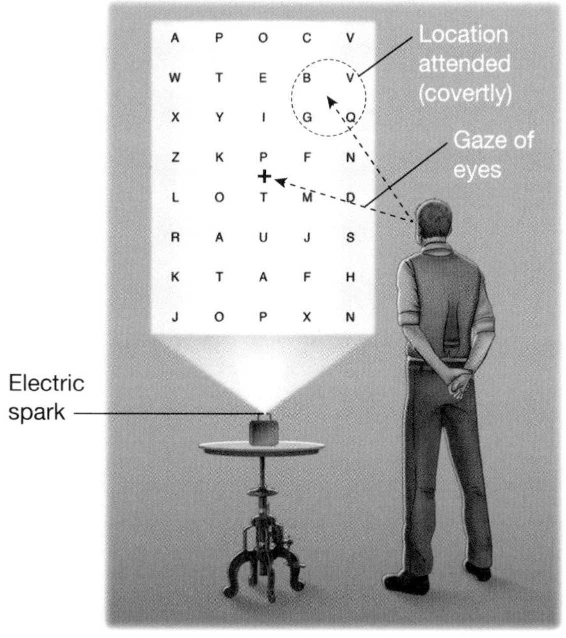

Carolina Hrejsa/Body Scientific Intl.

FIGURE 13.2

One image can command spatial, object, and feature attention, depending on the aspects of the scene on which you are focusing.

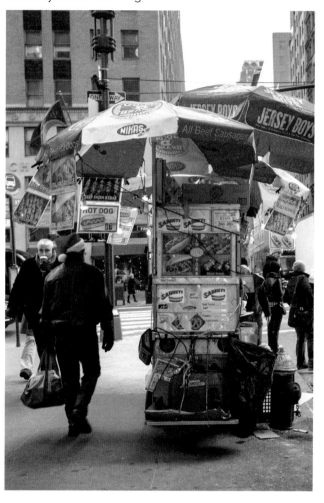

littleny/istockphoto

even if the entire array of letters was in his visual field, he could only read the letters in the area of the screen where his attention was directed (Figure 13.1).

Endogenous and Exogenous Attention

While sitting in class, you can choose either to listen to your professor or to engage in a whispered conversation with a classmate, which is not recommended because it is annoying to everyone. If you choose the conversation, you are focusing your attention on your classmate's words. However, if your professor suddenly says, "Okay, listen up!" the chances are that you will attend to what the professor has to say. Attending to what your classmate had to say, over the professor's words of wisdom, was voluntary and self-directed. Self-directed and voluntary attention to a stimulus is known as **endogenous attention**. However, when your professor said, "Okay, listen up!" your attention was reflexively drawn away from your classmate to your professor, in an automatic and involuntary manner. Attention that is drawn toward a stimulus in a reflexive and involuntary manner is known as **exogenous attention**.

Spatial, Object, and Feature Attention

Attention can be directed to different aspects of a scene. For example, you can direct your attention to the spatial location of particular stimuli, for example, the left side of the New York street scene in Figure 13.2. This is known as **spatial attention**. Directing your attention to a specific object in that location, such as the food stand, is known as **object attention**. In addition, you can focus on a specific feature of the food stand, such as the picture of a hot dog. Attention to a feature of an object is known as **feature attention**.

13.1.2 CONCEPTS IN THE STUDY OF ATTENTION

>> LO 13.1.2 **Describe and explain the various concepts in the study of attention.**

Key Terms

- **Selective attention:** The process that permits specific information to be picked voluntarily out of a number of stimuli.
- **Cocktail party effect:** The phenomenon in which selective attention is paid to a specific stimulus among a range of other stimuli.
- **Dichotic listening:** An experimental set-up in which a spoken message is played into a participant's ear while another message is played into the participant's other ear.
- **Early-selection models:** Selective attention models in which sensory information is selected before any perceptual analysis is completed.
- **Early-filtering model:** An early-selection model in which only sensory information that is selectively attended to makes it through a filter leading to further perceptual analysis.
- **Attenuator model:** An early-selection model in which some sensory information is attenuated rather than being completely filtered out from further perceptual analysis.
- **Late-filtering model:** A selective attention model in which perceptual systems process all the information that enters them, followed by an unconscious decision concerning which information to attend to.
- **Conjunction search:** A visual search based on focusing attention on a combination of specific features.
- **Feature search:** A visual search based on focusing attention on a specific feature.
- **Binding problem:** The question of how features of experience are processed by distinct brain areas and neural systems but experienced as a unified whole.
- **Feature integration theory (FIT):** A proposed solution to the binding problem, in which attention is the glue that binds the various features of objects.
- **Illusory conjunction:** A visual task from which FIT is derived, in which the features of two distinct stimuli are erroneously conjoined when presented briefly.

The Cocktail Party Effect

So far, our examples of attention involved visual attention. However, as you may have guessed, the same attentional processes exist for all senses. For example, have you ever noticed that while focusing on your friend's words during a conversation in a busy place, such as a café or cafeteria, you pay no attention to the background noise, even if it is quite loud? That is, if someone were to ask you what the people sitting right beside you were saying, you would likely draw a blank. This is the result of **selective attention**, which permits you to voluntarily pick specific information to focus on out of a number of stimuli. The phenomenon in which selective attention is paid to a specific stimulus among a range of other stimuli is known as the **cocktail party effect**. It was first investigated by British psychologist E. C. Cherry (1914–1979) in the early 1950s.

However, as you selectively attend to your friend's words, you retain the ability to covertly monitor auditory information that is going on around you. For example, if your friend is boring, you can start paying attention to a more interesting conversation between the people sitting beside you while seemingly hanging on to every one of your friend's words. Also, even if you are selectively attending to what your friend is saying while tuning out other people's conversations, should someone mention your name or other information of interest, you are likely to automatically turn your attention toward that person.

Cherry investigated the cocktail party effect in the laboratory by recreating it using **dichotic listening**, illustrated in Figure 13.3. A spoken message was played into a participant's right ear while a different message was played into the left ear. The participant was asked to repeat the message played into one ear while listening to it. This proved to be an easy task for most participants. However, participants failed to repeat much of what was played into the ear not attended to.

FIGURE 13.3

The dichotic-listening set-up used by Cherry.

Ignored input
The horses galloped across the field . . .
Attended input
President Lincoln often read by the light of the fire . . .
Headphones
Speech output
"President Lincoln often read by the light of the fire . . ."

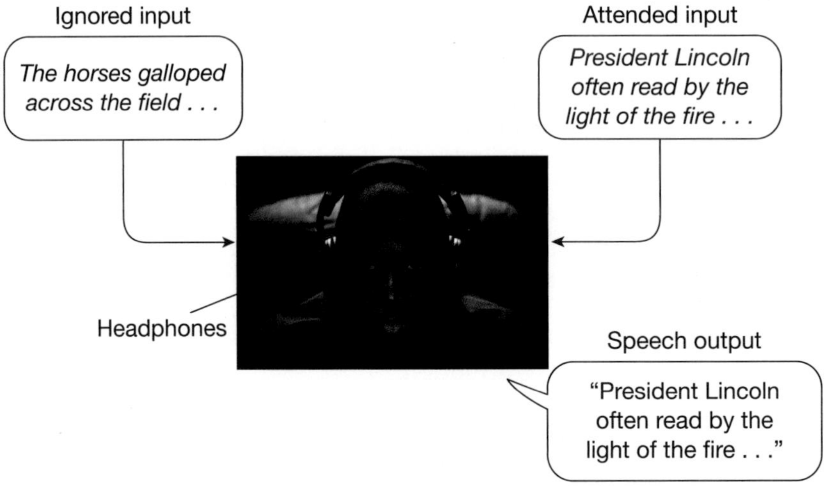

halbergman/istockphoto

These were fascinating results, but the mechanisms for how we can selectively attend to some stimuli while ignoring other stimuli going on simultaneously were still in need of an explanation.

Early- Versus Late-Selection Models

Imagine what life would be like without selective attention. Focusing on any one thing would be impossible. You would have great difficulty getting anything done, being distracted continuously with countless bits of information exciting every one of your senses. For this reason, information from our senses must enter a bottleneck or filtering process through which only a limited amount of information enters.

Psychologists have wondered about the nature of this filtering process and have come up with three models. The first two models illustrated in Figure 13.4 are **early-selection models**. Within these models, sensory information is selected early, that is, before any perceptual analysis is completed. According to the first of these models, proposed by psychologist Donald Broadbent (1957), sensory information is filtered out early in the nervous system and only the information selectively attended to makes it through the filter. This is known as an **early-filtering model** (Figure 13.4a). However, the problem with Broadbent's early-filtering model is that information not attended to is sometimes perceived. For example, this happens when, as mentioned earlier, you hear your name being said in background noise that, until your name was mentioned, you were not paying any attention to.

FIGURE 13.4

Models of selective attention: (a) early-filtering model, (b) attenuation model, (c) late-filtering model.

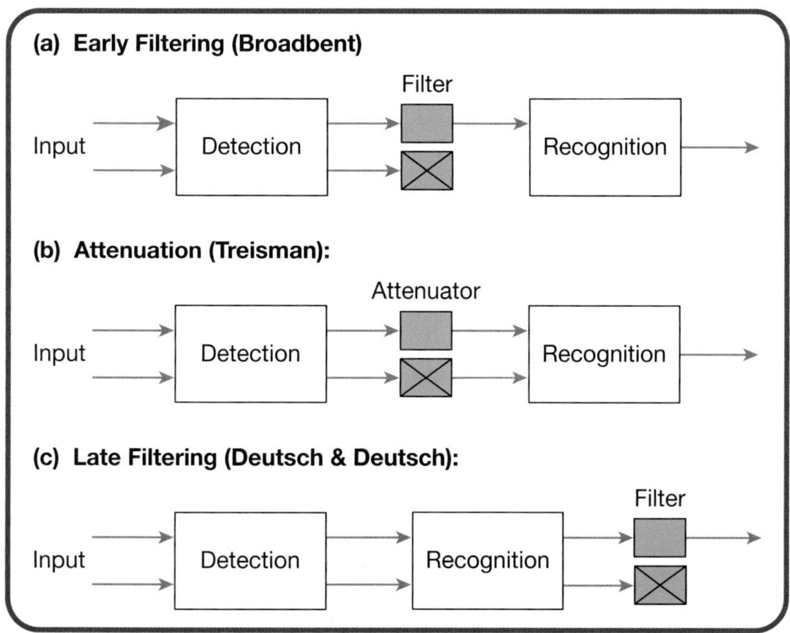

This problem was addressed by psychologist Anne Treisman, who proposed an alteration to Broadbent's early-filtering model. She proposed that unattended information is attenuated but not blocked out from further perceptual analysis (A. M. Treisman, 1964). This is known as the **attenuator model** (Figure 13.4b). She also proposed that certain types of information, such as your name, have a lower threshold for making it through the filter—that is, it makes it through more easily.

Finally, within the **late-filtering model** (Figure 13.4c), proposed by Deutsch and Deutsch (1963), perceptual systems process all the information that enters them. A later-occurring process then selects which information makes it to our conscious awareness or is stored in memory. This means that even if you are not consciously aware of things being said around you at the moment (because you are not paying attention to them), they may still influence your understanding of other information at a later time.

Visual Search

You are certainly familiar with the situation where you park your car in a shopping mall's parking lot, spend several hours shopping, and then spend several more minutes looking for your car. If your car is a black sedan of a certain make, then you're in trouble. This is because many cars in the parking lot fit that description. It may take you a long time to find your car, and you might even walk up to a car only to find that it is not yours. I once even got into someone else's car whose doors were unlocked. However, if your car is bright pink, you are likely to spot it soon after you exit the mall. Why is this so? The answer seems obvious . . . because it will appear to "pop out" among other cars.

Nevertheless, what you need to know is that looking for a specific black sedan among many others involves different attentional processes than spotting a bright pink car that looks like no other car in the lot. Looking for your black sedan requires that you discriminate it from the other black sedans by looking for the specific features that make up your car. For example, assume your black sedan is of a certain make, with mag wheels, and a "Baby on Board" sticker on the back window. In this case, you are focusing your attention on a combination of specific features, that is, a black sedan with mags and a "Baby on Board" sticker in the back window. This is known as a **conjunction search**. In a conjunction search, information is processed serially. Your attentional spotlight moves from car to car in the parking lot, looking for the combination

FIGURE 13.5

(a) In a feature search, a stimulus can be located based on a single feature, such as discriminating a red X among several green ones. (b) In a conjunction search, a stimulus is discriminated based on a combination of features, such as finding a red X among several green Xs and red Os. In this case, discrimination is based on both shape (X) and color (red).

(a) Feature search display

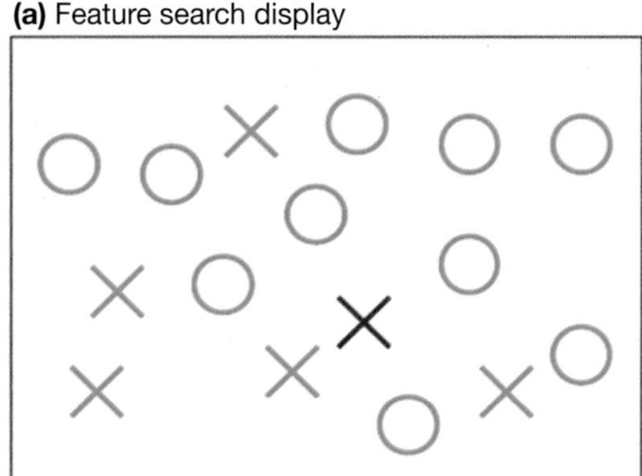

(b) Conjunction search display

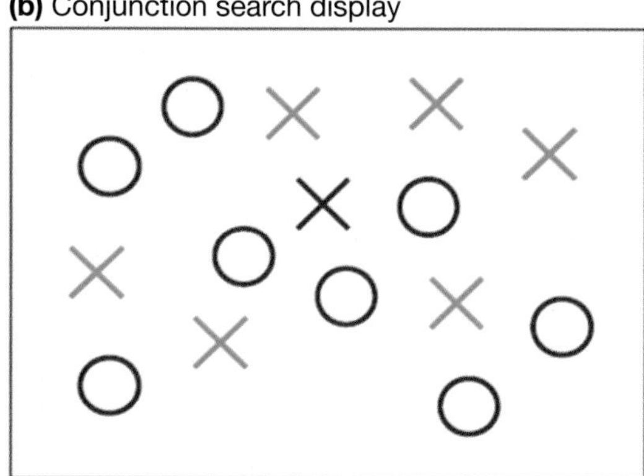

Robertson, L.C. (2003). Binding, spatial attention and perceptual awareness. *Nature Reviews of Neuroscience* 4(2): 93–102. With permission from Springer Nature.

of features that correspond to your car. In addition, the time it will take you to find your car will depend on the number of similar cars in the lot.

In contrast, if your car is bright pink, you can find it based on only one feature—"bright pink"—because there are not likely to be many bright pink cars in the lot. This is known as a **feature search**. Your pink car pops out among all the others automatically and no serial search is necessary.

Anne Treisman investigated the differences in attentional processing during feature and conjunction searches (A. Treisman, 1982). As shown in Figure 13.5, she found that study participants more readily identified a red X among several green Xs than a red X among several green Xs and red Os.

In Figure 13.5a (the feature search), finding the red X among several green Xs is done quickly because one's attention does not have to focus on each of the Xs in a serial manner. The red X appears to just pop out of the crowd of Xs, just like the bright pink car popped out of the sea of cars in the parking lot in the preceding example.

In contrast, in Figure 13.5b (the conjunction search), finding the red X takes significantly longer because it does not simply pop out at you. This is because "red" is not the only feature of the target letter X, as in Figure 13.5a. There are also red Os and several green Xs. In other words, the correct color must be combined with the correct letter. To do so, attention must be focused on each of the letters in a serial manner, which takes significantly longer.

FIGURE 13.6

Feature integration theory.

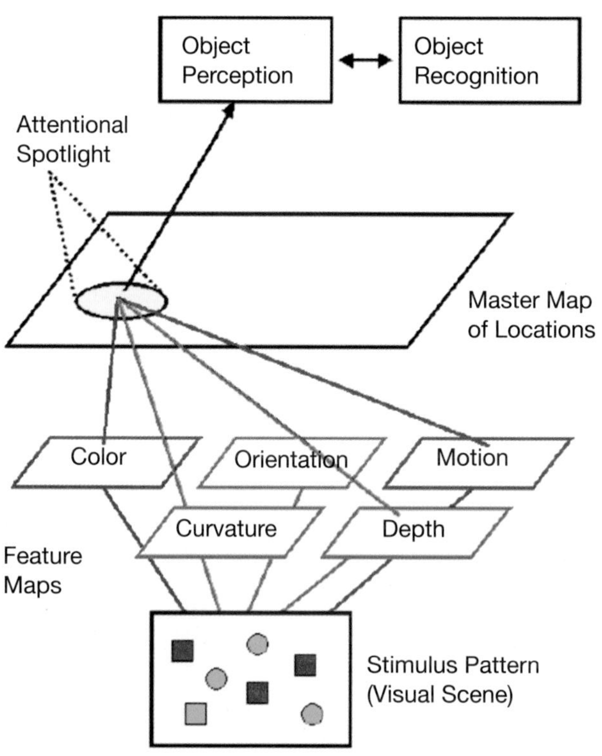

From Ch. 7: A Cognitive Basis for Friend-Foe Misidentification in Combat, Keebler, Sciarini, & Jentsch. In *Human Factors Issues in Combat Identification*, edited by Herz, Andrews & Wolf. Copyright © 2010. With permission from Taylor & Francis.

Feature Integration Theory

When you look at an object, you can perceive its color, shape, orientation, and distance and whether it is moving or stationary. Without hesitation, you attribute these qualities to the specific object to which you are paying attention, for example, a red ball rolling down a hill. However, these various features of objects are processed within distinct brain areas. The question of how different features of an object are perceived as a whole is known as the **binding problem**.

Several solutions to the binding problem have been proposed (see Revonsuo, 1999). One solution that has attracted much attention (pun intended) is known as the **feature integration theory (FIT)** (A. M. Treisman & Gelade, 1980). According to FIT, visual scenes are made up of stimulus patterns, consisting of features such as color, curvature, orientation, motion, and depth. As illustrated in Figure 13.6, Treisman proposed that these features compose a feature map. In this map, the features are unbound and not associated with a particular object. According to Treisman, the feature map is scanned by an attentional spotlight. Once under the spotlight, the features of an object are bound. At this point, the object is perceived and compared to representations of objects in memory and recognized.

Feature integration theory accounts for a phenomenon known as **illusory conjunction**, in which the features of two distinct stimuli are erroneously conjoined when presented briefly. For example, as illustrated in Figure 13.7, Anne Treisman and colleagues (A. Treisman & Schmidt, 1982) showed subjects a pair of letters, with each letter of the pair being in a different color (e.g., red A and blue X), for a very brief period. The subjects were then asked to report on what they had seen. Subjects frequently combined the letters with the wrong colors (i.e., blue A and red X), an illusory conjunction. Subjects sometimes reported seeing a letter or a color that was not part of the presented stimuli, known as a letter or color intrusion, respectively.

The explanation for these results is that, when presented for a brief period, the features of objects cannot be accurately bound, because there is not enough time for the attentional spotlight to zoom into the feature map.

FIGURE 13.7

Illusory conjunction. See text for details.

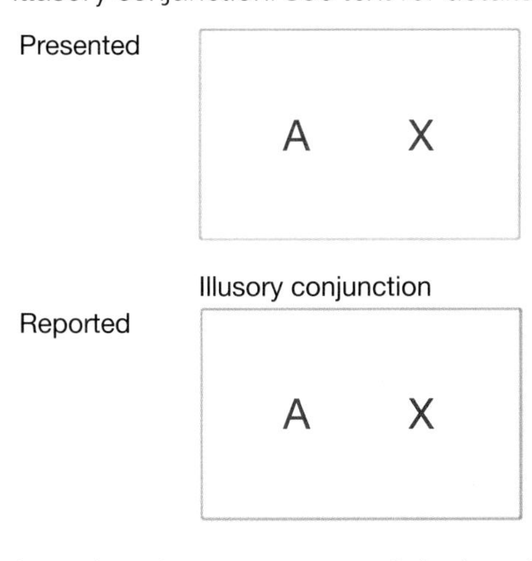

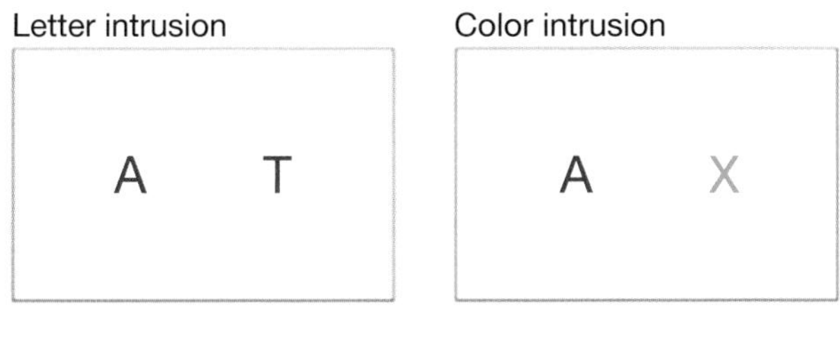

Robertson, L.C. (2003). Binding, spatial attention and perceptual awareness. *Nature Reviews of Neuroscience 4*(2): 93–102. With permission from Springer Nature.

13.1.3 ATTENTION: WHERE IN THE BRAIN?

>> LO 13.1.3 **Describe the main brain networks of attention and how they were discovered.**

Key Terms

- **Dorsal-frontoparietal system:** Includes areas of the dorsal-posterior parietal cortex along the intraparietal sulcus and the frontal eye field in the frontal cortex. It is involved in the top-down control of attention.
- **Ventral-frontoparietal system:** Includes the temporoparietal cortex (or temporoparietal junction [TPJ]) and the ventral frontal cortex. It is involved in the bottom-up control of attention.
- **Top-down control of attention:** When attention is voluntary and controlled by conscious thought, expectations, and goals.
- **Bottom-up control of attention:** Also known as stimulus-driven attention, in which stimuli that are currently unattended to, surprising, or unexpected shift your attention from what you are currently attending to.

So far, you have learned about some of the basic ideas and concepts that compose the study of attention. However, we have not yet mentioned the brain areas thought to be involved in attention. Researchers have investigated (and continue to investigate) many brain areas and how they interact in attention.

The Dorsal-Frontoparietal System and the Ventral-Frontoparietal System

In this section, we focus on two systems known to be involved in attention. These are the **dorsal-frontoparietal system** and the **ventral-frontoparietal system**. The dorsal-frontoparietal system includes areas of the dorsal-posterior parietal cortex along the intraparietal sulcus and the frontal eye field (FEF) in the frontal cortex. The ventral-frontoparietal system includes the temporoparietal cortex (or temporoparietal junction [TPJ]) and the ventral frontal cortex.

Each system is involved predominantly in one of the ways in which we use our ability to pay attention. The dorsal-frontoparietal system is activated during endogenous attention. Recall that, as mentioned in the first section of the chapter, endogenous attention is guided voluntarily, such as when you decide to pay attention to what your friend is saying rather than to conversations between other people. This requires what is known as the **top-down control of attention**, which refers to attention controlled by conscious thought, expectations, and goals.

In contrast, the ventral-frontoparietal system is involved in exogenous attention. Again, recall from the beginning of the chapter that exogenous attention is driven by stimuli that are outside of your current focus of attention, such as when a knock at the door causes you to momentarily abandon your textbook to see who is at the door. This involves the **bottom-up control of attention**, in which unexpected stimuli automatically shift your attention away from what you are currently attending to. This is also known as stimulus-driven attention.

Maurizio Corbetta (1998) discovered that different brain systems are involved in the top-down and bottom-up control of attention. He did so by conducting some ingenious experiments. To see how the brain was activated during the top-down control of attention, Corbetta and Shulman (2002) asked participants to stare at the middle of a screen, while their brains were being imaged by functional magnetic resonance imaging (fMRI). The participants then saw an arrow signaling them to covertly shift their attention to a location in the periphery of their visual field, where a visual stimulus would be presented. Remember the meaning of covert attention from the beginning of the chapter. Here it means that the participants had to direct their attention to where the arrow indicated but without moving their eyes. This is an example of covert spatial attention.

The procedure and results of this experiment are illustrated in Figure 13.8a. The top-down control of attention activated areas along the intraparietal sulcus, including the anterior, posterior, and ventral intraparietal sulcus (aPs, pPs and vPs, respectively) as well as the FEF. These are the areas, mentioned earlier, that are part of the dorsal-frontoparietal system of attention. This occurred whether the participants covertly attended to the right or to the left. Note that other brain areas, such as the fusiform gyrus and area MT+, were also activated. However, these were thought to be activated by the sensory analysis of the cue and were not attributed to attentional processes.

Remember that in addition to spatial attention, attention can also be focused on objects and features of objects. As mentioned earlier, features of objects include color, shape, and direction of motion. Corbetta (1998) also found that the same regions were activated when participants were told to pay attention to the direction of motion of objects (Figure 13.8b).

FIGURE 13.8

Top-down direction of attention. Areas activated (a) by covertly attending to a region of space and (b) by covertly attending to the direction of motion.

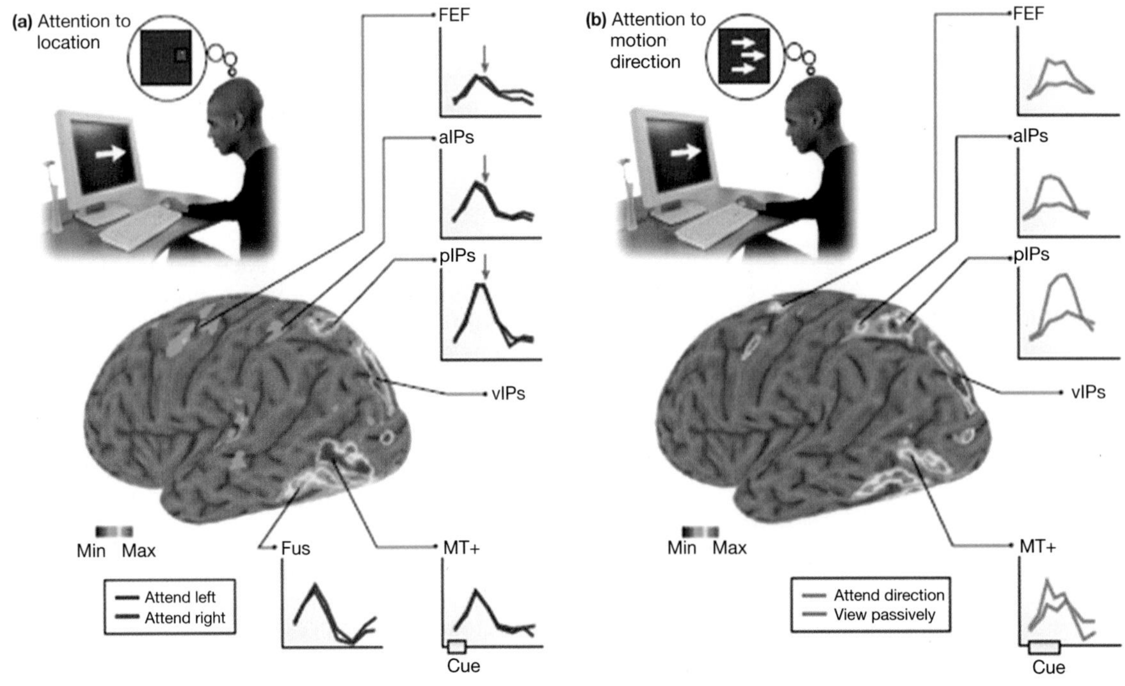

Corbetta, M & G.L. Shulman. Control of Goal-Directed and Stimulus-Driven Attention in the Brain. *Nature Reviews Neuroscience* 3(3): 201–215. With permission from Springer Nature.

As you just learned, we do not always direct our attention to stimuli in a top-down manner. Attention is often directed to stimuli that were previously unattended to or unexpected. That is, attention is often directed through a bottom-up or stimulus-driven process, such as when the sound of an incoming email interrupts your attention to an important research paper you were reading, or when someone taps you on the shoulder to ask you a question while you are immersed in listening to music through your earbuds. In each case, your attention is reoriented from focusing on one stimulus to another. Notice that this reorienting occurs across sensory modalities. For example, from visual (studying) to auditory (email notification) or from auditory (listening to music) to tactile (tap on the shoulder).

The brain areas involved in the reorientation of attention were investigated in an experiment conducted by Karen Davis and colleagues at the University of Toronto (Downar, Crawley, Mikulis, & Davis, 2000). The experimental procedure is illustrated in Figure 13.9a. While having their brain imaged by fMRI, participants were simultaneously stimulated in three different modalities: visual, auditory, and tactile. The participants were subjected to two types of stimuli for each modality. The visual stimuli consisted of either a blue or a red abstract figure, the auditory stimuli consisted of either the sound of running water or that of a croaking frog, and the tactile stimuli consisted of either circular brushing or the tapping of the right leg with a brush. Each of the stimuli is represented in the corresponding visual, auditory, and tactile rows in the figure.

The reorientation of the participants' attention was created by changing the stimulus type in one of the modalities (a transition) every 14 seconds. For example, at the far left of Figure 13.9a, a participant is stimulated by the blue abstract figure, the running water sound, and circular brushing of the leg simultaneously. After 14 seconds, a transition was made in the auditory stimulus only (represented by the capital A in the transition row). Fourteen seconds later, a transition was made only in the tactile stimulus, that is, from circular brushing to tapping. These transitions caused the participants to reorient their attention to the change.

Figure 13.9b shows the results of the experiment. The reorienting of attention at each transition was associated with activity in the ventral-frontoparietal attentional network, especially in the TPJ, independently of the modality in which the transition occurred. Activity was also shown to increase in the brain areas associated with each of the modalities when a transition in each of the respective modalities occurred. These results suggest that the TPJ, which is part of the frontoparietal attentional network, is involved in the reorienting of attention.

FIGURE 13.9

(a) Participants were subjected to two types of stimuli in three sensory modalities simultaneously: visual (blue or red abstract figures), auditory (sound of running water or of a croaking frog), and tactile (circular brushing or tapping on the right leg). A transition in only one type of stimulus was made every 14 seconds (top row). (b) Activation of the TPJ occurred at every transition, irrespective of modality.

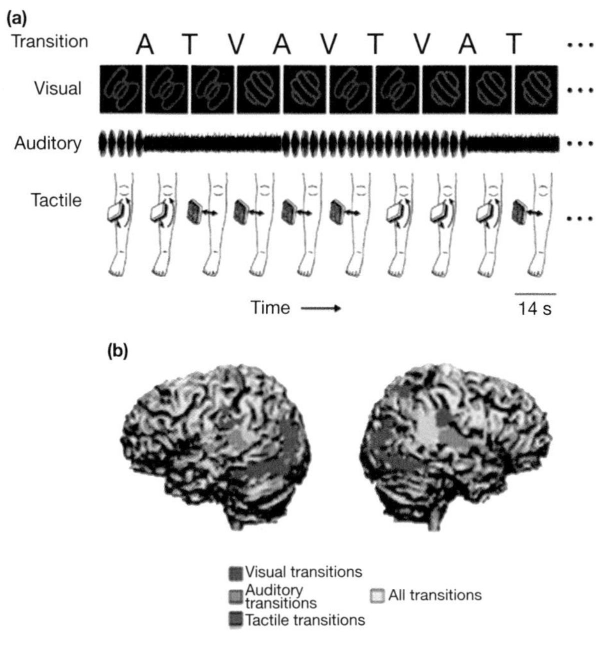

(a) Downar, J., et al. (2000). A multimodal cortical network for the detection of changes in the sensory environment. *Nature Neuroscience* 3(3), 277–283. With permission from Springer Nature; (b) Corbetta, M & G.L. Shulman. Control of Goal-Directed and Stimulus-Driven Attention in the Brain. *Nature Reviews Neuroscience* 3(3): 201–215. With permission from Springer Nature.

FIGURE 13.10

The thalamus is subdivided in many different areas. The pulvinar (green) is located at the posterior-most end of the thalamus.

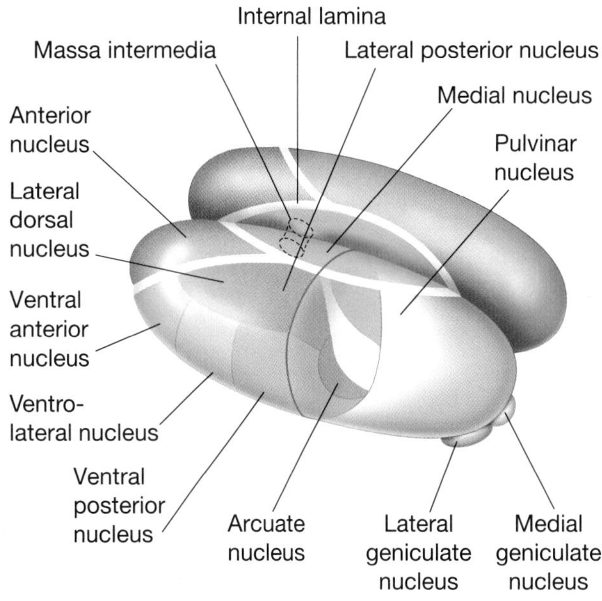

Amanda Tomasikiewicz/Body Scientific Intl.

The Thalamus

In addition to the two cortical networks of attention just discussed, attention is also controlled subcortically. Neuroscientists Steven Petersen and David Lee Robinson inactivated a region of the thalamus called the pulvinar on one side of the brain (Figure 13.10) in monkeys (Petersen, Robinson, & Keys, 1985).

The monkeys had difficulty in covertly orienting their attention to cued locations presented on the side of the screen that was opposite to the side of the thalamus that was inactivated. They were also less able to ignore distracting stimuli. Taken together, these findings meant that the pulvinar is important for both top-down and bottom-up processing of attention.

One idea about selective attention is that it depends on the synchronous firing of neurons in different brain areas. For example, selective attention has been associated with the synchronous firing of neurons in the FEF with those in the visual cortex (Gregoriou, Gotts, Zhou, & Desimone, 2009), as well as with the synchronous firing of neurons in the frontal cortex with those in the parietal cortex (Buschman & Miller, 2007). However, it was not known how the firing of neurons in different brain areas became synchronized. Neuroscientist Sabine Kastner and colleagues at Princeton University found that the synchronous firing of neurons across brain areas is driven by the pulvinar (Saalmann, Pinsk, Wang, Li, & Kastner, 2012).

13.1.4 DISORDERS OF ATTENTION

>> LO 13.1.4 **Describe two disorders of attention due to brain damage.**

Key Terms

- **Balint syndrome:** A syndrome characterized by simultanagnosia, optic ataxia, and oculomotor apraxia due to damage to the parieto-occipital region.
- **Simultanagnosia:** The inability to perceive multiple objects simultaneously in a visual scene.
- **Optic ataxia:** The inability to accurately reach for objects.
- **Oculomotor apraxia:** The inability to perform voluntary eye movements.
- **Unilateral neglect:** A syndrome characterized by the inability to attend to the side of visual space on the opposite side of unilateral damage to the parietal and temporal cortices (sometimes referred to as hemispatial neglect).

The brain processes associated with attention are taken for granted. In fact, we are not aware of them. However, damage to the brain areas involved in these processes can significantly affect the way we perceive the world. In this unit, we discuss two different patterns of damage to the brain's attentional systems. These patterns of brain damage are associated with attentional disorders such as Balint syndrome and unilateral neglect.

Balint Syndrome

Imagine not being able to perceive two objects at the same time. For example, suppose that both a fork and

FIGURE 13.11

Common tests of simultanagnosia. (a) Patients with Balint syndrome can focus their attention on only one object in a visual scene at a time, resulting in the inability to describe the context of the scene. (b) Balint syndrome patients also have difficulty disengaging their attention from an individual component of an object (e.g., they would likely perceive an individual W rather than the letter F, or an individual vegetable rather than a face).

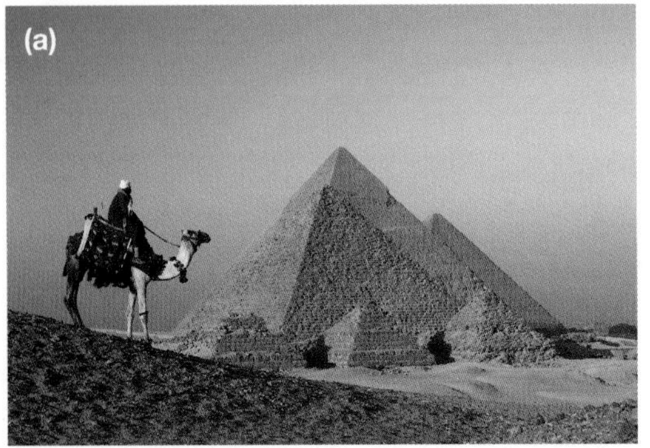

(b) WWWWWWWWWWWWW
W
W
W
W
WWWWWWWWWWWWW
W
W
W
W

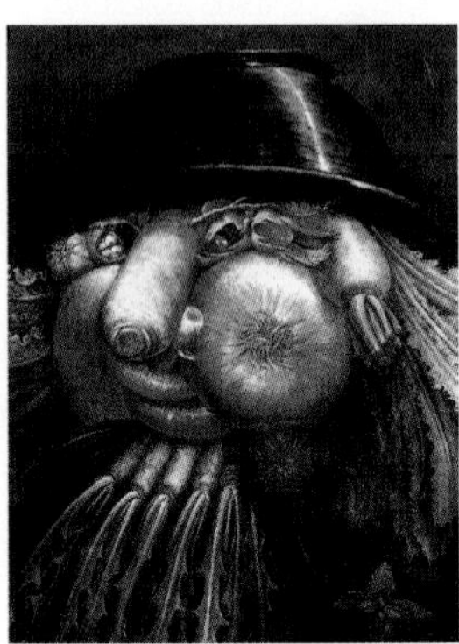

(a) sculpies/istockphoto

a key were presented within your visual field. When asked what you are seeing, you would report seeing only the fork or the key but not both. This means that you would be unable to grasp the relationship between objects in a visual scene. As reported by a patient with **Balint syndrome**, watching television can be a frustrating experience because she could focus her attention on only one character at a time.

Balint syndrome was named after Hungarian neurologist and psychiatrist Rezso Balint (1874–1929), who first observed it in a brain-damaged patient (Husain & Stein, 1988). Balint syndrome is associated with bilateral damage to the parieto-occipital region, which attests to the importance of the parietal and occipital cortices for visual attention. The damage to these regions can occur in many different ways, including through strokes, tumors, traumatic brain injury, or neurodegenerative diseases.

Balint syndrome is characterized by three primary symptoms. **Simultanagnosia**, as described previously, is the inability to perceive multiple objects in a visual scene. For example, while looking at the scene in Figure 13.11a, a Balint syndrome patient may be able to focus attention only on the man riding the camel, resulting in the failure to describe the context of the entire scene, which is a man riding a camel in the vicinity of the Egyptian pyramids.

This deficit also extends to individual objects. That is, they may focus on only one specific feature of an object without being able to process the whole. For example, a patient with Balint syndrome looking at Figure 13.11b (left) might focus on only a single W, failing to perceive that the collection of Ws forms the letter F. They may also fail to perceive that a collection of vegetables forms a face (Figure 13.11b, right).

Other symptoms of Balint syndrome include **optic ataxia**, which is the inability to accurately reach for objects, and **oculomotor apraxia**, which is the difficulty in voluntarily moving the eyes.

Unilateral Neglect

Spatial neglect refers to a condition in which brain-damaged patients can pay attention to only one side of visual space and completely ignore the other side. For example, a neglect patient may eat the food located on only one side of the plate. When asked to copy drawings of objects, patients typically copy only one side of the drawings (Figure 13.12). For this reason, it is often called **unilateral neglect** or hemispatial neglect.

FIGURE 13.12

Patients with unilateral neglect fail to attend to the side of visual space that is contralateral to the brain damage. When formally tested, patients with unilateral neglect copy only one side of the drawing and ignore the side of the drawing contralateral to the drawing to be copied.

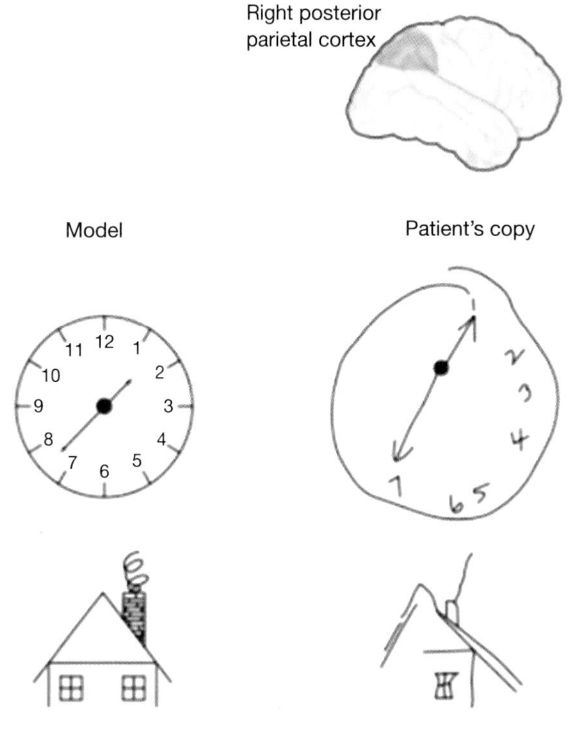

In contrast to Balint syndrome, unilateral neglect results from damage to only one hemisphere. This explains why the neglected side of visual space is contralateral to the brain damage. The damage observed in unilateral neglect is to the parietal and temporal cortices, usually in the right hemisphere, but is also sometimes observed in the left hemisphere.

MODULE SUMMARY

Attention is the ability to select a stimulus, focus on it, sustain that focus, and shift that focus at will. Attention can be subdivided in two broad types: overt attention and covert attention. Overt attention is the shifting of attention, which includes the reorienting of sensory receptors, whereas covert attention is the ability to shift attention from stimulus to stimulus without reorienting sensory receptors. Attention can also be endogenous, which is the self-directed and voluntary attention to a stimulus, or exogenous, which occurs when attention is drawn toward a stimulus in a reflexive and involuntary manner. Attention focused to a specific location in space is known as spatial attention. Object attention refers to attention directed at a specific object, and feature attention refers to attention directed at a specific feature of an object. During the process of selective attention, specific information to focus on is picked out of a number of stimuli. The phenomenon by which a specific stimulus, such as one's name, can be picked out of a range of other stimuli is known as the cocktail party effect.

Three models of selective attention have been proposed: an early-filtering model, in which only sensory information selectively attended to is analyzed; an attenuator model, in which some sensory information is attenuated rather than being completely filtered out; and a late-filtering model, in which perceptual systems process all incoming information followed by an unconscious decision concerning which information to attend to. Visual searches can involve focusing attention on a combination of features, in what is known as a conjunction search. Visual searches can also be done by focusing on one individual feature at a time, in what is known as a feature search.

Features of experience are processed by distinct brain areas and neural systems but are experienced as a unified whole. This is known as the binding problem. Feature integration theory was proposed as a solution to the binding problem. Support for feature integration theory comes from findings that features of two distinct stimuli are erroneously conjoined when presented briefly, in a phenomenon known as an illusory conjunction.

Two main attentional systems have been discovered in the brain. One of these systems is the dorsal-frontoparietal system, which is involved in the top-down control of attention, that is, when attention is controlled voluntarily by conscious thought. The other system is the ventral-frontoparietal system, which is involved in the bottom-up control of attention, that is, when stimuli that are currently unattended to, surprising, or unexpected shift attention away from what is currently being attended to. Attention is also controlled by the pulvinar, an area of the thalamus involved in both top-down and bottom-up control of attention. The pulvinar also synchronizes the activity of neurons across brain areas during focused attention. Damage to attentional systems can give rise to disorders of attention. Balint syndrome is characterized by simultanagnosia, optic ataxia, and oculomotor apraxia due to damage to the parieto-occipital region. Unilateral neglect (also known as hemispatial neglect) is characterized by the inability to attend to the side of visual space on the opposite side of unilateral damage to the parietal and temporal cortices.

TEST YOURSELF

13.1.1 Name the different types of attention and differentiate between the various types.

13.1.2 Explain the various concepts that are part of the study of attention.

13.1.3 Describe the main brain networks of attention. Describe the experiments by which they were discovered.

13.1.4 Name and describe two disorders of attention and the type of brain damage that characterizes them.

13.2 Consciousness

Module Contents

13.2.1 What Is Consciousness?

13.2.2 The Problems of Consciousness

13.2.3 The Neural Correlates and Contents of Consciousness

13.2.4 A Neurobiological Theory of Consciousness

13.2.5 Disorders of Consciousness

13.2.6 Hidden Consciousness

13.2.7 Free Will

Learning Objectives

13.2.1 Explain what scientists know about consciousness and describe its components.

13.2.2 Define and explain the hard and easy problems of consciousness.

13.2.3 Explain what is meant by neural correlates of consciousness.

13.2.4 Describe and explain the global workspace theory of consciousness.

13.2.5 Describe and explain some disorders of consciousness.

13.2.6 Explain how consciousness can be hidden.

13.2.7 Describe and explain experiments designed to test whether humans have free will.

13.2.1 WHAT IS CONSCIOUSNESS?

>> LO 13.2.1 Explain what scientists know about consciousness and describe its components.

Key Terms

- **Subjective experience:** The continuous flow of thoughts, feelings, and perceptions that one is privy to throughout life.
- **Intentionality:** The idea that consciousness includes mental states that are about something.

- **Chinese room:** A thought experiment designed to show that computers manipulate symbols by how they are organized and ordered but, unlike humans, do so without purpose, meaning, or understanding of what they are doing.

The mystery of consciousness has fascinated people for millennia and continues to baffle philosophers and scientists to this day. In the 1600s, philosopher and mathematician René Descartes (1596–1650) proposed that the mind and the brain were separate entities. Descartes thought that the immaterial and rational mind was what separated us from animals, which without a mind (or soul) were mere automatons. However, this raised the question of how an immaterial mind can interact with the physical body. Descartes's answer to this question was that the mind controlled the body through the pineal gland, situated between the two hemispheres of the brain (see Chapter 1).

Today, neuroscientists believe that the brain produces consciousness. However, the question of where and how consciousness is generated in the brain is the focus of much hypothesizing and heated debates. Some contemporary philosophers believe that this question will never be answered, whereas the most optimistic ones believe that we are close to an answer.

The study of consciousness is complex. This will become obvious to you as you read through the chapter. Defining consciousness is not an easy task. There is no universally accepted definition of consciousness. We can at least agree that consciousness has to do with **subjective experience**, which includes the continuous flow of thoughts, feelings, and perceptions that one is privy to throughout life. Subjective experiences often cannot be put into words for others to understand them. For example, imagine trying to explain to someone who is blind from birth the "redness" of an apple.

Is the Mind Like a Computer?

One question often asked by students is whether the mind or brain is like a computer. An answer to this question was proposed by philosopher John Rogers Searle. Searle rejects the idea that the mind is a computer-like, sophisticated information processor. To Searle, computers manipulate symbols by how they are organized and ordered, but they do so without **intentionality**, that is, with no purpose, meaning, or understanding of what they are doing. The computations they perform are about something to us but about nothing to them (J. R. Searle, 1983). To illustrate this idea, Searle proposed a thought experiment known as the **Chinese room** (J. Searle, 1980).

This thought experiment goes as follows: Imagine yourself alone, inside a room with nothing but a computer. Occasionally, a strip of paper with Chinese characters printed on it is slipped under the door. Your task is to respond to these characters, but you do not understand Chinese. Fortunately, you can feed the characters into the computer, which outputs the rules, written in your native language, for you to properly reply in Chinese (Figure 13.13). This would surely fool anyone on the outside that a Chinese speaker was in the room. The Chinese characters you thus produce would mean something to someone who can read Chinese but mean nothing to you. Searle's take-home message is that a computer can appear conscious simply because it can follow a set of instructions. But like you, in the Chinese room, the computer has no understanding of what its outputs mean.

FIGURE 13.13

The Chinese room. Examples of instructions given to non-Chinese speakers to properly reply to notes written in Chinese.

If you see this shape,	then produce this shape
"什麼"	"爲天"
followed by this shape,	followed by this shape,
"帶來"	"下式".
followed by this shape,	
"快樂"	

Why Study Consciousness?

Although neuroscientists have, so far, not been able to pinpoint the areas of the brain responsible for consciousness, research aimed at identifying these areas is definitely worthwhile (Michel et al., 2019). Aside from satisfying deep curiosity about the topic, which is the core of all scientific endeavors, finding out more about how the brain produces consciousness will provide a deeper understanding of various neurological disorders, such as unresponsive wakefulness, described in the chapter's opening vignette on Terri Schiavo.

13.2.2 THE PROBLEMS OF CONSCIOUSNESS

>> LO 13.2.2 **Define and explain the hard and easy problems of consciousness.**

Key Terms

- **Easy problem:** Explaining mental phenomena that are testable by standard methods of science.
- **Hard problem:** Explaining how brain activity produces subjective experience.
- **Explanatory gap:** The problem in explaining how neural mechanisms are linked to subjective experience.

Philosopher David Chalmers (1995) proposed what are known as the easy problem and the hard problem of consciousness. The **easy problem** refers to the explanation of mental phenomena that are testable by standard methods of science. This includes the recognition of stimuli, cognitive processes, and the processes involved in wakefulness and sleep. An easy problem is solved once its neurobiological mechanisms are specified. For example, visual experience is explained by the stimulation of photoreceptors by a specific range of wavelengths along the electromagnetic spectrum, which ultimately results in the activation of the visual cortex and extrastriate areas (see Chapter 6).

Chalmers proposed that the **hard problem** is what remains once the neurobiological mechanisms of a phenomenon have been explained. For example, we can explain the mechanisms by which visual experience occurs (through the sequence of events just described), but we cannot explain how these mechanisms give rise to the subjective experience of colors. Similarly, we can explain how potentially threatening stimuli activate the amygdala, which in turn activates the sympathetic nervous system through activation of the hypothalamus (see Chapter 11), but we cannot explain the feelings of fear and anxiety that emerge from this process.

Philosophers wonder why these mechanisms or processes give rise to subjective experience, and neuroscientists wonder about how the brain produces such experiences. Philosopher Joseph Levine (1983) calls the problem in explaining how neural mechanisms are linked to subjective experience the **explanatory gap**.

13.2.3 THE NEURAL CORRELATES AND CONTENTS OF CONSCIOUSNESS

>> LO 13.2.3 **Explain what is meant by neural correlates of consciousness.**

Key Terms

- **Neural correlates of consciousness:** The minimal neuronal events jointly sufficient for any one specific conscious percept.
- **Cortical blindness:** People for whom the source of blindness is damage to the primary visual cortex.
- **Blindsight:** The phenomenon observed in people with cortical blindness who can make accurate guesses about stimuli while at the same time not being visually aware of them.
- **Binocular rivalry:** The phenomenon in which perception spontaneously switches between two different images that are presented simultaneously to each eye.
- **Affective blindsight**: The phenomenon in which patients with blindsight react reliably to the emotional stimuli presented to their blind visual field.

Neuroscientists who study consciousness want to discover the brain processes that accompany conscious awareness. To do so, they conduct experiments in which stimuli are manipulated so that they can be processed in a conscious or an unconscious manner, while measuring the brain activity triggered in participants. The results of these experiments provide clues to the neurobiological basis of consciousness.

Neuroscientists Francis Crick, co-discoverer of DNA, and Christof Koch (1990) stated that "the problem of consciousness will, in the long run, be solved only by explanations at the neuronal level" (p. 263). To many scientists, great leaps in the understanding of consciousness will be made through discovering **neural correlates of consciousness** (NCCs). Crick and Koch (1990) define NCCs as the minimal neuronal events jointly sufficient for any one specific conscious percept. This is illustrated in Figure 13.14. In this example, the percept of a dog can be produced only once a

FIGURE 13.14

The neural correlates of consciousness (NCCs). For example, the percept of a dog can be achieved only once a minimal set of neuronal events have occurred.

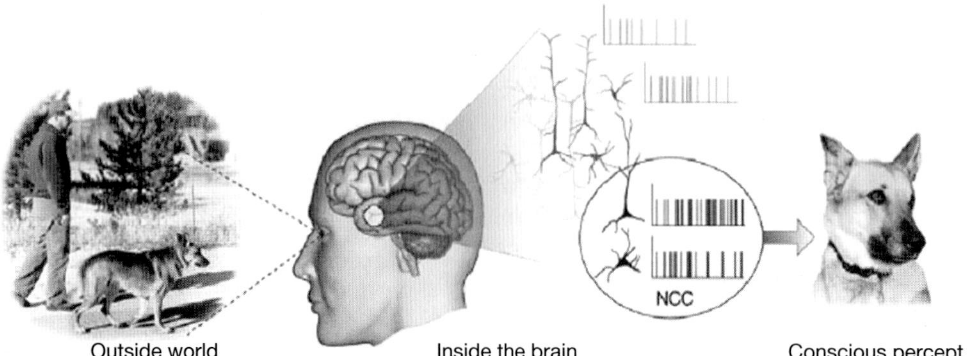

Adapted from *The Quest for Consciousness: A Neurobiological Approach*, Koch. Copyright © 2004 by Roberts and Company Publishers.

basic set of neural processes have occurred. In other words, it is the NCCs that differentiate conscious percepts from phenomena that remain unconscious.

Not all stimuli are consciously perceived. One goal of neuroscientists, in their quest to find the NCCs, is to distinguish between the brain processes involved when a subject is consciously aware of a stimulus from the processes involved when a subject is not consciously aware of a stimulus. A stimulus does not have to be consciously perceived to be acted upon. One striking example of this is found in patients with **cortical blindness**. These patients have intact retinas. The source of their blindness is damage to the primary visual cortex. In a phenomenon known as **blindsight**—a term coined by psychologist Lawrence Weiskrantz, who studied the phenomenon extensively—patients can make accurate guesses about a stimulus while at the same time not being visually aware of it. In another phenomenon, known as **binocular rivalry**, the brain processes involved in conscious and unconscious processing can be distinguished.

Blindsight

In a classic study, Weiskrantz and colleagues reported findings obtained from the study of a brain-damaged patient known as DB (Weiskrantz, Warrington, Sanders, & Marshall, 1974). DB was subjected to the ablation of the right occipital cortex (which contains the primary visual cortex) to remove a tumor. This left him blind to stimuli presented to him in his left visual field (you can read about the reasons for this crossover in Chapter 6). This is known as cortical blindness. Despite not being able to consciously perceive stimuli presented to his left, he was able to discriminate between different orientations of gratings and directions of movement when presented there. He was also able to reach out toward stimuli present in his left visual field.

More recently, Weiskrantz and colleagues studied a patient with cortical blindness, known as TN, who suffered damage to the primary visual cortex in both the left and right hemispheres, which means that he is blind to both the left and right visual fields. Remarkably, TN, who is totally blind, can navigate throughout his environment while avoiding objects (De Gelder, 2010).

How can this be happening? From the retina, visual information follows a path to the thalamus, from which information flows to the primary visual cortex and then through the "where" and "what" pathways of the parietal and temporal cortices, respectively (see Chapter 6). However, as shown in Figure 13.15, the retina also sends projections to the superior colliculus (SC), which in turn connects with the "where" pathway of the parietal cortex. In this way, the SC mediates reflexive responses to visual information, such as automatically orienting the eyes to objects moving around in the visual field (Tamietto et al., 2010).

Blindsight is but one example in which behavior is controlled without conscious perceptual awareness. Recall from Chapter 11 "the low road" and "the high road" of emotional processing proposed by psychologist Joseph LeDoux. On "the low road," the amygdala automatically triggers a fear response to potentially threatening stimuli through connections with the hypothalamus. You may also remember Antonio Damasio's somatic-marker hypothesis (also discussed in Chapter 11), according to which unconscious emotions can assist in decision making in times of uncertainty by giving you a hunch about which of several options you should choose or stay away from.

FIGURE 13.15

Visual pathways from the retina. Blindsight is mediated through a pathway from the retina to the superior colliculus and the "where" pathway of the parietal lobe.

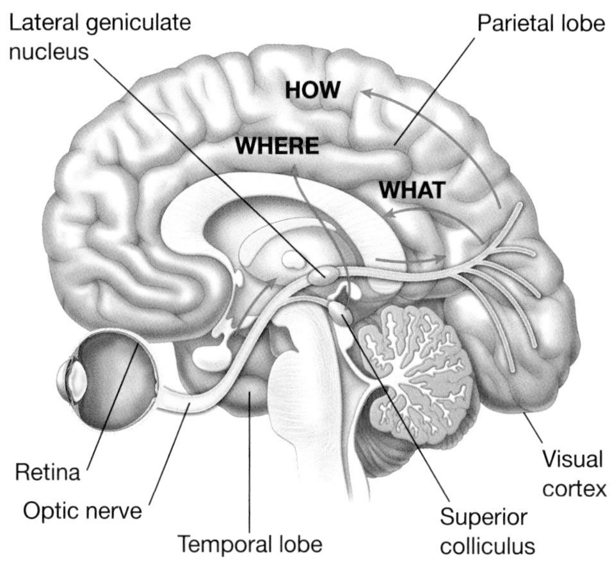

Amanda Tomasikiewicz/Body Scientific Intl.

FIGURE 13.16

Affective blindsight. Some patients with blindsight can reliably and appropriately react to faces with emotional expressions presented in their blind visual field, as measured by facial electromyography.

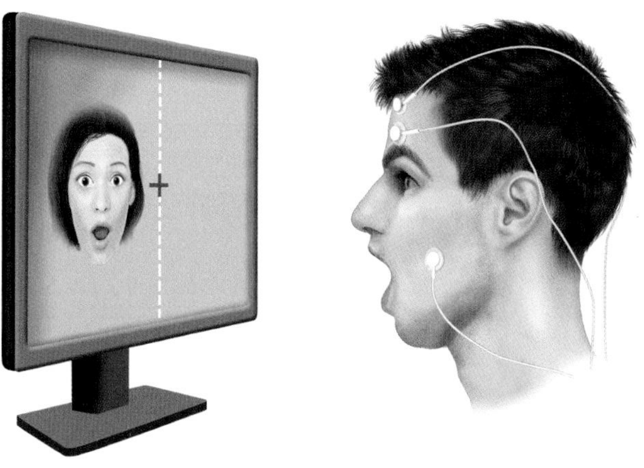

Liana Bauman/Body Scientific Intl.

FIGURE 13.17

(a) Binocular rivalry is induced by presenting each eye with a different image. Perception alternates between the two images. (b) Apparatus used in binocular rivalry experiments.

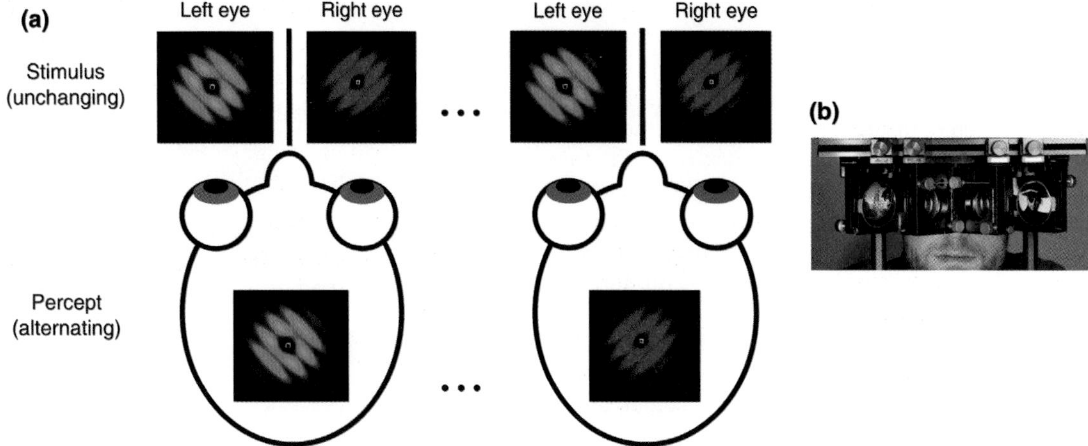

Vanderbilt University.

In fact, patients with blindsight can react to emotional expressions on the faces of people without being consciously aware of it, a phenomenon termed **affective blindsight**. Neuroscientist Beatrice De Gelder and colleagues (Tamietto et al., 2009) presented blindsight patients (including DB, mentioned earlier) with images of faces displaying various emotions in their blind visual field (Figure 13.16). At the same time, they measured the patients' facial reactions using facial electromyography, which measures muscle tension. Amazingly, even if the patients could not see the faces on the screen, the patients' facial expressions mimicked those presented on the screen. The authors took these findings as evidence that emotional contagion, which is the spreading of emotions from one person to another, occurs through visual pathways that do not include conscious visual awareness.

Binocular Rivalry

Binocular rivalry refers to the phenomenon in which visual perception spontaneously switches between two different images that are presented simultaneously to each eye, as illustrated in Figure 13.17. You can experience this on your own by looking at two different objects through a paper-towel roll held to each of your eyes.

Why is binocular rivalry important for neuroscientists who study consciousness? What is intriguing about binocular rivalry is that, although both images are stimulating each of the retinas simultaneously,

FIGURE 13.18

Binocular rivalry procedure used by Sheinberg and Logothetis (1997). Top row: Sequence of stimuli presented to the left and right eyes simultaneously during the procedure (stimulus). Middle row (top): Pattern of action potentials generated in the inferotemporal cortex (IT) neuron (Cell r105) from which electrical activity was recorded. Middle row (bottom): Histogram of the neuronal response from the IT neuron. Bottom row: Pattern of left and right chain pulls in response to faces or starburst patterns (Report).

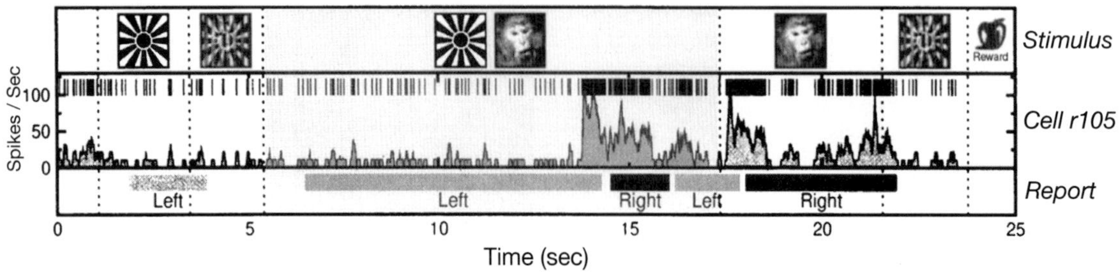

D. L. Sheinberg, D.L. & N. K. Logothetis. (1997). The role of temporal cortical areas inperceptualorganization. *Proceedings of the National Academy of Sciences U. S. A. 94*(7): 3408–3413. With permission from the National Academy of Sciences.

only one of them enters visual consciousness at a time. Neuroscientists realized that they could record brain activity to discover which brain area is active when one of the two images enters consciousness, providing them with an NCC for visual information. The results of such a study were reported by neuroscientists David Sheinberg and Nikos Logothetis (1997). The procedure is illustrated in Figure 13.18.

They recorded electrical activity from an individual neuron in the inferotemporal cortex (IT) of a monkey while subjected to a procedure meant to induce binocular rivalry. The IT neuron responded to images of human and animal faces but not to images of a starburst pattern. They trained the monkeys to pull a lever situated to the left when they saw a starburst pattern and a lever situated to the right when they saw a face, by giving them a food reward when they did so.

After having trained the monkeys to do this task, the experimenters put them through a rivalry test. Neither the image of a starburst nor the image of an ambiguous figure (top row) presented to the left eye triggered a response in IT neurons (middle row). However, the monkey pulled the left lever, as it was taught to do, in response to seeing the starburst image during training (bottom row).

Next, they observed that the monkey, while being presented simultaneously with a starburst pattern to the left eye and a face to the right eye, alternately pulled the left and right levers, indicating that it alternated between perceiving the face and the starburst pattern. Interestingly, electrical activity was recorded only from the IT neuron when the monkey pulled on the right lever, indicating that it perceived the face.

What does this mean? Because the neuron in area IT became active only when the monkey became consciously aware of the face, even if it was stimulating the retina of the monkey's right eye continuously, it was concluded that activation of area IT was an NCC for the visual perception of faces.

Binocular rivalry has also been studied in humans. For example, psychologist Frank Tong and colleagues induced binocular rivalry in study participants by having them view the image of a face with one eye and the image of a house with the other, through green-red glasses (Figure 13.19a) (Tong, Nakayama, Vaughan, & Kanwisher, 1998).

The fusiform face area (FFA) was found to be activated when the subjects reported being consciously aware of the face. In contrast, the parahippocampal place area (PPA) was activated when the subjects reported being consciously aware of the house (Figure 13.19b). A plot of the pattern of the alternating brain activation depending on whether the subjects consciously perceived the face or the house is shown in Figure 13.19c. The right side of the plot shows that activation of the FFA and PPA during conscious awareness of the face and house during the rivalry test did not differ from when subjects were made to fixate on either the face or house separately. This indicated that activation of the FFA and the PPA may be an NCC for perceiving faces and other objects, respectively.

FIGURE 13.19

(a) Viewing a superimposed face and a house, in different colors (green and red, respectively), through green-red glasses induces binocular rivalry. (b) fMRI image of the activation in the FFA when subjects reported being consciously aware of the face (left) and activation of the PPA when subjects reported being consciously aware of the house (right). (c) Plot of the activation (% MR Signal) in the FFA (blue) and PPA (red) with conscious awareness of the face (F) and house (H) during rivalry (left) and while fixating on only the image of the face or the house in a nonrivalrous condition (right).

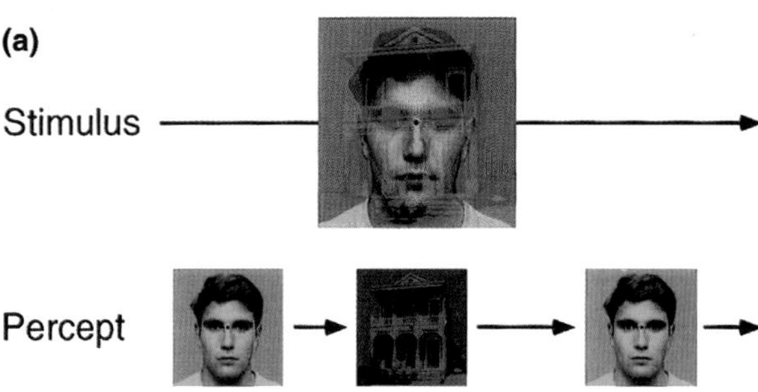

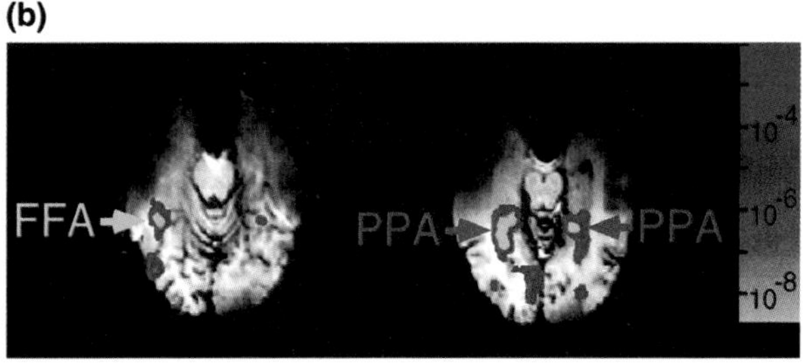

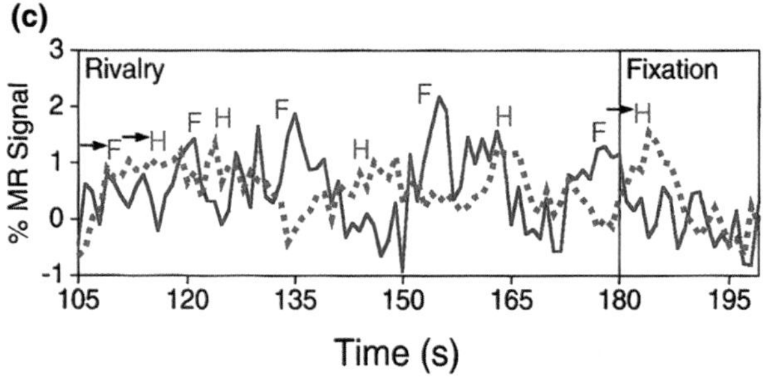

Tong, F. et al. (1998). Binocular Rivalry and Visual Awareness in Human Extrastriate Cortex. *Neuron 21*(4): 753–759. With permission from Elsevier.

13.2.4 A NEUROBIOLOGICAL THEORY OF CONSCIOUSNESS

>> LO 13.2.4 **Describe and explain the global workspace theory of consciousness.**

Key Terms

- **Global workspace theory:** The idea that consciousness arises from the activity of brain modules that process and bind the features of a specific kind of information, which is then broadcast throughout the brain.
- **Cortico-thalamic core:** Refers to the dense connectivity between the thalamus and the cortex.
- **Subliminal stimulus:** A stimulus that can affect behavior while remaining below the threshold of consciousness.
- **Preconscious stimulus:** A stimulus that does not give rise to conscious awareness despite its high strength.
- **Inattentional blindness**: A phenomenon by which a stimulus of high strength fails to be perceived due to the lack of attention to it.
- **Conscious stimulus:** A stimulus that gives rise to conscious awareness due to its high strength and the level of attention it elicits.

Several neurobiological theories of consciousness have been proposed, and several others are being developed (Mayner et al., 2018; Tononi, 2012; Zeman, Grayling, & Cowey, 1997). So far, none of them can explain all of what consciousness involves. For example, none can solve the hard problem of consciousness, that is, how the interaction between neurons gives rise to subjective experience. However, these theories do propose ways by which information processed by our senses either remains unconscious or enters conscious awareness.

Global Workspace Theory

The **global workspace theory** (GWT) of consciousness was proposed by neuroscientist Bernard Baars (Baars, 2005; Cho, Baars, & Newman, 1997). The basic idea of GWT is that the brain has several modules within the **cortico-thalamic core**, which refers to the dense connectivity between the thalamus and cortex. According to GWT, each of these modules processes and binds the features of a specific kind of information. This is illustrated in Figure 13.20a. Simple decontextualized visual information, such as viewing a single star against a dark sky, is processed in the primary visual cortex. Objects that incorporate several visual features such as color, shape, and size, such as a coffee cup, are processed within another module. Events within their context are processed within the medial temporal lobes (MTL) and hippocampal system. A module also exists in the prefrontal cortex for nonsensory experiences such as the feeling-of-knowing (the feeling that you are able to retrieve information about something), judgment, expectations, and beliefs (Baars, Franklin, & Ramsoy, 2013).

Figure 13.20b shows how features containing specific kinds of information, within modules, are bound to produce the conscious experience of an event. The information within the modules is represented by connector nodes or "hubs," which permit communication between the modules. Each hub represents a node of the global workspace and forms its connective core (Figure 13.20c).

FIGURE 13.20

(a) Possible modules and their location within the cortico-thalamic core. (b) Information contained within each module is represented within connector hubs by which the bound content of each module is broadcasted. (c) The interconnected hubs from each module form the connective core of the global workspace.

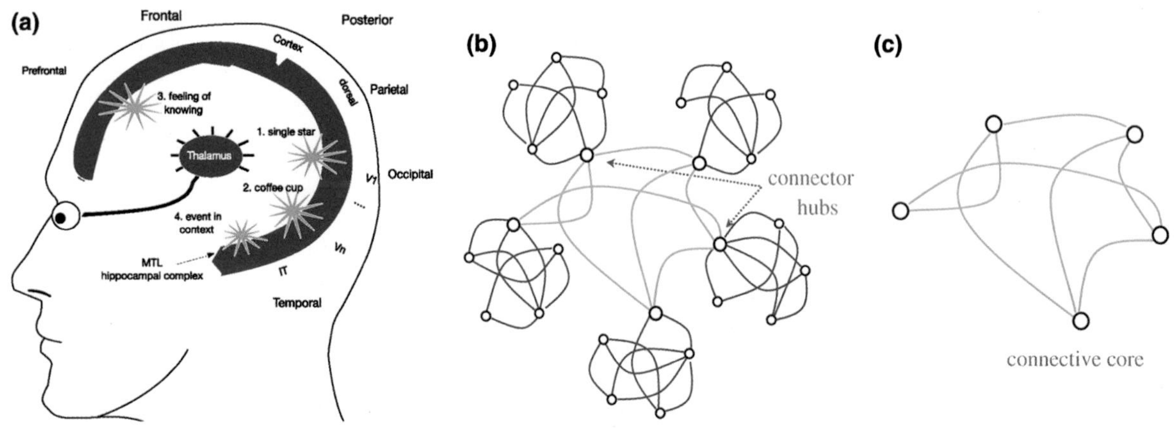

(a) Baars, B. J., S. Franklin, & T.Z. Ramsoy. (2013). Global workspace dynamics: cortical "binding and propagation" enables conscious contents. *Frontiers in Psychology 4*, 20; (b) & (c) Shanahan, M. (2012). The brain's connective core and its role in animal cognition. *Philosophical Transactions of the Royal Society B 367*(1603), 2704–2714.

The bound information contained within a module can thereby be broadcast to every other module in the global workspace (Shanahan, 2012).

How does information make it into the global workspace to begin with? The answer to this question is attention. The attentional spotlight, as described earlier, binds the features of whatever is being focused on to be entered in the appropriate module(s). Neuroscientist Stanislas Dehaene (an important contributor to GWT) suggests that if the strength of the stimulus crosses a certain threshold of neuronal activation, it "ignites" conscious awareness by being broadcast throughout the global workspace, where it can be combined with other information, giving rise to the unified quality of conscious experience (Dehaene, Changeux, Naccache, Sackur, & Sergent, 2006).

Dehaene and colleagues identified three types of stimuli, based on their ability to ignite conscious awareness: subliminal stimuli, preconscious stimuli, and conscious stimuli. A **subliminal stimulus** can affect behavior while remaining below the threshold of consciousness. For example, in one experiment, subjects were presented with a scene designed to induce either negative or positive emotions. However, the duration of the presentations was so brief that all the participants reported seeing was a flash of light. Nevertheless, the participants rated people associated with the positive scene more positively than people associated with the negative scene (Krosnick et al., 1992).

A **preconscious stimulus** is one that does not ignite conscious awareness despite its high strength. **Inattentional blindness** is a prime example of preconscious stimulation, where a strong stimulus does not enter conscious awareness due to the attentional spotlight being diverted to other stimuli. The most famous example of inattentional blindness is the invisible gorilla test by Harvard University psychologist Christopher Chabris (Chabris & Simons, 2010). In the invisible gorilla test, participants are asked to watch a video in which six people are passing around a basketball. Three of them are wearing black shirts, and the other three are wearing white shirts. The participants are asked to count the number of passes made by the people wearing white shirts. As the participants' attention is focused on counting the passes, a person dressed in a gorilla suit enters the scene, stands in the middle, pounds its chest for 9 seconds, and then leaves the scene. Half of the participants reported not seeing the gorilla.

A **conscious stimulus** is one that is of high strength and is paid attention to. As shown in Figure 13.21, subliminal and preconscious stimuli activate nodes only locally, within modules, but activation does not spread to a connector hub that would broadcast the information through the global workspace. Only stimuli that are powerful enough and to which attention is paid can do so. Through long-distance connections, conscious stimuli activate global workspace neurons situated in the parietal, cingulate, and prefrontal cortices.

FIGURE 13.21

Patterns of activation triggered by conscious, preconscious, and subliminal stimuli (T = visual target). Only high-strength stimuli that are paid attention to result in igniting conscious awareness, through long-distance connections that encompass parietal, cingulate, and prefrontal cortices (T1). Preconscious stimuli, which are of high strength but not paid attention to, and subliminal stimuli, which are of weak strength, result in activity that remains local (i.e., it does not spread through the global workspace).

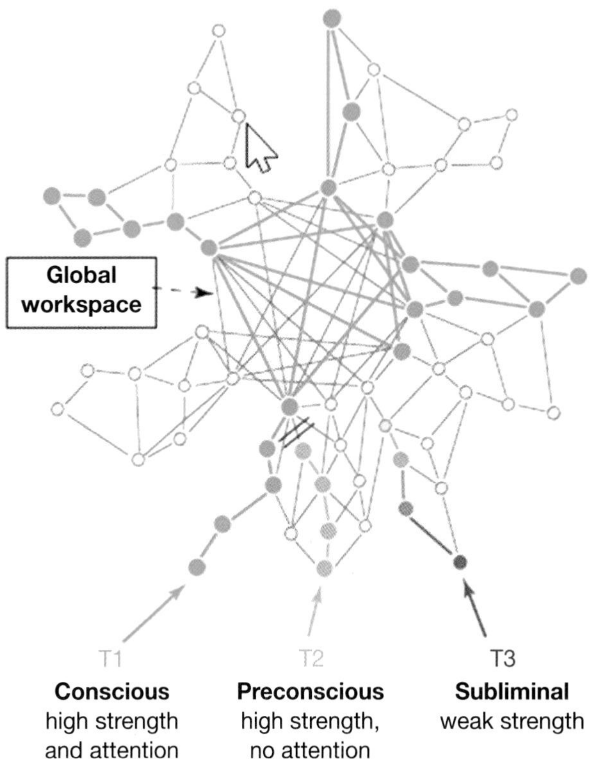

Dehaene, S., et al. (2006). Conscious, preconscious, and subliminal processing: a testable taxonomy. *Trends in Cognitive Sciences 10*(5), 204–211. With permission from Elsevier.

13.2.5 DISORDERS OF CONSCIOUSNESS

>> LO 13.2.5 **Describe and explain some disorders of consciousness.**

Key Terms

- **Level of consciousness:** The extent to which a person is awake.
- **Content of consciousness:** The extent to which ongoing stimuli are being processed.

- **Coma:** A state of unresponsiveness that results from brain injury. Patients in a coma have closed eyes, cannot be awakened, and do not respond to stimulation.
- **Glasgow coma scale:** A scale used to assess whether a patient has slipped into a coma. It measures the extent to which patients can open their eyes and perform verbal and motor responses.
- **Brain death:** A condition in which life-sustaining activity of the brainstem cannot be detected.
- **Unresponsive wakefulness:** A condition in which patients show high levels of wakefulness without any signs of consciousness (previously known as a persistent vegetative state).
- **Minimally conscious state:** A condition in which patients show high levels of wakefulness with some signs of consciousness.

Figure 13.22 illustrates how states of consciousness can be conceived as varying along two dimensions, that is, the **level of consciousness** (wakefulness) and the **content of consciousness** (awareness) (Laureys, 2005).

Coma

Coma is a state of unresponsiveness that results from brain injury. Patients in a coma have closed eyes, cannot be awakened, and do not respond to stimulation. However, painful stimuli may result in a stereotypical withdrawal response, which may disappear as the coma deepens. Contrary to popular belief, coma is not a state in which a person is simply sleeping. Comatose patients do not go through the sleep stages of NREM you learned about in Chapter 9. They do, however, show high-amplitude and low-frequency brain waves that resemble stages 3 and 4 of NREM sleep. They do not show the characteristic EEG patterns of REM sleep. Coma results from damage to the brain's ascending activating system, which includes areas in the brainstem such as the locus coeruleus, raphe nuclei, and pedunculopontine tegmental nucleus (see Chapter 9 to review). It can also occur with widespread damage to the cortex. The brain damage that results in coma can have several causes. These include stroke, where blood flow to the brain is cut off or significantly reduced, and physical trauma, such as may occur during an automobile accident. In that case, swelling of the brain may push down on the brainstem, which as you already know, contains the ascending activating system. Coma can also occur in people who are diabetic if brain levels of glucose get too low. Cardiac arrest stops blood flow to the brain, depriving it of oxygen and giving rise to hypoxia, as in the case of Terri Schiavo, recounted in the chapter's opening vignette.

Whether someone has slipped into a coma, as well as the depth of the coma, is typically measured using the **Glasgow coma scale** (Table 13.1). The Glasgow coma scale was developed by University of Glasgow professors of neurosurgery Graham Teasdale and Bryan J.

FIGURE 13.22

States of consciousness plotted in relation to their levels of wakefulness and awareness. The green ellipse contains normal states, whereas the red, orange, blue, and yellow ellipses contain abnormal disruptions in consciousness that are sometimes induced or occur through brain damage.

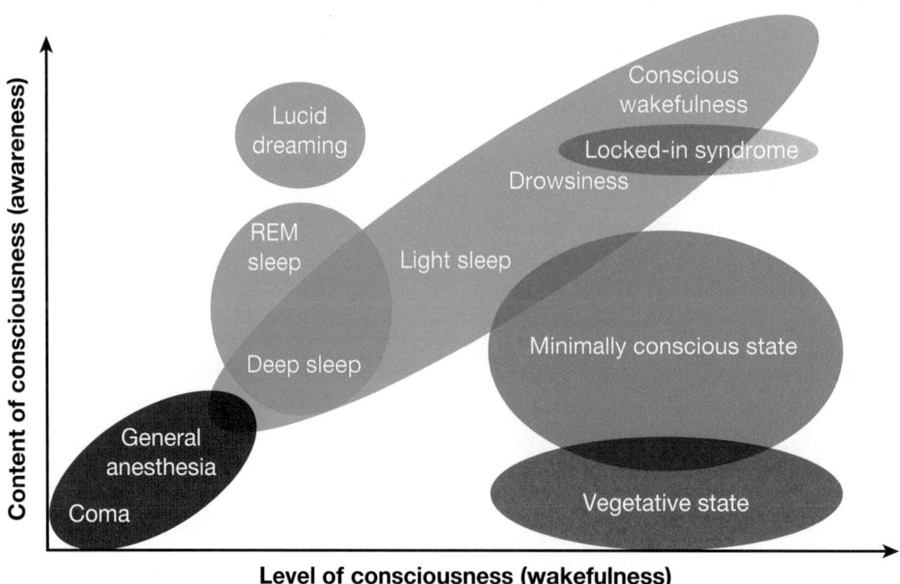

Adapted from Laureys, S. (2005). The Neural Correlate of (Un)awareness: Lessons From the Vegetative State. *Trends in Cognitive Sciences* 9(12): 556–559. With permission from Elsevier.

TABLE 13.1

The Glasgow coma scale. Patients are scored on their best response on criteria for eye opening (1–4), verbal response (1–5), and motor response (1–6). The maximum score is 15. A patient whose score is 8 or less is considered to be in a coma.

BEHAVIOR	RESPONSE	SCORE
Eye-opening response	Spontaneously	4
	To speech	3
	To pain	2
	No response	1
Best verbal response	Oriented to time, place, and person	5
	Confused	4
	Inappropriate words	3
	Incomprehensible sounds	2
	No response	1
Best motor response	Obeys commands	6
	Moves to localized pain	5
	Flexion withdrawal from pain	4
	Abnormal flexion (decorticate)	3
	Abnormal extension (decerebrate)	2
	No response	1
Total score:	*Best response*	15
	Comatose client	8 or less
	Totally unresponsive	3

Source: Based on Teasdale G. and B. Jennett. (1974). Assessment of coma and impaired consciousness. A practical scale. *The Lancet* 2(7872):81–4. With permission from Elsevier.

Jennet in the 1970s (Teasdale & Jennett, 1974). It is used to measure the extent to which patients open their eyes and can perform verbal and motor responses. Each of these components is given a maximum score of 4, 5, and 6, respectively, for a total maximum of 15. A patient is considered to be in a coma if his or her score is 8 or less.

Coma is a transitional stage, which can last from a few days to a few weeks. Many comatose patients recover, whereas others lose function of the brainstem in a condition called **brain death**. Still others will progress from coma to a state of unresponsive wakefulness and may then progress to a minimally conscious state, both of which are discussed in the sections that follow.

Unresponsive Wakefulness

Emergence from coma may mean that the person has recovered. Unfortunately, some patients instead make a transition to what is known as **unresponsive wakefulness** (see Figure 13.22). Patients in the state of unresponsive wakefulness show high levels of wakefulness but have no conscious awareness. They open their eyes but show no signs of being conscious. They can only perform reflexive responses. Also, contrary to what is observed in coma, patients in unresponsive wakefulness go through normal sleep-wake cycles. Unresponsive wakefulness is associated with normal life-sustaining functions of the brainstem and reestablishment of ascending activating system functioning. However, conscious awareness is prevented because of widespread cortical damage, including loss of connectivity between the frontal and parietal cortices as well as between primary sensory areas and association areas of the cortex.

There are two classes of association areas: unimodal association areas and multimodal association areas. Unimodal association areas are located adjacent to their respective primary sensory cortex and integrate the different types of sensory information processed by that area. For example, the visual association area is unimodal in that it only integrates different types of visual information, such as shape, color, and size. Multimodal association areas link information from different sources. There are three types of multimodal association areas, illustrated in Figure 13.23. Each of these multimodal association areas combines different kinds of information. These are (1) *the limbic association area*, which links emotions and memory to sensory inputs; (2) *the posterior association area*, which is at the junction of the occipital, temporal, and parietal lobes and links together information from the primary sensory areas and unimodal association areas; and (3) *the anterior association area of the prefrontal cortex*, which links information from all association areas and is involved in higher mental functions such as memory and planning.

In a related condition, known as **minimally conscious state**, patients show higher levels of responsiveness. That is, they can follow simple commands, can give simple verbal or gestural yes-or-no answers,

FIGURE 13.23

Association areas of the cortex as well as primary sensory areas.

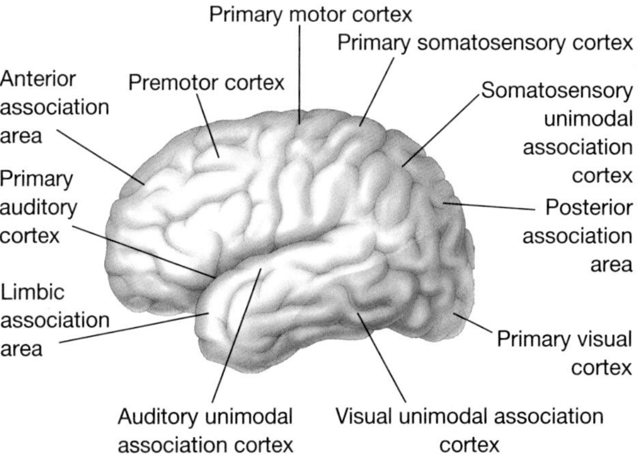

Amanda Tomasikiewicz/Body Scientific Intl.

FIGURE 13.24

PET scans showing the reduction of glucose metabolism in patients in a minimally conscious state (left) and patients in unresponsive wakefulness (right). Blue areas show significantly reduced metabolism compared to controls, whereas red shows areas with relatively preserved metabolism.

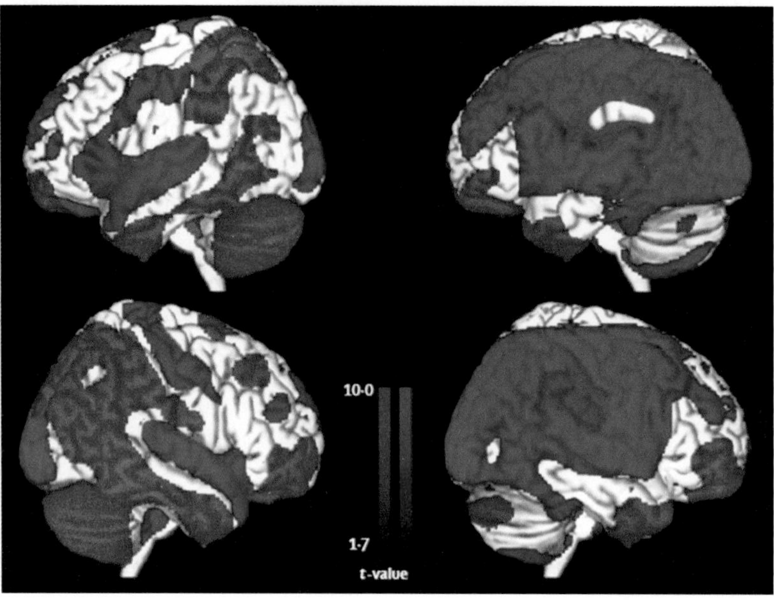

Stender, J., et al. (2014). Diagnostic precision of PET imaging and functional MRI in disorders of consciousness: a clinical validation study. *The Lancet 384*(9942): P514–522. With permission from Elsevier.

and show some purposeful behavior. Whether someone is in the state of unresponsive awareness or a minimally conscious state depends on the amount of brain damage and loss of connectivity between brain areas. Positron emission tomography (PET) scans performed on the brains of patients in both minimally conscious state and unresponsive wakefulness (Figures 13.24a and 13.24b, respectively) show significant reduction of metabolism in the associative cortices (Stender et al., 2014).

IT'S A MYTH!

General Anesthesia: It's Just Like Going to Sleep

The Myth

If you have ever undergone surgery, there is a good chance that it was done under general anesthesia. If so, you may have been told by a doctor, likely the anesthesiologist, that you were going to be put to sleep. In fact, this is not the case. Think about it. If you were just sleeping, you would certainly be awakened by the first cut of the knife or even by the noises going on around you. It is not as if the members of the surgical team are whispering and tippy-toeing around, being careful not to wake you.

FIGURE 1

Awake state

General Anesthesia

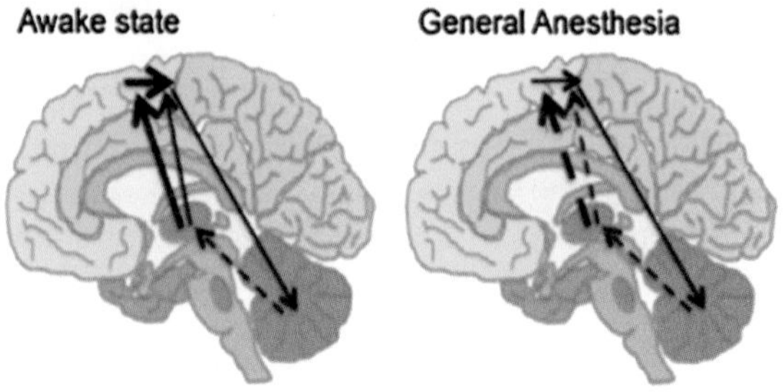

Uhrig, L. et al. (2014). Cerebral mechanisms of general anesthesia. Effets des agents d'anesthesie. Annales Francaises d'Anesthesie et de Reanimation 33. *Annales Françaises d'Anesthesie et de Réanimation 33*(2): 72–82. With permission from Elsevier.

So, What Is General Anesthesia?

General anesthesia is a drug-induced state of unconsciousness. While under general anesthesia people are insensitive to pain, are immobile, and have no memory of the event. As you can see in Figure 1, anesthesia is more akin to a coma than any phase of sleep in the associated levels of awareness. In fact, the patterns of EEG activity observed in general anesthesia have more similarities to unresponsive wakefulness, a minimally conscious state, and even brain death than they do with sleep.

General anesthesia has been described in some detail by Emery Brown and colleagues (Brown, Lydic, & Schiff, 2010). General anesthesia consists of three periods: induction, maintenance, and emergence, which are subdivided further into four phases:

Induction period (paradoxical excitation): This period is called *paradoxical* because patients show excitation when the anesthetic drug is meant to make the patient unconscious. Soon after induction, as the dose is increased, patients show excitation, which includes defensive movements, incoherent speech, and euphoria. *Phase 1:* Respiration becomes progressively irregular, and the patient requires ventilation. Beta activity gives way to alpha activity.

Maintenance period (surgery is performed during phases 2 and 3). *Phase 2:* This is the intermediate state of anesthesia. It is characterized by mostly alpha and delta activity and resembles stage 3 of sleep. *Phase 3:* Characterized by what is known as burst suppression, which consists of a flat EEG with periods of alpha and beta activity. *Phase 4:* The deepest phase of anesthesia, where the EEG is completely flat and is equivalent to brain death. Phase 4 is induced only to protect the brain during neurosurgery or to control seizures.

Emergence period: The patient emerges from general anesthesia by going through the four phases in reverse order.

General anesthetics interfere with the transfer of sensory information between the thalamus and the cortex in a thalamus-cortical loop. They also inhibit wake-promoting signals that emanate from the reticular activating system (see Chapter 9 for a review). In a study published in 2000, researcher Michael Alkire and colleagues scanned the brain of patients, under general anesthesia, using PET (Alkire, Haier, & Fallon, 2000). They found that the thalamo-cortical and cortico-thalamic loops were significantly disrupted in the brains of people who received a general anesthetic drug, compared to people who were awake.

So, why do doctors tell patients that they will simply go to sleep? Because telling them they will be going into a drug-induced coma might be scary for some patients and add unnecessary stress to that already associated with undergoing surgery. ●

13.2.6 HIDDEN CONSCIOUSNESS

>> LO 13.2.6 **Explain how consciousness can be hidden.**

Key Term

- **Locked-in syndrome:** A condition characterized by intact awareness, wakefulness, and cognitive function while the person is paralyzed and unable to speak.

The absence of signs of consciousness does not mean that consciousness is not present to some extent. In fact, Schnakers et al. (2009) found that out of 44 patients diagnosed to be in unresponsive wakefulness, 18 were actually in a minimally conscious state, which means that they showed signs of consciousness, such as purposeful eye movements. In addition, 4 out of 41 patients initially diagnosed with being in a minimally conscious state were found to have emerged from that state. Finally, signs of consciousness were found in another 16 patients who had received an uncertain diagnosis. These results as well as the criteria used to assess the patients are shown in Table 13.2.

TABLE 13.2

Criteria Used to Assess Consciousness

BEHAVIOR	VS	MCS	UNSURE OF DIAGNOSIS
1 – Response to verbal order	4	*	4
2 – Purposeful eye movements	8	*	6
3 – Automatic motor response	1	*	1
4 – Pain localization	1	*	1
5 – Several criteria for MCS	4	*	4
6 – Communication	*	1	*
7 – Functional object use	*	1	*
8 – Several criteria for EMCS	*	2	*
Total	18	4	16

Source: Schnakers, C., et al. (2009). Diagnostic accuracy of the vegetative and minimally conscious state: Clinical consensus versus standardized neurobehavioral assessment. *BMC Neurology* 2009:35.

Note: Number of patients initially diagnosed with unresponsive wakefulness (VS–formerly, vegetative state) and minimally conscious state (MCS), and those whose diagnosis was unsure, showing behaviors taken as signs of consciousness. EMCS = emergence from MCS. An asterisk (*) indicates that the criterion is nonapplicable.

FIGURE 13.25

(a) MRI scan showing the location of hemorrhage in a patient with locked-in syndrome. (b) PET scan showing intact cerebral metabolism (activity) in the cortex of a locked-in patient.

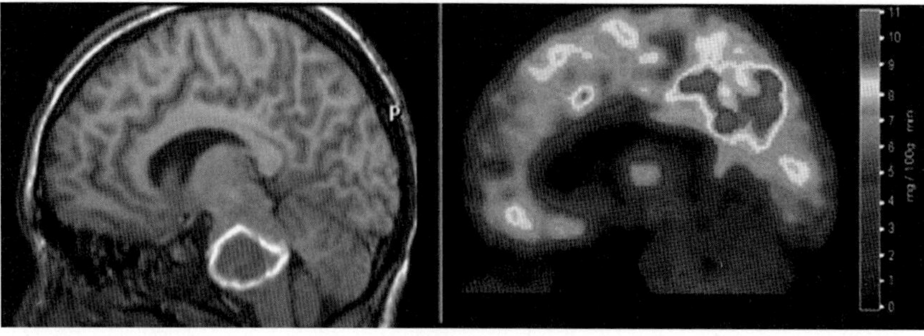

Laureys, S. et al. (2005). The locked-in syndrome: what is it like to be conscious but paralyzed and voiceless? *Progress in Brain Research, 150*: 495–511, 611. With permission from Elsevier.

In addition, fMRI scans of the brains of patients considered to be in unresponsive wakefulness demonstrated that some of them showed signs of consciousness. In a study performed by neuroscientist Adrian Owen and colleagues (Monti et al., 2010), patients considered to be in unresponsive wakefulness were asked to imagine themselves performing a motor task such as playing tennis and a spatial task such as mentally walking through their homes. When imagining the motor task, playing tennis, the supplementary motor area of 4 out of 23 patients was activated. When patients were asked to mentally walk through their homes, their parahippocampal area was activated, consistent with the role that this area plays in spatial memory. This pattern of activation for the motor and spatial tasks was also observed in control subjects.

However, this was not convincing evidence that these patients were indeed conscious. After all, it was possible that the observed brain activity was generated in response to stimuli evoked by the content of the instructions given to them without conscious awareness. To make certain that this was not what they were observing, Owen and colleagues asked the patients questions that can be answered by *yes* or *no* while their brains were being scanned. They also instructed the patients to imagine playing tennis if they wanted to answer yes and to picture themselves walking through their home to answer no. Owen and colleagues therefore expected that activation of the supplementary motor cortex would correspond to a yes and that activation of the parahippocampal gyrus would correspond to a no. One patient could answer questions using this method with 100% accuracy.

Another condition in which unresponsive wakefulness can mistakenly be assumed is **locked-in syndrome**. Locked-in syndrome is characterized by intact awareness, wakefulness, and cognitive function. However, people with locked-in syndrome are paralyzed and are unable to speak. They are, nevertheless, able to open, close, and move their eyes. Some can use vertical eye movements to communicate.

Locked-in syndrome occurs most commonly following damage to the brainstem and corticospinal tract due to a stroke, where blood flow to the brain is interrupted or restricted. In contrast, cortical function remains relatively intact. Brain imaging of the location of damage as well as intact cortical function in someone with locked-in syndrome is shown in Figure 13.25 (Laureys et al., 2005).

13.2.7 FREE WILL

>> LO 13.2.7 Describe and explain experiments designed to test whether humans have free will.

Key Terms

- **Sense of agency:** The feeling of initiating and controlling one's own actions.
- **Readiness potential:** Neuronal activity, measured by EEG, that preceded the urge to press a button by 500 ms in Benjamin Libet's free will experiment.

Another question related to consciousness is whether we have free will. That is, are people's actions consciously willed, or are they determined by unconscious brain processes (despite the feeling of initiating and controlling one's own actions, which is referred to as the **sense of agency**)?

In the 1980s, Benjamin Libet set out to answer this question in what was to become a famous experiment (Libet, Gleason, Wright, & Pearl, 1983). The experiment is illustrated in Figure 13.26. Participants were instructed to press a button, at any time, while observing a clock. At the same time, their brainwave activity was being measured by EEG. The participants' task was to note the time on the clock when they felt the urge to press the button. What Libet discovered

FIGURE 13.26

Top: The experimental set-up in Libet's study. Bottom: The readiness potential. Movement onset occurred 200 ms after the time participants reported they had the urge to press the button. The EEG activity in the SMA (the readiness potential) was detected 1 second, or more, prior to the reported urge to press the button.

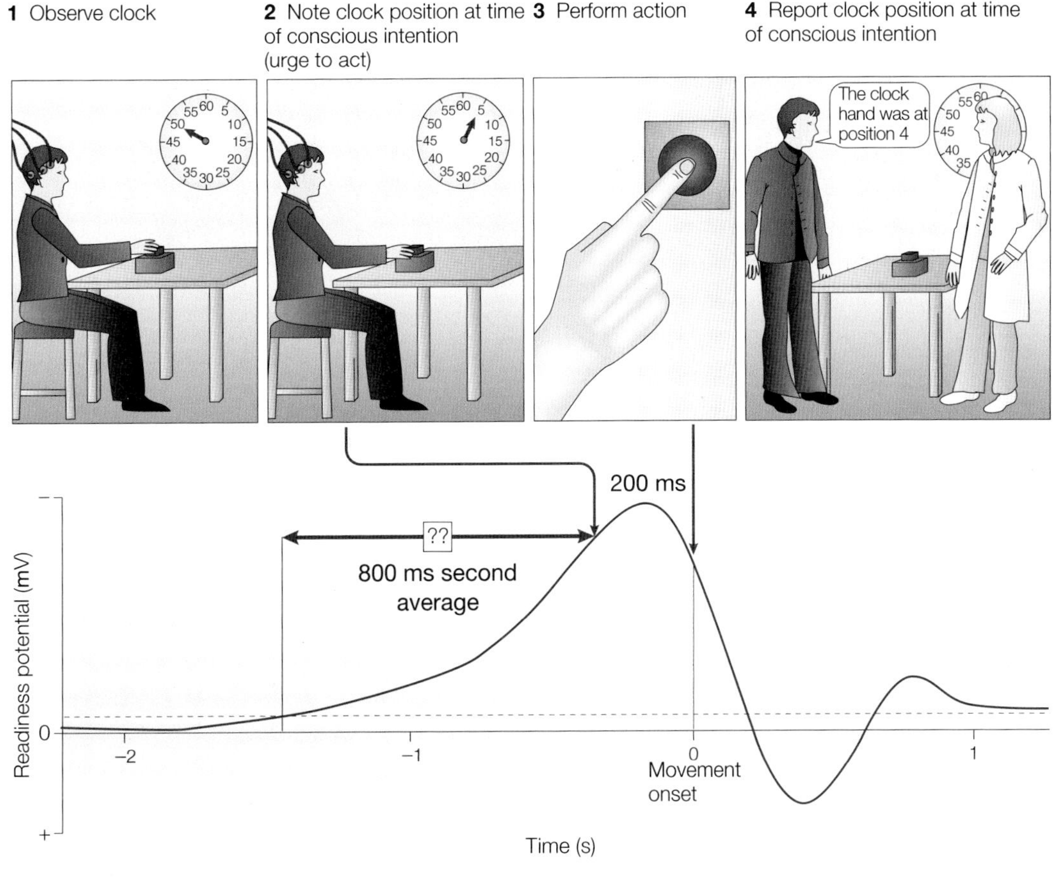
1 Observe clock
2 Note clock position at time of conscious intention (urge to act)
3 Perform action
4 Report clock position at time of conscious intention
The clock hand was at position 4
200 ms
??
800 ms second average
Readiness potential (mV)
Movement onset
Time (s)

Haggard, P. (2008). Human volition: towards a neuroscience of will. *Nature Reviews Neuroscience*, 9(12): 934–946. With permission from Springer Nature.

was that EEG activity in the supplementary motor area (SMA), which is involved in the preparation of motor actions, was detectable, on average, 800 ms before their reported urge to press the button. This neural activity, as measured by EEG, that preceded the urge to press the button became known as the **readiness potential**.

In a more recent study, Chun Siong Soon and colleagues (Soon, Brass, Heinze, & Haynes, 2008) presented participants with a stream of consonants each separated by 500 ms, on a screen, while their brains were imaged by fMRI (Figure 13.27a). The participants were told to press either a left or a right button with the corresponding index finger whenever they felt the urge to do so. They were then presented with the last three letters in the sequence and asked to indicate which letter was on the screen when they felt the urge to press a button.

As expected, left and right button presses were associated with activation of the right and left motor cortices, respectively, which occurred slightly after subjects reported feeling the urge to press a button. Activity was also detected in the pre-SMA and SMA (Figure 13.27b). The main finding was that activity in the lateral and medial frontopolar cortex, as well as activity in an area of the parietal cortex extending from the precuneus to the posterior cingulate cortex, was detected, at least 7 seconds before the time at which participants said they felt the urge to press a button (Figure 13.27c). This suggested that the intention to act had already been formulated by the brain before the participants felt the urge to press a button. This result supported Libet's findings but also extended them, in that brain activity that preceded the urge to press a button was detected in cortical areas involved in earlier motor planning.

Taken together, the results obtained by Libet and Soon suggest that motor actions may be the product of unconscious brain processes that precede the conscious decision to act. This also means that the sense of agency may arise only once a threshold of this subconscious brain activity has been crossed.

FIGURE 13.27

(a) Procedure followed by Soon and colleagues. (b) Activity in the pre-SMA, SMA, right and left motor cortex occurred after the urge to act had become conscious. (c) Activity that preceded the urge to act in the lateral and medial frontopolar cortex as well as in the parietal cortex extending from the precuneus to the posterior cingulate cortex was detected with above-chance accuracy at least 7 seconds before the conscious decision to act was made.

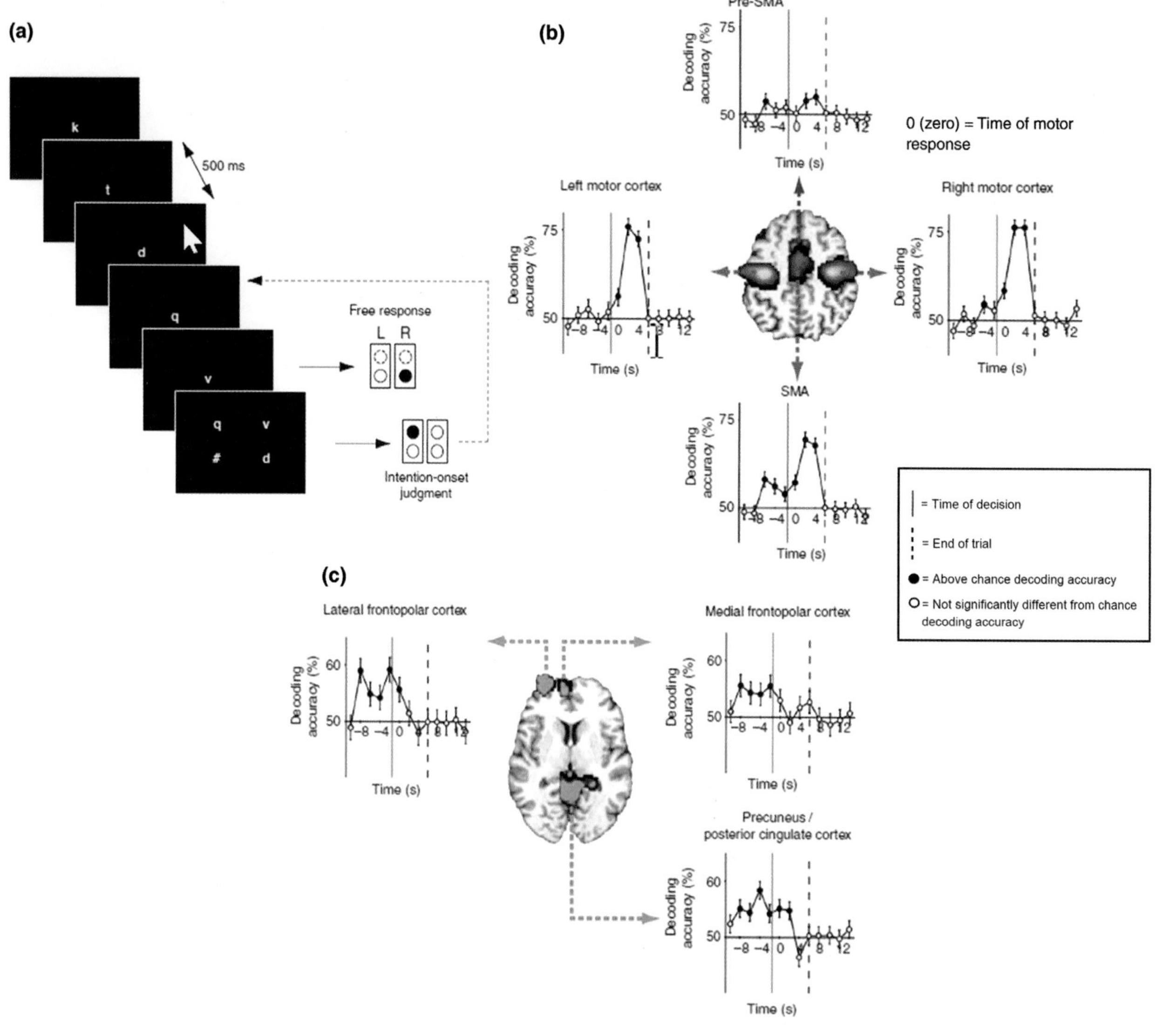

Adapted from Soon, C.S., et al. (2008). Unconscious determinants of free decisions in the human brain. *Nature Neuroscience, 11*(5): 543–545. With permission from Springer Nature.

MODULE SUMMARY

Consciousness can be defined as the flow of thoughts and feelings that are continuous throughout life. These are grounded in subjective experience. Contemporary philosopher David Chalmers differentiated between the easy and hard problem of consciousness. The easy problem concerns mental phenomena that are testable by standard methods of science, whereas the hard problem concerns how operations of the brain account for subjective experience. Neural correlates of consciousness (NCC) are the minimal neuronal events jointly sufficient for any one specific conscious percept. This differs from the constituents of consciousness, which are neural correlates of consciousness that are an integral part of consciousness or that directly cause it to occur.

Several neurobiological theories of consciousness have been proposed and several others are being developed, but so far, none of them can explain everything that consciousness involves. One of these theories is known as the global workspace theory (GWT) proposed by neuroscientist Bernard Baars in the 1980s. The basic idea of GWT is that the brain has several modules within the cortico-thalamic core. Each of these modules processes and binds the features of a specific kind of information. The bound information contained within a module can then be broadcast to every other module in the global workspace, which can then add their content to the experience, together giving rise to conscious awareness.

There are several disorders of consciousness. These include coma, which is a state in which patients cannot be awakened and do not respond to stimulation; unresponsive wakefulness, in which patients show high levels of wakefulness without any signs of consciousness; and minimally conscious state, in which patients show high levels of wakefulness with some signs of consciousness. Brain death is a condition in which life-sustaining activity of the brainstem cannot be detected. The absence of signs of consciousness does not mean that consciousness is not present to some extent. Brain scans of patients considered to be in unresponsive wakefulness demonstrated that some of them showed signs of consciousness. Locked-in syndrome is characterized by an inability to move but with intact awareness, wakefulness, and cognitive functions. Neuroscientists have investigated the question as to whether free will exists. The results of these experiments suggest that motor actions are the product of unconscious brain processes that precede the conscious decision to act.

TEST YOURSELF

13.2.1 Define consciousness. What are two key components of it?

13.2.2 Name and define the two problems of consciousness according to David Chalmers.

13.2.3 What is meant by the "neural correlates of consciousness"? Why are the phenomena of blindsight and binocular rivalry important to the study of neural correlates of consciousness?

13.2.4 Explain the global workspace theory of consciousness proposed by Bernard Baars.

13.2.5 Explain the conditions of coma, unresponsive wakefulness, and minimally conscious state.

13.2.6 What do the findings of Adrian Owen and colleagues mean regarding the treatment of people diagnosed with unresponsive wakefulness?

13.2.7 Describe the two experiments in this section regarding free will. How do they suggest that we may not have free will?

APPLICATIONS

Cellphone Use While Driving: Just Don't Do It!

Have you or someone you know ever texted or spoken on a cellphone while driving? The answer is likely to be yes. You probably already know that this is a bad idea. Driving involves dealing with many potential dangers that can put the life of the driver and others at risk. An easier question to answer is if you would consider driving after drinking alcohol. I hope the answer to this question is "No!" Even so, research shows that driving ability is just as impaired by distractions such as speaking on the phone or texting as it is by drinking (Leung, Croft, Jackson, Howard, & McKenzie, 2012).

Driving requires paying attention to multiple environmental stimuli occurring at the same time and through different sensory modalities (e.g., vision and hearing). When someone is engaged in distracting activities while driving, such as texting or speaking on the phone, attention is being switched from the vital information required for safe driving to reading and writing text or listening to or speaking to the person on the phone. Contrary to popular belief, attention is not efficiently divided among tasks (Ophir, Nass, & Wagner, 2009). Driving while texting or while speaking on the phone has been shown to significantly slow braking reaction and reduce driving speed. It also causes participants to have trouble staying in their own lane or adjusting their speed to that of a car directly ahead, it decreases the driver's peripheral detection, and it produces several other significant impairments (Consiglio, Driscoll, Witte, & Berg, 2003; Hosking, Young, & Regan, 2009; Strayer & Johnston, 2001).

Researchers are interested in finding how the brain allots attentional resources while driving. That is, does the brain allot attentional resources to distractors at the expense of resources allotted to the tasks relevant to driving? In one study, researchers challenged participants driving a car within a virtual reality

(Continued)

(Continued)

FIGURE 13.28

(a) Virtual reality driving task. Left: Straight country road with no traffic. Center: Making a left turn with no traffic. Right: Making a left turn with traffic. (b) fMRI images of the brains of participants in the regular-driving condition (left turn + traffic). (c) fMRI images of the brains of participants in the distracted-driving condition (left turn + traffic + distractor). Green circles show the shift in activation from posterior regions in the regular-driving condition to frontal regions in the distracted-driving condition.

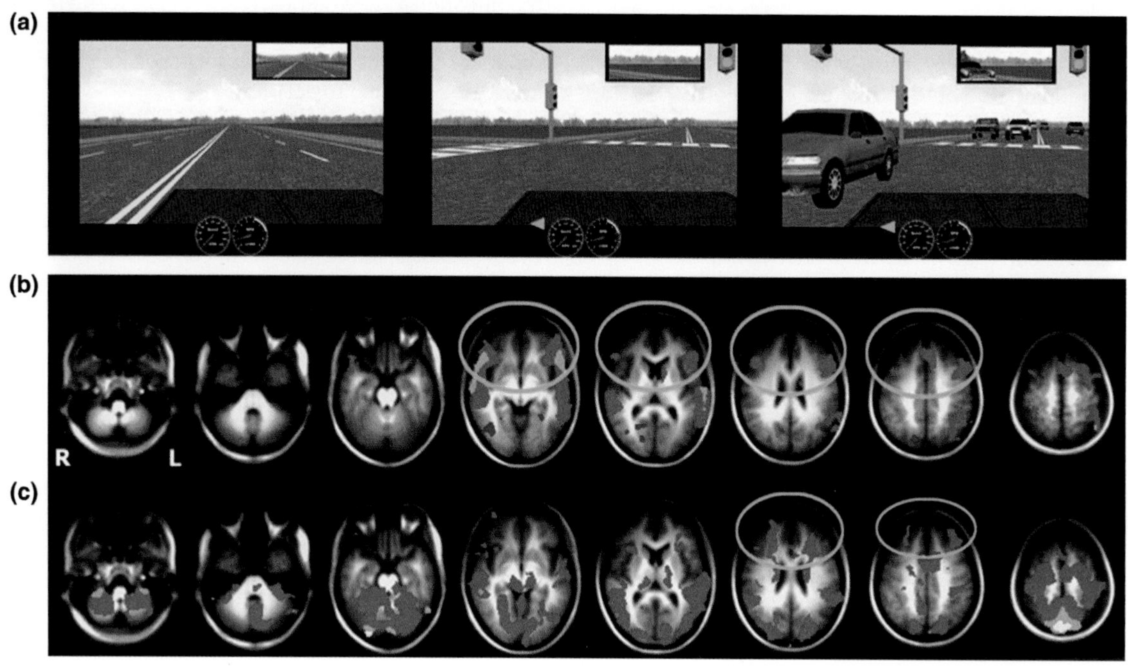

Schweizer, T.A., et al. (2013). Brain activity during driving with distraction: an immersive fMRI study. *Front. Hum. Neuroscience* 7:53.

computer program with distractors, while their brains were being imaged by fMRI (Schweizer et al., 2013). The virtual driving task is illustrated in Figure 13.28a.

In a regular-driving condition, participants were required to drive on a straight country road with no traffic, make a right or left turn with no traffic, and make a left turn with traffic (left, middle, and right, respectively [right turn not shown]). In each condition, participants also had to listen to yes-or-no questions and answer by pressing corresponding buttons on the steering wheel. This effectively mimics the use of a hands-free device to speak on a cellphone.

What Was Found?

Brain activation during regular (left turn + traffic) and distracted driving (left turn + traffic + audio) is shown in Figures 13.28b and 13.28c, respectively. Brain areas associated with motor, visuomotor, and visuospatial integration were activated during regular driving. This includes the somatosensory cortex, visual cortex, premotor cortex, and cerebellum. During distracted driving, areas involved in higher cognitive processes, such as the prefrontal cortex, were also activated.

Figures 13.28b and 13.28c indicate that there is a shift in activation from posterior regions to frontal regions. This means that the distractor caused a shift from the use of resources necessary for safe driving (e.g., visuospatial and motor skills) to the use of resources necessary for listening to and answering questions. This means that you should avoid speaking on your cellphone while driving, even if you use a legal and widely promoted hands-free device.

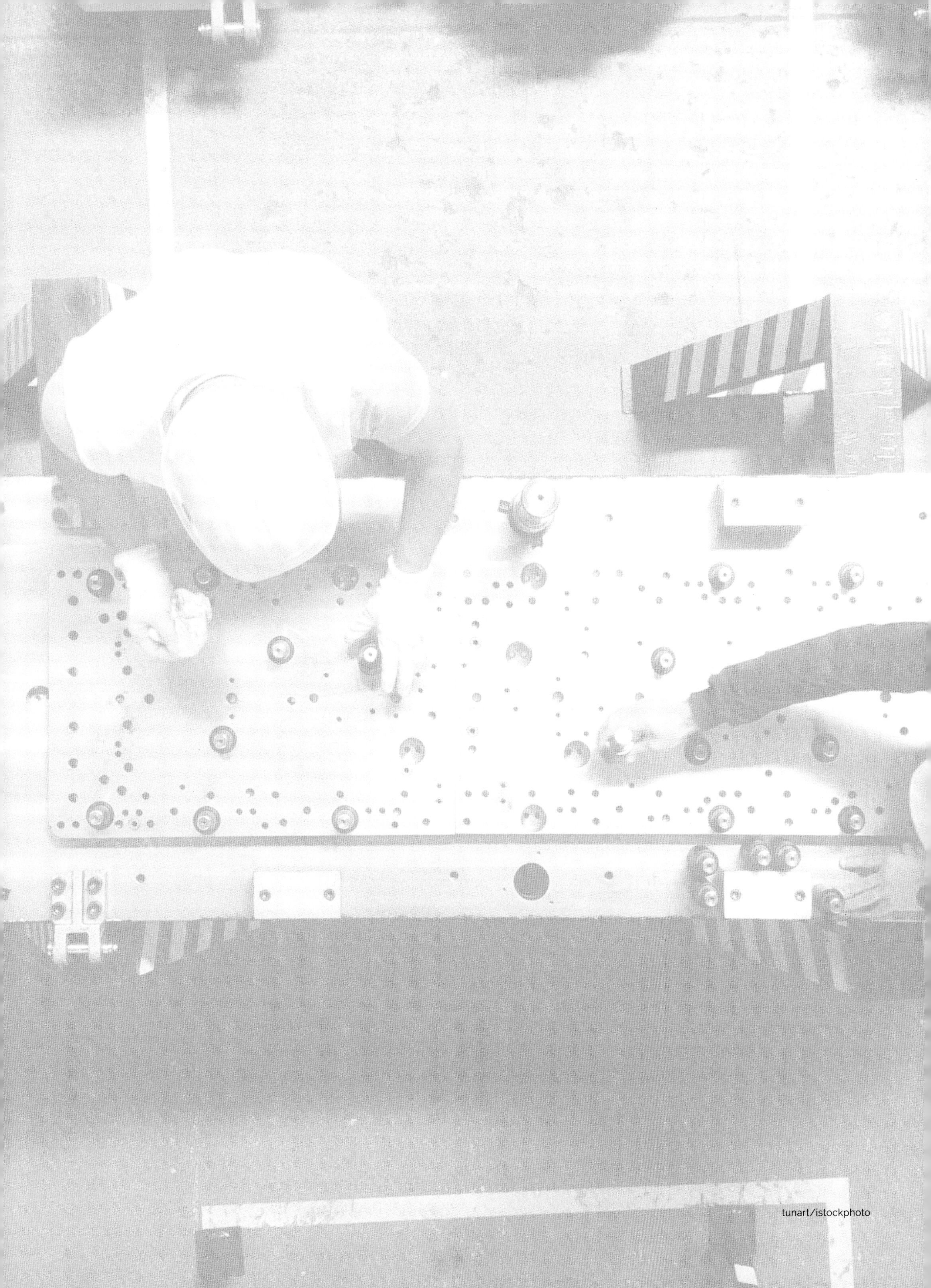

tunart/istockphoto

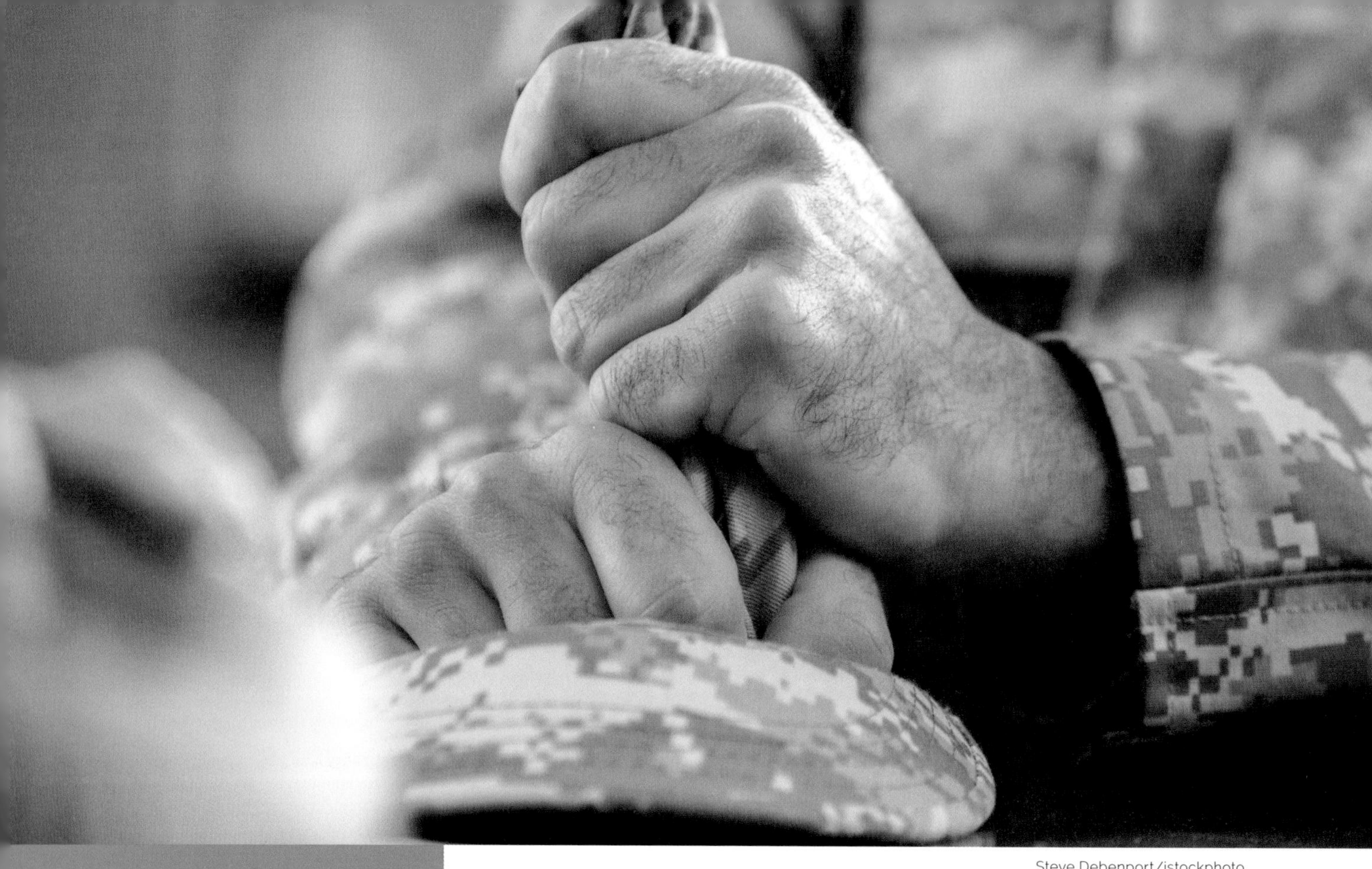

Steve Debenport/istockphoto

14 Psychological Disorders

Chapter Contents

Learning Objectives

14.1.1 Define and explain what a psychological disorder is.

14.1.2 Explain why psychological disorders cannot be attributed to any single cause.

14.2.1 Define anxiety, fear, and anxiety disorders.

14.2.2 Explain the neurobiological basis of anxiety and anxiety disorders.

14.2.3 Describe some of the symptoms of posttraumatic stress disorder.

14.2.4 Explain the neurobiological basis of posttraumatic stress disorder.

14.3.1 Describe the symptoms of obsessive-compulsive disorder.

14.3.2 Explain the neurobiological basis of obsessive-compulsive disorder.

14.4.1 Describe the symptoms of major depressive disorder.

14.4.2 Explain the neurobiological basis of major depressive disorder.

14.5.1 Describe the symptoms of schizophrenia.

14.5.2 Explain the neurobiological basis of schizophrenia.

Recalculate Your Possibilities

At the age of 21, Neil Marshall was diagnosed with schizophrenia. He suffered from hallucinations, which are perceptions of sensory events that are not occurring in reality, and delusions, which are false beliefs about oneself or about the world. Marshall was on medications, known as antipsychotics, to help control his symptoms. However, he felt discouraged and dropped out of his computer science degree program. Feeling lethargic from the antipsychotic drugs he was taking, he lay on the couch all day, and came to feel that he would never be able to do anything with his life. One day, his brother asked him to be the best man at his wedding. This is when things began to change for Marshall. Expected to give a toast, he was motivated to get up and back into shape. The toast at the wedding went well, and he realized that he could truly accomplish something if he put his mind to it. This also gave Marshall the confidence to enroll in a university mathematics program, giving himself the goal of "sticking it out" for an entire year. Contrary to his first stint at university, this time he had a strategy. He learned to anticipate his symptoms, completed his work well ahead of deadlines, took breaks, and built a social support system composed of family and friends. Marshall got 100% on a midterm exam that two-thirds of the class failed. Marshall no longer saw himself as a "weak and broken individual." He completed his honors thesis, got his bachelor's degree, and completed a master's degree. His supervisor and parents were extremely proud of him. Marshall has since presented his work at international conferences. Marshall's goal in telling his story is not to encourage other people to follow his exact path but to recalculate what they believe they are capable of.

INTRODUCTION

In 2017, approximately 46.6 million U.S. adults aged 18 or older (18.9% of that population) suffered from mental illness (Substance Abuse and Mental Health Services Administration, 2018). Mental illness includes disorders in which people suffer from exaggerated amounts of fear and anxiety; extremely depressed moods; and debilitating symptoms, such as delusions and hallucinations, in which the line between what is real and what is not is blurred. The exact causes of mental illness are largely unknown. In fact, they are thought to be due to complex interactions among biological, psychological, environmental, and social factors, sometimes referred to as biopsychosocial factors (Forero, Castro-Rodriguez, & Alonso, 2015), and not to any single cause. Understanding the neuroscience that underlies psychological disorders can go a long way toward understanding how differences in the brains of people suffering from psychological disorders contribute to their suffering, in the hope of developing better treatment options. In this chapter, we explore the neurobiological basis of the most prevalent psychological disorders worldwide: anxiety disorders, obsessive-compulsive disorder, and major depressive disorder. We also examine posttraumatic stress disorder and schizophrenia.

14.1 What Is a Psychological Disorder?

Module Contents

Learning Objectives

14.1.1 Define and explain what a psychological disorder is.

14.1.2 Explain why psychological disorders cannot be attributed to any single cause.

14.1.1 DEFINING PSYCHOLOGICAL DISORDER

>> LO 14.1.1 Define and explain what a psychological disorder is.

Key Terms

- **Psychological disorder:** A psychological dysfunction within an individual associated with distress or impairment in functioning and a response that is not typical or culturally expected.
- ***Diagnostic and Statistical Manual of Mental Disorders* (*DSM*):** The manual published by the American Psychiatric Association that provides diagnostic criteria for the various psychological disorders.

A **psychological disorder** can be defined as a psychological dysfunction within an individual associated with distress or impairment in functioning and a response that is not typical or culturally expected (Barlow, Durand, & Hofmann, 2018). Psychological disorders are classified in the ***Diagnostic and Statistical Manual of Mental Disorders* (*DSM*)** of the American Psychiatric Association, which provides diagnostic criteria for the various psychological disorders. The *DSM* is updated from time to time and is now in its fifth edition; therefore, it is officially referred to as the *DSM*-5. The categories of disorders defined in the *DSM*-5 include anxiety disorders, obsessive-compulsive and related disorders, mood disorders, somatic symptom/dissociative disorders, personality disorders, schizophrenia spectrum disorders, neurocognitive disorders, and several others (American Psychiatric Association, 2013).

14.1.2 THE INTERACTING FACTORS BEHIND PSYCHOLOGICAL DISORDERS

>> LO 14.1.2 Explain why psychological disorders cannot be attributed to any single cause.

Key Terms

- **Gene-environment interactions:** Interactions between genetic inheritance and environmental factors.
- **Animal studies:** In the context of gene-environment interactions, studies in which animals of different genetic strains are exposed to different environments.
- **Family studies**: Studies that compare individuals at high risk of developing a disorder, because they have relatives with the disorder, to individuals at low risk who do not have relatives with the disorder.
- **Adoption studies:** Studies that compare individuals who share the same parents but who were adopted into different families.
- **Twin studies:** Studies that compare identical twins who were reared in different environments in an effort to tease out the effects of genes versus those of the environment.
- **Molecular analysis:** A study that compares the effects of different environmental conditions across individuals with different genetic makeups.

Psychological disorders are determined by complex interactions among biological, environmental, and psychological factors. Therefore, the idea that psychological disorders develop from a single cause such as one's upbringing, genes, faulty brain mechanisms, or chemical imbalances is deeply flawed (see this chapter's "It's a Myth!" box).

Biological factors include genetic predispositions, that is, vulnerabilities to a disorder inherited from relatives. The chances of inheriting a disorder decrease with the degree of relatedness. For example, a child with a parent who has schizophrenia has a 6% chance of developing the disorder, compared to only a 2% chance for a child with an aunt or an uncle with schizophrenia. If one of two identical twins has schizophrenia, the likelihood of the other twin having schizophrenia is 48%

(Henriksen, Nordgaard, & Jansson, 2017). This last statistic about identical twins supports the idea that no one factor, such as genetic inheritance, can explain the development of psychological disorders. Why? Because identical twins (monozygotic) share 100% of their genes, the chances of one of the two twins having schizophrenia if the other has the disorder should also be 100%, not 48%. Clearly, other factors must be involved to explain the remaining 52%.

An individual's environment accounts for much of the interaction that occurs with genetic predispositions to result in a disorder. To name just a few environmental factors, negative life events, social isolation, drugs, exposure to chemicals, bacterial and viral infections, as well as family and work-related stressors can all play a role in triggering a disorder in the genetically predisposed person (Arnau-Soler et al., 2019; Morley, 1983).

Finally, psychological factors, which include cognitive, emotional, and behavioral factors, can interact with biological and environmental factors to contribute to the development of a psychological disorder. Cognitive factors include how people think about themselves, the world, the future, and life events. Emotional factors include reactivity and the ability to regulate one's emotions. Behavioral factors include how people learn from the consequences of their actions and the behaviors in which they engage in response to internal or environmental stimulation (Jacob et al., 2012).

FIGURE 14.1

Psychological disorders are determined by complex interactions among biological, environmental, and psychological factors.

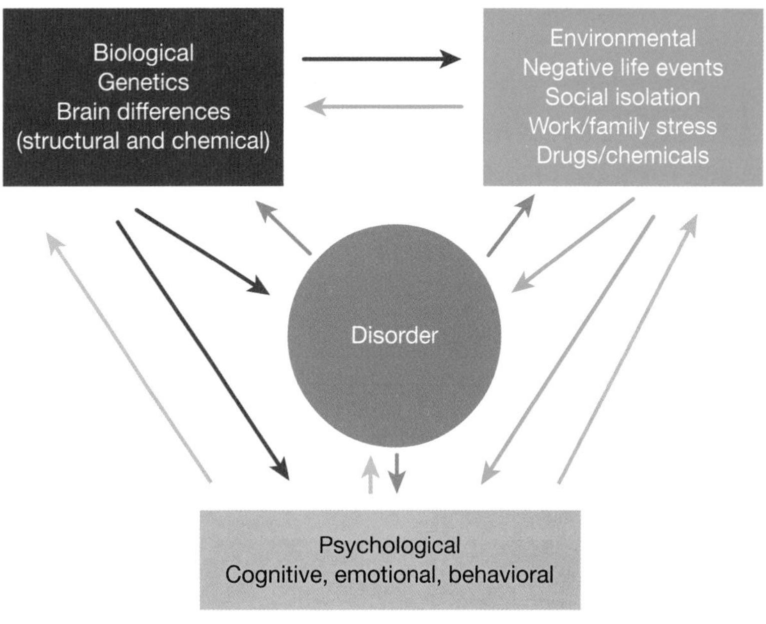

The Study of Gene-Environment Interactions

The interactions between genetic inheritance and environmental factors are known as **gene-environment interactions**. Evidence for such interactions comes from several different types of studies. These include animal studies, family studies, adoption studies, twin studies, and molecular analysis (Dick, 2011). **Animal studies** expose animals of different genetic strains to different environments. **Family studies** compare individuals at high risk of developing a disorder, because they have relatives with the disorder, to individuals at low risk who do not have relatives with the disorder. In addition, individuals who have migrated to a different environment, such as to another country, are compared to individuals of the same family who have not migrated. **Adoption studies** compare individuals who share the same parents but who were adopted into different families. **Twin studies** compare identical twins who have been reared in different environments in an effort to tease out the effects of genes versus those of the environment. Finally, using methods of **molecular analysis**, researchers can compare the effects of different environmental conditions across individuals with different genetic makeups. The idea that disorders are caused by multiple and complex interactions between these factors is illustrated in Figure 14.1.

MODULE SUMMARY

A psychological disorder can be defined as a psychological dysfunction within an individual associated with distress or impairment in functioning and a response that is not typical or culturally expected. Psychological disorders are classified in the American Psychiatric Association's *Diagnostic and Statistical Manual of Mental Disorders* (*DSM*). Many classes of disorders exist, including anxiety disorders, obsessive-compulsive and related disorders, mood disorders, somatic symptom/dissociative disorders, personality disorders, schizophrenia spectrum disorders, neurocognitive disorders, and several others. Psychological disorders are determined by complex interactions among biological, psychological, and environmental factors. The interactions between genetic inheritance and the environment are known as gene-environment interactions. Evidence for gene-environment interactions comes from several types of studies. These include animal studies, family studies, adoption studies, twin studies, and molecular analysis.

TEST YOURSELF

14.1.1 Define psychological disorder.

14.1.2 (a) Discuss the factors involved in the development of psychological disorders and why these disorders cannot be reduced to having a single cause. (b) Name and briefly describe the different types of studies that show evidence for gene-environment interactions.

14.2 Anxiety Disorders and Posttraumatic Stress Disorder

Module Contents

Learning Objectives

14.2.1 Define anxiety, fear, and anxiety disorders.

14.2.2 Explain the neurobiological basis of anxiety and anxiety disorders.

14.2.3 Describe some of the symptoms of posttraumatic stress disorder.

14.2.4 Explain the neurobiological basis of posttraumatic stress disorder.

14.2.1 ANXIETY, FEAR, AND ANXIETY DISORDERS

>> LO 14.2.1 Define anxiety, fear, and anxiety disorders.

Key Terms

- **Anxiety:** An adaptive emotional state characterized by a feeling of worry or nervousness directed toward a future event, accompanied by a state of hypervigilance.
- **Fear:** An adaptive emotional state triggered by an immediate and readily identifiable threat, which is associated with being startled, freezing, or escape.
- **Anxiety disorders:** A group of psychological disorders whose symptoms include excessive anxiety, fear, and worry, which give rise to abnormally strong avoidance and escapist tendencies.

Anxiety

Anxiety is an emotional state characterized by worry or nervousness directed toward a future event. It is often described as a feeling of unease, apprehension, or, in the worst cases, impending doom. The source of someone's anxiety is often unclear. However, anxiety leads to a hypervigilant state (being constantly on guard), which can help the individual recognize cues that signal potential dangers so that potentially threatening situations can be avoided. Moderate amounts of anxiety are normal and adaptive, as it helps people prepare for important or dangerous events. For example, it is normal to be anxious about an upcoming test, to the extent that it motivates you to prepare for it.

Fear

Although the terms *anxiety* and *fear* are often used interchangeably, they differ in important ways (Kastner-Dorn, Andreatta, Pauli, & Wieser, 2018). In contrast to anxiety, **fear** is triggered by an immediate and readily identifiable threat. The role of fear is to protect from immediate harm. Fear is associated with a range of responses, such as being startled, freezing, or attempting to escape an immediately threatening situation. As you read in Chapter 11, fear can also be conditioned. This was shown repeatedly in fear conditioning studies, in which a fear response is triggered by exposure to cues that have been associated with aversive or painful stimuli (Carneiro, Moulin, Macleod, & Amaral, 2018).

To summarize, anxiety and fear play complementary roles. Anxiety permits you to anticipate a potentially threatening future situation so that something can be done to prepare for or to avoid it. Fear permits you to do something about a situation that represents a clear and present danger.

Anxiety Disorders

Anxiety disorders are a group of psychological disorders whose symptoms include exaggerated levels of anxiety, fear, and worry, which give rise to abnormally strong avoidance and escapist tendencies. Anxiety disorders are among the most common psychological disorders in the United States. More than 42.5 million adults (more than 21% of the adult population) are affected by an anxiety disorder every year (Kessler, Petukhova, Sampson, Zaslavsky, & Wittchen, 2012). Anxiety disorders include phobias (social and specific), panic disorder, and generalized anxiety disorder. People who have these disorders have not lost touch with reality. They are, for the most part, aware that their thoughts and behaviors are irrational. This sets them apart from people who have disorders such as schizophrenia, in which people do lose touch with reality. In the next unit, we explore some of the neurobiological basis of anxiety disorders. We then briefly explore post-traumatic stress disorder, which is not classified as an anxiety disorder, although fear and anxiety play a significant role in the disorder (VanElzakker, Dahlgren, Davis, Dubois, & Shin, 2014).

14.2.2 THE NEUROBIOLOGY OF ANXIETY DISORDERS

>> LO 14.2.2 **Explain the neurobiological basis of anxiety and anxiety disorders.**

Key Term

- **Fear circuit:** The circuit of brain areas centered on the amygdala thought to be involved in the learning and expression of fear.

The neurobiology of anxiety disorders is complex. However, it is thought to include dysfunctions in the brain structures that process emotions. As discussed in Chapter 11, the amygdala processes potential environmental threats, and is thought to be at the center of a so-called **fear circuit**, which is involved in the learning and expression of fear (Wilensky, Schafe, Kristensen, & LeDoux, 2006). In response to these potential threats, the amygdala starts a chain reaction through its connections with the hypothalamus. This results in the activation of what is known as the hypothalamic-pituitary-adrenal (HPA) axis, illustrated in Figure 14.2. Within the HPA axis, neurons in the hypothalamus produce and secrete corticotropin-releasing factor (CRF), which binds to receptors in the pituitary gland, which results in the release of adrenocorticotropic hormone (ACTH) from the pituitary in the general circulation. ACTH then binds to receptors on the adrenal glands, situated on top of the kidneys. In turn, the adrenal glands release cortisol, which gives rise to the activation of the fight-or-flight response triggered by the sympathetic nervous system. At the same time, the medial prefrontal cortex analyzes the information about potential threats to either accentuate or dampen the amygdala's activity, depending on whether a real danger is present or not.

FIGURE 14.2

The hypothalamic-pituitary-adrenal (HPA) axis.

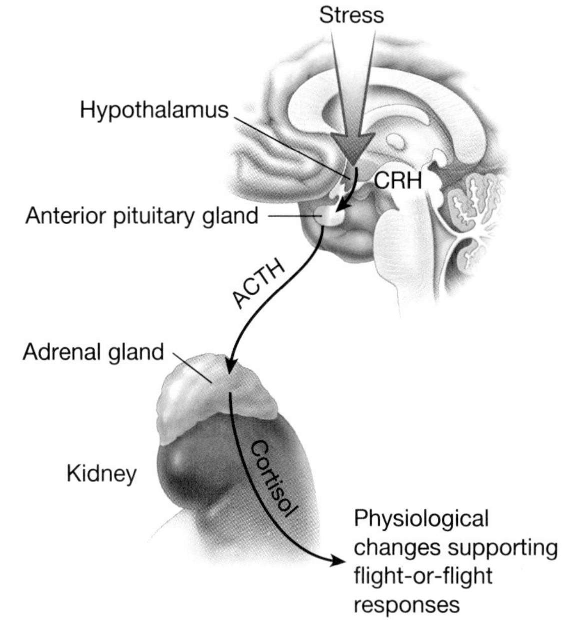

Amanda Tomasikiewicz/Body Scientific Intl.

The hippocampus dampens the stress response by inhibiting the release of CRH by the hypothalamus. In anxiety disorders, the amygdala's response is exaggerated, resulting in the inappropriate activation of the HPA axis. In addition, the hippocampus fails to respond appropriately to HPA overactivity by diminishing its activity.

Excessive activity of the amygdala has been found frequently in studies on anxiety disorders. For example, excessive activity of the amygdala was observed in an experiment involving participants with social anxiety disorder (also known as social phobia). Social anxiety disorder is characterized by the persistent concern of being judged, embarrassed, or humiliated. According to the *DSM*-5, symptoms of social anxiety include fear and anxiety in specific social settings, such as when interviewing for a job, going on a first date, giving an oral presentation, or speaking up in class. The fear experienced by the person with social anxiety is in disproportion to the actual situation.

Several studies have shown that people with social anxiety disorder have a hyperactive amygdala in response to situations that can be perceived as potentially threatening. For example, the amygdala of a person with social anxiety disorder will be significantly more active to the prospects of having to give an oral presentation than the amygdala of someone who does not have social anxiety disorder. This was demonstrated in a study in which participants with and without social anxiety disorder were shown an anxiety-arousing stimulus while their brains were being imaged by functional magnetic resonance imaging (fMRI) (Phan, Fitzgerald, Nathan, & Tancer, 2006).

The procedure of the study is illustrated in Figure 14.3a. Researchers presented subjects with and without social anxiety disorder with 20-second blocks of neutral, angry, and happy faces and different types of radios. The purpose of the study was to find out whether there were differences in reactivity between the amygdalas of participants with social anxiety disorder and healthy control subjects while being presented with angry faces versus neutral and happy ones. The different types of radios served as controls, and no difference in the response of the amygdala was expected with their presentation. As illustrated in Figure 14.3b, compared to healthy control subjects, participants with social anxiety disorder showed significantly higher levels of activation in their amygdalas in response to angry faces.

Anxiety: Beyond the Fear Circuit

As described in the preceding unit, fear and anxiety differ in important ways. Activity of the HPA axis triggered by the amygdala gives rise to startle, freezing, or escape reactions, in response to an immediate threat, that are characteristic of fear. However, we have not discussed the brain areas responsible for anxiety, which is characterized by feelings of unease and apprehension in response to a future potential threat. Although there is significant overlap between the areas responsible for fear and anxiety, some researchers have ventured beyond the fear circuit to explain anxiety.

For example, some researchers have found that anxiety is related to functional networks of brain areas (Sylvester et al., 2012). As illustrated in Figure 14.4a, these include (1) the cingulo-opercular network, which includes the anterior insula and the dorsal anterior cingulate cortex (dACC); (2) the frontoparietal network, which includes the anterior dorsolateral prefrontal cortex (aDLPFC), the medial cingulate cortex (MCC), and the inferior parietal sulcus (IPS); (3) the ventral attention network, which includes the ventrolateral prefrontal cortex (VLPFC) and the temporoparietal junction (TPJ); and (4) the default-mode network, which comprises the inferior-temporal cortex (IT), the lateral parietal cortex (LP), the posterior cingulate cortex (PCC), the subgenual anterior cingulate cortex (sgACC), and the medial prefrontal cortex (MPF). Dysfunctions in each of these networks are associated with particular behaviors observed in people with anxiety disorders.

The cingulo-opercular network is normally involved in the detection of conflicts such as when a strong tendency to respond in a certain way is in opposition to performing a correct response. For example, a conflict exists when a batter's tendency to swing his bat must be withheld when a ball is thrown out of the strike zone.

It is thought that this information about a conflict is passed on to the frontoparietal network, which is involved in cognitive control. Next time, a strong

FIGURE 14.3

Social anxiety disorder and the amygdala. (a) Stimuli presented to participants with both social anxiety disorder (generalized social phobia [GSP]) and healthy control (HC) participants. (b) fMRI image of the right amygdala. (c) Activation of the amygdala in both GSP and HC participants. GSP participants showed significantly higher activation levels of the amygdala than did HC participants.

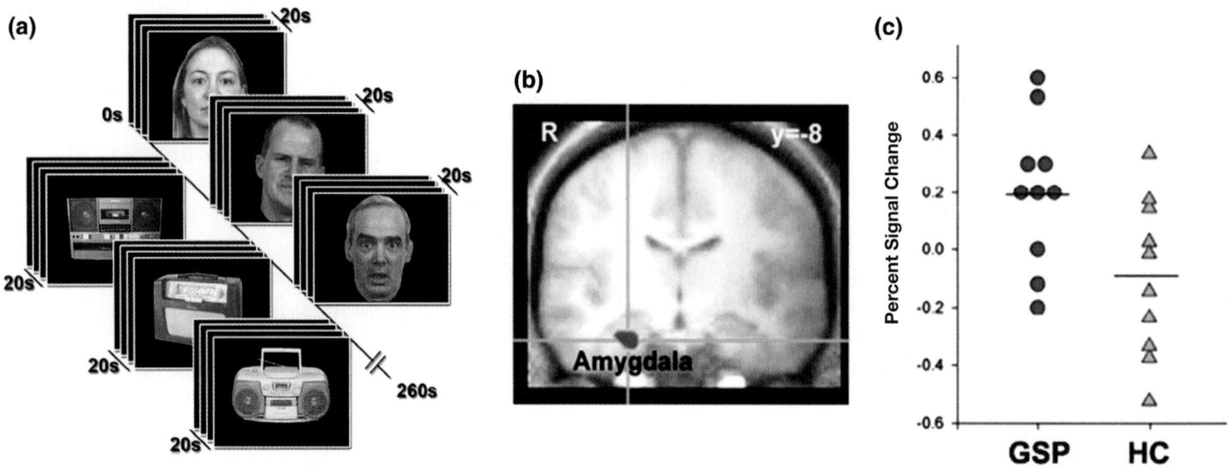

Phan, K.L., et al. (2006). Association between amygdala hyperactivity to harsh faces and severity of social anxiety in generalized social phobia. *Biological Psychiatry, 59*(5), 424–429. With permission from Elsevier.

FIGURE 14.4

(a) Networks of brain areas thought to be involved in anxiety disorders. These include the cingulo-opercular network (purple), frontoparietal network (yellow), ventral attentional network (blue), and default-mode network (red). (b) Behaviors associated with the dysfunctions in each network. (See p. 394 for explanation of abbreviations.)

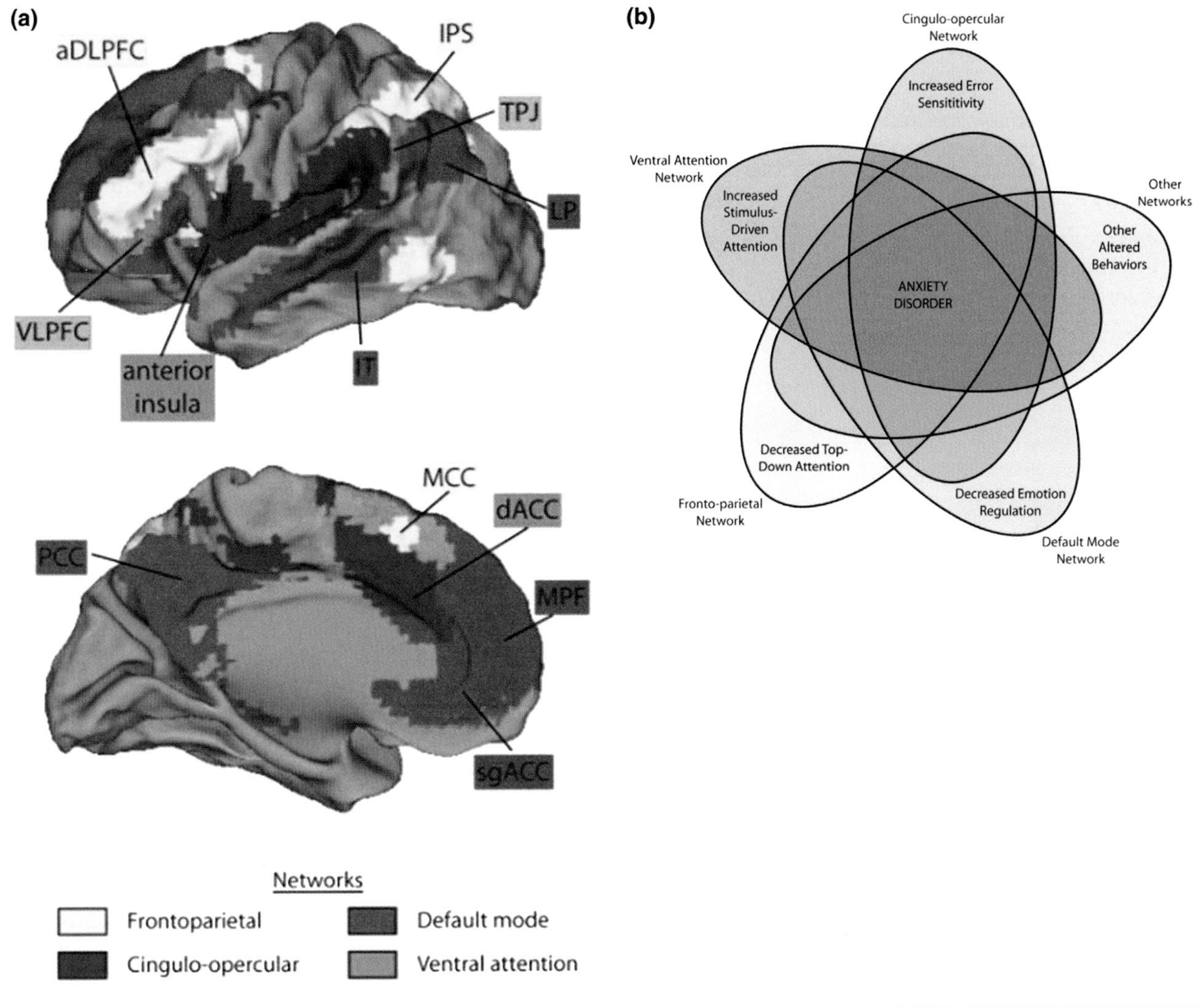

Sylvester, C.M., et al. (2012). Functional network dysfunction in anxiety and anxiety disorders. *Trends in Neuroscience* 35(9), 527–535. With permission from Elsevier.

tendency to respond in the wrong way is more likely to be inhibited by top-down processing—that is, through conscious thought—instead of responding in an habitual or automatic fashion (see Chapter 13 for a discussion of top-down versus bottom-up processing).

The ventral attentional network is thought to be involved in stimulus-driven attention, that is, when a stimulus automatically grabs your attention, as when your attention turns toward a loud noise in the hallway as you are focusing on the professor's illuminating words of wisdom.

Finally, the default-mode network is active when a person's mental activities are not focused on the external world, for example, when thinking about the past, planning for the future, engaging in self-reflection, or regulating one's emotions (Buckner, Andrews-Hanna, & Schacter, 2008; Raichle, 2015).

The relevance of these networks in anxiety disorders is illustrated in Figure 14.4b. The extent to which a person suffers from an anxiety disorder is related to the extent to which dysfunctions occur in these networks of brain areas. For example, someone suffering from an anxiety disorder may be more sensitive to conflicts and may detect them when none exists, giving the person the impression that something is wrong and leading to a strong drive to remedy the situation. Dysfunctions in the frontoparietal network may result in a person's decreased ability to engage in top-down processing, such as having difficulty inhibiting habitual actions when these are not appropriate. Dysfunctions in the ventral attentional network may lead someone to be easily distracted by irrelevant stimuli, leading to difficulties in focusing on the task at hand. Finally, dysfunctions in the default-mode network may lead to difficulties in regulating one's emotions. It is also thought that dysfunctions in other networks, yet to be identified, may be involved in anxiety disorders.

Neurotransmitters

The neurotransmitter gamma-aminobutyric acid (GABA) plays a major role in the regulation of anxiety. As you learned in Chapter 3, GABA is the major inhibitory neurotransmitter in the brain. Evidence indicates that GABA is important in regulating anxiety levels by keeping in check the activity of the amygdala, which as you just learned is hyperactive in anxiety disorders. For example, infusions of GABA antagonists in the amygdala increase fear and anxiety in animals (an anxiogenic effect). In contrast, infusions of GABA agonists decrease fear and anxiety (an anxiolytic effect) (Barbalho, Nunes-de-Souza, & Canto-de-Souza, 2009; Sanders & Shekhar, 1995). In addition, the administration of drugs known as benzodiazepines, which are GABA-receptor agonists, reduced activity in the amygdala and the anxiety felt by participants in a study where they were shown angry faces (Del-Ben et al., 2012).

Another neurotransmitter thought to be involved in anxiety is serotonin. As you will read later in the chapter, serotonin is also believed to be important for regulating mood and is the target of many antidepressant drugs. It has long been believed that dysfunctions in serotonergic function are also involved in the development of anxiety disorders (Baldwin & Rudge, 1995; Donaldson et al., 2014; Hoes, 1982).

The drugs of choice to treat anxiety disorders were for a long time benzodiazepines. As just mentioned, these are GABA-receptor agonists. However, because of their high addictive potential, they have for the most part been replaced by drugs that act on serotonin, namely, selective serotonin reuptake inhibitors, or SSRIs (Rickels & Moeller, 2018), which are discussed in some length in the module on major depression.

14.2.3 POSTTRAUMATIC STRESS DISORDER

>> LO 14.2.3 Describe some of the symptoms of posttraumatic stress disorder.

Key Terms

- **Posttraumatic stress disorder (PTSD):** A disorder observed in people having experienced a traumatic event that can be considered out of normal human experience.
- **Intrusive syndrome:** The intrusive thoughts, such as unwanted memories of events, and nightmares that a person with PTSD experiences.

Posttraumatic stress disorder (PTSD) is classified in the *DSM*-5 as a trauma- and stressor-related disorder. Kessler et al. (2005) found that 6.8% of the population have experienced PTSD at some point in their lives. PTSD is observed in people having experienced a traumatic event that can be considered out of normal human experience. Such experiences include living through war, rape, muggings, natural disasters, and other horrifying events. PTSD can also occur in people having indirectly experienced an event. For example, PTSD can be observed in rescuers dispatched to the sight of an airplane crash.

The symptoms of PTSD are wide ranging, so only a summary of them is given here. As defined in the *DSM*-5, a person with PTSD experiences what is known as the **intrusive syndrome**, which consists of intrusive thoughts, such as unwanted memories of the event, and nightmares. The person with PTSD may also experience intense distress and reactivity following exposure to stimuli that act as reminders of the traumatic event and may make great efforts to avoid those stimuli. This may be due to a reduced ability to process contextual information. For example, the sound of a helicopter overhead may signal danger in the context of war but not in the context of walking on a downtown street near one's home in a peaceful town.

Emotional and cognitive disturbances may also be observed. For example, the person with PTSD may experience intense negative emotions, such as fear and horror, with an inability to control them but not remember specific details of the event. PTSD patients may also become irritable, aggressive, and hypervigilant. Cognitive deficits may include difficulties in concentrating and in switching attention.

14.2.4 THE NEUROBIOLOGY OF POSTTRAUMATIC STRESS DISORDER

>> LO 14.2.4 Explain the neurobiological basis of posttraumatic stress disorder.

To some extent, the symptoms of PTSD can be attributed to either hypo- or hyperactivity in certain brain areas and circuits (Fenster, Lebois, Ressler, & Suh, 2018; Shalev, Liberzon, & Marmar, 2017). For example, people with PTSD have been shown to have reduced activity in the prefrontal cortex (which includes the medial, dorsolateral, and ventromedial prefrontal cortices) (Figure 14.5a). Reduced activity in these areas may account for the cognitive symptoms observed in PTSD, such as difficulties in concentration, attention, and emotional regulation (Etkin & Wager, 2007). Reduced activity in the prefrontal cortex may be responsible for the intrusive syndrome, due to its inability to dampen exaggerated fear responses triggered by the amygdala (Lanius et al., 2010). Excessive

FIGURE 14.5

Brain areas thought to be involved in PTSD. (a) Hypoactivity in the prefrontal cortex (medial, dorsolateral, and ventromedial) may account for the reduced ability to regulate emotions and impaired executive functioning. (b) Hyperactivity in the ACC, insula, and amygdala may account for exaggerated responses to potential threats. (c) Hypoactivity in a circuit that includes the hippocampus, medial prefrontal cortex, thalamus, and locus coeruleus may account for impaired contextual processing. (d) Hyperactivity in the amygdala may account for exaggerated fear reactions.

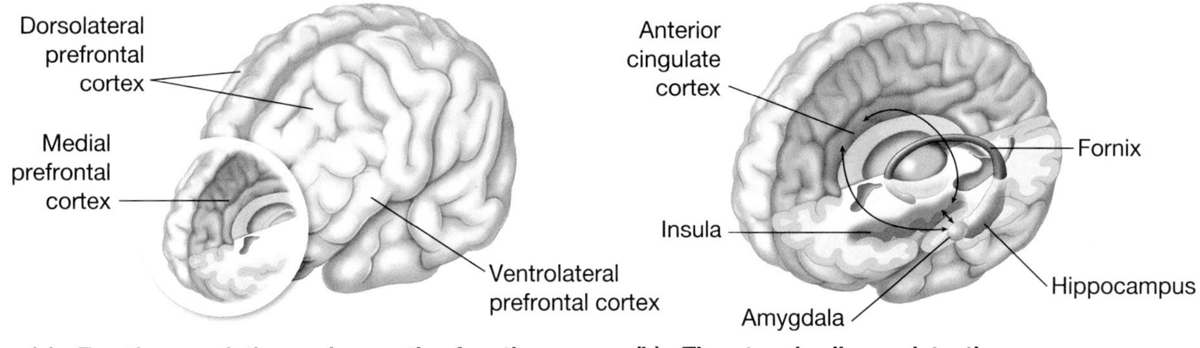

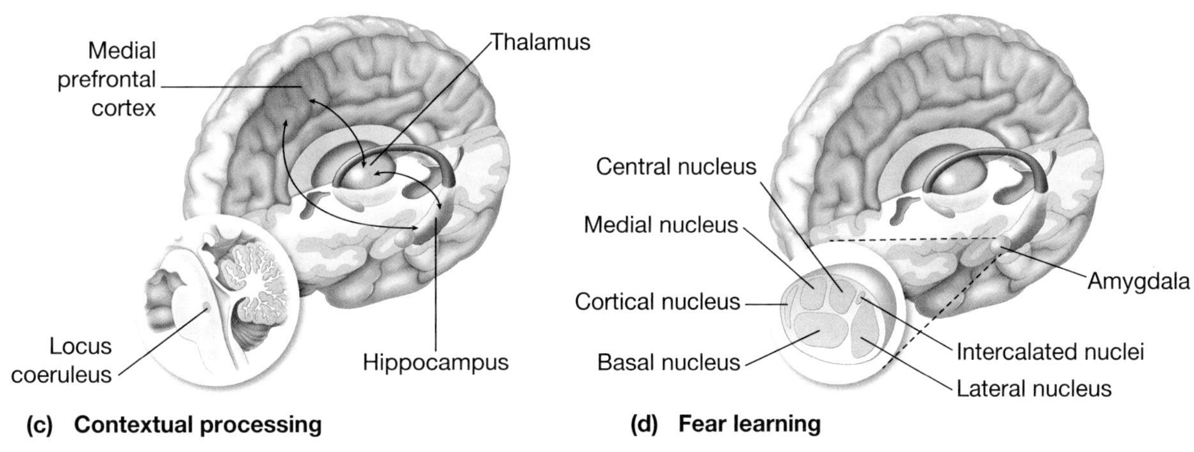

Carolina Hrejsa/Body Scientific Intl.

activity was also found in a circuit that includes the amygdala, insula, and ACC (Rosso et al., 2014), which, as mentioned earlier, is involved in the detection of conflicting information (Figure 14.5b).

The hippocampus is well known to play an important role in the memory for contextual information, for example, recognizing that the sound of a helicopter may be dangerous on a battlefield but not in the middle of a peaceful town. The hippocampus is smaller in volume in people who have PTSD (Logue et al., 2018). A circuit that includes the hippocampus, locus coeruleus, thalamus, and medial prefrontal cortex (Figure 14.5c) was found to be dysfunctional in PTSD (Liberzon & Abelson, 2016), which may account for the reduced ability to process contextual information. Contrary to the hippocampus, the amygdala (Figure 14.5d), which has for a long time been associated with emotional processing, was found to be of larger volume than normal (Pieper et al., 2019) and is overactive in people with PTSD, when exposed to anxiety-provoking stimuli, compared to healthy control subjects (Rauch et al., 2000).

Neurotransmitters

As you read earlier, the stress response includes the release of the hormone cortisol from the adrenal glands, and this leads to activation of the fight-or-flight response of the sympathetic nervous system. This response is ultrasensitive in people with anxiety disorders. However, some studies have found that cortisol levels are no different in people with PTSD compared to people who do not have PTSD and that there is no difference in the functioning of the HPA axis (Yehuda et al., 2000). Instead, people suffering from PTSD had elevated levels of norepinephrine (Pan, Kaminga, Wen, & Liu, 2018), which may be the result of amygdala overactivity (O'Donnell, Hegadoren, & Coupland, 2004).

MODULE SUMMARY

Anxiety is a negative mood state that is future oriented. Some people describe it as a feeling of unease, apprehension, or, in the worst cases, impending doom. Mental illness is on a continuum from what is normal and adaptive behavior to what can be considered abnormal and maladaptive. For example, it is normal and adaptive to be anxious about an upcoming test, to the extent that it motivates you to prepare for it. Anxiety disorders are characterized by exaggerated anxiety and fear. The terms *anxiety* and *fear* are sometimes used interchangeably, but they are not the same thing. Anxiety is about the possibility of a future threat, whereas fear is about a clear and present danger.

In people with anxiety disorders, the amygdala responds to potential threats in an exaggerated manner and the prefrontal cortex does not do a good job of keeping the amygdala in check. This has been shown in brain imaging studies of people suffering from social phobia. People with anxiety disorders also show overactivity of the hypothalamic-pituitary adrenal (HPA) axis in combination with environmental factors that can be a predisposition to anxiety disorders. Anxiety disorders have also been shown to be associated with functional networks of brain areas and with dysfunctional neurotransmitter systems, for example, those that involve GABA and serotonin. For a long time, benzodiazepines, which are GABA-receptor agonists, were used to treat anxiety disorders; however, because of their highly addictive potential, these have largely been replaced by drugs that act on serotonin, such as selective serotonin reuptake inhibitors, which are also used to treat major depressive disorder.

Posttraumatic stress disorder (PTSD) is associated with abnormalities in certain brain areas, such as the prefrontal cortex, anterior cingulate cortex, insula, hippocampus, and amygdala. In addition, people with PTSD are thought to have normal levels of the stress hormone cortisol but elevated levels of norepinephrine, which may be due to overactivation of the amygdala.

TEST YOURSELF

14.2.1 Differentiate fear from anxiety and briefly describe what constitutes an anxiety disorder.

14.2.2 Which brain areas, networks of brain areas, and neurotransmitter systems are thought to be involved in anxiety disorders?

14.2.3 Describe some of the symptoms of PTSD.

14.2.4 Name the brain regions thought to be dysfunctional in PTSD. Which hormone and neurotransmitter are thought to be involved in PTSD?

14.3 Obsessive-Compulsive Disorder

Module Contents

Learning Objectives

14.3.1 Describe the symptoms of obsessive-compulsive disorder.

14.3.2 Explain the neurobiological basis of obsessive-compulsive disorder.

Key Terms

- **Obsessive-compulsive disorder (OCD):** A psychological disorder characterized by intrusive and unwanted thoughts (obsessions) and repetitive behaviors that the person with OCD feels compelled to perform (compulsions).
- **Obsessions:** Intrusive and unwanted thoughts that give rise to high levels of anxiety.
- **Compulsions**: Behaviors that the person with obsessive-compulsive disorder feels compelled to perform.

14.3.1 WHAT IS OBSESSIVE-COMPULSIVE DISORDER?

>> LO 14.3.1 Describe the symptoms of obsessive-compulsive disorder.

Obsessive-compulsive disorder (OCD) is characterized by intrusive and unwanted thoughts (**obsessions**) and repetitive behaviors that the person with OCD feels compelled to perform (**compulsions**). It was classified as an anxiety disorder in previous versions of the *DSM* but now has a chapter of its own in the *DSM*-5, titled "Obsessive-Compulsive and Related Disorders." Obsessive-compulsive disorder is one of the most common of all mental illnesses. A study conducted in 2014 found that more than 2% of the population will suffer from OCD at some point in their lives (Goodman, Grice, Lapidus, & Coffey, 2014). People with OCD suffer significant personal distress as well as social and occupational limitations.

FIGURE 14.6

A hand-washing compulsion can lead to dry and painfully cracked skin.

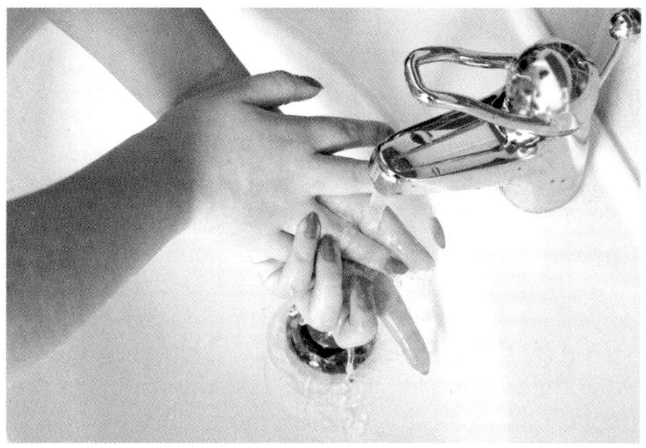

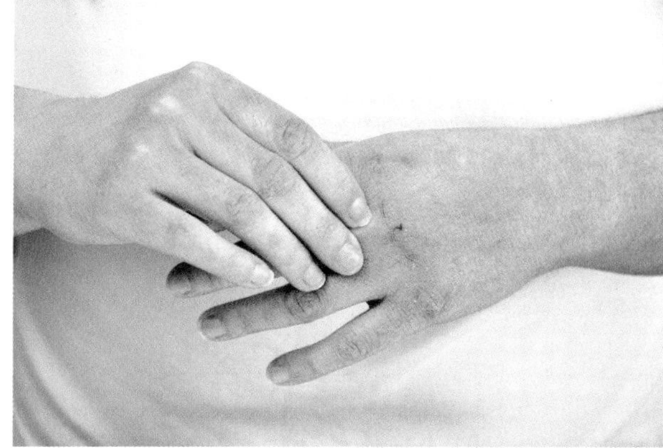

(left) Cunaplus_M.Faba/istockphoto; (right) Rhoberazzi/istockphoto

In OCD, obsessive thoughts give rise to anxiety. To reduce this anxiety, an action is performed that takes attention away from the thoughts or that is directly relevant in alleviating the anxiety provoked by these thoughts. For example, one may have the obsessive thought of being contaminated by germs. A compulsive response to this thought may be to repeatedly wash one's hands. People with a hand-washing compulsion may wash their hands so often that their skin becomes excessively dry with painful cracks (Figure 14.6).

In another type of obsession, a person may feel unsure that an important task was performed before leaving the house, such as shutting off the stove or locking the door. In response to this obsessive thought, the person may repeatedly go back to check the stove, door, or whatever else it might be. Checking behavior often becomes a ritualized process that must be accomplished before leaving the house. This may take up so much time that the person ends up late for school or work. Compulsions can also take the form of mental actions such as ritualized praying, without which the person with OCD feels that something horrible will happen to a loved one.

14.3.2 THE NEUROBIOLOGY OF OBSESSIVE-COMPULSIVE DISORDER

>> LO 14.3.2 **Explain the neurobiological basis of obsessive-compulsive disorder.**

Key Terms

- **CSTC model of OCD:** Dysfunction in a loop that includes brain areas in the prefrontal cortex, orbitofrontal cortex, basal ganglia, and thalamus is thought to contribute to the symptoms of OCD.
- **Vicious cycle of OCD:** Obsessive thoughts trigger significant amounts of anxiety, which is relieved temporarily by performing compulsive actions, until obsessive thoughts arise again, leading the person with OCD to repeat the cycle.

In this unit, we cover two major aspects of the neurobiology of OCD. First, we look at the brain areas thought to be implicated in OCD as well as how some of them may be dysfunctional or not communicating with one another properly. Then, we move to the molecular level of analysis so that you can gain a basic understanding of how OCD involves peculiarities in neurotransmitter systems.

OCD Circuit in the Brain

There is evidence that abnormal activity in a functional loop comprising brain areas in the prefrontal cortex (anterior cingulate cortex/medial prefrontal cortex, dorsolateral prefrontal cortex, orbitofrontal cortex), the basal ganglia (caudate, nucleus accumbens, and putamen), and the thalamus contributes significantly to the symptoms of OCD (Burguiere, Monteiro, Mallet, Feng, & Graybiel, 2015; Pauls, Abramovitch, Rauch, & Geller, 2014; Saxena & Rauch, 2000). This circuit of brain areas is known as the cortico-striatal-thalamic-cortical (CSTC) loop, illustrated in Figure 14.7. This has become known as the **CSTC model of OCD** (Saxena, Brody, Schwartz, & Baxter, 1998).

Information travels through this circuit along two pathways (Figure 14.8). These are the direct and indirect pathways. The direct pathway is excitatory, whereas the indirect pathway is inhibitory. In the excitatory direct pathway, the cortical regions (orbitofrontal cortex [OFC] and anterior cingulate cortex [ACC]) excite the striatum. In turn, the striatum inhibits the globus pallidus internal (GPi) and substantia nigra (SN), which

FIGURE 14.7

The cortical-striatal-thalamic-cortical (CSTC) loop.

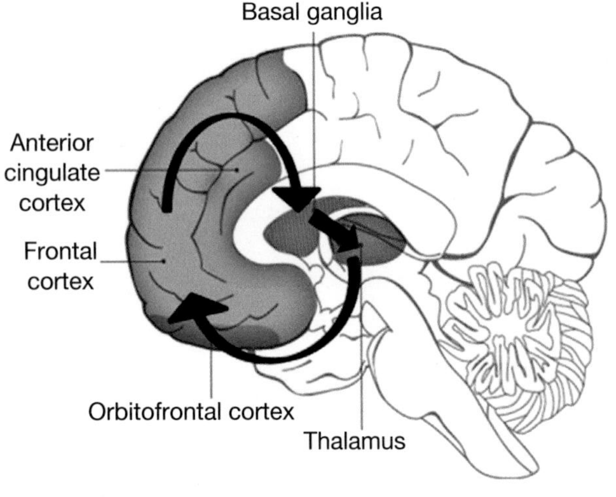

normally inhibit the thalamus. However, because the GPI and SN are themselves being inhibited by the striatum, their inhibitory action on the thalamus is removed, resulting in the thalamus being permitted to excite the cortical regions (OFC and ACC).

In the inhibitory indirect pathway, the cortical regions (OFC and ACC) also excite the striatum. However, in the indirect pathway, the striatum inhibits an area known as the global pallidus external (GPe). The GPe normally inhibits an area known as the subthalamic nucleus (STN). Without the inhibitory influence of the GPe, the STN is free to excite the GPi, which in turn can inhibit the thalamus. Inhibition of the thalamus prevents it from exciting the cortex. As we just described, activity in the direct pathway, which is excitatory, is kept in check by the indirect pathway, which is inhibitory (Figure 14.8a).

In OCD (Figure 14.8b), the direct pathway is more easily activated than the indirect pathway and therefore escapes the indirect pathway's inhibitory influence. This overactivity of the direct pathway compared to the indirect pathway is thought to account for the obsessive thoughts that characterize OCD. These thoughts, which create a significant amount of anxiety, are triggered by the cortical areas (OFC and ACC) and often take the form of exaggerated concerns about contamination, danger, or potential harm. Compulsive acts, such as excessive hand-washing, temporarily provide relief from the anxiety produced by these thoughts. However, this temporary relief from anxiety reinforces the compulsion, leading it to be repeated each time the obsessive thoughts arise. This is known as the **vicious cycle of OCD**, illustrated in Figure 14.9.

OCD and the Anterior Cingulate Cortex

As we saw for anxiety disorders, one potential factor involved in the cause of OCD is the generation of exaggerated error signals within a functional circuit that includes the anterior cingulate cortex (ACC). In OCD, exaggerated error signals may continually give the person with OCD the feeling of something being wrong, which may form the basis for obsessions, giving rise to high levels of anxiety.

FIGURE 14.8

(a) The direct and indirect pathways of the cortico-striatal-thalamic-cortical (CSTC) loop. Activity in the direct pathway is normally kept in check by inhibitory connections (hashed marks) in the indirect pathway. (b) In OCD, the direct pathway (now represented by thicker lines) is more easily excited than the indirect pathway, escaping the indirect pathway's inhibitory influence.

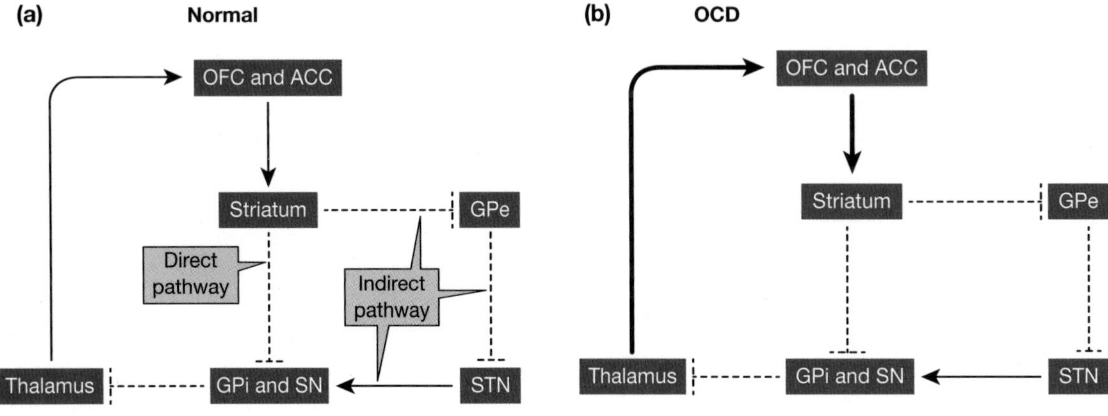

FIGURE 14.9

The vicious cycle of OCD.

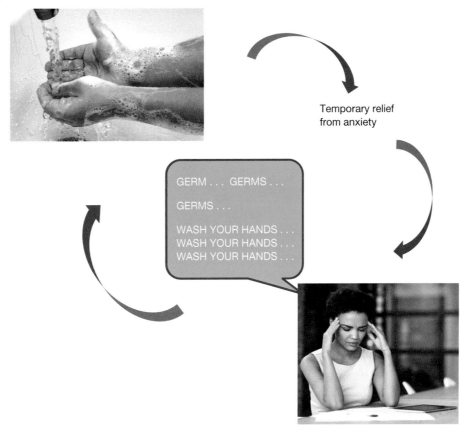

(top) mapodile/istockphoto; (bottom) HughStonelan/istockphoto

In an fMRI study published in 2003, neuroscientist Stefan Ursu and colleagues found greater activity in the ACC (Figure 14.9a) of OCD patients than in a control group when performing an AX-continuous response task (AX-CRT) (Ursu, Stenger, Shear, Jones, & Carter, 2003). This task was designed to induce conflict in responding. In this task, subjects are instructed to press a target button when a probe, X, presented on a computer screen, is preceded by a cue, A (AX trials), and to press another button when on other trials. Some of these cue-probe pairs are designed to create a conflict in responding and others are not. For example, cue-probe pairs containing an X or an A (e.g., BX or AY trials) generally cause more of a conflict than pairs that do not contain these letters, such as BY. The results are shown in Figure 14.10 (parts b–d). Conflict trials gave rise to greater activation in the ACC of OCD patients than in control subjects (Figure 14.10b). In contrast, no significant difference in activation was found during nonconflict trials, which consist of the AX (Figure 14.10c) and BY trials (Figure 14.10d).

Neurotransmitters

As mentioned earlier, many people who suffer from anxiety and depression benefit from taking selective serotonin reuptake inhibitors, or SSRIs. This may point to the involvement of dysfunctional serotonin neurotransmission in OCD. Evidence for this was found in a study by neuroscientist Daniela Perani and colleagues (2008). As illustrated in Figure 14.11, people with OCD had fewer serotonin receptors on postsynaptic neurons of the frontal lobes, cingulate cortex, and parietal and temporal cortices. In addition, they found an increase in dopamine activity in the basal ganglia, which as you learned earlier, is part of the CSTC loop thought to be at the center of the vicious cycle of OCD.

Normally, activity in the basal ganglia is driven by dopamine and inhibited by serotonin. Therefore, the deficiency of serotonin activity in people with OCD may result in the lack of inhibition in an already overactive basal ganglia due to abnormally high levels of dopamine. This in turn may be what gives rise to exaggerated activity in the CSTC loop.

FIGURE 14.10

(a) fMRI image showing activation of the ACC in OCD patients. (b) Change in fMRI signal across scanning sessions; ACC shows greater activation in conflict trials in OCD patients than in control subjects. (c and d) Change in fMRI signals across scanning sessions during nonconflict trials, showing no significant difference in activation between control subjects and OCD patients.

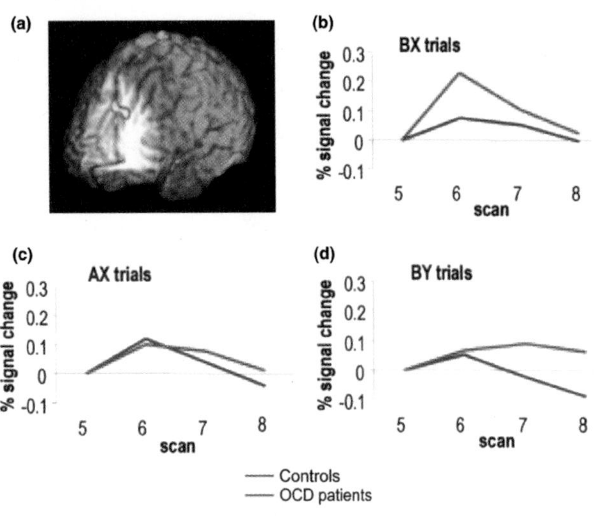

Ursu, S., et al. (2003). Overactive action monitoring in obsessive-compulsive disorder: evidence from functional magnetic resonance imaging. *Psychological Science 14*(4), 347–353. With permission from SAGE.

FIGURE 14.11

Areas of the brain with reduced numbers of serotonin receptors on postsynaptic neurons in the frontal lobes, cingulate cortex, and parietal and temporal cortices of people with OCD. Arrows point to these areas in both the left (L) and the right (R) hemispheres.

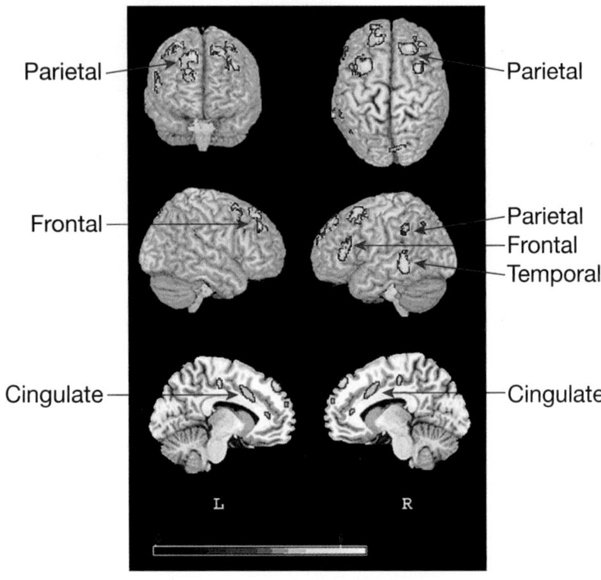

Perani, D., et al. (2008). In vivo PET study of 5HT(2A) serotonin and D(2) dopamine dysfunction in drug-naive obsessive-compulsive disorder. *Neuroimage 42*(1), 306–314. With permission from Elsevier.

MODULE SUMMARY

Obsessive-compulsive disorder (OCD) is characterized by intrusive and unwanted thoughts (obsessions) and repetitive behaviors that the person feels compelled to perform (compulsions). According to the cortico-striatal-thalamic-cortical (CSTC) model, OCD results from abnormal activity in the CSTC loop, which consists of cortical areas, the thalamus, and the basal ganglia. In OCD, people suffer from anxiety provoked by obsessive thoughts, and compulsive acts temporarily relieve the anxiety. However, the obsessions and the anxiety arise again, leading to more compulsive acts. This is known as the vicious cycle of OCD. In OCD, exaggerated error signals, within the cortical areas of the CSTC loop such as the ACC/mPFC, are generated. These error signals give rise, in the person with OCD, to the feeling of something being wrong, the basis for obsessions. Several neurotransmitter systems are implicated in OCD and other psychopathologies. People suffering from OCD have an abnormally low number of serotonin receptors in the frontal lobes, cingulate cortex, and parietal and temporal cortices. They also have abnormally high levels of dopamine in the basal ganglia.

TEST YOURSELF

14.3.1 Define obsessive-compulsive disorder.

14.3.2 Describe and explain the different neurobiological theories of obsessive-compulsive disorder.

14.4 Major Depressive Disorder

Module Contents

Learning Objectives

14.4.1 Describe the symptoms of major depressive disorder.

14.4.2 Explain the neurobiological basis of major depressive disorder.

14.4.1 WHAT IS MAJOR DEPRESSIVE DISORDER?

>> LO 14.4.1 Describe the symptoms of major depressive disorder.

Key Terms

- **Major depressive disorder (MDD):** A psychological disorder characterized by episodes of extremely sad moods accompanied by a loss of pleasure in usual activities. MDD may also include sleep disruptions, changes in appetite, agitation or psychomotor retardation, somatic symptoms, feelings of worthlessness, difficulty concentrating, and recurrent thoughts of suicide.
- **Psychomotor retardation:** A slowing down of thoughts and movement.
- **Multiply determined:** The idea that, like other psychological disorders, major depressive disorder is determined by many interacting factors.

Major depressive disorder (MDD), commonly known as depression, is one of several mood disorders described in the *DSM*-5. The chapter on mood disorders in the *DSM*-5 is subdivided into two categories. The first category describes disorders that include only depression as their main symptom. These are major depressive disorder, persistent depressive disorder (previously known as dysthymia), premenstrual depressive disorder, and disruptive mood dysregulation disorder. The other category involves disorders that include mania in addition to depressive symptoms. These are bipolar 1 and 2 disorder and cyclothymia. We focus only on the neurobiology of MDD.

Approximately 16.6% of the population has had depression at some point in their lives (Kessler et al., 2005). As described in the *DSM*-5, MDD is characterized by a sad mood accompanied by a loss of pleasure in usual activities. It may include sleep disturbances such as sleeping too little or too much. Weight loss and changes in appetite are also sometimes observed. The depressive person may also show agitation or **psychomotor retardation**, which is a slowing down of thoughts and movement. Some people who have MDD also experience somatic symptoms such as backaches, stomach pain, or musculoskeletal pain. The person with MDD may also feel worthless, have difficulty concentrating, and have recurrent thoughts of suicide.

Major depressive disorder is episodic. Episodes may last for five months or longer. The symptoms recur after a period during which the person with MDD is free of symptoms. It is important to distinguish between MDD and other types of depressive moods such as sadness or grief. For example, it is perfectly normal to feel depressed after the death of a loved one or after being emotionally hurt by someone. Most people successfully deal with these situations and are able to go on with their lives. Although negative life events can be contributing factors in the development of MDD, the causes of MDD, like all psychological disorders, are **multiply determined** and include biological factors, such as genetics, as well as structural and chemical differences within the brain. Psychological factors include cognitive, emotional, and behavioral problems. In addition to negative life events, such as the death of a loved one, environmental factors can include social isolation, work stress, and family stress.

14.4.2 THE NEUROBIOLOGY OF MAJOR DEPRESSIVE DISORDER

>> LO 14.4.2 Explain the neurobiological basis of major depressive disorder.

Key Terms

- **Rumination:** Repeatedly going over negative thoughts or problems.
- **Neuroinflammation:** The inflammation of nervous tissue.
- **Monoamine oxidase inhibitors:** Antidepressant drugs that prevent the degradation of monoamines by monoamine oxidase.

- **Monoamine hypothesis:** The idea that people with major depressive disorder have low levels of norepinephrine and serotonin.
- **Tricyclic antidepressants:** Antidepressant drugs that block the reuptake of serotonin and norepinephrine.
- **Serotonin reuptake inhibitors (SSRIs):** Antidepressant drugs that selectively block the reuptake of serotonin.
- **Atypical antidepressants:** Antidepressant drugs that inhibit the reuptake of both dopamine and norepinephrine as well as those that inhibit the reuptake of serotonin and norepinephrine.

Figure 14.12 shows some of the brain areas involved in MDD. These largely involve regions of the frontal lobes and include the orbitofrontal cortex (OFC), ventromedial prefrontal cortex (VMPFC), dorsolateral prefrontal cortex (DLPFC), hippocampus, amygdala, and anterior cingulate cortex (ACC) (Davidson, Pizzagalli, Nitschke, & Putnam, 2002).

FIGURE 14.12

Brain areas implicated in MDD. These include (a) the orbitofrontal cortex (green) and ventromedial prefrontal cortex (red), (b) the dorsolateral prefrontal cortex (blue), (c) the hippocampus (pink) and the amygdala (orange), and (d) the anterior cingulate cortex (yellow).

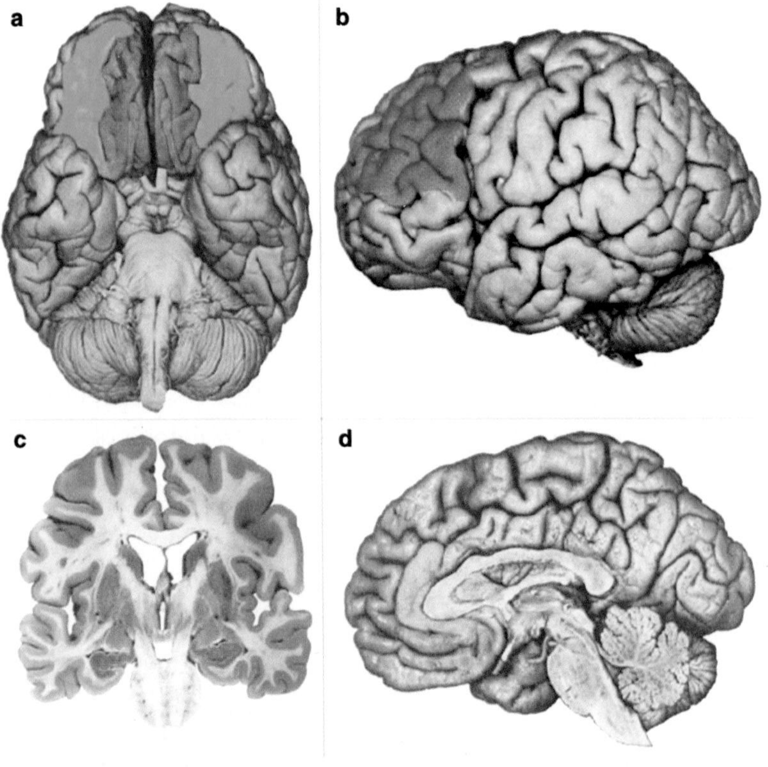

Davidson et al. (2002). Depression: Perspectives from Affective Neuroscience. *Annual Review of Psychology* 53: 545–574. With permission from Annual Reviews, Inc.

Orbitofrontal Cortex

Abnormalities or dysfunctions of the OFC are associated with depressed mood, anger, irritability, and anxiety, which are symptoms often observed in people with MDD and may be due partly to higher than normal activity in this area. In fact, studies show that the OFC of people with MDD is significantly more activated than the OFC of healthy control subjects. Dysfunctions in the OFC contribute to the maintenance of negative thoughts and emotions. In fact, disrupting the activity of the OFC, by electrical stimulation, leads to an improvement in the mood of people with MDD, possibly opening the way for new treatment strategies (Downar, 2019; Rao et al., 2018).

Ventromedial and Dorsolateral Prefrontal Cortices

The VMPFC and DLPFC show opposite patterns of activity during MDD. Studies have shown hyperactivity in the VMPFC and hypoactivity in the DLPFC in people with MDD (Koenigs & Grafman, 2009).

Hyperactivity of the VMPFC is also related to increased **rumination**, which consists of repeatedly going over negative thoughts or problems. Hypoactivity of the DLPFC is associated with psychomotor retardation and apathy. It may also relate to the deficits in working memory often seen in people with MDD. The DLPFC is also involved in reinterpreting negative stimuli as being less threatening. This function of the DLPFC seems to be impaired in some people with MDD (Park et al., 2019).

Hippocampus

Many studies have found that the hippocampus of people with MDD is reduced in volume (Roddy et al., 2019; Sheline, Liston, & McEwen, 2019). This reduction in volume is accounted for by the loss of gray matter. Psychiatrist Ian Anderson and colleagues at the University of Manchester (Arnone et al., 2013) showed that the longer a person with MDD goes without treatment, the greater the loss in gray matter in both the left and right hippocampi (Figure 14.13). However, the good news is that they also found increases in the amount of gray matter following treatment with antidepressants and remission of the depressive symptoms. Antidepressants may promote nerve growth by increasing levels of proteins known as brain-derived neurotrophic factor (BDNF) and nerve growth factors, which may be low in the hippocampus of people with MDD (Mondal & Fatima, 2019).

FIGURE 14.13

Relationship between duration of untreated depressive symptoms and the reduction in gray matter in the left and right hippocampi. The longer depressive symptoms go untreated, the less gray matter is observed.

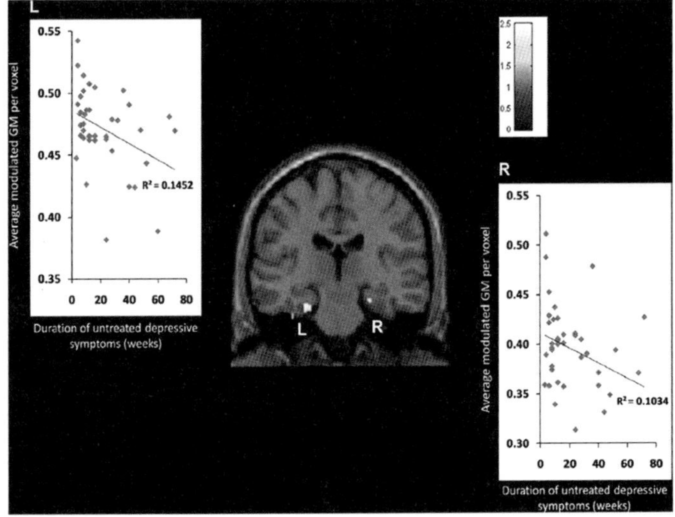

Arnone, D. et al. (2013). State-dependent changes in hippocampal grey matter in depression. *Molecular Psychiatry 18*(12): 1265–1272. With permission from Springer Nature.

The hippocampus plays an important role in regulating levels of glucocorticoids, which, as we saw in the module on anxiety, are elevated in people with MDD. Figure 14.14 illustrates the effects of high levels of glucocorticoids on the hippocampus (Maletic et al., 2007):

1. High levels of glucocorticoids, due to overactivity of the HPA axis, are toxic to the hippocampus, resulting in decreases of gray matter and smaller hippocampal volumes.
2. Smaller hippocampal volumes in people with MDD disrupt the hippocampus's ability to regulate levels of glucocorticoids.
3. Activation of the HPA axis results in the release of corticotropin-releasing hormone (CRH) from the hypothalamus. Activation of the HPA axis is triggered by activity in the amygdala.
4. The release of CRH from the hypothalamus causes the release of adrenocorticotropic hormone (ACTH) from the pituitary gland, which promotes the release of glucocorticoids from the adrenal glands.
5. Activation of the HPA axis also promotes the release of what are known as cytokines from macrophages. Cytokines are molecules that are part of the immune system. Microphages are white blood cells that engulf and digest cellular debris and potentially toxic substances.

This process further undermines the ability of the hippocampus to regulate glucocorticoid levels. Cytokines (tumor-necrosis factor [TNF], interleukin-1 and 6 [IL-1, IL6]) reduce the amount of BDNF in the brain and affect neurotransmission of the monoamines (dopamine [DA], serotonin [5-HT], and norepinephrine [NE] initiated in the ventral-tegmental area, locus coeruleus, and raphe nuclei, respectively). This can lead to the death of neurons and affect the brain's ability to turn off the stress response.

Amygdala

The amygdala is known to monitor threats in the environment. You already know this from having read the earlier module on anxiety in this chapter and about the "low road" and "high road" in Chapter 11. Similar to what can be observed in people with anxiety disorders, the amygdala of people with MDD shows heightened activity (Drevets, 2003; Drevets et al., 2002).

FIGURE 14.14

Process by which elevated activity in the HPA axis leads to the impaired ability of the hippocampus to regulate levels of glucocorticoids (red arrows indicate inhibition, and green arrows, excitation). See text for details.

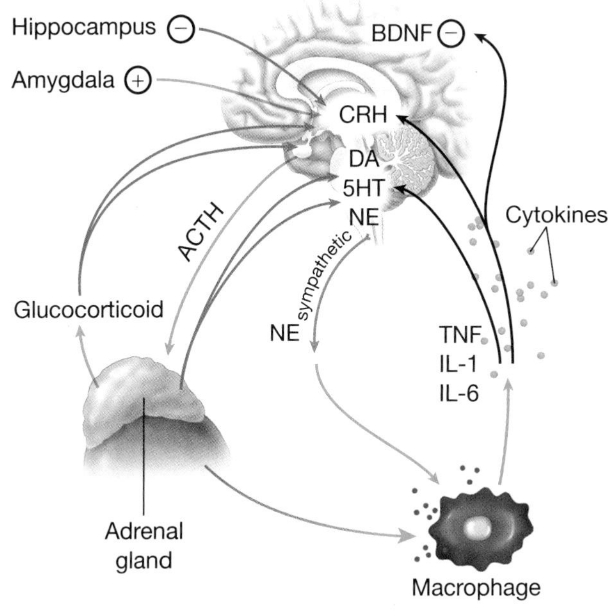

Amanda Tomasikiewicz/Body Scientific Intl.

Anterior Cingulate Cortex

Many studies have found dysfunctions of the ACC in people with MDD (Burger et al., 2017; Harada et al., 2018; Rolls et al., 2018). In addition to being involved in detecting conflicts (as you read earlier), the ACC is also important for linking emotions with attention. In fact, the rostral and ventral parts of the ACC have been found to process emotions, whereas the dorsal part is involved in cognitive processes (Stevens, Hurley, & Taber, 2011). This makes the ACC a prime area for emotional self-regulation (Park et al., 2019), which may occur through its connections with the DLPFC and motor areas of the cortex so that appropriate responses are selected based on the processing of the conscious appraisal of information.

Consistent with the findings that the ACC is dysfunctional in people with MDD, people with MDD also have difficulty taking corrective action in response to errors they have committed. This was shown by researcher Douglas Steele and colleagues (Steele, Kumar, & Ebmeier, 2007). Healthy control participants had slower reaction times in trials after which they had received negative feedback about their performance in a gambling task. This slowed reaction time is called "post-error slowing" and is thought to be due to cognitive processes involved in correcting errors. In healthy control subjects, post-error slowing was accompanied by activation of the ACC. Neither post-error slowing nor activation of the ACC was observed in the participants with MDD (Figure 14.15).

Neuroinflammation

Medical conditions that cause **neuroinflammation**, which refers to the inflammation of nervous tissue, are associated with MDD (Eswarappa, Neylan, Whooley, Metzler, & Cohen, 2019; Oh, Van Dam, Doucette, & Murrough, 2019; Whooley et al., 2007). Neuroscientists tracked the distribution of translocator protein (TSPO), which is a marker of inflammation, in the brains of healthy participants versus participants with MDD (Setiawan et al., 2015). They tracked levels of TSPO in the brain using positron emission tomography (PET).

Molecules of interest in the brain can be tracked by PET by attaching them to radiotracers. People differ in how well the radiotracer binds to different molecules. Therefore, the researchers were able to test how well the radiotracers bound to TSPO in all of the participants. They divided the participants into high-affinity binders (HAB) and mixed-affinity binders (MAB). In HAB, most TSPO molecules have high-affinity binding sites. In MAB, half of the TSPO molecules have high-affinity binding sites, whereas the other half of the TSPO molecules have low-affinity binding sites.

Participants with MDD had significantly higher levels of TSPO (the marker for inflammation) in the PFC, ACC, insula, dorsal putamen, thalamus, ventral striatum, and hippocampus, when compared with healthy control subjects. Also, levels of TSPO in the ACC were associated with symptoms of MDD as measured by scores on the Hamilton Depression Rating Scale (HAM-D).

FIGURE 14.15

Activity in the ACC of (a) healthy control subjects and (b) participants with MDD. In addition to post-error slowing (see text), healthy control subjects showed activity of the ACC with negative feedback. In contrast, no such activity was observed in the ACC of participants with MDD.

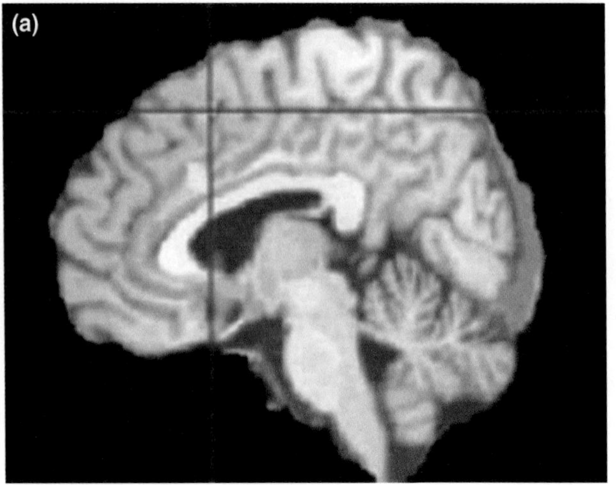

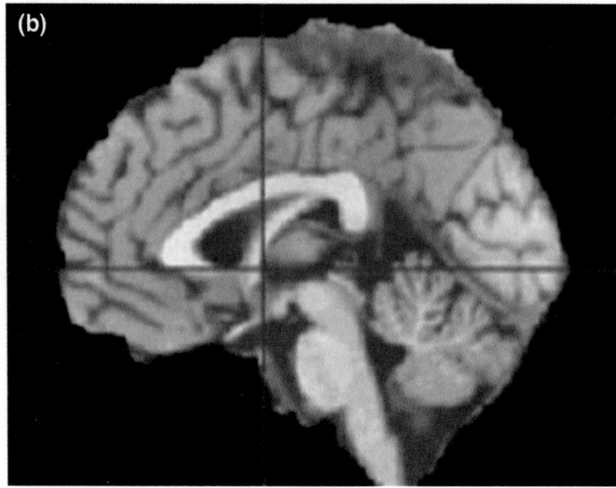

Steele, J.D., et al. (2007). Blunted response to feedback information in depressive illness. *Brain 130*(Pt 9): 2367–2374. With permission from Oxford University Press.

These findings were later supplemented by the results of another study (Setiawan et al., 2018). In that study, the levels of TSPO in participants with chronologically advanced MDD, with long periods (10 years or longer) of not having been treated with antidepressants, were compared to those who had short periods of antidepressant treatment. Participants with MDD who had not been treated for a long period had higher TSPO levels in the same brain areas as in the previous study, compared to participants who had short periods of treatment. In addition, increased TSPO levels did not persist in participants treated with antidepressant medications that inhibit the reuptake of serotonin, discussed in the next section.

Neurotransmitters in MDD and Antidepressant Medication

People suffering from MDD are widely believed to have depleted levels of monoamine neurotransmitters serotonin, norepinephrine, and dopamine. This is known as the **monoamine hypothesis** (Bunney & Davis, 1965; Schildkraut, 1965). The monoamine hypothesis is based on two lines of evidence. In the 1950s, researchers found that the antihypertensive drug reserpine caused depression by depleting the monoamines, a finding that has since been disproved (Baumeister, Hawkins, & Uzelac, 2003).

The second line of evidence is grounded in the discovery, in the 1960s, that the drug iproniazid, used to treat tuberculosis, had antidepressant effects by inhibiting monoamine oxidase, an enzyme that breaks down the monoamines (Kirshner, 1962; Weiner, Cloutier, Bjur, & Pfeffer, 1972). Iproniazid and similar drugs are referred to as **monoamine oxidase inhibitors**. It was later found that the drug imipramine and other drugs had antidepressant effects by inhibiting the reuptake of serotonin and norepinephrine. These are known as the **tricyclic antidepressants** (Domino, 1999).

In the late 1970s, researchers found that antidepressant effects could be achieved by focusing on the reuptake of serotonin. This led to the development of drugs that specifically inhibit the reuptake of serotonin. These drugs, which are widely in use today, are known as **selective serotonin reuptake inhibitors** (SSRIs) and are sometimes called second-generation antidepressants (Wong, Bymaster, Horng, & Molloy, 1975). The mechanisms of action of tricyclic antidepressants and SSRIs are illustrated in Figure 14.16.

Following the introduction of SSRIs, another class of drugs known as **atypical antidepressants**, some of which inhibit the reuptake of dopamine and norepinephrine, were approved for use in 1989 (Fava et al., 2005); others in this class inhibit the reuptake of serotonin and norepinephrine (Bymaster et al., 2001). The most recent atypical antidepressant, approved for use in 2013, is known as vortioxetine; it inhibits the reuptake of serotonin, norepinephrine, and dopamine (Mork et al., 2012).

Beyond the Monoamine Hypothesis

Depression may also be due to dysfunctions in glutaminergic neurotransmission. For example, people

FIGURE 14.16

Mechanisms of action of tricyclic antidepressants and selective serotonin reuptake inhibitors (second generation).

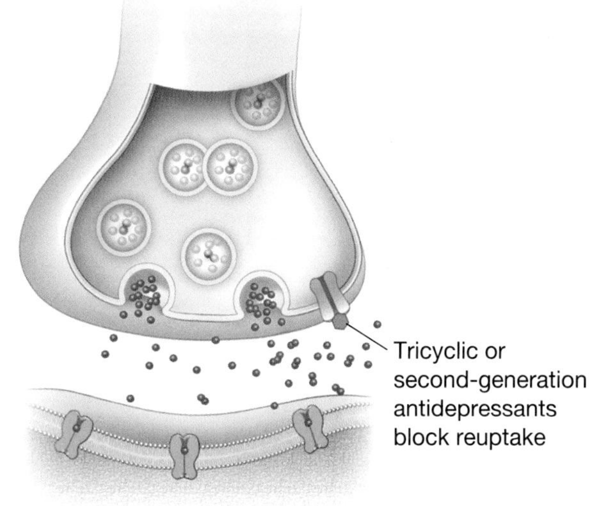

Amanda Tomasikiewicz/Body Scientific Intl.

suffering from MDD have higher levels of the neurotransmitter glutamate (J. Levine et al., 2000). In addition, the monoamine antidepressants reviewed earlier reduce the levels of glutamate, possibly accounting for their antidepressant effects (Garakani, Martinez, Yehuda, & Gorman, 2013). This has led to studies in which the antidepressant effects of drugs that reduce the neurotransmission of glutamate are being assessed. One such drug is the hallucinogenic drug ketamine, which is an NMDA-receptor antagonist (remember that the NMDA receptor is a subtype of glutamate receptor). The use of glutamate receptor antagonists has not been approved for use in the treatment of MDD, although it is the focus of intense study (Chen et al., 2018; Khakpai, Ebrahimi-Ghiri, Alijanpour, & Zarrindast, 2019; Li et al., 2019; Murrough et al., 2013).

MODULE SUMMARY

Major depressive disorder (MDD) is characterized by a sad mood accompanied by a loss of pleasure in usual activities. MDD is episodic, with episodes lasting for five months or longer. Like all other disorders, the causes of MDD are multiply determined and include biological factors, such as genetics, as well as structural and chemical differences within the brain. The hippocampus plays an important role in regulating levels of glucocorticoids, which are elevated in people with MDD. There may be many structural abnormalities in the brains of people with MDD, for example, in the anterior cingulate cortex, orbitofrontal cortex, ventromedial and dorsolateral prefrontal cortex, and hippocampus. Conditions that create inflammation in the brain are related to MDD.

Major depressive disorder is thought to involve dysfunctions in monoamine neurotransmitter systems. This is known as the monoamine hypothesis. Medications used to treat MDD involve several classes of drugs that interact with these systems. These include monoamine oxidase inhibitors, tricyclic antidepressants, and selective serotonin reuptake inhibitors (SSRIs), serotonin and norepinephrine reuptake inhibitors (SNRIs), and atypical antidepressants. MDD may also implicate dysfunctions in the neurotransmitter glutamate. Therefore, drugs that increase levels of glutamate, such as ketamine, are being tested for the treatment of MDD.

TEST YOURSELF

14.4.1 What are the symptoms of MDD?

14.4.2 (a) What are three groups of drugs that contributed to a neurobiological theory of MDD? Briefly trace their history and describe how they act in the brain. (b) How does elevated activity in the HPA axis contribute to the reduced ability of the hippocampus to regulate levels of glucocorticoids?

14.5 Schizophrenia

Module Contents

14.5.1 What Is Schizophrenia?

14.5.2 The Neurobiology of Schizophrenia

Learning Objectives

14.5.1 Describe the symptoms of schizophrenia.

14.5.2 Explain the neurobiological basis of schizophrenia.

14.5.1 WHAT IS SCHIZOPHRENIA?

>> LO 14.5.1 **Describe the symptoms of schizophrenia.**

Key Terms

- **Schizophrenia:** A psychological disorder characterized by the presence of symptoms that includes delusions, hallucinations, disorganized speech, disorganized behavior, diminished emotional expression, and cognitive impairments.
- **Positive symptoms:** The presence of symptoms that people do not normally experience, such as hallucinations and delusions.
- **Psychotic symptoms:** Positive symptoms of schizophrenia that are characterized as delusions and hallucinations.
- **Delusions:** Misrepresentations of reality. Some common delusions in schizophrenia are delusions of grandeur, delusions of persecution, and paranoid delusions.
- **Hallucinations:** Perceptions of sensory events that are not occurring in reality, which can involve any of the senses.
- **Negative symptoms:** Deficits in normal emotional expression as well as avolition and anhedonia.

Schizophrenia is a psychological disorder characterized by the presence of symptoms that include delusions, hallucinations, disorganized speech, disorganized behavior, diminished emotional expression, and cognitive impairments. Schizophrenia significantly impairs people's ability to think clearly, manage their emotions, make decisions, and relate to others. The lifetime prevalence of schizophrenia in the United States is approximately 1.2% (Erlich, Smith, Horwath, & Cournos, 2014). It is classified under "Schizophrenia Spectrum and Other Psychotic Disorders" in the *DSM*-5. That chapter of the *DSM*-5 includes disorders that are on a continuum of severity. These are schizotypal (personality) disorder, delusional disorder, brief psychotic disorder, and schizophreniform disorder. This module, however, focuses only on schizophrenia.

Positive and Negative Symptoms

Positive Symptoms. What are referred to as **positive symptoms** of schizophrenia include delusions and hallucinations, which are sometimes referred to as the **psychotic symptoms** of schizophrenia. **Delusions** are misrepresentations of reality. Some common delusions in schizophrenia are delusions of grandeur, delusions of persecution, and paranoid delusions. People with delusions of grandeur act as if they are someone they are not. For example, a woman may falsely believe she is a famous opera singer or actress. People with delusions of persecution falsely believe that someone is out to hurt them. People with paranoid delusions are overly suspicious of others in the most nonrealistic ways. For example, a woman with paranoid delusions may believe that aliens are monitoring her mind and sending information about her thoughts to the government.

Hallucinations are perceptions of sensory events that are not occurring in reality. Hallucinations can involve any of the senses. For example, in a visual hallucination, someone sees something that is not there. In an auditory hallucination, someone hears something that is not there. The most common types of hallucinations in schizophrenia are auditory. However, other types of hallucinations, such as visual, gustatory (taste), or tactile hallucinations, are sometimes observed.

Positive symptoms that are not considered psychotic include disorganized speech, which refers to speech that is poor or incoherent or that goes off onto a tangent or in unrelated directions. They also include disorganized behavior, which refers to behavior that is bizarre or unusual.

Negative Symptoms. The **negative symptoms** of schizophrenia include diminished emotional expressions, known as flat affect. Other negative symptoms include avolition, which is a reduction in motivations to engage in activities; anhedonia, which is an inability to feel pleasure; and alogia, which is a poverty of speech.

14.5.2 THE NEUROBIOLOGY OF SCHIZOPHRENIA

>> LO 14.5.2 Explain the neurobiological basis of schizophrenia.

Key Terms

- **Hypofrontality theory of schizophrenia:** The idea that people with schizophrenia have reduced activity in the prefrontal cortex.
- **Dopamine hypothesis:** The idea that a dysfunctional dopamine system is at the core of the symptoms observed in schizophrenia.
- **Aberrant salience hypothesis:** The hypothesis that excessive dopamine release results in external and internal stimuli that have no particular importance becoming exaggeratedly salient, giving rise to delusions and hallucinations.
- **NMDA-receptor-hypofunction hypothesis:** The hypothesis that NMDA receptors are dysfunctional in people with schizophrenia.

Various patterns of abnormalities in brain structures as well as in the connectivity between brain areas have been found in people who have schizophrenia. One often-cited finding is that some people with schizophrenia have enlarged ventricles. This difference in ventricular size has been shown in identical twins where one suffered from schizophrenia and the other did not. An MRI image of this ventricular enlargement is shown in Figure 14.17a. Figure 14.17b shows the results of an earlier study, in which patients with schizophrenia had ventricles that were enlarged in relation to the rest of their brains (ventricle-to-brain ratio) (Weinberger, Torrey, Neophytides, & Wyatt, 1979). Note, however, that not all patients had elevated ventricle-to-brain ratios. Many of the patients had the same ratio as control participants.

It is important to understand that this enlargement of the ventricles is not thought to be the cause of the symptoms of schizophrenia. It is more likely that some of the symptoms of schizophrenia are at least partly caused by the reduction of brain tissue, due to the extra space taken up by the ventricles.

In addition to enlarged ventricles, people with schizophrenia have shown a pattern of gray matter loss beginning in adolescence. Researchers Paul M. Thompson and colleagues followed adolescents with schizophrenia for a period of five years, scanning their brains with fMRI at two-year intervals (P. M. Thompson et al., 2001). As shown in Figure 14.18, gray matter loss was widespread in adolescents with schizophrenia compared with healthy control subjects. The greater losses, over the years, were observed in parietal, temporal, and frontal areas. The amount of gray matter loss was also associated with a progression in the severity of symptoms.

FIGURE 14.17

Difference in ventricular size in the brains of identical twins. (a) Image of the brain of the twin suffering from schizophrenia (left) compared to the brain of the twin who did not suffer from schizophrenia (right).
(b) Difference in the ventricle-to-brain ratios between patients with schizophrenia versus control subjects. Many of the patients have the same ratio as control subjects.

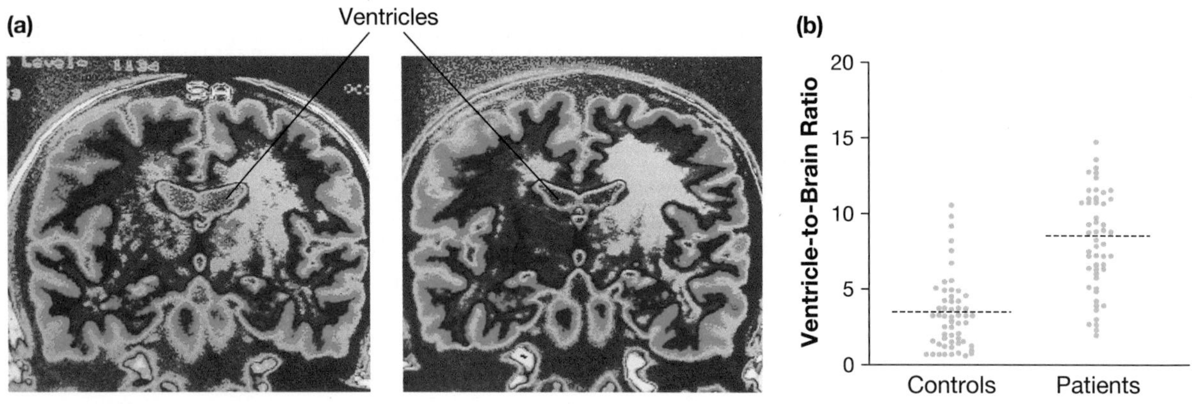

The cognitive deficits observed in people with schizophrenia resemble the deficits in people who have suffered damage to the frontal lobes. This may be due to lower than normal functioning of the prefrontal cortex. In the 1980s, neuroscientist Daniel R. Weinberger and colleagues administered the Wisconsin Card Sorting Test, shown in Figure 14.19, to people with schizophrenia and normal control subjects (Goldberg, Weinberger, Berman, Pliskin, & Podd, 1987). In this task, participants are asked to sort out a deck of cards by shape, color, or symbols. Once the cards have been sorted according to the rule (e.g., by shape) on several occasions, the rule changes (e.g., now sort by color). People with damage to the prefrontal cortex have great

FIGURE 14.18

Rate of gray matter loss over a five-year period in normal adolescents and adolescents with schizophrenia.

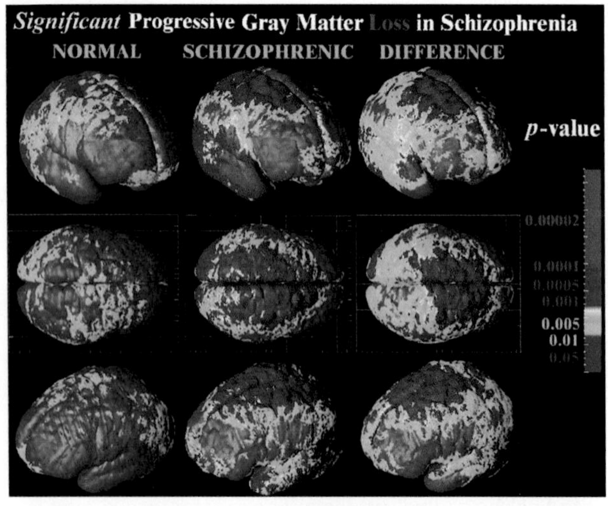

FIGURE 14.19

The Wisconsin Card Sorting Test. See text for details.

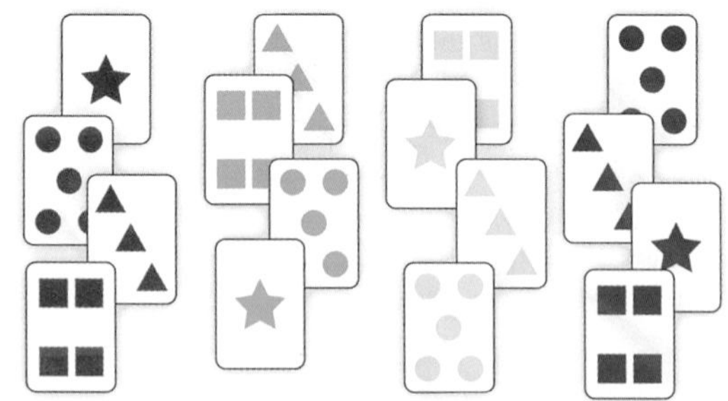

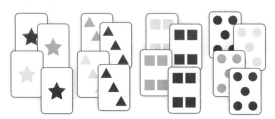

difficulty switching to sorting the cards according to the new rule and persevere on applying the old rule. This finding attests to the importance of the prefrontal cortex in working memory (remembering the cards and errors made to correct them) and behavioral flexibility (changing behavior according to a new rule).

Weinberger and colleagues found that people with schizophrenia were impaired at performing this task in a way that is similar to what is observed in people with damage to the prefrontal cortex. The same participants also had lower activity in the prefrontal cortex than control participants. The idea that the activity of prefrontal cortex is reduced in people with schizophrenia is called the **hypofrontality theory of schizophrenia** (Weinberger & Berman, 1988).

In 2005, researcher Vicente Molina and colleagues subjected men who had a first episode of psychosis to an attention task while being scanned by PET (Molina et al., 2005). At the beginning of the study, none of the men met all the criteria for schizophrenia. However, two years later, some of these men progressed to meeting the criteria for schizophrenia while the others did not. Only the men who had progressed to schizophrenia showed hypofrontality, compared to men who did not progress to schizophrenia and control subjects (Figure 14.20). These results suggested that hypofrontality can be used as a marker for the development of schizophrenia after a single episode of psychosis.

Neurotransmitters

Abnormalities in a variety of neurotransmitter systems are thought to be involved in the development and symptoms of schizophrenia. These include the dopaminergic, serotoninergic, glutamatergic, and cholinergic systems. Here we focus our attention on the dopaminergic and glutamatergic systems.

Dopamine. Of all of the neurotransmitters thought to be involved in schizophrenia, none has received as much attention as dopamine. The idea that a dysfunctional dopaminergic system is at the core of the symptoms observed in schizophrenia is known as the **dopamine hypothesis** (Seeman, 1987).

There are three versions of the dopamine hypothesis (O. D. Howes & Kapur, 2009). The first version is based on the observation that drugs that are effective in treating the symptoms of schizophrenia block dopamine receptors (specifically D_2 receptors) in the brain. As shown in Figure 14.21, many such drugs exist. Also illustrated is the relationship between the potency of these drugs and their efficacy in blocking D_2 receptors (Creese, Burt, & Snyder, 1996; Seeman, Lee, Chau-Wong, & Wong, 1976). Further support for this version of the dopamine hypothesis came from findings that drugs that increase dopamine levels, such as amphetamine and cocaine, can induce schizophrenic-like symptoms in people without schizophrenia and exacerbate these symptoms in people with schizophrenia (Angrist & Gershon, 1970).

However, there are problems with this version of the dopamine hypothesis. For example, it does not differentiate between the positive symptoms, characterized by hallucinations and delusions, and the negative symptoms such as flattened emotions and poverty of speech. It also provides no insight into which specific brain area contains dysfunctional dopamine transmission. This version also does not account for the possible interactions between a dysfunctional dopaminergic system and genetic and environmental factors.

In contrast to the first version, the second version of the dopamine hypothesis relates positive and negative symptoms to dopamine neurotransmission in particular brain areas (K. L. Davis, Kahn, Ko, & Davidson,

FIGURE 14.20

PET results showing the metabolic activity in the DLPFC of men who progressed to meet the criteria for schizophrenia, compared to men who did not and control subjects.

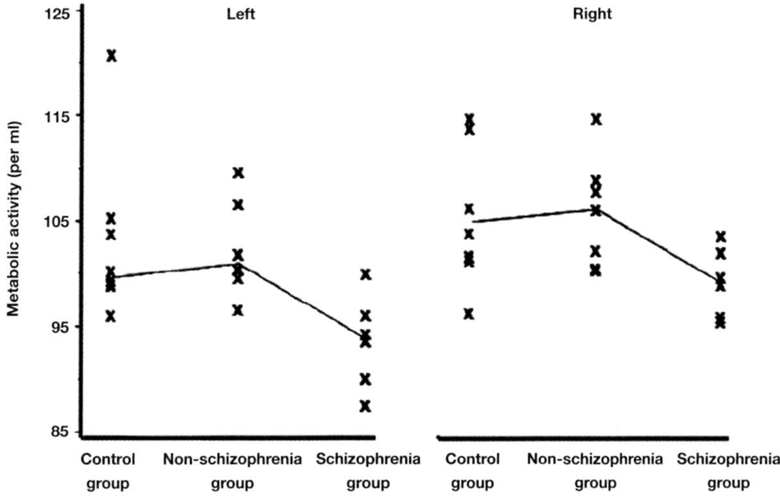

Molina, V., et al. (2005). Hypofrontality in men with first-episode psychosis. *The British Journal of Psychiatry 186*(3): 203–208. With permission from Cambridge University Press.

FIGURE 14.21

The relationship between the potency of several antipsychotic drugs and their effectiveness at blocking D_2 dopamine receptors.

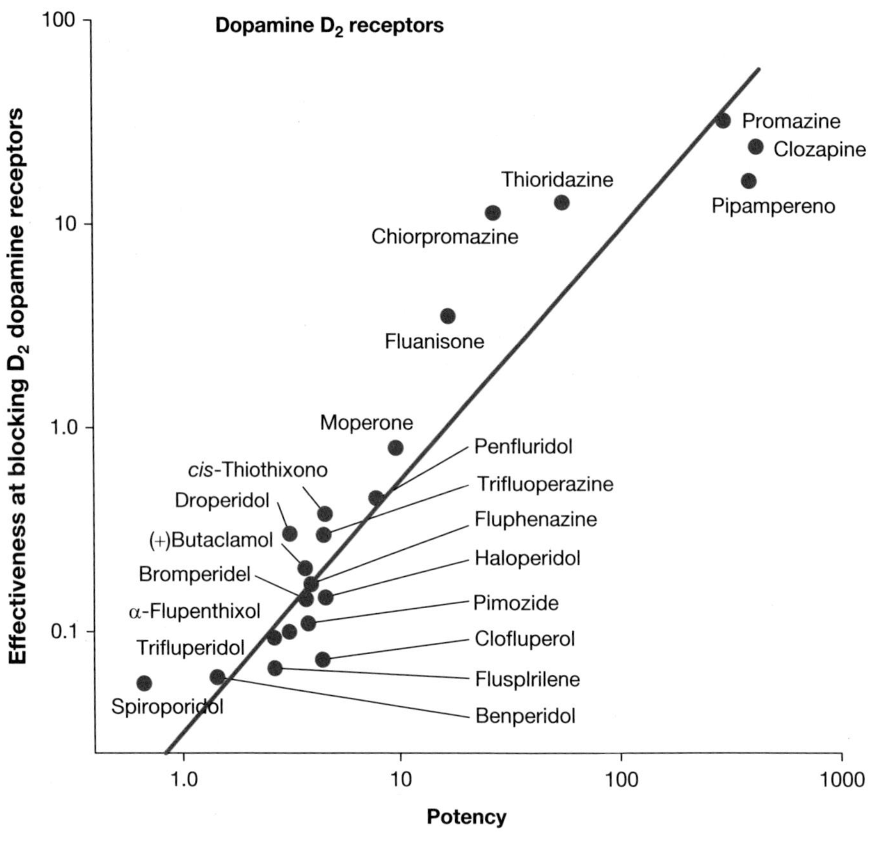

Adapted from *Molecular Neuropharmacology: A Foundation for Clinical Neuroscience*, 2nd Edition, Nestler, Hyman and Malenka, McGraw-Hill, 2009.

1991). According to this version, positive symptoms are due to excessive dopamine neurotransmission in the striatum, whereas negative symptoms are due to a lack of dopamine neurotransmission in the frontal lobes.

The third version of the dopamine hypothesis (O. D. Howes & Kapur, 2009; Kapur, 2003; Miyata, 2019) can be summarized in four points:

(1) The deregulation of dopamine in schizophrenia is induced by multiple interacting factors such as genetics, stress, drugs, and faulty interactions between brain areas such as the frontal and temporal cortices.

(2) Dopamine dysfunctions occur in presynaptic neurons rather than at postsynaptic D_2 receptors.

(3) Dopamine dysregulation is linked only to the psychotic symptoms of schizophrenia (i.e., hallucinations and delusions), and dopamine-receptor antagonists are effective in disorders other than schizophrenia. For example, psychotic symptoms are also sometimes observed in depression and dementia, such as Alzheimer's disease (see Chapter 5).

(4) Excessive dopamine release from neurons increases the salience of stimuli to the point where it becomes aberrant or exaggerated, giving rise to psychotic symptoms (note that the salience of a stimulus refers to the extent to which it is noticeable, prominent, or seems important).

The third version of the dopamine hypothesis of schizophrenia gave rise to what is known as the **aberrant salience hypothesis** (Kapur, 2003; Miyata, 2019). The aberrant salience hypothesis seeks to explain only the psychotic symptoms of schizophrenia, that is, hallucinations and delusions. The aberrant salience hypothesis is based on the incentive-salience theory you read about in Chapters 3 and 9. To recap, this hypothesis states that dopamine release causes stimuli that are associated with reward (e.g., food, sex, or drugs) to become excessively salient. According to the aberrant salience hypothesis, excessive dopamine release results in external and internal stimuli that have no particular importance becoming exaggeratedly salient, giving rise to delusions and hallucinations.

For example, a particular innocuous thought, such as thinking of a news story involving the police, in a person with schizophrenia may become the subject of intense

FIGURE 14.22

According to the third version of the dopamine hypothesis, the psychotic symptoms of schizophrenia are due to multiple interacting factors. These include frontotemporal dysfunction as well as genes, stress, and drugs. Excessive dopamine release leads to aberrant salience, which is dampened by antipsychotic medication.

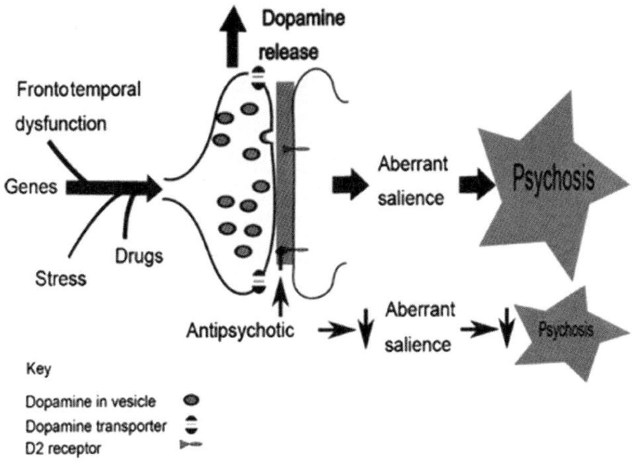

Howes, O. D., & S. Kapur. (2009). The dopamine hypothesis of schizophrenia: version III—the final common pathway. *Schizophrenia Bulletin 35*(3): 549–562. With permission from Oxford University Press.

and persistent focus, giving rise to the delusion of being pursued by the police. In addition, sights and sounds that are externally or internally generated may also be exaggeratedly focused on and result in visual or auditory hallucinations. Accordingly, it is suggested that antipsychotic medications that block D_2 receptors attenuate psychotic symptoms by attenuating the exaggerated salience awarded to stimuli. The third version of the dopamine hypothesis is illustrated in Figure 14.22.

Glutamate. The prevailing idea about the implication of glutamate in schizophrenia focuses on the function of glutamate receptors, specifically the N-methyl-D-aspartate (NMDA) receptor. (You read about glutamate and the NMDA receptor in Chapter 3.) The **NMDA-receptor-hypofunction hypothesis** of schizophrenia suggests that NMDA receptors are dysfunctional in people with schizophrenia. This idea came from the observation that drugs that block NMDA receptors (NMDA-receptor antagonists), such as phencyclidine (PCP) and ketamine, give rise to effects that are similar to the positive and negative symptoms observed in people with schizophrenia. Alternatively, drugs (NMDA receptor agonists) that increase glutaminergic neurotransmission in the brain alleviate these symptoms (Javitt, 1987; Javitt & Zukin, 1991). Abnormal glutamate neurotransmission has also been imaged, using PET, in the brains of schizophrenic patients. Stone (2011) found that patients with schizophrenia showed significantly less binding of glutamate to NMDA receptors in the hippocampus than control subjects. This is illustrated in Figure 14.23.

Hallucinations and Alterations in Brain Connectivity

Recent theories of auditory and verbal hallucinations (AVHs) in schizophrenia point to alterations in the connectivity between networks of brain areas responsible for language memory and auditory processing (Curcic-Blake et al., 2017; Di Biase et al., 2019). In one of these theories, AVHs are due to intrusive and unwanted memories that are irrelevant to the present context (Waters, Badcock, Michie, & Maybery, 2006). These memories fail to be suppressed by memory systems and other features of schizophrenia that include disordered thinking. It is thought that, in schizophrenia, memories translated into auditory and verbal images inappropriately intrude into consciousness. According to this model, AVHs are due to altered connectivity between the hippocampus (known to be important for processing memories, see Chapter 11), the superior temporal gyrus (STG, also known as the auditory cortex), Wernicke's area (important for understanding language), and Broca's area (which is involved in the production of language) through the striatum (Figure 14.24a).

FIGURE 14.23

The binding of glutamate to NMDA receptors in the left hippocampus of patients with schizophrenia and control subjects.

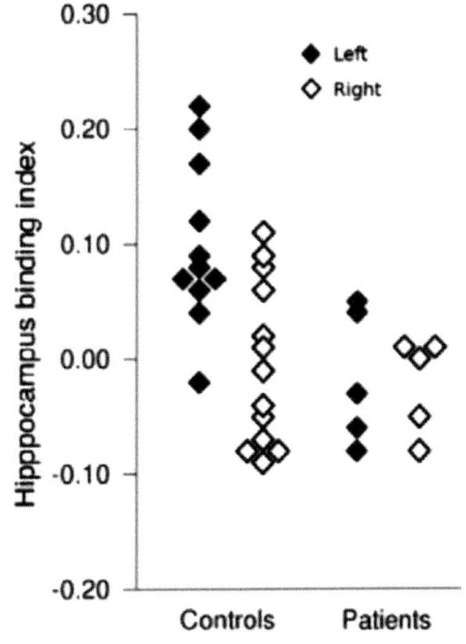

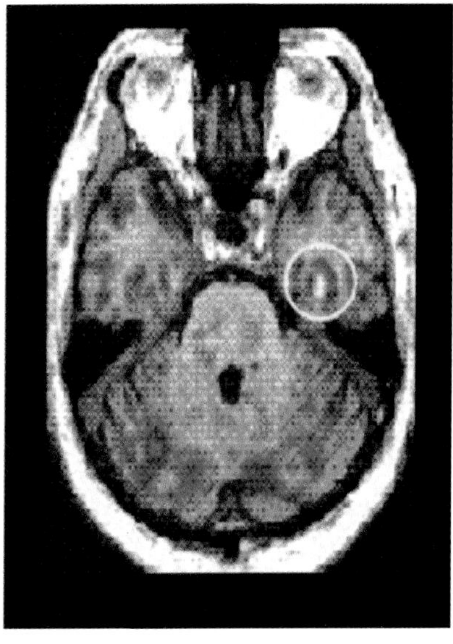

Stone, J.M. (2011). Glutamatergic antipsychotic drugs: a new dawn in the treatment of schizophrenia? *Therapeutic Advances in Psychopharmacology 1*(1): 5–18. With permission from SAGE.

In another theory, AVHs are thought to be due to deficits in self-monitoring. According to this theory, people with schizophrenia may perceive internally generated speech (inner speech) as being externally generated (P. Allen, Aleman, & McGuire, 2007). Normally, the brain makes a prediction about the sensory consequence of an action and suppresses the sensations that are a direct consequence of the action (P. Allen, Laroi, McGuire, & Aleman, 2008). That is why you cannot tickle yourself (for example, by gently stroking your forearm). As your brain generates the motor command to tickle yourself, a prediction is made that you will feel something on your forearm. When this prediction matches the sensory event (gentle stroking of the forearm), the perception is suppressed. One possibility is that this process is impaired in schizophrenia and that the brain fails to suppress the perception that speech is externally generated. As illustrated in Figure 14.24b, this deficit may be due to altered connectivity between frontal areas, such as the anterior cingulate cortex (ACC) and Broca's area, and temporal areas, such as Wernicke's area.

A third possibility is that AVHs are due to hyperconnectivity between auditory areas of both hemispheres through the corpus callosum, the bundle of nerve fibers that links both hemispheres of the brain (P. Allen et al., 2007). This theory is based on the findings that tinnitus, a condition in which sound is perceived without any external stimulation, is due to changes in the corpus callosum. The normal production and comprehension of speech depend on intact connectivity between both hemispheres via the corpus callosum, which may be altered in schizophrenia (Figure 14.24c).

Finally, AVHs may be caused by an alteration in the balance between bottom-up sensory processing and top-down mechanisms. Remember that top-down processing occurs when your perceptions are based on what you already know or when your perceptions are influenced by your thoughts. In contrast, bottom-up processing is when your perceptions or thoughts are influenced by incoming sensory information. In schizophrenia, it may be that top-down processing beginning with mental imagery dominates over bottom-up processing beginning with processing of auditory information stemming from the external world while monitoring reality (de Boer et al., 2019).

FIGURE 14.24

Four theories of auditory verbal hallucinations involving altered connectivity: (a) memory intrusion; (b) self-monitoring; (c) interhemispheric auditory pathway; and (d) two-hit bottom-up top-down (see text for explanations).

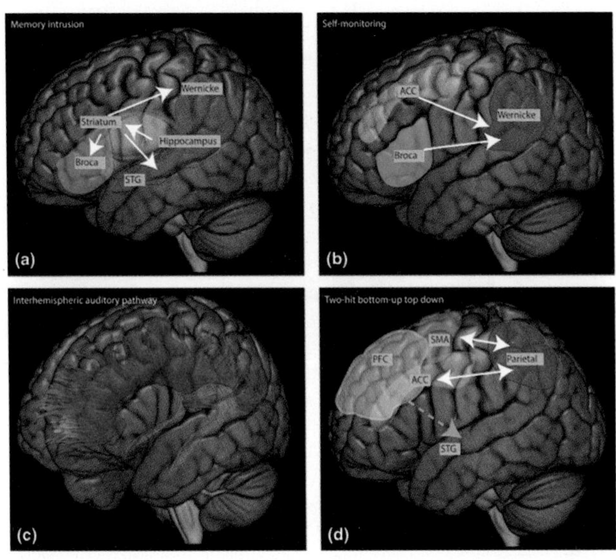

Curcic-Blake, B., et al. (2017). Interaction of language, auditory and memory brain networks in auditory verbal hallucinations. *Progress Neurobiology 148*: 1–20. With permission from Elsevier.

Remember from the module on anxiety that the default-mode network composed of frontal and parietal areas is activated while thinking about the past, planning for the future, engaging in self-reflection, or regulating one's emotions. However, the default-mode network is deactivated when monitoring reality. Monitoring the world for auditory stimulation requires the activation of the superior temporal gyrus. In schizophrenia, excessive top-down control over bottom-up processing may take the form of increased connectivity and control from frontal regions such as the prefrontal cortex (PFC) and supplementary motor area (SMA) as well as by higher perceptual regions, such as the parietal cortex (Figure 14.24d).

IT'S A MYTH!

Mental Illness = Chemical Imbalance

The Myth

You have probably heard from friends, family, and the media that psychological disorders are due to chemical imbalances in the brain. You may also have heard and even be convinced that the medication prescribed to treat psychological disorders restores this balance. Well, after reading this chapter, the hope is that you are now convinced that this is nothing but a myth. Indeed, there is not a shred of evidence that psychological disorders are caused by a chemical imbalance of any kind. Psychological disorders are caused by a combination of interacting factors, biological, environmental, and psychological.

Where Does the Myth Come From?

The source of this myth dates to the 1950s, when the drug reserpine was found to cause depression in about 15% of the people to whom it was administered. This effect was attributed to the reduced levels of the monoamine neurotransmitter norepinephrine. The idea that low levels of monoamines were part of the root causes of depression was bolstered by the finding, in the 1960s, that the drug iproniazid, used to treat tuberculosis, had antidepressant effects by inhibiting monoamine oxidase, an enzyme that breaks down monoamines. Another class of drugs, called tricyclic antidepressants, which block the reuptake of serotonin and norepinephrine, was also used to treat depression. In the 1980s, drugs known as selective serotonin reuptake inhibitors (SSRIs) were developed to treat depression. This eventually led to the catecholamine hypothesis of depression (Schildkraut, 1995). In the 1980s, the drug chlorpromazine was found to be effective in treating the positive symptoms of schizophrenia. The drug's ability to block dopamine receptors is thought to be responsible for alleviating these symptoms. This, in combination with the observation that drugs that increase levels of dopamine in the brain are associated with symptoms that resemble some of those observed in schizophrenia, led to the dopamine hypothesis of schizophrenia (Seeman, 1987). More recently, it was hypothesized that people with schizophrenia have hypofunctioning glutamate receptors. It was also observed that drugs that decrease levels of glutamate create symptoms that resemble some of the ones observed in schizophrenia. Therefore, drugs that increase levels of glutamate in the brain have been developed, leading to the NMDA-receptor hypofunction hypothesis of schizophrenia (Javitt, 1987; Javitt & Zukin, 1991, Stone, 2011). These findings were exploited extensively by the pharmaceutical industry, and the drugs manufactured and sold to address so-called chemical imbalances are aggressively marketed directly to consumers. The chemical imbalance theory of psychological disorders has become so popular with laypeople, and even some scientists and physicians, that the contributions of the interactions among myriad biological, environmental, and psychological factors are greatly overshadowed.

Why Is the Myth Wrong?

Mental illness comprises many psychological disorders, including a variety of anxiety, mood, and personality disorders and schizophrenia. No single cause for any one disorder has been identified. In fact, we know that psychological disorders are multiply determined. This means that a combination of factors, each interacting with the others, contributes to the development of psychological disorders. These factors include both biological and environmental factors. Biological factors include the genetics that can predispose an individual to structural and chemical abnormalities of the brain, as well as temperamental dispositions that can make the development of disorders more likely. Also, among biological factors are the possibilities of viral and bacterial infections during brain development. The presence of these factors is by no means a guarantee that a person possessing them will develop a disorder. Environmental influences such as exposure to toxins, environmental stressors such as those experienced at home or work, and the use of drugs are also known factors that can influence the development of psychological disorders. ●

MODULE SUMMARY

Schizophrenia is a psychological disorder characterized by the presence of symptoms that may include some of the following: delusion, hallucinations, disorganized speech, disorganized behavior, diminished emotional expression, and cognitive impairments. Hallucinations and delusions are referred to as positive symptoms. Diminished emotional expression, avolition, and anhedonia are negative symptoms. People with schizophrenia also show a range of cognitive impairments such as in working memory, planning, behavioral flexibility, and problem solving.

Many abnormalities in brain areas, structures, and connectivity have been found in people who have schizophrenia. It is also thought that schizophrenia may be due to a dysfunctional hippocampus due to inflammation. The idea that a dysfunctional dopamine system is at the core of the symptoms observed in schizophrenia is known as the dopamine hypothesis, which has three versions. The first version is based on the effects of blocking and activating dopamine D_2 receptors. The second version addresses the locations of dopamine dysfunctions in the brain. The third version focuses on the psychotic symptoms of schizophrenia and takes into account genetics and environmental factors. In the aberrant salience hypothesis, which is part of the third version, it is thought that the psychotic symptoms of schizophrenia are due to innocuous stimuli, externally or internally generated, being given exaggerated importance, driven by excessive activity of dopamine. The NMDA-receptor-hypofunction hypothesis of schizophrenia suggests that NMDA receptors are dysfunctional in people with schizophrenia. It is also thought that hallucinations and delusions in schizophrenia are due to dysfunctions in four networks of brain areas related to memory, self-monitoring, auditory perception, and top-down/bottom-up processing.

TEST YOURSELF

14.5.1 Describe the symptoms of schizophrenia.

14.5.2 (a) Define the dopamine hypothesis of schizophrenia and describe its three versions. (b) What abnormalities were found in the brains of people with schizophrenia? How can some of these abnormalities be linked to auditory and visual hallucinations?

APPLICATIONS

Neuromodulation and the Treatment of Depression

Major depressive disorder fails to remit in 60% of patients after treatment with antidepressant medication. Many of these patients will undergo subsequent courses of antidepressant medication, but in 32%–41% of those patients, MDD will again fail to remit. Patients with MDD that fails to remit after two courses of medication are said to have treatment-resistant depression.

For these patients, other types of therapy are considered. The aim of some of these therapies is to alter (modulate) neural activity in brain areas thought to be implicated in major depression, known as neuromodulation. These include electroconvulsive therapy (ECT), transcranial-magnetic stimulation (TMS), and vagus-nerve stimulation (VNS).

Electroconvulsive Therapy (ECT)

Electroconvulsive therapy was first used in the 1930s. It was the outcome of discovering that inducing seizures, through administration of various drugs, often relieved the symptoms of patients suffering from psychological disorders, including major depression (Alverno, 1990; Endler, 1988; Faedda et al., 2010). ECT is now reserved for patients whose symptoms are treatment resistant and who are at high risk for suicide.

You may have heard horrible things about ECT. This is largely because of its misuse during its early years. For example, the intensity of the shocks used resulted in severe convulsions that sometimes injured patients. The bad reputation of ECT was also perpetuated by its portrayal in movies and the media (Sienaert, 2016).

Today, ECT is considered a relatively safe procedure. Convulsions have been eliminated with the administration of muscle relaxants, and patients are put under general anesthesia during the procedure. This fact has pushed some observers to suggest changing the name from ECT to brain-synchronization therapy (BST) (Okasha & Okasha, 2014). ECT is administered by attaching electrodes to a patient's head. A current of approximately 150 volts is passed through the brain for less than one second. Treatments may be administered every second day for a period spanning several weeks. The most common side effect for most patients is temporary memory loss. However, more permanent memory loss for distant memories is observed in a minority of patients. Another drawback is the high probability of relapse after treatment, which can be prevented by closely following up on patients. This includes psychotherapy and the prescription of antidepressant drugs. Another course of ECT treatments is often required (Barlow, Durand, & Stewart, 2012).

How Does ECT Work?

The neurobiological mechanisms by which ECT alleviates the symptoms of major depression have for a long time been a mystery. However, recent research has begun to provide clues to the mystery. Hypotheses about the effects of ECT are based on three lines of evidence: neurophysiological, neuro-biochemical, and neuroplasticity (Singh & Kar, 2017).

Neurophysiological

Low glucose metabolism in the frontal cortex and anterior cingulate cortex has been found in patients with major depression. Electroconvulsive therapy may produce its effects by increasing blood flow and glucose metabolism.

Neuro-biochemical

Levels of brain-derived neurotrophic factor (BDNF), which affect the neurotransmission of monoamines (dopamine, norepinephrine, and serotonin), were found to be low in the hippocampus in patients with major depression. ECT increased levels of neurotrophic factors such as BDNF.

Neuroplasticity

The hippocampus in patients with major depression was found to be reduced in volume. The hippocampus plays an important role of regulating levels of glucocorticoids, which are elevated in people with major depression. ECT results in a significant increase in the volume of brain substructures such as the hippocampus, amygdala, anterior cingulate gyrus, and medial and inferior temporal cortices.

Transcranial-Magnetic Stimulation (TMS)

Over the years, other methods to stimulate the brain were devised. One of these methods uses technology invented in the 1980s, known as transcranial-magnetic stimulation (TMS) (Barker, Jalinous, & Freeston, 1985).

The goal was to achieve the same results as ECT but without the undesirable side effects.

In TMS, a rapidly alternating magnetic field is delivered to the cortex with magnetic coils placed on top of the patient's skull. One great advantage of TMS over ECT is that it does not create convulsions. Therefore, it does not require sedation. The side effects are also mild compared with ECT, and the patient can typically return to daily activities following treatment, which is given three to five times a week for approximately six weeks (Barlow et al., 2012; Holtzheimer & Mayberg, 2012).

How Does TMS Work?

The observed changes in neurocircuitry with TMS are comparable to those induced by ECT in terms of neurophysiology, neuro-biochemistry, and neuroplasticity (Baeken & De Raedt, 2011).

Vagus-Nerve Stimulation

The vagus nerve is a major component of the parasympathetic nervous system. It regulates the function of various organs in the body, bringing their level of activity back to normal following their activation by the sympathetic nervous system. However, the vagus nerve also carries information from the body to the brain. During the 1930s and 1940s, researchers found that electrical stimulation of the vagus nerve can suppress seizures and influence brain activity (Zabara, 1992). In 2005, the U.S. Food and Drug Administration (FDA) approved the use of vagus-nerve stimulation (VNS) for the treatment of treatment-resistant depression (Howland, Shutt, Berman, Spotts, & Denko, 2011).

In VNS, an electrical pulse generator is implanted under the skin of the patient's chest. Electrical signals move along a wire that extends from the pulse generator to attach to the vagus nerve. Side effects include voice alterations, cough, and neck pain, but these can be reduced by adjusting the current parameters.

How Does VNS Work?

Vagus-nerve stimulation was shown to increase activity in a network of brain areas known to regulate mood (Ruffoli et al., 2011). As with ECT and TMS, VNS also increases production of BDNF (Furmaga, Carreno, & Frazer, 2012) and promotes neurogenesis in the hippocampus (Gebhardt et al., 2013).

FIGURE 14.25

Neuromodulation in the treatment of depression. (a) A person undergoing TMS. (b) An illustration of VNS.

(a)

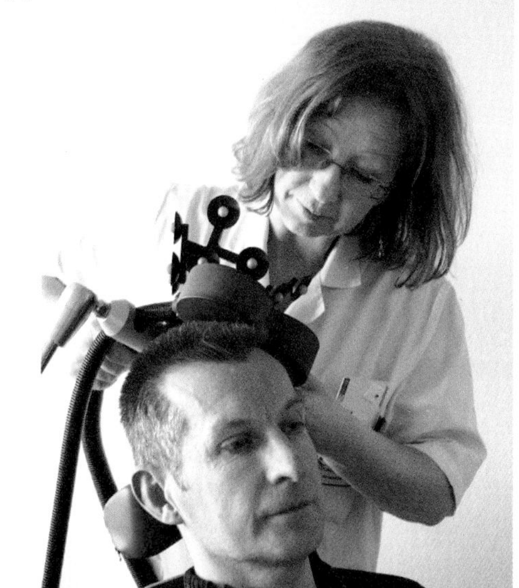

(b)

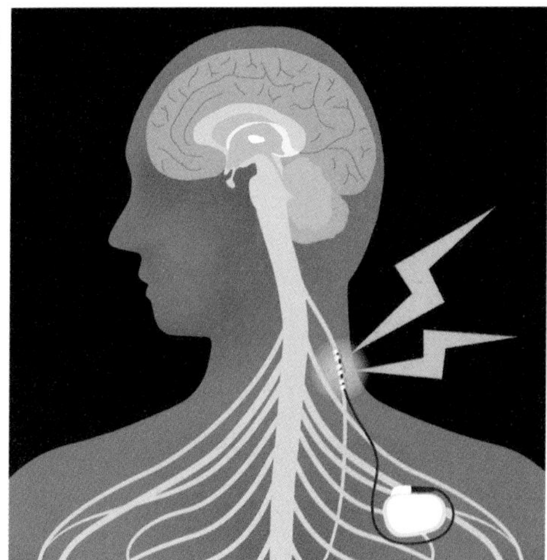

(a) Amélie Benoist/Science Source; (b) metamorworks/istockphoto

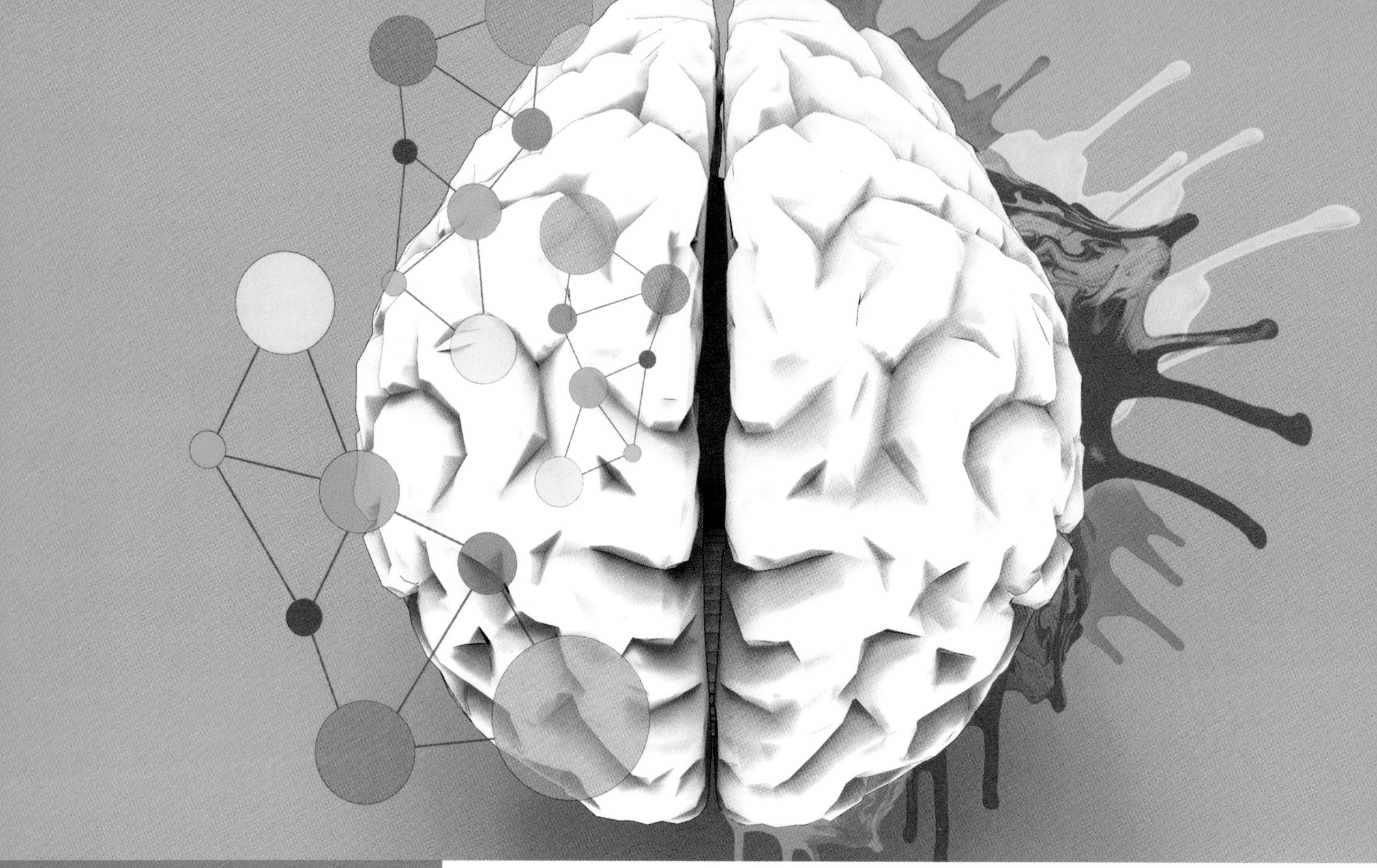

Gugurat/istockphoto

15 Social Neuroscience

Chapter Contents

Learning Objectives

15.1.1 Explain how neural mechanisms and environmental factors interact to determine how people behave in a social context.

15.1.2 Describe the perspective from which neuroscientists study social behavior.

15.2.1 Explain what is meant by self-awareness.

15.2.2 Identify the different components of self-awareness and the brain areas associated with each component.

15.3.1 Define theory of mind.

15.3.2 Identify the brain areas associated with each of the theories of mind.

15.3.3 Define empathy, its different types, and the brain areas associated with each type.

15.4.1 Explain the components of physical pain.

15.4.2 Explain what social pain is and how it is similar to physical pain.

15.5.1 Define altruism and explain how it may be a product of evolutionary adaptation.

15.5.2 Identify the brain areas associated with altruism and explain how they are associated with various altruistic behaviors.

15.6.1 Explain game theory, identify two examples, and describe what each is used for and why.

15.6.2 Identify the brain areas associated with trust and cooperation.

Extreme Altruism

Wesley Autrey saved the life of a 50-year-old man who had fallen onto subway tracks. Autrey jumped in and covered the man while subway cars rolled inches above his head. Richard Moore put his own life in danger to save a 20-year-old woman from a shark attack. Darryl Starnes pulled a 40-year-old woman from a burning car. These are but a few examples of altruistic behavior. The same can be said about health care workers putting their lives in danger to save the victims of dangerous epidemics, such as Ebola in West Africa. Although each of these examples differs, they all have one thing in common. In each one, someone put his or her own life in considerable danger to save the life of one person or of many people. These are examples of extreme altruism. Altruism is defined as selfless behavior with the aim of helping others at the cost of potential or actual harm to oneself. What drives such behavior has fascinated scientists for decades. When asked why he put his own life in danger to save another, Autrey simply replied, "I don't feel like I did something spectacular; I just saw someone who needed help" (Buckley, 2007). Moore said that it only dawned on him that he was in danger when the shark was around them and that the woman was bleeding. After saving the woman from certain death in the burning car, Starnes stated, "I just did what I felt like I needed to do" (Robson, 2015). Another commonality among these cases is that each of the heroes acted very quickly without giving much thought about what he should do. This may be because, in situations such as these, cooperation is time pressured. To save lives, there often is little time for deliberation or to think about one's own safety. However, in other situations, there is plenty of time to decide, such as when someone puts his or her health at risk by donating an organ. Because not everyone readily engages in such heroic actions, scientists have attempted to answer the question of whether the brains of such heroes differ from the brains of others.

INTRODUCTION

Social neuroscience is the field in which researchers investigate how the brain is involved in social behavior. It brings together the fields of social psychology and cognitive neuroscience. Social neuroscientists seek to understand the neurobiological underpinnings of social behavior at three broad levels: social perception, social cognition, and social regulation (Adolphs, 2010). Social perception refers to the study of how complex arrays of sensory stimuli are used for communication. Social cognition refers to the study of the cognitive operations performed on the information gathered through interacting with others. This includes recognizing other people's emotions, inferring their intentions, and looking at the world from their perspectives. Social regulation refers to the ability to be self-aware so as to control one's emotions, thinking, and behavior to act in a manner that is appropriate to the social context.

Each of these levels provides myriad topics to study, far more than can be covered in this chapter. However, an effort has been made to introduce you to some of the basic topics of interest in social neuroscience. After an introduction to what constitutes the social neuroscience perspective, you will learn how self-awareness forms the basis of all social interactions and how it is implemented in a circuit of structures within the brain. You will next learn about how taking the perspective of others so that we can better understand how they feel depends on the activity of certain brain areas. You will then be introduced to the concept of social pain, such as the kind of pain felt when being rejected, and how it seems to share neurobiological characteristics with physical pain. We will then examine how people can engage in acts of altruism as well as experiments that show which brain areas are associated with such actions. Finally, we will examine the neurobiological basis of cooperation and trust, which play a crucial role in establishing social structures.

15.1 What Is Social Neuroscience?

Module Contents

Learning Objectives

15.1.1 Explain how neural mechanisms and environmental factors interact to determine how people behave in a social context.

15.1.2 Describe the perspective from which neuroscientists study social behavior.

15.1.1 SOCIAL NEUROSCIENCE: THE CHICKEN OR THE EGG?

>> LO 15.1.1 Explain how neural mechanisms and environmental factors interact to determine how people behave in a social context.

Key Terms

- **Social psychology:** The study of how people's thoughts are influenced by the actual, inferred, or imagined presence of others.
- **Nature or nurture:** A once hotly debated question as to whether individual characteristics are entirely inherited or determined by environmental influences.

The term *social neuroscience* was coined by psychologists John Cacioppo and Gary Berntson (1992). It can be defined as the field that seeks to understand how brain activity relates to how people think, feel, and behave in social situations.

As mentioned in the introduction, social neuroscience brings together the study of **social psychology**, which is the study of how people's thoughts are influenced by the actual, inferred, or imagined presence of others, and cognitive neuroscience, which is the study of the neurobiological substrates of mental processes such as those involved in memory, attention, reasoning, and language.

The definition of social neuroscience provided here gives rise to a form of "the chicken or the egg" question. That is, what comes first? Are processes in the brain responsible for social behavior, or is the brain shaped by social experience? This question is akin to the age-old question: Do people become who they are due to **nature or nurture**? A modern version of this question would be: Are people's characteristics strictly a product of biological factors, such as genetics, or a product of their environment? Most behavioral scientists reject these either-or questions about why people behave the way they do. Most believe that people are the way they are due to interactions between biological factors and environmental influences. One of the challenges of social neuroscience is to understand how these interactions are related to social behavior.

15.1.2 THE SOCIAL-NEUROSCIENTIFIC PERSPECTIVE

>> LO 15.1.2 Describe the perspective from which neuroscientists study social behavior.

Key Terms

- **Reductionism:** The idea that complex phenomena can be explained by knowing their basic structure.
- **Social cognitive neuroscience prism:** A prism that represents interactions among four levels of analysis that result in social behavior.

It is important to understand that social neuroscientists do not use a reductionist approach. **Reductionism** is the idea that complex phenomena can be explained by knowing their basic structure. Instead, social neuroscientists think of social behavior as being an emergent property that stems from complex interactions among basic biological and environmental factors.

According to psychologists Kevin Ochsner and Matthew Lieberman (2001), the study of social neuroscience comprises four interacting levels of analysis. This is represented by what they called the **social cognitive neuroscience prism**, shown in Figure 15.1. The prism is meant to show how social behavior arises from interactions among several factors, which can be thought of as levels of analysis. These include neural mechanisms, cognition and information processing, behavior and experience, as well as the personal and social context.

The social cognitive neuroscience prism contains the areas of interest to both cognitive neuroscientists and social psychologists, which are put together by social neuroscientists. Cognitive neuroscience involves studying the underlying neural mechanisms of behavior, how it is influenced by experience and information processing. Significantly less emphasis is placed on the personal and social context of behavior. In contrast, social psychology emphasizes the study of the effects of personal and social contexts, experience, information processing, and behavior but is not concerned with its neural mechanisms.

FIGURE 15.1

The social cognitive neuroscience prism represents the idea that social neuroscience studies social behavior from the perspective of four interacting levels of analysis.

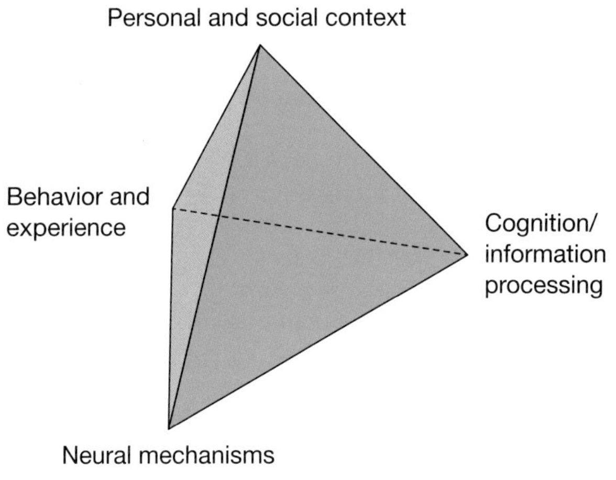

Based on Ochsner, K. N., & M. D. Lieberman. (2001). The emergence of social cognitive neuroscience. *American Psychologist 56*(9), 717–734.

MODULE SUMMARY

An age-old question concerns whether processes in the brain are responsible for social behavior or if the brain is itself shaped by social experience. One of the challenges of social neuroscience is to understand how the interplay between biology and environment gives rise to social behavior. Social neuroscientists think of social behavior as emergent properties stemming from complex interactions among basic components, both biological and environmental. Social neuroscience brings together the interests of cognitive neuroscientists and social psychologists. The combined interests of both fields are encapsulated in the social cognitive neuroscience prism.

TEST YOURSELF

15.1.1 Explain what is meant by "the chicken or the egg" question in the context of social neuroscience and explain how the different components of the social cognitive neuroscience prism interact.

15.1.2 Explain why and how social scientists do not use a reductionist approach.

15.2 Self-Awareness

Module Contents

Learning Objectives

15.2.1 Explain what is meant by self-awareness.

15.2.2 Identify the different components of self-awareness and the brain areas associated with each component.

15.2.1 WHAT IS SELF-AWARENESS?

>> LO 15.2.1 Explain what is meant by self-awareness.

Key Terms

- **Self-awareness:** The ability to reflect on one's traits, beliefs, abilities, and attitudes.
- **Mirror test:** A test designed to know whether animals and human babies are self-aware.

When engaged in social interactions, people are aware of their own presentation and are concerned about how others perceive them. People are also aware of their strengths and weaknesses and can monitor their thoughts and behavior so that they can act in a socially appropriate manner. People can also differentiate between stimuli that are self-generated, such as one's inner voice, and stimuli generated by external sources, such as another person's voice. The capacity to engage in all of the above depends on what is known as **self-awareness**, which can be defined as the ability to reflect on one's traits, beliefs, abilities, and attitudes.

In the 1970s, psychologist Gordon Gallup developed a test designed to find out whether animals were self-aware. This test became known as the **mirror test** (Gallup, 1970). The test consists of marking an animal, such as a chimpanzee, with a dye (e.g., a spot of rouge) and placing it in front of a mirror. Researchers can then observe whether the animal reacts in a way that shows it realizes that the mark is on its own body. Gallup noticed that chimpanzees frequently touched a marked area, such as the top of their eyebrow while looking at themselves in the mirror (Figure 15.2). This was taken as evidence that the chimpanzee recognized that the reflection in the mirror was its own and not that of another chimpanzee, hence, evidence of being self-aware.

Psychologist Beulah Amsterdam (1972) used the same kind of test on human children. A spot of lipstick was applied to the noses of children. The children were then made to look at their reflection in a mirror. Before age 2, toddlers reacted to their reflection in the mirror as if the lipstick had nothing to do with them. In contrast, most children around age 2 reacted as if they were aware that the lipstick was on their face and not on someone else's face. These children sometimes avoided their reflection, were self-admiring, or appeared embarrassed.

FIGURE 15.2

The mirror test. A chimpanzee's reaction to seeing rouge on its image in a mirror is taken as evidence that it is self-aware.

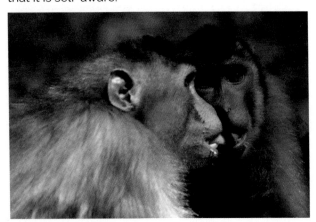

Michel Gunther/Science Source

Since these classic experiments, several other species have also passed the mirror test, including elephants (Plotnik, de Waal, & Reiss, 2006), dolphins (Reiss & Marino, 2001), and even fish (Kohda et al., 2019). Note, however, that the use of the mirror test and modified versions of it to determine self-awareness is controversial. One criticism is that mirror recognition may not provide a full picture of what is required to be considered self-aware (Suddendorf & Butler, 2013). Another criticism is that the mirror test is not relevant to species in which vision is not the primary sensory modality. This led to the development of an olfactory version of the mirror test for dogs. Based on this kind of test, dogs, which do not typically look at themselves in mirrors, were suggested to also possess self-awareness (Horowitz, 2017).

Others believe that claims of self-awareness in species other than humans and great apes are based on studies with flawed experimental procedures. It has also been suggested that alternative explanations for behaviors that suggest self-awareness are readily available (Gallup & Anderson, 2018).

15.2.2 SELF-AWARENESS: WHERE IN THE BRAIN?

>> LO 15.2.2 Identify the different components of self-awareness and the brain areas associated with each component.

Key Terms

- **Self-referential stimuli:** Stimuli that are perceived as being related to one's self.
- **Representation:** Organizing information as it is relevant to the self.
- **Evaluating:** Determining whether a stimulus is internally or externally generated.
- **Monitoring:** The ability to override habitual responses, choose among a variety of available responses, and detect errors.
- **Integration:** The integration of attitudes, goals, traits, memories, and values into a unified concept of self.
- **Agency:** The feeling that you are the cause of your own thoughts and actions.
- **Body ownership:** The perception that one's body belongs to the self.

British neurologist John Hughlings Jackson (1835–1911) suggested that self-awareness depends on the evolution of the prefrontal cortex (Meares, 1999). However, we now know that self-awareness depends

FIGURE 15.3

Cortical midline brain areas involved in four different components of self-awareness: representing, monitoring, evaluating, and integrating. OMPFC = orbitomedial prefrontal cortex; DMPFC = the dorsomedial prefrontal cortex; ACC = anterior cingulate cortex; PCC = posterior cingulate cortex.

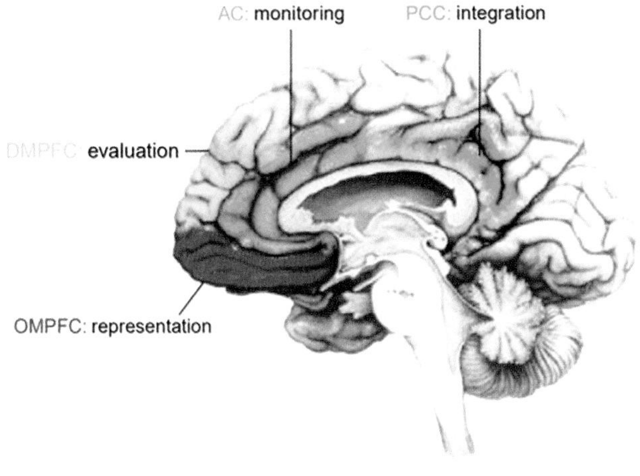

Northoff, G., & F. Bermpohl. (2004). Cortical midline structures and the self. *Trends in Cognitive Science 8*(3): 102–107. With permission from Elsevier.

on a network of brain areas. This includes brain areas in the center of the brain known as the cortical midline structures (Northoff & Bermpohl, 2004). As illustrated in Figure 15.3, they include the orbitomedial prefrontal cortex (OMPFC), the dorsomedial prefrontal cortex (DMPFC), the anterior cingulate cortex (ACC), and the posterior cingulate cortex (PCC).

Based on the results of brain imaging studies, neuroscientist Georg Northoff suggests that these areas are involved in processing what is known as **self-referential stimuli** (Northoff & Bermpohl, 2004). Self-referential stimuli are stimuli that are perceived as being related to one's self. According to Northoff, the processing of self-referential stimuli gives rise to a model of the self. He suggests that self-referential stimuli are represented, evaluated, monitored, and integrated and that each of these processes depends on a particular structure within the cortical midline structures.

The **representation** of self-referential stimuli—which involves attributing personality traits, talents, and skills to oneself—is thought to depend on the OMPFC. The DMPFC is important for **evaluating** stimuli on the basis of whether they are internally generated, such as one's internal voice, or externally generated, such as the voice of another person calling you. The ACC was found to be involved in **monitoring** and controlling one's actions. This includes the ability to override habitual responses, choose among a variety of available responses, and detect errors by comparing intended correct responses to an actual response. Finally, the PCC was shown to be involved in the **integration** of attitudes, goals, traits, memories, and values into a unified concept of self.

Keep in mind, however, that self-awareness includes more than the functions attributed to cortical midline structures. For example, the sense of **agency**, which is the feeling that you are the cause of your own thoughts and actions, was found to depend on the right temporoparietal junction (Decety & Lamm, 2007; Hughes, 2018), illustrated later in the chapter in Figure 15.5. The sense of **body ownership**, which is the perception that one's body belongs to the self, involves the right temporoparietal cortex (Smit, Van Stralen, Van den Munckhof, Snijders, & Dijkerman, 2018).

MODULE SUMMARY

Self-awareness can be defined as the ability to reflect on one's traits, beliefs, abilities, and attitudes. Self-awareness is inferred if an organism passes what is known as the mirror test, which several species did. However, the mirror test has been criticized on the grounds that not all animals have vision as their primary sensory modality. Others have criticized the mirror test on the grounds that, apart from the tests performed on humans and great apes, studies in which it was administered suffered from flawed methodology. A model of the self develops from the processing of self-referential stimuli, which includes representing, performed by the orbitomedial prefrontal cortex; evaluating, performed by the dorsomedial prefrontal cortex; monitoring, performed by the anterior cingulate cortex; and integrating, performed by the posterior cingulate cortex. Self-awareness also includes the sense of agency processed by the temporoparietal junction and the sense of body ownership, which involves the temporoparietal cortex.

TEST YOURSELF

15.2.1 Define self-awareness.

15.2.2 Name the areas of the cortical midline and how they each process self-referential stimuli.

15.3 Theory of Mind and Empathy

Module Contents

Learning Objectives

15.3.1 Define theory of mind.

15.3.2 Identify the brain areas associated with each of the theories of mind.

15.3.3 Define empathy, its different types, and the brain areas associated with each type.

15.3.1 WHAT IS THEORY OF MIND?

>> LO 15.3.1 **Define theory of mind.**

Key Terms

- **Theory of mind:** The ability to infer what is going on in the minds of others, such as their emotions, beliefs, and intentions, by observing their behaviors.
- **False-belief task:** A task that assesses whether a child realizes that another person can hold beliefs that differ from his or her own.

In our everyday encounters with other people, we can spontaneously infer what is going on in their minds by observing their behavior. This includes their emotions, beliefs, and intentions. This ability requires having what is known as a **theory of mind**. The following scenarios illustrate how we infer other people's states of mind from their behavior, thanks to our having a theory of mind:

- You are at your friend's house getting ready to go to a movie. However, just before leaving, your friend starts frantically looking in multiple locations all over the house. Her father enters the room you are in, sees his daughter, and smiles. Do you think you would be able to infer what is going on in the scenario? You may infer from your friend's behavior that she is worried about having lost her keys but that her father knows exactly where they are.
- You are waiting in line to order a beverage at a café. You observe that another customer is standing in front of the display of muffins and sandwiches without saying a word, letting other customers pass in front of him in the line. Because you have a theory of mind, you can infer that he is pondering whether to have a muffin or a sandwich.

The Development of Theory of Mind

Theory of mind is thought to develop at around 4 years of age (Callaghan et al., 2005; Perner, Leekam, & Wimmer, 1987). This is based on findings from studies that assessed children using what are known as **false-belief tasks**. In false-belief tasks, participants, usually children, are tested on whether they realize that another person can hold beliefs that differ from their own. Psychologists Heinz Wimmer and Josef Perner (1983) were the first to report the results of a study using a false-belief task. They presented children with stories that were enacted by the manipulation of dolls (Figure 15.4).

In one of these stories, the mother of a little boy named Maxi returns from a shopping trip with chocolate for baking a cake. In the first scene, the mother

FIGURE 15.4

Theory-of-mind task. In this version of the task, the participant in possession of a theory of mind takes the perspective of Maxi, who does not know that his mother has changed the location of the chocolate.

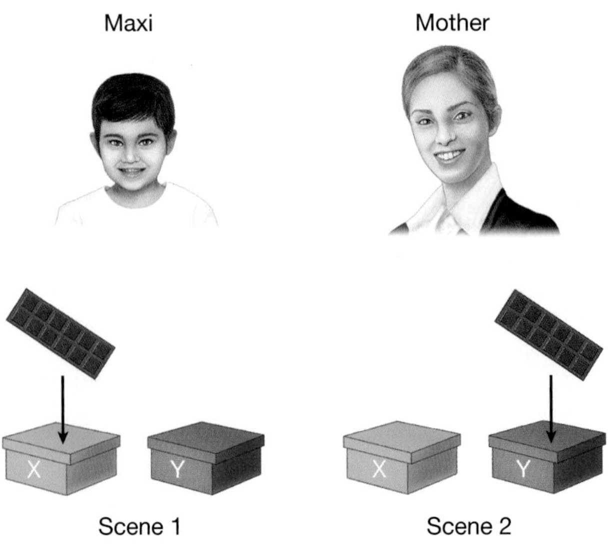

Amanda Tomasikiewicz/Body Scientific Intl.

decides to let Maxi help her put the groceries away. After being handed the chocolate by his mom, Maxi asks her where he should put it. Given the choice of two possible cupboards, represented by blue and green boxes, she tells Maxi to put the chocolate in the green cupboard. The experimenter enacts this by placing a toy chocolate in a green matchbox. In scene 2, Maxi is playing outside while the mother mixes the chocolate into the cake mix. However, once done, she puts the unused portion of the chocolate into the blue cupboard instead of the green one. The experimenter enacts this by moving the toy chocolate from the green matchbox to a blue one. The mother then realizes that she forgot to buy some eggs and leaves for the store. Upon his return from playing, Maxi is hungry and remembers the chocolate. In which cupboard (represented by the matchboxes) will he go look for it?

To give the correct response to this question, children must forgo their own perspective and answer from the point of view of Maxi. The correct answer, of course, is that Maxi will look in the green cupboard, where he placed the chocolate before he went to play outside. The incorrect response—that Maxi will look in the blue cupboard, where his mother moved it to—disregards Maxi's false belief since he did not benefit from the knowledge that his mother moved the chocolate to another cupboard while he was playing outside.

The correct response—that Maxi will incorrectly look in the original location, where he placed the chocolate—demonstrates that the child has developed a theory of mind. The incorrect response—that Maxi will look in the new location—demonstrates that the child can consider only his or her own point of view and has, therefore, not yet developed a theory of mind, by which the child would know that his or her thoughts can differ from the thoughts of others.

Although the results of studies using false-belief tasks, such as the one just described, suggest that theory of mind develops at around age 4, there is evidence that even 18- to 24-month-old toddlers can identify the false beliefs of others when tested with other types of tasks (Knudsen & Liszkowski, 2012a, 2012b).

15.3.2 THEORY OF MIND: WHERE IN THE BRAIN?

>> LO 15.3.2 Identify the brain areas associated with each of the theories of mind.

Key Terms

- **Modularity theories:** Theories that an innate module that specializes in the theory of mind exists within the brain.
- **Simulation theories:** Theories that a theory of mind is achieved through our ability to put ourselves in a person's mental "shoes" and imagine ("simulate") what we would experience in a similar situation.
- **Executive theory:** A theory that theory of mind is dependent on our ability to inhibit our own thoughts and behavior (inhibitory control), as well as take our own perspective when trying to attribute mental states to others.

There are several theories about the neurobiological nature of theory of mind. We discuss three of them: modularity, simulation, and executive theories.

Modularity Theories

Modularity theories propose that an innate module that specializes in theory of mind exists within the brain. The most thoroughly explained modularity theory was proposed by psychologist Allan Leslie and colleagues (Leslie, Friedman, & German, 2004). They suggested that theory of mind emanates from an innate brain module specialized in mentalizing about the intentions of others. They hypothesized the existence of this module because inferring the mental states of others does not have to be learned and once acquired it is quick and effortless. In addition, having a theory of mind is mandatory. That is, one cannot decide whether to have it or not.

Modularity: Where in the Brain?

One brain area that may be central to a theory of mind module is the temporoparietal junction (TPJ), illustrated in Figure 15.5. Evidence for the involvement of this area comes from neuroimaging studies. For example, the TPJ was activated when people listened to stories about people's mental states rather than their physical descriptions. Further studies showed that the right TPJ might be more implicated in theory of mind than the left TPJ. For example, the right TPJ was more active than the left TPJ during true-and-false belief reasoning in adults.

However, the TPJ is involved not just in theory of mind but also in broader social and cognitive functions. For example, using functional magnetic resonance imaging (fMRI), neuroscientists Jean Decety and Claus Lamm (2007) found that the TPJ plays a role in reorienting attention to important stimuli, empathy, and having a sense of agency. Each of these functions activated slightly different parts of the TPJ (Figure 15.5).

Simulation Theories

Simulation theories suggest that theory of mind is achieved through our ability to put ourselves in a person's "mental" shoes and imagine ("simulate") what we would experience in a similar situation. Simulation theory was proposed by neurophysiologist Vittorio Gallese and colleagues (Gallese, 2013; Gallese & Goldman,

FIGURE 15.5

fMRI images of the activation of various areas within the TPJ in reorienting, empathy, the feeling of agency, and theory of mind.

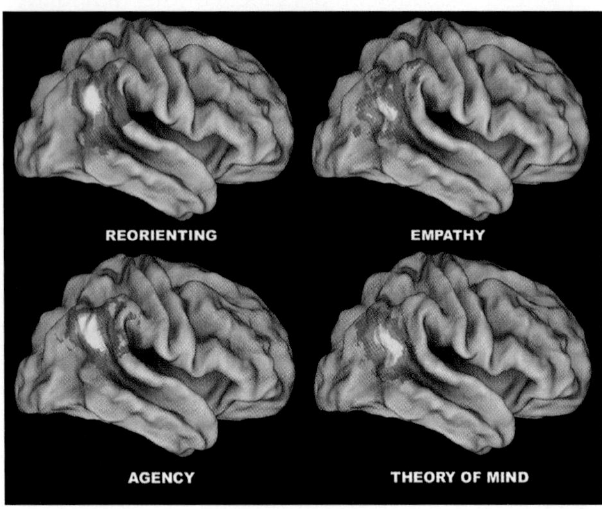

Decety, J. & C. Lamm. (2007). The role of the right temporoparietal junction in social interaction: how low-level computational processes contribute to meta-cognition. *Neuroscientist 13*(6), 580–593. With permission from SAGE.

1998). They suggest that our own mental mechanisms are used to predict the mental states of others. These mental mechanisms allow us to mimic the mental activity of others. This leads us to create in ourselves pretend desires, beliefs, and intentions that we attribute to other people (Gallese & Goldman, 1998). We then feed this information into our own decision-making system to infer what someone might decide to do but do not ourselves act on this decision. Figure 15.6 outlines the process of simulation, applying the steps involved to the earlier example in which a customer in a café is standing in front of the display of muffins and sandwiches.

Simulation: Where in the Brain?

Two possible systems have been proposed for simulation: one based on the medial prefrontal cortex and one based on the fascinating type of cells called mirror neurons (these are discussed in more detail in Chapter 8).

Medial Prefrontal Cortex. Neuroimaging studies showed that the medial prefrontal cortex was activated when participants focused on other people's mental states by taking their perspective (simulating). Interestingly, Jason P. Mitchell and colleagues found that different parts of the medial prefrontal cortex were activated depending on whether the simulation was directed toward a person perceived as being similar or dissimilar to the participants (J. P. Mitchell, Macrae, & Banaji, 2006). They had subjects infer the mental states of people they saw pictures of and read about. Simulation directed toward someone perceived as being similar activated the ventromedial prefrontal cortex (VMPFC), whereas simulation directed toward a person perceived as being dissimilar activated the dorsal medial prefrontal cortex (DMPFC) (Figure 15.7).

Mirror Neurons. Mirror neurons were described in Chapter 8. To recap, mirror neurons were discovered in the premotor cortex of macaque monkeys by neurophysiologist Giacomo Rizzolatti and colleagues in the 1990s (Rizzolatti, Fadiga, Fogassi, & Gallese, 1999). Using electrophysiological recordings, they found that these neurons responded both when a monkey performed an action and when the monkey observed another monkey perform the same action. The activity

FIGURE 15.6

The steps involved in the process of simulation. These include a pretend desire, a decision-making system, a pretend decision, not taking action, and predicting the decision of another person.

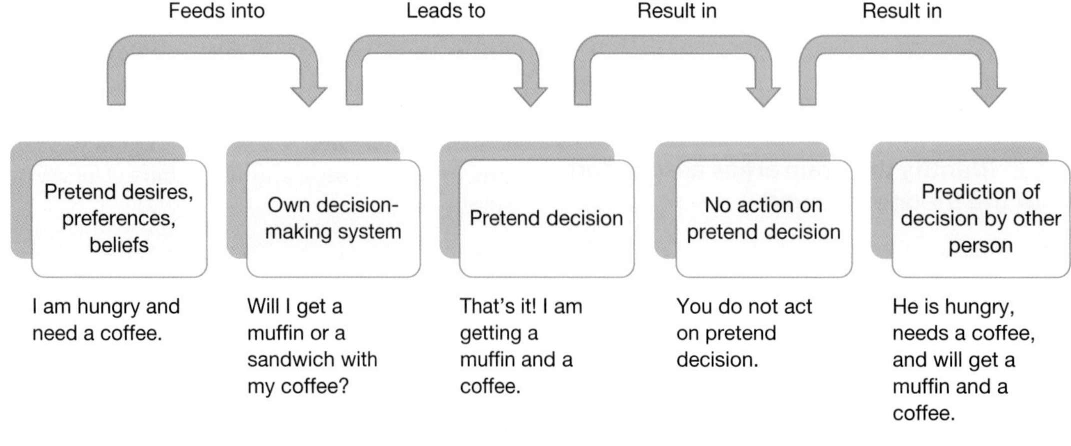

FIGURE 15.7

Activity in the prefrontal cortex (as imaged by fMRI) while participants focused on other people's mental states. (a) Greater activity in the VMPFC was observed when participants focused on the mental states of people they perceived as being similar to themselves. (b) Greater activity in the DMPFC was observed when participants focused on the mental states of people they perceived as being dissimilar to themselves.

A

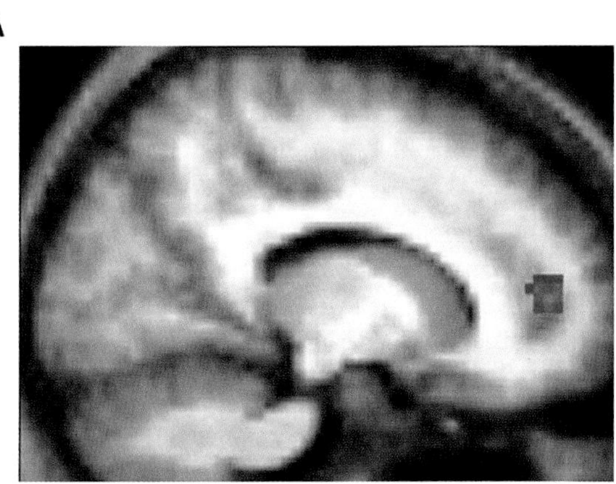

B

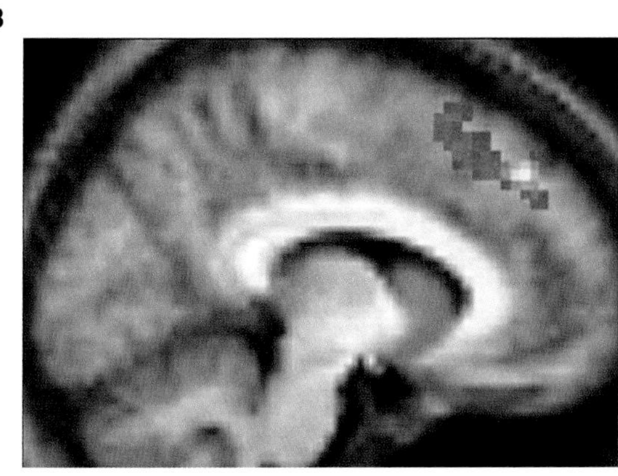

Mitchell, J. P., C.N. Macrae & M.R. Banaji. (2006). Dissociable medial prefrontal contributions to judgments of similar and dissimilar others. *Neuron 50*(4), 655–663. With permission from Elsevier.

of mirror neurons is both externally generated, by observing the actions of others, and internally generated, by the planning and performance of our own actions.

Vittorio Gallesse and colleagues outlined the steps in mirror neuron activity that led to the prediction of other people's actions and mental states (Gallese & Goldman, 1998). These steps are consistent with the steps thought to be involved in simulation, illustrated in Figure 15.6:

1. The same mirror neurons are activated whether we plan to execute an action ourselves or we observe other people execute the same action.
2. Through visual input, mirror neurons are activated by actions performed by another person.
3. The externally generated activity in motor neurons does not usually produce an action in the observer.
4. Belief and intention are attributed to the person being observed.

Executive Theory

Executive theory postulates that theory of mind is dependent on the ability to inhibit one's own thoughts and behavior (inhibitory control), including the taking of one's own perspective, when trying to attribute mental states to others. For example, in the false-belief task previously described, as well as in the task described in the next section, participants must inhibit responding according to their knowledge of where the object has been transferred so that they can respond from the perspective of the character in the story. Inhibitory control is an executive function of the brain. According to proponents of executive theory, theory of mind depends on the development of executive functions.

Executive Theory: Where in the Brain?

If having a theory of mind requires inhibitory control, then many of the same brain areas should be activated in tasks that require only inhibitory control (without false belief) and false-belief tasks, which, as you learned earlier, are solved by having a theory of mind.

Researcher Christoph Rothmayr and colleagues in Germany tested this idea by looking for brain areas activated both in a false-belief task and in what is known as a go/no-go task (Rothmayr et al., 2011). Go/no-go tasks are designed to assess the ability to inhibit responding to a stimulus. In the task used by Rothmayr and colleagues, participants were instructed to press a button when the number of children in a picture on a computer screen differed from the number of children in the previous picture (go condition), but they had to refrain from pressing the button when the number of children was the same (no-go condition).

Although some areas were activated during the false-belief task only, many areas were activated during both the false-belief task and the inhibitory-control task. These results showed that a strong relationship exists between false-belief reasoning and inhibitory control. Among the areas activated during both tasks were the right TPJ, the right medial prefrontal cortex, and the right dorsolateral prefrontal cortex. These are illustrated in Figure 15.8.

FIGURE 15.8

Brain areas activated during both the false-belief task and the go/no-go task. These include the right TPJ (rTPJ), the right medial prefrontal cortex (rMPFC), and the right dorsolateral prefrontal cortex (rDLPFC).

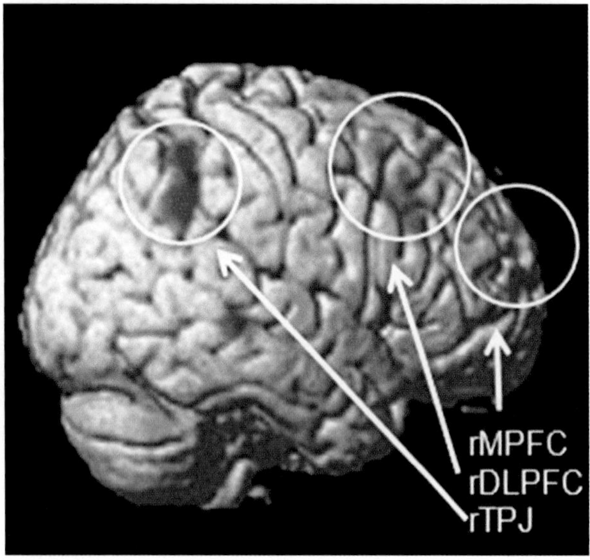

Rothmayr, C., et al. (2011). Common and distinct neural networks for false-belief reasoning and inhibitory control. *Neuroimage 56*(3), 1705–1713. With permission from Elsevier.

15.3.3 EMPATHY

>> LO 15.3.3 **Define empathy, its different types, and the brain areas associated with each type.**

Key Terms

- **Empathy:** The ability to understand or feel the emotions experienced by another person from that person's perspective.
- **Emotional empathy:** The ability to experience emotions automatically triggered by observing the emotional states of others.
- **Cognitive empathy:** The ability to cognitively engage in adopting another person's point of view to understand that person's experience.
- **Emotional contagion:** The spread of an emotion from one person to another.
- **Perception-action model:** A model that states that when one perceives another person's emotional state, both the representation related to that state and the actions related to it are triggered in one's own brain.

Empathy can be described as the ability to understand or feel the emotions experienced by another person from that person's perspective. This is often described as "putting yourself in someone else's shoes" to feel what they feel (A. Smith, 2006). It is believed that two types of empathy exist, each associated with a specific brain system. These are emotional empathy and cognitive empathy (Shamay-Tsoory, 2011). **Emotional empathy** occurs when observing another person experiencing an emotion automatically triggers the personal experience of the same emotion. **Cognitive empathy** refers to a cognitive process by which one adopts another person's point of view by making inferences about that person's emotional state.

Emotional empathy and cognitive empathy were found to depend on separate systems within the brain. Each of these systems is thought to differ in its basic mechanisms and processes.

Emotional Empathy and the Brain

The processes that underlie emotional empathy include emotional contagion, emotion recognition, and shared pain. **Emotional contagion** refers to the phenomenon by which emotions spread from one person to another. According to psychologists Stephanie Preston and Frans de Waal (2002), emotional contagion can be explained by what they called the **perception-action model**. Within this model, people share neural representations for perceiving and generating actions. For example, whenever you perceive an object, the representation of the body part relating to the use of that object is activated, as if you were preparing to use the object. According to the perception-action model, emotional contagion occurs through a similar process. That is, when you see that another person is experiencing a particular emotional state, a representation related to that state as well as the actions related to it are triggered in your own brain. It is thought that this process underlies emotional empathy.

This process is consistent with simulation theory, explained earlier as one of the theories proposed to explain theory of mind (Gallese, 2013). Remember that simulation theory is believed to involve the activity of mirror neurons, which were found to be activated whether one performs an action or watches another perform the same action (see Chapter 8 for a detailed discussion of mirror neurons). Emotional contagion was found to depend on a circuit of brain areas that includes the inferior parietal lobule and the inferior frontal gyrus.

Two other components are believed to be necessary for emotional empathy. These are emotional recognition and the feeling of shared pain. Both emotional contagion and emotional recognition were found to be impaired by damage to the inferior frontal gyrus, which, as you just read, is part of the emotional contagion system (Shamay-Tsoory, Aharon-Peretz, & Perry, 2009). Feelings of shared pain are related to the anterior cingulate cortex (ACC) and the anterior insula (Yesudas & Lee, 2015). The ACC is also activated when

FIGURE 15.9

Brain areas related to emotional empathy. Left: Areas involved in shared pain include the anterior cingulate cortex (ACC) and the anterior insula. Right: Areas involved in emotional contagion and emotional recognition involve the inferior parietal lobule (IPL) and the inferior frontal gyrus (IFG).

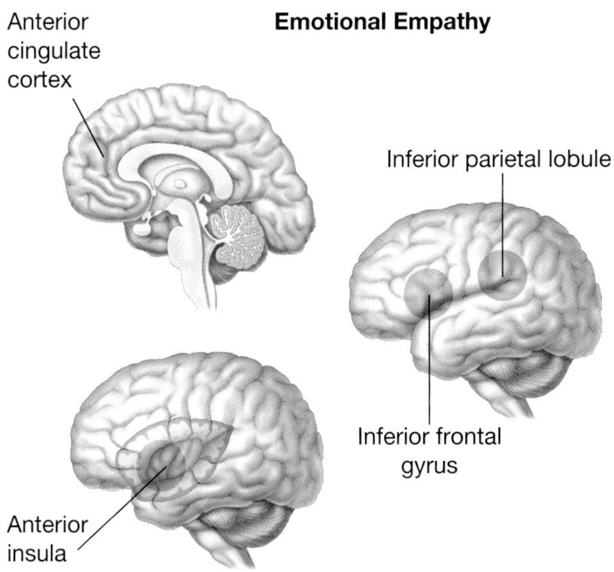

Amanda Tomasikiewicz/Body Scientific Intl.

FIGURE 15.10

The brain areas involved in cognitive empathy include the ventromedial prefrontal cortex (VMPFC), the dorsomedial prefrontal cortex (DMPFC), and the medial temporal lobe (MTL).

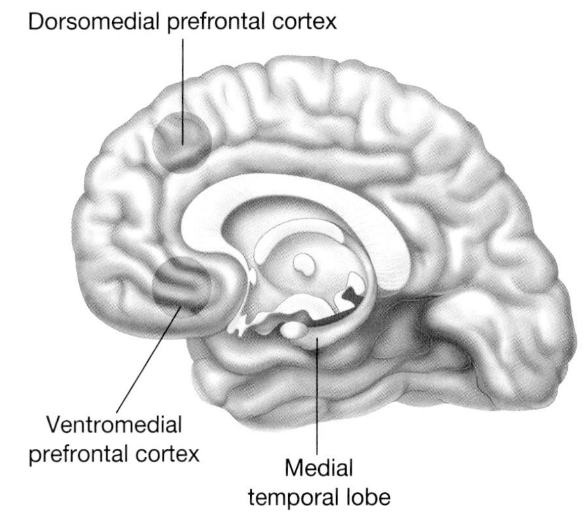

Amanda Tomasikiewicz/Body Scientific Intl.

one experiences physical pain or social pain, such as when one feels socially excluded (the role of the ACC in physical and social pain is explored in the next module). The brain areas related to emotional empathy are illustrated in Figure 15.9.

Cognitive Empathy and the Brain

As stated earlier, cognitive empathy includes making inferences about another person's emotional state. This requires one to create a theory of that person's mental state. This process involves theory of mind, which was discussed earlier. However, as emotional empathy is related to the brain areas associated with simulation theory, cognitive empathy is related to some of the same brain areas related to executive theory (see the preceding unit).

Cognitive empathy was found to be related to activity in the VMPFC, DMPFC, superior temporal sulcus, and temporal poles. As you read in the preceding unit, one of the roles of the VMPFC may be in the differentiation between self and others (J. P. Mitchell et al., 2006) and in the processing of the emotional aspects of empathy (affective mentalizing) (Shamay-Tsoory & Aharon-Peretz, 2007). The TPJ may be involved in the attribution of mental states to others (Van Overwalle & Baetens, 2009).

Cognitive empathy is also related to activity in the medial temporal lobe. Remember, from Chapter 12, that the medial temporal lobe is deeply involved in episodic memories, which are memories for events in one's past. In cognitive empathy, the medial temporal lobe, along with the DMPFC, may be involved in drawing from past experiences to better understand the mental states presently experienced by other people (cognitive mentalizing). The main areas involved in cognitive empathy are illustrated in Figure 15.10.

Although emotional and cognitive empathy are thought to be part of two different systems, in everyday life both of these systems are active and contribute to empathizing with others. Depending on the social context and the information available, one's emotional responses to the mental states of others may be more automatic and intuitive, therefore involving emotional empathy, which relies on simulation. On other occasions, cognitive effort may be required to decipher another person's mental states, therefore, involving cognitive empathy, which relies on executive functions. What is even more plausible is that both systems interact to varying degrees within the same situation (Bernhardt & Singer, 2012). The basic mechanisms and processes involved in producing an empathic response (emotional empathy or cognitive empathy) and how they may interact to produce a general empathetic response are illustrated in Figure 15.11.

FIGURE 15.11

The basic mechanisms and processes that give rise to emotional and cognitive empathy. ACC = anterior cingulate cortex; IFG = inferior frontal gyrus; IPL = inferior parietal lobule; MPFC = medial prefrontal cortex; MTL = medial temporal lobe; TPJ = temporoparietal junction; VMPFC = ventromedial prefrontal cortex. See text for details.

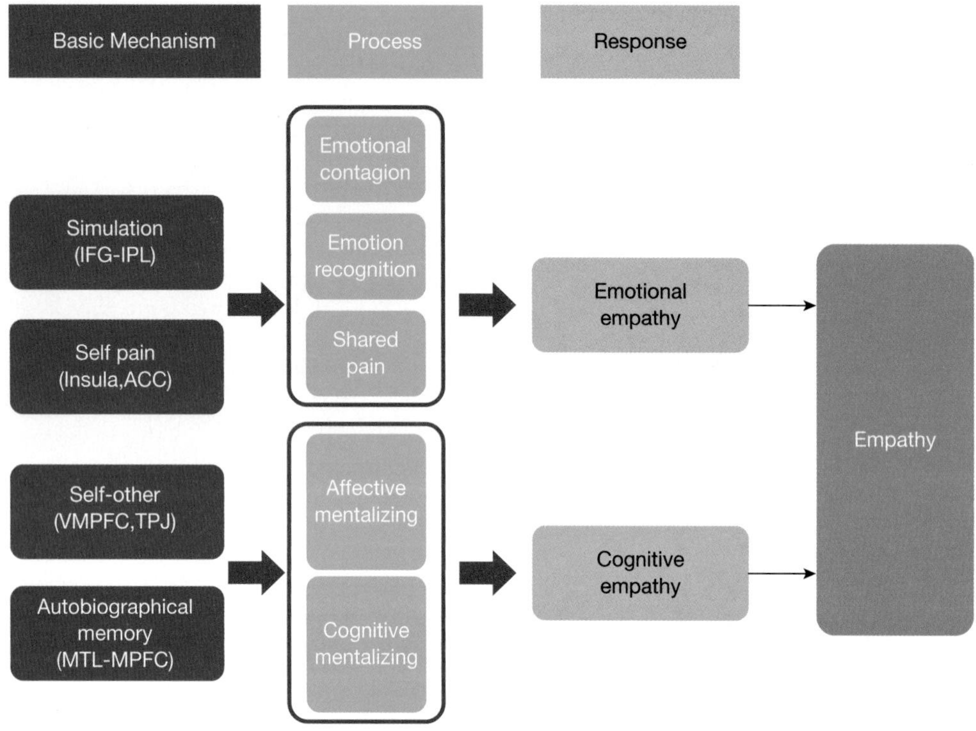

Tsoory, S.G. (2011). The neural bases for empathy. *Neuroscientist 17*(1): 18–24. With permission from SAGE.

IT'S A MYTH!

Autism: Lack of Empathy and the Broken-Mirror Theory

What Is Autism?

Autism, now known as autism spectrum disorder (ASD), is defined in the American Psychiatric Association's *Diagnostic and Statistical Manual of Mental Disorders* (*DSM*-5) as deficits in social-emotional reciprocity; nonverbal communicative behaviors used for social interaction; deficits in developing, maintaining, and understanding relationships; and restricted repetitive patterns of behavior, interests, or activities (American Psychiatric Association, 2013).

Individuals with ASD typically also have difficulties in executive function, such as inhibition of behavior, planning, and attention. Another challenge faced by individuals with ASD is related to their inability to have a theory of mind (Frith, 2001). Theory of mind refers to the ability to infer the mental states such as beliefs, desires, intentions, and emotions of others as distinct from their own, a phenomenon that became known as mindblindness (Baron-Cohen, Leslie, & Frith, 1985). Having an intact theory of mind has also often been attributed to having an intact mirror neuron system (MNS) (Gallese & Goldman, 1998). Mirror neurons were discovered in the promotor cortex of monkeys and were found to be active both when a monkey watched another monkey perform an action and when it performed the same action itself. Mirror neurons are thought by some researchers to be at the root of the ability to imitate and understand the actions of others as well as to infer their intentions (Rizzolatti & Craighero, 2004).

The Myth

You may have heard that people with ASD lack empathy, which refers to the ability to deeply understand the thoughts and emotions of others by genuinely imaging experiencing the world as they do. This supposed deficit has repeatedly been attributed to mindblindness, resulting from a malfunctioning MNS. This is known as the broken-mirror theory of autism (Ramachandran & Oberman, 2006).

Why Is the Myth Wrong?

The Lack of Empathy

Recent research shows what seems to be a lack of empathy may have to do more with the inability of individuals with ASD to read the facial expressions and body language of other people. It is also thought that people with ASD lack the social skills that one would normally use to express their empathy to other people. Another factor may be that people with ASD may not desire the same things as people without it, such as job aspirations or the intense willingness to pursue romantic relationships. However, researchers recently found that, when faced with a moral dilemma (i.e., when having to make decisions that take into account the well-being of others), people with ASD show just as much empathy as neurotypical persons (Patil, Melsbach, Hennig-Fast, & Silani, 2016).

The Broken-Mirror Theory

Because the MNS has repeatedly been associated with action understanding, it is no surprise that an association was readily proposed between a defective MNS and the apparent lack of empathy in ASD. However, the evidence linking the two is extremely weak. Numerous studies have failed to provide support for this idea, showing that the MNS in people with ASD is normal and that dysfunctions in areas outside of the MNS are more likely to be responsible for ASD symptoms. These studies have used a variety of methods to reach their findings, including electroencephalographic measures, transcranial magnetic stimulation, fMRI, magnetoencephalography, and eye tracking (A. F. Hamilton, 2013).

It is time to put this harmful myth to rest. ●

MODULE SUMMARY

Having a theory of mind permits us to infer what goes on in the minds of others: their expectations, beliefs, emotions, and intentions. In false-belief tasks, participants, usually children, are tested on whether they realize that another person can hold beliefs that differ from their own, that is, whether they have a theory of mind. Mastery in false-belief tasks appears to emerge around 4 years of age.

There are several theories about the neurobiological nature of theory of mind: Modularity theories state that an innate module that specializes in theory of mind exists within the brain and that this module is in the temporal parietal junction. Simulation theories explain that theory of mind is achieved through our ability to simulate what another person experiences in a given situation and that this ability depends on the medial prefrontal cortex and mirror neurons in the premotor cortex. Executive theory postulates that theory of mind is dependent on our ability to inhibit our own perspective when attributing mental states to others. This seems to depend on the right medial prefrontal cortex, the right temporal-parietal junction, and parts of the prefrontal cortex. Activity in mirror neurons is both externally generated, by observing the actions of others, and internally generated, by the planning and performance of our own actions.

Empathy is the ability to emotionally and cognitively react to another person's emotional state. Two systems of empathy are believed to exist: an emotional system and a cognitive system. The emotional system for empathy relies on simulation. The main brain areas related to simulation are the ones that are part of the mirror neuron system. These include the inferior parietal lobule and the inferior frontal gyrus. Emotional empathy also includes activity in the anterior cingulate cortex and insula. Cognitive empathy is related to the executive theory of theory of mind. The brain areas associated with cognitive empathy are the ventromedial prefrontal cortex, dorsomedial prefrontal cortex, superior temporal sulcus, temporoparietal junction, and medial temporal lobe.

TEST YOURSELF

15.3.1 What is meant by "theory of mind"? Give an example that shows that someone has a theory of mind.

15.3.2 What are the different theories that explain theory of mind? Describe the brain areas associated with each theory.

15.3.3 Define empathy and its different types. Name the brain areas associated with each type.

15.4 Social Pain

Module Contents

Learning Objectives

15.4.1 Explain the components of physical pain.

15.4.2 Explain what social pain is and how it is similar to physical pain.

15.4.1 TWO DIMENSIONS OF PHYSICAL PAIN

>> LO 15.4.1 **Explain the components of physical pain.**

Key Terms

- **Perceptual dimension of pain:** The detection of a painful stimulus.
- **Affective dimension of pain:** The perceived unpleasantness of the pain-inducing stimulus.
- **Pain regulation:** What is done to manage or cope with pain.

Figure 15.12 shows that there are two components to physical pain, a perceptual component and an affective (emotional) component. We also deal or cope with pain by regulating it. The **perceptual dimension of pain** relates to the detection of a painful stimulus. The main brain areas involved are the insula and the somatosensory cortex. The **affective dimension of pain** relates to the perceived unpleasantness of the pain-inducing stimulus. It was shown to involve the anterior cingulate cortex. **Pain regulation** is what people do to manage or cope with pain. This may include trying to focus on something other than the pain or engaging in other strategies that have worked in the past. Pain regulation involves the right ventral prefrontal cortex (RVPFC).

Neuropsychologist Pierre Rainville and colleagues showed that a relationship exists between activity in the ACC and the unpleasantness of pain (Rainville, Duncan, Price, Carrier, & Bushnell, 1997) (Figure 15.13a). To do so, they dissociated the sensory and affective dimensions of pain using hypnotic suggestions. They had subjects immerse their left hand in 45°C (113°F) water (this is painfully hot) while given the hypnotic suggestion of increased unpleasantness in one condition or decreased unpleasantness in another. Higher degrees of unpleasantness induced by the hypnotic suggestion were correlated with greater activity in the ACC as measured by positron emission tomography (PET). Figure 15.13b shows the PET image of activity in the ACC.

FIGURE 15.12

The components of pain. The perceptual component of pain is related to a sensory process, which is processed by the somatosensory cortex and insula. The affective component depends on the anterior cingulate cortex. Pain is also regulated through the right ventral prefrontal cortex (RVPFC).

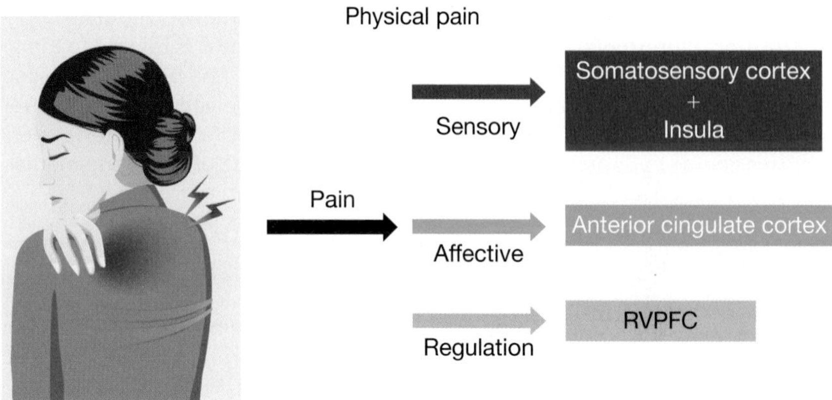

solar22/ istockphoto

FIGURE 15.13

(a) Relationship between ratings of unpleasantness of a painful stimulus and activity in the ACC. (b) PET image of activity in the ACC in response to a painful stimulus (yellow and red dots indicate low and high degrees of unpleasantness, respectively).

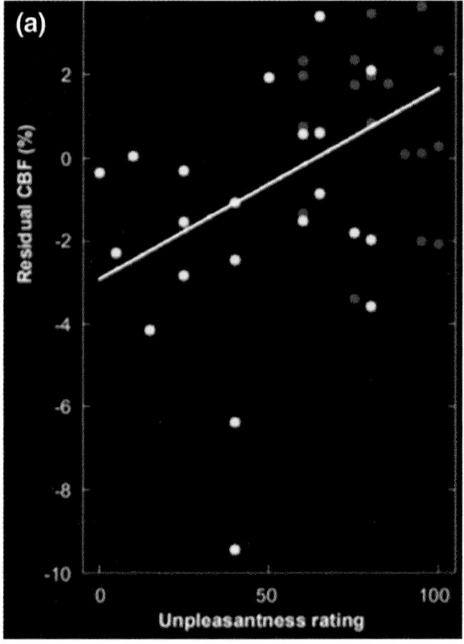

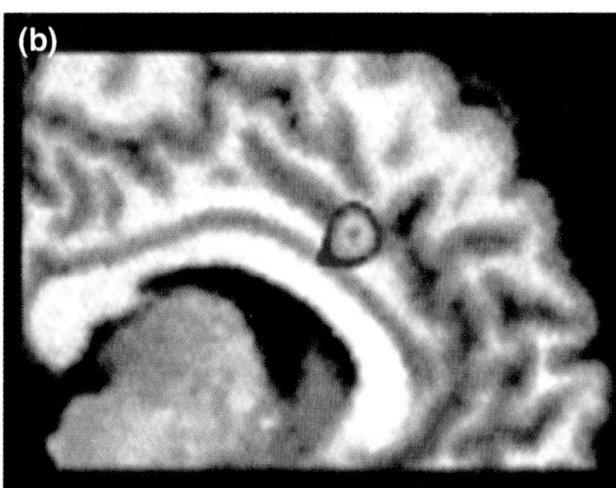

Rainville, P. (1997). Pain affect encoded in human anterior cingulate but not somatosensory cortex. *Science 277*(5328): 968–971. With permission from AAAS.

that your friend is doing this to you. You have just been subjected to **social exclusion**, in which a person is not permitted to participate socially with other people. Social exclusion is a source of social pain. Social neuroscientists believe that social pain is similar to physical pain and that this can be demonstrated by studying brain areas that are commonly activated during both physical and social pain.

Have you ever wondered why we use the same language for both physical pain and emotional pain? For example, we use the word *hurt* when experiencing both physical and emotional pain. Does emotional pain really "hurt"? In fact, in this unit you will learn that studies show that social pain—such as the pain induced by social exclusion, isolation, separation distress, romantic breakups, or the loss of a loved one—activates some of the same brain areas as physical pain.

15.4.2 SOCIAL PAIN: DOES IT REALLY HURT?

>> LO 15.4.2 **Explain what social pain is and how it is similar to physical pain.**

Key Terms

- **Social exclusion:** When a person is not permitted to participate socially with other people.
- **Cyberball:** A video game designed to test emotional and neurological reactions to social exclusion.
- **Social pain/physical pain overlap theory (spot):** The idea that there are overlapping neural mechanisms for physical and social pain.
- **Separation distress:** A mechanism that may have evolved in mammals to keep the young close to maternal contact and care.

You are at a party with your best friend when suddenly another one of her friends from the past approaches her. You are introduced briefly, but for the rest of the evening your best friend and her friend from the past spend hours catching up while completely ignoring you. You know no one else at the party and cannot believe

Now imagine that you are in an fMRI scanner and asked to participate in a video game called **cyberball**, illustrated in Figure 15.14. In this game, you are one of three participants throwing a ball around. You are at first an active participant in the game, but after several rounds of ball throwing, the other two participants (who are not real but are part of a computer program) exclude you from the game and start playing between themselves, not throwing you the ball again. How would you feel?

Such a study was actually conducted by psychologist Naomi Eisenberger and colleagues (Masten et al., 2011). Participants subjected to exclusion from the game reported that they felt ignored and indeed excluded and that the experience was distressing. The imaging results showed that the excluded participants had significantly greater amounts of activation of the ACC (Figure 15.15a), which, as you learned in the preceding unit, processes the affective component of physical pain, compared to participants who were not excluded. The amount of activation of the ACC also related to the social distress the participants felt. That is, the more social distress the participants felt, the greater the activity in the ACC (Figure 15.15b). In addition, the excluded participants showed significantly more activity in the RVPFC than nonexcluded participants, presumably because of an effort to regulate their pain by attempting to cope with their distress. Figure 15.15c shows the similarity of activation of the RVPFC during the regulation of physical and social pain.

FIGURE 15.14

Cyberball: In this game, participants play with two virtual partners while having their brain scanned. The object of the game is simply to throw the ball from participant to participant (left). In one condition (right), the two virtual participants omit passing the ball to the participant, resulting in a feeling of exclusion.

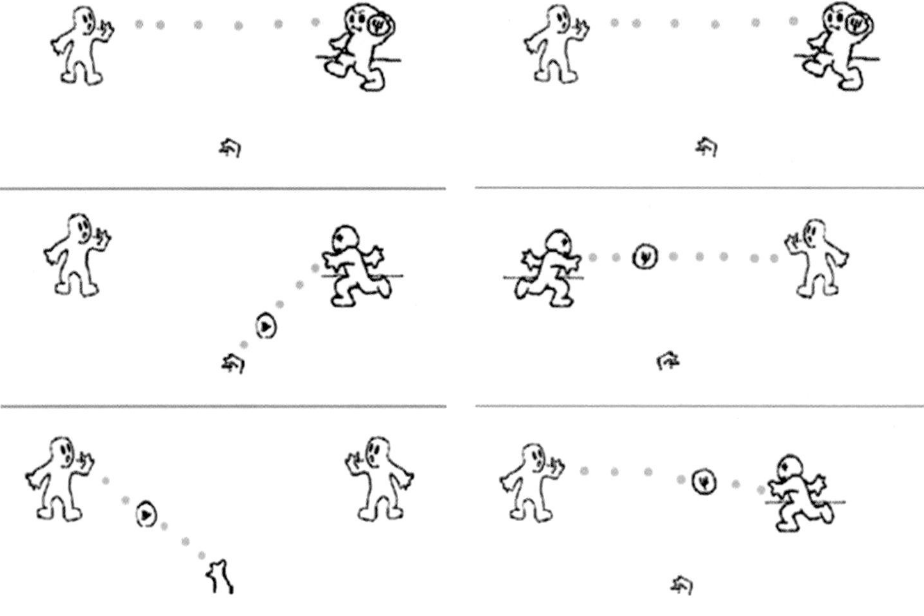

Eisenberger, N. I., & M.D. Lieberman. (2004). Why rejection hurts: a common neural alarm system for physical and social pain. *Trends in Cognitive Science 8*(7): 294–300. With permission from Elsevier.

Social Pain/Physical Pain Overlap Theory (SPOT)

The findings obtained from the cyberball study described in the preceding section and from other studies suggest that having overlapping neural mechanisms for physical and social pain may have adaptive value. This idea is embodied in what psychologists Naomi Eisenberger and Matthew Lieberman (2004) called the **social pain/physical pain overlap theory (SPOT)**. According to them, this overlap makes evolutionary sense. Having a mechanism that warns us about physical and social distress has tremendous survival value. They suggest that a social pain signal is activated during **separation distress**, which may have evolved in mammals to keep the young close to maternal contact and care. They also suggest that this pain signal "piggybacked" onto a signal for physical pain, which explains the overlap, and that the consequence of this overlap is that one type of pain (physical) relates to the other (social) and vice versa. They point to three lines of evidence to make this point:

1. When children experience physical pain, they experience more social pain in response to separation from a caregiver.
2. Increased social support reduces chronic physical pain.
3. Some drugs regulate both social pain and physical pain.

In a later study, Eisenberger and colleagues tested whether acetaminophen, a common pain reliever, was effective in relieving the social pain induced by being excluded in the cyberball game described earlier (Dewall et al., 2010). Participants were asked to take daily doses of acetaminophen (1,000 mg) or a placebo for three weeks. They were then subjected to the cyberball game while their brains were scanned by fMRI. Figures 15.16a and 15.16b show the results of the experiment. Participants in the exclusion group, who took acetaminophen, had significantly less activation of the ACC than the participants who took a placebo. However, the participants in both groups reported similar amounts of distress. In another experiment within the same study, participants who took daily doses of acetaminophen reported fewer occasions on which they felt their feelings were hurt over a 21-day period (Figure 15.16c). The experimenters verified that the acetaminophen did not increase the number of positive emotions felt by the participants.

The findings on the implication of the ACC in social pain indicate that the ACC can be thought of as part of a neural alarm system. An alarm system scans the environment and detects when something has gone wrong, such as when one is being rejected.

FIGURE 15.15

(a) fMRI image of the ACC of excluded participants during the game of cyberball. (b) Relationship between the level of distress reported by excluded participants and activity in the ACC during the cyberball game. (c) Similarity of activation of the RVPFC during the regulation of physical and social pain.

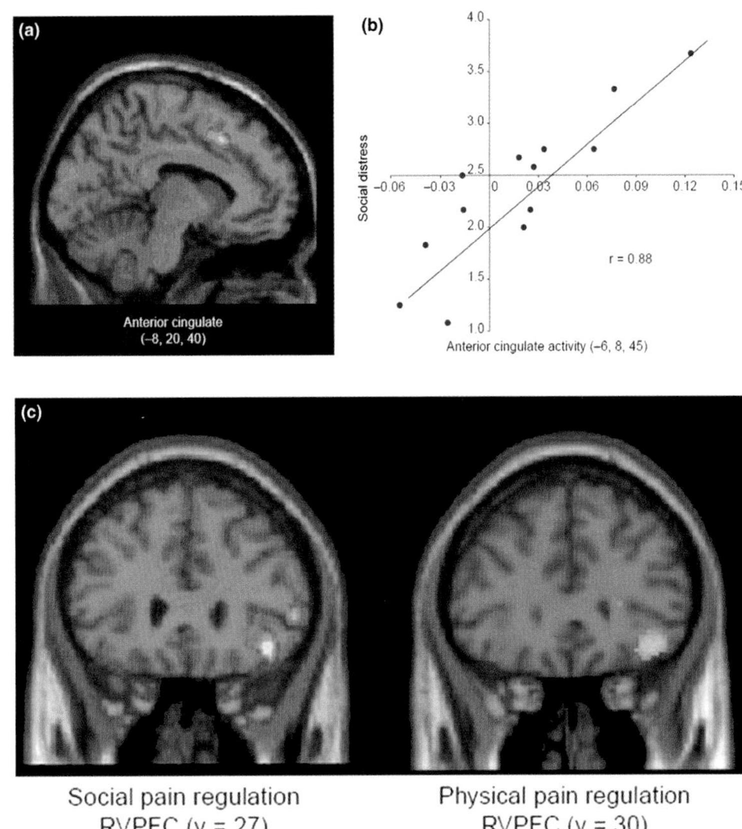

Eisenberger, N. I., & M.D. Lieberman. (2004). Why rejection hurts: a common neural alarm system for physical and social pain. *Trends in Cognitive Science* 8(7): 294–300. With permission from Elsevier.

FIGURE 15.16

(a) fMRI image of ACC activity in participants playing the cyberball game. (b) Activity in the ACC of participants in the cyberball game during the exclusion versus the inclusion condition. Activity in the ACC was significantly higher in the exclusion condition than in the inclusion condition. (c) Participants who took daily doses of acetaminophen reported fewer occasions of hurt feelings over a 21-day period, compared to those who took a placebo.

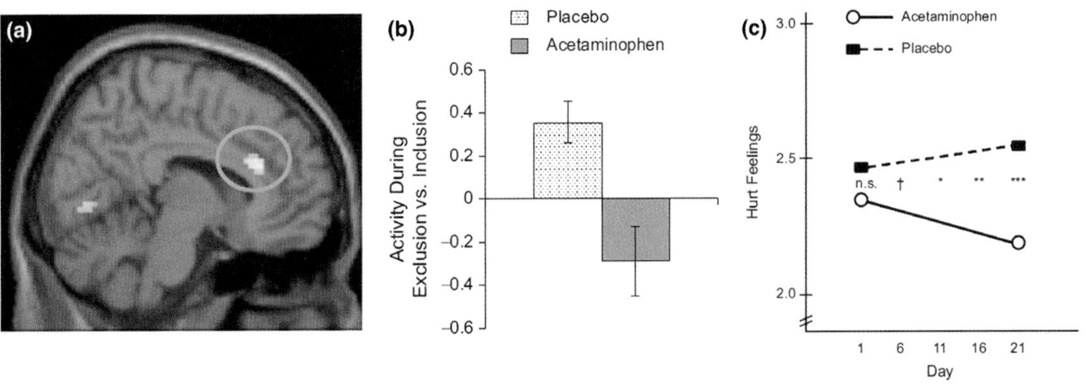

Dewall, C.N., et al. (2010). Acetaminophen reduces social pain: behavioral and neural evidence. *Psychological Science* 21(7): 931–937. With permission from SAGE.

MODULE SUMMARY

There are two dimensions to pain: a perceptual dimension and an affective dimension. The perceptual dimension relates to the detection of a painful stimulus, and the affective dimension relates to the perceived unpleasantness of the pain-inducing stimulus. The main brain areas involved in the perceptual dimension are the insula and the somatosensory cortex. The affective dimension of pain involves the anterior cingulate cortex (ACC).

Pain regulation is what you do to manage or cope with your pain. Pain regulation involves the right ventral prefrontal cortex. Studies show that social pain activates some of the same brain areas as physical pain. Cyberball is a video game used to study social exclusion. It can be played by participants while their brains are imaged by fMRI. Imaging results show that excluded participants have significantly more activation of the ACC, which also processes the affective component of physical pain.

Having overlapping neural mechanisms for physical and social pain may have adaptive value. This idea is embodied by the social pain/physical pain overlap theory (SPOT). It was further found that medication that is used to alleviate physical pain, such as acetaminophen, also alleviates social pain. The ACC is thought to act as a neural alarm system, which alerts you when subjected to events that induce social pain such as being socially excluded.

TEST YOURSELF

15.4.1 What brain areas are associated with social pain? How and why might they overlap with the brain areas involved in physical pain?

15.4.2 Which brain area has been called a neural alarm system and why?

15.5 Altruism

Module Contents

15.5.1 What Is Altruism?

15.5.2 Altruism: Where in the Brain?

Learning Objectives

15.5.1 Define altruism and explain how it may be a product of evolutionary adaptation.

15.5.2 Identify the brain areas associated with altruism and explain how they are associated with various altruistic behaviors.

15.5.1 WHAT IS ALTRUISM?

>> LO 15.5.1 Define altruism and explain how it may be a product of evolutionary adaptation.

Key Terms

- **Negative-state release model:** The idea that we help others to alleviate the negative feelings that come while observing others in distress.
- **Cost-benefit analysis theory of helping:** The idea that we may help others only if the cost of helping, such as any potential threat or danger, is not too high.
- **Altruism:** Giving or helping behavior strictly for the good of others. The behavior is often regarded to be selfless or without regard for any personal gain or satisfaction.
- **Kin selection:** The idea that we more readily choose to help others who are related to us.
- **Reciprocal altruism:** The idea that we help others with the expectation of getting help from them in the future.

Consider the chapter-opening story of David Starnes, who helped to pull a woman from a burning car, or think about volunteers who have exposed themselves to deadly viruses to help others during epidemics. What could have given rise to such selfless acts? In this section, we explore some possible answers.

Several models exist to explain why we help others. According to the **negative-state release model**, we help others to alleviate the negative feelings that come while observing others in distress (Cialdini & Kenrick, 1976). According to the **cost-benefit analysis theory of helping** (Piliavin & Rodin, 1969), we may help others only if the cost of helping, such as any potential threat or danger, is not too high. We also tend to help others who have helped us in the past and out of social responsibility.

Altruism refers to giving or helping behavior strictly for the good of others. The behavior is often regarded to be selfless or without regard for any personal gain or satisfaction. That is, altruistic behavior is often referred to as being selfless. Altruism may have arisen for evolutionary reasons. Two main ideas point in this direction: kin selection and reciprocal altruism.

Kin selection refers to the idea that we more readily choose to help others who are related to us than those who are unrelated. Evolutionary biologist William Hamilton (1964) describes kin selection as a mechanism that increases the probability that adaptive traits, which increase survivability of relatives, are passed on to the next generations.

In a famous example of kin selection, Warren G. Holmes and Paul Sherman (2015) found that ground squirrels, like the one illustrated in Figure 15.17, emit two types of alarm calls that alert their kin group to the presence of predators. A whistle signals the approach of an aerial predator, whereas trills signal the presence of a terrestrial predator. It turns out that whistles are not very costly, as the individual that whistles is highly likely to escape. However, the individual that trills in response to the presence of a ground predator increases the likelihood that the kin group will survive but increases its own likelihood of being devoured.

Reciprocal altruism, first described by evolutionary biologist Robert Trivers, is the idea that we help others with the expectation of getting help from them in the future (Trivers, 1971). Trivers explains that two people who risked their lives for each other will be selected for over those who must face a life-threatening situation on their own. In other words, if you do not reciprocate ("cheat"), you run the risk of the altruist no longer helping you in the future.

FIGURE 15.17

Ground squirrels emit two types of alarm calls that alert their kin group of the presence of predators. A whistle signals the approach of an aerial predator, whereas trills signal the presence of a terrestrial predator.

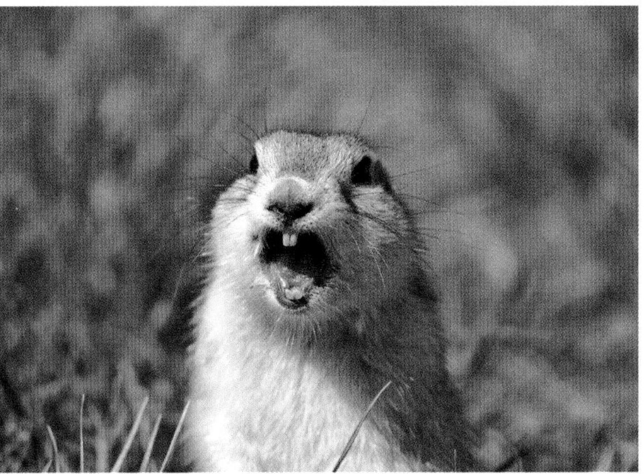

4loops/istockphoto

15.5.2 ALTRUISM: WHERE IN THE BRAIN?

>> LO 15.5.2 Identify the brain areas associated with altruism and explain how they are associated with various altruistic behaviors.

Key Terms

- **Psychopaths:** People who generally show disregard for the well-being of others as well as a lack of guilt, empathy, and remorse.
- **Joy of giving:** Giving was shown to have the same neurobiological basis as different types of rewards, such as money, drugs, and food.

Altruistic actions like the ones presented in the chapter's opening vignette are common occurrence. The reason may become clear when we consider reciprocal altruism. Social neuroscientists have wondered about which brain areas are responsible for altruism. In a 2014 study, social neuroscientist Abigail Marsh and colleagues showed kidney donors, who are obviously altruists, faces expressing fear or anger or neutral faces, while scanning their brains using fMRI. Kidney donors had larger right amygdalas, which also showed significantly more activity, compared to the amygdalas of control participants, who had never donated an organ. These results are shown in Figures 15.18a and 15.18b. Marsh found the opposite pattern (smaller amygdala and less responsive to fearful faces) in **psychopaths**, who generally show disregard for the well-being of others as well as a lack of guilt, empathy, and remorse (Marsh et al., 2014). You know from your reading of Chapter 11 that the amygdala is important for processing emotions. Therefore, it should not be surprising to you that the amygdala is activated to a higher degree in people who engage in altruistic behavior. You also learned in Chapter 11 that damage to the amygdala can impair emotional responses. Recall patient SM, who could not experience fear and who was also not able to recognize emotions in other people's faces.

The Joy of Giving

Neuropsychologist Jordan Grafman and colleagues wanted to answer the question of whether altruistic behaviors that take the form of giving to charitable organizations activated the same brain areas associated with obtaining rewards (Moll et al., 2006). They predicted that when people perceive that they are alleviating the suffering of others through giving, areas in the mesolimbic reward system (discussed in Chapters 3 and 9), would be activated.

The participants in the experiment had the choice of receiving $128 to either walk away from the experiment or to sacrifice part of the money by donating it to charitable organizations, while their brains were

FIGURE 15.18

Activity and size of the amygdala in altruists versus control participants. (a) fMRI imaging of the right amygdala, showing that the amygdala of altruists was significantly more active than that of control participants while viewing faces expressing emotions. (b) Altruists also had a significantly larger amygdala.

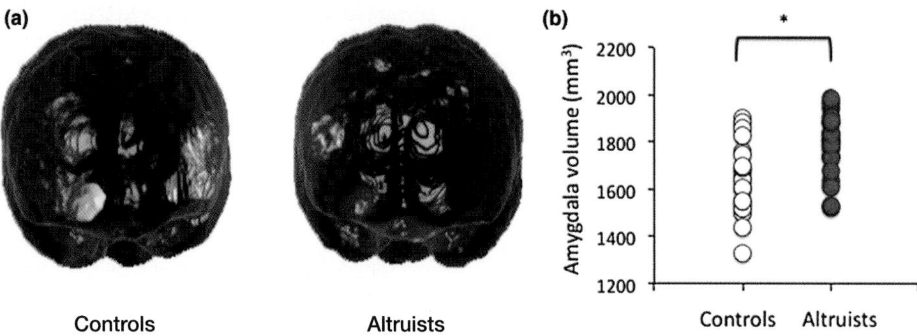

Marsh, A. A., et al. (2014). Neural and cognitive characteristics of extraordinary altruists. *Proceedings of the National Academy of Sciences U S A 111*(42): 15036–15041. With permission from the National Academy of Sciences.

being scanned using fMRI. The participants were given a choice of several organizations to donate to. The names of the organizations and the causes associated with them were given to each participant. The participants then had to decide whether to support the organization through a donation or to oppose it.

The researchers found that brain areas associated with reward were activated by both walking away with the monetary reward and by deciding to give. These areas were the ventral-tegmental area (VTA), dorsal striatum, and ventral striatum (Figure 15.19a). These results showed that the **joy of giving** has the same neurobiological basis as different types of rewards, such as money, drugs, and food. They also found that the amount of activity in the ventral striatum and the septal region (an area associated with the ventral striatum) was associated with the percentage of decisions to give. This means that the more people donated, the higher the activity in those areas. These results are shown in Figure 15.19b.

FIGURE 15.19

fMRI images of brain areas associated with giving (joy-of-giving effect) and the relationship between activity and the decision to give. (a) Activity in brain areas associated with reward: ventral-tegmental area (VTA) and striatum (STR). (b) Relationship between the decision to donate and activity in the ventral striatum (VS) and the septal region (SR).

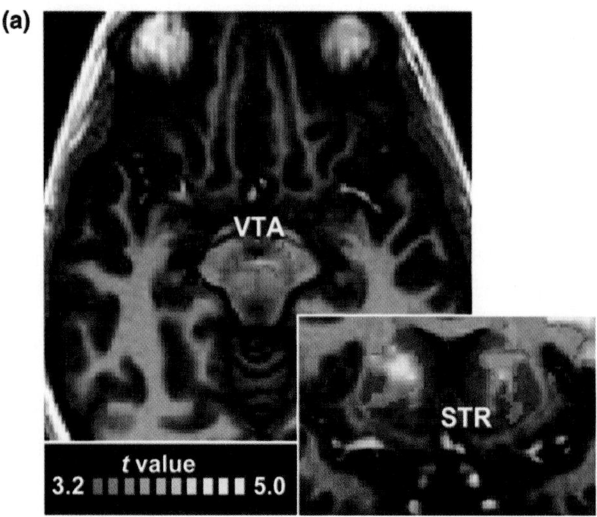

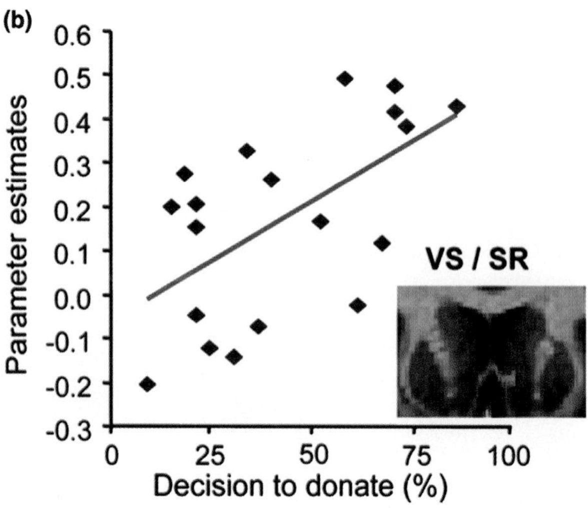

Moll, J., et al. (2006). Human fronto-mesolimbic networks guide decisions about charitable donation. *Proceedings of the National Academy of Sciences U S A, 103*(42), 15623–15628. With permission from the National Academy of Sciences.

MODULE SUMMARY

There are two main ideas for how altruism evolved. These are kin selection, which is the idea that we more readily choose to help others who are related to us, and reciprocal altruism, which is the idea that we help others with the expectation of getting help from them in the future. In one study, kidney donors, who were obviously altruists, had a larger right amygdala, which also showed significantly more activity, compared to the amygdalas of control participants. Psychopaths, who generally show disregard for the well-being of others as well as a lack of guilt, empathy, and remorse had smaller and less active right amygdalas. The joy of giving has the same neurobiological basis as different types of rewards, such as money, drugs, and food. In one study, the amounts of activity in the ventral striatum and the septal region were associated with the percentage of decisions to give.

TEST YOURSELF

15.5.1 Describe the models that seek to explain why we help people.

15.5.2 What brain areas were found to be involved in altruism. What might it mean that these areas are involved?

15.6 Cooperation and Trust

Module Contents

15.6.1 Game Theory

15.6.2 Game Theory and the Brain?

Learning Objectives

15.6.1 Explain game theory, identify two examples, and describe what each is used for and why.

15.6.2 Identify the brain areas associated with trust and cooperation.

15.6.1 GAME THEORY

>> LO 15.6.1 **Explain game theory, identify two examples, and describe what each is used for and why.**

Key Terms

- **Game theory:** A branch of mathematics devised to explain the behavior of animals in nature and of people in social or political contexts.
- **Prisoner's dilemma:** A game based on cooperation that shows that people's decisions are not always based on rational thought.
- **Defecting:** In the prisoner's dilemma, when a participant decides based only on his or her own best interest.
- **Cooperating:** In the prisoner's dilemma, a decision that has the good of both participants in mind.
- **Trust game:** A game based on trust in which an investor transfers a sum of money to a trustee with the expectancy of a return.

Cooperation refers to the actions of individuals or groups to maximize their mutual benefits. Reciprocal altruism is an example of cooperation, because, in addition to benefiting the person being helped, the very same action is associated with a probability that you will obtain help from that person in the future. However, as stated earlier, we can never be certain that others will cooperate by reciprocating with the common good in mind. It may sometimes be perceived as advantageous to obtain help from others but not to reciprocate when that other person needs help. So, the question is, "to cooperate or not to cooperate." Indeed, this is often a dilemma that needs to be solved.

An excellent way to study the ability of people to cooperate and to trust each other is through **game theory**, which is a branch of mathematics devised to explain the behavior of animals in nature and of people in social or political contexts. Game theory was used during the Cold War to help devise strategies in the case of nuclear conflict. In this module, we examine two of these games, the prisoner's dilemma and the trust game, as well as the brain areas thought to be involved in decisions that people make during those games.

The Prisoner's Dilemma

The **prisoner's dilemma** was invented by mathematicians Merrill Flood and Melvin Dresher in the 1950s. Imagine the following scenario: You and your friend are arrested for a crime. However, there is not enough evidence for a serious charge that would carry a five-year prison sentence. Because of this, you are facing only a one-year prison sentence. However, the prosecutor really needs to nab someone with a more serious charge, so you are offered a deal. You will receive a six-month reduced sentence if you squeal on your friend, while your friend serves the full five-year sentence.

This sounds good to you until you learn that your friend has been offered the same deal. That is, if he squeals (**defecting**) but you remain silent, he will get off with a six-month sentence, while you will be charged with the serious crime and receive the full five years. You also learn that if you both squeal on each other, both of you will receive a sentence of four and a half years. What to do? **Cooperating** among yourselves—by remaining silent and accepting your one-year sentence—is the best you can do for each other. This puts you in a real bind. If you knew that your friend would remain silent, you would do the same, but there is no way for you to know that.

The prisoner's dilemma shows that our decisions are not always rational. In this case, the best option is for both to remain silent. However, because neither can be certain that the other will remain silent, they face a dilemma. The questions are "to cooperate or not to cooperate" and "to trust or not to trust."

The Trust Game

Joyce Berg and colleagues devised an experiment to measure trust (Berg, Dickhaut, & McCabe, 1995). The **trust game** (Figure 15.20) is played between two participants, an investor and a trustee. The investor is given a sum of money and may transfer some of this money to a trustee. The experimenter triples the amount transferred to the trustee by the investor. The trustee may return some or the entire amount back to the investor. In a single-trial game, the best decision for the trustee, based on personal gain, would be to keep all the money. However, with multiple trials, the trustee risks that he will lose the investor's trust and no longer receive any money. It is, therefore, advantageous for the trustee to return some of the money to gain the investor's trust. From the investor's perspective, receiving some money back is an indication of the trustee's trustworthiness.

FIGURE 15.20

The trust game. In this game, an investor is given a sum of money and has the opportunity to invest some or all of it with a trustee. The trustee receives triple the sum invested. The trustee then has the choice of returning some of the money to the investor.

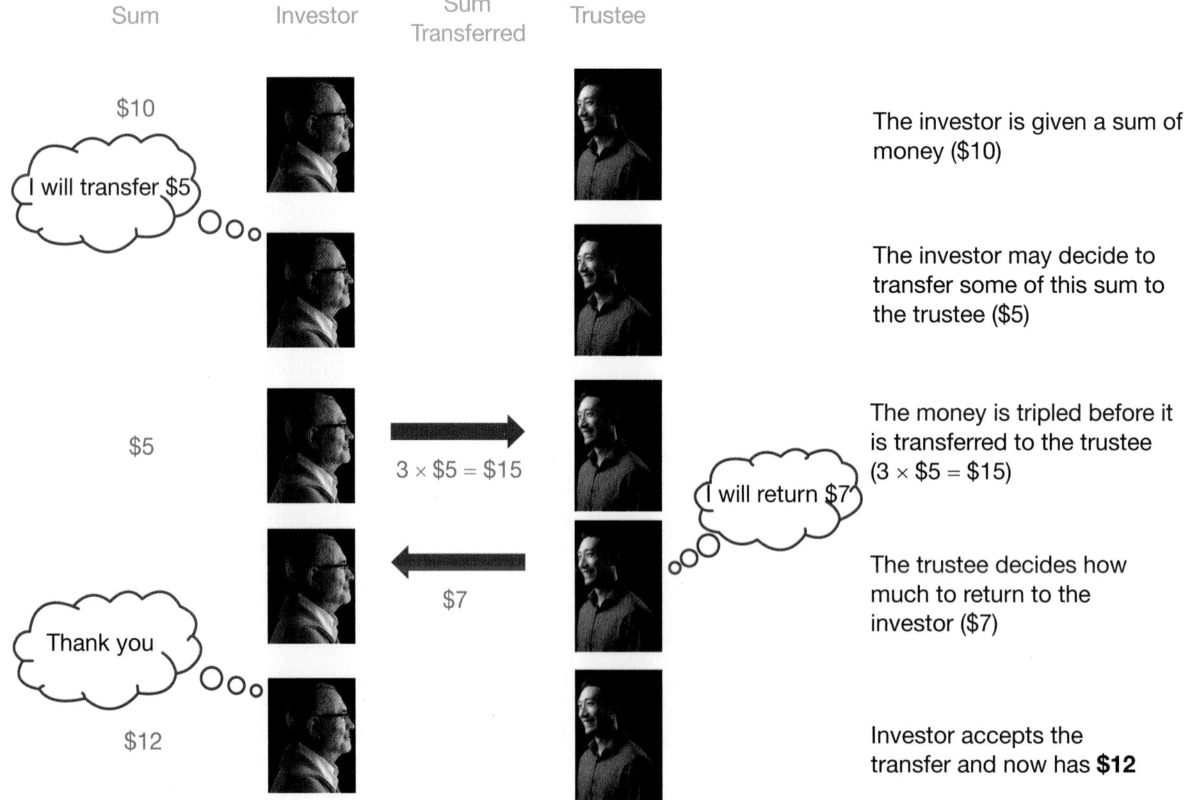

(left) curtoicurto/ istockphoto; (right) Ranta Images/ istockphoto

15.6.2 GAME THEORY AND THE BRAIN?

>> LO 15.6.2 Identify the brain areas associated with trust and cooperation.

Key Term

- **Hyper-scanning fMRI (h-fMRI):** A method in which the brains of multiple participants are imaged simultaneously to determine how they may influence each other.

James K. Rilling and colleagues conducted a study in which women engaged in a prisoner's dilemma game while their brains were being imaged by fMRI (Rilling et al., 2002). Each participant who was being scanned played with another who was not being scanned. The participants, designated Player A and Player B, were awarded a sum of money depending on how they interacted with each other. If Player A defected but Player B cooperated, Player A was awarded $3.00 and Player B was awarded nothing. If both players cooperated, each was awarded $2.00. If both players defected, each was awarded $1.00. Finally, if Player B defected and Player A cooperated, Player B was awarded $3.00 and Player A was awarded nothing.

The most rewarding situation, as measured by the level of activation of a network of brain areas associated with processing rewards, was when both players cooperated (Figure 15.21). Interestingly, this was not the situation that resulted in the biggest monetary payoff. That is, the biggest monetary payoff for a player occurred when she defected and the other cooperated.

FIGURE 15.21

fMRI images of the brain while cooperating in the prisoner's dilemma game. Cooperation between participants was associated with activity in brain areas associated with reward: the orbitofrontal cortex (OFC) and anteroventral striatum.

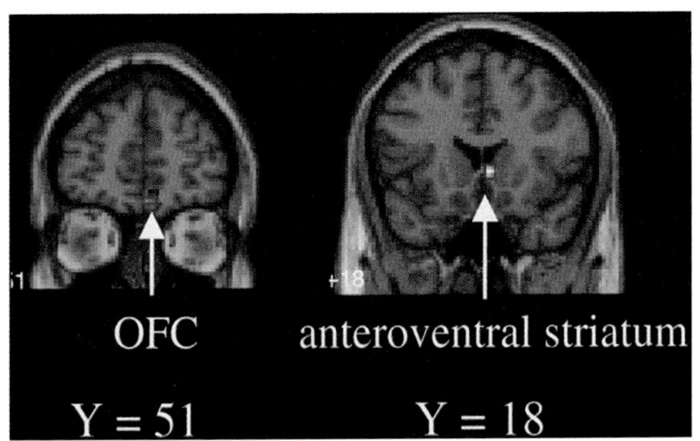

Rilling, J.K., et al. (2002). A Neural Basis for Social Cooperation. *Neuron* 35(2): 395–405. With permission from Elsevier.

These results were taken to indicate that, when activated, this network of brain areas, which includes the anteroventral striatum (nucleus accumbens and caudate nucleus) and orbitofrontal cortex, reinforces altruism in favor of actions that would be personally advantageous if an action is not reciprocated. By the same token, these results may also provide evidence for a network of brain areas that supports reciprocal altruism, discussed in the previous module.

In 2006, psychologist Brookes King-Casas and colleagues published a research article reporting their use of **hyper-scanning fMRI (h-fMRI)** to investigate the brain areas activated in participants while engaged in a trust game (Li, McClure, King-Casas, & Montague, 2006). Hyper scanning is a method in which the brains of more than one person, each in a separate fMRI scanner, are imaged simultaneously while engaged in the task. This method, developed by physicist Read Montague in the early 2000s (Montague et al., 2002), permits researchers to image the brain of one participant, while engaged in one behavior, and the brain of another participant at the same time, even if the participants are located in different geographic locations. It also permits researchers to image the second participant's brain in response to that behavior.

King-Casas subjected people to an iterated version of the trust game described in the preceding unit. This means that instead of a single round of the game where the investor and trustee could reciprocate according to the money received from each other, participants played multiple rounds of the game. This resulted in a more lifelike situation, since social and economic exchanges between people go on for several occasions as trust develops between them.

The procedure of their experiment was as follows: Pairs of participants were scanned by fMRI as they played multiple rounds of the trust game. A round started when the investor was presented with a cue to invest on a computer screen. After a delay period, the amount invested by the investor was visible to both players on their own screens. Following another delay, the trustee was presented with a cue to repay the investor.

The experimenters tracked the patterns of payments made by the investors to the trustees and classified them under three conditions: benevolent, neutral, and malevolent, based on the results of the two previous rounds of the game. This is shown in Figure 15.22a. In the benevolent condition, the investors increased the amounts invested despite the reduction in repayments made by the trustees. In the neutral condition, the amount paid by both the investors and the trustees remained constant throughout the rounds. Finally, in the malevolent condition, the investors reduced the amount invested despite increased repayments by the trustees.

They found that the caudate nucleus (Figure 15.22b), a brain area involved in processing reward, showed more activation in the trustee's brain in the

FIGURE 15.22

(a) Payments from the investor were classified under three conditions: benevolent, neutral, and malevolent, based on the results of the two previous rounds of the game. (b) fMRI images showing activity in the caudate nucleus (areas associated with reward) of the trustees. (c) Significantly greater activity was observed in the caudate nucleus of the trustees when the investor was benevolent (reciprocated) than when the investor was either neutral or malevolent.

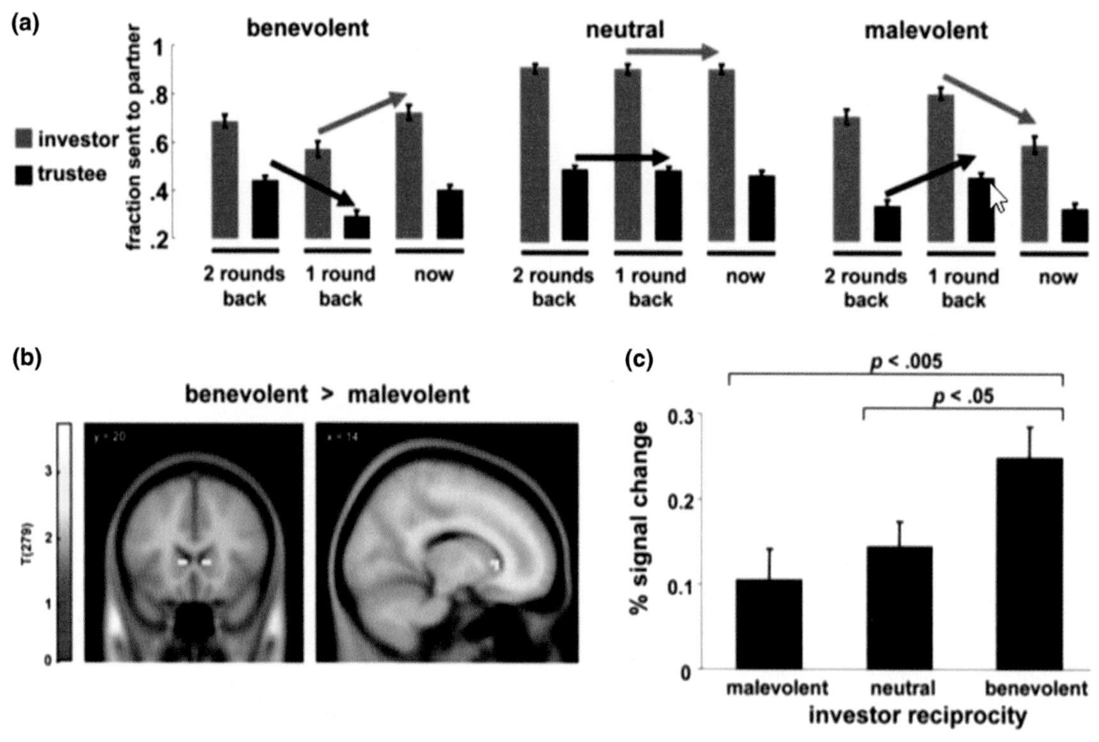

King-Casas, B., et al. (2005). Getting to Know You: Reputation and Trust in a Two-Person Economic Exchange. *Science 308*(5718): 78–83. With permission from AAAS.

benevolent condition than in either the neutral or malevolent conditions. These results are shown in Figure 15.22c.

The hyper-scanning results showed that the investor's decisions to invest correlated with activity in the middle cingulate cortex. However, in the trustee, the ACC was highly active when learning about the investor's decisions, indicating the trustee's intention to trust the investor. In addition, activity in the caudate nucleus increased with the trustee's decisions to trust the investor. The hyper-scanning images with activated brain areas are shown in Figure 15.23.

Another interesting result was that increased activation of the caudate in the trustee occurred progressively earlier with the number of rounds. For example, in the early rounds of the game, activity in the caudate increased only after the trustee learned about the investor's investment. In the middle and late rounds, activity in the trustee's caudate occurred before the investor's decision was revealed. To the authors, this meant that a model of the investor developed in the trustee's brain.

FIGURE 15.23

Hyper-scanning results. The investor's decision to invest was related to activity in the middle cingulate cortex. When learning about the investor's decision, activity increased in the trustee's ACC (green arrow). When the trustee decided to trust the investor, increased activity in the caudate nucleus was observed (blue arrow).

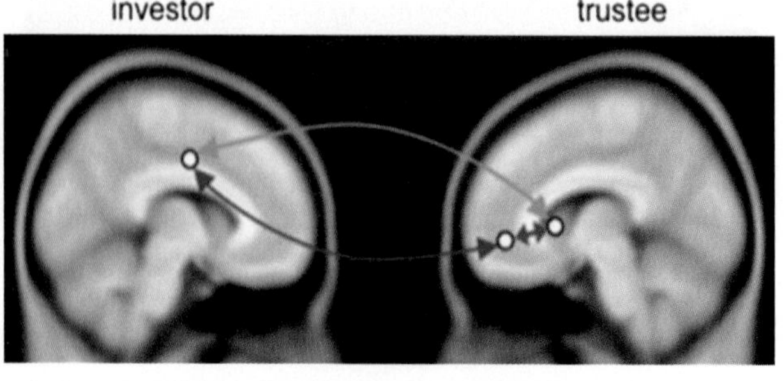

King-Casas, B., et al. (2005). Getting to Know You: Reputation and Trust in a Two-Person Economic Exchange. *Science 308*(5718): 78–83. With permission from AAAS.

MODULE SUMMARY

Game theory was devised to explain the behavior of animals in nature and of people in social or political contexts. Two widely used games are the prisoner's dilemma, based on cooperation, and the trust game, based on trust. In the prisoner's dilemma, the level of activation in brain areas associated with processing rewards, such as the orbitofrontal cortex and the striatum, was higher when the participants cooperated.

In the trust game, the caudate nucleus, also involved in processing rewards, showed more activation in the trustee's brain in a benevolent condition than in either the neutral or malevolent condition. Increased activation of the caudate in the trustee occurred progressively earlier with the number of rounds of the trust game. This meant that a model of the investor developed in the trustee's brain.

TEST YOURSELF

15.6.1 What is game theory? Describe two games, one based on cooperation and the other based on trust.

15.6.2 What has been learned about the relationships among brain activity, trust, and cooperation through the use of games?

APPLICATIONS

Neuroeconomics and Neuromarketing

Neuroeconomics

Neuroeconomics combines the fields of economics, psychology, and neuroscience in an effort to understand the neurobiological processes that underlie motivation, decision making under risk and uncertainty, and how people decide in a social context (Loewenstein et al., 2008). This is done mainly through the use of imaging methods such as fMRI, magnetoencephalography, electroencephalography, transcranial magnetic stimulation, and several other methods (Kable, 2011).

Neuroeconomists explore activity in the brain's reward system to understand how potential risks, costs, rewards, and benefits are processed in the nervous system when having to choose among several options. Neuroeconomists are also interested in understanding how some people are risk takers and others shy away from risks (risk-averse). They are also aware that decision making depends not just on rational processes but also on emotional responses triggered by having to choose among multiple options in times of uncertainty.

Neuroeconomists sometimes make use of games to study cooperative/noncooperative behaviors and selfish/altruistic behaviors and to evaluate risk taking. These games are typically played by study participants while their brains are being imaged so that the neural correlates of such behaviors can be determined. Neuroeconomists are also interested in how psychological disorders affect the brain's involvement in decision making through the evaluation of risks, potential rewards, and potential costs and benefits.

Neuromarketing

Neuromarketing can be considered the branch of economics that uses methods of brain imaging to understand consumer behavior (Lee, Broderick, & Chamberlain, 2007). Neuromarketing research involves studying the neurobiological mechanisms that underlie the reasons one might prefer one product over another or studying the brain's reward systems to provide clues into how to devise advertising campaigns so that products are difficult to resist. Neuromarketing research may also provide clues for how to devise commercials and other advertising tools to maximize activity in the brain's attentional systems so that specific information is being attended to. Neuromarketing research also can potentially uncover whether different patterns of brain activation exist between genders when viewing advertisements, in order to elicit gender-specific responses.

Neuromarketing research may also uncover the type and intensity of emotions aroused by certain products in consumers. For example, researchers showed that exposure to preferred brands may activate the

(Continued)

(Continued)

brain's reward system (Schaefer, Knuth, & Rumpel, 2011; Schaefer & Rotte, 2007). In one of these studies, participants were shown the trademark logos of different car manufacturers while their brains were being imaged by fMRI. The degree of activity in the striatum, a brain area activated when rewards are obtained, was positively correlated with the degree to which brands are associated with sports and luxury attributions. In contrast, brain activity in the striatum was negatively correlated with brands that are more easily chosen by rational choice (Schaefer & Rotte, 2007). The results of this study are shown in Figure 15.24.

FIGURE 15.24

(a) fMRI showing activation of the striatum, a brain area activated when subjects receive rewards. (b) Top: Positive correlation between the degree of activity in the striatum and the extent to which sports and luxury attributions are associated with a brand. Bottom: Negative correlation between the extent to which rational choice is attributed to a brand and the degree of activity in the striatum.

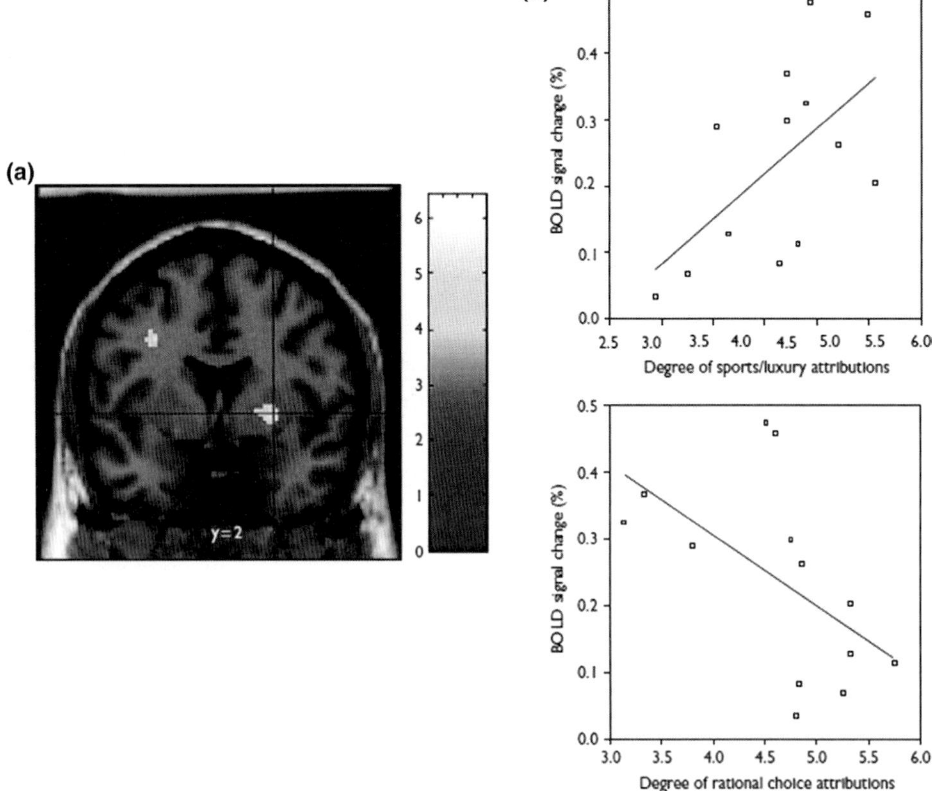

Schaefer, M., & M. Rotte. (2007). Favorite brands as cultural objects modulate reward circuit. *Neuroreport 18*(2): 141–145. With permission from Wolters Kluwer.

GLOSSARY

Abductors: Muscles that move body parts away from the midline of the body.

Aberrant salience hypothesis: The hypothesis that excessive dopamine release results in external and internal stimuli that have no particular importance becoming exaggeratedly salient, giving rise to delusions and hallucinations.

Absolute refractory period: The voltage at which further depolarization of the neuron is impossible and another action potential cannot be initiated in that neuron.

Accessory olfactory bulb: The part of the olfactory bulb that receives projections from the vomeronasal organ.

Accommodation: The eye's ability to keep objects in focus with changing distance.

Across-neuron response pattern theory: The idea that precise information about stimuli is encoded not by single neurons but by the response patterns of populations of neurons.

Actin filaments: Also called microfilaments; the smallest of the cytoskeletal elements.

Action potential: Also known as a nerve impulse; the conduction of an electrical charge within a neuron.

Activation threshold: The minimal amount of depolarization that must occur for an action potential to be initiated, which is about −55 mV.

Active zones: The areas of the presynaptic axon terminal where synaptic vesicles bind to the axon terminal's membrane.

Activity-dependent synaptic plasticity: The change in the strength of synapses that occurs as a result of repeated experience.

Addiction: Drug abuse that is characterized by the presence of tolerance and withdrawal symptoms.

Adductors: Muscles that bring body parts closer to the midline of the body.

Adoption studies: Studies that compare individuals who share the same parents but who were adopted into different families.

Adult growth hormone deficiency (AGHD): Abnormally low levels of growth hormone in adults with disease or trauma that affects the hypothalamus or pituitary.

Adult neural stem/progenitor cells (NSPCs): Cells that give rise to adult neurogenesis. They have been found mainly in the dentate gyrus of the hippocampus and the subventricular zone.

Affective blindsight: The phenomenon in which patients with blindsight react reliably to the emotional stimuli presented to their blind visual field.

Affective dimension of pain: The perceived unpleasantness of the pain-inducing stimulus.

Affective neuroscience: A branch of behavioral neuroscience in which researchers focus on the neurobiological processes that underlie emotions.

Afferent nerve fiber: Sensory nerve fibers that are associated with and stimulated by nonneuronal capsules.

Afferent pathway: A pathway through which trains of action potentials course through sensory neurons in the direction of the spinal cord.

Agency: The feeling that you are the cause of your own thoughts and actions.

Aggression: A type of hostile social behavior aimed at inflicting damage or harm on others.

Agonists: Drugs that bind to receptors to mimic the effects of the neurotransmitter that normally binds to it.

All-or-none law: The fact that more stimulation than is necessary for the neuron to be depolarized to threshold will not result in a stronger action potential.

Allosteric modulation: When different chemicals can regulate the activity of a channel by each having their own receptor site on that same channel.

Alpha, beta, theta, and delta: Brain waves that differ in amplitude and/or frequency; identified by EEG.

Altruism: Giving or helping behavior strictly for the good of others. The behavior is often regarded to be selfless or without regard for any personal gain or satisfaction.

Alzheimer's disease: A degenerative brain disease characterized by the severe and progressive loss of memory and other thinking skills to the point where self-care is no longer possible.

Amelioride-sensitive Na^+ channels: Sodium channels that are blocked by the drug amelioride.

Amnesia: Memory deficits resulting from brain damage or psychological trauma.

Amyloid hypothesis: The hypothesis that Alzheimer's disease results from an accumulation of the peptide beta-amyloid, which forms plaques that cause synaptic dysfunction, inflammation, and neuronal death.

Amyloid precursor protein: A transmembrane protein that is a precursor to beta-amyloid.

Anabolic-androgenic steroids: Drugs designed to mimic the muscle-building (anabolic) and masculinizing (androgenic) effects of male steroids.

Anhedonia: The inability to feel pleasure.

Animal studies: In the context of gene-environment interactions, studies in which animals of different genetic strains are exposed to different environments.

Anosmia: The loss of the sense of smell.

Antagonistic muscle: A muscle that directly counteracts the actions of another muscle.

Antagonists: Drugs that block the actions of a neurotransmitter by binding to its receptors.

Anterograde amnesia: The inability to form new memories since brain damage has occurred.

Antidromic conduction: Movement of an action potential toward the cell body.

Anxiety: An adaptive emotional state characterized by a feeling of worry or nervousness directed toward a future event, accompanied by a state of hypervigilance.

Anxiety disorders: A group of psychological disorders whose symptoms include excessive anxiety, fear, and worry, which give rise to abnormally strong avoidance and escapist tendencies.

Aphasia: The loss of an individual's ability to speak.

Apoptosis: Organized cell death that results from cellular injury.

Arcuate nucleus: A region of the hypothalamus involved in the regulation of food intake.

Arousal: The state of physiological activity of an organism.

Arousal continuum: The continuum of arousal states, associated with various activities, ranging from low to high.

Arousal theory (activation theory): The theory proposing that an organism's motivation to act is based on the organism's state of physiological activity.

Ascending arousal system (AAS): A wakefulness-promoting system that includes areas of the brainstem.

Ascending fibers: Nerves through which sensory information travels to the brain.

Associative learning: A change in behavior that results from the association between stimuli.

Attention: The ability to select a stimulus, focus on it, sustain that focus, and shift that focus at will.

Attentional set shifting task: A task that measures attention and cognitive flexibility.

Attenuator model: An early-selection model in which some sensory information is attenuated rather than being completely filtered out from further perceptual analysis.

Attractivity: A female's stimulus value in evoking a sexual response in a male.

Atypical antidepressants: Antidepressant drugs that inhibit the reuptake of both dopamine and norepinephrine as well as those that inhibit the reuptake of serotonin and norepinephrine.

Auditory nerve: Axons of ganglion cells (also called the vestibulocochlear nerve or cranial nerve VIII).

Autocrine hormone: A hormone that binds to receptors located on the cell that released it to regulate its function.

Autogenic inhibition reflex: A reflex that relaxes the muscle by inhibiting motor neurons in response to an overly strong muscle contraction.

Autonoetic consciousness: The ability to reflect upon past events while being aware that those are your own memories.

Axoaxonic synapse: A synapse between two axons.

Axodendritic synapse: A synapse between an axon and a dendrite.

Axon: An outgrowth of neurons through which action potentials are conducted.

Axon hillock: The point of contact between the soma and the beginning of the axon.

Axon terminal: The part of the axon farthest from the cell body; stores and releases neurotransmitters.

Axoplasmic transport: The transport of materials from one part of the cell to another via microtubules.

Axosomatic synapse: A synapse between an axon and a cell body.

Balint syndrome: A syndrome characterized by simultanagnosia, optic ataxia, and oculomotor apraxia due to damage to the parieto-occipital region.

Basal cells: Cells that remain undifferentiated and that can be incorporated into papillae to take the form of taste receptor cells when they need to be replenished.

Basic emotions: A subset of discrete emotions thought to be universal across cultures.

Basilar membrane: The membrane within the organ of Corti on which hair cells are situated.

Behavioral estrus: The period during which female animals mate, corresponding to vaginal proestrus, which is coordinated to occur just before ovulation when a mature egg is released from the ovary, ready to be fertilized.

Behavioral genetics: The field of study that seeks to understand how the variation of a trait in a population is related to the variation of genes within that population.

Behavioral neuroscience: The scientific study of how brain activity influences behavior.

Behavioral tolerance: When a person has learned to compensate for the drug's effects.

Beta-amyloid plaques: Plaques formed by an accumulation of the beta-amyloid peptide, which is derived from a larger protein called amyloid precursor protein.

Binding problem: The question of how features of experience are processed by distinct brain areas and neural systems but experienced as a unified whole.

Binocular rivalry: The phenomenon in which perception spontaneously switches between two different images that are presented simultaneously to each eye.

Bipolar neuron: A neuron that has a single dendrite and axon, each exiting opposite sides of the soma.

Blastocyst: A fluid-filled ball that contains a mass of cells.

Blindsight: The phenomenon observed in people with cortical blindness who can make accurate guesses about stimuli while at the same time not being visually aware of them.

Blood-brain barrier: The protective barrier formed by the cells of the brain's blood vessels, which block or slow the passage of harmful molecules to the brain.

Body ownership: The perception that one's body belongs to the self.

Border cells: Cells that record the location of boundaries in the rats' environment.

Bottom-up control of attention: Also known as stimulus-driven attention, in which stimuli that are currently unattended to, surprising, or unexpected shift your attention from what you are currently attending to.

Brain death: A condition in which life-sustaining activity of the brainstem cannot be detected.

Brain reward areas: Brain areas that provide a sense of pleasure when stimulated.

Broadly tuned: Refers to how neurons can respond to different types of stimuli.

Broca's area: The area of the third convolution of the left frontal lobe, associated with speech production.

cAMP-responsive element-binding protein (CREB): A protein that puts into motion the transcription of DNA by messenger ribonucleic acid (mRNA).

Cannon-Bard theory: A theory of emotions in which physiological arousal and emotional experience can occur at the same time and are independent of each other.

Categorization: The process by which signals from the body are labeled using knowledge about emotions, past experiences, and the current situation.

Cell assembly: A group of neurons that fire together in response to a stimulus.

Cell theory: The idea that the cell is the basic functional unit of all living things.

Cell-adaptation theory: The idea that functional tolerance occurs when neurons become progressively adjusted to the effects of a drug.

Cell-adhesion molecules (CAMs): Molecules that play a crucial role in synapse formation.

Cellular consolidation: The early and local (within the same brain area) molecular processes that occur shortly after learning.

Cellular level of analysis: The study of the morphology and physiological properties of cells within the nervous system.

Central canal: The hollow center of the spinal cord.

Central nervous system: The division of the nervous system that includes the brain and the spinal cord.

Cerebral dominance: The idea that the left hemisphere is dominant in the control of speech function.

Cerebrospinal fluid (CSF): Fluid that cushions the brain and spinal cord.

Chemical messengers: A substance that mediates effects within the cell that produces it or that affects the function of other cells.

Chemoaffinity hypothesis: The idea that axons find their way to their targets by following a chemical signal.

Chemoattraction: The attraction of growth cones toward chemical cues.

Chemorepulsion: The repulsion of growth cones away from a chemical source.

Chemotaxis: The guidance of growth cones by chemical cues.

Chemotopic organization: The concept that different areas within the gustatory cortex are dedicated to the perception of each taste.

Chinese room: A thought experiment designed to show that computers manipulate symbols by how they are organized and ordered but, unlike humans, do so without purpose, meaning, or understanding of what they are doing.

Chronesthesia: The awareness of the passage of subjective time.

Cilia: Hairlike projections on which olfactory receptors are located.

Circadian rhythm: Physiological, behavioral, or psychological events that occur over an approximate 24-hour cycle.

Circuit of addiction: A circuit of brain areas associated with the stages of the cycle of addiction.

Classical conditioning: A form of associative learning in which a neutral stimulus is associated with a meaningful stimulus to create a reflexive response.

Clostridium botulinum: A bacterium found in improperly conserved foods. It is better known as botulinum toxin.

Cochlea: The snail-shaped and fluid-filled organ of the inner ear.

Cocktail party effect: The phenomenon in which selective attention is paid to a specific stimulus among a range of other stimuli.

Cognitive empathy: The ability to cognitively engage in adopting another person's point of view to understand that person's experience.

Cognitive level of analysis: The study of the neurobiological basis of higher mental processes.

Cognitive map: A map within the brains of animals that stores associations among environmental cues.

Cognitive neuroscience: A branch of behavioral neuroscience that focuses on the processes within the brain that are associated with cognitive functions such as reasoning, problem solving, memory, and attention.

Cold defense: Output from the hypothalamus in response to potentially threatening cooling of the body.

Color afterimage: An image of an object that persists after having stared at it for several seconds.

Coma: A state of unresponsiveness that results from brain injury. Patients in a coma have closed eyes, cannot be awakened, and do not respond to stimulation.

Common progenitor cells: Cells that give rise to neuronal and glial progenitor cells, which differentiate into neurons and glia.

Compulsions: Behaviors that the person with obsessive-compulsive disorder feels compelled to perform.

Computed tomography (CT scan): A method in which X-ray images are taken from many angles and processed by a computer to produce virtual cross-sections, permitting the examination of structures deep within the brain.

Congenital adrenal hyperplasia (CAH): A genetic disorder in which people lack one of the enzymes used by the adrenal glands to produce cortisol and melanocorticoids and have higher than normal levels of testosterone.

Conjunction search: A visual search based on focusing attention on a combination of specific features.

Connexins: Proteins that allow the passage of ions from one neuron to the other at electrical synapses.

Conscious stimulus: A stimulus that gives rise to conscious awareness due to its high strength and the level of attention it elicits.

Contact attraction: The attraction of growth cones through direct contact with chemicals.

Contact guidance: The guidance of growth cones induced by direct contact with chemicals.

Contact repulsion: The repulsion of growth cones through direct contact with chemicals.

Content of consciousness: The extent to which ongoing stimuli are being processed.

Convergence: The ratio of connectivity between photoreceptors and retinal ganglion cells.

Cooperating: In the prisoner's dilemma, a decision that has the good of both participants in mind.

Corpus callosum: A bundle of nerve fibers that permits communication between both hemispheres.

Cortex: The outermost layer of the brain.

Cortical blindness: People for whom the source of blindness is damage to the primary visual cortex.

Corticogenesis: The process by which the cortex develops from the generation of neuronal and glial progenitor cells.

Cortico-thalamic core: Refers to the dense connectivity between the thalamus and the cortex.

Cortisol: A hormone released by the adrenal glands in response to stress.

Cost-benefit analysis theory of helping: The idea that we may help others only if the cost of helping, such as any potential threat or danger, is not too high.

Covert attention: The ability to shift attention from stimulus to stimulus without reorienting sensory receptors.

Covert behavior: Behavior that cannot readily be observed, such as thinking, remembering, paying attention, experiencing emotions, and a range of others.

Crystallized intelligence: Cognitive skills that depend on accumulated wisdom, knowledge, expertise, and vocabulary.

CSTC model of OCD: Dysfunction in a loop that includes brain areas in the prefrontal cortex, orbitofrontal cortex, basal ganglia, and thalamus is thought to contribute to the symptoms of OCD.

Cyberball: A video game designed to test emotional and neurological reactions to social exclusion.

Cycle: One complete oscillation of a wave.

Cycle of addiction: A theory that views addiction as progressing through three stages.

Cytoskeleton: The collection of filaments and tubules that gives the cell its shape, rigidity, and ability to move.

Dark adaptation: The eye's ability to adjust to low levels of light.

Dark current: The process that results in rods being constantly depolarized in the dark.

Decibels: A measure of the intensity of sound.

Decision neuroscience: A branch of behavioral neuroscience that focuses on the neurobiological basis of choice behavior; sometimes known as neuroeconomics.

Declarative memories: Long-term memories that require the conscious recollection of information.

Decortication: A procedure in which the cortex is removed to varying degrees.

Deep brain stimulation (DBS): Inferring the functions of a particular brain area through the administration of a low-voltage electrical current to that area.

Defecting: In the prisoner's dilemma, when a participant decides based only on his or her own best interest.

Defeminization: The loss of the ability of males to display behaviors that are characteristic of females.

Delayed nonmatching-to-place (DNMP) task: A test used to assess spatial memory.

Delayed nonmatching-to-sample (DNMS) task: A test used to assess object-recognition memory.

Delayed-response task: A behavioral task that requires holding a stimulus in working memory, after it has disappeared from view, to later make a correct choice.

Delusions: Misrepresentations of reality. Some common delusions in schizophrenia are delusions of grandeur, delusions of persecution, and paranoid delusions.

Dementia: An umbrella term used to designate a group of symptoms shared by several neurodegenerative diseases.

Dendrite: An outgrowth of the neuron at which connections between neurons are typically made.

Dendrodendritic synapse: A synapse between two dendrites.

Deoxyribonucleic acid (DNA): A molecule composed of sequences of smaller molecules called nucleotides, bound together by molecules of sugar and phosphate.

Depolarization: To reduce polarity (i.e., to make less negative); the inside of the neuron becomes less electrically negative relative to the outside.

Depressants: Drugs that slow activity in the central and peripheral nervous systems.

Dermatome: An area of the skin innervated by a segment of the spinal cord.

Descending fibers: Nerves that carry information from the brain.

Descent with modification: The idea that current forms of life evolved from preexisting forms.

Deuteranopia: A type of red-green color deficiency due to the absence of M-cones.

***Diagnostic and Statistical Manual of Mental Disorders* (*DSM*):** The manual published by the American Psychiatric

Association that provides diagnostic criteria for the various psychological disorders.

Dichotic listening: An experimental set-up in which a spoken message is played into a participant's ear while another message is played into the participant's other ear.

Differentiation: The process by which progenitor cells give rise to neurons and glia.

Diffusion: The process by which molecules tend to move from an area of high concentration to an area of low concentration.

Dimensional theories of emotions: Theories in which emotions can be broken down into basic elements and individual differences exist in the way people experience emotions.

Direct pathway (motor): Composed of the axons of neurons located in the motor cortex.

Direct pathway (to the amygdala): Also known as the low road and "quick and dirty road"; brings sensory information from the thalamus directly to the amygdala.

Directional selectivity: A property associated with complex cells in the primary visual cortex, which best respond when bars of light moving in a particular direction are projected onto the retina.

Disconnection hypothesis: The hypothesis that the normal cognitive declines that occur during aging are due to the degeneration of white fiber tracts that connect the brain areas relevant to cognitive functions.

Discrete theories of emotions: Theories in which a small set of emotions can be distinguished from one another and represented by particular response patterns in the brain, physiological processes, and facial expressions.

Dispositional tolerance: When the body becomes progressively better at breaking down and eliminating the drug.

Docking: The process by which synaptic vesicles align to the area from which they will release the neurotransmitters they contain.

Dopamine hypothesis: The idea that a dysfunctional dopamine system is at the core of the symptoms observed in schizophrenia.

Dopamine ramping: The way in which dopamine is released in increasing amounts as the steps required to obtain a reward are completed.

Dorsal column–medial lemniscus system (DCML): The pathway followed by afferent neurons that conduct information from mechanoreceptors to the somatosensory cortex.

Dorsal roots: Areas through which sensory neurons enter the spinal cord.

Dorsal-frontoparietal system: Includes areas of the dorsal-posterior parietal cortex along the intraparietal sulcus and the frontal eye field in the frontal cortex. It is involved in the top-down control of attention.

Drive: An internal state that pushes an organism to fulfill a deficiency.

Drug: A chemical or mixture of chemicals that alters physiological function.

Drug abuse: Using drugs in a way that causes physical and/or psychological harm to self or to others.

Dual hormone/serotonergic hypothesis: The hypothesis that impulsive aggression is related to high levels of testosterone in the presence of low cortisol and low serotonin.

Dualism: The philosophical position that mind and body are distinct and that they could exist independently of each other.

Early-filtering model: An early-selection model in which only sensory information that is selectively attended to makes it through a filter leading to further perceptual analysis.

Early-selection models: Selective attention models in which sensory information is selected before any perceptual analysis is completed.

Easy problem: Explaining mental phenomena that are testable by standard methods of science.

Ectoderm: The germ layer that develops into the nervous system and the skin.

Ectotherms: Animals that have no internal mechanisms to regulate their body temperature.

Edwin Smith Papyrus: A medical papyrus that seems to have been written around 1600 B.C.E., during the third dynasty of pharaohs.

Efferent copy: A copy of a motor command sent by the primary motor cortex to another brain area.

Efferent pathway: A pathway through which trains of action potentials course through motor neurons in the direction of the periphery.

Eight-arm radial maze: A maze consisting of an octagonal central platform with an arm radiating from each side.

Electroencephalography (EEG): A method in which brain function is inferred by detecting differences in the electrical energy emitted from different brain areas.

Electromagnetic energy: Light energy.

Electromagnetic spectrum: The range of all wavelengths of light.

Electromyography (EMG): Recording of movements of the body through measuring changes in the electrical activity of muscles.

Electrooculography (EOG): Recording of eye movements through changes in the electrical activity of eye muscles.

Electrostatic pressure: The phenomenon by which ions that are of the same charge repel each other and ions that are of opposite charge attract each other.

Embryonic disk: The mass of cells that develop within the blastocyst.

Emotion: An automatic physiological, behavioral, and cognitive reaction to external or internal events.

Emotional contagion: The spread of an emotion from one person to another.

Emotional empathy: The ability to experience emotions automatically triggered by observing the emotional states of others.

Emotional experience: Subjective feelings that are labeled to identify particular emotions.

Emotional expression: The covert and overt behaviors that accompany emotions.

Empathy: The ability to understand or feel the emotions experienced by another person from that person's perspective.

Encoding: Converting the information acquired by your senses into patterns of activity within groups of neurons within the brain.

Endocrine glands: Glands that produce and release hormones in various regions of the body.

Endocrine hormone: A hormone released into the bloodstream that affects the function of cells at some distance from the source of release.

Endocrine signaling: Communication mediated by hormones, having their effects by binding to receptors on cells at distant locations in the body.

Endocrine system: The system of glands that release hormones at various locations within the body.

Endocytosis: The process by which molecules are taken up into a cell.

Endoderm: The germ layer that gives rise to the digestive system, lungs, and glands.

Endogenous attention: Self-directed and voluntary attention to a stimulus.

Endogenous opioids: Opioids that are naturally present in the nervous system.

Endotherms: Animals that can regulate their body temperature through internal mechanisms.

Energy homeostasis: The process that maintains cellular metabolism.

Engram: The stable representation of the stimuli in the cell assembly.

Engram cells: Neurons that become active during learning and are reactivated with the presentation of cues related to the context of learning.

Entrained rhythm: A rhythm regulated by external cues, such as light or heat.

Epigenetics: The study of changes in gene expression with no changes in DNA sequences, which can occur naturally or through the influence of environmental factors.

Episodic memories: Declarative memories that comprise life events; rich in contextual details including the time and place in which an event occurred.

Equilibrium potential: The voltage across the membrane (V_m) at which the forces of electrostatic pressure and diffusion counteract each other.

Euphoria: An enhanced sense of pleasure, excitement, and well-being.

Evaluating: Determining whether a stimulus is internally or externally generated.

Event-related potentials (ERP): Small voltage changes, called waveforms, in brain areas responsive to specific events or stimuli.

Exaptation: The adaptation of a trait that differs from the one it was selected for.

Excitatory neurotransmitter: A neurotransmitter that binds to receptors that trigger the opening of Na^+ channels, which results in the depolarization of the neuronal membrane.

Excitatory postsynaptic potential (EPSP): A postsynaptic potential that causes the voltage of the membrane to move toward the activation threshold.

Executive functions: Brain functions, attributed to the frontal lobes, that include planning, judgment, attention, problem solving, working memory, and decision making.

Executive system for wakefulness: A system that includes orexinergic neurons in the lateral hypothalamus.

Executive theory: A theory that theory of mind is dependent on our ability to inhibit our own thoughts and behavior (inhibitory control), as well as take our own perspective when trying to attribute mental states to others.

Exocrine hormone: A hormone released into an organism's external environment.

Exocytosis: The process by which molecules are exported out of a cell.

Exogenous attention: Attention drawn toward a stimulus in a reflexive and involuntary manner.

Explanatory gap: The problem in explaining how neural mechanisms are linked to subjective experience.

Extensors: Muscles that move two body parts away from each other, such as the triceps, which move the forearm and upper arm away from each other.

Exteroception: The sensing of innocuous touch, pain, and itch.

Extracellular recording: A method by which a microelectrode is inserted into the fluid surrounding neurons to record electrical currents generated by the neurons in the electrode's vicinity.

Extrapyramidal tracts: Tracts of the indirect pathway.

False-belief task: A task that assesses whether a child realizes that another person can hold beliefs that differ from his or her own.

Family studies: Studies that compare individuals at high risk of developing a disorder, because they have relatives with the disorder, to individuals at low risk who do not have relatives with the disorder.

Fast-twitch muscle fibers: Muscle fibers that are strong but fatigue easily; important for brief, unsustained efforts.

Fear: An adaptive emotional state triggered by an immediate and readily identifiable threat, which is associated with being startled, freezing, or escape.

Fear circuit: The circuit of brain areas centered on the amygdala thought to be involved in the learning and expression of fear.

Fear conditioning: A procedure in which animals (typically rats) are exposed to a mild foot shock simultaneously to hearing a tone, resulting in the conditioning of a fear response.

Feature attention: Attention directed at a specific feature of an object.

Feature integration theory (FIT): A proposed solution to the binding problem, in which attention is the glue that binds the various features of objects.

Feature search: A visual search based on focusing attention on a specific feature.

Fetal alcohol spectrum disorders (FASDs): A group of disorders associated with a mother drinking alcohol during pregnancy, which affects the development of the baby; characterized by abnormal facial features, short height, low body weight, low intelligence, and behavioral problems.

Filopodia: Thin membranes that protrude from the axon's cytoplasm and are part of its growth cone.

First-order neurons: Afferent neurons associated with mechanoreceptors.

Fissures: Large grooves that can be used to delineate cortical areas.

Flavor: The total perceptual experience you get from food.

Flexors: Muscles that bring two body parts closer together, such as the biceps that bring together forearm and upper arm.

Fluid intelligence: The ability to think quickly and abstractly. It includes the capacity of working memory and processing speed.

Fluid-mechanical theory: The idea that movement can be explained by the movement of fluids, called animal spirits, through hollow tubes in the body.

Focal task-specific dystonia: A movement disorder that interferes with movements involved in highly practiced tasks.

Foliate papillae: The papillae located along the edges in the back of the tongue.

Foramen magnum: The hole at the base of the skull through which the spinal cord passes.

Forced restraint: A condition in which animals are forcibly restrained to measure the effects of chronic stress.

Forebrain, midbrain, hindbrain: The three primary brain vesicles.

Fraternal birth order effect: Derived from the observation that gay men have a greater number of older brothers than heterosexual men.

Free running rhythm: A rhythm that is self-regulated, not requiring any external cues.

Frontostriatal circuit: A network of brain areas highly involved in impulse control, which includes the inferior frontal gyrus and the ventrolateral prefrontal cortex and the striatum.

Functional brain imaging: An imaging technique that permits the measurement of subjects' brain activity while performing a task.

Functional magnetic resonance imaging (fMRI): Inferring brain function using MRI technology to image the brain in a way that detects the amount of oxygen used by neurons.

Functional plasticity: Functional changes in a brain area to compensate for damage to another area or changes in the body.

Functional tolerance: When neurons progressively become adjusted to the effects of a drug.

Fungiform papillae: The papillae located on the anterior surface of the tongue.

Game theory: A branch of mathematics devised to explain the behavior of animals in nature and of people in social or political contexts.

Ganglia: A collection of cell bodies.

Gap junctions: The points of connection between presynaptic and postsynaptic neurons at electrical synapses.

Gastrula: The structure that develops from the blastocyst and forms the germ layers.

Gastrulation: The process by which the blastocyst develops into the gastrula.

Gate control theory: The theory by which the transmission of nociceptive information to the brain can be inhibited by the activity of mechanoreceptors.

Gene-environment interactions: Interactions between genetic inheritance and environmental factors.

Genes: Once referred to as the basic functional units of heredity, genes are sequences of deoxyribonucleic acid (DNA), some of which code for proteins.

Genetics: The study of inherited traits and their variation.

Genotype: Every individual's unique genetic constitution.

Germ layers: Three layers of cells that develop into the different tissues of the body.

GH therapy: The therapeutic administration of growth hormone in individuals with abnormally low levels of the hormone.

Gill-withdrawal reflex: The reflexive withdrawal of the sea slug's gill as a defense mechanism when its siphon is touched.

Glabrous skin: Hairless skin.

Glasgow coma scale: A scale used to assess whether a patient has slipped into a coma. It measures the extent to which patients can open their eyes and perform verbal and motor responses.

Glia: Cells that support neuronal function and clear debris, toxins, and bacteria from the brain.

Glioblasts: Immature glial cells that differentiate from neuronal progenitor cells.

Global workspace theory: The idea that consciousness arises from the activity of brain modules that process and bind the features of a specific kind of information, which is then broadcast throughout the brain.

Glomeruli: Structures that contain different types of neurons.

Golgi tendon organ: A structure located in tendons that senses changes in muscle tension; responsible for the autogenic inhibition reflex.

G-protein: A protein that, when activated, travels on the inside of the neuron, where it can influence its function.

G-protein-coupled receptor: A type of receptor to which a G-protein is attached.

Grid cells: Cells located in the entorhinal cortex that record the metrics of space.

Growth cone: Processes at the tip of growing axons that possess a structure capable of changing its structure in response to chemical signals.

Grueneberg ganglion: An organ involved in detecting alarm signals from conspecifics.

Gustatory chemoreceptors: Taste receptor cells.

Gustatory cortex: The area of the brain that processes taste.

Gustatory pathway: The pattern of neuronal connections from taste receptor cells to the gustatory cortex.

Gyri: Ridges (or bumps) on the surface of the cortex.

Habituation: A decrease in response to a stimulus with its repeated occurrence.

Hair cells: Receptor cells responsible for hearing.

Hallucinations: Perceptions of sensory events that are not occurring in reality, which can involve any of the senses.

Hallucinogens: Drugs that alter perceptions to the point of creating hallucinations.

Handedness: The preferred usage of one hand over the other.

Hard problem: Explaining how brain activity produces subjective experience.

Head-direction cells: Cells located in the subiculum and other brain areas that indicate the orientation of the rat's head.

Heat defense: Output from the hypothalamus in response to potentially threatening heating of the body.

Hebbian modification: The process by which reverberating activity strengthens the connections between the neurons in a cell assembly.

Hedonic coldspots: Brain areas that enhance disgust reactions when stimulated with opioids.

Hedonic hotspots: Brain areas that enhance "liking" reactions when stimulated with opioids.

Hedonics of food: Whether a food is perceived to be pleasant or unpleasant.

Hemispheres: The two halves of the brain.

Hemispheric asymmetry: When functions are associated with either the right or left hemisphere.

Heritability estimates: The proportion of variation in a trait that can be accounted for by genetic variation in a population.

Hermann grid: An optical illusion often used to demonstrate lateral inhibition.

Hertz: The number of cycles per second.

High vocal center (HVC): The brain area at the center of a song-learning system in song birds.

High-threshold mechanoreceptors (HTMRs): Mechanoreceptors that respond to harmful stimulation such as pain.

Histology: The scientific study of cells and tissues.

Homeostasis: The tendency of biological systems to maintain a stable internal environment in response to stimuli that challenge stability.

Hormones: Substances released into the bloodstream that have their effects by binding to receptors on cells at distant locations.

Humoral theory of sleep regulation: The idea that sleep-inducing chemicals accumulate in the body during wakefulness.

Hyper-scanning fMRI (h-fMRI): A method in which the brains of multiple participants are imaged simultaneously to determine how they may influence each other.

Hyperthyroidism: A condition in which the thyroid gland produces too much thyroxine.

Hypertonic: When salt is overly concentrated relative to water inside blood cells.

Hypofrontality theory of schizophrenia: The idea that people with schizophrenia have reduced activity in the prefrontal cortex.

Hypophyseal portal system: The mesh of small blood vessels that connect the hypothalamus to the anterior pituitary.

Hypothalamic inhibiting hormones: Hormones that inhibit the release of hormones from the pituitary.

Hypothalamic releasing hormones: Hormones that cause the release of hormones from the pituitary.

Hypothalamic-pituitary-adrenal (HPA) axis: The hormonal link between the hypothalamus and the adrenal glands via the pituitary. The HPA axis is activated in the presence of environmental stressors.

Hypothyroidism: A condition in which the thyroid gland does not produce enough thyroxine.

Illusory conjunction: A visual task from which FIT is derived, in which the features of two distinct stimuli are erroneously conjoined when presented briefly.

Implicit racial prejudice: Prejudice shown in people who do not endorse any form of prejudice toward other groups but who demonstrate a negative bias on evaluation.

Impulse control: The ability to inhibit thoughts and actions that lead to immediate gratification in favor of those that are oriented toward the fulfillment of goals.

Impulsive aggression: Also known as defensive or affective aggression; occurs in response to perceived threats.

Inattentional blindness: A phenomenon by which a stimulus of high strength fails to be perceived due to the lack of attention to it.

Incentive-salience theory: The theory in which two components of motivated behaviors, "wanting" and "liking," are involved in the development of drug addiction and the stimulation of dopamine pathways is not responsible for the pleasurable effects of drugs.

Indirect pathway (motor): Composed of the axons of neurons originating in subcortical motor nuclei.

Indirect pathway (to the amygdala): Also known as the high road and "slow but accurate road"; brings sensory information from the thalamus indirectly through the cortex.

Inferior colliculus: A part of the tectum that plays a role in processing auditory information.

Inferior view: The brain as viewed from the bottom.

Inhibitory neurotransmitter: A neurotransmitter that binds to receptors that trigger the opening of Cl^- channels, which results in the hyperpolarization of the neuronal membrane.

Inhibitory postsynaptic potential (IPSP): A postsynaptic potential that causes the voltage of the neuronal membrane to move away from and below the activation threshold and even below the resting membrane potential.

Innocuous touch: A type of touch that does not include harmful stimulation such as pain or itch.

Instrumental aggression: Also known as predatory aggression; cold-blooded (unemotional), often premeditated actions directed toward others.

Integration: The integration of attitudes, goals, traits, memories, and values into a unified concept of self.

Intentionality: The idea that consciousness includes mental states that are about something.

Intermediate filaments: Also called neurofilaments; of intermediate size between microtubules and actin filaments.

Interneuron: A neuron that connects sensory neurons to motor neurons.

Interoception: The sensing of the body's physiological condition, such as hunger and thirst.

Intracellular recording: A method by which tiny electrodes are inserted directly inside neurons to record their electrical activity.

Intracranial self-stimulation: A procedure in which animals are trained to press a lever to receive electrical stimulation through electrodes implanted in these areas.

Intracrine hormone: A hormone that mediates effects within the same cell that synthesized it.

Intrusive syndrome: The intrusive thoughts, such as unwanted memories of events, and nightmares that a person with PTSD experiences.

Inverse agonists: Drugs that bind to a neurotransmitter receptor but exert opposite effects.

Involuntary muscles: Muscles that are not under conscious control.

Ion: An electrically charged particle.

Ionotropic receptors: Receptors located on ion channels that directly affect the cell's function.

Iowa gambling task: A task used to assess the role played by emotions in decision-making processes in brain-damaged patients.

Isotropic fractionation: A method by which the number of cells in a brain area of interest can be estimated.

James-Lange theory: A theory in which emotions arise from the brain's interpretation of bodily changes induced by sensory events.

Joy of giving: Giving was shown to have the same neurobiological basis as different types of rewards, such as money, drugs, and food.

Junctional folds: Deep indentations in the membranes of muscle cells that are rich in neurotransmitter receptors.

K-complexes: Slight negative deflections in brain waves (wave movement is exaggerated downward) followed by a positive deflection (exaggerated upward).

Kin selection: The idea that we more readily choose to help others who are related to us.

Klüver-Bucy syndrome: A set of symptoms, including a loss of fear and flattened emotions, that follow the removal of the temporal lobes.

Koniocellular (K-cells): Cells of the LGN that receive information from short-wavelength cones in the retina as well as from bistratified retinal ganglion cells, which convey information about spatial resolution.

Lamellipodia: A thin sheetlike membrane that is part of an axon's growth cone.

Late-filtering model: A selective attention model in which perceptual systems process all the information that enters them, followed by an unconscious decision concerning which information to attend to.

Lateral and ventral corticospinal tracts: The individual tracts of the direct pathway.

Lateral inhibition: How receptors in the surround of on-center receptive fields have inhibitory connections with receptors located in the center of the same receptive fields.

Lateral olfactory tract: Formed by the axons of mitral/tuft cells, which transmit olfactory information to the cortex.

Lateral parabrachial nucleus (LBN): The region of the brainstem involved in temperature regulation.

Lateral view: The surface of the brain as viewed from one of its sides.

LBN-POA pathway: The pathway through which body temperature is conveyed to the LBP and POA for temperature regulation.

Learning: The mechanisms by which new information is acquired through experience.

Lesioning: Creating brain damage in experimental animals to determine the functions of particular areas.

Level of analysis: Refers to the location, scale, or size of what is being studied.

Level of consciousness: The extent to which a person is awake.

Ligand: Neurotransmitters or other chemicals, such as drugs, that bind to neurotransmitter receptors.

Ligand-binding assay: Adding a radioactive label to a molecule to trace its location in the tissue.

Ligand-gated ion channels: Channels that open in response to the binding of ligands to their receptors.

Liking: Linked to the pleasurable sensations experienced by users when they have taken a drug.

Limbic system: A revised version of the Papez circuit that includes the amygdala, septum, and prefrontal cortex.

Lobes: Anatomical subdivisions of the brain.

Localization of function: The theory that individual brain areas are dedicated to distinct functions.

Locked-in syndrome: A condition characterized by intact awareness, wakefulness, and cognitive function while the person is paralyzed and unable to speak.

Long-term depression (LTD): The decrease in the efficiency of a synapse following low-frequency electrical stimulation.

Long-term memory: A memory register of potentially unlimited capacity for both the amount of information it can store and the time for which information is retained.

Long-term plasticity: Changes in synaptic efficacy that last more than a few minutes and are thought to be the basis for the formation of long-term memories.

Long-term potentiation (LTP): The increase in the efficiency of a synapse following high-frequency electrical stimulation.

Lordosis: The position observed when a female animal crouches so that the vagina is brought into a horizontal position with the tail deflected to the side.

Lordosis pathway: A set of neuroanatomical regions that, when activated, result in contraction of the appropriate set of muscles to result in lordosis.

Lower motor neurons: Motor neurons that innervate the muscles.

Low-threshold mechanoreceptors (LTMRs): Mechanoreceptors for innocuous touch. These are activated by stimuli of minimal intensity.

Lysosome: An organelle that contains digestive enzymes.

Mach bands: An illusion that makes it easier to determine where surfaces of different brightness meet.

Magnetic resonance imaging (MRI): A method by which an image of any part of the body can be created with the use of a powerful magnetic field and the emission of a resonant frequency.

Magnetoencephalography (MEG): A method in which brain function is inferred by detecting differences in the electromagnetic fields emitted from different brain areas.

Magnocellular (M-cells): Cells of the LGN that receive contrast information from the parasol ganglion cells.

Major depressive disorder (MDD): A psychological disorder characterized by episodes of extremely sad moods accompanied by a loss of pleasure in usual activities. MDD may also include sleep disruptions, changes in appetite, agitation or psychomotor retardation, somatic symptoms, feelings of worthlessness, difficulty concentrating, and recurrent thoughts of suicide.

Manipulation technique: A technique in which the structure or function of the brain is altered and the resulting effects on behavior are observed.

Maternal immune hypothesis (MIH): A hypothesis aimed at explaining the fraternal birth order effect, which states that some mothers develop an immune response to a specific substance, important for determining sexual orientation, on the Y chromosome of the male fetus.

Measurement technique: A technique in which the brain activity of subjects is measured while they are engaged in some behavioral task with the aim of identifying brain areas that might be involved in its performance.

Mechanoreceptors: Sensory receptors that detect mechanical deformations of the skin.

Melanopsin: A pigment in certain photoreceptor cells of the retina, which influences the light-dark cycle through projections to the suprachiasmatic nucleus.

Melatonin: A hormone, released by the pineal gland, that induces sleepiness.

Membrane differentiations: The combination of the active zones of the presynaptic axon terminals and postsynaptic densities of the postsynaptic dendrites.

Memory: The processes by which information is encoded, stored, and retrieved for the purposes of remembering the past, informing current behavior, and planning the future.

Memory consolidation: The process by which memories go from a temporary and fragile state to a more stable and long-lasting form.

Meninges: Three membranes that envelop the brain (and spinal cord): the pia mater, the arachnoid mater, and the dura mater.

Menstrual cycle: The regular changes that occur in the female reproductive system that make pregnancy possible.

Mental time travel: The ability to travel back in time, in your mind's eye, to reexperience an event.

Mesocortical pathway: The part of the mesocorticolimbic pathway that runs from the ventral-tegmental area to the prefrontal cortex.

Mesocorticolimbic pathway: The pathway through which dopaminergic neurons project from the ventral-tegmental area. It is subdivided into the mesocortical and mesolimbic pathways.

Mesoderm: The germ layer that gives rise to the muscles, skeleton, some of the internal organs, and the circulatory system.

Mesolimbic pathway: The part of the mesocorticolimbic pathway that runs from the ventral-tegmental area to the nucleus accumbens, amygdala, and hippocampus.

Metabolism hypothesis: The hypothesis that Alzheimer's disease and type-2 diabetes share common characteristics.

Metabotropic receptors: Receptors located on proteins embedded in the neuronal membrane that do not form channels but indirectly affect the cell's function.

Microelectrode: A tiny electrode used to measure the electrical activity of neurons.

Microscopy: The field that uses microscopes to see objects that are not visible to the naked eye.

Microtome: A laboratory instrument used to cut extremely thin sections of tissue.

Microtubules: The largest of the cytoskeletal elements.

Migration: The process during which young neurons make their way to the superficial layers of the cortex.

Mild cognitive impairment: A condition marked by short-term memory problems that worsen over about a seven-year period. These problems are associated with a progressive degeneration of the medial temporal lobes.

Mind-body problem: The age-old philosophical question concerning how the mind, which is immaterial, interacts with the material body.

Minimally conscious state: A condition in which patients show high levels of wakefulness with some signs of consciousness.

Mirror neurons: Neurons in the premotor cortex that are activated when performing an action or when watching another individual perform the same action.

Mirror test: A test designed to know whether animals and human babies are self-aware.

Mitral/tuft cells: The first neurons contacted by olfactory receptor neurons within glomeruli.

Modularity theories: Theories that an innate module that specializes in the theory of mind exists within the brain.

Molecular analysis: A study that compares the effects of different environmental conditions across individuals with different genetic makeups.

Molecular coincidence detector: A receptor that regulates the activity of a channel by detecting two events that are occurring in temporal proximity.

Molecular level of analysis: The study of the workings of the nervous system using methods that permit the study of the genes and the chemistry of proteins within neurons.

Monitoring: The ability to override habitual responses, choose among a variety of available responses, and detect errors.

Monoamine hypothesis: The idea that people with major depressive disorder have low levels of norepinephrine and serotonin.

Monoamine oxidase inhibitors: Antidepressant drugs that prevent the degradation of monoamines by monoamine oxidase.

Monochromacy: Color blindness due to the absence or failure of two of the three types of cones.

Monosynaptic pathway: A pathway to a response that requires only one synapse.

Morris water maze: A pool of water in which animals search for a submerged platform.

Motivation: The processes that determine the initiation, maintenance, direction, and termination of behavior.

Motor end plate: The area where acetylcholine receptors are located on a muscle cell.

Motor homunculus: A representation of the body mapped onto the primary motor cortex.

Motor neuron: A neuron that carries movement information from the central nervous system to the peripheral nervous system.

Motor neuron pool: All the motor neurons that innervate a single muscle.

Motor programs: Neural networks situated in the brainstem that initiate automatic and rhythmic movements such as walking; also known as central pattern generators.

Motor unit: A single motor neuron as well as all the muscle cells it innervates.

Mouth-feel: What the food feels like in your mouth.

M-pathway: The visual information pathway from the retina to the visual cortex that connects parasol retinal ganglion cells to P-cells of the LGN.

Multicomponent working memory model: A model in which working memory is thought to depend on the operations of several components: a visuospatial sketch pad, a phonological loop, an episodic buffer, and a central executive.

Multiple sclerosis: An autoimmune disease in which the myelin sheath is destroyed.

Multiple-trace theory: The idea that the hippocampus is always involved in the storage and retrieval of memories.

Multiply determined: The idea that, like other psychological disorders, major depressive disorder is determined by many interacting factors.

Multipolar neuron: A neuron that has many dendrites sticking out of one side of the soma and an axon sticking out of the other side.

Muscle spindles: Bundles of tiny muscle fibers encircled by sensory axons inside a capsule; responsible for the stretch reflex.

Myasthenia gravis: An autoimmune disease in which the body's immune system destroys the receptors for acetylcholine at the neuromuscular junction.

Myelin sheath: Fatty tissue that insulates axons.

Natural reinforcers: Activities or events that naturally provide pleasure, such as food, sex, or having a good time with friends.

Natural selection: The process by which evolution can be explained.

Nature or nurture: A once hotly debated question as to whether individual characteristics are entirely inherited or determined by environmental influences.

Need reduction theory: The theory that states that organisms are motivated by the fulfillment of needs.

Negative feedback: A mechanism by which a stimulus input causes a system to react by causing an opposite output to maintain a desired set point.

Negative reinforcement: When a behavior removes an aversive or unwanted outcome, increasing the probability that it will be repeated.

Negative symptoms: Deficits in normal emotional expression as well as avolition and anhedonia.

Negative-state release model: The idea that we help others to alleviate the negative feelings that come while observing others in distress.

***Nervenkitt*:** German word for "nerve cement"; used by Rudolf Virchow to describe the role of glia.

Nervous tissue: Tissue that makes up the nervous system. It is composed of neurons and glia.

Network of parental care: A network of brain areas known to be involved in generating and maintaining parental behavior, which consists of the median preoptic area, the amygdala, and the dopamine reward pathway.

Neural correlates of consciousness: The minimal neuronal events jointly sufficient for any one specific conscious percept.

Neural crest: Made from migrating cells of the ectoderm; gives rise to the peripheral nervous system.

Neural folds: Risen edges of the ectoderm, which fuse together to form the neural tube.

Neural groove: The depression in the central region of the ectoderm caused by the neural folds.

Neural plate: The region that spans the neural folds along with the neural groove.

Neural stem cells: Cells that emerge from the ectoderm and produce progenitor cells.

Neuroanatomy: The scientific study of the structures and organization of the nervous system.

Neuroanatomy of long-term memory: The collection of brain structures known to be involved in long-term memory.

Neuroblasts: Immature neurons that differentiate from neuronal progenitor cells.

Neurochemistry: The scientific study of how chemicals in the brain are synthesized and involved in brain function.

Neuroecology: The field that studies relationships between the brain and ecologically relevant behaviors and how they may have evolved through natural selection.

Neuroendocrinology: The scientific study of how hormones, which are chemicals that control important bodily functions, interact with the nervous system.

Neurofibrillary tangles: Abnormal aggregates of a protein known as tau, which is normally essential in maintaining the structural integrity of microtubules.

Neurogenesis: The creation of new neurons, which first occurs during embryological development and then continues throughout life.

Neuroinflammation: The inflammation of nervous tissue.

Neuromuscular junction: The synapse between a motor neuron and a muscle cell.

Neuron doctrine: The idea that the cell theory is applicable to neurons.

Neuronal membrane: The cellular membrane of neurons.

Neurons: Cells that perform the major computational functions of the nervous system.

Neuropathology: The scientific study of the changes in the brain that occur when it becomes diseased.

Neuropeptides: Molecules that can act as neurotransmitters or hormones.

Neuropharmacology: The scientific study of how drugs and other agents already inside the brain affect the function of cells.

Neurophysiology: The scientific study of brain function by using various methods to stimulate, measure, or record the activity of individual brain cells or entire brain areas.

Neuroplasticity: The brain's ability to change with experience.

Neuropsychology: The scientific study of how psychological functions are localized in certain brain areas.

Neuropsychopharmacology: The scientific study of how drugs produce psychotropic effects.

Neurosecretory cells: Cells of the hypothalamus that synthesize and release hormones.

Neurosecretory granules: Membrane-bound vesicles that contain large-molecule neurotransmitters.

Neurotransmitter: A chemical messenger released from neurons; used to communicate with other neurons and other types of cells in the body.

Neurotransmitter-gated ion channels: Channels that open in response to the binding of a neurotransmitter to receptors located on the channel.

Neurulation: The process by which the neural tube is formed, which gives rise to the central nervous system.

Nigrostriatal pathway: The pathway through which dopaminergic neurons project from the substantia nigra to the striatum.

NMDA-receptor-hypofunction hypothesis: The hypothesis that NMDA receptors are dysfunctional in people with schizophrenia.

Nociception: The neurobiological process that leads to the perception of pain.

Nonassociative learning: A type of learning in which a change in behavior does not involve associations between stimuli or between a stimulus and any kind of reward or punishment.

Nondeclarative memories: Memories that are expressed only through the performance of tasks and habits, without the need for conscious recollection of information.

Nonhomeostatic drive: A drive that is not aimed at fulfilling a physiological need.

Nonneuronal capsules: Receptors that are not neurons.

Nonsteroid hormones: Also known as peptide or protein-like hormones; short chains of amino acids. Nonsteroid hormones cannot cross the cell membrane; they act through second messenger cascades.

Notochord: A flexible, rodlike structure made out of cells from the mesoderm, which serves as the skeleton of the embryo until the formation of the vertebrae.

Novel-object-preference (NOP) paradigm: Object-recognition memory test that takes advantage of an animal's preference for novelty.

NREM sleep: Non–rapid eye movement sleep. Sleep that is subdivided into four stages of progressively deeper sleep.

Nucleus: The part of the cell that contains deoxyribonucleic acid (DNA), which codes for proteins.

Nucleus of the solitary tract (NST): A bundle of nerve fibers that carries excitatory messages from the stomach to the hypothalamus.

Object attention: Attention directed at a specific object.

Obsessions: Intrusive and unwanted thoughts that give rise to high levels of anxiety.

Obsessive-compulsive disorder (OCD): A psychological disorder characterized by intrusive and unwanted thoughts (obsessions) and repetitive behaviors that the person with OCD feels compelled to perform (compulsions).

Oculomotor apraxia: The inability to perform voluntary eye movements.

Oculomotor delayed-response task: A delayed-response task in which the location of a stimulus on a screen has to be held in short-term memory to later perform a correct response, as demonstrated by moving the eyes toward the area in which the stimulus previously appeared.

Odorants: Chemical molecules from the air that bind to specialized receptors within the nasal cavity, ultimately giving rise to the perception of odors.

Odotopic mapping: The mapping of odors in the olfactory bulb.

Off-center receptive field: A receptive field in which illumination of its center inhibits activity in its associated retinal ganglion cell.

Olfactory epithelium: Layer of cells deep inside the nostrils made up of olfactory receptor neurons and supporting cells.

Olfactory receptor neurons (ORNs): Cells on which olfactory sensory receptors are located.

Oligodendrocytes: Myelin-producing glia in the central nervous system.

On-center receptive field: A receptive field in which illumination of its center activates its associated retinal ganglion cell.

Operant conditioning: A form of associative learning in which an association is created between a behavior and its consequence.

Opiates: Powerful painkillers that also provide feelings of intense feelings of pleasure, well-being, and calm.

Opioid: Any drug that interacts with opiate receptors.

Optic ataxia: The inability to accurately reach for objects.

Optogenetics: The field in which genetics and optics are combined to use light-sensitive molecules to control cellular activity.

Orexigenic: An agent such as a drug or a hormone that stimulates appetite.

Organ of Corti: The organ within the cochlea that contains the necessary components for hearing.

Organizational-activation hypothesis: The idea that hormones have organizing effects on the brain by acting on neuronal circuits soon after conception and that action on those circuits determines gender-typical sexual behavior.

Orientation selectivity: A property associated with simple cells in the primary visual cortex, which best respond when bars of a particular orientation are projected onto the retina.

Orthodromic conduction: Movement of an action potential from the soma to the axon terminal.

Orthonasal route: The pathway to the olfactory bulb followed by airborne molecules that have entered the nostrils.

Ossicles: Three tiny bones that connect the tympanic membrane to the inner ear.

Overt attention: The shifting of attention that includes the reorienting of sensory receptors.

Overt behavior: Behavior that is readily observable such as reaching out for a cup of coffee.

Pain regulation: What is done to manage or cope with pain.

Pair bonding: A monogamous relationship between a male and a female (sometimes between individuals of the same sex) of the same species that leads to reproduction and a lifelong bond.

Papez circuit: The circuit of brain areas once thought to be dedicated to processing emotions.

Papillae: Small rounded structures that contain the taste buds.

Paracrine hormone: A hormone that affects cells in the immediate vicinity of the cell that released it.

Paradoxical sleep: Another name given to REM sleep because brain activity during REM resembles that of wakefulness.

Paraplegia: Loss of the use of and sensation in the lower limbs that results from damage to the lower parts of the spinal cord.

Parasympathetic nervous system: Counters the activity of the sympathetic nervous system by slowing things down; often referred to as the "rest-and-digest" system.

Parenting: The process that promotes and supports the development of offspring through caregiving. Depending on the species, this may include physical, emotional, behavioral, intellectual, and social development.

Parkinson's disease: A neurodegenerative brain disease in which dopamine neurons in the substantia nigra die, giving rise to the inability of affected individuals to smoothly control their movements.

Parvocellular (P-cells): Cells of the LGN that receive color information from the axons of midget ganglion cells of the retina

Perception: What the brain makes of stimuli that activate receptors.

Perception-action model: A model that states that when one perceives another person's emotional state, both the representation related to that state and the actions related to it are triggered in one's own brain.

Perceptual dimension of pain: The detection of a painful stimulus.

Peripheral nervous system: The nervous tissue that connects to the muscles and organs of the body.

Phagocytosis: The engulfing of particles by the membrane of a cell.

Phantom limb: The phenomenon in which amputees report retaining sensation of a missing limb.

Phantom pain: The phenomenon in which a patient experiences pain in a phantom limb.

Phenotype: The characteristic traits observed in individuals resulting from the interactions between their genotype and the environment.

Pheromones: Chemicals (hormones) that are secreted outside of an individual's body, which can trigger specific reactions in other individuals of the same species.

Phineas Gage: A historical and prototypical case of prefrontal cortex function.

Phosphatidylserine: A chemical marker that appears on dying cells, marking them for engulfment by microglia.

Photons: Particles that create light and travel in waves.

Photopigment: A pigment that undergoes chemical changes when it absorbs light.

Photoreceptors: Sensory receptors that convert energy from the electromagnetic spectrum into electrical impulses.

Phototransduction: The process by which light rays are converted into nerve impulses.

Phrenology: The idea that bumps on the skull reflect the size of the underlying brain region, which is associated with a particular faculty.

Pigment epithelium: The layer of cells that nourishes the photoreceptors.

Pimozide: A dopamine receptor antagonist used as an antipsychotic.

Place cells: Cells located in the hippocampus that indicate a rat's position in its environment.

Polymodal nociceptors: Nociceptors, such as C nerve fibers, that respond to intense thermal, mechanical, and chemical stimulation.

Polysomnography: A set of physiological measures that includes electroencephalography, electrooculography, and electromyography.

Polysynaptic pathway: A pathway to a response that requires more than one synapse.

Positive reinforcement: When a behavior produces a pleasurable or desirable outcome, increasing the probability that the behavior that produced the outcome will be repeated.

Positive symptoms: The presence of symptoms that people do not normally experience, such as hallucinations and delusions.

Positron emission tomography (PET): An imaging method in which brain function is inferred by detecting the consumption of glucose by neurons.

Postabsorptive state: A state in which nutrients are no longer entering the bloodstream and when the body relies on the release of stored energy from the liver as glucose and from fat cells as fatty acids and ketones.

Postganglionic fibers: Fibers that exit ganglia and enter the spinal cord.

Postsynaptic densities: Areas of the dendrite on which receptors are located.

Postsynaptic element: The area that contains neurotransmitter receptors on the post-synaptic neuron.

Postsynaptic neuron: The neuron located across the synaptic cleft.

Postsynaptic potential: The change in voltage of the neuronal membrane due to the entry of Na^+ or Cl^- into a neuron.

Posttraumatic stress disorder (PTSD): A disorder observed in people having experienced a traumatic event that can be considered out of normal human experience.

P-pathway: The visual information pathway from the retina to the visual cortex that connects midget retinal ganglion cells to P-cells of the LGN.

Prandial state: A state in which energy stores are replenished as nutrients are absorbed in the bloodstream and stored.

Preconscious stimulus: A stimulus that does not give rise to conscious awareness despite its high strength.

Prediction error: The extent to which the conditioned stimulus predicts the presence of the unconditioned stimulus.

Preganglionic fibers: Fibers that exit the spinal cord and enter ganglia.

Preoptic area (POA): The region of the hypothalamus involved in temperature regulation.

Presynaptic element: The axon terminals of the presynaptic neuron.

Presynaptic neuron: The neuron that releases neurotransmitter molecules into the synaptic cleft.

Primary motive: An innate need that must be fulfilled to ensure survival.

Primer effects: Effects that affect development, such as the acceleration of puberty in young females.

Priming: A type of nondeclarative memory, in which exposure to a stimulus influences response to a later stimulus.

Prisoner's dilemma: A game based on cooperation that shows that people's decisions are not always based on rational thought.

Procedural memories: A type of nondeclarative memory that leads to the performance of skills and habit without the need for conscious recollection of information.

Processing speed: The speed at which information can be analyzed and at which mental tasks are performed.

Proliferation: The stage during which neural stem cells multiply.

Proprioception: The ability to know the relative position of one's own body parts.

Protanopia: A type of red-green color deficiency due to the absence of L-cones.

Psychoactive drugs: Drugs that can give rise to feelings of euphoria and altered perceptions.

Psychological disorder: A psychological dysfunction within an individual associated with distress or impairment in functioning and a response that is not typical or culturally expected.

Psychomotor retardation: A slowing down of thoughts and movement.

Psychopaths: People who generally show disregard for the well-being of others as well as a lack of guilt, empathy, and remorse.

Psychotic symptoms: Positive symptoms of schizophrenia that are characterized as delusions and hallucinations.

Pyramidal neuron: A type of neuron that has the appearance of a pyramid.

Pyramidal tracts: Tracts of the direct pathway.

Quadriplegia (also known as tetraplegia): Loss of the use of and sensation in both upper and lower limbs that results from damage to the upper spinal cord.

Radial migration: The process by which cells reach their destination by sliding along processes extended by radial glia.

Rapidly adapting fibers: Sensory nerve fibers that respond at the initial contact with a stimulus, as well as with its removal, but will quickly stop responding with continuous stimulation.

Readiness potential: Neuronal activity, measured by EEG, that preceded the urge to press a button by 500 ms in Benjamin Libet's free will experiment.

Receptive field: An area of the body where a stimulus can elicit a reflex. In vision, it is a spot on the retina, which, when illuminated, activates a single retinal ganglion cell and other cells in the visual system.

Receptivity: Actions performed by a female that are necessary for copulation.

Reciprocal altruism: The idea that we help others with the expectation of getting help from them in the future.

Reconsolidation: The idea that consolidated memories return to a fragile state when reactivated and require another round of consolidation to be stabilized.

Reductionism: The idea that complex phenomena can be explained by knowing their basic structure.

Reflex arc: A loop of information that begins with the activation of sensory neurons and ends with muscle contraction, through the activation of motor neurons.

Refraction: The change in direction of light rays as they travel from one medium to another.

Relative refractory period: The period when initiation of another action potential is possible but is difficult to induce.

Releaser effects: Effects that trigger stereotypic behaviors, such as emotional responses or anxiety in other individuals as well as the attraction of females by males.

REM sleep: Rapid eye movement sleep. Sleep stage mostly associated with dreaming; characterized by relative muscle paralysis and eye movements.

Representation: Organizing information as it is relevant to the self.

Reproductive behavior: Any behavioral pattern that results in sperm and egg being brought together to produce offspring.

Resting membrane potential: The difference in charge between the inside and the outside of the neuron when not conducting action potentials.

Reticular theory: The idea that the neurites (axons and dendrites) of neurons fuse with the neurites of other neurons in a neural net.

Retina: The cell layer at the back of the eye that contains photoreceptors.

Retinohypothalamic projections: The projections of photoreceptors containing melanopsin from the retina to the hypothalamus.

Retinotopic mapping: The preservation of the relative location of neurons from the retina to the cortex.

Retrieval: The recollection of information stored in memory.

Retrograde amnesia: Memory loss for information acquired before brain damage.

Retrograde signaling: The process by which the activity of a neuron is regulated by a chemical messenger released by its postsynaptic target neuron.

Retronasal route: The pathway to the olfactory bulb followed by molecules that have entered the mouth.

Reuptake inhibitors: Drugs that inhibit the reuptake of a neurotransmitter by the neuron that released it.

Reverberating activity: The continuous firing of the neurons in a cell assembly.

Reward deficiency syndrome: A proposed syndrome in which high sensation seekers have inherited a low number of a type of dopamine receptors in the striatum and prefrontal cortex.

Risk-taking behaviors: Behaviors that carry potential for harm such as unprotected sexual activity, sexting, smoking, alcohol and illegal substance use, dangerous driving, and various illegal activities.

Rod monochromacy: Color blindness due to the absence of cones.

Roid rage: A condition associated with users of anabolic-androgenic steroids, characterized by the loss of impulse control and overreaction to stimuli that do not usually provoke a reaction.

Rosehip neuron: A recently discovered type of neuron with unknown function that is found in humans but not in rodents.

Rumination: Repeatedly going over negative thoughts or problems.

Sagittal view: A lateral view of the brain with one of the hemispheres missing.

Saltatory conduction: Propagation of an action potential down an axon by jumping from one node of Ranvier to another.

Schachter and Singer's two-factor theory: A theory of emotions in which physiological changes triggered by stimuli are accompanied by an interpretation of what these changes mean.

Schizophrenia: A psychological disorder characterized by the presence of symptoms that includes delusions, hallucinations, disorganized speech, disorganized behavior, diminished emotional expression, and cognitive impairments.

Schwann cells: Myelin-producing glia in the peripheral nervous system.

Second messenger cascade: The process by which a G-protein activates an effector enzyme, which in turn can synthesize molecules known as second messengers.

"Second wind" effect: Periods of alertness interspersed with periods of sleepiness after being sleep deprived.

Second-order neurons: Neurons located in the medulla in the brainstem to which first-order neurons synapse.

Secretin: Pancreatic secretions triggered by the release of an agent from the intestines in response to the applications of hydrochloric acid.

Sedative hypnotics: Drugs that can relieve anxiety as well as having the potential to induce sleep.

Selective attention: The process that permits specific information to be picked voluntarily out of a number of stimuli.

Self-awareness: The ability to reflect on one's traits, beliefs, abilities, and attitudes.

Self-referential stimuli: Stimuli that are perceived as being related to one's self.

Semantic memories: Declarative memories that comprise learned facts and life events.

Sensation: The detection of external or internal stimuli through the stimulation of specialized receptors.

Sense of agency: The feeling of initiating and controlling one's own actions.

Sensitization: An increase in response to an innocuous stimulus after being exposed to an aversive stimulus.

Sensorimotor retuning: A neuromuscular treatment used to reduce abnormal movements during instrument play in musicians with focal hand dystonia.

Sensorineural hearing loss: A type of deafness caused by damage to hair cells within the inner ear.

Sensory homunculus: Map of the entire body in the somatosensory cortex.

Sensory memory: The persisting representation of a sensory stimulus for a brief period after it is no longer physically present.

Sensory neuron: A neuron that carries sensory information from the peripheral nervous system to the central nervous system.

Separation distress: A mechanism that may have evolved in mammals to keep the young close to maternal contact and care.

Septal organ of Masera: An organ for which the function is still a mystery, but it is suspected to serve alerting functions.

Serotonin reuptake inhibitors (SSRIs): Antidepressant drugs that selectively block the reuptake of serotonin.

Set point: The desired target value of a system.

Sex-determining region Y protein: A protein made from the instruction of the *SRY* gene located on the Y chromosome that causes the fetus to produce male gonads and inhibits the formation of female gonads.

Sexual behavior: A component of reproductive behavior that includes responses directly associated with genital stimulation and copulation.

Sexual orientation: The term used to define sexual identity, attraction, and behavior.

Sham rage: A range of autonomic and motor reactions associated with rage devoid of accompanying subjective feelings.

Shivering: Shaking of skeletal muscles that generate heat through the expenditure of energy.

Shortcut pathway: A pathway by which activated G-proteins can bind to ion channels from inside the cell.

Short-term plasticity: Changes in synaptic strength that occur within a matter of milliseconds to a few minutes and are thought to be the basis for short-term memory and decision making.

Simulation theories: Theories that a theory of mind is achieved through our ability to put ourselves in a person's mental "shoes" and imagine ("simulate") what we would experience in a similar situation.

Simultanagnosia: The inability to perceive multiple objects simultaneously in a visual scene.

Single-unit recording: A method by which the electrical activity of a single neuron can be recorded.

Sleep spindles: Series of high-frequency spikes of activity lasting anywhere from 0.5 to 1.0 seconds.

Sliding filament model: A model proposed to explain how muscles contract.

Slowly adapting fibers: Sensory nerve fibers that keep responding to continuous contact with a stimulus.

Slow-twitch muscle fibers: Muscle fibers that do not fatigue easily; effective in long, sustained efforts, such as in long-distance running.

Social behavior: Behavioral interactions between individuals of the same species that are beneficial to one or more individuals of the species.

Social behavior neural network: A network of interconnected brain areas that are thought to underlie the neurobiological basis of social behaviors.

Social cognitive neuroscience prism: A prism that represents interactions among four levels of analysis that result in social behavior.

Social exclusion: When a person is not permitted to participate socially with other people.

Social level of analysis: The study of how neurobiological processes are involved in social behavior.

Social neuroscience: A branch of behavioral neuroscience that focuses on the neurobiological processes of social behaviors such as those involved in empathy, affiliation, and morality.

Social pain/physical pain overlap theory (spot): The idea that there are overlapping neural mechanisms for physical and social pain.

Social psychology: The study of how people's thoughts are influenced by the actual, inferred, or imagined presence of others.

Social recognition: The ability to recognize individuals to determine how to act with them.

Solitary nucleus: A collection of cell bodies located in the medulla oblongata within the brainstem.

Soma: Also called the cell body or perikaryon; contains the nucleus and organelles found in other cell types.

Somatic marker: The perception of physiological changes that act as a biasing mechanism in decision making.

Somatic-marker hypothesis: The hypothesis that the unconscious activation of past emotional experiences informs decision making.

Somites: Protrusions on either side of the neural tube formed by the mesoderm, which give rise to the vertebrae and associated skeletal muscles.

Somnogens: Substances in the body that produce sleep.

Spatial attention: Attention directed to the spatial location of stimuli.

Spatial memory: The encoding, storage, and retrieval of spatial information that results in successful navigation toward goals in the environment.

Spatial summation: When several postsynaptic potentials that occur at the same time but at different synapses are added together.

Spinal nerves: Pairs of nerves that carry information to and from parts of the body.

Spinothalamocortical pathway (STC pathway): The pathway through which body temperature is conveyed to the somatosensory cortex for the perception of temperature.

Spiral ganglion cells: Cells that contact hair cells to bring auditory information to the brain.

Split-brain patients: Patients who have been subjected to the removal of the corpus callosum.

Standard model: The idea that the hippocampus is needed only temporarily as the cortex gradually stores memories.

Stellate cell: A neuron in which the disposition of the dendrites gives it a star-shaped appearance.

Steroid hormones: Hormones synthesized from cholesterol; produced in the adrenal glands, ovaries (in women), and testes (in men). Steroid hormones can cross the cell membrane and can cause DNA to synthesize proteins.

Stimulants: Drugs that speed activity in the central and peripheral nervous systems.

Storage: The retention of information acquired by your senses.

Stretch reflex: A contraction initiated in response to the stretch of a muscle to prevent it from tearing.

Stretch-sensitive channels: Ion channels that open in response to indentation, stretch, or vibration of the skin.

Structural brain imaging: Imaging techniques that permit the detection of brain injury.

Structural plasticity: Changes in brain structure that occur in response to the extensive practice of motor or cognitive skills.

Structural remodeling: Changes in the structure of neurons in response to the activity of other neurons or stimulation from the external environment.

Subgranular zone (SGZ): The area located near the dentate gyrus (DG) of the hippocampus, which contains NSPCs that generate neurons that migrate to the DG and differentiate into what are known as granule cells.

Subjective experience: The continuous flow of thoughts, feelings, and perceptions that one is privy to throughout life.

Subliminal stimuli: Stimuli that are not consciously perceived but that can nevertheless influence behavior.

Subliminal stimulus: A stimulus that can affect behavior while remaining below the threshold of consciousness.

Subventricular zone (SVZ): The area that lines the walls of the lateral ventricles and contains NSPCs that generate neurons that migrate to the olfactory bulb.

Sulci: Grooves that separate the gyri.

Summation: The processes of summing the input of neurons in the form of EPSPs or IPSPs, which may or may not result in the firing of action potentials.

Superior colliculus: Also referred to as the optic tectum because it plays an important role in controlling eye movements.

Superior view: The brain as viewed from the top.

Suprachiasmatic nucleus (SCN): The region of the hypothalamus thought to control circadian rhythms (sometimes called the master clock).

Sylvian fissure: The fissure that separates the frontal lobe from the temporal lobe.

Sympathetic nervous system: Gets your body ready for action; often referred to as the "fight-or-flight" system.

Synapse: The site of communication between neurons or between neurons and other types of cells.

Synaptic cleft: The tiny gap that exists between neurons.

Synaptic integration: The computational process that a neuron performs to determine whether it will be more or less likely to fire an action potential.

Synaptic plasticity: Changes in the efficacy of synapses.

Synaptic signaling: Communication mediated by neurotransmitters at a local level.

Synaptic vesicles: Membrane-bound vesicles that contain small-molecule neurotransmitters.

Synaptogenesis: The formation of new synapses in developing and adult brains.

Synergy: The co-contraction of body parts as a unit due to a lack of inhibition of adjacent cortical representations.

Systems consolidation: The reorganization in systems throughout the brain that are involved in the storage of memories.

Systems level of analysis: The study of how the activity in patterns of neuronal connections gives rise to overt and covert behaviors and how information is encoded and stored in the patterns of connections between neurons that are part of functional systems.

T/CRT ratio: The ratio of testosterone to cortisol.

Tangential migration: The process by which cells reach their destination by sliding across one glial cell to another.

Taste: The perception generated when chemicals are dissolved in saliva and bind to gustatory chemoreceptors.

Taste buds: Structures that contain taste receptor cells.

Tau hypothesis: A hypothesis based on the observation that the progression of Alzheimer's disease is related more to the effects of changes in tau than to the formation of beta-amyloid plaques and that the formation of neurofibrillary tangles precedes the formation of beta-amyloid plaques.

Tectospinal, vestibulospinal, rubrospinal, and reticulospinal tracts: The individual tracts of the indirect pathway.

Tectum: A subdivision of the mesencephalon involved in producing reflexive eye movements, pitch perception, and the spatial localization of sounds.

Tegmentum: A subdivision of the midbrain involved in motor coordination and the regulation of pain. It also contains the ventral-tegmental area, which is part of the brain's reward system.

Telencephalon, diencephalon, mesencephalon, metencephalon, myelencephalon: The five secondary brain vesicles.

Temporal summation: When several postsynaptic potentials that follow each other with little delay are added together at the same synapse.

Temporally graded retrograde amnesia: A type of amnesia in which information acquired shortly before brain damage is lost but memories formed at a more remote period are preserved.

Teratogens: Factors that can cause malformations of the embryo.

Theory of constructed emotions: The theory that emotions are not hardwired entities but emerge into consciousness from interoception and categorization.

Theory of mind: The ability to infer what is going on in the minds of others, such as their emotions, beliefs, and intentions, by observing their behaviors.

Third-order neurons: Neurons located in the thalamus to which second-order neurons synapse and that send sensory information to the somatosensory cortex.

Thyroxine: A hormone released by the thyroid gland that is important for maintaining the body's metabolic rate, muscle control, and brain development.

"Tip of the tongue" phenomenon: A type of retrieval failure accompanied by the strong feeling that temporarily forgotten information is on the verge of being recalled.

Tolerance: The phenomenon by which a person needs to take increasingly large amounts of a drug to experience the same effects.

Tonotopic mapping: The preservation of the relative spatial organization of frequency processing on the basilar membrane and within the cortex.

Top-down control of attention: When attention is voluntary and controlled by conscious thought, expectations, and goals.

Topographical map: A map, within the brain, that represents different areas of the body in an orderly way.

Transcranial magnetic stimulation (TMS): Inferring the functions of a particular brain area through the application of a magnetic field over a brain area of interest from the top of the skull.

Transcutaneous electrical nerve stimulation (TENS): A device that reduces pain through electrical stimulation.

Transducers: Devices that convert one form of energy into another.

Transporters: Proteins that transport neurotransmitters and other molecules across cellular membranes.

Traumatic brain injury: An injury that results from a blow to the head or from an object penetrating the skull.

Trichromatic theory: The theory that the brain produces our perception of colors by reading out the combined input of three types of cones, each responding best to a specific wavelength.

Tricyclic antidepressants: Antidepressant drugs that block the reuptake of serotonin and norepinephrine.

Tritanomaly: A type of blue-yellow color deficiency due to a limited number of functioning S-cones.

Tritanopia: A type of blue-yellow color deficiency due to the complete absence of S-cones.

Trust game: A game based on trust in which an investor transfers a sum of money to a trustee with the expectancy of a return.

Tuberoinfundibular pathway: The pathway through which dopaminergic neurons project from the arcuate nucleus of the hypothalamus.

Twin studies: Studies that compare identical twins who were reared in different environments in an effort to tease out the effects of genes versus those of the environment.

Two-point discrimination test: Test that assesses a person's ability to discriminate between two contact points on the skin.

Unified theory (or "C" theory): The memory consolidation theory in which learning induces cellular consolidation in both the cortex and the hippocampus rapidly and simultaneously.

Unilateral neglect: A syndrome characterized by the inability to attend to the side of visual space on the opposite side of unilateral damage to the parietal and temporal cortices (sometimes referred to as hemispatial neglect).

Unipolar neuron: A neuron with only one process that flows uninterrupted by the soma.

Unresponsive wakefulness: A condition in which patients show high levels of wakefulness without any signs of consciousness (previously known as a persistent vegetative state).

Upper motor neurons: Motor neurons that carry information from the brain.

Urbach-Wiethe disease: A disease that causes the temporal lobes to degenerate because of a calcium build-up in the brain.

Vallate papillae: The papillae forming a "V" in the center of the back of the tongue.

Ventral roots: Areas through which motor neurons exit the spinal cord.

Ventral-frontoparietal system: Includes the temporoparietal cortex (or temporoparietal junction [TPJ]) and the ventral frontal cortex. It is involved in the bottom-up control of attention.

Ventral-posterior medial nucleus: The area of the thalamus that processes gustatory information.

Ventricles: Hollow areas of the brain in which cerebrospinal fluid is produced.

Ventromedial prefrontal cortex: A part of the prefrontal cortex important for planning and judgment.

Vicious cycle of OCD: Obsessive thoughts trigger significant amounts of anxiety, which is relieved temporarily by performing compulsive actions, until obsessive thoughts arise again, leading the person with OCD to repeat the cycle.

Visible spectrum: The narrow band of the electromagnetic spectrum, ranging from 400 nm to 700 nm, that can be perceived as colors.

Vomeronasal organ: Also known as Jacobson's organ; part of the accessory olfactory system that sends information about pheromones to the accessory olfactory bulb.

Wanting: Strong cravings and drug-seeking behavior observed in the addicted person when exposed to environmental cues associated with taking the drug.

White light: What is perceived when all the wavelengths of the visual spectrum are mixed.

Withdrawal: Occurs with the cessation of the use of a drug once the nervous system has adjusted to the drug's presence. Depending on the drug, withdrawal symptoms may include nausea, headaches, weakness, and body aches.

Working memory: A memory register of limited capacity for both the amount of information it can store and the time for which information is retained.

Yerkes-Dodson law: The relationship between performance and levels of arousal.

Zeitgebers: Factors in the environment that influence circadian rhythms.

REFERENCES

Abraira, V. E., & Ginty, D. D. (2013). The sensory neurons of touch. *Neuron, 79*(4), 618–639. Retrieved from https://www.ncbi.nlm.nih.gov/pubmed/23972592. doi:10.1016/j.neuron.2013.07.051

Adams, J. A. (1987). Historical review and appraisal of research on the learning, retention, and transfer of human motor skills. *Psychological Bulletin, 101*(1), 41–74.

Adan, R. A. H., Vanderschuren, L. J. M. J., & la Fleur, S. E. (2008). Anti-obesity drugs and neural circuits of feeding. *Trends in Pharmacological Sciences, 29*(4), 208–217. Retrieved from https://www.ncbi.nlm.nih.gov/pubmed/18353447

Adolphs, R. (2010). Conceptual challenges and directions for social neuroscience. *Neuron, 65*(6), 752–767. Retrieved from https://www.ncbi.nlm.nih.gov/pubmed/20346753. doi:10.1016/j.neuron.2010.03.006

Adolphs, R., Tranel, D., Damasio, H., & Damasio, A. (1994). Impaired recognition of emotion in facial expressions following bilateral damage to the human amygdala. *Nature, 372*(6507), 669–672. Retrieved from https://www.ncbi.nlm.nih.gov/pubmed/7990957. doi:10.1038/372669a0

Aggleton, J. P. (1992). *The amygdala: Neurobiological aspects of emotion, memory and mental dysfunction*. New York, NY: Wiley-Liss.

Ahmari, S. E., & Smith, S. J. (2002). Knowing a nascent synapse when you see it. *Neuron, 34*(3), 333–336. Retrieved from https://www.ncbi.nlm.nih.gov/pubmed/11988164

Aizpurua-Olaizola, O., Soydaner, U., Ozturk, E., Schibano, D., Simsir, Y., Navarro, P., . . . Usobiaga, A. (2016). Evolution of the cannabinoid and terpene content during the growth of cannabis sativa plants from different chemotypes. *Journal of Natural Products, 79*(2), 324–331. Retrieved from https://www.ncbi.nlm.nih.gov/pubmed/26836472. doi:10.1021/acs.jnatprod.5b00949

Alain, C., Woods, D. L., & Knight, R. T. (1998). A distributed cortical network for auditory sensory memory in humans. *Brain Research, 812*(1–2), 23–37. Retrieved from https://www.ncbi.nlm.nih.gov/pubmed/9813226

Alkire, M. T., Haier, R. J., & Fallon, J. H. (2000). Toward a unified theory of narcosis: Brain imaging evidence for a thalamocortical switch as the neurophysiologic basis of anesthetic-induced unconsciousness. *Consciousness and Cognition, 9*(3), 370–386. Retrieved from http://www.ncbi.nlm.nih.gov/pubmed/10993665. doi:10.1006/ccog.1999.0423

Allen, J. S., Damasio, H., & Grabowski, T. J. (2002). Normal neuroanatomical variation in the human brain: An MRI-volumetric study. *American Journal of Physical Anthropology, 118*(4), 341–358. Retrieved from https://www.ncbi.nlm.nih.gov/pubmed/12124914. doi:10.1002/ajpa.10092

Allen, L. S., Hines, M., Shryne, J. E., & Gorski, R. A. (1989). Two sexually dimorphic cell groups in the human brain. *The Journal of Neuroscience, 9*(2), 497–506. Retrieved from https://www.ncbi.nlm.nih.gov/pubmed/2918374

Allen, N. J. (2014). Synaptic plasticity: Astrocytes wrap it up. *Current Biology, 24*(15), R697–R699. Retrieved from http://www.ncbi.nlm.nih.gov/pubmed/25093563. doi:10.1016/j.cub.2014.06.030

Allen, P., Aleman, A., & McGuire, P. K. (2007). Inner speech models of auditory verbal hallucinations: Evidence from behavioural and neuroimaging studies. *International Review of Psychiatry, 19*(4), 407–415. Retrieved from https://www.ncbi.nlm.nih.gov/pubmed/17671873. doi:10.1080/09540260701486498

Allen, P., Laroi, F., McGuire, P. K., & Aleman, A. (2008). The hallucinating brain: A review of structural and functional neuroimaging studies of hallucinations. *Neuroscience & Biobehavioral Reviews, 32*(1), 175–191. Retrieved from http://www.ncbi.nlm.nih.gov/pubmed/17884165. doi:10.1016/j.neubiorev.2007.07.012

Altman, J. (1962). Are new neurons formed in the brains of adult mammals? *Science, 135*(3509), 1127–1128. Retrieved from https://www.ncbi.nlm.nih.gov/pubmed/13860748

Altman, J., & Das, G. D. (1967). Postnatal neurogenesis in the guinea-pig. *Nature, 214*(5093), 1098–1101. Retrieved from https://www.ncbi.nlm.nih.gov/pubmed/6053066. doi:10.1038/2141098a0

Alvarez, P., & Squire, L. R. (1994). Memory consolidation and the medial temporal lobe: A simple network model. *Proceedings of the National Academy of Sciences of the United States of America, 91*(15), 7041–7045. Retrieved from https://www.ncbi.nlm.nih.gov/pubmed/8041742. doi:10.1073/pnas.91.15.7041

Alvarez-Buylla, A., Ling, C. Y., & Nottebohm, F. (1992). High vocal center growth and its relation to neurogenesis, neuronal replacement and song acquisition in juvenile canaries. *Journal of Neurobiology, 23*(4), 396–406. Retrieved from https://www.ncbi.nlm.nih.gov/pubmed/1634887. doi:10.1002/neu.480230406

Alverno, L. (1990). The origins of electroconvulsive therapy. *Wisconsin Medical Journal, 89*(2), 54–56. Retrieved from https://www.ncbi.nlm.nih.gov/pubmed/2408251

Alzheimer's Association. (2018). 2018 Alzheimer's disease facts and figures. *Alzheimer's & Dementia, 14*(3), 367–429.

American Psychiatric Association. (2013). *Diagnostic and statistical manual of mental disorders: DSM-5* (5th ed.). Washington, DC: American Psychiatric Association.

Amsterdam, B. (1972). Mirror self-image reactions before age two. *Developmental Psychobiology, 5*(4), 297–305. Retrieved from http://www.ncbi.nlm.nih.gov/pubmed/4679817. doi:10.1002/dev.420050403

Amunts, K., Schlaug, G., Jancke, L., Steinmetz, H., Schleicher, A., Dabringhaus, A., & Zilles, K. (1997). Motor cortex and hand motor skills: Structural compliance in the human brain. *Human Brain Mapping, 5*(3), 206–215. Retrieved from https://www.ncbi.nlm.nih.gov/pubmed/20408216. doi:10.1002/(SICI)1097-0193(1997)5:3<206::AID-HBM5>3.0.CO;2-7

Anacker, C. (2014). Adult hippocampal neurogenesis in depression: Behavioral implications and regulation by the stress system. *Current Topics in Behavioral Neurosciences, 18*, 25–43. Retrieved from https://www.ncbi.nlm.nih.gov/pubmed/24478038. doi:10.1007/7854_2014_275

Andersen, R. A., & Buneo, C. A. (2002). Intentional maps in posterior parietal cortex. *Annual Review of Neuroscience, 25*, 189–220. Retrieved from https://www.ncbi.nlm.nih.gov/pubmed/12052908. doi:10.1146/annurev.neuro.25.112701.142922

Andersen, R. A., & Buneo, C. A. (2003). Sensorimotor integration in posterior parietal cortex. *Advances in Neurology, 93*, 159–177. Retrieved from https://www.ncbi.nlm.nih.gov/pubmed/12894407

Anderson, A. K., Spencer, D. D., Fulbright, R. K., & Phelps, E. A. (2000). Contribution of the anteromedial temporal lobes to the evaluation of facial emotion. *Neuropsychology, 14*(4), 526–536. Retrieved from https://www.ncbi.nlm.nih.gov/pubmed/11055255

Angrist, B. M., & Gershon, S. (1970). The phenomenology of experimentally induced amphetamine psychosis—preliminary observations. *Biological Psychiatry*, *2*(2), 95–107. Retrieved from http://www.ncbi.nlm.nih.gov/pubmed/5459137

Arnau-Soler, A., Adams, M. J., Clarke, T. K., MacIntyre, D. J., Milburn, K., Navrady, L., . . . Thomson, P. A. (2019). A validation of the diathesis-stress model for depression in Generation Scotland. *Translational Psychiatry*, *9*(1), 25. Retrieved from https://www.ncbi.nlm.nih.gov/pubmed/30659167. doi:10.1038/s41398-018-0356-7

Arnaud, L., Gracco, V., & Menard, L. (2018). Enhanced perception of pitch changes in speech and music in early blind adults. *Neuropsychologia*, *117*, 261–270. Retrieved from https://www.ncbi.nlm.nih.gov/pubmed/29906457. doi:10.1016/j.neuropsychologia.2018.06.009

Arnone, D., McKie, S., Elliott, R., Juhasz, G., Thomas, E. J., Downey, D., . . . Anderson, I. M. (2013). State-dependent changes in hippocampal grey matter in depression. *Molecular Psychiatry*, *18*(12), 1265–1272. Retrieved from http://www.ncbi.nlm.nih.gov/pubmed/23128153. doi:10.1038/mp.2012.150

Asbridge, M., Hayden, J. A., & Cartwright, J. L. (2012). Acute cannabis consumption and motor vehicle collision risk: Systematic review of observational studies and meta-analysis. *British Medical Journal*, *344*, e536. Retrieved from https://www.ncbi.nlm.nih.gov/pubmed/22323502. doi:10.1136/bmj.e536

Aschoff, J. (1967). Human circadian rhythms in activity, body temperature and other functions. *Life Sciences and Space Research*, *5*, 159–173. Retrieved from https://www.ncbi.nlm.nih.gov/pubmed/11973844

Aserinsky, E., & Kleitman, N. (1953). Regularly occurring periods of eye motility, and concomitant phenomena, during sleep. *Science*, *118*(3062), 273–274. Retrieved from https://www.ncbi.nlm.nih.gov/pubmed/13089671

Augustinack, J. C., van der Kouwe, A. J., Salat, D. H., Benner, T., Stevens, A. A., Annese, J., . . . Corkin, S. (2014). H.M.'s contributions to neuroscience: A review and autopsy studies. *Hippocampus*, *24*(11), 1267–1286. Retrieved from https://www.ncbi.nlm.nih.gov/pubmed/25154857. doi:10.1002/hipo.22354

Azevedo, F. A., Carvalho, L. R., Grinberg, L. T., Farfel, J. M., Ferretti, R. E., Leite, R. E., . . . Herculano-Houzel, S. (2009). Equal numbers of neuronal and nonneuronal cells make the human brain an isometrically scaled-up primate brain. *The Journal of Comparative Neurology*, *513*(5), 532–541. Retrieved from https://www.ncbi.nlm.nih.gov/pubmed/19226510. doi:10.1002/cne.21974

Baars, B. J. (2005). Global workspace theory of consciousness: Toward a cognitive neuroscience of human experience. *Progress in Brain Research*, *150*, 45–53. Retrieved from http://www.ncbi.nlm.nih.gov/pubmed/16186014. doi:10.1016/S0079-6123(05)50004-9

Baars, B. J., Franklin, S., & Ramsoy, T. Z. (2013). Global workspace dynamics: Cortical "binding and propagation" enables conscious contents. *Frontiers in Psychology*, *4*, 200. Retrieved from http://www.ncbi.nlm.nih.gov/pubmed/23974723. doi:10.3389/fpsyg.2013.00200

Baars, B. J., & Gage, N. M. (2010). *Cognition, brain, and consciousness: Introduction to cognitive neuroscience* (2nd ed.). Burlington, MA: Academic Press/Elsevier.

Baddeley, A. D., & Hitch, D. (1974). Working memory. In H. G. Bower (Ed.), *Psychology of learning and motivation* (Vol. 8, pp. 47–89). New York, NY: Academic Press.

Baddeley, A. D., & Larsen, J. D. (2007). The phonological loop unmasked? A comment on the evidence for a "perceptual-gestural" alternative. *Quarterly Journal of Experimental Psychology*, *60*(4), 497–504. Retrieved from https://www.ncbi.nlm.nih.gov/pubmed/17455059. doi:10.1080/17470210601147572

Baeken, C., & De Raedt, R. (2011). Neurobiological mechanisms of repetitive transcranial magnetic stimulation on the underlying neurocircuitry in unipolar depression. *Dialogues in Clinical Neuroscience*, *13*(1), 139–145. Retrieved from https://www.ncbi.nlm.nih.gov/pubmed/21485753

Bagyinszky, E., Giau, V. V., Shim, K., Suk, K., An, S. S. A., & Kim, S. (2017). Role of inflammatory molecules in the Alzheimer's disease progression and diagnosis. *Journal of the Neurological Sciences*, *376*, 242–254. Retrieved from https://www.ncbi.nlm.nih.gov/pubmed/28431620. doi:10.1016/j.jns.2017.03.031

Baldwin, D., & Rudge, S. (1995). The role of serotonin in depression and anxiety. *International Clinical Psychopharmacology*, *9*(Suppl 4), 41–45. Retrieved from https://www.ncbi.nlm.nih.gov/pubmed/7622823

Barak, O., Tsodyks, M., & Romo, R. (2010). Neuronal population coding of parametric working memory. *Journal of Neuroscience*, *30*(28), 9424–9430. Retrieved from https://www.ncbi.nlm.nih.gov/pubmed/20631171. doi:10.1523/JNEUROSCI.1875-10.2010

Barbalho, C. A., Nunes-de-Souza, R. L., & Canto-de-Souza, A. (2009). Similar anxiolytic-like effects following intra-amygdala infusions of benzodiazepine receptor agonist and antagonist: Evidence for the release of an endogenous benzodiazepine inverse agonist in mice exposed to elevated plus-maze test. *Brain Research*, *1267*, 65–76. Retrieved from https://www.ncbi.nlm.nih.gov/pubmed/19268657. doi:10.1016/j.brainres.2009.02.042

Barber, M., & Pierani, A. (2016). Tangential migration of glutamatergic neurons and cortical patterning during development: Lessons from Cajal-Retzius cells. *Developmental Neurobiology*, *76*(8), 847–881. Retrieved from https://www.ncbi.nlm.nih.gov/pubmed/26581033. doi:10.1002/dneu.22363

Bard, P. (1928). A diencephalic mechanism for the expression of rage with special reference to the sympathetic nervous system. *American Journal of Physiology*, *84*, 490–515.

Barker, A. T., Jalinous, R., & Freeston, I. L. (1985). Non-invasive magnetic stimulation of human motor cortex. *The Lancet*, *1*(8437), 1106–1107. Retrieved from https://www.ncbi.nlm.nih.gov/pubmed/2860322

Barlow, D. H., Durand, V. M., & Hofmann, S. G. (2018). *Abnormal psychology: An integrative approach*. Boston, MA: Cengage Learning.

Barlow, D. H., Durand, V. M., & Stewart, S. H. (2012). *Abnormal psychology: An integrative approach* (3rd Canadian ed.). Toronto, Canada: Nelson Education.

Baron-Cohen, S., Leslie, A. M., & Frith, U. (1985). Does the autistic child have a "theory of mind"? *Cognition*, *21*(1), 37–46. Retrieved from https://www.ncbi.nlm.nih.gov/pubmed/2934210

Barr, R. L., Llanwyn Jones, D., & Rodger, C. J. (2000). ELF and VLF radio waves. *Journal of Atmospheric and Solar-Terrestrial Physics*, *62*(17–18).

Barratt, E. S., & Slaughter, L. (1998). Defining, measuring, and predicting impulsive aggression: A heuristic model. *Behavioral Sciences & the Law*, *16*(3), 285–302. Retrieved from https://www.ncbi.nlm.nih.gov/pubmed/9768462

Barrett, L. F. (2006a). Are emotions natural kinds? *Perspectives on Psychological Science*, *1*(1), 28–58. Retrieved from https://www.ncbi.nlm.nih.gov/pubmed/26151184. doi:10.1111/j.1745-6916.2006.00003.x

Barrett, L. F. (2006b). Solving the emotion paradox: Categorization and the experience of emotion. *Personality and Social Psychology Review*, *10*(1), 20–46. Retrieved from https://www.ncbi.nlm.nih.gov/pubmed/16430327. doi:10.1207/s15327957pspr1001_2

Barrett, L. F., Mesquita, B., Ochsner, K. N., & Gross, J. J. (2007). The experience of emotion. *The Annual Review of Psychology*, *58*,

373–403. Retrieved from https://www.ncbi.nlm.nih.gov/pubmed/17002554. doi:10.1146/annurev.psych.58.110405.085709

Barrett, L. F., & Satpute, A. B. (2013). Large-scale brain networks in affective and social neuroscience: Towards an integrative functional architecture of the brain. *Current Opinion in Neurobiology, 23*(3), 361–372. Retrieved from https://www.ncbi.nlm.nih.gov/pubmed/23352202. doi:10.1016/j.conb.2012.12.012

Barry, C., Lever, C., Hayman, R., Hartley, T., Burton, S., O'Keefe, J., ... Burgess, N. (2006). The boundary vector cell model of place cell firing and spatial memory. *Reviews in the Neurosciences, 17*(1–2), 71–97. Retrieved from https://www.ncbi.nlm.nih.gov/pubmed/16703944

Basso, J. C., & Suzuki, W. A. (2017). The effects of acute exercise on mood, cognition, neurophysiology, and neurochemical pathways: A review. *Brain Plasticity, 2*(2), 127–152. Retrieved from https://www.ncbi.nlm.nih.gov/pubmed/29765853. doi:10.3233/BPL-160040

Baumeister, A. A., Hawkins, M. F., & Uzelac, S. M. (2003). The myth of reserpine-induced depression: Role in the historical development of the monoamine hypothesis. *Journal of the History of the Neurosciences, 12*(2), 207–220. Retrieved from https://www.ncbi.nlm.nih.gov/pubmed/12953623. doi:10.1076/jhin.12.2.207.15535

Bayliss, W. M., & Starling, E. H. (1902). The mechanism of pancreatic secretion. *The Journal of Physiology, 28*(5), 325–353. Retrieved from https://www.ncbi.nlm.nih.gov/pubmed/16992627

Beach, F. A. (1976). Sexual attractivity, proceptivity, and receptivity in female mammals. *Hormones and Behavior, 7*(1), 105–138. Retrieved from https://www.ncbi.nlm.nih.gov/pubmed/819345

Bechara, A., & Damasio, A. R. (2005). The somatic marker hypothesis: A neural theory of economic decision. *Games and Economic Behavior, 52*, 336–372. doi:10.1016/j.geb.2004.06.010

Bechara, A., Damasio, A. R., Damasio, H., & Anderson, S. W. (1994). Insensitivity to future consequences following damage to human prefrontal cortex. *Cognition, 50*(1–3), 7–15. Retrieved from https://www.ncbi.nlm.nih.gov/pubmed/8039375

Bechara, A., Damasio, H., & Damasio, A. R. (2000). Emotion, decision making and the orbitofrontal cortex. *Cerebral Cortex, 10*(3), 295–307. Retrieved from https://www.ncbi.nlm.nih.gov/pubmed/10731224

Bechara, A., Tranel, D., & Damasio, H. (2000). Characterization of the decision-making deficit of patients with ventromedial prefrontal cortex lesions. *Brain, 123*(Pt. 11), 2189–2202. Retrieved from https://www.ncbi.nlm.nih.gov/pubmed/11050020. doi:10.1093/brain/123.11.2189

Bechara, A., Tranel, D., Damasio, H., & Damasio, A. R. (1996). Failure to respond autonomically to anticipated future outcomes following damage to prefrontal cortex. *Cerebral Cortex, 6*(2), 215–225. Retrieved from https://www.ncbi.nlm.nih.gov/pubmed/8670652. doi:10.1093/cercor/6.2.215

Becker, B., Mihov, Y., Scheele, D., Kendrick, K. M., Feinstein, J. S., Matusch, A., ... Hurlemann, R. (2012). Fear processing and social networking in the absence of a functional amygdala. *Biological Psychiatry, 72*(1), 70–77. Retrieved from https://www.ncbi.nlm.nih.gov/pubmed/22218285. doi:10.1016/j.biopsych.2011.11.024

Bekkers, J. M., & Suzuki, N. (2013). Neurons and circuits for odor processing in the piriform cortex. *Trends in Neurosciences, 36*(7), 429–438. Retrieved from https://www.ncbi.nlm.nih.gov/pubmed/23648377. doi:10.1016/j.tins.2013.04.005

Berg, J., Dickhaut, J., & McCabe, K. (1995). Trust, reciprocity, and social history. *Games and Economic Behavior, 10*(10), 122–142. Retrieved from http://www.sciencedirect.com/science/article/pii/S0899825685710275. doi: 10.1006/game.1995.1027

Bergles, D. E., Diamond, J. S., & Jahr, C. E. (1999). Clearance of glutamate inside the synapse and beyond. *Current Opinion in Neurobiology, 9*(3), 293–298. Retrieved from https://www.ncbi.nlm.nih.gov/pubmed/10395570

Berk, L. E. (2018). *Development through the lifespan* (7th ed.). Hoboken, NJ: Pearson Education, Inc.

Berlucchi, G., & Buchtel, H. A. (2009). Neuronal plasticity: Historical roots and evolution of meaning. *Experimental Brain Research, 192*(3), 307–319. Retrieved from https://www.ncbi.nlm.nih.gov/pubmed/19002678. doi:10.1007/s00221-008-1611-6

Bernhardt, B. C., & Singer, T. (2012). The neural basis of empathy. *The Annual Review of Neuroscience, 35*, 1–23. Retrieved from https://www.ncbi.nlm.nih.gov/pubmed/22715878. doi:10.1146/annurev-neuro-062111-150536

Berridge, K. C. (2009). "Liking" and "wanting" food rewards: Brain substrates and roles in eating disorders. *Physiology & Behavior, 97*(5), 537–550. Retrieved from https://www.ncbi.nlm.nih.gov/pubmed/19336238. doi:10.1016/j.physbeh.2009.02.044

Berridge, K. C., & Kringelbach, M. L. (2015). Pleasure systems in the brain. *Neuron, 86*(3), 646–664. Retrieved from https://www.ncbi.nlm.nih.gov/pubmed/25950633. doi:10.1016/j.neuron.2015.02.018

Berridge, K. C., & Robinson, T. E. (1998). What is the role of dopamine in reward: Hedonic impact, reward learning, or incentive salience? *Brain Research Reviews, 28*(3), 309–369. Retrieved from https://www.ncbi.nlm.nih.gov/pubmed/9858756

Berridge, K. C., & Robinson, T. E. (2016). Liking, wanting, and the incentive-sensitization theory of addiction. *American Psychologist, 71*(8), 670–679. Retrieved from https://www.ncbi.nlm.nih.gov/pubmed/27977239. doi:10.1037/amp0000059

Berthold, A. A. (1849). Transplantation der Hoden. *Archiv für Anatomie, Physiologie und wissenschaftliche Medicin*, 42–46.

Bhimji, S. S., & Sinha, V. (2018). *Adrenal, congenital hyperplasia*. Treasure Island, FL: StatPearls.

Binder, J. R. (2017). Current controversies on Wernicke's area and its role in language. *Current Neurology and Neuroscience Reports, 17*(8), 58. Retrieved from https://www.ncbi.nlm.nih.gov/pubmed/28656532. doi:10.1007/s11910-017-0764-8

Blanchard, R. (1997). Birth order and sibling sex ratio in homosexual versus heterosexual males and females. *Annual Review of Sex Research, 8*, 27–67. Retrieved from https://www.ncbi.nlm.nih.gov/pubmed/10051890

Blanchard, R., & Bogaert, A. F. (1996). Homosexuality in men and number of older brothers. *American Journal of Psychiatry, 153*(1), 27–31. Retrieved from https://www.ncbi.nlm.nih.gov/pubmed/8540587. doi:10.1176/ajp.153.1.27

Blanchard, R., Zucker, K. J., Siegelman, M., Dickey, R., & Klassen, P. (1998). The relation of birth order to sexual orientation in men and women. *Journal of Biosocial Science, 30*(4), 511–519. Retrieved from https://www.ncbi.nlm.nih.gov/pubmed/9818557

Blennow, K., de Leon, M. J., & Zetterberg, H. (2006). Alzheimer's disease. *The Lancet, 368*(9533), 387–403. Retrieved from https://www.ncbi.nlm.nih.gov/pubmed/16876668. doi:10.1016/S0140-6736(06)69113-7

Bliss, T. V., & Lømo, T. (1973). Long-lasting potentiation of synaptic transmission in the dentate area of the anaesthetized rabbit following stimulation of the perforant path. *The Journal of Physiology, 232*(2), 331–356. Retrieved from https://www.ncbi.nlm.nih.gov/pubmed/4727084

Bloomfield, M. A., Ashok, A. H., Volkow, N. D., & Howes, O. D. (2016). The effects of Delta9-tetrahydrocannabinol on the dopamine system. *Nature, 539*(7629), 369–377. Retrieved from https://www.ncbi.nlm.nih.gov/pubmed/27853201. doi:10.1038/nature20153

Blum, K., Sheridan, P. J., Wood, R. C., Braverman, E. R., Chen, T. J., Cull, J. G., & Comings, D. E. (1996). The D2 dopamine receptor gene as a determinant of reward deficiency syndrome. *Journal of the Royal Society of Medicine, 89*(7), 396–400. Retrieved from https://www.ncbi.nlm.nih.gov/pubmed/8774539

Bogen, J. E., & Bogen, G. M. (1976). Wernicke's region—Where is it? *Annals of the New York Academy of Sciences, 280*, 834–843. Retrieved from https://www.ncbi.nlm.nih.gov/pubmed/1070943

Boguszewski, C. L. (2017). Update on GH therapy in adults. *F1000Research, 6*, 2017. Retrieved from https://www.ncbi.nlm.nih.gov/pubmed/29225782. doi:10.12688/f1000research.12057.1

Bojanowski, V., & Hummel, T. (2012). Retronasal perception of odors. *Physiology & Behavior, 107*(4), 484–487. Retrieved from https://www.ncbi.nlm.nih.gov/pubmed/22425641. doi:10.1016/j.physbeh.2012.03.001

Boldog, E., Bakken, T. E., Hodge, R. D., Novotny, M., Aevermann, B. D., Baka, J., . . . Tamas, G. (2018). Transcriptomic and morphophysiological evidence for a specialized human cortical GABAergic cell type. *Nature Neuroscience, 21*(9), 1185–1195. Retrieved from https://www.ncbi.nlm.nih.gov/pubmed/30150662. doi:10.1038/s41593-018-0205-2

Boldrini, M., Fulmore, C. A., Tartt, A. N., Simeon, L. R., Pavlova, I., Poposka, V., . . . Mann, J. J. (2018). Human Hippocampal Neurogenesis Persists throughout Aging. *Cell Stem Cell, 22*(4), 589–599.e585. Retrieved from https://www.ncbi.nlm.nih.gov/pubmed/29625071. doi:10.1016/j.stem.2018.03.015

Boring, E. G. (1930). A new ambiguous figure. *The American Journal of Psychology, 42*, 444–445. doi:10.2307/1415447

Boring, E. G. (1942). *Sensation and perception in the history of experimental psychology*. New York/London: D. Appleton-Century Company, Incorporated.

Bornstein, M. H., Putnick, D. L., Rigo, P., Esposito, G., Swain, J. E., Suwalsky, J. T. D., . . . Venuti, P. (2017). Neurobiology of culturally common maternal responses to infant cry. *Proceedings of the National Academy of Sciences, 114*(45), E9465–E9473. Retrieved from https://www.ncbi.nlm.nih.gov/pubmed/29078366. doi:10.1073/pnas.1712022114

Borodovitsyna, O., Flamini, M., & Chandler, D. (2017). Noradrenergic modulation of cognition in health and disease. *Neural Plasticity, 2017*, 6031478. Retrieved from https://www.ncbi.nlm.nih.gov/pubmed/28596922. doi:10.1155/2017/6031478

Bossong, M. G., Jager, G., Bhattacharyya, S., & Allen, P. (2014). Acute and non-acute effects of cannabis on human memory function: A critical review of neuroimaging studies. *Current Pharmaceutical Design, 20*(13), 2114–2125. Retrieved from https://www.ncbi.nlm.nih.gov/pubmed/23829369

Broadbent, D. E. (1957). A mechanical model for human attention and immediate memory. *Psychological Review, 64*(3), 205–215. Retrieved from https://www.ncbi.nlm.nih.gov/pubmed/13441856

Broadbent, D. E. (1958). *Perception and communication*. New York, NY: Pergamon Press.

Broadbent, N. J., Gaskin, S., Squire, L. R., & Clark, R. E. (2010). Object recognition memory and the rodent hippocampus. *Learning Memory, 17*(1), 5–11. Retrieved from https://www.ncbi.nlm.nih.gov/pubmed/20028732. doi:10.1101/lm.1650110

Brody, A. L., Mandelkern, M. A., London, E. D., Olmstead, R. E., Farahi, J., Scheibal, D., . . . Mukhin, A. G. (2006). Cigarette smoking saturates brain alpha 4 beta 2 nicotinic acetylcholine receptors. *Archives of General Psychiatry, 63*(8), 907–915. Retrieved from https://www.ncbi.nlm.nih.gov/pubmed/16894067. doi:10.1001/archpsyc.63.8.907

Brown, A. S. (1991). A review of the tip-of-the-tongue experience. *Psychological Bulletin, 109*(2), 204–223. Retrieved from https://www.ncbi.nlm.nih.gov/pubmed/2034750

Brown, E. N., Lydic, R., & Schiff, N. D. (2010). General anesthesia, sleep, and coma. *The New England Journal of Medicine, 363*(27), 2638–2650. Retrieved from http://www.ncbi.nlm.nih.gov/pubmed/21190458. doi:10.1056/NEJMra0808281

Brown, G. C., & Neher, J. J. (2014). Microglial phagocytosis of live neurons. *Nature Reviews Neuroscience, 15*(4), 209–216. Retrieved from http://www.ncbi.nlm.nih.gov/pubmed/24646669. doi:10.1038/nrn3710

Brown, G. T. (1911). The intrinsic factors in the act of progression in the mammal. *Proceedings of the Royal Society of London Series B, 84*, 308–319.

Brown, R. E., Basheer, R., McKenna, J. T., Strecker, R. E., & McCarley, R. W. (2012). Control of sleep and wakefulness. *Physiological Reviews, 92*(3), 1087–1187. Retrieved from https://www.ncbi.nlm.nih.gov/pubmed/22811426. doi:10.1152/physrev.00032.2011

Brown, S. R. (2000). Tip-of-the-tongue phenomena: An introductory phenomenological analysis. *Consciousness and Cognition, 9*(4), 516–537. Retrieved from https://www.ncbi.nlm.nih.gov/pubmed/11150221. doi:10.1006/ccog.2000.0421

Buckley, C. (2007). Man is rescued by stranger on subway tracks. *New York Times*, January 3. Retrieved from https://www.nytimes.com/2007/01/03/nyregion/03life.html

Buckner, R. L. (2013). The cerebellum and cognitive function: 25 years of insight from anatomy and neuroimaging. *Neuron, 80*(3), 807–815. Retrieved from https://www.ncbi.nlm.nih.gov/pubmed/24183029. doi:10.1016/j.neuron.2013.10.044

Buckner, R. L., Andrews-Hanna, J. R., & Schacter, D. L. (2008). The brain's default network: Anatomy, function, and relevance to disease. *Annals of the New York Academy of Sciences, 1124*, 1–38. Retrieved from https://www.ncbi.nlm.nih.gov/pubmed/18400922. doi:10.1196/annals.1440.011

Budde, H., Wegner, M., Soya, H., Voelcker-Rehage, C., & McMorris, T. (2016). Neuroscience of exercise: Neuroplasticity and its behavioral consequences. *Neural Plasticity, 2016*, 3643879. Retrieved from https://www.ncbi.nlm.nih.gov/pubmed/27818802. doi:10.1155/2016/3643879

Bunney, W. E., Jr., & Davis, J. M. (1965). Norepinephrine in depressive reactions. A review. *Archives of General Psychiatry, 13*(6), 483–494. Retrieved from https://www.ncbi.nlm.nih.gov/pubmed/5320621

Burger, C., Redlich, R., Grotegerd, D., Meinert, S., Dohm, K., Schneider, I., . . . Dannlowski, U. (2017). Differential abnormal pattern of anterior cingulate gyrus activation in unipolar and bipolar depression: An fMRI and pattern classification approach. *Neuropsychopharmacology, 42*(7), 1399–1408. Retrieved from https://www.ncbi.nlm.nih.gov/pubmed/28205606. doi:10.1038/npp.2017.36

Burgess, N. (2014). The 2014 nobel prize in physiology or medicine: A spatial model for cognitive neuroscience. *Neuron, 84*(6), 1120–1125. Retrieved from https://www.ncbi.nlm.nih.gov/pubmed/25521374. doi:10.1016/j.neuron.2014.12.009

Burguiere, E., Monteiro, P., Mallet, L., Feng, G., & Graybiel, A. M. (2015). Striatal circuits, habits, and implications for obsessive-compulsive disorder. *Current Opinion in Neurobiology, 30*, 59–65. Retrieved from http://www.ncbi.nlm.nih.gov/pubmed/25241072. doi:10.1016/j.conb.2014.08.008

Busardo, F. P., Pellegrini, M., Klein, J., & di Luca, N. M. (2017). Neurocognitive correlates in driving under the influence of cannabis. *CNS & Neurological Disorders Drug Targets, 16*(5), 534–540. Retrieved from https://www.ncbi.nlm.nih.gov/pubmed/28440193. doi:10.2174/1871527316666170424115455

Buschman, T. J., & Miller, E. K. (2007). Top-down versus bottom-up control of attention in the prefrontal and posterior parietal cortices. *Science, 315*(5820), 1860–1862. Retrieved from https://www.ncbi.nlm.nih.gov/pubmed/17395832. doi:10.1126/science.1138071

Bushdid, C., Magnasco, M. O., Vosshall, L. B., & Keller, A. (2014). Humans can discriminate more than 1 trillion olfactory stimuli. *Science, 343*(6177), 1370–1372. Retrieved from https://www.ncbi.nlm.nih.gov/pubmed/24653035. doi:10.1126/science.1249168

Bymaster, F. P., Dreshfield-Ahmad, L. J., Threlkeld, P. G., Shaw, J. L., Thompson, L., Nelson, D. L., . . . Wong, D. T. (2001). Comparative affinity of duloxetine and venlafaxine for serotonin and norepinephrine transporters in vitro and in vivo, human serotonin receptor subtypes, and other neuronal receptors. *Neuropsychopharmacology, 25*(6), 871–880. Retrieved from https://www.ncbi.nlm.nih.gov/pubmed/11750180. doi:10.1016/S0893-133X(01)00298-6

Bystron, I., Blakemore, C., & Rakic, P. (2008). Development of the human cerebral cortex: Boulder Committee revisited. *Nature Reviews Neuroscience, 9*(2), 110–122. Retrieved from https://www.ncbi.nlm.nih.gov/pubmed/18209730. doi:10.1038/nrn2252

Cacioppo, J. T., & Berntson, G. G. (1992). Social psychological contributions to the decade of the brain. Doctrine of multilevel analysis. *American Psychologist, 47*(8), 1019–1028. Retrieved from https://www.ncbi.nlm.nih.gov/pubmed/1510329

Caldwell, H. K. (2017). Oxytocin and vasopressin: Powerful regulators of social behavior. *The Neuroscientist, 23*(5):517–528. Retrieved from https://www.ncbi.nlm.nih.gov/pubmed/28492104. doi:10.1177/1073858417708284

Callaghan, T., Rochat, P., Lillard, A., Claux, M. L., Odden, H., Itakura, S., . . . Singh, S. (2005). Synchrony in the onset of mental-state reasoning: Evidence from five cultures. *Psychological Science, 16*(5), 378–384. Retrieved from https://www.ncbi.nlm.nih.gov/pubmed/15869697. doi:10.1111/j.0956-7976.2005.01544.x

Camchong, J., Lim, K. O., & Kumra, S. (2017). Adverse effects of cannabis on adolescent brain development: A longitudinal study. *Cerebral Cortex, 27*(3), 1922–1930. Retrieved from https://www.ncbi.nlm.nih.gov/pubmed/26912785. doi:10.1093/cercor/bhw015

Cameron, J., & Doucet, E. (2007). Getting to the bottom of feeding behaviour: Who's on top? *Applied Physiology, Nutrition, and Metabolism, 32*(2), 177–189. Retrieved from https://www.ncbi.nlm.nih.gov/pubmed/17486158. doi:10.1139/h06-072

Candia, V., Schafer, T., Taub, E., Rau, H., Altenmuller, E., Rockstroh, B., & Elbert, T. (2002). Sensory motor retuning: A behavioral treatment for focal hand dystonia of pianists and guitarists. *Archives of Physical Medicine and Rehabilitation, 83*(10), 1342–1348. Retrieved from https://www.ncbi.nlm.nih.gov/pubmed/12370865

Cannon, W. B. (1987). The James-Lange theory of emotions: A critical examination and an alternative theory. By Walter B. Cannon, 1927. *The American Journal of Psychology, 100*(3–4), 567–586. Retrieved from https://www.ncbi.nlm.nih.gov/pubmed/3322057

Canseco, J. (2005). *Juiced: Wild times, rampant 'roids, smash hits, and how baseball got big*. New York: Harper.

Cappelletti, M., & Wallen, K. (2016). Increasing women's sexual desire: The comparative effectiveness of estrogens and androgens. *Hormones and Behavior, 78*, 178–193. Retrieved from https://www.ncbi.nlm.nih.gov/pubmed/26589379. doi:10.1016/j.yhbeh.2015.11.003

Cardinal, R. N. (2006). Neural systems implicated in delayed and probabilistic reinforcement. *Neural Networks, 19*(8), 1277–1301. Retrieved from https://www.ncbi.nlm.nih.gov/pubmed/16938431. doi:10.1016/j.neunet.2006.03.004

Carew, T. J., Castellucci, V. F., & Kandel, E. R. (1971). An analysis of dishabituation and sensitization of the gill-withdrawal reflex in Aplysia. *International Journal of Neuroscience, 2*(2), 79–98. Retrieved from https://www.ncbi.nlm.nih.gov/pubmed/4347410

Carew, T. J., Hawkins, R. D., & Kandel, E. R. (1983). Differential classical conditioning of a defensive withdrawal reflex in Aplysia californica. *Science, 219*(4583), 397–400. Retrieved from https://www.ncbi.nlm.nih.gov/pubmed/6681571

Carlson, C., & Devinsky, O. (2009). The excitable cerebral cortex Fritsch G, Hitzig E. Uber die elektrische Erregbarkeit des Grosshirns. Arch Anat Physiol Wissen 1870;37:300-32. *Epilepsy & Behavior, 15*(2), 131–132. Retrieved from https://www.ncbi.nlm.nih.gov/pubmed/19269348. doi:10.1016/j.yebeh.2009.03.002

Carneiro, C. F. D., Moulin, T. C., Macleod, M. R., & Amaral, O. B. (2018). Effect size and statistical power in the rodent fear conditioning literature - A systematic review. *PLoS One, 13*(4), e0196258. Retrieved from https://www.ncbi.nlm.nih.gov/pubmed/29698451. doi:10.1371/journal.pone.0196258

Carr, G. D., Phillips, A. G., & Fibiger, H. C. (1988). Independence of amphetamine reward from locomotor stimulation demonstrated by conditioned place preference. *Psychopharmacology (Berl), 94*(2), 221–226. Retrieved from https://www.ncbi.nlm.nih.gov/pubmed/3127848

Carter, C. S., & Getz, L. L. (1993). Monogamy and the prairie vole. *Scientific American, 268*(6), 100–106. Retrieved from https://www.ncbi.nlm.nih.gov/pubmed/8516669

Casey, B. J., Jones, R. M., & Hare, T. A. (2008). The adolescent brain. *Annals of the New York Academy of Sciences, 1124*, 111–126. Retrieved from https://www.ncbi.nlm.nih.gov/pubmed/18400927. doi:10.1196/annals.1440.010

Castellucci, V., Pinsker, H., Kupfermann, I., & Kandel, E. R. (1970). Neuronal mechanisms of habituation and dishabituation of the gill-withdrawal reflex in Aplysia. *Science, 167*(3926), 1745–1748. Retrieved from https://www.ncbi.nlm.nih.gov/pubmed/5416543

Centonze, D., Siracusano, A., Calabresi, P., & Bernardi, G. (2004). The Project for a Scientific Psychology (1895): A Freudian anticipation of LTP-memory connection theory. *Brain Research Reviews, 46*(3), 310–314. Retrieved from https://www.ncbi.nlm.nih.gov/pubmed/15571772. doi:10.1016/j.brainresrev.2004.07.006

Chabris, C. F., & Simons, D. J. (2010). *The invisible gorilla: And other ways our intuitions deceive us* (1st ed.). New York: Crown.

Chadwick, B., Miller, M. L., & Hurd, Y. L. (2013). Cannabis use during adolescent development: Susceptibility to psychiatric illness. *Frontiers in Psychiatry, 4*, 129. Retrieved from https://www.ncbi.nlm.nih.gov/pubmed/24133461. doi:10.3389/fpsyt.2013.00129

Chalmers, D. J. (1995). The puzzle of conscious experience. *Scientific American, 273*(6), 80–86. Retrieved from http://www.ncbi.nlm.nih.gov/pubmed/8525350

Chandra, A., Mosher, W. D., Copen, C., & Sionean, C. (2011). Sexual behavior, sexual attraction, and sexual identity in the United States: Data from the 2006-2008 National Survey of Family Growth. *National Health Statistics Reports, 36*(36), 1–36. Retrieved from https://www.ncbi.nlm.nih.gov/pubmed/21560887

Chandrashekar, J., Kuhn, C., Oka, Y., Yarmolinsky, D. A., Hummler, E., Ryba, N. J., & Zuker, C. S. (2010). The cells and peripheral representation of sodium taste in mice. *Nature, 464*(7286), 297–301. Retrieved from https://www.ncbi.nlm.nih.gov/pubmed/20107438. doi:10.1038/nature08783

Charnigo, R., Noar, S. M., Garnett, C., Crosby, R., Palmgreen, P., & Zimmerman, R. S. (2013). Sensation seeking and impulsivity:

Combined associations with risky sexual behavior in a large sample of young adults. *Journal of Sex Research, 50*(5), 480–488. Retrieved from https://www.ncbi.nlm.nih.gov/pubmed/22456443. doi:10.1080/00224499.2011.652264

Chaudhari, N., Landin, A. M., & Roper, S. D. (2000). A metabotropic glutamate receptor variant functions as a taste receptor. *Nature Neuroscience, 3*(2), 113–119. Retrieved from https://www.ncbi.nlm.nih.gov/pubmed/10649565. doi:10.1038/72053

Chaudhari, N., Pereira, E., & Roper, S. D. (2009). Taste receptors for umami: The case for multiple receptors. *The American Journal of Clinical Nutrition, 90*(3), 738S–742S. Retrieved from https://www.ncbi.nlm.nih.gov/pubmed/19571230. doi:10.3945/ajcn.2009.27462H

Chavkin, C., Shoemaker, W. J., McGinty, J. F., Bayon, A., & Bloom, F. E. (1985). Characterization of the prodynorphin and proenkephalin neuropeptide systems in rat hippocampus. *The Journal of Neuroscience, 5*(3), 808–816. Retrieved from https://www.ncbi.nlm.nih.gov/pubmed/3838345

Chen, M. H., Li, C. T., Lin, W. C., Hong, C. J., Tu, P. C., Bai, Y. M., . . . Su, T. P. (2018). Rapid inflammation modulation and antidepressant efficacy of a low-dose ketamine infusion in treatment-resistant depression: A randomized, double-blind control study. *Psychiatry Research, 269*, 207–211. Retrieved from https://www.ncbi.nlm.nih.gov/pubmed/30153598. doi:10.1016/j.psychres.2018.08.078

Cheng, C. H., & Detrich, H. W., 3rd. (2007). Molecular ecophysiology of Antarctic notothenioid fishes. *Philosophical Transactions of the Royal Society of London Series B, Biological Sciences, 362*(1488), 2215–2232. Retrieved from https://www.ncbi.nlm.nih.gov/pubmed/17553777. doi:10.1098/rstb.2006.1946

Cheng, D. T., Knight, D. C., Smith, C. N., Stein, E. A., & Helmstetter, F. J. (2003). Functional MRI of human amygdala activity during Pavlovian fear conditioning: Stimulus processing versus response expression. *Behavioral Neuroscience, 117*(1), 3–10. Retrieved from https://www.ncbi.nlm.nih.gov/pubmed/12619902

Cheng, G., Huang, C., Deng, H., & Wang, H. (2012). Diabetes as a risk factor for dementia and mild cognitive impairment: A meta-analysis of longitudinal studies. *Internal Medicine Journal, 42*(5), 484–491. Retrieved from https://www.ncbi.nlm.nih.gov/pubmed/22372522. doi:10.1111/j.1445-5994.2012.02758.x

Cherniak, C. (1990). The bounded brain: Toward quantitative neuroanatomy. *Journal of Cognitive Neuroscience, 2*(1), 58–68. Retrieved from https://www.ncbi.nlm.nih.gov/pubmed/23964724. doi:10.1162/jocn.1990.2.1.58

Chiao, C. C., Chubb, C., & Hanlon, R. T. (2015). A review of visual perception mechanisms that regulate rapid adaptive camouflage in cuttlefish. *Journal of Comparative Physiology A, Neuroethology, Sensory, Neural, and Behavioral Physiology, 201*(9), 933–945. Retrieved from https://www.ncbi.nlm.nih.gov/pubmed/25701389. doi:10.1007/s00359-015-0988-5

Chieng, B., & Williams, J. T. (1998). Increased opioid inhibition of GABA release in nucleus accumbens during morphine withdrawal. *The Journal of Neuroscience, 18*(17), 7033–7039. Retrieved from https://www.ncbi.nlm.nih.gov/pubmed/9712672

Cho, S. B., Baars, B. J., & Newman, J. (1997). A neural global workspace model for conscious attention. *Neural Networks, 10*(7), 1195–1206. Retrieved from http://www.ncbi.nlm.nih.gov/pubmed/12662511

Choudhury, M. N., Uddin, A., & Chakraborty, S. (2018). Nucleotide composition and codon usage bias of SRY gene. *Andrologia, 50*(1). Retrieved from https://www.ncbi.nlm.nih.gov/pubmed/28124482. doi:10.1111/and.12787

Christou, G. A., & Kiortsis, D. N. (2015). The efficacy and safety of the naltrexone/bupropion combination for the treatment of obesity: An update. *Hormones (Athens), 14*(3), 370–375. Retrieved from https://www.ncbi.nlm.nih.gov/pubmed/26188223. doi:10.14310/horm.2002.1600

Cialdini, R. B., & Kenrick, D. T. (1976). Altruism as hedonism: A social development perspective on the relationship of negative mood state and helping. *Journal of Personality and Social Psychology, 34*(5), 907–914. Retrieved from http://www.ncbi.nlm.nih.gov/pubmed/993985

Cilz, N. I., Cymerblit-Sabba, A., & Young, W. S. (2019). Oxytocin and vasopressin in the rodent hippocampus. *Genes, Brain and Behavior, 18*(1), e12535. Retrieved from https://www.ncbi.nlm.nih.gov/pubmed/30378258. doi:10.1111/gbb.12535

Clark, L., Lawrence, A. J., Astley-Jones, F., & Gray, N. (2009). Gambling near-misses enhance motivation to gamble and recruit win-related brain circuitry. *Neuron, 61*(3), 481–490. Retrieved from https://www.ncbi.nlm.nih.gov/pubmed/19217383. doi:10.1016/j.neuron.2008.12.031

Clark, R. E., Broadbent, N. J., & Squire, L. R. (2005). Hippocampus and remote spatial memory in rats. *Hippocampus, 15*(2), 260–272. Retrieved from https://www.ncbi.nlm.nih.gov/pubmed/15523608. doi:10.1002/hipo.20056

Clarke, D. D., & Sokoloff, L. (1999). Circulation and energy metabolism of the brain. In G. J. Sigel, B. W. Agrano, R. W. Albers, S. K. Fisher, & M. D. Uhler (Eds.), *Basic neurochemistry: Molecular, cellular and medical aspects* (pp. 637–669). Philadelphia, PA: Lippincott-Raven

Clarke, E., & Stannard, J. (1963). Aristotle on the anatomy of the brain. *Journal of the History of Medicine and Allied Sciences, 18*, 130–148. Retrieved from https://www.ncbi.nlm.nih.gov/pubmed/14021565

Cohen, N. J., Poldrack, R. A., & Eichenbaum, H. (1997). Memory for items and memory for relations in the procedural/declarative memory framework. *Memory, 5*(1–2), 131–178. Retrieved from https://www.ncbi.nlm.nih.gov/pubmed/9156097. doi:10.1080/741941149

Collings, V. B. (1974). Human taste response as a function of locus of stimulation on the tongue and soft palate. *Perception & Psychophysics, 16*(1), 169–174.

Comery, T. A., Harris, J. B., Willems, P. J., Oostra, B. A., Irwin, S. A., Weiler, I. J., & Greenough, W. T. (1997). Abnormal dendritic spines in fragile X knockout mice: Maturation and pruning deficits. *Proceedings of the National Academy of Sciences of the United States of America, 94*(10), 5401–5404. Retrieved from http://www.ncbi.nlm.nih.gov/pubmed/9144249

Conel, J. L. (1939). *The postnatal development of the human cerebral cortex*. Cambridge, MA: Harvard University Press.

Connor, S. A., & Wang, Y. T. (2016). A place at the Table: LTD as a mediator of memory genesis. *The Neuroscientist, 22*(4), 359–371. Retrieved from https://www.ncbi.nlm.nih.gov/pubmed/25993993. doi:10.1177/1073858415588498

Consiglio, W., Driscoll, P., Witte, M., & Berg, W. P. (2003). Effect of cellular telephone conversations and other potential interference on reaction time in a braking response. *Accident Analysis & Prevention, 35*(4), 495–500. Retrieved from https://www.ncbi.nlm.nih.gov/pubmed/12729813

Cooper, S., Robison, A. J., & Mazei-Robison, M. S. (2017). Reward circuitry in addiction. *Neurotherapeutics, 14*(3), 687–697. Retrieved from https://www.ncbi.nlm.nih.gov/pubmed/28324454. doi:10.1007/s13311-017-0525-z

Corballis, M. C. (2009). The evolution and genetics of cerebral asymmetry. *Philosophical Transactions of the Royal Society of London Series B, Biological Sciences, 364*(1519), 867–879. Retrieved from https://www.ncbi.nlm.nih.gov/pubmed/19064358. doi:10.1098/rstb.2008.0232

Corbetta, M. (1998). Frontoparietal cortical networks for directing attention and the eye to visual locations: Identical, independent, or overlapping neural systems? *Proceedings of the National Academy of Sciences of the United States of America, 95*(3), 831–838. Retrieved from https://www.ncbi.nlm.nih.gov/pubmed/9448248

Corbetta, M., & Shulman, G. L. (2002). Control of goal-directed and stimulus-driven attention in the brain. *Nature Reviews Neuroscience, 3*(3), 201–215.

Cordaro, D. T., Sun, R., Keltner, D., Kamble, S., Huddar, N., & McNeil, G. (2018). Universals and cultural variations in 22 emotional expressions across five cultures. *Emotion, 18*(1), 75–93. Retrieved from https://www.ncbi.nlm.nih.gov/pubmed/28604039. doi:10.1037/emo0000302

Corder, E. H., Woodbury, M. A., Volkmann, I., Madsen, D. K., Bogdanovic, N., & Winblad, B. (2000). Density profiles of Alzheimer disease regional brain pathology for the Huddinge brain bank: Pattern recognition emulates and expands upon Braak staging. *Experimental Gerontology, 35*(6–7), 851–864. Retrieved from https://www.ncbi.nlm.nih.gov/pubmed/11053676

Corfield, E. C., Yang, Y., Martin, N. G., & Nyholt, D. R. (2017). A continuum of genetic liability for minor and major depression. *Translational Psychiatry, 7*(5), e1131. Retrieved from https://www.ncbi.nlm.nih.gov/pubmed/28509901. doi:10.1038/tp.2017.99

Cosic, K., Popovic, S., Kukolja, D., Dropuljic, B., Ivanec, D., & Tonkovic, M. (2016). Multimodal analysis of startle type responses. *Computer Methods and Programs in Biomedicine, 129*, 186–202. Retrieved from https://www.ncbi.nlm.nih.gov/pubmed/26826902. doi:10.1016/j.cmpb.2016.01.002

Coutinho, V., & Knopfel, T. (2002). Metabotropic glutamate receptors: Electrical and chemical signaling properties. *The Neuroscientist, 8*(6), 551–561. Retrieved from https://www.ncbi.nlm.nih.gov/pubmed/12467377. doi:10.1177/1073858402238514

Cowan, N. (1984). On short and long auditory stores. *Psychological Bulletin, 96*(2), 341–370. Retrieved from https://www.ncbi.nlm.nih.gov/pubmed/6385047

Cowan, W. M., & Kandel, E. R. (2001). A brief history of synapses and synaptic transmission. In W. M. Cowan, T. C. Südhof, & C. F. Davies (Eds.), *Synapses*. Baltimore, MD: Johns Hopkins University Press.

Creese, I., Burt, D. R., & Snyder, S. H. (1996). Dopamine receptor binding predicts clinical and pharmacological potencies of antischizophrenic drugs. *The Journal of Neuropsychiatry and Clinical Neurosciences, 8*(2), 223–226. Retrieved from http://www.ncbi.nlm.nih.gov/pubmed/9081563. doi:10.1176/jnp.8.2.223

Crestani, F., Lorez, M., Baer, K., Essrich, C., Benke, D., Laurent, J. P., . . . Mohler, H. (1999). Decreased GABAA-receptor clustering results in enhanced anxiety and a bias for threat cues. *Nature Neuroscience, 2*(9), 833–839. Retrieved from https://www.ncbi.nlm.nih.gov/pubmed/10461223. doi:10.1038/12207

Crick, F., & Koch, C. (1990). Towards a neurobiological theory of consciousness. *Seminars in the Neurosciences, 2*, 263–275.

Cui, H., & Andersen, R. A. (2007). Posterior parietal cortex encodes autonomously selected motor plans. *Neuron, 56*(3), 552–559. Retrieved from https://www.ncbi.nlm.nih.gov/pubmed/17988637. doi:10.1016/j.neuron.2007.09.031

Curcic-Blake, B., Ford, J. M., Hubl, D., Orlov, N. D., Sommer, I. E., Waters, F., . . . Aleman, A. (2017). Interaction of language, auditory and memory brain networks in auditory verbal hallucinations. *Progress in Neurobiology, 148*, 1–20. Retrieved from https://www.ncbi.nlm.nih.gov/pubmed/27890810. doi:10.1016/j.pneurobio.2016.11.002

Czeisler, C. A., Weitzman, E., Moore-Ede, M. C., Zimmerman, J. C., & Knauer, R. S. (1980). Human sleep: Its duration and organization depend on its circadian phase. *Science, 210*(4475), 1264–1267. Retrieved from https://www.ncbi.nlm.nih.gov/pubmed/7434029

Dalgleish, T. (2004). The emotional brain. *Nature Reviews Neuroscience, 5*(7), 583–589. Retrieved from https://www.ncbi.nlm.nih.gov/pubmed/15208700. doi:10.1038/nrn1432

Dalley, J. W., Mar, A. C., Economidou, D., & Robbins, T. W. (2008). Neurobehavioral mechanisms of impulsivity: Fronto-striatal systems and functional neurochemistry. *Pharmacology Biochemistry and Behavior, 90*(2), 250–260. Retrieved from https://www.ncbi.nlm.nih.gov/pubmed/18272211. doi:10.1016/j.pbb.2007.12.021

Daly, M. (2018). Partitioning aggression. *Proceedings of the National Academy of Sciences of the United States of America, 115*(4), 633–634. Retrieved from https://www.ncbi.nlm.nih.gov/pubmed/29326233. doi:10.1073/pnas.1720838115

Damasio, A. R. (1994). *Descartes' error: Emotion, reason, and the human brain*. New York, NY: Putnam.

Damasio, A. R. (1996). The somatic marker hypothesis and the possible functions of the prefrontal cortex. *Philosophical Transactions of the Royal Society of London Series B, Biological Sciences, 351*(1346), 1413–1420. Retrieved from https://www.ncbi.nlm.nih.gov/pubmed/8941953. doi:10.1098/rstb.1996.0125

Damier, P., Hirsch, E. C., Agid, Y., & Graybiel, A. M. (1999). The substantia nigra of the human brain. II. Patterns of loss of dopamine-containing neurons in Parkinson's disease. *Brain, 122*(Pt. 8), 1437–1448. Retrieved from https://www.ncbi.nlm.nih.gov/pubmed/10430830

D'Arcangelo, G., Triossi, T., Buglione, A., Melchiorri, G., & Tancredi, V. (2017). Modulation of synaptic plasticity by short-term aerobic exercise in adult mice. *Behavioural Brain Research, 332*, 59–63. Retrieved from https://www.ncbi.nlm.nih.gov/pubmed/28559180. doi:10.1016/j.bbr.2017.05.058

Darnell, D., & Gilbert, S. F. (2017). Neuroembryology. *Wiley Interdisciplinary Reviews: Developmental Biology, 6*(1). Retrieved from https://www.ncbi.nlm.nih.gov/pubmed/27906497. doi:10.1002/wdev.215

Darwin, C. (1859). *On the origin of species by means of natural selection: Or, the preservation of favoured races in the struggle for life*. London: J. Murray.

Darwin, C. (1873). *The expression of the emotions in man and animals*. New York: D. Appleton.

da Silva Alves, F., Figee, M., van Amelsvoort, T., Veltman, D., & de Haan, L. (2008). The revised dopamine hypothesis of schizophrenia: Evidence from pharmacological MRI studies with atypical antipsychotic medication. *Psychopharmacology Bulletin, 41*(1), 121–132. Retrieved from https://www.ncbi.nlm.nih.gov/pubmed/18362875

Dash, P. K., Hebert, A. E., & Runyan, J. D. (2004). A unified theory for systems and cellular memory consolidation. *Brain Research Reviews, 45*(1), 30–37. Retrieved from https://www.ncbi.nlm.nih.gov/pubmed/15063098. doi:10.1016/j.brainresrev.2004.02.001

Davidson, R. J., Pizzagalli, D., Nitschke, J. B., & Putnam, K. (2002). Depression: Perspectives from affective neuroscience. *Annual Review of Psychology, 53*, 545–574. Retrieved from http://www.ncbi.nlm.nih.gov/pubmed/11752496. doi:10.1146/annurev.psych.53.100901.135148

Davis, E. C., Popper, P., & Gorski, R. A. (1996). The role of apoptosis in sexual differentiation of the rat sexually dimorphic nucleus of the preoptic area. *Brain Research, 734*(1–2), 10–18. Retrieved from https://www.ncbi.nlm.nih.gov/pubmed/8896803

Davis, H. P., & Squire, L. R. (1984). Protein synthesis and memory: A review. *Psychological Bulletin, 96*(3), 518–559. Retrieved from https://www.ncbi.nlm.nih.gov/pubmed/6096908

Davis, K. L., Kahn, R. S., Ko, G., & Davidson, M. (1991). Dopamine in schizophrenia: A review and reconceptualization. *The American*

Journal of Psychiatry, *148*(11), 1474–1486. Retrieved from http://www.ncbi.nlm.nih.gov/pubmed/1681750. doi:10.1176/ajp.148.11.1474

Davis, M. (1992). The role of the amygdala in fear and anxiety. *Annual Review of Neuroscience*, *15*, 353–375. Retrieved from https://www.ncbi.nlm.nih.gov/pubmed/1575447. doi:10.1146/annurev.ne.15.030192.002033

de Boer, J. N., Linszen, M. M. J., de Vries, J., Schutte, M. J. L., Begemann, M. J. H., Heringa, S. M., . . . Sommer, I. E. C. (2019). Auditory hallucinations, top-down processing and language perception: A general population study. *Psychological Medicine*, 1–9. Retrieved from https://www.ncbi.nlm.nih.gov/pubmed/30606279. doi:10.1017/S003329171800380X

De Felice, F. G., & Benedict, C. (2015). A key role of insulin receptors in memory. *Diabetes*, *64*(11), 3653–3655. Retrieved from https://www.ncbi.nlm.nih.gov/pubmed/26494219. doi:10.2337/dbi15-0011

De Gelder, B. (2010). Uncanny sight in the blind. *Scientific American*, *302*(5), 60–65. Retrieved from http://www.ncbi.nlm.nih.gov/pubmed/20443379

de Nazareth, A. M. (2017). Type 2 diabetes mellitus in the pathophysiology of Alzheimer's disease. *Dementia e Neuropsychologia*, *11*(2), 105–113. Retrieved from https://www.ncbi.nlm.nih.gov/pubmed/29213501. doi:10.1590/1980-57642016dn11-020002

De Valois, R. L., Smith, C. J., Kitai, S. T., & Karoly, A. J. (1958). Response of single cells in monkey lateral geniculate nucleus to monochromatic light. *Science*, *127*(3292), 238–239. Retrieved from https://www.ncbi.nlm.nih.gov/pubmed/13495504

De Wit, H., & Wise, R. A. (1977). Blockade of cocaine reinforcement in rats with the dopamine receptor blocker pimozide, but not with the noradrenergic blockers phentolamine or phenoxybenzamine. *Canadian Journal of Psychology*, *31*(4), 195–203. Retrieved from https://www.ncbi.nlm.nih.gov/pubmed/608135

Deahl, M. (1991). Cannabis and memory loss. *British Journal of Addiction*, *86*(3), 249–252. Retrieved from https://www.ncbi.nlm.nih.gov/pubmed/2025687

Decety, J., & Keenan, J. P. (2006). Social neuroscience: A new journal. *Social Neuroscience*, *1*(1), 1–4. Retrieved from https://www.ncbi.nlm.nih.gov/pubmed/18633771. doi:10.1080/17470910601117463

Decety, J., & Lamm, C. (2007). The role of the right temporoparietal junction in social interaction: How low-level computational processes contribute to meta-cognition. *Neuroscientist*, *13*(6), 580–593. Retrieved from https://www.ncbi.nlm.nih.gov/pubmed/17911216. doi:10.1177/1073858407304654

Deco, G., Rolls, E. T., & Romo, R. (2010). Synaptic dynamics and decision making. *Proceedings of the National Academy of Sciences of the United States of America*, *107*(16), 7545–7549. Retrieved from https://www.ncbi.nlm.nih.gov/pubmed/20360555. doi:10.1073/pnas.1002333107

Defoe, I. N., Dubas, J. S., Figner, B., & van Aken, M. A. (2015). A meta-analysis on age differences in risky decision making: Adolescents versus children and adults. *Psychological Bulletin*, *141*(1), 48–84. Retrieved from https://www.ncbi.nlm.nih.gov/pubmed/25365761. doi:10.1037/a0038088

Dehaene, S., Changeux, J. P., Naccache, L., Sackur, J., & Sergent, C. (2006). Conscious, preconscious, and subliminal processing: A testable taxonomy. *Trends in Cognitive Sciences*, *10*(5), 204–211. Retrieved from http://www.ncbi.nlm.nih.gov/pubmed/16603406. doi:10.1016/j.tics.2006.03.007

Del Valle, M. E., Cobo, T., Cobo, J. L., & Vega, J. A. (2012). Mechanosensory neurons, cutaneous mechanoreceptors, and putative mechanoproteins. *Microsc Res Tech*, *75*(8), 1033–1043. doi:10.1002/jemt.22028

Del-Ben, C. M., Ferreira, C. A., Sanchez, T. A., Alves-Neto, W. C., Guapo, V. G., de Araujo, D. B., & Graeff, F. G. (2012). Effects of diazepam on BOLD activation during the processing of aversive faces. *Journal of Psychopharmacology*, *26*(4), 443–451. Retrieved from https://www.ncbi.nlm.nih.gov/pubmed/21106607. doi:10.1177/0269881110389092

DeLong, M. R., & Wichmann, T. (2007). Circuits and circuit disorders of the basal ganglia. *Archives of Neurology*, *64*(1), 20–24. Retrieved from https://www.ncbi.nlm.nih.gov/pubmed/17210805. doi:10.1001/archneur.64.1.20

DeLuca, R. S. (2017). *The hormone myth: How junk science, gender politics & lies about PMS keep women down*. Oakland, CA: New Harbinger Publications, Inc.

Demonbreun, A. R., Biersmith, B. H., & McNally, E. M. (2015). Membrane fusion in muscle development and repair. *Seminars in Cell and Developmental Biology*, *45*, 48–56. Retrieved from http://www.ncbi.nlm.nih.gov/pubmed/26537430. doi:10.1016/j.semcdb.2015.10.026

Deng, F., Jiang, X., Zhu, D., Zhang, T., Li, K., Guo, L., & Liu, T. (2014). A functional model of cortical gyri and sulci. *Brain Structure and Function*, *219*(4), 1473–1491. Retrieved from https://www.ncbi.nlm.nih.gov/pubmed/23689502. doi:10.1007/s00429-013-0581-z

Deng, W., Aimone, J. B., & Gage, F. H. (2010). New neurons and new memories: How does adult hippocampal neurogenesis affect learning and memory? *Nature Reviews Neuroscience*, *11*(5), 339–350. Retrieved from https://www.ncbi.nlm.nih.gov/pubmed/20354534. doi:10.1038/nrn2822

Dent, E. W., & Gertler, F. B. (2003). Cytoskeletal dynamics and transport in growth cone motility and axon guidance. *Neuron*, *40*(2), 209–227. Retrieved from https://www.ncbi.nlm.nih.gov/pubmed/14556705

Descartes, R., & Schuyl, F. (1662). *De homine, figuris*. Lugduni Batavorum: Apud Franciscum Moyardum & Petrum Leffen.

Desmurget, M., Richard, N., Harquel, S., Baraduc, P., Szathmari, A., Mottolese, C., & Sirigu, A. (2014). Neural representations of ethologically relevant hand/mouth synergies in the human precentral gyrus. *Proceedings of the National Academy of Sciences of the United States of America*, *111*(15), 5718–722. Retrieved from https://www.ncbi.nlm.nih.gov/pubmed/24706796. doi:10.1073/pnas.1321909111

Deutsch, J. A., & Deutsch, D. (1963). Some theoretical considerations. *Psychological Review*, *70*, 80–90. Retrieved from https://www.ncbi.nlm.nih.gov/pubmed/14027390

Dewall, C. N., Macdonald, G., Webster, G. D., Masten, C. L., Baumeister, R. F., Powell, C., . . . Eisenberger, N. I. (2010). Acetaminophen reduces social pain: Behavioral and neural evidence. *Psychological Science*, *21*(7), 931–937. Retrieved from http://www.ncbi.nlm.nih.gov/pubmed/20548058. doi:10.1177/0956797610374741

DeYoe, E. A., Carman, G. J., Bandettini, P., Glickman, S., Wieser, J., Cox, R., . . . Neitz, J. (1996). Mapping striate and extrastriate visual areas in human cerebral cortex. *Proceedings of the National Academy of Sciences of the United States of America*, *93*(6), 2382–2386. Retrieved from https://www.ncbi.nlm.nih.gov/pubmed/8637882

Di Biase, M. A., Zhang, F., Lyall, A., Kubicki, M., Mandl, R. C. W., Sommer, I. E., & Pasternak, O. (2019). Neuroimaging auditory verbal hallucinations in schizophrenia patient and healthy populations. *Psychological Medicine*, 1–10. Retrieved from https://www.ncbi.nlm.nih.gov/pubmed/30782233. doi:10.1017/S0033291719000205

Dias, B. G., & Ressler, K. J. (2014). Parental olfactory experience influences behavior and neural structure in subsequent generations. *Nature Neuroscience*, *17*(1), 89–96. Retrieved from https://www.ncbi.nlm.nih.gov/pubmed/24292232. doi:10.1038/nn.3594

Dick, D. M. (2011). Gene-environment interaction in psychological traits and disorders. *Annual Review of Clinical Psychology, 7*, 383–409. Retrieved from https://www.ncbi.nlm.nih.gov/pubmed/21219196. doi:10.1146/annurev-clinpsy-032210-104518

Dickinson, A., Smith, J., & Mirenowicz, J. (2000). Dissociation of Pavlovian and instrumental incentive learning under dopamine antagonists. *Behavioral Neuroscience, 114*(3), 468–483. Retrieved from https://www.ncbi.nlm.nih.gov/pubmed/10883798

Dickson, D. W. (2018). Neuropathology of Parkinson disease. *Parkinsonism & Related Disorders, 46*(Suppl. 1), S30–S33. Retrieved from https://www.ncbi.nlm.nih.gov/pubmed/28780180. doi:10.1016/j.parkreldis.2017.07.033

Dobolyi, A., Grattan, D. R., & Stolzenberg, D. S. (2014). Preoptic inputs and mechanisms that regulate maternal responsiveness. *Journal of Neuroendocrinology, 26*(10), 627–640. Retrieved from https://www.ncbi.nlm.nih.gov/pubmed/25059569. doi:10.1111/jne.12185

Dodge, K. A., & Coie, J. D. (1987). Social-information-processing factors in reactive and proactive aggression in children's peer groups. *Journal of Personality and Social Psychology, 53*(6), 1146–1158. Retrieved from https://www.ncbi.nlm.nih.gov/pubmed/3694454

Doetsch, F. (2003). The glial identity of neural stem cells. *Nature Neuroscience, 6*(11), 1127–1134. Retrieved from https://www.ncbi.nlm.nih.gov/pubmed/14583753. doi:10.1038/nn1144

Doetsch, G. S. (2000). Patterns in the brain. Neuronal population coding in the somatosensory system. *Physiology & Behavior, 69*(1–2), 187–201. Retrieved from https://www.ncbi.nlm.nih.gov/pubmed/10854929

Domino, E. F. (1999). History of modern psychopharmacology: A personal view with an emphasis on antidepressants. *Psychosomatic Medicine, 61*(5), 591–598. Retrieved from https://www.ncbi.nlm.nih.gov/pubmed/10511010

Domjan, M., & Grau, J. W. (2015). *The principles of learning and behavior* (7th ed.). Stamford, CT: Cengage Learning.

Donaldson, Z. R., Piel, D. A., Santos, T. L., Richardson-Jones, J., Leonardo, E. D., Beck, S. G., . . . Hen, R. (2014). Developmental effects of serotonin 1A autoreceptors on anxiety and social behavior. *Neuropsychopharmacology, 39*(2), 291–302. Retrieved from https://www.ncbi.nlm.nih.gov/pubmed/23907404. doi:10.1038/npp.2013.185

Dong, A., Liu, S., & Li, Y. (2018). Gap junctions in the nervous system: Probing functional connections using new imaging approaches. *Frontiers in Cellular Neuroscience, 12*, 320. Retrieved from https://www.ncbi.nlm.nih.gov/pubmed/30283305. doi:10.3389/fncel.2018.00320

Dotti, C. G., Sullivan, C. A., & Banker, G. A. (1988). The establishment of polarity by hippocampal neurons in culture. *Journal of Neuroscience, 8*(4), 1454–1468. Retrieved from https://www.ncbi.nlm.nih.gov/pubmed/3282038

Doty, R. L. (2018). Age-related deficits in Taste and Smell. *Otolaryngologic Clinics of North America, 51*(4), 815–825. Retrieved from https://www.ncbi.nlm.nih.gov/pubmed/30001793. doi:10.1016/j.otc.2018.03.014

Douglas, R. M., & Goddard, G. V. (1975). Long-term potentiation of the perforant path-granule cell synapse in the rat hippocampus. *Brain Research, 86*(2), 205–215. Retrieved from https://www.ncbi.nlm.nih.gov/pubmed/163667

Downar, J. (2019). Orbitofrontal cortex: A 'Non-rewarding' new treatment target in depression? *Current Biology, 29*(5), 896. Retrieved from https://www.ncbi.nlm.nih.gov/pubmed/30836077. doi:10.1016/j.cub.2019.02.015

Downar, J., Crawley, A. P., Mikulis, D. J., & Davis, K. D. (2000). A multimodal cortical network for the detection of changes in the sensory environment. *Nature Neuroscience, 3*(3), 277–283. Retrieved from https://www.ncbi.nlm.nih.gov/pubmed/10700261. doi:10.1038/72991

Doya, K. (2008). Modulators of decision making. *Nature Neuroscience, 11*(4), 410–416. Retrieved from https://www.ncbi.nlm.nih.gov/pubmed/18368048. doi:10.1038/nn2077

Drachman, D. A. (2005). Do we have brain to spare? *Neurology, 64*(12), 2004–2005. Retrieved from https://www.ncbi.nlm.nih.gov/pubmed/15985565. doi:10.1212/01.WNL.0000166914.38327.BB

Draganski, B., Gaser, C., Busch, V., Schuierer, G., Bogdahn, U., & May, A. (2004). Neuroplasticity: Changes in grey matter induced by training. *Nature, 427*(6972), 311–312. Retrieved from https://www.ncbi.nlm.nih.gov/pubmed/14737157. doi:10.1038/427311a

Drevets, W. C. (2003). Neuroimaging abnormalities in the amygdala in mood disorders. *Annals of the New York Academy of Sciences, 985*, 420–444. Retrieved from http://www.ncbi.nlm.nih.gov/pubmed/12724175

Drevets, W. C., Price, J. L., Bardgett, M. E., Reich, T., Todd, R. D., & Raichle, M. E. (2002). Glucose metabolism in the amygdala in depression: Relationship to diagnostic subtype and plasma cortisol levels. *Pharmacology, Biochemistry and Behavior, 71*(3), 431–447. Retrieved from http://www.ncbi.nlm.nih.gov/pubmed/11830178

Drobisz, D., & Damborska, A. (2019). Deep brain stimulation targets for treating depression. *Behavioural Brain Research, 359*, 266–273. Retrieved from https://www.ncbi.nlm.nih.gov/pubmed/30414974. doi:10.1016/j.bbr.2018.11.004

Du, X., Wang, X., & Geng, M. (2018). Alzheimer's disease hypothesis and related therapies. *Translational Neurodegeneration, 7*, 2. Retrieved from https://www.ncbi.nlm.nih.gov/pubmed/29423193. doi:10.1186/s40035-018-0107-y

Duncan, C. P. (1949). The retroactive effect of electroshock on learning. *Journal of Comparative and Physiological Psychology, 42*(1), 32–44. Retrieved from https://www.ncbi.nlm.nih.gov/pubmed/18111554

Dursteler, M. R., & Wurtz, R. H. (1988). Pursuit and optokinetic deficits following chemical lesions of cortical areas MT and MST. *Journal of Neurophysiology, 60*(3), 940–965. Retrieved from https://www.ncbi.nlm.nih.gov/pubmed/3171667. doi:10.1152/jn.1988.60.3.940

Edwards, A., & Abizaid, A. (2017). Clarifying the Ghrelin system's ability to regulate feeding behaviours despite enigmatic spatial separation of the GHSR and its endogenous ligand. *International Journal of Molecular Sciences, 18*(4). Retrieved from https://www.ncbi.nlm.nih.gov/pubmed/28422060. doi:10.3390/ijms18040859

Eisenberger, N. I., & Lieberman, M. D. (2004). Why rejection hurts: A common neural alarm system for physical and social pain. *Trends in Cognitive Sciences, 8*(7), 294–300. Retrieved from http://www.ncbi.nlm.nih.gov/pubmed/15242688. doi:10.1016/j.tics.2004.05.010

Ekman, P. (1982). *Emotion in the human face* (2nd ed.). Cambridge Cambridgeshire/New York; Paris: Cambridge University Press; Editions de la Maison des Sciences de l'Homme.

Ekman, P. (1992). An argument for basic emotions. *Cognition and Emotion, 6*(3–4), 169–200. Retrieved from https://doi.org/10.1080/02699939208411068. doi:10.1080/02699939208411068

Ekman, P., & Cordaro, D. (2011). What is meant by calling emotions basic. *Emotion Review, 3*(4), 364–370. Retrieved from https://journals.sagepub.com/doi/abs/10.1177/1754073911410740. doi:10.1177/1754073911410740

Ellis, L., & Blanchard, R. (2001). Birth order, sibling sex ratio, and maternal miscarriages in homosexual and heterosexual men and women. *Personality and Individual Differences, 30*, 543–552.

ElSohly, M. A., Radwan, M. M., Gul, W., Chandra, S., & Galal, A. (2017). Phytochemistry of Cannabis sativa L. *Progress in the Chemistry of Organic Natural Products, 103*, 1–36. Retrieved from https://www.ncbi.nlm.nih.gov/pubmed/28120229. doi:10.1007/978-3-319-45541-9_1

Endler, N. S. (1988). The origins of electroconvulsive therapy (ECT). *Convulsive Therapy, 4*(1), 5–23. Retrieved from https://www.ncbi.nlm.nih.gov/pubmed/11940939

Engeroff, T., Ingmann, T., & Banzer, W. (2018). Physical activity throughout the adult life span and domain-specific cognitive function in old age: A systematic review of cross-sectional and longitudinal data. *Sports Medicine, 48*(6), 1405–1436. Retrieved from https://www.ncbi.nlm.nih.gov/pubmed/29667159. doi:10.1007/s40279-018-0920-6

Enke, A. M., & Poskey, G. A. (2018). Neuromuscular re-education programs for musicians with focal hand dystonia: A systematic review. *Medical Problems of Performing Artists, 33*(2), 137–145. Retrieved from https://www.ncbi.nlm.nih.gov/pubmed/29868689. doi:10.21091/mppa.2018.2014

Epp, J. R., Chow, C., & Galea, L. A. (2013). Hippocampus-dependent learning influences hippocampal neurogenesis. *Frontiers in Neuroscience, 7*, 57. Retrieved from https://www.ncbi.nlm.nih.gov/pubmed/23596385. doi:10.3389/fnins.2013.00057

Epstein, L. H., Truesdale, R., Wojcik, A., Paluch, R. A., & Raynor, H. A. (2003). Effects of deprivation on hedonics and reinforcing value of food. *Physiology & Behavior, 78*(2), 221–227. Retrieved from https://www.ncbi.nlm.nih.gov/pubmed/12576119

Erickson, K. I., Voss, M. W., Prakash, R. S., Basak, C., Szabo, A., Chaddock, L., . . . Kramer, A. F. (2011). Exercise training increases size of hippocampus and improves memory. *Proceedings of the National Academy of Sciences of the United States of America, 108*(7), 3017–3022. Retrieved from https://www.ncbi.nlm.nih.gov/pubmed/21282661. doi:10.1073/pnas.1015950108

Erlanson-Albertsson, C. (2005). Appetite regulation and energy balance. *Acta paediatrica. Supplementum, 94*(448), 40–41. Retrieved from https://www.ncbi.nlm.nih.gov/pubmed/16175806

Erlich, M. D., Smith, T. S., Horwath, E., & Cournos, F. (2014). Schizophrenia and other psychotic disorders. In Janis L. Cutler (Ed.), *Psychiatry*, 3rd ed. New York: Oxford University Press.

Eswarappa, M., Neylan, T. C., Whooley, M. A., Metzler, T. J., & Cohen, B. E. (2019). Inflammation as a predictor of disease course in posttraumatic stress disorder and depression: A prospective analysis from the Mind Your Heart Study. *Brain, Behavior, and Immunity, 75*, 220–227. Retrieved from https://www.ncbi.nlm.nih.gov/pubmed/30389462. doi:10.1016/j.bbi.2018.10.012

Etkin, A., & Wager, T. D. (2007). Functional neuroimaging of anxiety: A meta-analysis of emotional processing in PTSD, social anxiety disorder, and specific phobia. *The American Journal of Psychiatry, 164*(10), 1476–1488. Retrieved from http://www.ncbi.nlm.nih.gov/pubmed/17898336. doi:10.1176/appi.ajp.2007.07030504

Evarts, E. V. (1966). Pyramidal tract activity associated with a conditioned hand movement in the monkey. *Journal of Neurophysiology, 29*(6), 1011–1027. Retrieved from https://www.ncbi.nlm.nih.gov/pubmed/4961643

Everitt, B. J. (1990). Sexual motivation: A neural and behavioural analysis of the mechanisms underlying appetitive and copulatory responses of male rats. *Neuroscience & Biobehavioral Reviews, 14*(2), 217–232. Retrieved from https://www.ncbi.nlm.nih.gov/pubmed/2190121

Ezzyat, Y., Wanda, P. A., Levy, D. F., Kadel, A., Aka, A., Pedisich, I., . . . Kahana, M. J. (2018). Closed-loop stimulation of temporal cortex rescues functional networks and improves memory. *Nature Communications, 9*(1), 365. Retrieved from https://www.ncbi.nlm.nih.gov/pubmed/29410414. doi:10.1038/s41467-017-02753-0

Faedda, G. L., Becker, I., Baroni, A., Tondo, L., Aspland, E., & Koukopoulos, A. (2010). The origins of electroconvulsive therapy: Prof. Bini's first report on ECT. *Journal of Affective Disorders, 120*(1–3), 12–15. Retrieved from https://www.ncbi.nlm.nih.gov/pubmed/19268370. doi:10.1016/j.jad.2009.01.023

Farah, M. J., Hutchinson, J. B., Phelps, E. A., & Wagner, A. D. (2014). Functional MRI-based lie detection: Scientific and societal challenges. *Nature Reviews Neuroscience, 15*(2), 123–131. Retrieved from https://www.ncbi.nlm.nih.gov/pubmed/24588019

Fava, M., Rush, A. J., Thase, M. E., Clayton, A., Stahl, S. M., Pradko, J. F., & Johnston, J. A. (2005). 15 years of clinical experience with bupropion HCl: From bupropion to bupropion SR to bupropion XL. *The Primary Care Companion to the Journal of Clinical Psychiatry, 7*(3), 106–113. Retrieved from https://www.ncbi.nlm.nih.gov/pubmed/16027765

Feindel, W. (1982). The contributions of Wilder Penfield to the functional anatomy of the human brain. *Human Neurobiology, 1*(4), 231–234. Retrieved from https://www.ncbi.nlm.nih.gov/pubmed/6764468

Feinstein, J. S., Adolphs, R., Damasio, A., & Tranel, D. (2011). The human amygdala and the induction and experience of fear. *Current Biology, 21*(1), 34–38. Retrieved from https://www.ncbi.nlm.nih.gov/pubmed/21167712. doi:10.1016/j.cub.2010.11.042

Feinstein, J. S., Buzza, C., Hurlemann, R., Follmer, R. L., Dahdaleh, N. S., Coryell, W. H., . . . Wemmie, J. A. (2013). Fear and panic in humans with bilateral amygdala damage. *Nature Neuroscience, 16*(3), 270–272. Retrieved from https://www.ncbi.nlm.nih.gov/pubmed/23377128. doi:10.1038/nn.3323

Feldman, L. A. (1995). Valence focus and arousal focus: Individual differences in the structure of affective experience. *Journal of Personality and Social Psychology, 69*(1), 153–166. doi:http://dx.doi.org/10.1037/0022-3514.69.1.153

Fellows, L. K., & Farah, M. J. (2007). The role of ventromedial prefrontal cortex in decision making: Judgment under uncertainty or judgment per se? *Cerebral Cortex, 17*(11), 2669–2674. Retrieved from https://www.ncbi.nlm.nih.gov/pubmed/17259643. doi:10.1093/cercor/bhl176

Fenster, R. J., Lebois, L. A. M., Ressler, K. J., & Suh, J. (2018). Brain circuit dysfunction in post-traumatic stress disorder: From mouse to man. *Nature Reviews Neuroscience, 19*(9), 535–551. Retrieved from https://www.ncbi.nlm.nih.gov/pubmed/30054570. doi:10.1038/s41583-018-0039-7

Ferrario, C. R., & Reagan, L. P. (2018). Insulin-mediated synaptic plasticity in the CNS: Anatomical, functional and temporal contexts. *Neuropharmacology, 136*(Pt. B), 182–191. Retrieved from https://www.ncbi.nlm.nih.gov/pubmed/29217283. doi:10.1016/j.neuropharm.2017.12.001

Fettiplace, R., & Hackney, C. M. (2006). The sensory and motor roles of auditory hair cells. *Nature Reviews Neuroscience, 7*(1), 19–29. Retrieved from https://www.ncbi.nlm.nih.gov/pubmed/16371947. doi:10.1038/nrn1828

Finger, S. (2000). *Minds behind the brain: A history of the pioneers and their discoveries*. Oxford/New York: Oxford University Press.

Flegal, K. M., Kruszon-Moran, D., Carroll, M. D., Fryar, C. D., & Ogden, C. L. (2016). Trends in obesity among adults in the United States, 2005 to 2014. *The Journal of the American Medical Association*, 315(21), 2284–2291. Retrieved from https://www.ncbi.nlm.nih.gov/pubmed/27272580. doi:10.1001/jama.2016.6458

Fleischer, J., & Krieger, J. (2018). Insect Pheromone Receptors - Key Elements in Sensing Intraspecific Chemical Signals. *Frontiers in Cellular Neuroscience*, *12*, 425. Retrieved from https://www.ncbi.nlm.nih.gov/pubmed/30515079. doi:10.3389/fncel.2018.00425

Fleischman, J. (2002). *Phineas Gage: A gruesome but true story about brain science*. Boston: Houghton Mifflin.

Flinker, A., Korzeniewska, A., Shestyuk, A. Y., Franaszczuk, P. J., Dronkers, N. F., Knight, R. T., & Crone, N. E. (2015). Redefining the role of Broca's area in speech. *Proceedings of the National Academy of Sciences of the United States of America*, *112*(9), 2871–2875. Retrieved from https://www.ncbi.nlm.nih.gov/pubmed/25730850. doi:10.1073/pnas.1414491112

Flo, F. J., Kanu, O., Teleb, M., Chen, Y., & Siddiqui, T. (2018). Anabolic androgenic steroid-induced acute myocardial infarction with multiorgan failure. *Proceedings (Baylor University. Medical Center)*, *31*(3), 334–336. Retrieved from https://www.ncbi.nlm.nih.gov/pubmed/29904303. doi:10.1080/08998280.2018.1460130

Fogassi, L., Ferrari, P. F., Gesierich, B., Rozzi, S., Chersi, F., & Rizzolatti, G. (2005). Parietal lobe: From action organization to intention understanding. *Science*, *308*(5722), 662–667. Retrieved from https://www.ncbi.nlm.nih.gov/pubmed/15860620. doi:10.1126/science.1106138

Fontaine, J. R., Scherer, K. R., Roesch, E. B., & Ellsworth, P. C. (2007). The world of emotions is not two-dimensional. *Psychological Science*, *18*(12), 1050–1057. Retrieved from https://www.ncbi.nlm.nih.gov/pubmed/18031411. doi:10.1111/j.1467-9280.2007.02024.x

Forero, C. G., Castro-Rodriguez, J. I., & Alonso, J. (2015). Towards a biopsychosocial nosology of mental illness: Challenges and opportunities for psychiatric epidemiology. *Journal of Epidemiology & Community Health*, *69*(4), 301–302. Retrieved from https://www.ncbi.nlm.nih.gov/pubmed/25311478. doi:10.1136/jech-2014-203900

Fowler, J. S., Volkow, N. D., Kassed, C. A., & Chang, L. (2007). Imaging the addicted human brain. *Science & Practice Perspectives*, *3*(2), 4–16. Retrieved from https://www.ncbi.nlm.nih.gov/pubmed/17514067

Fraigne, J. J., Torontali, Z. A., Snow, M. B., & Peever, J. H. (2015). REM sleep at its core - circuits, neurotransmitters, and pathophysiology. *Frontiers in Neurology*, *6*, 123. Retrieved from https://www.ncbi.nlm.nih.gov/pubmed/26074874. doi:10.3389/fneur.2015.00123

Franke, W. W., & Berendonk, B. (1997). Hormonal doping and androgenization of athletes: A secret program of the German Democratic Republic government. *Clinical Chemistry*, *43*(7), 1262–1279. Retrieved from https://www.ncbi.nlm.nih.gov/pubmed/9216474

Frankle, W. G., Lombardo, I., New, A. S., Goodman, M., Talbot, P. S., Huang, Y., . . . Siever, L. J. (2005). Brain serotonin transporter distribution in subjects with impulsive aggressivity: A positron emission study with [11C]McN 5652. *The American Journal of Psychiatry*, *162*(5), 915–923. Retrieved from https://www.ncbi.nlm.nih.gov/pubmed/15863793. doi:10.1176/appi.ajp.162.5.915

Frati, P., Busardo, F. P., Cipolloni, L., Dominicis, E. D., & Fineschi, V. (2015). Anabolic Androgenic Steroid (AAS) related deaths: Autoptic, histopathological and toxicological findings. *Current Neuropharmacology*, *13*(1), 146–159. Retrieved from https://www.ncbi.nlm.nih.gov/pubmed/26074749. doi:10.2174/1570159X13666141210225414

Frith, U. (2001). Mind blindness and the brain in autism. *Neuron*, *32*(6), 969–979. Retrieved from https://www.ncbi.nlm.nih.gov/pubmed/11754830

Frohlich, J., & Van Horn, J. D. (2014). Reviewing the ketamine model for schizophrenia. *Journal of Psychopharmacology*, *28*(4), 287–302. Retrieved from https://www.ncbi.nlm.nih.gov/pubmed/24257811. doi:10.1177/0269881113512909

Funahashi, S., Bruce, C. J., & Goldman-Rakic, P. S. (1989). Mnemonic coding of visual space in the monkey's dorsolateral prefrontal cortex. *Journal of Neurophysiology*, *61*(2), 331–349. Retrieved from https://www.ncbi.nlm.nih.gov/pubmed/2918358. doi:10.1152/jn.1989.61.2.331

Furmaga, H., Carreno, F. R., & Frazer, A. (2012). Vagal nerve stimulation rapidly activates brain-derived neurotrophic factor receptor TrkB in rat brain. *PLoS One*, *7*(5), e34844. Retrieved from https://www.ncbi.nlm.nih.gov/pubmed/22563458. doi:10.1371/journal.pone.0034844

Furmark, T., Fischer, H., Wik, G., Larsson, M., & Fredrikson, M. (1997). The amygdala and individual differences in human fear conditioning. *Neuroreport*, *8*(18), 3957–3960. Retrieved from https://www.ncbi.nlm.nih.gov/pubmed/9462473

Fuster, J. M., & Alexander, G. E. (1971). Neuron activity related to short-term memory. *Science*, *173*(3997), 652–654. Retrieved from https://www.ncbi.nlm.nih.gov/pubmed/4998337

Gaetz, W., Kessler, S. K., Roberts, T. P. L., Berman, J. I., Levy, T. J., Hsia, M., . . . Levin, L. S. (2018). Massive cortical reorganization is reversible following bilateral transplants of the hands: Evidence from the first successful bilateral pediatric hand transplant patient. *Annals of Clinical and Translational Neurology*, *5*(1), 92–97. Retrieved from https://www.ncbi.nlm.nih.gov/pubmed/29376095. doi:10.1002/acn3.501

Gallace, A., & Spence, C. (2009). The cognitive and neural correlates of tactile memory. *Psychological Bulletin*, *135*(3), 380–406. Retrieved from https://www.ncbi.nlm.nih.gov/pubmed/19379022. doi:10.1037/a0015325

Gallese, V. (2013). Mirror neurons, embodied simulation and a second-person approach to mindreading. *Cortex*, *49*(10), 2954–2956. Retrieved from https://www.ncbi.nlm.nih.gov/pubmed/24209736. doi:10.1016/j.cortex.2013.09.008

Gallese, V., & Goldman, A. (1998). Mirror neurons and the simulation theory of mind-reading. *Trends in Cognitive Sciences*, *2*(12), 493–501. Retrieved from https://www.ncbi.nlm.nih.gov/pubmed/21227300

Gallup, G. G., Jr. (1970). Chimpanzees: Self-recognition. *Science*, *167*(3914), 86–87. Retrieved from http://www.ncbi.nlm.nih.gov/pubmed/4982211

Gallup, G. G., Jr., & Anderson, J. R. (2018). The "olfactory mirror" and other recent attempts to demonstrate self-recognition in non-primate species. *Behavioural Processes*, *148*, 16–19. Retrieved from https://www.ncbi.nlm.nih.gov/pubmed/29274762. doi:10.1016/j.beproc.2017.12.010

Galvan, A., Hare, T. A., Parra, C. E., Penn, J., Voss, H., Glover, G., & Casey, B. J. (2006). Earlier development of the accumbens relative to orbitofrontal cortex might underlie risk-taking behavior in adolescents. *The Journal of Neuroscience*, *26*(25), 6885–6892. Retrieved from https://www.ncbi.nlm.nih.gov/pubmed/16793895. doi:10.1523/JNEUROSCI.1062-06.2006

Gamer, M., Klimecki, O., Bauermann, T., Stoeter, P., & Vossel, G. (2012). fMRI-activation patterns in the detection of concealed information rely on memory-related effects. *Social Cognitive and Affective Neuroscience*, *7*(5), 506–515. Retrieved from https://www.ncbi.nlm.nih.gov/pubmed/19258375. doi:10.1093/scan/nsp005

Garakani, A., Martinez, J. M., Yehuda, R., & Gorman, J. M. (2013). Cerebrospinal fluid levels of glutamate and corticotropin releasing hormone in major depression before and after treatment. *Journal of Affective Disorders*, *146*(2), 262–265. Retrieved from https://www.ncbi.nlm.nih.gov/pubmed/22840611. doi:10.1016/j.jad.2012.06.037

Garber, G. (2009). *Doctors: Wrestler had brain damage*. Retrieved from http://www.espn.com/espn/otl/news/story?id=4724912

Garcia, M. C., Bastian, B., Rossen, L. M., Anderson, R., Minino, A., Yoon, P. W., . . . Iademarco, M. F. (2016). Potentially preventable deaths among the five leading causes of death - United States, 2010 and 2014. *MMWR Morbidity and Mortality Weekly Report*, *65*(45), 1245–1255. Retrieved from https://www.ncbi.nlm.nih.gov/pubmed/27855145. doi:10.15585/mmwr.mm6545a1

Garcia Pardo, M. P., Roger Sanchez, C., De la Rubia Orti, J. E., & Aguilar Calpe, M. A. (2017). Animal models of drug addiction. *Adicciones*, *29*(4), 278–292. Retrieved from https://www.ncbi.nlm.nih.gov/pubmed/28170057. doi:10.20882/adicciones.862

Gaskin, S., Tardif, M., & Mumby, D. G. (2011). Prolonged inactivation of the hippocampus reveals temporally graded retrograde amnesia for unreinforced spatial learning in rats. *Neurobiology of Learning and Memory*, *96*(2), 288–296. Retrieved from https://www.ncbi.nlm.nih.gov/pubmed/21704177. doi:10.1016/j.nlm.2011.06.001

Gaskin, S., Tremblay, A., & Mumby, D. G. (2003). Retrograde and anterograde object recognition in rats with hippocampal lesions. *Hippocampus*, *13*(8), 962–969. Retrieved from https://www.ncbi.nlm.nih.gov/pubmed/14750658. doi:10.1002/hipo.10154

Gasparini, R., Panatto, D., Lai, P. L., & Amicizia, D. (2015). The "rban myth" of the association between neurological disorders and vaccinations. *Journal of Preventive Medicine and Hygiene*, *56*(1), E1–E8. Retrieved from https://www.ncbi.nlm.nih.gov/pubmed/26789825

Gaston, L. K., Shorey, H. H., & Saario, C. A. (1967). Insect population control by the use of sex pheromones to inhibit orientation between the sexes. *Nature*, *213*(5081), 155. Retrieved from https://www.ncbi.nlm.nih.gov/pubmed/6029808

Gawel, R., Smith, P. A., Cicerale, S., & Keast, R. (2018). The mouthfeel of white wine. *Critical Reviews in Food Science and Nutrition*, *58*(17), 2939–2956. Retrieved from https://www.ncbi.nlm.nih.gov/pubmed/28678530. doi:10.1080/10408398.2017.1346584

Gebhardt, N., Bar, K. J., Boettger, M. K., Grecksch, G., Keilhoff, G., Reichart, R., & Becker, A. (2013). Vagus nerve stimulation ameliorated deficits in one-way active avoidance learning and stimulated hippocampal neurogenesis in bulbectomized rats. *Brain Stimulation*, *6*(1), 78–83. Retrieved from https://www.ncbi.nlm.nih.gov/pubmed/22405742. doi:10.1016/j.brs.2012.01.009

Georgopoulos, A. P., Kettner, R. E., & Schwartz, A. B. (1988). Primate motor cortex and free arm movements to visual targets in three-dimensional space. II. Coding of the direction of movement by a neuronal population. *The Journal of Neuroscience*, *8*(8), 2928–2937. Retrieved from https://www.ncbi.nlm.nih.gov/pubmed/3411362

Gilbert, A. N. (2008). *What the nose knows: The science of scent in everyday life* (1st ed.). New York: Crown Publishers.

Giuliano, F., Rampin, O., Brown, K., Courtois, F., Benoit, G., & Jardin, A. (1996). Stimulation of the medial preoptic area of the hypothalamus in the rat elicits increases in intracavernous pressure. *Neuroscience Letters*, *209*(1), 1–4. Retrieved from https://www.ncbi.nlm.nih.gov/pubmed/8734895

Godlee, F., Smith, J., & Marcovitch, H. (2011). Wakefield's article linking MMR vaccine and autism was fraudulent. *The British Medical Journal*, *342*, c7452. Retrieved from https://www.ncbi.nlm.nih.gov/pubmed/21209060. doi:10.1136/bmj.c7452

Golby, A. J., Gabrieli, J. D. E., Chiao, J. Y., & Eberhardt, J. L. (2001). Differential responses in the fusiform region to same-race and other-race faces. *Nature Neuroscience*, *4*(8), 845–850. Retrieved from https://doi.org/10.1038/90565. doi:10.1038/90565

Goldberg, A. D., Allis, C. D., & Bernstein, E. (2007). Epigenetics: A landscape takes shape. *Cell*, *128*(4), 635–638. Retrieved from https://www.ncbi.nlm.nih.gov/pubmed/17320500. doi:10.1016/j.cell.2007.02.006

Goldberg, E. M., Wang, K., Goldberg, J., & Aliani, M. (2018). Factors affecting the ortho- and retronasal perception of flavors: A review. *Critical Reviews in Food Science and Nutrition*, *58*(6), 913–923. Retrieved from https://www.ncbi.nlm.nih.gov/pubmed/27646486. doi:10.1080/10408398.2016.1231167

Goldberg, T. E., Weinberger, D. R., Berman, K. F., Pliskin, N. H., & Podd, M. H. (1987). Further evidence for dementia of the prefrontal type in schizophrenia? A controlled study of teaching the Wisconsin Card Sorting Test. *Archives of General Psychiatry*, *44*(11), 1008–1014. Retrieved from http://www.ncbi.nlm.nih.gov/pubmed/3675128

Goldman, S. A., & Nottebohm, F. (1983). Neuronal production, migration, and differentiation in a vocal control nucleus of the adult female canary brain. *Proceedings of the National Academy of Sciences of the United States of America*, *80*(8), 2390–2394. Retrieved from https://www.ncbi.nlm.nih.gov/pubmed/6572982

Goodale, M. A., & Milner, A. D. (1992). Separate visual pathways for perception and action. *Trends in Neuroscience*, *15*(1), 20–25. Retrieved from https://www.ncbi.nlm.nih.gov/pubmed/1374953

Goodman, W. K., Grice, D. E., Lapidus, K. A., & Coffey, B. J. (2014). Obsessive-compulsive disorder. *Psychiatric Clinics of North America*, *37*(3), 257–267. Retrieved from http://www.ncbi.nlm.nih.gov/pubmed/25150561. doi:10.1016/j.psc.2014.06.004

Gordon, J. L., Rubinow, D. R., Eisenlohr-Moul, T. A., Xia, K., Schmidt, P. J., & Girdler, S. S. (2018). Efficacy of transdermal estradiol and micronized progesterone in the prevention of depressive symptoms in the menopause transition: A randomized clinical trial. *JAMA Psychiatry*, *75*(2), 149–157. Retrieved from https://www.ncbi.nlm.nih.gov/pubmed/29322164. doi:10.1001/jamapsychiatry.2017.3998

Gorski, R. A., Gordon, J. H., Shryne, J. E., & Southam, A. M. (1978). Evidence for a morphological sex difference within the medial preoptic area of the rat brain. *Brain Research*, *148*(2), 333–346. Retrieved from https://www.ncbi.nlm.nih.gov/pubmed/656937

Gougoux, F., Lepore, F., Lassonde, M., Voss, P., Zatorre, R. J., & Belin, P. (2004). Neuropsychology: Pitch discrimination in the early blind. *Nature*, *430*(6997), 309. Retrieved from https://www.ncbi.nlm.nih.gov/pubmed/15254527. doi:10.1038/430309a

Gould, S. J., & Vrba, E. S. (1982). Exaptation—a missing term in the science of form. *Paleobiology*, *8*(1), 4–15. doi:10.1017/S0094837300004310

Gracheva, E. O., Ingolia, N. T., Kelly, Y. M., Cordero-Morales, J. F., Hollopeter, G., Chesler, A. T., . . . Julius, D. (2010). Molecular basis of infrared detection by snakes. *Nature*, *464*(7291), 1006–1011. Retrieved from https://www.ncbi.nlm.nih.gov/pubmed/20228791. doi:10.1038/nature08943

Graziano, M. S., Aflalo, T. N., & Cooke, D. F. (2005). Arm movements evoked by electrical stimulation in the motor cortex of monkeys. *Journal of Neurophysiology*, *94*(6), 4209–4223. Retrieved from https://www.ncbi.nlm.nih.gov/pubmed/16120657. doi:10.1152/jn.01303.2004

Greenberg, B. D., Gabriels, L. A., Malone, D. A., Jr., Rezai, A. R., Friehs, G. M., Okun, M. S., . . . Nuttin, B. J. (2010). Deep brain stimulation of the ventral internal capsule/ventral striatum for obsessive-compulsive disorder: Worldwide experience. *Molecular*

Psychiatry, 15(1), 64–79. Retrieved from https://www.ncbi.nlm.nih.gov/pubmed/18490925. doi:10.1038/mp.2008.55

Greenwald, A. G., & Krieger, L. H. (2006). Implicit bias: Scientific foundations. *California Law Review, 94*(4), 945–967. Retrieved from http://www.jstor.org/stable/20439056. doi:10.2307/20439056

Greenwald, A. G., McGhee, D. E., & Schwartz, J. L. (1998). Measuring individual differences in implicit cognition: The implicit association test. *Journal of Personality and Social Psychology, 74*(6), 1464–1480. Retrieved from https://www.ncbi.nlm.nih.gov/pubmed/9654756

Greenwald, A. G., Smith, C. T., Sriram, N., Bar-Anan, Y., & Nosek, B. A. (2009). Implicit Race Attitudes Predicted Vote in the 2008 U.S. Presidential Election. *Analyses of Social Issues and Public Policy, 9*(1), 241–253. Retrieved from https://spssi.onlinelibrary.wiley.com/doi/abs/10.1111/j.1530-2415.2009.01195.x. doi:10.1111/j.1530-2415.2009.01195.x

Gregoriou, G. G., Gotts, S. J., Zhou, H., & Desimone, R. (2009). High-frequency, long-range coupling between prefrontal and visual cortex during attention. *Science, 324*(5931), 1207–1210. Retrieved from https://www.ncbi.nlm.nih.gov/pubmed/19478185. doi:10.1126/science.1171402

Grothe, M. J., Schuster, C., Bauer, F., Heinsen, H., Prudlo, J., & Teipel, S. J. (2014). Atrophy of the cholinergic basal forebrain in dementia with Lewy bodies and Alzheimer's disease dementia. *Journal of Neurology, 261*(10), 1939–1948. Retrieved from https://www.ncbi.nlm.nih.gov/pubmed/25059393. doi:10.1007/s00415-014-7439-z

Guerri, C., Bazinet, A., & Riley, E. P. (2009). Foetal alcohol spectrum disorders and alterations in brain and behaviour. *Alcohol Alcohol, 44*(2), 108–114. Retrieved from https://www.ncbi.nlm.nih.gov/pubmed/19147799. doi:10.1093/alcalc/agn105

Guler, A. D., Lee, H., Iida, T., Shimizu, I., Tominaga, M., & Caterina, M. (2002). Heat-evoked activation of the ion channel, TRPV4. *The Journal of Neuroscience, 22*(15), 6408–6414. Retrieved from https://www.ncbi.nlm.nih.gov/pubmed/12151520. doi:20026679

Gunn, J. K., Rosales, C. B., Center, K. E., Nunez, A., Gibson, S. J., Christ, C., & Ehiri, J. E. (2016). Prenatal exposure to cannabis and maternal and child health outcomes: A systematic review and meta-analysis. *BMJ Open, 6*(4), e009986. Retrieved from https://www.ncbi.nlm.nih.gov/pubmed/27048634. doi:10.1136/bmjopen-2015-009986

Gurtubay-Antolin, A., & Rodriguez-Fornells, A. (2017). Neurophysiological evidence for enhanced tactile acuity in early blindness in some but not all haptic tasks. *Neuroimage, 162*, 23–31. Retrieved from https://www.ncbi.nlm.nih.gov/pubmed/28843538. doi:10.1016/j.neuroimage.2017.08.054

Haam, J., & Yakel, J. L. (2017). Cholinergic modulation of the hippocampal region and memory function. *Journal of Neurochemistry, 142*(Suppl 2), 111–121. Retrieved from https://www.ncbi.nlm.nih.gov/pubmed/28791706. doi:10.1111/jnc.14052

Hafting, T., Fyhn, M., Molden, S., Moser, M. B., & Moser, E. I. (2005). Microstructure of a spatial map in the entorhinal cortex. *Nature, 436*(7052), 801–806. Retrieved from https://www.ncbi.nlm.nih.gov/pubmed/15965463. doi:10.1038/nature03721

Hakim, J. D., & Keay, K. A. (2018). Prolonged ad libitum access to low-concentration sucrose changes the neurochemistry of the nucleus accumbens in male Sprague-Dawley rats. *Physiology & Behavior, 201*, 95–103. Retrieved from https://www.ncbi.nlm.nih.gov/pubmed/30553896. doi:10.1016/j.physbeh.2018.12.016

Hamilton, A. F. (2013). Reflecting on the mirror neuron system in autism: A systematic review of current theories. *Developmental Cognitive Neuroscience, 3*, 91–105. Retrieved from https://www.ncbi.nlm.nih.gov/pubmed/23245224. doi:10.1016/j.dcn.2012.09.008

Hamilton, W. D. (1964). The genetical evolution of social behaviour. I. *Journal of Theoretical Biology, 7*(1), 1–16. Retrieved from http://www.ncbi.nlm.nih.gov/pubmed/5875341

Han, K., Chen, H., Gennarino, V. A., Richman, R., Lu, H. C., & Zoghbi, H. Y. (2015). Fragile X-like behaviors and abnormal cortical dendritic spines in cytoplasmic FMR1-interacting protein 2-mutant mice. *Human Molecular Genetics, 24*(7), 1813–1823. Retrieved from http://www.ncbi.nlm.nih.gov/pubmed/25432536. doi:10.1093/hmg/ddu595

Han, Y., Yang, H., Lv, Y. T., Zhu, C. Z., He, Y., Tang, H. H., . . . Dong, Q. (2009). Gray matter density and white matter integrity in pianists' brain: A combined structural and diffusion tensor MRI study. *Neuroscience Letters, 459*(1), 3–6. Retrieved from https://www.ncbi.nlm.nih.gov/pubmed/18672026. doi:10.1016/j.neulet.2008.07.056

Hanig, D. P. (1901). Zur Psychophysik des Geschmackssinnes. *Philosophische Studien, 17*, 576–623.

Hannum, M., Stegman, M. A., Fryer, J. A., & Simons, C. T. (2018). Different olfactory percepts evoked by orthonasal and retronasal odorant delivery. *Chemical Senses, 43*(7), 515–521. Retrieved from https://www.ncbi.nlm.nih.gov/pubmed/29982522. doi:10.1093/chemse/bjy043

Harada, K., Ikuta, T., Nakashima, M., Watanuki, T., Hirotsu, M., Matsubara, T., . . . Matsuo, K. (2018). Altered connectivity of the anterior cingulate and the posterior superior temporal gyrus in a longitudinal study of later-life depression. *Frontiers in Aging Neuroscience, 10*, 31. Retrieved from https://www.ncbi.nlm.nih.gov/pubmed/29472854. doi:10.3389/fnagi.2018.00031

Harlow, J. M. (1999). Passage of an iron rod through the head. *The Journal of Neuropsychiatry and Clinical Neurosciences, 11*(2), 281–283. Retrieved from https://neuro.psychiatryonline.org/doi/abs/10.1176/jnp.11.2.281. doi:10.1176/jnp.11.2.281

Harper-Harrison, G., & Shanahan, M. M. (2018). Hormone replacement therapy. Treasure Island, FL: StatPearls.

Hartley, I. E., Liem, D. G., & Keast, R. (2019). Umami as an 'alimentary' taste. A new perspective on taste classification. *Nutrients, 11*(1). Retrieved from https://www.ncbi.nlm.nih.gov/pubmed/30654496. doi:10.3390/nu11010182

Hartline, H. K., Wagner, H. G., & Ratliff, F. (1956). Inhibition in the eye of Limulus. *Journal of General Physiology, 39*(5), 651–673. Retrieved from https://www.ncbi.nlm.nih.gov/pubmed/13319654

Hasselmo, M. E. (2006). The role of acetylcholine in learning and memory. *Current Opinion in Neurobiology, 16*(6), 710–715. Retrieved from https://www.ncbi.nlm.nih.gov/pubmed/17011181. doi:10.1016/j.conb.2006.09.002

Hastings, M. H., Brancaccio, M., & Maywood, E. S. (2014). Circadian pacemaking in cells and circuits of the suprachiasmatic nucleus. *Journal of Neuroendocrinology, 26*(1), 2–10. Retrieved from https://www.ncbi.nlm.nih.gov/pubmed/24329967. doi:10.1111/jne.12125

Haubrich, J., & Nader, K. (2018). Memory reconsolidation. *Current Topics in Behavioral Neurosciences, 37*, 151–176. Retrieved from https://www.ncbi.nlm.nih.gov/pubmed/27885549. doi:10.1007/7854_2016_463

Hebb, D. O. (1949). *The organization of behavior: A neuropsychological theory*. New York: Wiley.

Heidinger, B., Gorgens, K., & Morgenstern, J. (2015). The effects of sexual sensation seeking and alcohol use on risky sexual behavior among men who have sex with men. *AIDS and Behavior, 19*(3), 431–439. Retrieved from https://www.ncbi.nlm.nih.gov/pubmed/25096894. doi:10.1007/s10461-014-0871-3

Henriksen, M. G., Nordgaard, J., & Jansson, L. B. (2017). Genetics of schizophrenia: Overview of methods, findings and limitations. *Frontiers in Human Neuroscience, 11*, 322. Retrieved from https://www.ncbi.nlm.nih.gov/pubmed/28690503. doi:10.3389/fnhum.2017.00322

Herculano-Houzel, S. (2014). The glia/neuron ratio: How it varies uniformly across brain structures and species and what that means for brain physiology and evolution. *Glia, 62*(9), 1377–1391. Retrieved from http://www.ncbi.nlm.nih.gov/pubmed/24807023. doi:10.1002/glia.22683

Herculano-Houzel, S., Mota, B., Wong, P., & Kaas, J. H. (2010). Connectivity-driven white matter scaling and folding in primate cerebral cortex. *Proceedings of the National Academy of Sciences of the United States of America, 107*(44), 19008–19013. Retrieved from https://www.ncbi.nlm.nih.gov/pubmed/20956290. doi:10.1073/pnas.1012590107

Hering, E. (1964). *Outlines of a theory of the light sense*. Cambridge, MA, US: Harvard University Press.

Herman, M. A., & Roberto, M. (2015). The addicted brain: Understanding the neurophysiological mechanisms of addictive disorders. *Frontiers in Integrative Neuroscience, 9*, 18. Retrieved from https://www.ncbi.nlm.nih.gov/pubmed/25852502. doi:10.3389/fnint.2015.00018

Hermann, L. (1870). Eine Erscheinung des simultanen Kontrastes. *Pflugers Archiv fur die gesamte Physiologie des Menschen und der Tiere, 3*, 13–45.

Hess, W. R. (1932). *Beiträge zur Physiologie des Hirnstammes*. Leipzig: Thieme.

Heyn, P., Abreu, B. C., & Ottenbacher, K. J. (2004). The effects of exercise training on elderly persons with cognitive impairment and dementia: A meta-analysis. *Archives of Physical Medicine and Rehabilitation, 85*(10), 1694–1704. Retrieved from https://www.ncbi.nlm.nih.gov/pubmed/15468033

Hill, R. W., Wyse, G. A., & Anderson, M. (2012). *Animal physiology* (3rd ed.). Sunderland, MA: Sinauer Associates, Inc. Publishers.

Hines, M. (2011). Prenatal endocrine influences on sexual orientation and on sexually differentiated childhood behavior. *Frontiers in Neuroendocrinology, 32*(2), 170–182. Retrieved from https://www.ncbi.nlm.nih.gov/pubmed/21333673. doi:10.1016/j.yfrne.2011.02.006

Hiyoshi, A., Miyahara, K., Kato, C., & Ohshima, Y. (2011). Does a DNA-less cellular organism exist on Earth? *Genes to Cells, 16*(12), 1146–1158. Retrieved from https://www.ncbi.nlm.nih.gov/pubmed/22093146. doi:10.1111/j.1365-2443.2011.01558.x

Ho, V. M., Lee, J. A., & Martin, K. C. (2011). The cell biology of synaptic plasticity. *Science, 334*(6056), 623–628. Retrieved from https://www.ncbi.nlm.nih.gov/pubmed/22053042. doi:10.1126/science.1209236

Hochberg, L. R., Bacher, D., Jarosiewicz, B., Masse, N. Y., Simeral, J. D., Vogel, J., . . . Donoghue, J. P. (2012). Reach and grasp by people with tetraplegia using a neurally controlled robotic arm. *Nature, 485*(7398), 372–375. Retrieved from https://www.ncbi.nlm.nih.gov/pubmed/22596161. doi:10.1038/nature11076

Hodgkin, A. L., & Katz, B. (1949). The effect of temperature on the electrical activity of the giant axon of the squid. *The Journal of Physiology, 109*(1–2), 240–249. Retrieved from https://www.ncbi.nlm.nih.gov/pubmed/15394322

Hoes, M. J. (1982). Monoamines in Psychiatry: The role of serotonin in depression, anxiety and stress. *Acta Psychiatrica Belgica, 82*(3), 287–309. Retrieved from https://www.ncbi.nlm.nih.gov/pubmed/7164838

Hofman, M. A., & Swaab, D. F. (1989). The sexually dimorphic nucleus of the preoptic area in the human brain: A comparative morphometric study. *Journal of Anatomy, 164*, 55–72. Retrieved from https://www.ncbi.nlm.nih.gov/pubmed/2606795

Holland, P. C., & Gallagher, M. (1999). Amygdala circuitry in attentional and representational processes. *Trends in Cognitive Sciences, 3*(2), 65–73. Retrieved from https://www.ncbi.nlm.nih.gov/pubmed/10234229

Holmes, W. G., & Sherman, P. W. (2015). The ontogeny of Kin recognition in two species of ground squirrels1. *Integrative and Comparative Biology, 22*(3), 491–517. Retrieved from https://doi.org/10.1093/icb/22.3.491

Holtzheimer, P. E., & Mayberg, H. S. (2012). Neuromodulation for treatment-resistant depression. *F1000 Medicine Reports, 4*, 22. Retrieved from https://www.ncbi.nlm.nih.gov/pubmed/23189091. doi:10.3410/M4-22

Hong, Y. P., Lee, H. C., & Kim, H. T. (2015). Treadmill exercise after social isolation increases the levels of NGF, BDNF, and synapsin I to induce survival of neurons in the hippocampus, and improves depression-like behavior. *Journal of Exercise Nutrition & Biochemistry, 19*(1), 11–18. Retrieved from https://www.ncbi.nlm.nih.gov/pubmed/25960950. doi:10.5717/jenb.2015.19.1.11

Hori, T., Sugita, Y., Koga, E., Shirakawa, S., Inoue, K., Uchida, S., . . . Sleep Computing Committee of the Japanese Society of Sleep Research, S. (2001). Proposed supplements and amendments to 'A Manual of Standardized Terminology, Techniques and Scoring System for Sleep Stages of Human Subjects', the Rechtschaffen & Kales (1968) standard. *Psychiatry and Clinical Neurosciences, 55*(3), 305–310. Retrieved from https://www.ncbi.nlm.nih.gov/pubmed/11422885. doi:10.1046/j.1440-1819.2001.00810.x

Horowitz, A. (2017). Smelling themselves: Dogs investigate their own odours longer when modified in an "olfactory mirror" test. *Behavioural Processes, 143*, 17–24. Retrieved from https://www.ncbi.nlm.nih.gov/pubmed/28797909. doi:10.1016/j.beproc.2017.08.001

Hosking, S. G., Young, K. L., & Regan, M. A. (2009). The effects of text messaging on young drivers. *Human Factors: The Journal of the Human Factors and Ergonomics Society, 51*(4), 582–592. Retrieved from https://www.ncbi.nlm.nih.gov/pubmed/19899366. doi:10.1177/0018720809341575

Hotting, K., & Roder, B. (2013). Beneficial effects of physical exercise on neuroplasticity and cognition. *Neuroscience & Biobehavioral Reviews, 37*(9 Pt. B), 2243–2257. Retrieved from https://www.ncbi.nlm.nih.gov/pubmed/23623982. doi:10.1016/j.neubiorev.2013.04.005

Howe, M. W., Tierney, P. L., Sandberg, S. G., Phillips, P. E., & Graybiel, A. M. (2013). Prolonged dopamine signalling in striatum signals proximity and value of distant rewards. *Nature, 500*(7464), 575–579. Retrieved from https://www.ncbi.nlm.nih.gov/pubmed/23913271. doi:10.1038/nature12475

Howes, O. D., & Kapur, S. (2009). The dopamine hypothesis of schizophrenia: Version III—the final common pathway. *Schizophrenia Bulletin, 35*(3), 549–562. Retrieved from http://www.ncbi.nlm.nih.gov/pubmed/19325164. doi:10.1093/schbul/sbp006

Howland, R. H., Shutt, L. S., Berman, S. R., Spotts, C. R., & Denko, T. (2011). The emerging use of technology for the treatment of depression and other neuropsychiatric disorders. *Annals of Clinical Psychiatry, 23*(1), 48–62. Retrieved from https://www.ncbi.nlm.nih.gov/pubmed/21318196

Hu, S. S., & Mackie, K. (2015). Distribution of the endocannabinoid system in the central nervous system. *Handbook of Experimental Pharmacology, 231*, 59–93. Retrieved from https://www.ncbi.nlm.nih.gov/pubmed/26408158. doi:10.1007/978-3-319-20825-1_3

Huart, C., Rombaux, P., & Hummel, T. (2019). Neural plasticity in developing and adult olfactory pathways - focus on the human olfactory bulb. *Journal of Bioenergetics, 51*(7): 1–11. Retrieved from https://www.ncbi.nlm.nih.gov/pubmed/30604090. doi:10.1007/s10863-018-9780-x

Hubel, D. H., & Wiesel, T. N. (1959). Receptive fields of single neurones in the cat's striate cortex. *The Journal of Physiology*, *148*, 574–591. Retrieved from https://www.ncbi.nlm.nih.gov/pubmed/14403679

Hubel, D. H., & Wiesel, T. N. (2009). Republication of The Journal of Physiology (1959) 148, 574-591: Receptive fields of single neurones in the cat's striate cortex. 1959. *The Journal of Physiology*, *587*(Pt. 12), 2721–2732. Retrieved from https://www.ncbi.nlm.nih.gov/pubmed/19525558. doi:10.1113/jphysiol.2009.174151

Huettel, S. A., Song, A. W., & McCarthy, G. (2014). *Functional magnetic resonance imaging* (3rd ed.). Sunderland, MA: Sinauer Associates, Inc., Publishers.

Hughes, G. (2018). The role of the temporoparietal junction in implicit and explicit sense of agency. *Neuropsychologia*, *113*, 1–5. Retrieved from https://www.ncbi.nlm.nih.gov/pubmed/29567107. doi:10.1016/j.neuropsychologia.2018.03.020

Hughes, V. (2010). Science in court: Head case. *Nature*, *464*(7287), 340–342. Retrieved from https://www.ncbi.nlm.nih.gov/pubmed/20237536. doi:10.1038/464340a

Hull, C. L. (1943). *Principles of behavior, an introduction to behavior theory*. New York: D. Appleton-Century.

Hull, E. M., Du, J., Lorrain, D. S., & Matuszewich, L. (1995). Extracellular dopamine in the medial preoptic area: Implications for sexual motivation and hormonal control of copulation. *The Journal of Neuroscience*, *15*(11), 7465–7471. Retrieved from https://www.ncbi.nlm.nih.gov/pubmed/7472498

Hull, E. M., Wood, R. I., & McKenna, K. E. (2006). The neurobiology of male sexual behavior. In J. Neill & D. Pfaff (Ed.), *The physiology of reproduction* (pp. 1729–1824). New York: Elseveir Press.

Hung, H. C., Hsiao, Y. H., & Gean, P. W. (2014). Learning induces sonic hedgehog signaling in the amygdala which promotes neurogenesis and long-term memory formation. *International Journal of Neuropsychopharmacology*, *18*(3). Retrieved from https://www.ncbi.nlm.nih.gov/pubmed/25522410. doi:10.1093/ijnp/pyu071

Hupbach, A., Gomez, R., Hardt, O., & Nadel, L. (2007). Reconsolidation of episodic memories: A subtle reminder triggers integration of new information. *Learning & Memory*, *14*(1–2), 47–53. Retrieved from https://www.ncbi.nlm.nih.gov/pubmed/17202429. doi:10.1101/lm.365707

Husain, M., & Stein, J. (1988). Rezso Balint and his most celebrated case. *Archives of Neurology*, *45*(1), 89–93. Retrieved from https://www.ncbi.nlm.nih.gov/pubmed/3276300

Huxley, A. F., & Niedergerke, R. (1954). Structural changes in muscle during contraction: Interference microscopy of living muscle fibres. *Nature*, *173*(4412), 971–973. Retrieved from http://www.ncbi.nlm.nih.gov/pubmed/13165697

Huxley, H., & Hanson, J. (1954). Changes in the cross-striations of muscle during contraction and stretch and their structural interpretation. *Nature*, *173*(4412), 973–976. Retrieved from http://www.ncbi.nlm.nih.gov/pubmed/13165698

Hynes, T. R., Block, S. M., White, B. T., & Spudich, J. A. (1987). Movement of myosin fragments in vitro: Domains involved in force production. *Cell*, *48*(6), 953–963. Retrieved from http://www.ncbi.nlm.nih.gov/pubmed/3548997

Iacoboni, M., & Dapretto, M. (2006). The mirror neuron system and the consequences of its dysfunction. *Nature Reviews Neuroscience*, *7*(12), 942–951. Retrieved from https://www.ncbi.nlm.nih.gov/pubmed/17115076. doi:10.1038/nrn2024

Iacoboni, M., Molnar-Szakacs, I., Gallese, V., Buccino, G., Mazziotta, J. C., & Rizzolatti, G. (2005). Grasping the intentions of others with one's own mirror neuron system. *PLoS Biology*, *3*(3), e79. Retrieved from https://www.ncbi.nlm.nih.gov/pubmed/15736981. doi:10.1371/journal.pbio.0030079

Iliff, J. J., Wang, M., Liao, Y., Plogg, B. A., Peng, W., Gundersen, G. A., ... Nedergaard, M. (2012). A paravascular pathway facilitates CSF flow through the brain parenchyma and the clearance of interstitial solutes, including amyloid beta. *Science Translational Medicine*, *4*(147), 147ra111. Retrieved from http://www.ncbi.nlm.nih.gov/pubmed/22896675. doi:10.1126/scitranslmed.3003748

Inagaki, H., Kiyokawa, Y., Tamogami, S., Watanabe, H., Takeuchi, Y., & Mori, Y. (2014). Identification of a pheromone that increases anxiety in rats. *Proceedings of the National Academy of Sciences of the United States of America*, *111*(52), 18751–18756. Retrieved from https://www.ncbi.nlm.nih.gov/pubmed/25512532. doi:10.1073/pnas.1414710112

Ip, E. J., Lu, D. H., Barnett, M. J., Tenerowicz, M. J., Vo, J. C., & Perry, P. J. (2012). Psychological and physical impact of anabolic-androgenic steroid dependence. *Pharmacotherapy*, *32*(10), 910–919. Retrieved from https://www.ncbi.nlm.nih.gov/pubmed/23033230. doi:10.1002/j.1875-9114.2012.01123

Ito, M. (2008). Control of mental activities by internal models in the cerebellum. *Nature Reviews Neuroscience*, *9*(4), 304–313. Retrieved from https://www.ncbi.nlm.nih.gov/pubmed/18319727. doi:10.1038/nrn2332

Ito, M., & Kano, M. (1982). Long-lasting depression of parallel fiber-Purkinje cell transmission induced by conjunctive stimulation of parallel fibers and climbing fibers in the cerebellar cortex. *Neuroscience Letters*, *33*(3), 253–258. Retrieved from https://www.ncbi.nlm.nih.gov/pubmed/6298664

Izuma, K., Aoki, R., Shibata, K., & Nakahara, K. (2019). Neural signals in amygdala predict implicit prejudice toward an ethnic outgroup. *Neuroimage*, *189*, 341–352. Retrieved from https://www.ncbi.nlm.nih.gov/pubmed/30654171. doi:10.1016/j.neuroimage.2019.01.019

Jacini, W. F., Cannonieri, G. C., Fernandes, P. T., Bonilha, L., Cendes, F., & Li, L. M. (2009). Can exercise shape your brain? Cortical differences associated with judo practice. *Journal of Science and Medicine in Sport*, *12*(6), 688–690. Retrieved from https://www.ncbi.nlm.nih.gov/pubmed/19147406. doi:10.1016/j.jsams.2008.11.004

Jackson, J. H. (1958). *Selected writings*. New York: Basic Books.

Jacob, M. L., Morelen, D., Suveg, C., Brown Jacobsen, A. M., & Whiteside, S. P. (2012). Emotional, behavioral, and cognitive factors that differentiate obsessive-compulsive disorder and other anxiety disorders in youth. *Anxiety Stress Coping*, *25*(2), 229–237. Retrieved from https://www.ncbi.nlm.nih.gov/pubmed/21512917. doi:10.1080/10615806.2011.571255

Jacobsen, C. F., & Nissen, H. W. (1937). Studies of cerebral function in primates. IV. The effects of frontal lobe lesions on the delayed alternation habit in monkeys. *Journal of Comparative Psychology*, *23*(1), 101–112. doi:10.1037/h0056632

Jacobson, M. L., Kim, L. A., Patro, R., Rosati, B., & McKinnon, D. (2018). Common and differential transcriptional responses to different models of traumatic stress exposure in rats. *Translational Psychiatry*, *8*(1), 165. Retrieved from https://www.ncbi.nlm.nih.gov/pubmed/30139969. doi:10.1038/s41398-018-0223-6

James, E. L., Bonsall, M. B., Hoppitt, L., Tunbridge, E. M., Geddes, J. R., Milton, A. L., & Holmes, E. A. (2015). Computer Game Play Reduces Intrusive Memories of Experimental Trauma via Reconsolidation-Update Mechanisms. *Psychological Science*, *26*(8), 1201–1215. Retrieved from https://www.ncbi.nlm.nih.gov/pubmed/26133572. doi:10.1177/0956797615583071

James, W. (1890). *The principles of psychology*. New York: Holt.

James, W., & Richardson, R. D. (2010). *The heart of William James*. Cambridge, MA: Belknap Press of Harvard University Press.

Janak, P. H., & Tye, K. M. (2015). From circuits to behaviour in the amygdala. *Nature*, *517*(7534), 284–292. Retrieved from https://www.ncbi.nlm.nih.gov/pubmed/25592533. doi:10.1038/nature14188

Janson, J., Laedtke, T., Parisi, J. E., O'Brien, P., Petersen, R. C., & Butler, P. C. (2004). Increased risk of type 2 diabetes in Alzheimer disease. *Diabetes, 53*(2), 474–481. Retrieved from https://www.ncbi.nlm.nih.gov/pubmed/14747300

Javitt, D. C. (1987). Negative schizophrenic symptomatology and the PCP (phencyclidine) model of schizophrenia. *The Hillside Journal of Clinical Psychiatry, 9*(1), 12–35. Retrieved from http://www.ncbi.nlm.nih.gov/pubmed/2820854

Javitt, D. C., & Zukin, S. R. (1991). Recent advances in the phencyclidine model of schizophrenia. *The American Journal of Psychiatry, 148*(10), 1301–1308. Retrieved from http://www.ncbi.nlm.nih.gov/pubmed/1654746. doi:10.1176/ajp.148.10.1301

Jaworska, N., & MacQueen, G. (2015). Adolescence as a unique developmental period. *Journal of Psychiatry & Neuroscience, 40*(5), 291–293. Retrieved from https://www.ncbi.nlm.nih.gov/pubmed/26290063

Ji, L., Zhang, H., Potter, G. G., Zang, Y. F., Steffens, D. C., Guo, H., & Wang, L. (2017). Multiple neuroimaging measures for examining exercise-induced neuroplasticity in older adults: A quasi-experimental study. *Frontiers in Aging Neuroscience, 9*, 102. Retrieved from https://www.ncbi.nlm.nih.gov/pubmed/28473767. doi:10.3389/fnagi.2017.00102

Kable, J. W. (2011). The cognitive neuroscience toolkit for the neuroeconomist: A functional overview. *Journal of Neuroscience Psychology and Economics, 4*(2), 63–84. Retrieved from https://www.ncbi.nlm.nih.gov/pubmed/21796272. doi:10.1037/a0023555

Kadohisa, M. (2013). Effects of odor on emotion, with implications. *Frontiers in Systems Neuroscience, 7*, 66. Retrieved from https://www.ncbi.nlm.nih.gov/pubmed/24124415. doi:10.3389/fnsys.2013.00066

Kalichman, S. C., Heckman, T., & Kelly, J. A. (1996). Sensation seeking as an explanation for the association between substance use and HIV-related risky sexual behavior. *Archives of Sexual Behavior, 25*(2), 141–154. Retrieved from https://www.ncbi.nlm.nih.gov/pubmed/8740520

Kandel, E. R. (2013). *Principles of neural science* (5th ed.). New York: McGraw-Hill Medical.

Kandel, E. R., Schwartz, J. H., & Jessell, T. M. (2000). *Principles of neural science* (4th ed.). New York: McGraw-Hill, Health Professions Division.

Kapur, S. (2003). Psychosis as a state of aberrant salience: A framework linking biology, phenomenology, and pharmacology in schizophrenia. *The American Journal of Psychiatry, 160*(1), 13–23. Retrieved from https://www.ncbi.nlm.nih.gov/pubmed/12505794. doi:10.1176/appi.ajp.160.1.13

Kasparson, A. A., Badridze, J., & Maximov, V. V. (2013). Colour cues proved to be more informative for dogs than brightness. *Proceedings of the Royal Society B: Biological Sciences, 280*(1766), 20131356. Retrieved from https://www.ncbi.nlm.nih.gov/pubmed/23864600. doi:10.1098/rspb.2013.1356

Kastner-Dorn, A. K., Andreatta, M., Pauli, P., & Wieser, M. J. (2018). Hypervigilance during anxiety and selective attention during fear: Using steady-state visual evoked potentials (ssVEPs) to disentangle attention mechanisms during predictable and unpredictable threat. *Cortex, 106*, 120–131. Retrieved from https://www.ncbi.nlm.nih.gov/pubmed/29929061. doi:10.1016/j.cortex.2018.05.008

Kawamoto, T., & Endo, T. (2015). Genetic and environmental contributions to personality trait stability and change across adolescence: Results from a Japanese twin sample. *Twin Research and Human Genetics, 18*(5), 545–556. Retrieved from https://www.ncbi.nlm.nih.gov/pubmed/26206267. doi:10.1017/thg.2015.47

Keebaugh, A. C., Barrett, C. E., Laprairie, J. L., Jenkins, J. J., & Young, L. J. (2015). RNAi knockdown of oxytocin receptor in the nucleus accumbens inhibits social attachment and parental care in monogamous female prairie voles. *Social Neuroscience, 10*(5), 561–570. Retrieved from https://www.ncbi.nlm.nih.gov/pubmed/25874849. doi:10.1080/17470919.2015.1040893

Kendrick, K. M., Keverne, E. B., & Baldwin, B. A. (1987). Intracerebroventricular oxytocin stimulates maternal behaviour in the sheep. *Neuroendocrinology, 46*(1), 56–61. Retrieved from https://www.ncbi.nlm.nih.gov/pubmed/3614555. doi:10.1159/000124796

Kessler, R. C., Berglund, P., Demler, O., Jin, R., Merikangas, K. R., & Walters, E. E. (2005). Lifetime prevalence and age-of-onset distributions of DSM-IV disorders in the National Comorbidity Survey Replication. *Archives of General Psychiatry, 62*(6), 593–602. Retrieved from https://www.ncbi.nlm.nih.gov/pubmed/15939837. doi:10.1001/archpsyc.62.6.593

Kessler, R. C., Petukhova, M., Sampson, N. A., Zaslavsky, A. M., & Wittchen, H. U. (2012). Twelve-month and lifetime prevalence and lifetime morbid risk of anxiety and mood disorders in the United States. *International Journal of Methods in Psychiatric Research, 21*(3), 169–184. Retrieved from https://www.ncbi.nlm.nih.gov/pubmed/22865617. doi:10.1002/mpr.1359

Keverne, E. B. (2004). Importance of olfactory and vomeronasal systems for male sexual function. *Physiology & Behavior, 83*(2), 177–187. Retrieved from https://www.ncbi.nlm.nih.gov/pubmed/15488538. doi:10.1016/j.physbeh.2004.08.013

Keverne, E. B., & Kendrick, K. M. (1992). Oxytocin facilitation of maternal behavior in sheep. *Annals of the New York Academy of Sciences, 652*, 83–101. Retrieved from https://www.ncbi.nlm.nih.gov/pubmed/1385685

Keysers, C., Xiao, D. K., Földiák, P., & Perrett, D. I. (2005). Out of sight but not out of mind: The neurophysiology of iconic memory in the superior temporal sulcus. *Cognitive Neuropsychology, 22*(3–4), 316–332. Retrieved from https://doi.org/10.1080/02643290442000103. doi:10.1080/02643290442000103

Khakpai, F., Ebrahimi-Ghiri, M., Alijanpour, S., & Zarrindast, M. R. (2019). Ketamine-induced antidepressant like effects in mice: A possible involvement of cannabinoid system. *Biomedicine & Pharmacotherapy, 112*, 108717. Retrieved from https://www.ncbi.nlm.nih.gov/pubmed/30970516. doi:10.1016/j.biopha.2019.108717

Kim, J. J., & Jung, M. W. (2006). Neural circuits and mechanisms involved in Pavlovian fear conditioning: a critical review. *Neuroscience and Biobehavioral Reviews, 30*(2), 188–202. doi:10.1016/j.neubiorev.2005.06.005

Kirkham, T. C. (2005). Endocannabinoids in the regulation of appetite and body weight. *Behavioural Pharmacology, 16*(5–6), 297–313. Retrieved from https://www.ncbi.nlm.nih.gov/pubmed/16148436

Kirshner, N. (1962). Uptake of catecholamines by a particulate fraction of the adrenal medulla. *Journal of Biological Chemistry, 237*, 2311–2317. Retrieved from https://www.ncbi.nlm.nih.gov/pubmed/14456353

Kisler, K., Nelson, A. R., Rege, S. V., Ramanathan, A., Wang, Y., Ahuja, A., . . . Zlokovic, B. V. (2017). Pericyte degeneration leads to neurovascular uncoupling and limits oxygen supply to brain. *Nature Neuroscience, 20*(3), 406–416. Retrieved from https://www.ncbi.nlm.nih.gov/pubmed/28135240. doi:10.1038/nn.4489

Kitamura, T., Ogawa, S. K., Roy, D. S., Okuyama, T., Morrissey, M. D., Smith, L. M., . . . Tonegawa, S. (2017). Engrams and circuits crucial for systems consolidation of a memory. *Science, 356*(6333), 73–78. Retrieved from https://www.ncbi.nlm.nih.gov/pubmed/28386011. doi:10.1126/science.aam6808

Kleiman, D. G. (1977). Monogamy in mammals. *The Quarterly Review of Biology, 52*(1), 39–69. Retrieved from https://www.ncbi.nlm.nih.gov/pubmed/857268

Klein, C., Metz, S. I., Elmer, S., & Jancke, L. (2018). The interpreter's brain during rest - Hyperconnectivity in the frontal lobe. *PLoS One, 13*(8), e0202600. Retrieved from https://www.ncbi.nlm.nih.gov/pubmed/30138477. doi:10.1371/journal.pone.0202600

Klein, M., Shapiro, E., & Kandel, E. R. (1980). Synaptic plasticity and the modulation of the Ca2+ current. *Journal of Experimental Biology, 89*, 117–157. Retrieved from https://www.ncbi.nlm.nih.gov/pubmed/6110691

Klein, S. B., Cosmides, L., Tooby, J., & Chance, S. (2002). Decisions and the evolution of memory: Multiple systems, multiple functions. *Psychological Review, 109*(2), 306–329. Retrieved from https://www.ncbi.nlm.nih.gov/pubmed/11990320

Klinkenberg, I., Sambeth, A., & Blokland, A. (2011). Acetylcholine and attention. *Behavioural Brain Research, 221*(2), 430–442. Retrieved from https://www.ncbi.nlm.nih.gov/pubmed/21108972. doi:10.1016/j.bbr.2010.11.033

Klopfer, P. H. (1971). Mother love: What turns it on? *American Scientist, 59*(4), 404–407. Retrieved from https://www.ncbi.nlm.nih.gov/pubmed/5089199

Knudsen, B., & Liszkowski, U. (2012a). 18-month-olds predict specific action mistakes through attribution of false belief, not ignorance, and intervene accordingly. *Infancy, 17*(6), 672–691. Retrieved from https://onlinelibrary.wiley.com/doi/abs/10.1111/j.1532-7078.2011.00105.x. doi:10.1111/j.1532-7078.2011.00105.x

Knudsen, B., & Liszkowski, U. (2012b). Eighteen- and 24-month-old infants correct others in anticipation of action mistakes. *Developmental Science, 15*(1), 113–122. Retrieved from https://www.ncbi.nlm.nih.gov/pubmed/22251297. doi:10.1111/j.1467-7687.2011.01098.x

Ko, H. G., Jang, D. J., Son, J., Kwak, C., Choi, J. H., Ji, Y. H., . . . Kaang, B. K. (2009). Effect of ablated hippocampal neurogenesis on the formation and extinction of contextual fear memory. *Molecular Brain, 2*, 1. Retrieved from https://www.ncbi.nlm.nih.gov/pubmed/19138433. doi:10.1186/1756-6606-2-1

Kober, H., Barrett, L. F., Joseph, J., Bliss-Moreau, E., Lindquist, K., & Wager, T. D. (2008). Functional grouping and cortical-subcortical interactions in emotion: A meta-analysis of neuroimaging studies. *Neuroimage, 42*(2), 998–1031. Retrieved from https://www.ncbi.nlm.nih.gov/pubmed/18579414. doi:10.1016/j.neuroimage.2008.03.059

Koenigs, M., & Grafman, J. (2009). The functional neuroanatomy of depression: Distinct roles for ventromedial and dorsolateral prefrontal cortex. *Behavioural Brain Research, 201*(2), 239–243. Retrieved from https://www.ncbi.nlm.nih.gov/pubmed/19428640. doi:10.1016/j.bbr.2009.03.004

Kofuji, P., & Newman, E. A. (2004). Potassium buffering in the central nervous system. *Neuroscience, 129*(4), 1045–1056. Retrieved from http://www.ncbi.nlm.nih.gov/pubmed/15561419. doi:10.1016/j.neuroscience.2004.06.008

Kohda, M., Hotta, T., Takeyama, T., Awata, S., Tanaka, H., Asai, J. Y., & Jordan, A. L. (2019). If a fish can pass the mark test, what are the implications for consciousness and self-awareness testing in animals? *PLoS Biology, 17*(2), e3000021. Retrieved from https://www.ncbi.nlm.nih.gov/pubmed/30730878. doi:10.1371/journal.pbio.3000021

Kohl, J., Babayan, B. M., Rubinstein, N. D., Autry, A. E., Marin-Rodriguez, B., Kapoor, V., . . . Dulac, C. (2018). Functional circuit architecture underlying parental behaviour. *Nature, 556*(7701), 326–331. Retrieved from https://www.ncbi.nlm.nih.gov/pubmed/29643503. doi:10.1038/s41586-018-0027-0

Kohl, J., & Dulac, C. (2018). Neural control of parental behaviors. *Current Opinion in Neurobiology, 49*, 116–122. Retrieved from https://www.ncbi.nlm.nih.gov/pubmed/29482085. doi:10.1016/j.conb.2018.02.002

Kometer, M., & Vollenweider, F. X. (2018). Serotonergic Hallucinogen-Induced Visual Perceptual Alterations. *Current Opinion in Neurobiology, 36*, 257–282. Retrieved from https://www.ncbi.nlm.nih.gov/pubmed/27900674. doi:10.1007/7854_2016_461

Kondo, Y., & Arai, Y. (1995). Functional association between the medial amygdala and the medial preoptic area in regulation of mating behavior in the male rat. *Physiology & Behavior, 57*(1), 69–73. Retrieved from https://www.ncbi.nlm.nih.gov/pubmed/7878127

Kozlov, A. S., Risler, T., & Hudspeth, A. J. (2007). Coherent motion of stereocilia assures the concerted gating of hair-cell transduction channels. *Nature Neuroscience, 10*(1), 87–92. Retrieved from https://www.ncbi.nlm.nih.gov/pubmed/17173047. doi:10.1038/nn1818

Kraehenmann, R., Pokorny, D., Vollenweider, L., Preller, K. H., Pokorny, T., Seifritz, E., & Vollenweider, F. X. (2017). Dreamlike effects of LSD on waking imagery in humans depend on serotonin 2A receptor activation. *Psychopharmacology (Berl), 234*(13), 2031–2046. Retrieved from https://www.ncbi.nlm.nih.gov/pubmed/28386699. doi:10.1007/s00213-017-4610-0

Kramer, A. F., & Colcombe, S. (2018). Fitness effects on the cognitive function of older adults: A meta-analytic study-revisited. *Perspectives on Psychological Science, 13*(2), 213–217. Retrieved from https://www.ncbi.nlm.nih.gov/pubmed/29592650. doi:10.1177/1745691617707316

Krosnick, J. A., Betz, A. L., Jussim, L. J., & Lynn, A. R. (1992). Subliminal conditioning of attitudes. *Personality and Social Psychology Bulletin, 18*(2), 152–162.

Kubota, J. T., Banaji, M. R., & Phelps, E. A. (2012). The neuroscience of race. *Nature Neuroscience, 15*(7), 940–948. Retrieved from https://www.ncbi.nlm.nih.gov/pubmed/22735516. doi:10.1038/nn.3136

Kubota, K. (1989). Kuniomi Ishimori and the first discovery of sleep-inducing substances in the brain. *Neuroscience Research, 6*(6), 497–518. Retrieved from https://www.ncbi.nlm.nih.gov/pubmed/2677843

Kuca, K., Bajgar, J., & Kassa, J. (2019). Some possibilities to study new prophylactics against nerve agents. *Mini-Reviews in Medicinal Chemistry, 19*(12), 970–979. Retrieved from https://www.ncbi.nlm.nih.gov/pubmed/30827238. doi:10.2174/1389557519666190301112530

Kucewicz, M. T., Berry, B. M., Miller, L. R., Khadjevand, F., Ezzyat, Y., Stein, J. M., . . . Worrell, G. A. (2018). Evidence for verbal memory enhancement with electrical brain stimulation in the lateral temporal cortex. *Brain, 141*(4), 971–978. Retrieved from https://www.ncbi.nlm.nih.gov/pubmed/29324988. doi:10.1093/brain/awx373

Kuffler, S. W. (1953). Discharge patterns and functional organization of mammalian retina. *Journal of Neurophysiology, 16*(1), 37–68. Retrieved from https://www.ncbi.nlm.nih.gov/pubmed/13035466

Kumar, V. J., van Oort, E., Scheffler, K., Beckmann, C. F., & Grodd, W. (2017). Functional anatomy of the human thalamus at rest. *Neuroimage, 147*, 678–691. Retrieved from https://www.ncbi.nlm.nih.gov/pubmed/28041978. doi:10.1016/j.neuroimage.2016.12.071

Lacerte, M., & Mesfin, F. B. (2019). *Hypoxic brain injury*. Treasure Island, FL: StatPearls.

Lampe, L., Kharabian-Masouleh, S., Kynast, J., Arelin, K., Steele, C. J., Loffler, M., . . . Bazin, P. L. (2017). Lesion location matters: The relationships between white matter hyperintensities on cognition in the healthy elderly. *Journal of Cerebral Blood Flow & Metabolism*, 271678X17740501. Retrieved from https://www.ncbi.nlm.nih.gov/pubmed/29106319. doi:10.1177/0271678X17740501

Lamsa, K., & Lau, P. (2018). Long-term plasticity of hippocampal interneurons during in vivo memory processes. *Current Opinion in Neurobiology*, *54*, 20–27. Retrieved from https://www.ncbi.nlm.nih.gov/pubmed/30195105. doi:10.1016/j.conb.2018.08.006

Langen, C. D., Zonneveld, H. I., White, T., Huizinga, W., Cremers, L. G. M., de Groot, M., . . . Vernooij, M. W. (2017). White matter lesions relate to tract-specific reductions in functional connectivity. *Neurobiology of Aging*, *51*, 97–103. Retrieved from https://www.ncbi.nlm.nih.gov/pubmed/28063366. doi:10.1016/j.neurobiolaging.2016.12.004

Langleben, D. D., Schroeder, L., Maldjian, J. A., Gur, R. C., McDonald, S., Ragland, J. D., . . . Childress, A. R. (2002). Brain activity during simulated deception: An event-related functional magnetic resonance study. *Neuroimage*, *15*(3), 727–732. Retrieved from https://www.ncbi.nlm.nih.gov/pubmed/11848716. doi:10.1006/nimg.2001.1003

Lanius, R. A., Vermetten, E., Loewenstein, R. J., Brand, B., Schmahl, C., Bremner, J. D., & Spiegel, D. (2010). Emotion modulation in PTSD: Clinical and neurobiological evidence for a dissociative subtype. *The American Journal of Psychiatry*, *167*(6), 640–647. Retrieved from https://www.ncbi.nlm.nih.gov/pubmed/20360318. doi:10.1176/appi.ajp.2009.09081168

Lanska, D. J. (2018). The Kluver-Bucy syndrome. *Frontiers of Neurology and Neuroscience*, *41*, 77–89. Retrieved from https://www.ncbi.nlm.nih.gov/pubmed/29145186. doi:10.1159/000475721

Lau, A., & Tymianski, M. (2010). Glutamate receptors, neurotoxicity and neurodegeneration. *Pflügers Archiv - European Journal of Physiology*, *460*(2), 525–542. Retrieved from https://www.ncbi.nlm.nih.gov/pubmed/20229265. doi:10.1007/s00424-010-0809-1

Laureys, S. (2005). The neural correlate of (un)awareness: Lessons from the vegetative state. *Trends in Cognitive Sciences*, *9*(12), 556–559. Retrieved from http://www.ncbi.nlm.nih.gov/pubmed/16271507. doi:10.1016/j.tics.2005.10.010

Laureys, S., Pellas, F., Van Eeckhout, P., Ghorbel, S., Schnakers, C., Perrin, F., . . . Goldman, S. (2005). The locked-in syndrome: What is it like to be conscious but paralyzed and voiceless? *Progress in Brain Research*, *150*, 495–511. Retrieved from http://www.ncbi.nlm.nih.gov/pubmed/16186044. doi:10.1016/S0079-6123(05)50034-7

Lebedev, M. A., & Nicolelis, M. A. (2017). Brain-machine interfaces: From basic science to neuroprostheses and neurorehabilitation. *Physiological Reviews*, *97*(2), 767–837. Retrieved from https://www.ncbi.nlm.nih.gov/pubmed/28275048. doi:10.1152/physrev.00027.2016

Leboucher, A., Ahmed, T., Caron, E., Tailleux, A., Raison, S., Joly-Amado, A., . . . Blum, D. (2019). Brain insulin response and peripheral metabolic changes in a Tau transgenic mouse model. *Neurobiology of Disease*, *125*, 14–22. Retrieved from https://www.ncbi.nlm.nih.gov/pubmed/30665005. doi:10.1016/j.nbd.2019.01.008

LeDoux, J. E. (1996). *The emotional brain: The mysterious underpinnings of emotional life*. New York, NY: Simon & Schuster.

LeDoux, J. E. (2002). *Synaptic self: How our brains become who we are*. New York/London: Viking.

LeDoux, J. E., Sakaguchi, A., & Reis, D. J. (1984). Subcortical efferent projections of the medial geniculate nucleus mediate emotional responses conditioned to acoustic stimuli. *Journal of Neuroscience*, *4*(3), 683–698. Retrieved from https://www.ncbi.nlm.nih.gov/pubmed/6707732

Lee, D. A., Bedont, J. L., Pak, T., Wang, H., Song, J., Miranda-Angulo, A., . . . Blackshaw, S. (2012). Tanycytes of the hypothalamic median eminence form a diet-responsive neurogenic niche. *Nature Neuroscience*, *15*(5), 700–702. Retrieved from https://www.ncbi.nlm.nih.gov/pubmed/22446882. doi:10.1038/nn.3079

Lee, H. G., Casadesus, G., Zhu, X., Joseph, J. A., Perry, G., & Smith, M. A. (2004). Perspectives on the amyloid-beta cascade hypothesis. *J Alzheimers Dis*, *6*(2), 137–145. Retrieved from https://www.ncbi.nlm.nih.gov/pubmed/15096697

Lee, J. L. C., Nader, K., & Schiller, D. (2017). An update on memory reconsolidation updating. *Trends in Cognitive Sciences*, *21*(7), 531–545. Retrieved from https://www.ncbi.nlm.nih.gov/pubmed/28495311. doi:10.1016/j.tics.2017.04.006

Lee, N., Broderick, A. J., & Chamberlain, L. (2007). What is "neuromarketing"? A discussion and agenda for future research. *International Journal of Psychophysiology*, *63*(2), 199–204. Retrieved from https://www.ncbi.nlm.nih.gov/pubmed/16769143. doi:10.1016/j.ijpsycho.2006.03.007

Lefevre, J., & Mangin, J. F. (2010). A reaction-diffusion model of human brain development. *PLoS Computational Biology*, *6*(4), e1000749. Retrieved from https://www.ncbi.nlm.nih.gov/pubmed/20421989. doi:10.1371/journal.pcbi.1000749

Lehericy, S., Sharman, M. A., Dos Santos, C. L., Paquin, R., & Gallea, C. (2012). Magnetic resonance imaging of the substantia nigra in Parkinson's disease. *Movement Disorders*, *27*(7), 822–830. Retrieved from https://www.ncbi.nlm.nih.gov/pubmed/22649063. doi:10.1002/mds.25015

Lerch, J. P., van der Kouwe, A. J., Raznahan, A., Paus, T., Johansen-Berg, H., Miller, K. L., . . . Sotiropoulos, S. N. (2017). Studying neuroanatomy using MRI. *Nature Neuroscience*, *20*(3), 314–326. Retrieved from https://www.ncbi.nlm.nih.gov/pubmed/28230838. doi:10.1038/nn.4501

Leslie, A. M., Friedman, O., & German, T. P. (2004). Core mechanisms in "theory of mind". *Trends in Cognitive Sciences*, *8*(12), 528–533. Retrieved from http://www.ncbi.nlm.nih.gov/pubmed/15556021. doi:10.1016/j.tics.2004.10.001

Letinic, K., Zoncu, R., & Rakic, P. (2002). Origin of GABAergic neurons in the human neocortex. *Nature*, *417*(6889), 645–649. Retrieved from https://www.ncbi.nlm.nih.gov/pubmed/12050665. doi:10.1038/nature00779

Leung, S., Croft, R. J., Jackson, M. L., Howard, M. E., & McKenzie, R. J. (2012). A comparison of the effect of mobile phone use and alcohol consumption on driving simulation performance. *Traffic Injury Prevention*, *13*(6), 566–574. Retrieved from https://www.ncbi.nlm.nih.gov/pubmed/23137086. doi:10.1080/15389588.2012.683118

LeVay, S. (1991). A difference in hypothalamic structure between heterosexual and homosexual men. *Science*, *253*(5023), 1034–1037. Retrieved from https://www.ncbi.nlm.nih.gov/pubmed/1887219

Lever, C., Burton, S., Jeewajee, A., O'Keefe, J., & Burgess, N. (2009). Boundary vector cells in the subiculum of the hippocampal formation. *The Journal of Neuroscience*, *29*(31), 9771–9777. Retrieved from https://www.ncbi.nlm.nih.gov/pubmed/19657030. doi:10.1523/JNEUROSCI.1319-09.2009

Levine, D. N. (2007). Sherrington's "The Integrative action of the nervous system": A centennial appraisal. *The Journal of Neuroscience*, *253*(1–2), 1–6. Retrieved from https://www.ncbi.nlm.nih.gov/pubmed/17223135. doi:10.1016/j.jns.2006.12.002

Levine, J. (1983). Materialism and qualia: The explanatory gap. *Pacific Philosophical Quaterly*, *64*, 354–361.

Levine, J., Panchalingam, K., Rapoport, A., Gershon, S., McClure, R. J., & Pettegrew, J. W. (2000). Increased cerebrospinal fluid glutamine levels in depressed patients. *Biological Psychiatry*, *47*(7), 586–593. Retrieved from https://www.ncbi.nlm.nih.gov/pubmed/10745050

Levy, R., & Goldman-Rakic, P. S. (1999). Association of storage and processing functions in the dorsolateral prefrontal cortex of the nonhuman primate. *The Journal of Neuroscience, 19*(12), 5149–5158. Retrieved from https://www.ncbi.nlm.nih.gov/pubmed/10366648

Li, J., McClure, S. M., King-Casas, B., & Montague, P. R. (2006). Policy adjustment in a dynamic economic game. *PLoS One, 1*, e103. Retrieved from https://www.ncbi.nlm.nih.gov/pubmed/17183636. doi:10.1371/journal.pone.0000103

Li, J. M., Liu, L. L., Su, W. J., Wang, B., Zhang, T., Zhang, Y., & Jiang, C. L. (2019). Ketamine may exert antidepressant effects via suppressing NLRP3 inflammasome to upregulate AMPA receptors. *Neuropharmacology, 146*, 149–153. Retrieved from https://www.ncbi.nlm.nih.gov/pubmed/30496753. doi:10.1016/j.neuropharm.2018.11.022

Li, X., & Lui, F. (2019). *Anosmia*. Treasure Island, FL: StatPearls.

Liberzon, I., & Abelson, J. L. (2016). Context processing and the neurobiology of post-traumatic stress disorder. *Neuron, 92*(1), 14–30. Retrieved from https://www.ncbi.nlm.nih.gov/pubmed/27710783. doi:10.1016/j.neuron.2016.09.039

Libet, B., Gleason, C. A., Wright, E. W., & Pearl, D. K. (1983). Time of conscious intention to act in relation to onset of cerebral activity (readiness-potential). The unconscious initiation of a freely voluntary act. *Brain, 106*(Pt. 3), 623–642. Retrieved from http://www.ncbi.nlm.nih.gov/pubmed/6640273

Limanowski, J., & Blankenburg, F. (2016). Integration of visual and proprioceptive limb position information in human posterior parietal, premotor, and extrastriate cortex. *The Journal of Neuroscience, 36*(9), 2582–2589. Retrieved from https://www.ncbi.nlm.nih.gov/pubmed/26937000. doi:10.1523/JNEUROSCI.3987-15.2016

Lind, O., Mitkus, M., Olsson, P., & Kelber, A. (2013). Ultraviolet sensitivity and colour vision in raptor foraging. *Journal of Experimental Biology, 216*(Pt. 10), 1819–1826. Retrieved from https://www.ncbi.nlm.nih.gov/pubmed/23785106. doi:10.1242/jeb.082834

Lind, O., Mitkus, M., Olsson, P., & Kelber, A. (2014). Ultraviolet vision in birds: The importance of transparent eye media. *Proceedings of the Royal Society B: Biological Sciences, 281*(1774), 20132209. Retrieved from https://www.ncbi.nlm.nih.gov/pubmed/24258716. doi:10.1098/rspb.2013.2209

Lindquist, K. A., Siegel, E. H., Quigley, K. S., & Barrett, L. F. (2013). The hundred-year emotion war: Are emotions natural kinds or psychological constructions? Comment on Lench, Flores, and Bench (2011). *Psychological Bulletin, 139*(1), 255–263. Retrieved from https://www.ncbi.nlm.nih.gov/pubmed/23294094. doi:10.1037/a0029038

Lindquist, K. A., Wager, T. D., Kober, H., Bliss-Moreau, E., & Barrett, L. F. (2012). The brain basis of emotion: A meta-analytic review. *Behavioral and Brain Sciences, 35*(3), 121–143. Retrieved from https://www.ncbi.nlm.nih.gov/pubmed/22617651. doi:10.1017/S0140525X11000446

Lindsley, D. B. (1952). Psychological phenomena and the electroencephalogram. *Electroencephalography & Clinical Neurophysiology, 4*(4), 443–456. Retrieved from https://www.ncbi.nlm.nih.gov/pubmed/12998592

Lisman, J., Yasuda, R., & Raghavachari, S. (2012). Mechanisms of CaMKII action in long-term potentiation. *Nature Reviews Neuroscience, 13*(3), 169–182. Retrieved from https://www.ncbi.nlm.nih.gov/pubmed/22334212. doi:10.1038/nrn3192

Liston, C., Miller, M. M., Goldwater, D. S., Radley, J. J., Rocher, A. B., Hof, P. R., . . . McEwen, B. S. (2006). Stress-induced alterations in prefrontal cortical dendritic morphology predict selective impairments in perceptual attentional set-shifting. *The Journal of Neuroscience, 26*(30), 7870–7874. Retrieved from https://www.ncbi.nlm.nih.gov/pubmed/16870732. doi:10.1523/JNEUROSCI.1184-06.2006

Little, T. J., Horowitz, M., & Feinle-Bisset, C. (2005). Role of cholecystokinin in appetite control and body weight regulation. *Obesity Reviews, 6*(4), 297–306. Retrieved from https://www.ncbi.nlm.nih.gov/pubmed/16246215. doi:10.1111/j.1467-789X.2005.00212.x

Loewenstein, G., Rick, S., & Cohen, J. D. (2008). Neuroeconomics. *Annual Review of Psychology, 59*, 647–672. doi:10.1146/annurev.psych.59.103006.093710

Logue, M. W., van Rooij, S. J. H., Dennis, E. L., Davis, S. L., Hayes, J. P., Stevens, J. S., . . . Morey, R. A. (2018). Smaller hippocampal volume in posttraumatic stress disorder: A multisite ENIGMA-PGC study: Subcortical volumetry results from posttraumatic stress disorder consortia. *Biological Psychiatry, 83*(3), 244–253. Retrieved from https://www.ncbi.nlm.nih.gov/pubmed/29217296. doi:10.1016/j.biopsych.2017.09.006

Loomis, A., & Newton, H. (1937). Cerebral states during sleep as studied by human brain potentials. *Journal of Experimental Psychology, 21*, 127–144.

Lorenzetti, V., Solowij, N., & Yucel, M. (2016). The role of cannabinoids in neuroanatomic alterations in cannabis users. *Biological Psychiatry, 79*(7), e17–e31. Retrieved from https://www.ncbi.nlm.nih.gov/pubmed/26858212. doi:10.1016/j.biopsych.2015.11.013

Lu, H. C., & Mackie, K. (2016). An Introduction to the Endogenous Cannabinoid System. *Biological Psychiatry, 79*(7), 516–525. Retrieved from https://www.ncbi.nlm.nih.gov/pubmed/26698193. doi:10.1016/j.biopsych.2015.07.028

Lu, J., Sherman, D., Devor, M., & Saper, C. B. (2006). A putative flip-flop switch for control of REM sleep. *Nature, 441*(7093), 589–594. Retrieved from https://www.ncbi.nlm.nih.gov/pubmed/16688184. doi:10.1038/nature04767

Lu, Z. L., Williamson, S. J., & Kaufman, L. (1992). Behavioral lifetime of human auditory sensory memory predicted by physiological measures. *Science, 258*(5088), 1668–1670. Retrieved from https://www.ncbi.nlm.nih.gov/pubmed/1455246

Lum, J. A., & Conti-Ramsden, G. (2013). Long-term memory: A review and meta-analysis of studies of declarative and procedural memory in specific language impairment. *Topics in Language Disorders, 33*(4), 282–297. Retrieved from https://www.ncbi.nlm.nih.gov/pubmed/24748707

Lundholm, L., Frisell, T., Lichtenstein, P., & Langstrom, N. (2015). Anabolic androgenic steroids and violent offending: Confounding by polysubstance abuse among 10,365 general population men. *Addiction, 110*(1), 100–108. Retrieved from https://www.ncbi.nlm.nih.gov/pubmed/25170826. doi:10.1111/add.12715

Lunetta, P., Ohberg, A., & Sajantila, A. (2002). Suicide by intracerebellar ballpoint pen. *The American Journal of Forensic Medicine and Pathology, 23*(4), 334–337. Retrieved from https://www.ncbi.nlm.nih.gov/pubmed/12464807. doi:10.1097/01.PAF.0000040432.69175.E8

Lyons, K. (2016). 1 in 100 babies: The fetal alcohol spectrum disorder pathway. *Nursing Standard, 31*(13), 18–20. Retrieved from https://www.ncbi.nlm.nih.gov/pubmed/27892236. doi:10.7748/ns.31.13.18.s22

Ma, M., Grosmaitre, X., Iwema, C. L., Baker, H., Greer, C. A., & Shepherd, G. M. (2003). Olfactory signal transduction in the mouse septal organ. *The Journal of Neuroscience, 23*(1), 317–324. Retrieved from https://www.ncbi.nlm.nih.gov/pubmed/12514230

Maccioni, R. B., Farias, G., Morales, I., & Navarrete, L. (2010). The revitalized tau hypothesis on Alzheimer's disease. *Archives of Medical Research, 41*(3), 226–231. Retrieved from https://www.ncbi.nlm.nih.gov/pubmed/20682182. doi:10.1016/j.arcmed.2010.03.007

Macherey, O., & Carlyon, R. P. (2014). Cochlear implants. *Current Biology, 24*(18), R878–R884. Retrieved from https://www.ncbi.nlm.nih.gov/pubmed/25247367. doi:10.1016/j.cub.2014.06.053

MacLean, P. D. (1990). *The triune brain in evolution: Role in paleocerebral functions*. New York: Plenum Press.

Macmillan, M. (2001). John Martyn Harlow: "Obscure country physician"? *Journal of the History of the Neurosciences, 10*(2), 149–162. Retrieved from https://www.ncbi.nlm.nih.gov/pubmed/11512426. doi:10.1076/jhin.10.2.149.7254

Madsen, M. K., Fisher, P. M., Burmester, D., Dyssegaard, A., Stenbaek, D. S., Kristiansen, S., . . . Knudsen, G. M. (2019). Psychedelic effects of psilocybin correlate with serotonin 2A receptor occupancy and plasma psilocin levels. *Neuropsychopharmacology*. Retrieved from https://www.ncbi.nlm.nih.gov/pubmed/30685771. doi:10.1038/s41386-019-0324-9

Maguire, E. A. (2014). Memory consolidation in humans: New evidence and opportunities. *Experimental Physiology, 99*(3), 471–486. Retrieved from https://www.ncbi.nlm.nih.gov/pubmed/24414174. doi:10.1113/expphysiol.2013.072157

Maguire, E. A., Woollett, K., & Spiers, H. J. (2006). London taxi drivers and bus drivers: A structural MRI and neuropsychological analysis. *Hippocampus, 16*(12), 1091–1101. Retrieved from https://www.ncbi.nlm.nih.gov/pubmed/17024677. doi:10.1002/hipo.20233

Mahar, I., Bambico, F. R., Mechawar, N., & Nobrega, J. N. (2014). Stress, serotonin, and hippocampal neurogenesis in relation to depression and antidepressant effects. *Neuroscience & Biobehavioral Reviews, 38*, 173–192. Retrieved from https://www.ncbi.nlm.nih.gov/pubmed/24300695. doi:10.1016/j.neubiorev.2013.11.009

Mahler, S. V., Smith, K. S., & Berridge, K. C. (2007). Endocannabinoid hedonic hotspot for sensory pleasure: Anandamide in nucleus accumbens shell enhances 'liking' of a sweet reward. *Neuropsychopharmacology, 32*(11), 2267–2278. Retrieved from https://www.ncbi.nlm.nih.gov/pubmed/17406653. doi:10.1038/sj.npp.1301376

Makin, S. (2018). The amyloid hypothesis on trial. *Nature, 559*(7715), S4–S7. Retrieved from https://www.ncbi.nlm.nih.gov/pubmed/30046080. doi:10.1038/d41586-018-05719-4

Maletic, V., Robinson, M., Oakes, T., Iyengar, S., Ball, S. G., & Russell, J. (2007). Neurobiology of depression: An integrated view of key findings. *International Journal of Clinical Practice, 61*(12), 2030–2040. Retrieved from http://www.ncbi.nlm.nih.gov/pubmed/17944926. doi:10.1111/j.1742-1241.2007.01602.x

Malinow, R., Schulman, H., & Tsien, R. W. (1989). Inhibition of postsynaptic PKC or CaMKII blocks induction but not expression of LTP. *Science, 245*(4920), 862–866. Retrieved from https://www.ncbi.nlm.nih.gov/pubmed/2549638

Malsbury, C. W. (1971). Facilitation of male rat copulatory behavior by electrical stimulation of the medial preoptic area. *Physiology & Behavior, 7*(6), 797–805. Retrieved from https://www.ncbi.nlm.nih.gov/pubmed/5134017

Mani, S. K., & Oyola, M. G. (2012). Progesterone signaling mechanisms in brain and behavior. *Frontiers in Endocrinology (Lausanne), 3*, 7. Retrieved from https://www.ncbi.nlm.nih.gov/pubmed/22649404. doi:10.3389/fendo.2012.00007

Marco, L. A., Reed, T. F., Aldes, L. D., Chronister, R. B., Brown, C. B., & White, L. E. (1989). Cortical control of tongue contractility in the rat under ketamine anaesthesia. *Clinical and Experimental Pharmacology and Physiology, 16*(5), 395–401. Retrieved from https://www.ncbi.nlm.nih.gov/pubmed/2766581

Maren, S. (2001). Neurobiology of Pavlovian fear conditioning. *Annual Review of Neuroscience, 24*, 897–931. Retrieved from https://www.ncbi.nlm.nih.gov/pubmed/11520922. doi:10.1146/annurev.neuro.24.1.897

Maren, S., & Fanselow, M. S. (1996). The amygdala and fear conditioning: Has the nut been cracked? *Neuron, 16*(2), 237–240. Retrieved from https://www.ncbi.nlm.nih.gov/pubmed/8789938

Margolis, E. B., Hjelmstad, G. O., Fujita, W., & Fields, H. L. (2014). Direct bidirectional mu-opioid control of midbrain dopamine neurons. *The Journal of Neuroscience, 34*(44), 14707–14716. Retrieved from https://www.ncbi.nlm.nih.gov/pubmed/25355223. doi:10.1523/JNEUROSCI.2144-14.2014

Marsh, A. A., Stoycos, S. A., Brethel-Haurwitz, K. M., Robinson, P., VanMeter, J. W., & Cardinale, E. M. (2014). Neural and cognitive characteristics of extraordinary altruists. *Proceedings of the National Academy of Sciences of the United States of America, 111*(42), 15036–15041. Retrieved from https://www.ncbi.nlm.nih.gov/pubmed/25225374. doi:10.1073/pnas.1408440111

Marsicano, G., & Lafenetre, P. (2009). Roles of the endocannabinoid system in learning and memory. *Current Topics in Behavioral Neurosciences, 1*, 201–230. Retrieved from https://www.ncbi.nlm.nih.gov/pubmed/21104385. doi:10.1007/978-3-540-88955-7_8

Marvan, M. L., & Cortes-Iniestra, S. (2001). Women's beliefs about the prevalence of premenstrual syndrome and biases in recall of premenstrual changes. *Health Psychology, 20*(4), 276–280. Retrieved from https://www.ncbi.nlm.nih.gov/pubmed/11515739

Masten, C. L., Colich, N. L., Rudie, J. D., Bookheimer, S. Y., Eisenberger, N. I., & Dapretto, M. (2011). An fMRI investigation of responses to peer rejection in adolescents with autism spectrum disorders. *Developmental Cognitive Neuroscience, 1*(3), 260–270. Retrieved from http://www.ncbi.nlm.nih.gov/pubmed/22318914. doi:10.1016/j.dcn.2011.01.004

Matsuzawa, S., & Suzuki, T. (2002). [Psychological stress and rewarding effect of alcohol]. *Nihon Arukoru Yakubutsu Igakkai Zasshi, 37*(3), 143–152. Retrieved from https://www.ncbi.nlm.nih.gov/pubmed/12138720

Mattavelli, G., Sormaz, M., Flack, T., Asghar, A. U., Fan, S., Frey, J., . . . Andrews, T. J. (2014). Neural responses to facial expressions support the role of the amygdala in processing threat. *Social Cognitive and Affective Neuroscience, 9*(11), 1684–1689. Retrieved from https://www.ncbi.nlm.nih.gov/pubmed/24097376. doi:10.1093/scan/nst162

Max, D. T. (2007). *The family that couldn't sleep: A medical mystery* (Random House Trade Paperback ed.). New York: Random House Trade Paperbacks.

Mayford, M., Siegelbaum, S. A., & Kandel, E. R. (2012). Synapses and memory storage. *Cold Spring Harbor Perspectives in Biology, 4*(6). Retrieved from https://www.ncbi.nlm.nih.gov/pubmed/22496389. doi:10.1101/cshperspect.a005751

Mayner, W. G. P., Marshall, W., Albantakis, L., Findlay, G., Marchman, R., & Tononi, G. (2018). PyPhi: A toolbox for integrated information theory. *PLoS Computational Biology, 14*(7), e1006343. Retrieved from https://www.ncbi.nlm.nih.gov/pubmed/30048445. doi:10.1371/journal.pcbi.1006343

Mayor-Dubois, C., Maeder, P., Zesiger, P., & Roulet-Perez, E. (2010). Visuo-motor and cognitive procedural learning in children with basal ganglia pathology. *Neuropsychologia, 48*(7), 2009–2017. Retrieved from https://www.ncbi.nlm.nih.gov/pubmed/20362601. doi:10.1016/j.neuropsychologia.2010.03.022

McFarland, C., Ross, M., & DeCourville, N. (1989). Women's theories of menstruation and biases in recall of menstrual symptoms. *Journal of Personality and Social Psychology, 57*(3), 522–531. Retrieved from https://www.ncbi.nlm.nih.gov/pubmed/2778636

McGinnis, M. Y. (2004). Anabolic androgenic steroids and aggression: Studies using animal models. *Annals of the New York Academy of Sciences, 1036*, 399–415. Retrieved from https://www.ncbi.nlm.nih.gov/pubmed/15817752. doi:10.1196/annals.1330.024

Meares, R. (1999). The contribution of Hughlings Jackson to an understanding of dissociation. *The American Journal of Psychiatry*, *156*(12), 1850–1855. Retrieved from http://www.ncbi.nlm.nih.gov/pubmed/10588396. doi:10.1176/ajp.156.12.1850

Meier, M. H., Caspi, A., Cerda, M., Hancox, R. J., Harrington, H., Houts, R., . . . Moffitt, T. E. (2016). Associations between cannabis use and physical health problems in early midlife: A longitudinal comparison of persistent cannabis vs tobacco users. *JAMA Psychiatry*, *73*(7), 731–740. Retrieved from https://www.ncbi.nlm.nih.gov/pubmed/27249330. doi:10.1001/jamapsychiatry.2016.0637

Melzack, R., & Wall, P. D. (1965). Pain mechanisms: A new theory. *Science*, *150*(3699), 971–979. Retrieved from https://www.ncbi.nlm.nih.gov/pubmed/5320816

Menardo, E., Balboni, G., & Cubelli, R. (2017). Environmental factors and teenagers' personalities: The role of personal and familial socio-cultural level. *Behavioural Brain Research*, *325*(Pt. B), 181–187. Retrieved from https://www.ncbi.nlm.nih.gov/pubmed/28238826. doi:10.1016/j.bbr.2017.02.038

Meruelo, A. D., Castro, N., Cota, C. I., & Tapert, S. F. (2017). Cannabis and alcohol use, and the developing brain. *Behavioural Brain Research*, *325*(Pt. A), 44–50. Retrieved from https://www.ncbi.nlm.nih.gov/pubmed/28223098. doi:10.1016/j.bbr.2017.02.025

Meston, C. M., & Buss, D. M. (2007). Why humans have sex. *Archives of sexual behavior*, *36*(4), 477–507. Retrieved from https://www.ncbi.nlm.nih.gov/pubmed/17610060. doi:10.1007/s10508-007-9175-2

Meunier, M., Bachevalier, J., Mishkin, M., & Murray, E. A. (1993). Effects on visual recognition of combined and separate ablations of the entorhinal and perirhinal cortex in rhesus monkeys. *The Journal of Neuroscience*, *13*(12), 5418–5432. Retrieved from https://www.ncbi.nlm.nih.gov/pubmed/8254384

Meyer, J. M. (2008). Sexual dysfunction in patients treated with atypical antipsychotics. *The Journal of Clinical Psychiatry*, *69*(9), e26. Retrieved from https://www.ncbi.nlm.nih.gov/pubmed/19026271

Meyer-Bahlburg, H. F., Dolezal, C., Baker, S. W., & New, M. I. (2008). Sexual orientation in women with classical or non-classical congenital adrenal hyperplasia as a function of degree of prenatal androgen excess. *Archives of Sexual Behavior*, *37*(1), 85–99. Retrieved from https://www.ncbi.nlm.nih.gov/pubmed/18157628. doi:10.1007/s10508-007-9265-1

Micevych, P. E., & Meisel, R. L. (2017). Integrating neural circuits controlling female sexual behavior. *Frontiers in Systems Neuroscience*, *11*, 42. Retrieved from https://www.ncbi.nlm.nih.gov/pubmed/28642689. doi:10.3389/fnsys.2017.00042

Micevych, P. E., Mermelstein, P. G., & Sinchak, K. (2017). Estradiol Membrane-Initiated Signaling in the Brain Mediates Reproduction. *Trends in Neurosciences*, *40*(11), 654–666. Retrieved from https://www.ncbi.nlm.nih.gov/pubmed/28969926. doi:10.1016/j.tins.2017.09.001

Michel, M., Beck, D., Block, N., Blumenfeld, H., Brown, R., Carmel, D., . . . Yoshida, M. (2019). Opportunities and challenges for a maturing science of consciousness. *Nature Human Behaviour*, *3*(2), 104–107. Retrieved from https://doi.org/10.1038/s41562-019-0531-8. doi:10.1038/s41562-019-0531-8

Miczek, K. A., Fish, E. W., De Bold, J. F., & De Almeida, R. M. (2002). Social and neural determinants of aggressive behavior: Pharmacotherapeutic targets at serotonin, dopamine and gamma-aminobutyric acid systems. *Psychopharmacology (Berl)*, *163*(3–4), 434–458. Retrieved from https://www.ncbi.nlm.nih.gov/pubmed/12373445. doi:10.1007/s00213-002-1139-6

Miller, G., Tybur, J. M., & Jordan, B. D. (2007). Ovulatory cycle effects on tip earnings by lap dancers: Economic evidence for human estrus? *Evolution and Human Behavior*, *28*, 375–381.

Miller, P. E., & Murphy, C. J. (1995). Vision in dogs. *Journal of the American Veterinary Medical Association*, *207*(12), 1623–1634. Retrieved from https://www.ncbi.nlm.nih.gov/pubmed/7493905

Milner, B. (1972). Disorders of learning and memory after temporal lobe lesions in man. *Clinical Neurosurgery*, *19*, 421–446. Retrieved from https://www.ncbi.nlm.nih.gov/pubmed/4637561

Misanin, J. R., Miller, R. R., & Lewis, D. J. (1968). Retrograde amnesia produced by electroconvulsive shock after reactivation of a consolidated memory trace. *Science*, *160*(3827), 554–555. Retrieved from https://www.ncbi.nlm.nih.gov/pubmed/5689415

Mishkin, M., & Ungerleider, L. G. (1982). Contribution of striate inputs to the visuospatial functions of parieto-preoccipital cortex in monkeys. *Behavioural Brain Research*, *6*(1), 57–77. Retrieved from https://www.ncbi.nlm.nih.gov/pubmed/7126325

Mitchell, D. C., Knight, C. A., Hockenberry, J., Teplansky, R., & Hartman, T. J. (2014). Beverage caffeine intakes in the U.S. *Food and Chemical Toxicology*, *63*, 136–142. Retrieved from https://www.ncbi.nlm.nih.gov/pubmed/24189158. doi:10.1016/j.fct.2013.10.042

Mitchell, G. J. (2007). *Report to the commissioner of baseball of an independent investigation into the illegal use of steroids and other performance enhancing substances by players in Major League Baseball.*

Mitchell, J. P., Macrae, C. N., & Banaji, M. R. (2006). Dissociable medial prefrontal contributions to judgments of similar and dissimilar others. *Neuron*, *50*(4), 655–663. Retrieved from http://www.ncbi.nlm.nih.gov/pubmed/16701214. doi:10.1016/j.neuron.2006.03.040

Mitchell, M. R., Berridge, K. C., & Mahler, S. V. (2018). Endocannabinoid-enhanced "Liking" in nucleus accumbens shell hedonic hotspot requires endogenous opioid signals. *Cannabis and Cannabinoid Research*, *3*(1), 166–170. Retrieved from https://www.ncbi.nlm.nih.gov/pubmed/30069500. doi:10.1089/can.2018.0021

Miyata, J. (2019). Toward integrated understanding of salience in psychosis. *Neurobiology of Disease*. In press. Retrieved from https://www.ncbi.nlm.nih.gov/pubmed/30849509. doi:10.1016/j.nbd.2019.03.002

Mohammed, A., Bayford, R., & Demosthenous, A. (2018). Toward adaptive deep brain stimulation in Parkinson's disease: A review. *Neurodegenerative Disease Management*, *8*(2), 115–136. Retrieved from https://www.ncbi.nlm.nih.gov/pubmed/29693485. doi:10.2217/nmt-2017-0050

Molina, V., Sanz, J., Reig, S., Martinez, R., Sarramea, F., Luque, R., . . . Desco, M. (2005). Hypofrontality in men with first-episode psychosis. *The British Journal of Psychiatry*, *186*, 203–208. Retrieved from http://www.ncbi.nlm.nih.gov/pubmed/15738500. doi:10.1192/bjp.186.3.203

Moll, J., Krueger, F., Zahn, R., Pardini, M., de Oliveira-Souza, R., & Grafman, J. (2006). Human fronto-mesolimbic networks guide decisions about charitable donation. *Proceedings of the National Academy of Sciences of the United States of America*, *103*(42), 15623–15628. Retrieved from https://www.ncbi.nlm.nih.gov/pubmed/17030808

Mondal, A. C., & Fatima, M. (2019). Direct and indirect evidences of BDNF and NGF as key modulators in depression: Role of antidepressants treatment. *International Journal of Neuroscience*, *129*(3), 283–296. Retrieved from https://www.ncbi.nlm.nih.gov/pubmed/30235967. doi:10.1080/00207454.2018.1527328

Montague, P. R., Berns, G. S., Cohen, J. D., McClure, S. M., Pagnoni, G., Dhamala, M., . . . Fisher, R. E. (2002). Hyperscanning: Simultaneous fMRI during linked social interactions.

Neuroimage, 16(4), 1159–1164. Retrieved from https://www.ncbi.nlm.nih.gov/pubmed/12202103

Monti, M. M., Vanhaudenhuyse, A., Coleman, M. R., Boly, M., Pickard, J. D., Tshibanda, L., . . . Laureys, S. (2010). Willful modulation of brain activity in disorders of consciousness. *The New England Journal of Medicine, 362*(7), 579–589. Retrieved from http://www.ncbi.nlm.nih.gov/pubmed/20130250. doi:10.1056/NEJMoa0905370

Montoya, E. R., Terburg, D., Bos, P. A., & van Honk, J. (2012). Testosterone, cortisol, and serotonin as key regulators of social aggression: A review and theoretical perspective. *Motivation and Emotion, 36*(1), 65–73. Retrieved from https://www.ncbi.nlm.nih.gov/pubmed/22448079. doi:10.1007/s11031-011-9264-3

Mooney, R. A., Coxon, J. P., Cirillo, J., Glenny, H., Gant, N., & Byblow, W. D. (2016). Acute aerobic exercise modulates primary motor cortex inhibition. *Experimental Brain Research, 234*(12), 3669–3676. Retrieved from https://www.ncbi.nlm.nih.gov/pubmed/27590480. doi:10.1007/s00221-016-4767-5

Moore, D. S., & Shenk, D. (2017). The heritability fallacy. *Wiley Interdisciplinary Reviews Cognitive Science, 8*(1–2). Retrieved from https://www.ncbi.nlm.nih.gov/pubmed/27906501. doi:10.1002/wcs.1400

Moore, E. M., Migliorini, R., Infante, M. A., & Riley, E. P. (2014). Fetal Alcohol Spectrum Disorders: Recent Neuroimaging Findings. *Current Developmental Disorders Reports, 1*(3), 161–172. Retrieved from https://www.ncbi.nlm.nih.gov/pubmed/25346882. doi:10.1007/s40474-014-0020-8

Moore, K. L., Persaud, T. V. N., & Torchia, M. G. (2016). *The developing human: Clinically oriented embryology* (10th ed.). Philadelphia, PA: Elsevier.

Morales, J., Benavides-Piccione, R., Dar, M., Fernaud, I., Rodriguez, A., Anton-Sanchez, L., . . . Yuste, R. (2014). Random positions of dendritic spines in human cerebral cortex. *The Journal of Neuroscience, 34*(30), 10078–10084. Retrieved from http://www.ncbi.nlm.nih.gov/pubmed/25057209. doi:10.1523/JNEUROSCI.1085-14.2014

Moran, C., Beare, R., Phan, T. G., Bruce, D. G., Callisaya, M. L., Srikanth, V., & Alzheimer's Disease Neuroimaging, I. (2015). Type 2 diabetes mellitus and biomarkers of neurodegeneration. *Neurology, 85*(13), 1123–1130. Retrieved from https://www.ncbi.nlm.nih.gov/pubmed/26333802. doi:10.1212/WNL.0000000000001982

Moret, C., & Briley, M. (2011). The importance of norepinephrine in depression. *Neuropsychiatric Disease and Treatment, 7*(Suppl. 1), 9–13. Retrieved from https://www.ncbi.nlm.nih.gov/pubmed/21750623. doi:10.2147/NDT.S19619

Mork, A., Pehrson, A., Brennum, L. T., Nielsen, S. M., Zhong, H., Lassen, A. B., . . . Stensbol, T. B. (2012). Pharmacological effects of Lu AA21004: A novel multimodal compound for the treatment of major depressive disorder. *The Journal of Pharmacology and Experimental Therapeutics, 340*(3), 666–675. Retrieved from https://www.ncbi.nlm.nih.gov/pubmed/22171087. doi:10.1124/jpet.111.189068

Morley, S. (1983). The stress-diathesis model of illness. *Journal of Psychosomatic Research, 27*(1), 86–87. Retrieved from https://www.ncbi.nlm.nih.gov/pubmed/6834304

Morris, J. S., Öhman, A., & Dolan, R. J. (1998). Conscious and unconscious emotional learning in the human amygdala. *Nature, 393*(6684), 467–470. Retrieved from https://www.ncbi.nlm.nih.gov/pubmed/9624001. doi:10.1038/30976

Morris, R. (1984). Developments of a water-maze procedure for studying spatial learning in the rat. *Journal of Neuroscience Methods, 11*(1), 47–60. Retrieved from https://www.ncbi.nlm.nih.gov/pubmed/6471907

Morrison, S. F. (2016). Central control of body temperature. *F1000Research, 5*. Retrieved from https://www.ncbi.nlm.nih.gov/pubmed/27239289. doi:10.12688/f1000research.7958.1

Morrison, S. F., & Nakamura, K. (2011). Central neural pathways for thermoregulation. *Frontiers in bioscience (Landmark edition), 16*, 74–104. Retrieved from https://www.ncbi.nlm.nih.gov/pubmed/21196160

Mortimer, D., Fothergill, T., Pujic, Z., Richards, L. J., & Goodhill, G. J. (2008). Growth cone chemotaxis. *Trends in Neurosciences, 31*(2), 90–98. Retrieved from https://www.ncbi.nlm.nih.gov/pubmed/18201774. doi:10.1016/j.tins.2007.11.008

Moruzzi, G., & Magoun, H. W. (1949). Brain stem reticular formation and activation of the EEG. *Electroencephalography Clinical Neurophysiology, 1*(4), 455–473. Retrieved from https://www.ncbi.nlm.nih.gov/pubmed/18421835

Moser, E. I., Kropff, E., & Moser, M. B. (2008). Place cells, grid cells, and the brain's spatial representation system. *Annual Review of Neuroscience, 31*, 69–89. Retrieved from https://www.ncbi.nlm.nih.gov/pubmed/18284371. doi:10.1146/annurev.neuro.31.061307.090723

Mostafavi, S., Gaiteri, C., Sullivan, S. E., White, C. C., Tasaki, S., Xu, J., . . . De Jager, P. L. (2018). A molecular network of the aging human brain provides insights into the pathology and cognitive decline of Alzheimer's disease. *Nature Neuroscience, 21*(6), 811–819. Retrieved from https://www.ncbi.nlm.nih.gov/pubmed/29802388. doi:10.1038/s41593-018-0154-9

Motzkin, J. C., Philippi, C. L., Wolf, R. C., Baskaya, M. K., & Koenigs, M. (2015). Ventromedial prefrontal cortex is critical for the regulation of amygdala activity in humans. *Biological Psychiatry, 77*(3), 276–284. Retrieved from https://www.ncbi.nlm.nih.gov/pubmed/24673881. doi:10.1016/j.biopsych.2014.02.014

Mulkey, R. M., & Malenka, R. C. (1992). Mechanisms underlying induction of homosynaptic long-term depression in area CA1 of the hippocampus. *Neuron, 9*(5), 967–975. Retrieved from https://www.ncbi.nlm.nih.gov/pubmed/1419003

Muller, G. E., & Pilzecker, A. (Eds.). (1900). *Experimentelle Beiträge Zur Lehre Vom Gedächtniss* (Vol. 1). Leipzig, Germany: J.A. Barth.

Mumby, D. G., Gaskin, S., Glenn, M. J., Schramek, T. E., & Lehmann, H. (2002). Hippocampal damage and exploratory preferences in rats: Memory for objects, places, and contexts. *Learning & Memory, 9*(2), 49–57. Retrieved from https://www.ncbi.nlm.nih.gov/pubmed/11992015. doi:10.1101/lm.41302

Murillo-Rodriguez, E., Pastrana-Trejo, J. C., Salas-Crisostomo, M., & de-la-Cruz, M. (2017). The endocannabinoid system modulating levels of consciousness, emotions and likely dream contents. *CNS & Neurological Disorders Drug Targets, 16*(4), 370–379. Retrieved from https://www.ncbi.nlm.nih.gov/pubmed/28240187. doi:10.2174/1871527316666170223161908

Murrough, J. W., Iosifescu, D. V., Chang, L. C., Al Jurdi, R. K., Green, C. E., Perez, A. M., . . . Mathew, S. J. (2013). Antidepressant efficacy of ketamine in treatment-resistant major depression: A two-site randomized controlled trial. *The American Journal of Psychiatry, 170*(10), 1134–1142. Retrieved from https://www.ncbi.nlm.nih.gov/pubmed/23982301. doi:10.1176/appi.ajp.2013.13030392

Mushiake, H., Inase, M., & Tanji, J. (1991). Neuronal activity in the primate premotor, supplementary, and precentral motor cortex during visually guided and internally determined sequential movements. *Journal of Neurophysiology, 66*(3), 705–718. Retrieved from https://www.ncbi.nlm.nih.gov/pubmed/1753282

Nadel, L., & Moscovitch, M. (1997). Memory consolidation, retrograde amnesia and the hippocampal complex. *Current Opinion in Neurobiology, 7*(2), 217–227. Retrieved from https://www.ncbi.nlm.nih.gov/pubmed/9142752

Nader, K., Schafe, G. E., & Le Doux, J. E. (2000). Fear memories require protein synthesis in the amygdala for reconsolidation after retrieval. *Nature, 406*(6797), 722–726. Retrieved from https://www.ncbi.nlm.nih.gov/pubmed/10963596. doi:10.1038/35021052

Nakajima, K. (2007). Control of tangential/non-radial migration of neurons in the developing cerebral cortex. *Neurochem Int, 51*(2–4), 121–131. doi:10.1016/j.neuint.2007.05.006

Narayanan, N. S., & Laubach, M. (2006). Top-down control of motor cortex ensembles by dorsomedial prefrontal cortex. *Neuron, 52*(5), 921–931. Retrieved from https://www.ncbi.nlm.nih.gov/pubmed/17145511. doi:10.1016/j.neuron.2006.10.021

Narayanasetti, N., & Thomas, A. (2017). Exercise and neural plasticity: A review study. *Journal of Neurology and Neuroscience, 8*(5), 216. doi:10.21767/2171-6625.1000216

Nas, K., Yazmalar, L., Sah, V., Aydin, A., & Ones, K. (2015). Rehabilitation of spinal cord injuries. *World Journal of Orthopedics, 6*(1), 8–16. Retrieved from https://www.ncbi.nlm.nih.gov/pubmed/25621206. doi:10.5312/wjo.v6.i1.8

National Center on Birth Defects and Developmental Disabilities, Centers for Disease Control and Prevention, U.S. Department of Health and Human Services; National Task Force on Fetal Alcohol Syndrome and Fetal Alcohol Effect. (2004). *Fetal alcohol syndrome: Guidelines for referral and diagnosis*. Retrieved from http://www.cdc.gov/ncbddd/fasd/documents/FAS_guidelines_accessible.pdf

National Spinal Cord Injury Statistical Center. (2018). *Spinal cord injury: Facts and figures at a glance*. Birmingham, AL: National Spinal Cord Injury Statistical Center.

Nederkoorn, C., Houben, K., & Havermans, R. C. (2019). Taste the texture. The relation between subjective tactile sensitivity, mouthfeel and picky eating in young adults. *Appetite, 136*, 58–61. Retrieved from https://www.ncbi.nlm.nih.gov/pubmed/30664910. doi:10.1016/j.appet.2019.01.015

Neitz, J., Geist, T., & Jacobs, G. H. (1989). Color vision in the dog. *Visual Neuroscience, 3*(2), 119–125. Retrieved from https://www.ncbi.nlm.nih.gov/pubmed/2487095

Newman, S. W. (1999). The medial extended amygdala in male reproductive behavior. A node in the mammalian social behavior network. *Annals of the New York Academy of Sciences, 877*, 242–257. Retrieved from https://www.ncbi.nlm.nih.gov/pubmed/10415653

Newton, I. (1671). A letter of Mr. Isaac Newton, Professor of the Mathematicks in the University of Cambridge; containing his new theory about light and colors: Sent by the author to the publisher from Cambridge, Febr. 6. 1671/72; in order to be communicated to the R. Society. *Philosophical Transactions of the Royal Society of London, 6*(80), 3075–3087. doi:10.1098/rstl.1671.0072

Nicholls, M. E. R., Churches, O., & Loetscher, T. (2018). Perception of an ambiguous figure is affected by own-age social biases. *Scientific Reports, 8*(1), 12661. Retrieved from https://doi.org/10.1038/s41598-018-31129-7. doi:10.1038/s41598-018-31129-7

Nicola, S. M., & Malenka, R. C. (1997). Dopamine depresses excitatory and inhibitory synaptic transmission by distinct mechanisms in the nucleus accumbens. *The Journal of Neuroscience, 17*(15), 5697–5710. Retrieved from https://www.ncbi.nlm.nih.gov/pubmed/9221769

Nielsen, J. A., Zielinski, B. A., Ferguson, M. A., Lainhart, J. E., & Anderson, J. S. (2013). An evaluation of the left-brain vs. right-brain hypothesis with resting state functional connectivity magnetic resonance imaging. *PLoS One, 8*(8), e71275. Retrieved from https://www.ncbi.nlm.nih.gov/pubmed/23967180. doi:10.1371/journal.pone.0071275

Niimura, Y., & Nei, M. (2007). Extensive gains and losses of olfactory receptor genes in mammalian evolution. *PLoS One, 2*(8), e708. Retrieved from https://www.ncbi.nlm.nih.gov/pubmed/17684554. doi:10.1371/journal.pone.0000708

Nithianantharajah, J., & Hannan, A. J. (2006). Enriched environments, experience-dependent plasticity and disorders of the nervous system. *Nature Reviews Neuroscience, 7*(9), 697–709. Retrieved from https://www.ncbi.nlm.nih.gov/pubmed/16924259. doi:10.1038/nrn1970

Noctor, S. C., Martinez-Cerdeno, V., Ivic, L., & Kriegstein, A. R. (2004). Cortical neurons arise in symmetric and asymmetric division zones and migrate through specific phases. *Nature Neuroscience, 7*(2), 136–144. Retrieved from https://www.ncbi.nlm.nih.gov/pubmed/14703572. doi:10.1038/nn1172

Norman, A. L., Crocker, N., Mattson, S. N., & Riley, E. P. (2009). Neuroimaging and fetal alcohol spectrum disorders. *Developmental Disabilities Research Reviews, 15*(3), 209–217. Retrieved from https://www.ncbi.nlm.nih.gov/pubmed/19731391. doi:10.1002/ddrr.72

Noroozian, M. (2014). The role of the cerebellum in cognition: Beyond coordination in the central nervous system. *Neurologic Clinics, 32*(4), 1081–1104. Retrieved from https://www.ncbi.nlm.nih.gov/pubmed/25439295. doi:10.1016/j.ncl.2014.07.005

Northoff, G., & Bermpohl, F. (2004). Cortical midline structures and the self. *Trends in Cognitive Sciences, 8*(3), 102–107. Retrieved from http://www.ncbi.nlm.nih.gov/pubmed/15301749. doi:10.1016/j.tics.2004.01.004

Nortje, J., & Menon, D. K. (2004). Traumatic brain injury: Physiology, mechanisms, and outcome. *Current Opinion in Neurology, 17*(6), 711–718. Retrieved from https://www.ncbi.nlm.nih.gov/pubmed/15542980

Nottebohm, F. (1989). From bird song to neurogenesis. *Scientific American, 260*(2), 74–79. Retrieved from https://www.ncbi.nlm.nih.gov/pubmed/2643827

Nottebohm, F. (2005). The neural basis of birdsong. *PLoS Biology, 3*(5), e164. Retrieved from https://www.ncbi.nlm.nih.gov/pubmed/15884976. doi:10.1371/journal.pbio.0030164

Nottebohm, F., Stokes, T. M., & Leonard, C. M. (1976). Central control of song in the canary, Serinus canarius. *The Journal of Comparative Neurology, 165*(4), 457–486. Retrieved from https://www.ncbi.nlm.nih.gov/pubmed/1262540. doi:10.1002/cne.901650405

Nummenmaa, L., Glerean, E., Hari, R., & Hietanen, J. K. (2014). Bodily maps of emotions. *Proceedings of the National Academy of Sciences of the United States of America, 111*(2), 646–651. Retrieved from https://www.ncbi.nlm.nih.gov/pubmed/24379370. doi:10.1073/pnas.1321664111

Nyberg, L., McIntosh, A. R., & Tulving, E. (1998). Functional brain imaging of episodic and semantic memory with positron emission tomography. *Journal of Molecular Medicine (Berlin, Germany), 76*(1), 48–53. Retrieved from https://www.ncbi.nlm.nih.gov/pubmed/9462867

Ochsner, K. N., & Lieberman, M. D. (2001). The emergence of social cognitive neuroscience. *The American Psychologist, 56*(9), 717–734. Retrieved from https://www.ncbi.nlm.nih.gov/pubmed/11558357

O'Donnell, T., Hegadoren, K. M., & Coupland, N. C. (2004). Noradrenergic mechanisms in the pathophysiology of post-traumatic stress disorder. *Neuropsychobiology, 50*(4), 273–283. Retrieved from https://www.ncbi.nlm.nih.gov/pubmed/15539856. doi:10.1159/000080952

Oh, K. Y., Van Dam, N. T., Doucette, J. T., & Murrough, J. W. (2019). Effects of chronic physical disease and systemic inflammation on suicide risk in patients with depression: A hospital-based case-control study. *Psychological Medicine*, 1–9. Retrieved from https://www.ncbi.nlm.nih.gov/pubmed/30606276. doi:10.1017/S0033291718003902

Ohloff, G. (1994). *Scent and fragrances: The fascination of odors and their chemical perspectives*. Berlin/New York: Springer-Verlag.

Öhman, A. (2005). Psychology. Conditioned fear of a face: A prelude to ethnic enmity? *Science, 309*(5735), 711–713. Retrieved from https://www.ncbi.nlm.nih.gov/pubmed/16051776. doi:10.1126/science.1116710

Ohsu, T., Amino, Y., Nagasaki, H., Yamanaka, T., Takeshita, S., Hatanaka, T., . . . Eto, Y. (2010). Involvement of the calcium-sensing receptor in human taste perception. *The Journal of Biological Chemistry, 285*(2), 1016–1022. Retrieved from https://www.ncbi.nlm.nih.gov/pubmed/19892707. doi:10.1074/jbc.M109.029165

Okabe, S., Yoshida, M., Takayanagi, Y., & Onaka, T. (2015). Activation of hypothalamic oxytocin neurons following tactile stimuli in rats. *Neuroscience Letters, 600*, 22–27. Retrieved from https://www.ncbi.nlm.nih.gov/pubmed/26033183. doi:10.1016/j.neulet.2015.05.055

Okada, N., Yahata, N., Koshiyama, D., Morita, K., Sawada, K., Kanata, S., ... Kasai, K. (2019). Neurometabolic and functional connectivity basis of prosocial behavior in early adolescence. *Scientific Reports, 9*(1), 732. Retrieved from https://www.ncbi.nlm.nih.gov/pubmed/30679738. doi:10.1038/s41598-018-38355-z

Okasha, A., & Okasha, T. (2014). A plea to change the misnomer ECT. *World Psychiatry, 13*(3), 327. Retrieved from https://www.ncbi.nlm.nih.gov/pubmed/25273312. doi:10.1002/wps.20143

O'Keefe, J., Burgess, N., Donnett, J. G., Jeffery, K. J., & Maguire, E. A. (1998). Place cells, navigational accuracy, and the human hippocampus. *Philosophical Transactions of the Royal Society of London. Series B, Biological Sciences, 353*(1373), 1333–1340. Retrieved from https://www.ncbi.nlm.nih.gov/pubmed/9770226. doi:10.1098/rstb.1998.0287

O'Keefe, J., & Nadel, L. (1978). *The hippocampus as a cognitive map*. Oxford/New York: Clarendon Press;Oxford University Press.

Okun, M. S. (2012). Deep-brain stimulation for Parkinson's disease. *The New England Journal of Medicine, 367*(16), 1529–1538. Retrieved from https://www.ncbi.nlm.nih.gov/pubmed/23075179. doi:10.1056/NEJMct1208070

Olds, J., & Milner, P. (1954). Positive reinforcement produced by electrical stimulation of septal area and other regions of rat brain. *Journal of Comparative and Physiological Psychology, 47*(6), 419–427. Retrieved from https://www.ncbi.nlm.nih.gov/pubmed/13233369

Olivares-Banuelos, T. N., Chi-Castaneda, D., & Ortega, A. (2019). Glutamate transporters: Gene expression regulation and signaling properties. *Neuropharmacology*. In press. Retrieved from https://www.ncbi.nlm.nih.gov/pubmed/30822498. doi:10.1016/j.neuropharm.2019.02.032

Olkowicz, S., Kocourek, M., Lucan, R. K., Portes, M., Fitch, W. T., Herculano-Houzel, S., & Nemec, P. (2016). Birds have primate-like numbers of neurons in the forebrain. *Proc Natl Acad Sci U S A, 113*(26), 7255–7260. doi:10.1073/pnas.1517131113

Olton, D. S., & Papas, B. C. (1979). Spatial memory and hippocampal function. *Neuropsychologia, 17*(6), 669–682. Retrieved from https://www.ncbi.nlm.nih.gov/pubmed/522981

Olton, D. S., & Samuelson, R. J. (1976). Remembrance of places passed: Spatial memory in rats. *Journal of Experimental Psychology: Animal Behavior Processes, 2*(2), 97–116. http://dx.doi.org/10.1037/0097-7403.2.2.97

Ophir, E., Nass, C., & Wagner, A. D. (2009). Cognitive control in media multitaskers. *Proceedings of the National Academy of Sciences of the United States of America, 106*(37), 15583–15587. Retrieved from https://www.ncbi.nlm.nih.gov/pubmed/19706386. doi:10.1073/pnas.0903620106

O'Rourke, N. A., Sullivan, D. P., Kaznowski, C. E., Jacobs, A. A., & McConnell, S. K. (1995). Tangential migration of neurons in the developing cerebral cortex. *Development, 121*(7), 2165–2176. Retrieved from https://www.ncbi.nlm.nih.gov/pubmed/7635060

Ott, T., & Nieder, A. (2019). Dopamine and cognitive control in prefrontal cortex. *Trends in Cognitive Sciences, 23*(3), 213–234. Retrieved from https://www.ncbi.nlm.nih.gov/pubmed/30711326. doi:10.1016/j.tics.2018.12.006

Otto, T., & Eichenbaum, H. (1992). Complementary roles of the orbital prefrontal cortex and the perirhinal-entorhinal cortices in an odor-guided delayed-nonmatching-to-sample task. *Behavioral Neuroscience, 106*(5), 762–775. Retrieved from https://www.ncbi.nlm.nih.gov/pubmed/1445656

Ozawa, T., Yamada, K., & Ichitani, Y. (2017). Differential requirements of hippocampal de novo protein and mRNA synthesis in two long-term spatial memory tests: Spontaneous place recognition and delay-interposed radial maze performance in rats. *PLoS One, 12*(2), e0171629. Retrieved from https://www.ncbi.nlm.nih.gov/pubmed/28178292. doi:10.1371/journal.pone.0171629

Pacher, P., Batkai, S., & Kunos, G. (2006). The endocannabinoid system as an emerging target of pharmacotherapy. *Pharmacological Reviews, 58*(3), 389–462. Retrieved from https://www.ncbi.nlm.nih.gov/pubmed/16968947. doi:10.1124/pr.58.3.2

Pan, X., Kaminga, A. C., Wen, S. W., & Liu, A. (2018). Catecholamines in post-traumatic stress disorder: A systematic review and meta-analysis. *Frontiers in Molecular Neuroscience, 11*, 450. Retrieved from https://www.ncbi.nlm.nih.gov/pubmed/30564100. doi:10.3389/fnmol.2018.00450

Papez, J. W. (1995). A proposed mechanism of emotion. 1937. *The Journal of Neuropsychiatry and Clinical Neurosciences, 7*(1), 103–112. Retrieved from https://www.ncbi.nlm.nih.gov/pubmed/7711480. doi:10.1176/jnp.7.1.103

Parekh, R., & Ascoli, G. A. (2013). Neuronal morphology goes digital: A research hub for cellular and system neuroscience. *Neuron, 77*(6), 1017–1038. Retrieved from http://www.ncbi.nlm.nih.gov/pubmed/23522039. doi:10.1016/j.neuron.2013.03.008

Park, C., Rosenblat, J. D., Lee, Y., Pan, Z., Cao, B., Iacobucci, M., & McIntyre, R. S. (2019). The neural systems of emotion regulation and abnormalities in major depressive disorder. *Behavioural Brain Research, 367*, 181–188. Retrieved from https://www.ncbi.nlm.nih.gov/pubmed/30951753. doi:10.1016/j.bbr.2019.04.002

Pascual-Leone, A., & Torres, F. (1993). Plasticity of the sensorimotor cortex representation of the reading finger in Braille readers. *Brain, 116*(Pt. 1), 39–52. Retrieved from https://www.ncbi.nlm.nih.gov/pubmed/8453464

Pathan, H., & Williams, J. (2012). Basic opioid pharmacology: An update. *British Journal of Pain, 6*(1), 11–16. Retrieved from https://www.ncbi.nlm.nih.gov/pubmed/26516461. doi:10.1177/2049463712438493

Patil, I., Melsbach, J., Hennig-Fast, K., & Silani, G. (2016). Divergent roles of autistic and alexithymic traits in utilitarian moral judgments in adults with autism. *Scientific Reports, 6*, 23637. Retrieved from https://www.ncbi.nlm.nih.gov/pubmed/27020307. doi:10.1038/srep23637

Pauls, D. L., Abramovitch, A., Rauch, S. L., & Geller, D. A. (2014). Obsessive-compulsive disorder: An integrative genetic and neurobiological perspective. *Nature Reviews Neuroscience, 15*(6), 410–424. Retrieved from https://www.ncbi.nlm.nih.gov/pubmed/24840803. doi:10.1038/nrn3746

Pavlov, I. P., & Anrep, G. V. (1927). *Conditioned reflexes: An investigation of the physiological activity of the cerebral cortex*. London: Oxford University Press.

Pear, T. H. (1948). Professor Bartlett on skill. *Occupational Psychology, 22*(2), 92. Retrieved from https://www.ncbi.nlm.nih.gov/pubmed/18915340

Pearce, A. J., Thickbroom, G. W., Byrnes, M. L., & Mastaglia, F. L. (2000). Functional reorganisation of the corticomotor projection to the hand in skilled racquet players. *Experimental Brain Research, 130*(2), 238–243. Retrieved from https://www.ncbi.nlm.nih.gov/pubmed/10672477

Pearce, J. M. (2009). Marie-Jean-Pierre Flourens (1794-1867) and cortical localization. *European Neurology, 61*(5), 311–314. Retrieved from https://www.ncbi.nlm.nih.gov/pubmed/19295220. doi:10.1159/000206858

Penfield, W., & Rasmussen, T. (1968). *The cerebral cortex of man: A clinical study of localization of function*. New York: Hafner Publishing Company.

Pennisi, E. (2012). Genomics. ENCODE project writes eulogy for junk DNA. *Science, 337*(6099), 1159, 1161. Retrieved from https://www.ncbi.nlm.nih.gov/pubmed/22955811. doi:10.1126/science.337.6099.1159

Perani, D., Garibotto, V., Gorini, A., Moresco, R. M., Henin, M., Panzacchi, A., . . . Fazio, F. (2008). In vivo PET study of 5HT(2A) serotonin and D(2) dopamine dysfunction in drug-naive obsessive-compulsive disorder. *Neuroimage, 42*(1), 306–314. Retrieved from http://www.ncbi.nlm.nih.gov/pubmed/18511303. doi:10.1016/j.neuroimage.2008.04.233

Perner, J., Leekam, S. R., & Wimmer, H. (1987). Three-year-olds' difficulty with false belief: The case for a conceptual deficit. *British Journal of Developmental Psychology, 5*(2), 125–137. Retrieved from https://onlinelibrary.wiley.com/doi/abs/10.1111/j.2044-835X.1987.tb01048.x. doi:10.1111/j.2044-835X.1987.tb01048.x

Perry, A., Saunders, S. N., Stiso, J., Dewar, C., Lubell, J., Meling, T. R., . . . Knight, R. T. (2017). Effects of prefrontal cortex damage on emotion understanding: EEG and behavioural evidence. *Brain, 140*(4), 1086–1099. Retrieved from https://www.ncbi.nlm.nih.gov/pubmed/28334943. doi:10.1093/brain/awx031

Perry, P. J., Lund, B. C., Deninger, M. J., Kutscher, E. C., & Schneider, J. (2005). Anabolic steroid use in weightlifters and bodybuilders: An internet survey of drug utilization. *Clinical Journal of Sport Medicine, 15*(5), 326–330. Retrieved from https://www.ncbi.nlm.nih.gov/pubmed/16162991

Pertea, M., Shumate, A., Pertea, G., Varabyou, A., Breitwieser, F. P., Chang, Y. C., . . . Salzberg, S. L. (2018). CHESS: A new human gene catalog curated from thousands of large-scale RNA sequencing experiments reveals extensive transcriptional noise. *Genome Biology, 19*(1), 208. Retrieved from https://www.ncbi.nlm.nih.gov/pubmed/30486838. doi:10.1186/s13059-018-1590-2

Petersen, S. E., Robinson, D. L., & Keys, W. (1985). Pulvinar nuclei of the behaving rhesus monkey: Visual responses and their modulation. *Journal of Neurophysiology, 54*(4), 867–886. Retrieved from https://www.ncbi.nlm.nih.gov/pubmed/4067625. doi:10.1152/jn.1985.54.4.867

Petrulis, A., Alvarez, P., & Eichenbaum, H. (2005). Neural correlates of social odor recognition and the representation of individual distinctive social odors within entorhinal cortex and ventral subiculum. *Neuroscience, 130*(1), 259–274. Retrieved from https://www.ncbi.nlm.nih.gov/pubmed/15561442. doi:10.1016/j.neuroscience.2004.09.001

Pfaff, D. W. (2009). *Hormones, brain, and behavior* (2nd ed.). Amsterdam/Boston: Elsevier/Academic Press.

Phan, K. L., Fitzgerald, D. A., Nathan, P. J., & Tancer, M. E. (2006). Association between amygdala hyperactivity to harsh faces and severity of social anxiety in generalized social phobia. *Biological Psychiatry, 59*(5), 424–429. Retrieved from https://www.ncbi.nlm.nih.gov/pubmed/16256956. doi:10.1016/j.biopsych.2005.08.012

Phillips, K. T., Phillips, M. M., Lalonde, T. L., & Tormohlen, K. N. (2015). Marijuana use, craving, and academic motivation and performance among college students: An in-the-moment study. *Addictive Behaviors, 47*, 42–47. Retrieved from https://www.ncbi.nlm.nih.gov/pubmed/25864134. doi:10.1016/j.addbeh.2015.03.020

Phoenix, C. H. (2009). Organizing action of prenatally administered testosterone propionate on the tissues mediating mating behavior in the female guinea pig. *Hormones and Behavior, 55*(5), 566. Retrieved from https://www.ncbi.nlm.nih.gov/pubmed/19302826. doi:10.1016/j.yhbeh.2009.01.004

Phoenix, C. H., Goy, R. W., Gerall, A. A., & Young, W. C. (1959). Organizing action of prenatally administered testosterone propionate on the tissues mediating mating behavior in the female guinea pig. *Endocrinology, 65*, 369–382. Retrieved from https://www.ncbi.nlm.nih.gov/pubmed/14432658. doi:10.1210/endo-65-3-369

Pickles, J. O. (2015). Auditory pathways: Anatomy and physiology. *Handbook of Clinical Neurology, 129*, 3–25. Retrieved from https://www.ncbi.nlm.nih.gov/pubmed/25726260. doi:10.1016/B978-0-444-62630-1.00001-9

Pieper, J., Chang, D. G., Mahasin, S. Z., Swan, A. R., Quinto, A. A., Nichols, S. L., . . . Huang, M. (2019). Brain amygdala volume increases in veterans and active-duty military personnel with combat-related posttraumatic stress disorder and mild traumatic brain injury. *The Journal of Head Trauma Rehabilitation*. Retrieved from https://www.ncbi.nlm.nih.gov/pubmed/31033749. doi:10.1097/HTR.0000000000000492

Piliavin, I. M., & Rodin, J. (1969). Good samaritanism: An underground phenomenon? *Journal of Personality and Social Psychology, 13*(4), 289–299. Retrieved from http://www.ncbi.nlm.nih.gov/pubmed/5359227

Pinsker, H., Kupfermann, I., Castellucci, V., & Kandel, E. (1970). Habituation and dishabituation of the gill-withdrawal reflex in Aplysia. *Science, 167*(3926), 1740–1742. Retrieved from https://www.ncbi.nlm.nih.gov/pubmed/5416541

Pitzalis, S., Fattori, P., & Galletti, C. (2015). The human cortical areas V6 and V6A. *Visual Neuroscience, 32*, E007. Retrieved from https://www.ncbi.nlm.nih.gov/pubmed/26241369. doi:10.1017/S0952523815000048

Platkiewicz, J., & Brette, R. (2010). A threshold equation for action potential initiation. *PLoS Computational Biology, 6*(7), e1000850. Retrieved from https://www.ncbi.nlm.nih.gov/pubmed/20628619. doi:10.1371/journal.pcbi.1000850

Pliquett, R. U., Fuhrer, D., Falk, S., Zysset, S., von Cramon, D. Y., & Stumvoll, M. (2006). The effects of insulin on the central nervous system—focus on appetite regulation. *Hormone and Metabolic Research, 38*(7), 442–446. Retrieved from https://www.ncbi.nlm.nih.gov/pubmed/16933179. doi:10.1055/s-2006-947840

Plog, B. A., & Nedergaard, M. (2018). The glymphatic system in central nervous system health and sisease: Past, present, and future. *Annual Review of Pathology, 13*, 379–394. Retrieved from https://www.ncbi.nlm.nih.gov/pubmed/29195051. doi:10.1146/annurev-pathol-051217-111018

Plotnik, J. M., de Waal, F. B., & Reiss, D. (2006). Self-recognition in an Asian elephant. *Proceedings of the National Academy of Sciences of the United States of America, 103*(45), 17053–17057. Retrieved from http://www.ncbi.nlm.nih.gov/pubmed/17075063. doi:10.1073/pnas.0608062103

Pogarell, O., Koch, W., Karch, S., Dehning, S., Muller, N., Tatsch, K., . . . Moller, H. J. (2012). Dopaminergic neurotransmission in patients with schizophrenia in relation to positive and negative symptoms. *Pharmacopsychiatry*, 45(Suppl. 1), S36–S41. Retrieved from https://www.ncbi.nlm.nih.gov/pubmed/22565233. doi:10.1055/s-0032-1306313

Poremba, A., Saunders, R. C., Crane, A. M., Cook, M., Sokoloff, L., & Mishkin, M. (2003). Functional mapping of the primate auditory system. *Science, 299*(5606), 568–572. Retrieved from https://www.ncbi.nlm.nih.gov/pubmed/12543977. doi:10.1126/science.1078900

Portin, P., & Wilkins, A. (2017). The evolving definition of the term "gene." *Genetics, 205*(4), 1353–1364. Retrieved from https://www.ncbi.nlm.nih.gov/pubmed/28360126. doi:10.1534/genetics.116.196956

Preston, S. D., & de Waal, F. B. (2002). Empathy: Its ultimate and proximate bases. *The Behavioral and Brain Sciences, 25*(1), 1–20; discussion 20-71. Retrieved from http://www.ncbi.nlm.nih.gov/pubmed/12625087

Price, D. J. (2011). *Building brains: An introduction to neural development*. Chichester, West Sussex, UK/Hoboken, NJ: Wiley-Blackwell.

Prospero-Garcia, O., Amancio-Belmont, O., Becerril Melendez, A. L., Ruiz-Contreras, A. E., & Mendez-Diaz, M. (2016). Endocannabinoids and sleep. *Neuroscience & Biobehavioral Reviews, 71*, 671–679. Retrieved from https://www.ncbi.nlm.nih.gov/pubmed/27756691. doi:10.1016/j.neubiorev.2016.10.005

Putnam, S. K., Du, J., Sato, S., & Hull, E. M. (2001). Testosterone restoration of copulatory behavior correlates with medial preoptic dopamine release in castrated male rats. *Hormones and Behavior, 39*(3), 216–224. Retrieved from https://www.ncbi.nlm.nih.gov/pubmed/11300712. doi:10.1006/hbeh.2001.1648

Qu, L., Akbergenova, Y., Hu, Y., & Schikorski, T. (2009). Synapse-to-synapse variation in mean synaptic vesicle size and its relationship with synaptic morphology and function. *The Journal of Comparative Neurology, 514*(4), 343–352. Retrieved from https://www.ncbi.nlm.nih.gov/pubmed/19330815. doi:10.1002/cne.22007

Quinn, D. M. (2018). Resurrection biology: Aged acetylcholinesterase brought back to life. *Journal of Medicinal Chemistry, 61*(16), 7032–7033. Retrieved from https://www.ncbi.nlm.nih.gov/pubmed/30110162. doi:10.1021/acs.jmedchem.8b01122

Raam, T., McAvoy, K. M., Besnard, A., Veenema, A. H., & Sahay, A. (2017). Hippocampal oxytocin receptors are necessary for discrimination of social stimuli. *Nature Communications, 8*(1), 2001. Retrieved from https://www.ncbi.nlm.nih.gov/pubmed/29222469. doi:10.1038/s41467-017-02173-0

Raichle, M. E. (2015). The brain's default mode network. *Annual Review of Neuroscience, 38*, 433–447. Retrieved from https://www.ncbi.nlm.nih.gov/pubmed/25938726. doi:10.1146/annurev-neuro-071013-014030

Rainville, P., Duncan, G. H., Price, D. D., Carrier, B., & Bushnell, M. C. (1997). Pain affect encoded in human anterior cingulate but not somatosensory cortex. *Science, 277*(5328), 968–971. Retrieved from http://www.ncbi.nlm.nih.gov/pubmed/9252330

Rajagopal, L., Huang, M., Michael, E., Kwon, S., & Meltzer, H. Y. (2018). TPA-023 attenuates subchronic phencyclidine-induced declarative and reversal learning deficits via GABAA receptor agonist mechanism: Possible therapeutic target for cognitive deficit in schizophrenia. *Neuropsychopharmacology, 43*(12), 2468–2477. Retrieved from https://www.ncbi.nlm.nih.gov/pubmed/30093697. doi:10.1038/s41386-018-0160-3

Rajmohan, V., & Mohandas, E. (2007). The limbic system. *Indian Journal of Psychiatry, 49*(2), 132–139. Retrieved from https://www.ncbi.nlm.nih.gov/pubmed/20711399. doi:10.4103/0019-5545.33264

Rakic, P. (1972). Mode of cell migration to the superficial layers of fetal monkey neocortex. *The Journal of Comparative Neurology, 145*(1), 61–83. Retrieved from http://www.ncbi.nlm.nih.gov/pubmed/4624784. doi:10.1002/cne.901450105

Ramachandran, V. S. (1993). Behavioral and magnetoencephalographic correlates of plasticity in the adult human brain. *Proceedings of the National Academy of Sciences of the United States of America, 90*(22), 10413–10420. Retrieved from https://www.ncbi.nlm.nih.gov/pubmed/8248123

Ramachandran, V. S., & Hirstein, W. (1998). The perception of phantom limbs. The D. O. Hebb lecture. *Brain, 121*(Pt. 9), 1603–1630. Retrieved from https://www.ncbi.nlm.nih.gov/pubmed/9762952

Ramachandran, V. S., & Oberman, L. M. (2006). Broken mirrors: A theory of autism. *Scientific American, 295*(5), 62–69. Retrieved from https://www.ncbi.nlm.nih.gov/pubmed/17076085

Ramanujam, A., Momeni, K., Husain, S. R., Augustine, J., Garbarini, E., Barrance, P., . . . Forrest, G. F. (2018). Mechanisms for improving walking speed after longitudinal powered robotic exoskeleton training for individuals with spinal cord injury. *Conference Proceedings: . . . Annual International Conference of the IEEE Engineering in Medicine and Biology Society, 2018*, 2805–2808. Retrieved from https://www.ncbi.nlm.nih.gov/pubmed/30440984. doi:10.1109/EMBC.2018.8512821

Ramón y Cajal, S. (1995). *Histology of the nervous system of man and vertebrates*. New York: Oxford University Press.

Ramón y Cajal, S., DeFelipe, J., & Jones, E. G. (1991). *Cajal's degeneration and regeneration of the nervous system*. New York: Oxford University Press.

Ranasinghe, N., Cheok, A., Nakatsu, R. (2012, October 22–26). *Taste/IP: The sensation of taste for digital communication*. Paper presented at the Proceedings of the 14th ACM international conference on Multimodal interaction, Santa Monica, California, USA.

Ranasinghe, N., Cheok, A. D., Fernando, O. N. N., Nii, H., & Gopalakrishnakone P. (2011). Electronic stimulation of taste sensations. In D. V. Keyson, M. L. Maher, N. Streitz, A. Cheok, J. Carlos Augusto, et al. (Eds.), *Ambient Intelligence. AmI 2011. Lecture notes in Computer Science* (Vol. 7040). Berlin, Heidelberg: Springer.

Rao, V. R., Sellers, K. K., Wallace, D. L., Lee, M. B., Bijanzadeh, M., Sani, O. G., . . . Chang, E. F. (2018). Direct electrical stimulation of lateral orbitofrontal cortex acutely improves mood in individuals with symptoms of depression. *Current Bioliogy, 28*(24), 3893–390.e3894. Retrieved from https://www.ncbi.nlm.nih.gov/pubmed/30503621. doi:10.1016/j.cub.2018.10.026

Rapoport, M., van Reekum, R., & Mayberg, H. (2000). The role of the cerebellum in cognition and behavior: A selective review. *The Journal of Neuropsychiatry and Clinical Neurosciences, 12*(2), 193–198. Retrieved from https://www.ncbi.nlm.nih.gov/pubmed/11001597. doi:10.1176/jnp.12.2.193

Rasmussen, J. J., Schou, M., Madsen, P. L., Selmer, C., Johansen, M. L., Ulriksen, P. S., . . . Kistorp, C. (2018). Cardiac systolic dysfunction in past illicit users of anabolic androgenic steroids. *American Heart Journal, 203*, 49–56. Retrieved from https://www.ncbi.nlm.nih.gov/pubmed/30015068. doi:10.1016/j.ahj.2018.06.010

Rasmussen, T., & Milner, B. (1977). The role of early left-brain injury in determining lateralization of cerebral speech functions. *Annals of the New York Academy of Sciences, 299*, 355–369. Retrieved from https://www.ncbi.nlm.nih.gov/pubmed/101116

Ratliff, F., Knight, B. W., Jr., Dodge, F. A., Jr., & Hartline, H. K. (1974). Fourier analysis of dynamics of excitation and inhibition in the eye of Limulus: Amplitude, phase and distance. *Vision Research, 14*(11), 1155–1168. Retrieved from https://www.ncbi.nlm.nih.gov/pubmed/4428622

Rauch, S. L., Whalen, P. J., Shin, L. M., McInerney, S. C., Macklin, M. L., Lasko, N. B., . . . Pitman, R. K. (2000). Exaggerated amygdala response to masked facial stimuli in posttraumatic stress disorder: A functional MRI study. *Biological Psychiatry, 47*(9), 769–776. Retrieved from https://www.ncbi.nlm.nih.gov/pubmed/10812035

Rauschecker, J. P., & Scott, S. K. (2009). Maps and streams in the auditory cortex: Nonhuman primates illuminate human speech processing. *Nature Neuroscience, 12*(6), 718–724. Retrieved from https://www.ncbi.nlm.nih.gov/pubmed/19471271. doi:10.1038/nn.2331

Ravichandran, K. S. (2010). Find-me and eat-me signals in apoptotic cell clearance: Progress and conundrums. *The Journal of Experimental Medicine, 207*(9), 1807–1817. Retrieved from http://www.ncbi.nlm.nih.gov/pubmed/20805564. doi:10.1084/jem.20101157

Recabal, A., Caprile, T., & Garcia-Robles, M. L. A. (2017). Hypothalamic neurogenesis as an adaptive metabolic mechanism. *Frontiers in Neuroscience, 11*, 190. Retrieved from https://www.ncbi.nlm.nih.gov/pubmed/28424582. doi:10.3389/fnins.2017.00190

Rechtschaffen, A., & Kales, A. (1968). *A manual of standardized terminology, techniques and scoring system for sleep stages of human subjects*. Bethesda, MD: U. S. National Institute of Neurological Diseases and Blindness, Neurological Information Network.

Regehr, W. G. (2012). Short-term presynaptic plasticity. *Cold Spring Harbor Perspectives in Biology, 4*(7), a005702. Retrieved from https://www.ncbi.nlm.nih.gov/pubmed/22751149. doi:10.1101/cshperspect.a005702

Reiss, D., & Marino, L. (2001). Mirror self-recognition in the bottlenose dolphin: A case of cognitive convergence. *Proceedings of the National Academy of Sciences of the United States of America, 98*(10), 5937–5942. Retrieved from http://www.ncbi.nlm.nih.gov/pubmed/11331768. doi:10.1073/pnas.101086398

Rempel-Clower, N. L., Zola, S. M., Squire, L. R., & Amaral, D. G. (1996). Three cases of enduring memory impairment after bilateral damage limited to the hippocampal formation. *The Journal of Neuroscience, 16*(16), 5233–5255. Retrieved from https://www.ncbi.nlm.nih.gov/pubmed/8756452

Rensink, R. A. (2014). Limits to the usability of iconic memory. *Frontiers in Psychology, 5*, 971. Retrieved from https://www.ncbi.nlm.nih.gov/pubmed/25221539. doi:10.3389/fpsyg.2014.00971

Revonsuo, A. (1999). Binding and the phenomenal unity of consciousness. *Consciousness and Cognition, 8*(2), 173–185. Retrieved from http://www.ncbi.nlm.nih.gov/pubmed/10448000. doi:10.1006/ccog.1999.0384

Ricci, L. A., Morrison, T. R., & Melloni, R. H., Jr. (2013). Adolescent anabolic/androgenic steroids: Aggression and anxiety during exposure predict behavioral responding during withdrawal in Syrian hamsters (Mesocricetus auratus). *Hormones and Behavior, 64*(5), 770–780. Retrieved from https://www.ncbi.nlm.nih.gov/pubmed/24126136. doi:10.1016/j.yhbeh.2013.10.002

Ricciarelli, R., & Fedele, E. (2017). The amyloid cascade hypothesis in Alzheimer's disease: It's time to change our mind. *Current Neuropharmacology, 15*(6), 926–935. Retrieved from https://www.ncbi.nlm.nih.gov/pubmed/28093977. doi:10.2174/1570159X15666170116143743

Richeson, J. A., Baird, A. A., Gordon, H. L., Heatherton, T. F., Wyland, C. L., Trawalter, S., & Shelton, J. N. (2003). An fMRI investigation of the impact of interracial contact on executive function. *Nature Neuroscience, 6*(12), 1323–1328. Retrieved from https://www.ncbi.nlm.nih.gov/pubmed/14625557. doi:10.1038/nn1156

Rickels, K., & Moeller, H. J. (2018). Benzodiazepines in anxiety disorders: Reassessment of usefulness and safety. *The World Journal of Biological Psychiatry*, 1–5. Retrieved from https://www.ncbi.nlm.nih.gov/pubmed/30252578. doi:10.1080/15622975.2018.1500031

Riedel, B. C., Thompson, P. M., & Brinton, R. D. (2016). Age, APOE and sex: Triad of risk of Alzheimer's disease. *The Journal of Steroid Biochemistry and Molecular Biology, 160*, 134–147. Retrieved from https://www.ncbi.nlm.nih.gov/pubmed/26969397. doi:10.1016/j.jsbmb.2016.03.012

Riffell, J. A., & Rowe, A. H. (2016). Neuroecology: Neural Mechanisms of Sensory and Motor Processes that Mediate Ecologically Relevant Behaviors: An Introduction to the Symposium. *Integrative and Comparative Biology, 56*(5), 853–855. Retrieved from https://www.ncbi.nlm.nih.gov/pubmed/27880677. doi:10.1093/icb/icw109

Rilling, J., Gutman, D., Zeh, T., Pagnoni, G., Berns, G., & Kilts, C. (2002). A neural basis for social cooperation. *Neuron, 35*(2), 395–405. Retrieved from https://www.ncbi.nlm.nih.gov/pubmed/12160756

Rizzolatti, G., & Craighero, L. (2004). The mirror-neuron system. *Annual Review of Neuroscience, 27*, 169–192. Retrieved from https://www.ncbi.nlm.nih.gov/pubmed/15217330. doi:10.1146/annurev.neuro.27.070203.144230

Rizzolatti, G., Fadiga, L., Fogassi, L., & Gallese, V. (1999). Resonance behaviors and mirror neurons. *Archives Italiennes de Biologie, 137*(2–3), 85–100. Retrieved from http://www.ncbi.nlm.nih.gov/pubmed/10349488

Rizzolatti, G., Fadiga, L., Gallese, V., & Fogassi, L. (1996). Premotor cortex and the recognition of motor actions. *Brain Research Cognitive Brain Research, 3*(2), 131–141. Retrieved from https://www.ncbi.nlm.nih.gov/pubmed/8713554

Robertson, S. A., Leinninger, G. M., & Myers, M. G., Jr. (2008). Molecular and neural mediators of leptin action. *Physiology & Behavior, 94*(5), 637–642. Retrieved from https://www.ncbi.nlm.nih.gov/pubmed/18501391. doi:10.1016/j.physbeh.2008.04.005

Robinson, T. E., & Berridge, K. C. (1993). The neural basis of drug craving: An incentive-sensitization theory of addiction. *Brain Research Brain Research Reviews, 18*(3), 247–291. Retrieved from https://www.ncbi.nlm.nih.gov/pubmed/8401595

Robinson, T. E., & Berridge, K. C. (2008). Review. The incentive sensitization theory of addiction: Some current issues. *Philosophical transactions of the Royal Society of London. Series B, Biological sciences, 363*(1507), 3137–3146. Retrieved from https://www.ncbi.nlm.nih.gov/pubmed/18640920. doi:10.1098/rstb.2008.0093

Robson, D. (2015). The reason why "everyday heroes" emerge in atrocities. BBC, November 17. Retrieved from http://www.bbc.com/future/story/20151117-the-reason-why-everyday-heroes-emerge-in-atrocities

Rocca, J. (2003). Galen on the brain: Anatomical knowledge and physiological speculation in the second century AD. *Studies in Ancient Medicine, 26*, 1–313. Retrieved from https://www.ncbi.nlm.nih.gov/pubmed/12848196

Rockland, K. S. (2002). Non-uniformity of extrinsic connections and columnar organization. *Journal of Neurocytology, 31*(3–5), 247–253. Retrieved from https://www.ncbi.nlm.nih.gov/pubmed/12815244

Roddy, D. W., Farrell, C., Doolin, K., Roman, E., Tozzi, L., Frodl, T., . . . O'Hanlon, E. (2019). The hippocampus in depression: More than the sum of its parts? Advanced hippocampal substructure segmentation in depression. *Biological Psychiatry, 85*(6), 487–497. Retrieved from https://www.ncbi.nlm.nih.gov/pubmed/30528746. doi:10.1016/j.biopsych.2018.08.021

Rolls, E. T., Cheng, W., Gong, W., Qiu, J., Zhou, C., Zhang, J., . . . Feng, J. (2018). Functional connectivity of the anterior cingulate cortex in depression and in health. *Cerebral Cortex*. In press. Retrieved from https://www.ncbi.nlm.nih.gov/pubmed/30418547. doi:10.1093/cercor/bhy236

Romans, S., Clarkson, R., Einstein, G., Petrovic, M., & Stewart, D. (2012). Mood and the menstrual cycle: A review of prospective data studies. *Gender Medicine, 9*(5), 361–384. Retrieved from https://www.ncbi.nlm.nih.gov/pubmed/23036262. doi:10.1016/j.genm.2012.07.003

Ronay, R., & von Hippel, W. (2010). The presence of an attractive woman elevates testosterone and physical risk taking in young men. *Social Psychological and Personality Science, 1*(1), 57–64. doi:10.1177/1948550609352807

Roney, J. R., & Simmons, Z. L. (2013). Hormonal predictors of sexual motivation in natural menstrual cycles. *Hormones and Behavior, 63*(4), 636–645. Retrieved from https://www.ncbi.nlm.nih.gov/pubmed/23601091. doi:10.1016/j.yhbeh.2013.02.013

Ross, C. A., & Tabrizi, S. J. (2011). Huntington's disease: From molecular pathogenesis to clinical treatment. *Lancet Neurology, 10*(1), 83–98. Retrieved from https://www.ncbi.nlm.nih.gov/pubmed/21163446. doi:10.1016/S1474-4422(10)0245-3

Ross, H. E., Freeman, S. M., Spiegel, L. L., Ren, X., Terwilliger, E. F., & Young, L. J. (2009). Variation in oxytocin receptor density in the nucleus accumbens has differential effects on affiliative behaviors in monogamous and polygamous voles. *The Journal of Neuroscience, 29*(5), 1312–1318. Retrieved from https://www.ncbi.nlm.nih.gov/pubmed/19193878. doi:10.1523/JNEUROSCI.5039-08.2009

Rosso, I. M., Weiner, M. R., Crowley, D. J., Silveri, M. M., Rauch, S. L., & Jensen, J. E. (2014). Insula and anterior cingulate GABA levels in posttraumatic stress disorder: Preliminary findings using magnetic resonance spectroscopy. *Depression and Anxiety, 31*(2), 115–123. Retrieved from https://www.ncbi.nlm.nih.gov/pubmed/23861191. doi:10.1002/da.22155

Rothmayr, C., Sodian, B., Hajak, G., Dohnel, K., Meinhardt, J., & Sommer, M. (2011). Common and distinct neural networks for false-belief reasoning and inhibitory control. *Neuroimage, 56*(3), 1705–1713. Retrieved from http://www.ncbi.nlm.nih.gov/pubmed/21195194. doi:10.1016/j.neuroimage.2010.12.052

Rozental, R., Giaume, C., & Spray, D. C. (2000). Gap junctions in the nervous system. *Brain Research Brain Research Reviews, 32*(1), 11–15. Retrieved from https://www.ncbi.nlm.nih.gov/pubmed/10928802

Ruffoli, R., Giorgi, F. S., Pizzanelli, C., Murri, L., Paparelli, A., & Fornai, F. (2011). The chemical neuroanatomy of vagus nerve stimulation. *Journal of Chemical Neuroanatomy, 42*(4), 288–296. Retrieved from https://www.ncbi.nlm.nih.gov/pubmed/21167932. doi:10.1016/j.jchemneu.2010.12.002

Ruiz, R., Roque, A., Pineda, E., Licona-Limon, P., Jose Valdez-Alarcon, J., & Lajud, N. (2018). Early life stress accelerates age-induced effects on neurogenesis, depression, and metabolic risk. *Psychoneuroendocrinology, 96*, 203–211. Retrieved from https://www.ncbi.nlm.nih.gov/pubmed/30048914. doi:10.1016/j.psyneuen.2018.07.012

Running, C. A., Craig, B. A., & Mattes, R. D. (2015). Oleogustus: The unique taste of fat. *Chemical Senses, 40*(7), 507–516. Retrieved from https://www.ncbi.nlm.nih.gov/pubmed/26142421. doi:10.1093/chemse/bjv036

Runyan, J. D., Moore, A. N., & Dash, P. K. (2019). Coordinating what we've learned about memory consolidation: Revisiting a unified theory. *Neuroscience & Biobehavioral Reviews, 100*, 77–84. Retrieved from https://www.ncbi.nlm.nih.gov/pubmed/30790633. doi:10.1016/j.neubiorev.2019.02.010

Saalmann, Y. B., Pinsk, M. A., Wang, L., Li, X., & Kastner, S. (2012). The pulvinar regulates information transmission between cortical areas based on attention demands. *Science, 337*(6095), 753–756. Retrieved from https://www.ncbi.nlm.nih.gov/pubmed/22879517. doi:10.1126/science.1223082

Sacher, J., Neumann, J., Okon-Singer, H., Gotowiec, S., & Villringer, A. (2013). Sexual dimorphism in the human brain: Evidence from neuroimaging. *Magnetic Resonance Imaging, 31*(3), 366–375. Retrieved from https://www.ncbi.nlm.nih.gov/pubmed/22921939. doi:10.1016/j.mri.2012.06.007

Sachser, R. M., Haubrich, J., Lunardi, P. S., & de Oliveira Alvares, L. (2017). Forgetting of what was once learned: Exploring the role of postsynaptic ionotropic glutamate receptors on memory formation, maintenance, and decay. *Neuropharmacology, 112*(Pt. A), 94–103. Retrieved from https://www.ncbi.nlm.nih.gov/pubmed/27425202. doi:10.1016/j.neuropharm.2016.07.015

Salzberg, S. L. (2018). Open questions: How many genes do we have? *BMC Biology, 16*(1), 94. Retrieved from https://www.ncbi.nlm.nih.gov/pubmed/30124169. doi:10.1186/s12915-018-0564-x

Samuelson, K. W., Krueger, C. E., & Wilson, C. (2012). Relationships between maternal emotion regulation, parenting, and children's executive functioning in families exposed to intimate partner violence. *Journal of Interpersonal Violence, 27*(17), 3532–3550. Retrieved from https://www.ncbi.nlm.nih.gov/pubmed/22610834. doi:10.1177/0886260512445385

Sanders, L. (2010). Rare brain disorder prevents all fears. *Wired*. Retrieved from https://www.wired.com/2010/12/fear-brain-amygdala/

Sanders, S. K., & Shekhar, A. (1995). Regulation of anxiety by GABAA receptors in the rat amygdala. *Pharmacology, Biochemistry, and Behavior, 52*(4), 701–706. Retrieved from https://www.ncbi.nlm.nih.gov/pubmed/8587908

Saneyoshi, A., Niimi, R., Suetsugu, T., Kaminaga, T., & Yokosawa, K. (2011). Iconic memory and parietofrontal network: fMRI study using temporal integration. *Neuroreport, 22*(11), 515–519. Retrieved from https://www.ncbi.nlm.nih.gov/pubmed/21673607. doi:10.1097/WNR.0b013e328348aa0c

Santello, M., Cali, C., & Bezzi, P. (2012). Gliotransmission and the tripartite synapse. *Advances in Experimental Medicine and Biology, 970*, 307–331. Retrieved from http://www.ncbi.nlm.nih.gov/pubmed/22351062. doi:10.1007/978-3-7091-0932-8_14

Saper, C. B., Chou, T. C., & Scammell, T. E. (2001). The sleep switch: Hypothalamic control of sleep and wakefulness. *Trends in Neurosciences, 24*(12), 726–731. Retrieved from https://www.ncbi.nlm.nih.gov/pubmed/11718878

Sara, S. J. (2010). Reactivation, retrieval, replay and reconsolidation in and out of sleep: Connecting the dots. *Frontiers in Behavioral Neuroscience, 4*, 185. Retrieved from https://www.ncbi.nlm.nih.gov/pubmed/21179586. doi:10.3389/fnbeh.2010.00185

Saravia, R., Ten-Blanco, M., Julia-Hernandez, M., Gagliano, H., Andero, R., Armario, A., . . . Berrendero, F. (2019). Concomitant THC and stress adolescent exposure induces impaired fear extinction and related neurobiological changes in adulthood. *Neuropharmacology, 144*, 345–357. Retrieved from https://www.ncbi.nlm.nih.gov/pubmed/30439419. doi:10.1016/j.neuropharm.2018.11.016

Sato, N., Sakata, H., Tanaka, Y. L., & Taira, M. (2006). Navigation-associated medial parietal neurons in monkeys. *Proceedings of the National Academy of Sciences of the United States of America, 103*(45), 17001–17006. Retrieved from https://www.ncbi.nlm.nih.gov/pubmed/17068129. doi:10.1073/pnas.0604277103

Saxena, S., Brody, A. L., Schwartz, J. M., & Baxter, L. R. (1998). Neuroimaging and frontal-subcortical circuitry in obsessive-compulsive disorder. *The British Journal of Psychiatry. Supplement*, 35, 26–37. Retrieved from https://www.ncbi.nlm.nih.gov/pubmed/9829024

Saxena, S., & Rauch, S. L. (2000). Functional neuroimaging and the neuroanatomy of obsessive-compulsive disorder. *The Psychiatric Clinics of North America, 23*(3), 563–586. Retrieved from https://www.ncbi.nlm.nih.gov/pubmed/10986728

Schachter, S., & Singer, J. E. (1962). Cognitive, social, and physiological determinants of emotional state. *Psychological Review, 69*, 379–399. Retrieved from https://www.ncbi.nlm.nih.gov/pubmed/14497895

Schacter, D. L. (1987). Implicit memory: History and current status. *Journal of Experimental Psychology: Learning, memory and Cognition, 13*(3), 501–518.

Schaefer, M., Knuth, M., & Rumpel, F. (2011). Striatal response to favorite brands as a function of neuroticism and extraversion. *Brain Research, 1425*, 83–89. Retrieved from https://www.ncbi.nlm.nih.gov/pubmed/22035566. doi:10.1016/j.brainres.2011.09.055

Schaefer, M., & Rotte, M. (2007). Favorite brands as cultural objects modulate reward circuit. *Neuroreport, 18*(2), 141–145. Retrieved from https://www.ncbi.nlm.nih.gov/pubmed/17301679. doi:10.1097/WNR.0b013e328010ac84

Schildkraut, J. J. (1965). The catecholamine hypothesis of affective disorders: A review of supporting evidence. *The American Journal of Psychiatry, 122*(5), 509–522. Retrieved from https://www.ncbi.nlm.nih.gov/pubmed/5319766. doi:10.1176/ajp.122.5.509

Schildkraut, J. J. (1995). The catecholamine hypothesis of affective disorders: A review of supporting evidence. 1965 [classical article]. *Journal of Neuropsychiatry and Clinical Neurosciences, 7*(4), 524–533. doi:10.1176/jnp.7.4.524

Schlicker, E., & Feuerstein, T. (2017). Human presynaptic receptors. *Pharmacology & Therapeutics, 172*, 1–21. Retrieved from https://www.ncbi.nlm.nih.gov/pubmed/27902931. doi:10.1016/j.pharmthera.2016.11.005

Schmahmann, J. D. (1991). An emerging concept. The cerebellar contribution to higher function. *Archives of Neurology, 48*(11), 1178–1187. Retrieved from https://www.ncbi.nlm.nih.gov/pubmed/1953406

Schmahmann, J. D., & Pandya, D. N. (1997). The cerebrocerebellar system. *International Review of Neurobiology, 41*, 31–60. Retrieved from https://www.ncbi.nlm.nih.gov/pubmed/9378595

Schmitz, T. W., Nathan Spreng, R., & Alzheimer's Disease Neuroimaging Initiative. (2016). Basal forebrain degeneration precedes and predicts the cortical spread of Alzheimer's pathology. *Nature Communications, 7*, 13249. Retrieved from https://www.ncbi.nlm.nih.gov/pubmed/27811848. doi:10.1038/ncomms13249

Schnakers, C., Vanhaudenhuyse, A., Giacino, J., Ventura, M., Boly, M., Majerus, S., . . . Laureys, S. (2009). Diagnostic accuracy of the vegetative and minimally conscious state: Clinical consensus versus standardized neurobehavioral assessment. *BMC Neurology, 9*, 35. Retrieved from http://www.ncbi.nlm.nih.gov/pubmed/19622138. doi:10.1186/1471-2377-9-35

Schneider, G. E. (1969). Two visual systems. *Science, 163*(3870), 895–902. Retrieved from https://www.ncbi.nlm.nih.gov/pubmed/5763873

Schoeler, T., & Bhattacharyya, S. (2013). The effect of cannabis use on memory function: An update. *Substance Abuse and Rehabilitation, 4*, 11–27. Retrieved from https://www.ncbi.nlm.nih.gov/pubmed/24648785. doi:10.2147/SAR.S25869

Schoenfeld, M. A., Neuer, G., Tempelmann, C., Schussler, K., Noesselt, T., Hopf, J. M., & Heinze, H. J. (2004). Functional magnetic resonance tomography correlates of taste perception in the human primary taste cortex. *Neuroscience, 127*(2), 347–353. Retrieved from https://www.ncbi.nlm.nih.gov/pubmed/15262325. doi:10.1016/j.neuroscience.2004.05.024

Schott, B. H., Richardson-Klavehn, A., Henson, R. N., Becker, C., Heinze, H. J., & Duzel, E. (2006). Neuroanatomical dissociation of encoding processes related to priming and explicit memory. *J Neurosci, 26*(3), 792–800. doi:10.1523/JNEUROSCI.2402-05.2006

Schott, G. D. (1993). Penfield's homunculus: A note on cerebral cartography. *Journal of Neurology, Neurosurgery, and Psychiatry, 56*(4), 329–333. Retrieved from https://www.ncbi.nlm.nih.gov/pubmed/8482950

Schultz, W. (1986). Responses of midbrain dopamine neurons to behavioral trigger stimuli in the monkey. *Journal of Neurophysiology, 56*(5), 1439–1461. Retrieved from https://www.ncbi.nlm.nih.gov/pubmed/3794777. doi:10.1152/jn.1986.56.5.1439

Schultz, W., Dayan, P., & Montague, P. R. (1997). A neural substrate of prediction and reward. *Science, 275*(5306), 1593–1599. Retrieved from https://www.ncbi.nlm.nih.gov/pubmed/9054347

Schulz, P. E. (1997). Long-term potentiation involves increases in the probability of neurotransmitter release. *Proceedings of the National Academy of Sciences of the United States of America, 94*(11), 5888–5893. Retrieved from https://www.ncbi.nlm.nih.gov/pubmed/9159170

Schuster, R. M., Gilman, J., Schoenfeld, D., Evenden, J., Hareli, M., Ulysse, C., . . . Evins, A. E. (2018). One month of cannabis abstinence in adolescents and young adults is associated with improved memory. *Journal of Clinical Psychiatry, 79*(6). In press. Retrieved from https://www.ncbi.nlm.nih.gov/pubmed/30408351. doi:10.4088/JCP.17m11977

Schuster, R. M., Hoeppner, S. S., Evins, A. E., & Gilman, J. M. (2016). Early onset marijuana use is associated with learning inefficiencies. *Neuropsychology, 30*(4), 405–415. Retrieved from https://www.ncbi.nlm.nih.gov/pubmed/26986749. doi:10.1037/neu0000281

Schweizer, T. A., Kan, K., Hung, Y., Tam, F., Naglie, G., & Graham, S. J. (2013). Brain activity during driving with distraction: An immersive fMRI study. *Frontiers in Human Neuroscience, 7*, 53. Retrieved from https://www.ncbi.nlm.nih.gov/pubmed/23450757. doi:10.3389/fnhum.2013.00053

Scoville, W. B., & Milner, B. (1957). Loss of recent memory after bilateral hippocampal lesions. *Journal of Neurology, Neurosurgery, and Psychiatry, 20*(1), 11–21. Retrieved from https://www.ncbi.nlm.nih.gov/pubmed/13406589

Searle, J. (1980). Minds, Brains and Programs. *Behavioral and Brain Sciences, 3*, 417–424.

Searle, J. R. (1983). *Intentionality, an essay in the philosophy of mind*. Cambridge Cambridgeshire/New York: Cambridge University Press.

Seeman, P. (1987). Dopamine receptors and the dopamine hypothesis of schizophrenia. *Synapse, 1*(2), 133–152. Retrieved from http://www.ncbi.nlm.nih.gov/pubmed/2905529. doi:10.1002/syn.890010203

Seeman, P., Lee, T., Chau-Wong, M., & Wong, K. (1976). Antipsychotic drug doses and neuroleptic/dopamine receptors. *Nature, 261*(5562), 717–719. Retrieved from http://www.ncbi.nlm.nih.gov/pubmed/945467

Setiawan, E., Attwells, S., Wilson, A. A., Mizrahi, R., Rusjan, P. M., Miler, L., . . . Meyer, J. H. (2018). Association of translocator protein total distribution volume with duration of untreated major depressive disorder: A cross-sectional study. *Lancet Psychiatry, 5*(4), 339–347. Retrieved from https://www.ncbi.nlm.nih.gov/pubmed/29496589. doi:10.1016/S2215-0366(18)30048-8

Setiawan, E., Wilson, A. A., Mizrahi, R., Rusjan, P. M., Miler, L., Rajkowska, G., . . . Meyer, J. H. (2015). Role of translocator protein density, a marker of neuroinflammation, in the brain during major depressive episodes. *JAMA Psychiatry, 72*(3), 268–275. Retrieved from https://www.ncbi.nlm.nih.gov/pubmed/25629589. doi:10.1001/jamapsychiatry.2014.2427

Shah, A. A., Dar, T. A., Dar, P. A., Ganie, S. A., & Kamal, M. A. (2017). A current perspective on the inhibition of cholinesterase by natural and synthetic inhibitors. *Current Drug Metabolism, 18*(2), 96–111. Retrieved from https://www.ncbi.nlm.nih.gov/pubmed/27890007. doi:10.2174/1389200218666161123122734

Shalev, A., Liberzon, I., & Marmar, C. (2017). Post-traumatic stress disorder. *The New England Journal of Medicine, 376*(25), 2459–2469. Retrieved from https://www.ncbi.nlm.nih.gov/pubmed/28636846. doi:10.1056/NEJMra1612499

Shamay-Tsoory, S. G. (2011). The neural bases for empathy. *Neuroscientist, 17*(1), 18–24. Retrieved from https://www.ncbi.nlm.nih.gov/pubmed/21071616. doi:10.1177/1073858410379268

Shamay-Tsoory, S. G., & Aharon-Peretz, J. (2007). Dissociable prefrontal networks for cognitive and affective theory of mind: A lesion study. *Neuropsychologia, 45*(13), 3054–3067. Retrieved from https://www.ncbi.nlm.nih.gov/pubmed/17640690. doi:10.1016/j.neuropsychologia.2007.05.021

Shamay-Tsoory, S. G., Aharon-Peretz, J., & Perry, D. (2009). Two systems for empathy: A double dissociation between emotional and cognitive empathy in inferior frontal gyrus versus ventromedial prefrontal lesions. *Brain, 132*(Pt. 3), 617–627. Retrieved from https://www.ncbi.nlm.nih.gov/pubmed/18971202. doi:10.1093/brain/awn279

Shanahan, M. (2012). The brain's connective core and its role in animal cognition. *Philosophical Transactions of the Royal Society of London. Series B, Biological Sciences, 367*(1603), 2704–2714. Retrieved from http://www.ncbi.nlm.nih.gov/pubmed/22927569. doi:10.1098/rstb.2012.0128

Sheinberg, D. L., & Logothetis, N. K. (1997). The role of temporal cortical areas in perceptual organization. *Proceedings of the National Academy of Sciences of the United States of America,*

94(7), 3408–3413. Retrieved from http://www.ncbi.nlm.nih.gov/pubmed/9096407

Sheline, Y. I., Liston, C., & McEwen, B. S. (2019). Parsing the hippocampus in depression: chronic stress, hippocampal volume, and major depressive disorder. *Biological Psychiatry, 85*(6), 436–438. Retrieved from https://www.ncbi.nlm.nih.gov/pubmed/30777168. doi:10.1016/j.biopsych.2019.01.011

Sherrington, C. S. (1906a). *The integrative action of the nervous system*. New York: C. Scribner's sons.

Sherrington, C. S. (1906b). Observations on the scratch-reflex in the spinal dog. *The Journal of Physiology, 34*(1–2), 1–50. Retrieved from https://www.ncbi.nlm.nih.gov/pubmed/16992835

Sherrington, C. S. (1911). *The integrative action of the nervous system*. New Haven, CT: Yale University Press.

Sherry, D. F. (2006). Neuroecology. *Annual Review of Psychology, 57*, 167–197. Retrieved from https://www.ncbi.nlm.nih.gov/pubmed/16318593. doi:10.1146/annurev.psych.56.091103.070324

Sherry, D. F., & Hoshooley, J. S. (2010). Seasonal hippocampal plasticity in food-storing birds. *Philosophical Transactions of the Royal Society of London. Series B, Biological Sciences, 365*(1542), 933–943. Retrieved from https://www.ncbi.nlm.nih.gov/pubmed/20156817. doi:10.1098/rstb.2009.0220

Sherry, D. F., & Schacter, D. L. (1987). The evolution of multiple memory systems. *Psychological Review, 94*(4), 439–454. doi:10.1037/0033-295X.94.4.439

Sherwin, B. B., Gelfand, M. M., & Brender, W. (1985). Androgen enhances sexual motivation in females: A prospective, crossover study of sex steroid administration in the surgical menopause. *Psychosomatic Medicine, 47*(4), 339–351. Retrieved from https://www.ncbi.nlm.nih.gov/pubmed/4023162

Sheth, B. R., Sharma, J., Rao, S. C., & Sur, M. (1996). Orientation maps of subjective contours in visual cortex. *Science, 274*(5295), 2110–2115. Retrieved from https://www.ncbi.nlm.nih.gov/pubmed/8953048

Shiell, M. M., Champoux, F., & Zatorre, R. J. (2014). Enhancement of visual motion detection thresholds in early deaf people. *PLoS One, 9*(2), e90498. Retrieved from https://www.ncbi.nlm.nih.gov/pubmed/24587381. doi:10.1371/journal.pone.0090498

Shih, R., Dubrowski, A., & Carnahan, H. (2009). *Evidence for haptic memory*. Paper presented at the World Haptics 2009 - Third Joint EuroHaptics conference and Symposium on Haptic Interfaces for Virtual Environment and Teleoperator Systems, Salt Lake City, UT.

Shik, M. L., Severin, F. V., & Orlovsky, G. N. (1969). Control of walking and running by means of electrical stimulation of the mesencephalon. *Electroencephalography and Clinical Neurophysiology, 26*(5), 549. Retrieved from https://www.ncbi.nlm.nih.gov/pubmed/4181500

Sidi, H., Asiff, M., Kumar, J., Das, S., Hatta, N. H., & Alfonso, C. (2017). Hypersexuality as a Neuropsychiatric Disorder: The neurobiology and treatment options. *Current Drug Targets, 18*(12). Retrieved from https://www.ncbi.nlm.nih.gov/pubmed/28325146. doi:10.2174/1389450118666170321144931

Sienaert, P. (2016). Based on a true story? The portrayal of ECT in international movies and television programs. *Brain Stimulation, 9*(6), 882–891. Retrieved from https://www.ncbi.nlm.nih.gov/pubmed/27522170. doi:10.1016/j.brs.2016.07.005

Sierra, A., Abiega, O., Shahraz, A., & Neumann, H. (2013). Janus-faced microglia: Beneficial and detrimental consequences of microglial phagocytosis. *Frontiers in Cellular Neuroscience, 7*, 6. Retrieved from http://www.ncbi.nlm.nih.gov/pubmed/23386811. doi:10.3389/fncel.2013.00006

Silverthorn, D. U., Johnson, B. R., Ober, W. C., Ober, C. E., & Silverthorn, A. C. (2016). *Human physiology: An integrated approach* (7th ed.). San Francisco, CA: Pearson.

Simpson, D. (2005). Phrenology and the neurosciences: Contributions of F. J. Gall and J. G. Spurzheim. *ANZ Journal of Surgery, 75*(6), 475–482. Retrieved from https://www.ncbi.nlm.nih.gov/pubmed/15943741. doi:10.1111/j.1445-2197.2005.03426.x

Singh, A., & Kar, S. K. (2017). How electroconvulsive therapy works?: Understanding the neurobiological mechanisms. *Clinical Psychopharmacology and Neuroscience, 15*(3), 210–221. Retrieved from https://www.ncbi.nlm.nih.gov/pubmed/28783929. doi:10.9758/cpn.2017.15.3.210

Sirvio, J., & MacDonald, E. (1999). Central alpha1-adrenoceptors: Their role in the modulation of attention and memory formation. *Pharmacology & Therapeutics, 83*(1), 49–65. Retrieved from https://www.ncbi.nlm.nih.gov/pubmed/10501595

Sligte, I. G., Scholte, H. S., & Lamme, V. A. (2009). V4 activity predicts the strength of visual short-term memory representations. *The Journal of Neuroscience, 29*(23), 7432–7438. Retrieved from https://www.ncbi.nlm.nih.gov/pubmed/19515911. doi:10.1523/JNEUROSCI.0784-09.2009

Sliney, D. H. (2016). What is light? The visible spectrum and beyond. *Eye (London), 30*(2), 222–229. Retrieved from https://www.ncbi.nlm.nih.gov/pubmed/26768917. doi:10.1038/eye.2015.252

Small, D. M., & Prescott, J. (2005). Odor/taste integration and the perception of flavor. *Experimental Brain Research, 166*(3–4), 345–357. Retrieved from https://www.ncbi.nlm.nih.gov/pubmed/16028032. doi:10.1007/s00221-005-2376-9

Smeltzer, M. D., Curtis, J. T., Aragona, B. J., & Wang, Z. (2006). Dopamine, oxytocin, and vasopressin receptor binding in the medial prefrontal cortex of monogamous and promiscuous voles. *Neuroscience Letters, 394*(2), 146–151. Retrieved from https://www.ncbi.nlm.nih.gov/pubmed/16289323. doi:10.1016/j.neulet.2005.10.019

Smit, M., Van Stralen, H. E., Van den Munckhof, B., Snijders, T. J., & Dijkerman, H. C. (2018). The man who lost his body: Suboptimal multisensory integration yields body awareness problems after a right temporoparietal brain tumour. *Journal of Neuropsychology*. In press. Retrieved from https://www.ncbi.nlm.nih.gov/pubmed/29532598. doi:10.1111/jnp.12153

Smith, A. (2006). Cognitive empathy and emotional empathy in human behavior and evolution. *The Psychological Record, 56*(1), 3–21. Retrieved from https://doi.org/10.1007/BF03395534. doi:10.1007/bf03395534

Smith, A. S., Williams Avram, S. K., Cymerblit-Sabba, A., Song, J., & Young, W. S. (2016). Targeted activation of the hippocampal CA2 area strongly enhances social memory. *Molecular Psychiatry, 21*(8), 1137–144. Retrieved from https://www.ncbi.nlm.nih.gov/pubmed/26728562. doi:10.1038/mp.2015.189

Smith, C. N., Frascino, J. C., Hopkins, R. O., & Squire, L. R. (2013). The nature of anterograde and retrograde memory impairment after damage to the medial temporal lobe. *Neuropsychologia, 51*(13), 2709–2714. Retrieved from https://www.ncbi.nlm.nih.gov/pubmed/24041667. doi:10.1016/j.neuropsychologia.2013.09.015

Smith, C. U. (2010). The triune brain in antiquity: Plato, Aristotle, Erasistratus. *Journal of the History of the Neurosciences, 19*(1), 1–14. Retrieved from https://www.ncbi.nlm.nih.gov/pubmed/20391097. doi:10.1080/09647040802601605

Snyder, S. H., & Pasternak, G. W. (2003). Historical review: Opioid receptors. *Trends in Pharmacological Sciences, 24*(4), 198–205. Retrieved from https://www.ncbi.nlm.nih.gov/pubmed/12707007. doi:10.1016/S0165-6147(03)00066-X

Soares, C. N. (2017). Tailoring strategies for the management of depression in midlife years. *Menopause, 24*(6), 699–701. Retrieved from https://www.ncbi.nlm.nih.gov/pubmed/28291028. doi:10.1097/GME.0000000000000853

Sohn, J. W. (2015). Network of hypothalamic neurons that control appetite. *BMB Reports, 48*(4), 229–233. Retrieved from https://www.ncbi.nlm.nih.gov/pubmed/25560696

Solstad, T., Moser, E. I., & Einevoll, G. T. (2006). From grid cells to place cells: A mathematical model. *Hippocampus, 16*(12), 1026–1031. Retrieved from https://www.ncbi.nlm.nih.gov/pubmed/17094145. doi:10.1002/hipo.20244

Somerville, L. H., Hare, T., & Casey, B. J. (2011). Frontostriatal maturation predicts cognitive control failure to appetitive cues in adolescents. *Journal of Cognitive Neuroscience, 23*(9), 2123–2134. Retrieved from https://www.ncbi.nlm.nih.gov/pubmed/20809855. doi:10.1162/jocn.2010.21572

Soon, C. S., Brass, M., Heinze, H. J., & Haynes, J. D. (2008). Unconscious determinants of free decisions in the human brain. *Nature Neuroscience, 11*(5), 543–545. Retrieved from http://www.ncbi.nlm.nih.gov/pubmed/18408715. doi:10.1038/nn.2112

Sorrells, S. F., Paredes, M. F., Cebrian-Silla, A., Sandoval, K., Qi, D., Kelley, K. W., . . . Alvarez-Buylla, A. (2018). Human hippocampal neurogenesis drops sharply in children to undetectable levels in adults. *Nature, 555*(7696), 377–381. Retrieved from https://www.ncbi.nlm.nih.gov/pubmed/29513649. doi:10.1038/nature25975

Soudry, Y., Lemogne, C., Malinvaud, D., Consoli, S. M., & Bonfils, P. (2011). Olfactory system and emotion: Common substrates. *European Annals of Otorhinolaryngology, Head and Neck Diseases, 128*(1), 18–23. Retrieved from https://www.ncbi.nlm.nih.gov/pubmed/21227767. doi:10.1016/j.anorl.2010.09.007

Spence, C. J. F. (2015). Just how much of what we taste derives from the sense of smell?, *Flavour, 4*(1), 30. Retrieved from https://doi.org/10.1186/s13411-015-0040-2. doi:10.1186/s13411-015-0040-2

Sperling, G. (1960). The information available in brief visual presentations. *Psychological Monographs: General and Applied, 74*(11), 1–29. doi:10.1037/h0093759

Sperry, R. W. (1944a). Optic nerve regeneration with return of vision in anurans. *Journal of Neurophysiology, 7*(57–69).

Sperry, R. W. (1944b). Restoration of vision after crossing of the optic nerves and after contralateral transplantation of eye. *Journal of Neurophysiology, 8*, 15–28.

Sperry, R. W. (1956). The eye and the brain. *Scientific American, 194*(5), 48–52.

Sperry, R. W. (1961). Cerebral Organization and Behavior: The split brain behaves in many respects like two separate brains, providing new research possibilities. *Science, 133*(3466), 1749–1757. Retrieved from https://www.ncbi.nlm.nih.gov/pubmed/17829720. doi:10.1126/science.133.3466.1749

Spudich, J. A. (2001). The myosin swinging cross-bridge model. *Nature reviews. Molecular Cell Biology, 2*(5), 387–392. Retrieved from http://www.ncbi.nlm.nih.gov/pubmed/11331913. doi:10.1038/35073086

Squire, L. R. (2004). Memory systems of the brain: A brief history and current perspective. *Neurobiology of Learning and Memory, 82*(3), 171–177. Retrieved from https://www.ncbi.nlm.nih.gov/pubmed/15464402. doi:10.1016/j.nlm.2004.06.005

Squire, L. R., Amaral, D. G., Zola-Morgan, S., Kritchevsky, M., & Press, G. (1989). Description of brain injury in the amnesic patient N.A. based on magnetic resonance imaging. *Experimental Neurology, 105*(1), 23–35. Retrieved from https://www.ncbi.nlm.nih.gov/pubmed/2744126

Squire, L. R., Genzel, L., Wixted, J. T., & Morris, R. G. (2015). Memory consolidation. *Cold Spring Harbor Perspectives in Biology, 7*(8), a021766. Retrieved from https://www.ncbi.nlm.nih.gov/pubmed/26238360. doi:10.1101/cshperspect.a021766

Squire, L. R., & Moore, R. Y. (1979). Dorsal thalamic lesion in a noted case of human memory dysfunction. *Annals of Neurology, 6*(6), 503–506. Retrieved from https://www.ncbi.nlm.nih.gov/pubmed/119481. doi:10.1002/ana.410060607

Squire, L. R., & Zola, S. M. (1996). Structure and function of declarative and nondeclarative memory systems. *Proceedings of the National Academy of Sciences of the United States of America, 93*(24), 13515–13522. Retrieved from https://www.ncbi.nlm.nih.gov/pubmed/8942965

Stanley, D., Phelps, E., & Banaji, M. (2008). The neural basis of implicit attitudes. *Current Directions in Psychological Science, 17*(2), 164–170. Retrieved from https://journals.sagepub.com/doi/abs/10.1111/j.1467-8721.2008.00568.x. doi:10.1111/j.1467-8721.2008.00568.x

Stanley, D. A., Sokol-Hessner, P., Fareri, D. S., Perino, M. T., Delgado, M. R., Banaji, M. R., & Phelps, E. A. (2012). Race and reputation: Perceived racial group trustworthiness influences the neural correlates of trust decisions. *Philosophical transactions of the Royal Society of London. Series B, Biological sciences, 367*(1589), 744–753. Retrieved from https://www.ncbi.nlm.nih.gov/pubmed/22271789. doi:10.1098/rstb.2011.0300

Steele, J. D., Kumar, P., & Ebmeier, K. P. (2007). Blunted response to feedback information in depressive illness. *Brain, 130*(Pt. 9), 2367–2374. Retrieved from http://www.ncbi.nlm.nih.gov/pubmed/17586866. doi:10.1093/brain/awm150

Steinvorth, S., Levine, B., & Corkin, S. (2005). Medial temporal lobe structures are needed to re-experience remote autobiographical memories: Evidence from H.M. and W.R. *Neuropsychologia, 43*(4), 479–496. Retrieved from https://www.ncbi.nlm.nih.gov/pubmed/15716139. doi:10.1016/j.neuropsychologia.2005.01.001

Stender, J., Gosseries, O., Bruno, M. A., Charland-Verville, V., Vanhaudenhuyse, A., Demertzi, A., . . . Laureys, S. (2014). Diagnostic precision of PET imaging and functional MRI in disorders of consciousness: A clinical validation study. *The Lancet, 384*(9942), 514–522. Retrieved from http://www.ncbi.nlm.nih.gov/pubmed/24746174. doi:10.1016/S0140-6736(14)60042-8

Sternberg, R. (1998). *In search of the human mind* (2nd ed.). Fort Worth, TX: Harcourt Brace.

Stettler, D. D., & Axel, R. (2009). Representations of odor in the piriform cortex. *Neuron, 63*(6), 854–864. Retrieved from https://www.ncbi.nlm.nih.gov/pubmed/19778513. doi:10.1016/j.neuron.2009.09.005

Stevens, F. L., Hurley, R. A., & Taber, K. H. (2011). Anterior cingulate cortex: Unique role in cognition and emotion. *The Journal of Neuropsychiatry and Clinical Neurosciences, 23*(2), 121–125. Retrieved from https://www.ncbi.nlm.nih.gov/pubmed/21677237. doi:10.1176/appi.neuropsych.23.2.121, 10.1176/jnp.23.2.jnp121

Stiefel, K., Merrifield, A., & Holcombe, A. (2014). The claustrum's proposed role in consciousness is supported by the effect and target localization of Salvia divinorum. *Frontiers in Integrative Neuroscience, 8*(20). Retrieved from https://www.frontiersin.org/article/10.3389/fnint.2014.00020. doi:10.3389/fnint.2014.00020

Stinnett, T. J., & Zabel, M. K. (2018). *Neuroanatomy, Broca Area*. Treasure Island, FL: StatPearls.

Stone, J. M. (2011). Glutamatergic antipsychotic drugs: A new dawn in the treatment of schizophrenia? *Therapeutic Advances in Psychopharmacology, 1*(1), 5–18. Retrieved from http://www.ncbi.nlm.nih.gov/pubmed/23983922. doi:10.1177/2045125311400779

Strayer, D. L., & Johnston, W. A. (2001). Driven to distraction: Dual-Task studies of simulated driving and conversing on a cellular telephone. *Psychological Science, 12*(6), 462–466. Retrieved from https://www.ncbi.nlm.nih.gov/pubmed/11760132. doi:10.1111/1467-9280.00386

Subbaraman, M. S., & Kerr, W. C. (2018). Alcohol use and risk of related problems among cannabis users is lower among those with medical cannabis recommendations, though not due to health. *Journal of Studies on Alcohol and Drugs, 79*(6), 935–942. Retrieved from https://www.ncbi.nlm.nih.gov/pubmed/30573025

Substance Abuse and Mental Health Services Administration. (2018). Key substance use and mental health indicators in the United States: Results from the 2017 National Survey on Drug Use and Health (HHS Publication No. SMA 18-5068, NSDUH Series H-53). Rockville, MD: SAMHSA. Retrieved from https://www. samhsa.gov/data/

Suddendorf, T., & Butler, D. L. (2013). The nature of visual self-recognition. *Trends in Cognitive Sciences, 17*(3), 121–127. Retrieved from http://www.ncbi.nlm.nih.gov/pubmed/23410584. doi:10.1016/j.tics.2013.01.004

Sundstrom Poromaa, I., & Gingnell, M. (2014). Menstrual cycle influence on cognitive function and emotion processing-from a reproductive perspective. *Frontiers in Neuroscience, 8*, 380. Retrieved from https://www.ncbi.nlm.nih.gov/pubmed/25505380. doi:10.3389/fnins.2014.00380

Sur, S., & Sinha, V. K. (2009). Event-related potential: An overview. *Industrial Psychiatry Journal, 18*(1), 70–73. Retrieved from https://www.ncbi.nlm.nih.gov/pubmed/21234168. doi:10.4103/0972-6748.57865

Surmeier, D. J., & Foehring, R. (2004). A mechanism for homeostatic plasticity. *Nature Neuroscience, 7*(7), 691–692. Retrieved from https://www.ncbi.nlm.nih.gov/pubmed/15220926. doi:10.1038/nn0704-691

Sutherland, R. J., Kolb, B., & Whishaw, I. Q. (1982). Spatial mapping: Definitive disruption by hippocampal or medial frontal cortical damage in the rat. *Neuroscience Letters, 31*(3), 271–276. Retrieved from https://www.ncbi.nlm.nih.gov/pubmed/7133562. doi:10.1016/0304-3940(82)90032-5

Svaetichin, G., & Macnichol, E. F., Jr. (1959). Retinal mechanisms for chromatic and achromatic vision. *Annals of the New York Academy of Sciences, 74*(2), 385–404. Retrieved from https://www.ncbi.nlm.nih.gov/pubmed/13627867

Svob Strac, D., Pivac, N., & Muck-Seler, D. (2016). The serotonergic system and cognitive function. *Translational Neuroscience, 7*(1), 35–49. Retrieved from https://www.ncbi.nlm.nih.gov/pubmed/28123820. doi:10.1515/tnsci-2016-0007

Swaab, D. F., & Hofman, M. A. (1990). An enlarged suprachiasmatic nucleus in homosexual men. *Brain Research, 537*(1–2), 141–148. Retrieved from https://www.ncbi.nlm.nih.gov/pubmed/2085769

Sylvester, C. M., Corbetta, M., Raichle, M. E., Rodebaugh, T. L., Schlaggar, B. L., Sheline, Y. I., . . . Lenze, E. J. (2012). Functional network dysfunction in anxiety and anxiety disorders. *Trends in Neurosciences, 35*(9), 527–535. Retrieved from https://www.ncbi.nlm.nih.gov/pubmed/22658924. doi:10.1016/j.tins.2012.04.012

Szczepanski, S. M., & Knight, R. T. (2014). Insights into human behavior from lesions to the prefrontal cortex. *Neuron, 83*(5), 1002–1018. Retrieved from https://www.ncbi.nlm.nih.gov/pubmed/25175878. doi:10.1016/j.neuron.2014.08.011

Tallinen, T., Chung, J. Y., Biggins, J. S., & Mahadevan, L. (2014). Gyrification from constrained cortical expansion. *Proceedings of the National Academy of Sciences of the United States of America, 111*(35), 12667–12672. Retrieved from https://www.ncbi.nlm.nih.gov/pubmed/25136099. doi:10.1073/pnas.1406015111

Tamietto, M., Castelli, L., Vighetti, S., Perozzo, P., Geminiani, G., Weiskrantz, L., & de Gelder, B. (2009). Unseen facial and bodily expressions trigger fast emotional reactions. *Proceedings of the National Academy of Sciences of the United States of America, 106*(42), 17661–17666. Retrieved from http://www.ncbi.nlm.nih.gov/pubmed/19805044. doi:10.1073/pnas.0908994106

Tamietto, M., Cauda, F., Corazzini, L. L., Savazzi, S., Marzi, C. A., Goebel, R., . . . de Gelder, B. (2010). Collicular vision guides nonconscious behavior. *Journal of Cognitive Neuroscience, 22*(5), 888–902. Retrieved from http://www.ncbi.nlm.nih.gov/pubmed/19320547. doi:10.1162/jocn.2009.21225

Taube, J. S., Muller, R. U., & Ranck, J. B., Jr. (1990). Head-direction cells recorded from the postsubiculum in freely moving rats. I. Description and quantitative analysis. *The Journal of Neuroscience, 10*(2), 420–435. Retrieved from https://www.ncbi.nlm.nih.gov/pubmed/2303851

Taylor, L. E., Swerdfeger, A. L., & Eslick, G. D. (2014). Vaccines are not associated with autism: An evidence-based meta-analysis of case-control and cohort studies. *Vaccine, 32*(29), 3623–3629. Retrieved from https://www.ncbi.nlm.nih.gov/pubmed/24814559. doi:10.1016/j.vaccine.2014.04.085

Teasdale, G., & Jennett, B. (1974). Assessment of coma and impaired consciousness. A practical scale. *The Lancet, 2*(7872), 81–84. Retrieved from https://www.ncbi.nlm.nih.gov/pubmed/4136544

Terburg, D., Morgan, B., & van Honk, J. (2009). The testosterone-cortisol ratio: A hormonal marker for proneness to social aggression. *International Journal of Law and Psychiatry, 32*(4), 216–223. Retrieved from https://www.ncbi.nlm.nih.gov/pubmed/19446881. doi:10.1016/j.ijlp.2009.04.008

Teyler, T. J., & Rudy, J. W. (2007). The hippocampal indexing theory and episodic memory: Updating the index. *Hippocampus, 17*(12), 1158–1169. Retrieved from https://www.ncbi.nlm.nih.gov/pubmed/17696170. doi:10.1002/hipo.20350

Thach, W. T. (1998). What is the role of the cerebellum in motor learning and cognition? *Trends in Cognitive Sciences, 2*(9), 331–337. Retrieved from https://www.ncbi.nlm.nih.gov/pubmed/21227229

Thompson, P. M., Vidal, C., Giedd, J. N., Gochman, P., Blumenthal, J., Nicolson, R., . . . Rapoport, J. L. (2001). Mapping adolescent brain change reveals dynamic wave of accelerated gray matter loss in very early-onset schizophrenia. *Proceedings of the National Academy of Sciences of the United States of America, 98*(20), 11650–11655. Retrieved from http://www.ncbi.nlm.nih.gov/pubmed/11573002. doi:10.1073/pnas.201243998

Thompson, R. F. (1986). The neurobiology of learning and memory. *Science, 233*(4767), 941–947. Retrieved from https://www.ncbi.nlm.nih.gov/pubmed/3738519

Tolman, E. C. (1948). Cognitive maps in rats and men. *Psychol Rev, 55*(4), 189–208. doi:10.1037/h0061626

Tomkins, S. S. (2008). *Affect imagery consciousness: The complete edition*. New York: Springer Pub.

Tong, F., Nakayama, K., Vaughan, J. T., & Kanwisher, N. (1998). Binocular rivalry and visual awareness in human extrastriate cortex. *Neuron, 21*(4), 753–759. Retrieved from http://www.ncbi.nlm.nih.gov/pubmed/9808462

Toni, N., Buchs, P. A., Nikonenko, I., Bron, C. R., & Muller, D. (1999). LTP promotes formation of multiple spine synapses between a single axon terminal and a dendrite. *Nature, 402*(6760), 421–425. Retrieved from https://www.ncbi.nlm.nih.gov/pubmed/10586883. doi:10.1038/46574

Tonn Eisinger, K. R., Larson, E. B., Boulware, M. I., Thomas, M. J., & Mermelstein, P. G. (2018). Membrane estrogen receptor signaling impacts the reward circuitry of the female brain to influence motivated behaviors. *Steroids, 133*, 53–59. Retrieved from https://www.ncbi.nlm.nih.gov/pubmed/29195840. doi:10.1016/j.steroids.2017.11.013

Tononi, G. (2012). Integrated information theory of consciousness: An updated account. *Archives Italiennes de Biologie, 150*(2–3),

56–90. Retrieved from https://www.ncbi.nlm.nih.gov/pubmed/23165867. doi:10.4449/aib.v149i5.1388

Tracy, R. L., & Walsberg, G. E. (2000). Prevalence of cutaneous evaporation in Merriam's kangaroo rat and its adaptive variation at the subspecific level. *The Journal of Experimental Biology, 203*(Pt. 4), 773–781. Retrieved from https://www.ncbi.nlm.nih.gov/pubmed/10648219

Tranel, D., Bechara, A., & Denburg, N. L. (2002). Asymmetric functional roles of right and left ventromedial prefrontal cortices in social conduct, decision-making, and emotional processing. *Cortex, 38*(4), 589–612. Retrieved from https://www.ncbi.nlm.nih.gov/pubmed/12465670

Tranel, D., Gullickson, G., Koch, M., & Adolphs, R. (2006). Altered experience of emotion following bilateral amygdala damage. *Cognitive Neuropsychiatry, 11*(3), 219–232. Retrieved from https://www.ncbi.nlm.nih.gov/pubmed/17354069. doi:10.1080/13546800444000281

Treisman, A. (1982). Perceptual grouping and attention in visual search for features and for objects. *Journal of Experimental Psychology. Human Perception and Performance, 8*(2), 194–214. Retrieved from https://www.ncbi.nlm.nih.gov/pubmed/6461717

Treisman, A., & Schmidt, H. (1982). Illusory conjunctions in the perception of objects. *Cognitive Psychology, 14*(1), 107–141. Retrieved from http://www.ncbi.nlm.nih.gov/pubmed/7053925

Treisman, A. M. (1964). The effect of irrelevant material on the efficiency of selective listening. *The American Journal of Psychology, 77*, 533–546. Retrieved from https://www.ncbi.nlm.nih.gov/pubmed/14251963

Treisman, A. M., & Gelade, G. (1980). A feature-integration theory of attention. *Cognitive Psychology, 12*(1), 97–136. Retrieved from http://www.ncbi.nlm.nih.gov/pubmed/7351125

Tripathy, S. J., Burton, S. D., Geramita, M., Gerkin, R. C., & Urban, N. N. (2015). Brain-wide analysis of electrophysiological diversity yields novel categorization of mammalian neuron types. *Journal of Neurophysiology, 113*(10), 3474–3489. Retrieved from https://www.ncbi.nlm.nih.gov/pubmed/25810482. doi:10.1152/jn.00237.2015

Trivers, R. L. (1971). The evolution of reciprocal altruism. *The Quarterly Review of Biology, 46*(1), 35–57. Retrieved from https://www.journals.uchicago.edu/doi/abs/10.1086/406755. doi:10.1086/406755

Trotta, D. (2007). Brain injury, not steroids, seen in wrestler death. *Reuters*. Retrieved from https://www.reuters.com/article/us-usa-wrestler/brain-injury-not-steroids-seen-in-wrestler-death-idUSN0523057520070905

Tsao, A., Sugar J., Lu, L., Wang, C., Knierim, J. J., Moser, M. B., & Moser, E. I. (2018). Integrating time from experience in the lateral entorhinal cortex. *Nature, 561*(7721):57–62. doi:https://doi.org/10.1038/s41586-018-0459-6

Tschudin, S., Bertea, P. C., & Zemp, E. (2010). Prevalence and predictors of premenstrual syndrome and premenstrual dysphoric disorder in a population-based sample. *Archives of Women's Mental Health, 13*(6), 485–494. Retrieved from https://www.ncbi.nlm.nih.gov/pubmed/20449618. doi:10.1007/s00737-010-0165-3

Tse, D., Langston, R. F., Kakeyama, M., Bethus, I., Spooner, P. A., Wood, E. R., . . . Morris, R. G. (2007). Schemas and memory consolidation. *Science, 316*(5821), 76–82. Retrieved from https://www.ncbi.nlm.nih.gov/pubmed/17412951. doi:10.1126/science.1135935

Tuiten, A., Van Honk, J., Koppeschaar, H., Bernaards, C., Thijssen, J., & Verbaten, R. (2000). Time course of effects of testosterone administration on sexual arousal in women. *Archives of General Psychiatry, 57*(2), 149–153; discussion 155-146. Retrieved from https://www.ncbi.nlm.nih.gov/pubmed/10665617

Tulving, E. (1983). *Elements of episodic memory*. Oxford Oxfordshire/New York: Clarendon Press;Oxford University Press.

Tulving, E., & Schacter, D. L. (1990). Priming and human memory systems. *Science, 247*(4940), 301–306. Retrieved from https://www.ncbi.nlm.nih.gov/pubmed/2296719

Turner, A. M., & Greenough, W. T. (1985). Differential rearing effects on rat visual cortex synapses. I. Synaptic and neuronal density and synapses per neuron. *Brain Research, 329*(1–2), 195–203. Retrieved from https://www.ncbi.nlm.nih.gov/pubmed/3978441

Turrigiano, G. G., & Nelson, S. B. (2004). Homeostatic plasticity in the developing nervous system. *Nature Reviews Neuroscience, 5*(2), 97–107. Retrieved from https://www.ncbi.nlm.nih.gov/pubmed/14735113. doi:10.1038/nrn1327

Ursu, S., Stenger, V. A., Shear, M. K., Jones, M. R., & Carter, C. S. (2003). Overactive action monitoring in obsessive-compulsive disorder: Evidence from functional magnetic resonance imaging. *Psychological Science, 14*(4), 347–353. Retrieved from http://www.ncbi.nlm.nih.gov/pubmed/12807408

Valyear, K. F., & Frey, S. H. (2015). Human posterior parietal cortex mediates hand-specific planning. *Neuroimage, 114*, 226–238. Retrieved from https://www.ncbi.nlm.nih.gov/pubmed/25842294. doi:10.1016/j.neuroimage.2015.03.058

van Anders, S. M., Hamilton, L. D., & Watson, N. V. (2007). Multiple partners are associated with higher testosterone in North American men and women. *Hormones and Behavior, 51*(3), 454–459. Retrieved from https://www.ncbi.nlm.nih.gov/pubmed/17316638. doi:10.1016/j.yhbeh.2007.01.002

van der Meij, L., Buunk, A. P., van de Sande, J. P., & Salvador, A. (2008). The presence of a woman increases testosterone in aggressive dominant men. *Hormones and Behavior, 54*(5), 640–644. Retrieved from https://www.ncbi.nlm.nih.gov/pubmed/18675269. doi:10.1016/j.yhbeh.2008.07.001

Van Overwalle, F., & Baetens, K. (2009). Understanding others' actions and goals by mirror and mentalizing systems: A meta-analysis. *Neuroimage, 48*(3), 564–584. Retrieved from https://www.ncbi.nlm.nih.gov/pubmed/19524046. doi:10.1016/j.neuroimage.2009.06.009

VanElzakker, M. B., Dahlgren, M. K., Davis, F. C., Dubois, S., & Shin, L. M. (2014). From Pavlov to PTSD: The extinction of conditioned fear in rodents, humans, and anxiety disorders. *Neurobiology of Learning and Memory, 113*, 3–18. Retrieved from https://www.ncbi.nlm.nih.gov/pubmed/24321650. doi:10.1016/j.nlm.2013.11.014

Vemuri, P., & Jack, C. R., Jr. (2010). Role of structural MRI in Alzheimer's disease. *Alzheimer's Research & Therapy, 2*(4), 23. Retrieved from https://www.ncbi.nlm.nih.gov/pubmed/20807454. doi:10.1186/alzrt47

Verhulst, B., Neale, M. C., & Kendler, K. S. (2015). The heritability of alcohol use disorders: A meta-analysis of twin and adoption studies. *Psychological Medicine, 45*(5), 1061–1072. Retrieved from https://www.ncbi.nlm.nih.gov/pubmed/25171596. doi:10.1017/S0033291714002165

Verkhratsky, A., & Nedergaard, M. (2018). Physiology of astroglia. *Physiological Reviews, 98*(1), 239–389. Retrieved from https://www.ncbi.nlm.nih.gov/pubmed/29351512. doi:10.1152/physrev.00042.2016

Vijayraghavan, S., Major, A. J., & Everling, S. (2017). Neuromodulation of prefrontal cortex in non-human primates by dopaminergic receptors during rule-guided flexible behavior and cognitive control. *Frontiers in Neural Circuits, 11*, 91. Retrieved from https://www.ncbi.nlm.nih.gov/pubmed/29259545. doi:10.3389/fncir.2017.00091

Volkmar, F. R., & Greenough, W. T. (1972). Rearing complexity affects branching of dendrites in the visual cortex of the rat. *Science, 176*(4042), 1445–1447. Retrieved from https://www.ncbi.nlm.nih.gov/pubmed/5033647

Volkow, N. D., Baler, R. D., Compton, W. M., & Weiss, S. R. (2014). Adverse health effects of marijuana use. *The New England Journal of Medicine, 370*(23), 2219–2227. Retrieved from https://www.ncbi.nlm.nih.gov/pubmed/24897085. doi:10.1056/NEJMra1402309

Volkow, N. D., Wise, R. A., & Baler, R. (2017). The dopamine motive system: Implications for drug and food addiction. *Nature Reviews Neuroscience, 18*(12), 741–752. Retrieved from https://www.ncbi.nlm.nih.gov/pubmed/29142296. doi:10.1038/nrn.2017.130

Von Békésy, G., & Wever, E. G. (1960). *Experiments in hearing.* New York: McGraw-Hill.

Vukasovic, T., & Bratko, D. (2015). Heritability of personality: A meta-analysis of behavior genetic studies. *Psychological Bulletin, 141*(4), 769–785. Retrieved from https://www.ncbi.nlm.nih.gov/pubmed/25961374. doi:10.1037/bul0000017

Vytal, K., & Hamann, S. (2010). Neuroimaging support for discrete neural correlates of basic emotions: A voxel-based meta-analysis. *Journal of Cognitive Neuroscience, 22*(12), 2864–2885. Retrieved from https://www.ncbi.nlm.nih.gov/pubmed/19929758. doi:10.1162/jocn.2009.21366

Wada, J., & Rasmussen, T. (2007). Intracarotid injection of sodium amytal for the lateralization of cerebral speech dominance. 1960. *Journal of Neurosurgery, 106*(6), 1117–1133. Retrieved from https://www.ncbi.nlm.nih.gov/pubmed/17564192. doi:10.3171/jns.2007.106.6.1117

Walker, M. P., Brakefield, T., Hobson, J. A., & Stickgold, R. (2003). Dissociable stages of human memory consolidation and reconsolidation. *Nature, 425*(6958), 616–620. Retrieved from https://www.ncbi.nlm.nih.gov/pubmed/14534587. doi:10.1038/nature01930

Wall, P. D. (1978). The gate control theory of pain mechanisms. A re-examination and re-statement. *Brain, 101*(1), 1–18. Retrieved from https://www.ncbi.nlm.nih.gov/pubmed/205314

Wallis, J. D. (2011). Cross-species studies of orbitofrontal cortex and value-based decision-making. *Nature Neuroscience, 15*(1), 13–19. Retrieved from https://www.ncbi.nlm.nih.gov/pubmed/22101646. doi:10.1038/nn.2956

Wang, H. L., Zhang, S., Qi, J., Wang, H., Cachope, R., Mejias-Aponte, C. A., . . . Morales, M. (2019). Dorsal raphe dual serotonin-glutamate neurons drive reward by establishing excitatory synapses on VTA mesoaccumbens dopamine neurons. *Cell Reports, 26*(5), 1128–1142.e1127. Retrieved from https://www.ncbi.nlm.nih.gov/pubmed/30699344. doi:10.1016/j.celrep.2019.01.014

Warrington, E. K., & Weiskrantz, L. (1970). Amnesic syndrome: Consolidation or retrieval? *Nature, 228*(5272), 628–630. Retrieved from https://www.ncbi.nlm.nih.gov/pubmed/4990853

Wasman, M., & Flynn, J. P. (1962). Directed attack elicited from hypothalamus. *Archives of Neurology, 6*, 220–227. Retrieved from https://www.ncbi.nlm.nih.gov/pubmed/14005120

Watanabe, N., Sakagami, M., & Haruno, M. (2013). Reward prediction error signal enhanced by striatum-amygdala interaction explains the acceleration of probabilistic reward learning by emotion. *The Journal of Neuroscience, 33*(10), 4487–4493. Retrieved from https://www.ncbi.nlm.nih.gov/pubmed/23467364. doi:10.1523/JNEUROSCI.3400-12.2013

Watanabe, Y., Gould, E., & McEwen, B. S. (1992). Stress induces atrophy of apical dendrites of hippocampal CA3 pyramidal neurons. *Brain Research, 588*(2), 341–345. Retrieved from https://www.ncbi.nlm.nih.gov/pubmed/1393587

Waters, F. A., Badcock, J. C., Michie, P. T., & Maybery, M. T. (2006). Auditory hallucinations in schizophrenia: Intrusive thoughts and forgotten memories. *Cognitive Neuropsychiatry, 11*(1), 65–83. Retrieved from https://www.ncbi.nlm.nih.gov/pubmed/16537234. doi:10.1080/13546800444000191

Waters, P. D., Wallis, M. C., & Marshall Graves, J. A. (2007). Mammalian sex—Origin and evolution of the Y chromosome and SRY. *Seminars in Cell & Developmental Biology, 18*(3), 389–400. Retrieved from https://www.ncbi.nlm.nih.gov/pubmed/17400006. doi:10.1016/j.semcdb.2007.02.007

Weaver, I. C., Cervoni, N., Champagne, F. A., D'Alessio, A. C., Sharma, S., Seckl, J. R., . . . Meaney, M. J. (2004). Epigenetic programming by maternal behavior. *Nature Neuroscience, 7*(8), 847–854. Retrieved from https://www.ncbi.nlm.nih.gov/pubmed/15220929. doi:10.1038/nn1276

Weilburg, J. B. (2004). An overview of SSRI and SNRI therapies for depression. *Managed Care, 13*(6 Suppl Depression), 25–33. Retrieved from https://www.ncbi.nlm.nih.gov/pubmed/15293768

Weinberger, D. R., & Berman, K. F. (1988). Speculation on the meaning of cerebral metabolic hypofrontality in schizophrenia. *Schizophrenia Bulletin, 14*(2), 157–168. Retrieved from http://www.ncbi.nlm.nih.gov/pubmed/3059465

Weinberger, D. R., Torrey, E. F., Neophytides, A. N., & Wyatt, R. J. (1979). Lateral cerebral ventricular enlargement in chronic schizophrenia. *Archives of General Psychiatry, 36*(7), 735–739. Retrieved from https://www.ncbi.nlm.nih.gov/pubmed/36863

Weiner, N., Cloutier, G., Bjur, R., & Pfeffer, R. I. (1972). Modification of norepinephrine synthesis in intact tissue dy drugs and during short-term adrenergic nerve stimulation. *Pharmacological Reviews, 24*(2), 203–221. Retrieved from https://www.ncbi.nlm.nih.gov/pubmed/4405385

Weingarten, E., Chen, Q., McAdams, M., Yi, J., Hepler, J., & Albarracin, D. (2016). From primed concepts to action: A meta-analysis of the behavioral effects of incidentally presented words. *Psychological Bulletin, 142*(5), 472–497. Retrieved from https://www.ncbi.nlm.nih.gov/pubmed/26689090. doi:10.1037/bul0000030

Weiskrantz, L., Warrington, E. K., Sanders, M. D., & Marshall, J. (1974). Visual capacity in the hemianopic field following a restricted occipital ablation. *Brain, 97*(4), 709–728. Retrieved from http://www.ncbi.nlm.nih.gov/pubmed/4434190

White, N. M. (1997). Mnemonic functions of the basal ganglia. *Current Opinion in Neurobiology, 7*(2), 164–169. Retrieved from https://www.ncbi.nlm.nih.gov/pubmed/9142761

Whitlock, J. R., Sutherland, R. J., Witter, M. P., Moser, M. B., & Moser, E. I. (2008). Navigating from hippocampus to parietal cortex. *Proceedings of the National Academy of Sciences of the United States of America, 105*(39), 14755–14762. Retrieved from https://www.ncbi.nlm.nih.gov/pubmed/18812502. doi:10.1073/pnas.0804216105

Whooley, M. A., Caska, C. M., Hendrickson, B. E., Rourke, M. A., Ho, J., & Ali, S. (2007). Depression and inflammation in patients with coronary heart disease: Findings from the Heart and Soul Study. *Biological Psychiatry, 62*(4), 314–320. Retrieved from https://www.ncbi.nlm.nih.gov/pubmed/17434456. doi:10.1016/j.biopsych.2006.10.016

Wiech, K., Lin, C. S., Brodersen, K. H., Bingel, U., Ploner, M., & Tracey, I. (2010). Anterior insula integrates information about salience into perceptual decisions about pain. *The Journal of Neuroscience, 30*(48), 16324–16331. Retrieved from https://www.ncbi.nlm.nih.gov/pubmed/21123578. doi:10.1523/JNEUROSCI.2087-10.2010

Wiener, S. I., & Taube, J. S. (2005). *Head direction cells and the neural mechanisms of spatial orientation.* Cambridge, MA: MIT Press.

Wild, J. M. (1997). Neural pathways for the control of birdsong production. *Journal of Neurobiology, 33*(5), 653–670. Retrieved from https://www.ncbi.nlm.nih.gov/pubmed/9369465

Wilensky, A. E., Schafe, G. E., Kristensen, M. P., & LeDoux, J. E. (2006). Rethinking the fear circuit: The central nucleus of the amygdala is required for the acquisition, consolidation, and expression of Pavlovian fear conditioning. *The Journal of neuroscience, 26*(48), 12387–12396. Retrieved from https://www.ncbi.nlm.nih.gov/pubmed/17135400. doi:10.1523/JNEUROSCI.4316-06.2006

Wilhoit, L. F., Scott, D. A., & Simecka, B. A. (2017). Fetal alcohol spectrum disorders: Characteristics, complications, and treatment. *Community Mental Health Journal, 53*(6), 711–718. Retrieved from https://www.ncbi.nlm.nih.gov/pubmed/28168434. doi:10.1007/s10597-017-0104-0

Williams, J. R., Insel, T. R., Harbaugh, C. R., & Carter, C. S. (1994). Oxytocin administered centrally facilitates formation of a partner preference in female prairie voles (Microtus ochrogaster). *Journal of Neuroendocrinology, 6*(3), 247–250. Retrieved from https://www.ncbi.nlm.nih.gov/pubmed/7920590

Wimmer, H., & Perner, J. (1983). Beliefs about beliefs: Representation and constraining function of wrong beliefs in young children's understanding of deception. *Cognition, 13*(1), 103–128. Retrieved from http://www.ncbi.nlm.nih.gov/pubmed/6681741

Winslow, J. T., Hastings, N., Carter, C. S., Harbaugh, C. R., & Insel, T. R. (1993). A role for central vasopressin in pair bonding in monogamous prairie voles. *Nature, 365*(6446), 545–548. Retrieved from https://www.ncbi.nlm.nih.gov/pubmed/8413608. doi:10.1038/365545a0

Wise, R. A. (2002). Brain reward circuitry: Insights from unsensed incentives. *Neuron, 36*(2), 229–ss240. Retrieved from https://www.ncbi.nlm.nih.gov/pubmed/12383779

Wise, R. A., & Koob, G. F. (2014). The development and maintenance of drug addiction. *Neuropsychopharmacology, 39*(2), 254–262. Retrieved from https://www.ncbi.nlm.nih.gov/pubmed/24121188. doi:10.1038/npp.2013.261

Wisniewski, L., Epstein, L. H., & Caggiula, A. R. (1992). Effect of food change on consumption, hedonics, and salivation. *Physiology & Behavior, 52*(1), 21–26. Retrieved from https://www.ncbi.nlm.nih.gov/pubmed/1529009

Wixted, J. T., Goldinger, S. D., Squire, L. R., Kuhn, J. R., Papesh, M. H., Smith, K. A., . . . Steinmetz, P. N. (2018). Coding of episodic memory in the human hippocampus. *Proceedings of the National Academy of Sciences of the United States of America, 115*(5), 1093–1098. Retrieved from https://www.ncbi.nlm.nih.gov/pubmed/29339476. doi:10.1073/pnas.1716443115

Wolff, M., Wells, B., Ventura-DiPersia, C., Renson, A., & Grov, C. (2017). Measuring sexual orientation: A review and critique of U.S. data collection efforts and implications for health policy. *Journal of Sex Research, 54*(4–5), 507–531. Retrieved from https://www.ncbi.nlm.nih.gov/pubmed/28010119. doi:10.1080/00224499.2016.1255872

Wong, D. T., Bymaster, F. P., Horng, J. S., & Molloy, B. B. (1975). A new selective inhibitor for uptake of serotonin into synaptosomes of rat brain: 3-(p-trifluoromethylphenoxy). N-methyl-3-phenylpropylamine. *The Journal of Pharmacology and Experimental Therapeutics, 193*(3), 804–811. Retrieved from https://www.ncbi.nlm.nih.gov/pubmed/1151730

World Health Organization. (2013). *Spinal cord injury fact sheet No 384*. Retrieved from http://www.who.int/mediacentre/factsheets/fs384/en/

Wrangham, R. W. (2018). Two types of aggression in human evolution. *Proceedings of the National Academy of Sciences of the United States of America, 115*(2), 245–253. Retrieved from https://www.ncbi.nlm.nih.gov/pubmed/29279379. doi:10.1073/pnas.1713611115

Wrighten, S. A., Piroli, G. G., Grillo, C. A., & Reagan, L. P. (2009). A look inside the diabetic brain: Contributors to diabetes-induced brain aging. *Biochimica et Biophysica Acta, 1792*(5), 444–453. Retrieved from https://www.ncbi.nlm.nih.gov/pubmed/19022375. doi:10.1016/j.bbadis.2008.10.013

Wyatt, T. S. (2003). *Pheromones and animal behavior: Communication by smell and taste*. New York: Cambridge University Press.

Xu, G., Knutsen, A. K., Dikranian, K., Kroenke, C. D., Bayly, P. V., & Taber, L. A. (2010). Axons pull on the brain, but tension does not drive cortical folding. *Journal of Biomechanical Engineering, 132*(7), 071013. Retrieved from https://www.ncbi.nlm.nih.gov/pubmed/20590291. doi:10.1115/1.4001683

Xu, T., Yu, X., Perlik, A. J., Tobin, W. F., Zweig, J. A., Tennant, K., . . . Zuo, Y. (2009). Rapid formation and selective stabilization of synapses for enduring motor memories. *Nature, 462*(7275), 915–919. Retrieved from https://www.ncbi.nlm.nih.gov/pubmed/19946267. doi:10.1038/nature08389

Yahiro, T., Kataoka, N., Nakamura, Y., & Nakamura, K. (2017). The lateral parabrachial nucleus, but not the thalamus, mediates thermosensory pathways for behavioural thermoregulation. *Scientific Reports, 7*(1), 5031. Retrieved from https://www.ncbi.nlm.nih.gov/pubmed/28694517. doi:10.1038/s41598-017-05327-8

Yamaguchi, T., Wang, H. L., Li, X., Ng, T. H., & Morales, M. (2011). Mesocorticolimbic glutamatergic pathway. *The Journal of Neuroscience, 31*(23), 8476–8490. Retrieved from https://www.ncbi.nlm.nih.gov/pubmed/21653852. doi:10.1523/JNEUROSCI.1598-11.2011

Yanagisawa, N. (2018). Functions and dysfunctions of the basal ganglia in humans. *Proceedings of the Japan Academy. Series B, Physical and Biological Sciences, 94*(7), 275–304. Retrieved from https://www.ncbi.nlm.nih.gov/pubmed/30078828. doi:10.2183/pjab.94.019

Yasunami, T., Kuno, M., & Matsuura, S. (1988). Voltage-clamp analysis of taurine-induced suppression of excitatory postsynaptic potentials in frog spinal motoneurons. *Journal of Neurophysiology, 60*(4), 1405–1418. Retrieved from https://www.ncbi.nlm.nih.gov/pubmed/3264017. doi:10.1152/jn.1988.60.4.1405

Yehuda, R., Bierer, L. M., Schmeidler, J., Aferiat, D. H., Breslau, I., & Dolan, S. (2000). Low cortisol and risk for PTSD in adult offspring of holocaust survivors. *The American Journal of Psychiatry, 157*(8), 1252–1259. Retrieved from https://www.ncbi.nlm.nih.gov/pubmed/10910787. doi:10.1176/appi.ajp.157.8.1252

Yehuda, R., Daskalakis, N. P., Bierer, L. M., Bader, H. N., Klengel, T., Holsboer, F., & Binder, E. B. (2016). Holocaust exposure induced intergenerational effects on FKBP5 methylation. *Biological Psychiatry, 80*(5), 372–380. Retrieved from https://www.ncbi.nlm.nih.gov/pubmed/26410355. doi:10.1016/j.biopsych.2015.08.005

Yeo, C. H. (1991). Cerebellum and classical conditioning of motor responses. *Annals of the New York Academy of Sciences, 627*, 292–304. Retrieved from https://www.ncbi.nlm.nih.gov/pubmed/1883140

Yerkes, R. M., & Dodson, J. D. (1908). The relation of strength of stimulus to rapidity of habit-formation. *Journal of Comparative Neurology & Psychology, 18*, 18, 459–482.

Yesudas, E. H., & Lee, T. M. (2015). The role of cingulate cortex in vicarious pain. *BioMed Research International, 2015*, 719615. Retrieved from https://www.ncbi.nlm.nih.gov/pubmed/25815331. doi:10.1155/2015/719615

Yeung, A. W. K., Tzvetkov, N. T., & Atanasov, A. G. (2018). When neuroscience meets pharmacology: A neuropharmacology literature analysis. *Frontiers in Neuroscience, 12*, 852. Retrieved from https://www.ncbi.nlm.nih.gov/pubmed/30505266. doi:10.3389/fnins.2018.00852

Yoest, K. E., Cummings, J. A., & Becker, J. B. (2014). Estradiol, dopamine and motivation. *Central Nervous System Agents in Medicinal Chemistry, 14*(2), 83–89. Retrieved from https://www.ncbi.nlm.nih.gov/pubmed/25540977

Yong, E. (2010). *Meet the woman without fear*. Retrieved from http://blogs.discovermagazine.com/notrocketscience/2010/12/16/meet-the-woman-without-fear/

Young, T. (1802, January). The Bakerian Lecture: On the theory of light and colours. *Philosophical Transactions of the Royal Society of London, 1*(92), 12–48. doi:10.1098/rstl.1802.0004

Zabara, J. (1992). Inhibition of experimental seizures in canines by repetitive vagal stimulation. *Epilepsia, 33*(6), 1005–1012. Retrieved from https://www.ncbi.nlm.nih.gov/pubmed/1464256

Zeman, A. Z., Grayling, A. C., & Cowey, A. (1997). Contemporary theories of consciousness. *Journal of Neurology, Neurosurgery, and Psychiatry, 62*(6), 549–552. Retrieved from https://www.ncbi.nlm.nih.gov/pubmed/9219736

Zhang, S., Schonfeld, F., Wiskott, L., & Manahan-Vaughan, D. (2014). Spatial representations of place cells in darkness are supported by path integration and border information. *Frontiers in Behavioral Neuroscience, 8*, 222. Retrieved from https://www.ncbi.nlm.nih.gov/pubmed/25009477. doi:10.3389/fnbeh.2014.00222

Zheng, W., & Yuan, X. (2008). Guidance of cortical radial migration by gradient of diffusible factors. *Cell Adhesion & Migration, 2*(1), 48–50. Retrieved from http://www.ncbi.nlm.nih.gov/pubmed/19262126

Zhou, Y. D., & Fuster, J. M. (1996). Mnemonic neuronal activity in somatosensory cortex. *Proceedings of the National Academy of Sciences of the United States of America, 93*(19), 10533–10537. Retrieved from https://www.ncbi.nlm.nih.gov/pubmed/8927629

Zhou, Y. D., & Fuster, J. M. (1997). Neuronal activity of somatosensory cortex in a cross-modal (visuo-haptic) memory task. *Experimental Brain Research, 116*(3), 551–555. Retrieved from https://www.ncbi.nlm.nih.gov/pubmed/9372304

Zilles, K. (1992). Neuronal plasticity as an adaptive property of the central nervous system. *Annals of Anatomy, 174*(5), 383–391. Retrieved from https://www.ncbi.nlm.nih.gov/pubmed/1333175

Zmudzka, E., Salaciak, K., Sapa, J., & Pytka, K. (2018). Serotonin receptors in depression and anxiety: Insights from animal studies. *Life Sciences, 210*, 106–124. Retrieved from https://www.ncbi.nlm.nih.gov/pubmed/30144453. doi:10.1016/j.lfs.2018.08.050

Zuckerman, M. (1979). *Sensation seeking: Beyond the optimal level of arousal*. Hillsdale, NJ/New York: L. Erlbaum Associates; distributed by the Halsted Press Division of Wiley.

Zuckerman, M., & Neeb, M. (1979). Sensation seeking and psychopathology. *Psychiatry Research, 1*(3), 255–264. Retrieved from https://www.ncbi.nlm.nih.gov/pubmed/298353

AUTHOR INDEX

SUBJECT INDEX